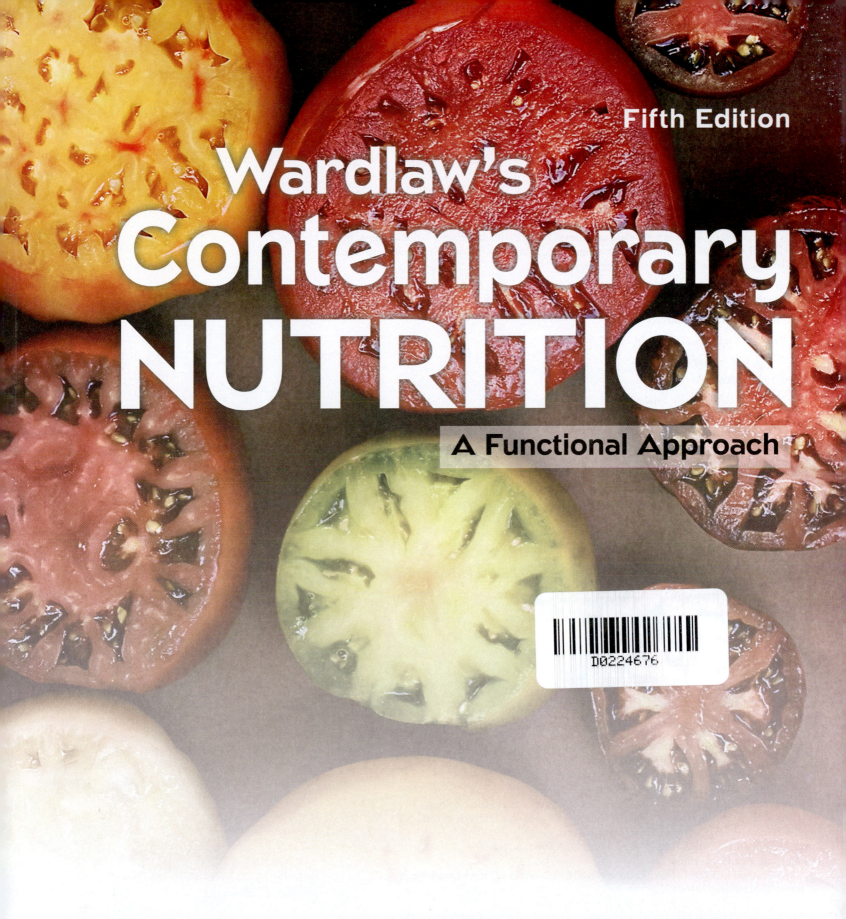

Fifth Edition

Wardlaw's
Contemporary
NUTRITION

A Functional Approach

D0224676

WARDLAW'S CONTEMPORARY NUTRITION: A FUNCTIONAL APPROACH,
FIFTH EDITION

Published by McGraw-Hill Education, 2 Penn Plaza, New York, NY 10121. Copyright © 2018 by
McGraw-Hill Education. All rights reserved. Printed in the United States of America. Previous
editions © 2015 and 2013. No part of this publication may be reproduced or distributed in any form
or by any means, or stored in a database or retrieval system, without the prior written consent of
McGraw-Hill Education, including, but not limited to, in any network or other electronic storage or
transmission, or broadcast for distance learning.

Some ancillaries, including electronic and print components, may not be available to customers
outside the United States.

This book is printed on acid-free paper.

1 2 3 4 5 6 7 8 9 LMN 21 20 19 18 17

ISBN 978-1-259-70660-8

MHID 1-259-70660-5

Chief Product Officer, SVP Products & Markets: *G. Scott Virkler*
Vice President, General Manager, Products & Markets: *Marty Lange*
Managing Director: *Lynn Breithaupt*
Brand Manager: *Marija Magner*
Director, Product Development: *Rose Koos*
Product Developer: *Darlene M. Schueller*
Marketing Manager: *Jessica Cannavo*
Market Development Manager: *Kristine Rellihan*
Digital Product Developer: *Michael Koot, Ph.D.*
Digital Product Analyst: *Christine Carlson*
Director, Content Design & Delivery: *Linda Avenarius*
Program Manager: *Angela R. FitzPatrick*
Content Project Managers: *April R. Southwood/Jane Mohr/Danielle Clement*
Buyer: *Jennifer Pickel*
Design: *Tara McDermott*
Content Licensing Specialists: *Lori Hancock/Lorraine Buczek*
Cover Image: © *Catherine Murray/Shutterstock*
Compositor: *SPi Global*
Printer: *LSC Communications*

All credits appearing on page or at the end of the book are considered to be an extension of the
copyright page.

Library of Congress Cataloging-in-Publication Data

Names: Wardlaw, Gordon M. | Smith, Anne M., 1955. | Collene, Angela.
Title: Wardlaw's contemporary nutrition : a functional approach.
Other titles: Contemporary nutrition : a functional approach
Description: Fifth edition / Anne M. Smith Ph.D., R.D.N., L.D.,
    Department of Human Sciences, College of Education and Human Ecology,
    The Ohio State University, Angela L. Collene M.S., R.D.N., L.D. | New York, NY :
    McGraw-Hill Education, [2018] | Includes index.
Identifiers: LCCN 2016042223 | ISBN 9781259706608 (alk. paper)
Subjects: LCSH: Nutrition.
Classification: LCC QP141 .W377 2018 | DDC 613.2—dc23 LC record available at
https://lccn.loc.gov/2016042223

The Internet addresses listed in the text were accurate at the time of publication. The inclusion of a
website does not indicate an endorsement by the authors or McGraw-Hill Education, and McGraw-
Hill Education does not guarantee the accuracy of the information presented at these sites.

mheducation.com/highered

Brief Contents

Breakfast: ©Corbis/Punchstock; bowl of cereal: ©Medioimages/Photodisc/Getty Images; citrus fruit: ©Creatas/PunchStock; woman hitting volleyball: ©Purestock/SuperStock; pregnant woman: ©Getty Images

Dear Students,

Welcome to the fascinating world of nutrition! Nutrition is our favorite area of science because it is so relevant—we all eat several times a day and the choices we make can have a dramatic influence on health. At the same time, though, the science of nutrition can seem a bit confusing. One reason for all the confusion is that it seems like "good nutrition" is a moving target; different authorities have different ideas of how we should eat, and nutrition recommendations are subject to change! Do carbohydrates cause weight gain? Do I need to limit saturated fat? Should we eat foods that contain gluten or not? Second, there are so many choices. Did you know that the average supermarket carries about 40,000 food and beverage products? The manufacturers of all those products are vying for your attention, but typically, the most aggressively marketed items are not the healthiest. How can you identify a healthy product? Third, as a nation, we eat many of our meals and snacks away from home. When we eat foods that someone else has prepared for us, we surrender control over what is in our food, where the food came from, and how much of it goes on our plates. Undoubtedly, you are interested in what you should be eating and how the food you eat affects you.

__Wardlaw's Contemporary Nutrition: A Functional Approach__ is designed to accurately convey changing and seemingly conflicting messages to all kinds of students. Our students commonly have misconceptions about nutrition, and many have a limited background in biology or chemistry. We teach complex scientific concepts at a level that will enable you to apply the material to your own life.

This marks the fifth edition of __Wardlaw's Contemporary Nutrition: A Functional Approach__. We are very excited to introduce you to our newest author, Dr. Colleen Spees! Like our other authors, she is a Registered Dietitian Nutritionist, which means she will help you to translate nutrition science into practical advice. At The Ohio State University, Dr. Spees is a valued expert on cancer, nutritional genomics, and food security. We are thrilled that she brings her unique perspective and contemporary ideas to our team.

As in previous editions, we have written this book to help you make informed choices about the food you eat. We will take you through explanations of the nutrients in food and their relationship to health but will also make you aware of the multitude of other factors that drive food choices. To guide you, we refer to many reputable research studies, books, policies, and websites throughout the book. With this information at your fingertips, you will be well equipped to make your own informed choices about what and how much to eat. There is much to learn, so let's get started!

Anne Smith
Angela Collene
Colleen Spees

Fifth Edition

Wardlaw's Contemporary NUTRITION

A Functional Approach

Anne M. Smith Ph.D., R.D.N., L.D.
Department of Human Sciences,
College of Education and Human Ecology
The Ohio State University

Angela L. Collene M.S., R.D.N., L.D.
Department of Human Sciences,
College of Education and Human Ecology
The Ohio State University

Colleen K. Spees Ph.D., M.Ed., R.D.N., L.D., FAND
Division of Medical Dietetics and Health Sciences,
College of Medicine
The Ohio State University

Mc
Graw
Hill
Education

About the Authors

ANNE M. SMITH, Ph.D., R.D.N., L.D., is an associate professor emeritus at The Ohio State University. She was the recipient of the 1995 Outstanding Teacher Award from the College of Human Ecology, the 2008 Outstanding Dietetic Educator Award from the Ohio Dietetic Association, the 2006 Outstanding Faculty Member Award from the Department of Human Nutrition, and the 2011 Distinguished Service Award from the College of Education and Human Ecology for her commitment to undergraduate education in nutrition. Dr. Smith's research in the area of vitamin and mineral metabolism has appeared in prominent nutrition journals, and she was awarded the 1996 Research Award from the Ohio Agricultural Research and Development Center. She is a member of the American Society for Nutrition and the Academy of Nutrition and Dietetics.

ANGELA L. COLLENE, M.S., R.D.N., L.D., began her career at her alma mater, The Ohio State University, as a research dietitian for studies related to diabetes and aging. Other professional experiences include community nutrition lecturing and counseling, owner of a personal chef business, and many diverse and rewarding science writing and editing projects. Her interests include novel approaches to glycemic control, weight management, and—quite predictably for the mother of three little girls—maternal and child nutrition. Mrs. Collene currently teaches nutrition at The Ohio State University and Ohio Northern University. She is a member of the Academy of Nutrition and Dietetics.

COLLEEN K. SPEES, Ph.D., M.Ed., R.D.N., L.D., FAND is an academic instructor and researcher at The Ohio State University College of Medicine. She earned her Doctorate in Health Sciences at Ohio State with a research focus on Nutritional Genomics and Cancer and her Master's degree in Exercise Science and Health Promotion from Vanderbilt University. Her primary focus of teaching and research involves interventions aimed at providing optimal nutrition for vulnerable populations (http://go.osu.edu/hope). In addition to teaching nutrition at The Ohio State University and Columbus State Community College, Dr. Spees also developed and teaches a graduate level Nutritional Genomics course. She is the recipient of several national awards from the Academy of Nutrition and Dietetics, including the 2016 Distinguished Practice Award; 2015 Award for Excellence in Oncology Nutrition Research; 2015 Outstanding Dietetic Educator Award; 2013 Nutrition Informatics Video Challenge Teaching Award; 2009 Top Innovator in Education Teaching Award; and has been a Content Expert and Reviewer for the Nutritional Genomics & Food Security Academy Position Papers. Dr. Spees is also a recognized Fellow of the Academy of Nutrition and Dietetics.

Acknowledgements

Special Acknowledgements

It is because of the tireless efforts of a cohesive team of talented professionals that we can bring you the fifth edition of *Wardlaw's Contemporary Nutrition: A Functional Approach*. We consider ourselves massively blessed to work with the top-notch staff at McGraw-Hill Education. We are grateful to Marija Magner, our Brand Manager, for her strategic leadership and vast knowledge of the higher education market. We value the efforts of our Marketing Manager, Jessica Cannavo, who connects instructors across the nation with our work and brings us constructive feedback from the field. We thank our award-winning Product Developer, Darlene Schueller, who coordinated the editorial team with her keen eye for detail, strong work ethic, and organizational expertise. We are grateful to our Content Project Managers, April Southwood and Jane Mohr, and their staff for the careful coordination of the numerous production efforts needed to create the very appealing and accurate fifth edition. We appreciate the meticulous work of our copyeditor, Carey Lange; proofreaders, David Staloch and Gina Delaney; our content licensing specialists, Lorraine Buczek and Lori Slattery; and photo editors, Lori Hancock and Mary Reeg. We thank our designer, Tara McDermott, who ensured that every aspect of our work is visually appealing—not just on the printed page, but also in a variety of digital formats. Finally, we are indebted to our colleagues, friends, and families for their constant encouragement, honest feedback, and shared passion for the science of nutrition.

In the preparation of each edition, we have been guided by the collective wisdom of reviewers who are excellent teachers. They represent experience in community colleges, liberal arts colleges, institutions, and universities. We have followed their recommendations, while remaining true to our overriding goal of writing a readable, student-centered text.

Also with this edition, we are very pleased to have been able to incorporate real student data points and input, derived from thousands of our LearnSmart users, to help guide our revision. LearnSmart heat maps provided a quick visual snapshot of usage of portions of the text and the relative difficulty students experienced in mastering the content. With these data, we were able to hone not only our text content but also the LearnSmart probes.

With the fifth edition of *Wardlaw's Contemporary Nutrition: A Functional Approach,* we remember its founding author, Gordon M. Wardlaw. We are saddened that he lost his battle with cancer on January 19, 2014. He was a brilliant example of a man who acted decisively, followed his dreams, and created a legacy of learning.

Dr. Wardlaw had a passion for the science of nutrition and the research that supports it. With his clear teaching style and no-nonsense nutrition advice, he demonstrated an exceptional ability to translate scientific principles into practical knowledge both inside and outside the classroom. This skill is what made his book truly "contemporary." He was tireless when it came to staying current and relevant to a changing world. Each edition benefited from his genuine interest in responding to feedback from students, colleagues, and instructors. He retired from teaching and writing in 2005 to pursue another passion—building his dream home in California. There, in a home he built with his own two hands, he spent the last years of his life with his family and friends.

It has been a privilege for all of us to join Dr. Wardlaw as coauthors of this textbook. For Anne Smith, he was an extraordinary colleague, mentor, and friend, who patiently taught her every step of the textbook writing process, beginning with the sixth edition of *Contemporary Nutrition*. Angela Collene was blessed to have been one of his graduate students at The Ohio State University, when she first began to assist with revisions to his books. Colleen Spees was a student in Dr. Wardlaw's first nutrition class at The Ohio State University and now holds his previous tenure-track position. Like so many other students, colleagues, and friends, we remember Dr. Wardlaw as a source of vast knowledge, good humor, and inspiration. The best way we know to honor our dear friend and mentor is to carry on his legacy of outstanding textbooks in introductory nutrition. *Wardlaw's Contemporary Nutrition: A Functional Approach* will continue to evolve and reflect current trends and breakthroughs in nutrition science, but Dr. Wardlaw's fingerprints will remain on every page.

McGraw-Hill Connect®
Learn Without Limits

Connect is a teaching and learning platform that is proven to deliver better results for students and instructors.

Connect empowers students by continually adapting to deliver precisely what they need, when they need it, and how they need it, so your class time is more engaging and effective.

73% of instructors who use Connect require it; instructor satisfaction increases by 28% when Connect is required.

Connect's Impact on Retention Rates, Pass Rates, and Average Exam Scores

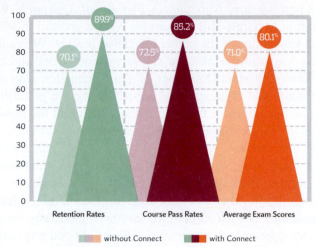

without Connect · with Connect

Using **Connect** improves retention rates by **19.8%**, passing rates by **12.7%**, and exam scores by **9.1%**.

Analytics

Connect Insight®

Connect Insight is Connect's new one-of-a-kind visual analytics dashboard—now available for both instructors and students—that provides at-a-glance information regarding student performance, which is immediately actionable. By presenting assignment, assessment, and topical performance results together with a time metric that is easily visible for aggregate or individual results, Connect Insight gives the user the ability to take a just-in-time approach to teaching and learning, which was never before available. Connect Insight presents data that empowers students and helps instructors improve class performance in a way that is efficient and effective.

Impact on Final Course Grade Distribution

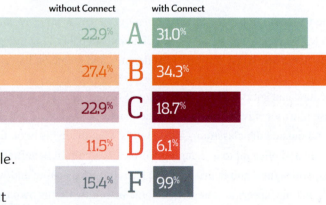

	without Connect	with Connect
A	22.9%	31.0%
B	27.4%	34.3%
C	22.9%	18.7%
D	11.5%	6.1%
F	15.4%	9.9%

Students can view their results for any Connect course.

Mobile

Connect's new, intuitive mobile interface gives students and instructors flexible and convenient, anytime–anywhere access to all components of the Connect platform.

Adaptive

THE **ADAPTIVE** **READING EXPERIENCE** DESIGNED TO TRANSFORM THE WAY STUDENTS READ

> More students earn **A's** and **B's** when they use McGraw-Hill Education **Adaptive** products.

SmartBook®

Proven to help students improve grades and study more efficiently, SmartBook contains the same content within the print book, but actively tailors that content to the needs of the individual. SmartBook's adaptive technology provides precise, personalized instruction on what the student should do next, guiding the student to master and remember key concepts, targeting gaps in knowledge and offering customized feedback, and driving the student toward comprehension and retention of the subject matter. Available on tablets, SmartBook puts learning at the student's fingertips—anywhere, anytime.

> Over **8 billion questions** have been answered, making McGraw-Hill Education products more intelligent, reliable, and precise.

www.mheducation.com

Connect® Improves Performance

Easily assign key features from the book to increase engagement and learning.

McGraw-Hill **Connect**® is a digital teaching and learning environment that saves students and instructors time while improving performance over a variety of critical outcomes. From in-site tutorials, to tips and best practices, to live help from colleagues and specialists—you are never left alone to maximize Connect's potential.

- **Auto-graded assessments and tutorials**

You can easily create customized assessments that will be automatically graded. All Connect content is created by the authors, so it is pedagogical, instructional, and at the appropriate level. Interactive questions using high-quality art from the textbook and animations and videos from a variety of sources take you way beyond multiple choice. Assignable features from the book, such as *Newsworthy Nutrition, What Would You Choose?,* and *Rate Your Plate,* increase student engagement and understanding.

- **Gather assessment information**

All Connect questions are tagged to a learning outcome, specific section and topic, and Bloom's level so you can easily track assessment data!

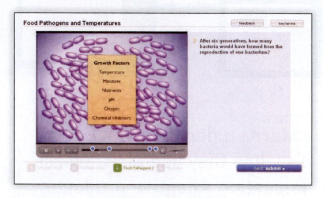

▲ Connect Assessment: Animation Tutorial

▲ Connect Assessment: Labeling Interactive

NutritionCalc Plus is an online dietary analysis tool fueled by the ESHA database of well over 30,000 foods. NutritionCalc Plus allows your students to track their food and activity, and then analyze their choices with a robust selection of reports. This tool is provided complimentary in Connect with *Wardlaw's Contemporary Nutrition: A Functional Approach.*

McGraw-Hill Campus® is a groundbreaking service that puts world-class digital learning resources just a click away for all your faculty and students. All your faculty—whether or not they use a McGraw-Hill Education title—can instantly browse, search, and access the entire library of McGraw-Hill Education instructional resources and services including eBooks, test banks, PowerPoint slides, animations, and learning objects—from any Learning Management System (LMS), at no additional cost to your institution. Users also have single sign-on access to McGraw-Hill Education digital platforms, including Connect, ALEKS, Create, and Tegrity.

McGraw-Hill Create™ is a self-service website that allows you to create customized course materials using McGraw-Hill Education's comprehensive, cross-disciplinary content and digital products. You can even access third-party content such as readings, articles, cases, videos, and more. Arrange the content you've selected to match the scope and sequence of your course. Personalize your book with a cover design and choose the best format for your students—eBook, color print, or black-and-white print. And, when you are done, you'll receive a PDF review copy in just minutes!

Tegrity® is a fully automated lecture capture solution used in traditional, hybrid, "flipped classes," and online courses to record lessons, lectures, and skills.

Fueled by LearnSmart—the most widely used and intelligent adaptive learning resource—**LearnSmart Prep®** is designed to get students ready for a forthcoming course by quickly and effectively addressing prerequisite knowledge gaps that may cause problems down the road.

Connecting Students to Today's Nutrition

Why the Functional Approach?

Wardlaw's Contemporary Nutrition: A Functional Approach is organized somewhat differently than the traditional nutrition textbook (as seen in the contents of *Contemporary Nutrition* shown on the right) in that Part Three presents information on vitamins, minerals, and water using "a functional approach." Instead of describing these nutrients in their traditional categories (e.g., water-soluble vitamins), we discuss them in groups based on their roles in fluid and electrolyte balance, body defenses, bone health, energy metabolism, blood health, and brain health. This format enables students to understand how these nutrients interact in food and in our bodies to support key functions that sustain our health.

Understanding Our Audience

We have written *Wardlaw's Contemporary Nutrition: A Functional Approach* assuming that our students have a limited background in college-level biology, chemistry, or physiology. We have been careful to include the essential science foundation needed to adequately comprehend certain topics in nutrition, such as protein synthesis in Chapter 6. The science in this text has been presented in a simple, straightforward manner so that undergraduate students can master the material and apply it to their own lives. The Concept Maps and detailed, annotated figures bring complex topics into view for students from any major.

Wardlaw's Contemporary Nutrition: A Functional Approach

Wardlaw's Contemporary Nutrition

Featuring the Latest Guidelines and Research

Nutrition is a dynamic field. A vast quantity of research constantly reshapes our knowledge of nutritional science. The fifth edition has been carefully updated to reflect current scientific understanding, as well as the latest health and nutrition guidelines. For everyday diet planning, students will learn about the 2015–2020 Dietary Guidelines for Americans, MyPlate, and Healthy People 2020. In discussions about specific nutrition concerns, the most recent data and recommendations from the Academy of Nutrition and Dietetics, American Heart Association, American Diabetes Association, Institute of Medicine, and American Psychological Association have been included in this edition.

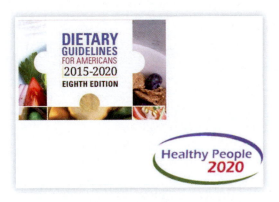

Newsworthy Nutrition, a feature in each chapter, highlights the use of the scientific method in recently published research studies that relate to the chapter topics. In addition, assignable questions in Connect take learning a step further by asking students to read primary literature and apply what they have learned.

Newsworthy Nutrition

No Change in Obesity Prevalence in Youth or Adults Between 2003 and 2012

The prevalence of obesity in the United States is high, with 30% of adults and 17% of children estimated to be obese. Despite its high occurrence, an earlier study found that the prevalence of obesity remained stable between 2003 and 2010. Because of this leveling off rate, scientists at the National Center for Health Statistics developed a hypothesis that the prevalence of obesity in youth and adults would also have remained stable between 2003 and 2012. The purpose of this study was to analyze trends in childhood and adult obesity between 2003 and 2012. The analyses were based on measurements of weight and height in 9120 participants from the 2011–2012 National Health and Nutrition Examination Survey (NHANES). Childhood obesity was defined as a body mass index (BMI) at or above the 95th percentile of the CDC BMI-for-age growth charts in children and adolescents aged 2 to 19 years. In adults, obesity was defined as a BMI greater than or equal to 30. Trends in obesity prevalence were analyzed across five periods (2003–2004, 2005–2006, 2007–2008, 2009–2010, and 2011–2012). Overall, the results of this study indicate no significant change for obesity from 2003–2004 through 2011–2012 in 2- to 19-year-olds or adults. Results for prevalence of obesity in 2011–2012 were 16.9% in youth and 34.9% in adults. There was a significant decrease in obesity from 13.9% to 8.4% among 2- to 5-year-olds and a significant increase in obesity from 31.5% to 38.1% among women aged 60 years and older. Based on these results, the authors of this study conclude that, while not increasing overall, the prevalence of obesity remains high in youth and adults, and thus should continue to be under surveillance.

Source: Ogden CL and others: Prevalence of childhood and adult obesity in the United States, 2011-2012. *Journal of the American Medical Association* 311:806. 2014 (see Further Reading 16).

Ask the RDN is a new feature in every chapter to answer questions about topics that may seem to have conflicting viewpoints. The Registered Dietitian Nutritionist is a qualified nutrition expert who is trained to help you separate facts from fads, and optimize your health with better food choices. This feature will highlight the ability of the RDN to translate the latest scientific findings into easy-to-understand nutrition information.

ASK THE RDN: Who's the Expert?

Dear RDN: *I am interested in making positive changes to my eating pattern to reach a healthy weight and feel better. How can I find a qualified nutrition expert who will give me personalized nutrition advice?*

You have already made a big step toward better nutrition by taking this nutrition course! The information in this textbook is written by authors who are all qualified nutrition experts, namely *registered dietitian nutritionists* (RDN). The textbook and your instructor will provide a solid foundation in nutrition, but be aware that some people call themselves "nutritionists" without qualified training in nutrition. The best approach to finding answers about your personal nutritional state is to consult your primary care provider, **registered dietitian (RD), or registered dietitian nutritionist (RDN).** The RD/RDN has been certified by the Commission on Dietetic Registration of the Academy of Nutrition and Dietetics (AND) after completing rigorous classroom and clinical training in nutrition. The RD/RDN must also complete continuing education. The RD credential was recently updated to RDN to better reflect the scope of practice of dietitians. While both titles signify the same credential, we will use RDN when referring to dietitians in this book.

You can begin your search for a local RDN by asking your primary care provider or calling your health insurance company for a referral. You can also find an RDN by using the AND national referral service, called *Find a Registered Dietitian Nutritionist.* This service links consumers with qualified nutrition practitioners who provide reliable, objective nutrition information. Visit the website, www.eatright.org, and click on "Find an Expert." (In Canada, visit the Dietitians of Canada website, www.dietitians.ca, and click on "Find a Dietitian.") Enter your ZIP code or state to display the providers in your area. Select additional specialties that may apply to your specific needs. The website will display a list of providers. A professional with the RD or RDN credential after his or her name is a qualified nutrition expert who is trained to help you separate facts from fads, and optimize your health with better food choices. You can trust an RDN to translate the latest scientific findings into easy-to-understand nutrition information that you can sink your teeth into.

I hope this answer was helpful. We will use this feature, "Ask the RDN," in every chapter to answer questions about topics that may seem to have conflicting viewpoints.

Your nutrition expert,

Anne M. Smith, PhD, RDN, LD (author)

The *Medicine Cabinet* feature presents information on common medications used to treat diseases that have a nutrition connection. These features highlight the ways medications can affect nutritional status, as well as ways food and nutrients can affect how medications work.

Medicine Cabinet

Proton pump inhibitors (PPIs) are medications that inhibit the ability of gastric cells to secrete hydrogen ions (i.e., protons). Low doses of this class of medications may be available without a prescription. Because stomach acid is important for the absorption of vitamin B-12, prolonged use of PPIs could impair vitamin B-12 status.

Examples:

- Omeprazole (Prilosec OTC®)
- Lansoprazole (Prevacid®)
- Rabeprazole (Aciphex®)
- Esomeprazole (Nexium®)

Connecting with a
Personal Focus

Applying Nutrition on a Personal Level

Throughout the fifth edition, we reinforce the fact that each person responds differently to nutrients. To further convey the importance of applying nutrition to their personal lives, we include many examples of people and situations that resonate with college students. We also stress the importance of learning to intelligently sort through the seemingly endless range of nutrition messages to recognize reliable information and to sensibly apply it to their own lives. Our goal is to provide students the tools they need to eat healthfully and make informed nutrition decisions after they complete the class. Many of these features can be assigned and graded through Connect to help students learn and apply the information and engage with the text.

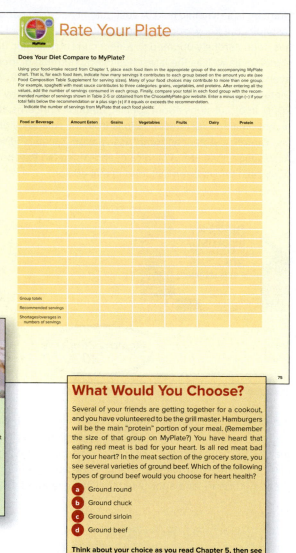

Rate Your Plate

Does Your Diet Compare to MyPlate?

Using your food-intake record from Chapter 1, place each food item in the appropriate group of the accompanying MyPlate chart. That is, for each food item, indicate how many servings it contributes to each group based on the amount you ate (see Food Composition Table Supplement for serving sizes). Many of your food choices may contribute to more than one group. For example, spaghetti with meat sauce contributes to three categories: grains, vegetables, and proteins. After entering all the values, add the number of servings consumed in each group. Finally, compare your total in each food group with the recommended number of servings shown in Table 2-5 or obtained from the ChooseMyPlate.gov website. Enter a minus sign (−) if your total falls below the recommendation or a plus sign (+) if it equals or exceeds the recommendation. Indicate the number of servings from MyPlate that each food yields:

Food or Beverage	Amount Eaten	Grains	Vegetables	Fruits	Dairy	Protein
Group totals						
Recommended servings						
Shortages/overages in numbers of servings						

75

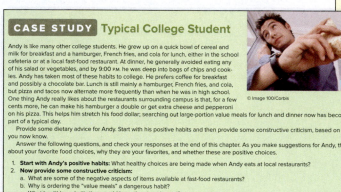

CASE STUDY **Typical College Student**

Andy is like many other college students. He grew up on a quick bowl of cereal and milk for breakfast and a hamburger, French fries, and cola for lunch, either in the school cafeteria or at a local fast-food restaurant. At dinner, he generally avoided eating any of his salad or vegetables, and by 9:00 P.M. he was deep into bags of chips and cookies. Andy has taken most of these habits to college. He prefers coffee for breakfast and possibly a chocolate bar. Lunch is still mainly a hamburger, French fries, and cola, but pizza and tacos now alternate more frequently than when he was in high school. One thing Andy really likes about the restaurants surrounding campus is that, for a few cents more, he can make his hamburger a double or get extra cheese and pepperoni on his pizza. This helps him stretch his food dollar; searching out large-portion value meals for lunch and dinner now has become part of a typical day.

© Image 100/Corbis

Provide some dietary advice for Andy. Start with his positive habits and then provide some constructive criticism, based on what you now know.

Answer the following questions, and check your responses at the end of this chapter. As you make suggestions for Andy, think about your favorite food choices, why they are your favorites, and whether these are positive choices.

1. **Start with Andy's positive habits:** What healthy choices are being made when Andy eats at local restaurants?
2. **Now provide some constructive criticism:**
   a. What are some of the negative aspects of items available at fast-food restaurants?
   b. Why is ordering the "value meals" a dangerous habit?
   c. What healthier substitutions could he make at each meal?
   d. List some healthier choices he could make at fast-food restaurants on campus.

What Would You Choose?

Several of your friends are getting together for a cookout, and you have volunteered to be the grill master. Hamburgers will be the main "protein" portion of your meal. (Remember the size of that group on MyPlate?) You have heard that eating red meat is bad for your heart. Is all red meat bad for your heart? In the meat section of the grocery store, you see several varieties of ground beef. Which of the following types of ground beef would you choose for heart health?

a Ground round
b Ground chuck
c Ground sirloin
d Ground beef

Think about your choice as you read Chapter 5, then see What the Dietitian Chose at the end of the chapter.

Challenging Students to Think Critically

The pages of *Wardlaw's Contemporary Nutrition: A Functional Approach* contain numerous opportunities for students to learn more about themselves and their diet and to use their new knowledge of nutrition to improve their health. These pedagogical elements include Critical Thinking, Ask the RDN, Case Studies, Nutrition and Your Health, What Would You Choose?, and Newsworthy Nutrition. Many of the thought-provoking topics highlighted in these features are expanded upon in the online resources found in Connect.

5.8 Nutrition and Your Health
Lipids and Cardiovascular Disease

The typical forms of cardiovascular disease—coronary heart disease and strokes—are associated with inadequate blood circulation in the heart and brain related to buildup of this plaque. Blood supplies the heart muscle, brain, and other body organs with oxygen and nutrients. When blood flow via the coronary arteries surrounding the heart is interrupted, the heart muscle can be damaged. A heart attack, or **myocardial infarction,** may result (review Fig. 5-17). This may cause the heart to beat irregularly or to stop. About 25% of people do not survive their first heart attack. If blood flow to parts of the brain is interrupted long enough, part of the brain dies, causing a **cerebrovascular accident,** or stroke.

A heart attack can strike with the sudden force of a sledgehammer, with pain radiating up the neck or down the arm. It can sneak up at night, masquerading as indigestion, with slight pain or pressure in the chest. Crushing chest pain is a more common symptom in men (see Further Reading 11). Many times, the symptoms are so subtle in women that death occurs before she or the health professional realizes that a heart attack is taking place. If there is any suspicion that a heart attack is taking place, the person should first

Connecting to Engaging Visuals

Attractive, Accurate Artwork

Illustrations, photographs, and tables in the text were created to help students more easily master complex scientific concepts.

- Many illustrations were updated or replaced to inspire student inquiry and comprehension and to promote interest and retention of information. Many were also redesigned to use brighter colors and a more attractive, contemporary style.
- In many figures, color-coding and directional arrows make it easier to follow events and reinforce interrelationships. Process descriptions appear in the body of the figures. This pairing of the action and an explanation walks students step-by-step through the process and increases teaching effectiveness.

The final result is a striking visual program that holds readers' attention and supports the goals of clarity, ease of comprehension, and critical thinking. The attractive layout and design of this edition are clean, bright, and inviting. This creative presentation of the material is geared toward engaging today's visually oriented students.

(a)

(b)

	Food Item and Amount	Vitamin C (milligrams)	% RDA for Adult Males (90 milligrams)	% RDA for Adult Females (75 milligrams)
Grains	Whole Grain Total® cereal, 1 cup	60	67%	80%
Grains	Tortellini with cheese filling, ½ cup	0	0%	0%
Grains	Brown rice, cooked, ½ cup	0	0%	0%
Vegetables	Red peppers, raw, 1 cup	190	211%	253%
Vegetables	Brussels sprouts, cooked, 1 cup	97	108%	129%
Vegetables	Spinach, raw, 2 cups	17	19%	23%
Fruits	Strawberries, 1 cup	89	99%	119%
Fruits	Orange, 1 medium	83	92%	111%
Fruits	Grapefruit juice, canned, 1 cup	72	80%	96%

FIGURE 10-11 Food sources of vitamin C. (a) The fill of the background color (none, 1/3, 2/3, or completely covered) within each food group on MyPlate indicates the average nutrient density for vitamin C in that group. (b) The bar graph shows the vitamin C content of several foods compared to the RDA for adult males and females. Overall, fruits and vegetables are the richest sources of vitamin C. Foods in the dairy and protein groups (not shown) are poor sources of vitamin C.

Source: *Nutrition data from USDA National Nutrient Database for Standard Reference, Release 26.*

Connecting with the Latest Updates

Global Changes

- To help our readers locate cross-references in the text, we have added section numbers when referring to other chapters/sections of text. This will be especially helpful when using the digital text because these references are hot links that will take you right to that section!

- Throughout this new edition we have replaced the term "diet" in most cases with the term "eating pattern" or "dietary pattern." This reflects the emphasis on "healthy eating patterns" in the new 2015–2020 Dietary Guidelines for Americans.

- In addition, we have replaced the term "calorie" with "kilocalorie" when referring to specific energy amounts. For example, the Concept Check for Section 1.4 now reads: What are the energy (kilocalorie) values for each of the "energy nutrients"?

- Images of the Nutrition Facts Label have been updated to the newly approved format.

- One of the most noticeable changes in this new edition is the inclusion of the new feature, *"Ask the RDN (Registered Dietitian Nutritionist)"* in every chapter. We have used this feature to address questions we frequently hear students asking about food and nutrition topics covered in the popular media. We use the *"Ask the RDN"* in Chapter 1 to set the stage, answering the most important question "How can I find a qualified nutrition expert who will give me personalized nutrition advice?" The feature is answered and signed by one of the authors, who are all Registered Dietitian Nutritionists! Along these same lines, we have emphasized RDNs as the nutrition experts and integral part of the health care team throughout the text.

- The last section of each chapter, *Nutrition and Your Health,* is now a numbered section (e.g., Section 1.8 in Chapter 1) for easier navigating especially within the digital components of the text.

- As we discuss healthy eating patterns throughout the text, you will notice more emphasis on the problems of overconsumption of added sugars and less emphasis on problems from the consumption of dietary cholesterol.

Chapter-by-Chapter Revisions

Chapter 1: *Nutrition, Food Choices, and Health*

- Section 1.1 has been updated with the latest statistics on fast-food restaurant advertising to children as well as a discussion of the increase in marketing of fast food via mobile devices and social media.

- Figure 1-3 now illustrates the 10 leading causes of death in the United States as reported by the Centers for Disease Control and Prevention in August 2015 (see Further Reading 15).

- The ingredient list on the Nutrition Facts panel shown in Figure 1-4 has been updated to reflect the inclusion of only whole wheat flour.

- Section 1.6, "What Is the Current State of the North American Diet and Health?" has been updated extensively to reflect recent changes in obesity trends. Figure 1-7 showing the percentage of adults who were obese in 2013, as well as other obesity statistics, has been updated. The most recent report, *F as in Fat: How Obesity Threatens America's Future 2013,* is discussed. The *Newsworthy Nutrition* feature has been updated to "No change in obesity prevalence in youth or adults between 2003 and 2012," summarizing research published in the *Journal of the American Medical Association* in 2014 (Further Reading 16).

- Further Readings have been updated with three new articles and all Further Readings are now linked to the end of chapter list in the digital text.

Chapter 2: *Designing a Healthy Dietary Pattern*

- Significant changes in Chapter 2 revolve around the newly released 2015–2020 Dietary Guidelines for Americans. In Section 2.2, the entire subsection, "Dietary Guidelines—The Basis for Menu Planning" has been revised. To help students understand the political issues surrounding the Guidelines, we have included a discussion of the process used to establish them. The five foundational guidelines of the 2015–2020 Dietary Guidelines are outlined and Key Recommendations are illustrated in Figure 2-2.

- Section 2.2 also highlights the Guidelines' new emphasis on "Healthy Eating Patterns" with the following new subsections: Shifting to Healthy Eating Patterns; Importance of Calorie Balance Within Healthy Eating Patterns; Food Components to Include in Your Healthy Eating Pattern; and Food Components to Limit in Your Healthy Eating Pattern. The new Figure 2-3, Comparing current eating patterns in the United States to the Dietary Guidelines, is directly from the Guidelines report.

- Section 2.3, MyPlate—A Menu-Planning Tool, has been updated to reflect the new Dietary Guidelines and includes the new *Ask the RDN* feature, which answers the question of how to follow the Mediterranean Diet eating plan.

- A new box on Diet and Nutrition Apps has been added to Section 2.7 and includes a link to the Academy of Nutrition and Dietetics' science-based reviews of the most popular diet and nutrition apps for phones and tablets.

Chapter 3: *The Human Body: A Nutrition Perspective*

- Figure 3-10 has been updated to illustrate the location of the pharynx.

- In Section 3.9, the *Newsworthy Nutrition* feature has been updated to present recent research on the effects of probiotics on bowel regularity.

- Section 3.11 has been updated with current terminology and the latest statistics on the relationships between nutrition and genetics. Readers will find an expanded and updated collection of web resources for further information on genetics.

- The *Nutrition and Your Health* feature in Section 3.12 includes updated information on treatments for irritable bowel syndrome. The new *Ask the RDN* feature explores the question of whether a gluten-free diet is an effective weight-loss method.

- In the *Rate Your Plate* activity, we now provide a link to an interactive tool to generate a medical family tree.

Chapter 4: *Carbohydrates*

- In Section 4.3, the idea of consuming fruits and vegetables as juice is discussed as an answer to the *Ask the RDN* question, Is juicing healthier than eating whole fruits or vegetables?

- *What Are FODMAPs?* is a new information box in Section 4.4 and explains this group of fermentable carbohydrates and lists several websites that provide practical information on foods to avoid and foods to include when restricting FODMAPs.

- Section 4.6 provides a list of the new 2015–2020 Dietary Guidelines' recommendations for carbohydrate intake as part of a healthy eating pattern.

- Also featured in Section 4.6 is a new *Newsworthy Nutrition*, "Americans are decreasing consumption of sugar-sweetened beverages," based on research published in 2013.

- The CDC *National Diabetes Statistics Report, 2014,* as well as the *Position of the Academy of Nutrition and Dietetics: Health implications of dietary fiber, 2015,* have been updated in the Further Readings.

Chapter 5: *Lipids*

- On the whole, Chapter 5 has been reorganized to improve flow of information. Some figures and text content have been moved so that all of the information on food sources of lipids appears in Section 5.3 and all of the recommendations for fat intake appear in Section 5.7.

- Throughout the chapter, to reflect updated advice from the 2015–2020 Dietary Guidelines and the American Heart Association's Diet and Lifestyle Recommendations, we emphasize that the quality of fat in the diet is just as important as the total amount of fat in the diet. In addition, we have removed any outdated recommendations about specific limits for dietary cholesterol intake.

- Section 5.1 has been expanded to introduce students to some of the core terminology in the chapter.

- Figure 5-3 has been revised to more accurately represent the relationships among key omega-3 and omega-6 fatty acids. Likewise, the Lipids Concept Map, now in Section 5.2, has been simplified to show how the various forms of lipids are related to each other.

- In Section 5.3, we point out that partially hydrogenated oils are no longer generally recognized as safe for use in food products.

- In Section 5.6, we have added a new subsection on the role of lipids in regulating body processes. Information about eicosanoids, which had previously existed elsewhere in the chapter, is now presented in this section.

- Table 5-5 has been updated with the latest Diet and Lifestyle Recommendations from the American Heart Association, which were released in 2013.

- A new subheading within Section 5.7 summarizes the advice of public health authorities on fish consumption. Also, a new subsection discusses dietary patterns that promote cardiovascular health.

- In Section 5.7 we have included a new *Ask the RDN* feature about the health benefits of coconut oil.

Chapter 6: *Proteins*

- The steady drop in U.S. meat and poultry consumption is highlighted in Section 6.3 with new statistics from 2014 and contrasted with the significant increase in dairy production and consumption in China and India.

- The new protein intake recommendations from the 2015–2020 Dietary Guidelines are outlined in Section 6.6, including the shifts recommended to increase variety in protein food choices and to make more nutrient-dense choices. Section 6.6 also includes a discussion of current research showing that a more equal distribution of protein at each meal is important in maintaining body composition and bone health and in regulating glucose.

- The association between the consumption of high levels of red and processed meat and the increased risk of colorectal cancer, including the findings of the 2015 report of the World Health Organization, is discussed in more detail in Section 6.7.

- Section 6.7 also includes a discussion of the Paleo Diet™ in the form of an answer to the *Ask the RDN* question: Is the Paleo Diet™ a healthy way to include a good amount of high-quality protein into my eating plan?

- The graphic of "The New American Plate" in Section 6.9 has been replaced with a new photo published by the American Institute for Cancer Research.

- Section 6.9 also includes a new *Newsworthy Nutrition*, Vegetarian Dietary Patterns Decrease Risk of Colorectal Cancers, based on research published in 2015.

Chapter 7: *Energy Balance and Weight Control*

- The CDC obesity prevalence and trends have been updated throughout to reflect the most current data.

- The components of a healthy body weight have been revised throughout the chapter to emphasize the importance of dietary patterns and positive lifestyle behaviors in successful weight management and align with the 2015–2020 Dietary Guidelines for Americans.

- Non-HDL cholesterol has been added as a risk factor for nutrition-related chronic disease in Section 7.3.

- Evidence-based updates for Health Problems Associated with Excess Body Fat have been revised in Table 7-2.

- Information on the DEXA-specific software that was developed to assess visceral body fat distribution has now been added in Section 7.3.
- Revisions aligning with the 2015–2020 Dietary Guidelines for Americans have been made to Table 7-3 to describe factors that encourage excess body fat stores and obesity.
- The weight-loss triad, Figure 7-17, has been updated to emphasize the interrelated components of successful weight loss.
- The Biggest Loser Eating Plan has been added in the new *Ask the RDN* feature in Section 7.5.
- The *Newsworthy Nutrition* article in Section 7.6 has been updated to a 2015 publication documenting the link between a plant-based dietary pattern and healthy body weight.
- Table 7-5 has been condensed to include most popular physical activities and estimated calorie costs associated with each activity.
- The Section 7.8 title has been altered (Behavioral Strategies for Weight Management) to emphasize the importance of modifiable lifestyle behaviors in successful weight management and control.
- Section 7.8 has also been updated throughout to reflect 2015–2020 DGA updates and recommended shifts in dietary patterns to promote a healthy lifestyle. The DGA Strategies for Action with guiding principles and societal efforts help to combat obesity.
- The title for Table 7-6 has been updated to Behavioral Tactics for Weight Loss.
- Updates to weight-loss medications, recommendations, and contraindications have been made in Section 7.9.
- Information on intermittent fasting has been added to Section 7.9 as a strategy for obesity treatment.
- Figure 7-20 has been condensed to reflect the most current bariatric procedures along with updated patient selection criteria.
- The Summary of Popular Diet Approaches to Weight Control has been condensed and updated in Table 7-7.
- Further Readings have been updated with three new references.

Chapter 8: *Overview of Micronutrients and Phytochemicals*

- The chapter title now includes phytochemicals and reflects that this information has been moved and updated in this chapter.
- A newly redesigned Figure 8-1 has been revised to reflect the key micronutrients contributing to bodily functions throughout the functional chapters.
- Summary Tables 8-1 through 8-4 have been updated to enhance readability and quickly summarize pertinent information on the functions, requirements, food sources, deficiency, and toxicity of vitamins and minerals detailed throughout the functional chapters.

- Sections have been renamed throughout Section 8.3 to reflect current research. New titles include Body Defenses, Bone Health, and Blood and Brain Health.
- The new *Ask the RDN* in Section 8.3 features the Raw Food Plant Diet.
- The Top 5 Dietary Supplements has been updated from 2012 to 2014 data in Section 8.5.
- A new *Newsworthy News* feature has been updated with a 2015 study documenting increased emergency department visits for dietary supplement users.
- The Chapter Summary reflects updates throughout and now includes functional foods. In addition, a new study question on phytochemicals has been added.
- Further Readings have been updated to include three new articles.

Chapter 9: *Fluid and Electrolyte Balance*

- Newly redesigned food source figures in this chapter (Figs. 9-14 and 9-15 for sodium and potassium) and throughout the text include both the nutrient density for the nutrients for foods in each food group on MyPlate and a bar graph showing the nutrient content of several foods from each food group compared to the AI for adult males and females.
- The discussion of bottled water has been expanded in Section 9.2 with new statistics for the consumption of bottled water in 2014, as well as a link to the Natural Resources Defense Council website where students can read more about bottled water.
- Questions about limiting the amount of salt in the diet are answered in the new *Ask the RDN* feature in Section 9.6, which concludes with a new *Newsworthy Nutrition*, No Evidence for Extreme Sodium Restrictions for Older Adults, based on research published in 2015.
- Several updates have been made to Section 9.9 on Minerals and Hypertension. The importance of balancing sodium and potassium to control blood pressure is highlighted in a new *Newsworthy Nutrition*, and medications used to lower blood pressure are now outlined in the *Medicine Cabinet* feature. We recommend the DASH diet and point out that it was named the best overall eating plan for the sixth year in a row on the *U.S. News & World Report's* 2016 Best Diets list.
- *What the Dietitian Chose* includes updates on the class action lawsuits filed by a number of U.S. consumers against the Coca-Cola® Bottling Company for false marketing of its popular vitaminwater® brand.
- There are six new *Further Readings*.

Chapter 10: *Nutrients Involved in Body Defenses*

- In this edition, discussions of nutrients that function as antioxidants and nutrients that support immunity have been combined into one revised chapter that focuses on body defenses. New pedagogical elements reflect this reorganization of content.

- Section 10.1 now presents an overview of the immune system and the immune response. Table 10-1 summarizes the nutrients that support immune function.

- Whereas they existed in separate chapters in the fourth edition of *Contemporary Nutrition: A Functional Approach,* vitamin A and carotenoids are now discussed in tandem in Section 10.3.

- Throughout the chapters on micronutrients, we have made the presentation of vitamins and minerals consistent to include subsections on functions, deficiency, dietary requirements, and toxicity (if applicable). Section 10.5 on vitamin E was one that we revised to ensure this consistent navigation of content.

- Formerly a *Nutrition and Your Health* feature, emerging evidence on the importance of probiotics for immune health is now presented in Section 10.9.

- Section 10.10 on Nutrition and Cancer contains updated statistics and a revised discussion of the progression of cancer. The link between excess body fat and cancer is explored in further detail. In the discussion of cancer prevention, we have emphasized the importance of overall dietary patterns and whole foods rather than individual nutrients.

Chapter 11: *Nutrients Involved In Bone Health*

- Table 11-1, Biological Factors Associated with Bone Status, has been expanded to include estrogen.

- Section 11.2, Factors That Influence Bone Health, has been reorganized and includes an update on the debate over the impact of protein intake and acid load on bone health. A critical review of this topic published in 2014 has been added to the Further Readings.

- A discussion of the effect of coffee and colas on bone health has been added to Section 11.3 in the answer to the *Ask the RDN* question, "Could the caffeine in these drinks be damaging my bones and leading to osteoporosis?"

- The functions of vitamin D are now presented in two subsections: (1) Blood Calcium Regulation; and (2) Gene Expression and Cell Growth. Figure 11-8 is a new illustration depicting how vitamin D regulates blood calcium.

- In Section 11.9, we have included updated 2014 prevalence statistics from the National Osteoporosis Foundation (see Further Reading 17), as well as a simplified Figure 11-16 depicting the relationship between peak bone mass and the ultimate risk of developing osteoporosis and related bone fractures.

- You will find more current information on the increasing sales of nondairy milk beverages and on the availability of new products such as cashew milk in Section 11.11. Cashew milk is now listed in Table 11-6, which also has updated values on the nutrient content of nondairy milk beverages. A new bulleted list, Dairy-Free Shopping Guide: Things to Consider, is also available in Section 11.11.

- The Further Readings have been updated with five new articles.

Chapter 12: *Micronutrient Function in Energy Metabolism*

- In Section 12.8, the term *iodine* is now used instead of *iodide* to be consistent with Dietary Reference Intakes. The link between mild iodine deficiency during pregnancy and decreased IQ in offspring is discussed based on recent studies published in 2013. To further explore this topic, a new *Newsworthy Nutrition* feature presents research published in 2015 on marginal iodine status among women of childbearing years in the United States.

- Tips that will help boost metabolism, burn more calories, and reduce extra body fat are listed in Section 12.10 in the answer to the *Ask the RDN* question "Are there things I can do that will increase my metabolism and help prevent my weight from creeping up?"

- There are three new Further Readings.

Chapter 13: *Nutrients That Support Blood and Brain Health*

- In the fifth edition, we have incorporated state-of-the-science research about the role of nutrition in brain health into Chapter 13. The chapter title has been updated to "Nutrients That Support Blood and Brain Health." The first part of the chapter now reviews the roles of vitamin K, folate, vitamin B-12, iron, and copper in synthesizing and maintaining the health of red blood cells. A new *Nutrition and Your Health* feature in Section 13.7 reviews the functions of nutrients in brain health. Content on the roles of nutrients and probiotics in immune health has been moved to Chapter 10.

- *What Would You Choose?* was revised to focus on the recent WHO report linking red meat consumption with cancer.

- The title of Section 13.2 has been updated to "Hemostasis and Vitamin K" to reflect revisions related to blood loss and vitamin K.

- Figure 13-5 has been updated to include arrows highlighting the importance of prothrombin activator in the conversion from prothrombin to thrombin.

- Information regarding parental refusal of vitamin K supplementation by parents has been added to Section 13.2 (also see Further Reading 18).

- The new *Ask the RDN* features reviews Peter D'Adamo's book *Eat Right for Your Type (4 Blood Types, 4 Diets): The Individualized Diet Solution to Staying Healthy, Living Longer & Achieving Your Ideal Weight.*

- In Section 13.3, a more detailed explanation of the functions of folate covers its roles in neurotransmission, depression, and cancer protection.

- Section 13.7 contains new information on *Brain Health: Food for Thought.* This novel addition details nutrients related to the formation of brain tissue, fuel for the brain, the nervous system, and brain health protection. The section also covers the latest research on the ways in which nutritional status during gestation and infancy, childhood, adolescence, and adulthood may affect cognition, learning abilities, behavior, migraines, depression, and neurodegenerative diseases. The MIND Diet, a dietary intervention that shows promising results for protecting the brain against cognitive decline, is detailed in Section 13.7 and supported by Further Reading 11.

- Seventeen new Further Readings have been added to reinforce the new concepts in this chapter.

Chapter 14: *Nutrition: Fitness and Sports*

- Sports nutrition advice throughout the chapter has been updated to align with the revised joint position statement on nutrition and athletic performance from the Academy of Nutrition and Dietetics, Dietitians of Canada, and the American College of Sports Medicine, released in March 2016.

- Figure 14-5 illustrates the general concept of energy storage in the chemical bonds of ATP.

- Throughout the chapter, especially in Table 14-5 and Table 14-9, references to sports nutrition products have been updated to reflect the current market.

- In Section 14.4, the discussion of the controversial topic of protein needs of athletes, including the amount and timing of protein intake, has been updated with the latest research.

- The *Newsworthy Nutrition* feature now focuses on research on a link between sports drinks and weight gain among adolescents and young adults.

- Section 14.6 has been updated with the latest statistics and data on commonly used ergogenic aids.

- The Further Readings have been updated with 10 new resources on sports nutrition.

Chapter 15: *Eating Disorders*

- In Section 15.2, we have added information about the two subtypes of anorexia nervosa: restricting type and binge-eating/purging type. This information reinforces the point that a person with an eating disorder exists on a spectrum of disordered eating behaviors and may migrate from one disorder to another.

- The discussion of physical effects of anorexia nervosa has been updated and expanded.

- In Section 15.3, a new *Newsworthy Nutrition* feature looks at the relationship between bulimia nervosa and binge drinking or substance abuse.

- Section 15.4 has been updated with information on lisdexamfetamine, the first drug to be approved for treatment of binge-eating disorder.

- A new *Ask the RDN* feature in Section 15.4 describes the science behind intermittent fasting, but cautions readers that this weight-loss method can be a gateway to disordered eating behavior.

- In Section 15.5, the various types of subthreshold eating disorders are explained in greater detail.

- Sixteen new articles have been incorporated into the listing of Further Readings.

Chapter 16: *Undernutrition Throughout the World*

- Targets and progress towards the eight United Nations Millennium Development Goals (MDGs) have been updated throughout the chapter and highlighted in Table 16-1.

- Statistics on both domestic and global poverty and hunger from the FAO and U.S. Census Bureau have been updated with 2015 data.

- The prevalence of hunger, nutrient-deficiency diseases, and related health outcomes have also been updated to reflect the current literature.

- Updates of the characteristics of users and impact of the federally subsidized nutrition programs, including SNAP, WIC, and Senior Nutrition Services that supply food for people in the United States, has been updated in Section 16.2.

- Section 16.3 now includes expanded information available related to the nutritional impact of war and political unrest in the Middle East and specific to refugees, those internally displaced, or those seeking political or religious asylum.

- A section on the Global Hunger Index (GHI), a tool designed to measure and track hunger worldwide, is discussed in Section 16.3. Climate change, the green revolution, and sustainable agriculture and their impact are also expanded in this section.

- The 17 United Nations Sustainable Development Goals, a blueprint for global health, have been updated in the text and Figure 16-5 added.

- Updates of the positive impact of global efforts to combat HIV/AIDS has been added.

- The Non-GMO Project initiative promoting GMO food labeling has been added.

- The *Ask the RDN* features the non-GMO diet.

- A 2014 global analysis on GMO crops and pesticide exposure is included in the text and as a Further Reading.

- Undernutrition throughout all life stages (pregnancy through older adults) has been updated to reflect current prevalence and associated health outcomes.

- The Further Readings include eight new references.

Chapter 17: *Safety of Our Food Supply*

- In Section 17.1, many recent examples of foodborne illness outbreaks have been added throughout the text and in Table 17-1.

- Table 17-2, which summarizes the agencies responsible for monitoring the food supply in the United States, has been streamlined to improve readability.

- The discussion of overuse of antibiotics in animal feeds in Section 17-1 has been revised and expanded.

- In Section 17-2, ultra-high temperature (UHT) processing has been added to the discussion of food preservation methods.

- A new Figure 17-2 illustrates the settings of Norovirus outbreaks in the United States.

- The *Ask the RDN* feature weighs the pros and cons of "clean" eating.

- To match the layout of other sections, we have added Table 17-7 to summarize natural substances in foods that can cause foodborne illness.

- Table 17-8 has been revised to include a greater variety of common sources of caffeine.

- Table 17-9 now includes bisphenol A.

- A new margin note in Section 17.6 highlights the ongoing public health crisis that surfaced when high levels of lead were detected in the drinking water in Flint, Michigan.

- In Section 17.6, we have included information about USDA's Pesticide Data Program.

- Table 17-10 has been updated with the Environmental Working Group's 2015 Dirty Dozen™ and Clean Fifteen.

- We have included the latest evidence on organic food production in Section 17.7.

- Ten new resources have been added to the Further Readings.

Chapter 18: *Nutrition During Pregnancy and Breastfeeding*

- The content about nutrition and fertility in Section 18.1 has been organized under the headings, "Hormonal Balance," "Key Nutrients," and "Alcohol."

- *Ask the RDN* reviews *The Fertility Diet.*

- Section 18.3 now includes updated statistics about low birthweight, preterm birth, teenage pregnancy, and prenatal care.

- In several places throughout the chapter, we point out some useful online resources to plan healthy dietary patterns during pregnancy.

- Section 18.4 has been revised to reflect the most recent recommendations of the 2015–2020 Dietary Guidelines and the American Heart Association. We also reiterate the importance of adequate hydration during exercise.

- In Section 18.5, we have expanded our discussion of a healthy dietary pattern during pregnancy to offer advice on food choices within each food group.

- A new margin note in Section 18.7 summarizes the striking results of a 2016 analysis of the economic benefits of breastfeeding.

- The listing of Further Readings now includes 13 updated resources.

Chapter 19: *Nutrition from Infancy Through Adolescence*

- In Table 19-2, the descriptions of infant nutrition products have been updated to reflect the current market.

- In Section 19.3, the paragraph on safe preparation and storage of infant formula has been expanded and updated. Information about BPA in baby bottles has been revised.

- A new Table 19-4 presents typical formula intake by infants across a range of ages.

- Updated information about kilocalories, sodium, and added sugars from the 2015–2020 Dietary Guidelines for Americans

has been incorporated throughout the recommendations for infant, child, and adolescent dietary planning.

- A new margin note in Section 19.4 highlights current events pertaining to lead contamination of the water supply in Flint, Michigan.

- In Section 19.4, the content on vegetarian diet planning for children has been expanded and revised.

- A new *Ask the RDN* feature explores the connections between nutrition and autism.

- In Section 19.5, we have included information from the 2016 WHO Report of the Commission on Ending Childhood Obesity.

- In Section 19.7, information pertaining to food allergies and intolerances has been updated with new statistics and terminology to reflect current medical literature. A new *Newsworthy Nutrition* feature explains the ramifications of the LEAP study for children at risk of peanut allergies.

- Fifteen new resources have been added to the Further Readings.

Chapter 20: *Nutrition During Adulthood*

- Some of the content related to brain health (e.g., depression, Alzheimer's disease) has been moved from this chapter to the new *Nutrition and Your Health* feature in Section 13.7. Because of this reorganization, we have combined the two sections that discussed physiological and psychosocial changes that affect nutritional status. Now, Section 20.3 is called "Factors Related to Nutritional Status of Adults."

- In Section 20.1, a new *Newsworthy Nutrition* feature highlights research on the relationship between animal protein intake and mortality.

- In Section 20.2, nutrition recommendations for the adult years have been updated to reflect the 2015–2020 Dietary Guidelines for Americans. In this section, we also present the latest research on protein needs of older adults.

- Figure 20-3 has been updated to match the most recent version of the Nutrition Screening Initiative's Nutrition Checklist for Older Adults, which utilizes the DETERMINE mnemonic.

- Table 20-2 has been revised and expanded to provide more comprehensive array of strategies to cope with the physiological changes of aging.

- In Section 20.3, we have expanded our discussion of nutritional strategies to cope with arthritis. To further expand upon this topic, the new *Ask the RDN* feature reviews the potential benefits of an anti-inflammatory diet.

- Table 20-3 has been updated with the latest research on popular herbal remedies used by American adults. Referrals to some current and relevant online resources pertaining to complementary and alternative medicine are provided.

- In Section 20.4, we have included the recent MyPlate for Older Adults from Tufts University. Information related to the use of community nutrition services by older Americans has been updated.

- In Section 20.5, we have incorporated new research about alcohol intake and cancer risk. Recommendations regarding alcohol use now reflect the 2015–2020 Dietary Guidelines for Americans.
- Eleven recent resources have been added to the Further Readings.

List of Key Digital Updates*

2015–2020 Dietary Guidelines for Americans updates across Question Bank, Test Bank, and LearnSmart/SmartBook

Connect Question Banks Updates

- Addition of *case studies* for every chapter as assignable content
- Addition of dietary analysis assignment (from Appendix C) as assignable content
- NEW *Newsworthy Nutrition* integrated concept questions from text
  - Chapter 1: No change in obesity prevalence in youth or adults between 2003 and 2012.
  - Chapter 3: Probiotics provide relief from constipation.
  - Chapter 4: Americans are decreasing consumption of sugar-sweetened beverages.
  - Chapter 7: Plant-based dietary pattern promotes healthy body weight.
  - Chapter 8: Increased emergency department visits for dietary supplement users.
  - Chapter 9: No evidence for extreme sodium restrictions for older adults/sodium, but step up potassium to control blood pressure.

  - Chapter 12: Marginal iodine status in women planning pregnancies.
  - Chapter 14: Sports drinks cause weight gain among adolescents and young adults.
  - Chapter 15: Substance use among adolescents with eating disorders.
  - Chapter 19: Glycemic index of food choices may influence acne, early introduction of peanut protein reduces peanut allergy.
  - Chapter 20: Low animal protein intake is associated with a major reduction in mortality.
- Revised *What Would You Choose* integrated concept question, Chapter 13: Reducing red meat intake

Instructor Resources Updates

- PowerPoint slides updates to include:
  - What Would You Choose from text
  - NEW **Case Studies** from each chapter
  - Accessibility updates
- Updated Teaching Strategies include a variety of classroom discussion topics and activities for student learning. With this edition, we have included many new ideas that make use of digital resources and social media to engage millennial learners. This "buffet" of teaching strategies will provide options that are adaptable for face-to-face, hybrid, or online learning environments.
- "Dietary Analysis Assignment" available as a Word document.

*One of the many benefits of digital tools is the ability for live/real-time improvements to benefit the modern students' learning. This list is updated at the time it was first available for purchase; there may be more anytime after.

Contents

Preface iv

Part One: Nutrition: A Key to Health

Part Two: Energy Nutrients and Energy Balance

Breakfast: ©Corbis/Punchstock; oriental woman: ©BloomImage RF/Getty Images; salad, pizza: ©Getty Images/Jonelle Weaver; bowl of cereal: ©Medioimages/Photodisc/Getty Images; salmon: ©Ingram Publishing/SuperStock; beans/rice: ©Digital Vision/age footstock; picnic basket: ©Ingram Publishing

Part Three: Vitamins, Minerals, and Water

Part Four: Nutrition: Beyond the Nutrients

Part Five: Nutrition: A Focus on Life Stages

© Corbis/Punchstock

Student Learning Outcomes

Chapter 1 is designed to allow you to:

1.1 Describe how our food choices are affected by the flavor, texture, and appearance of food; routines and habits; early experiences and customs; advertising; nutrition and health concerns; restaurants; social changes; economics; and physiological processes affected by meal size and composition.

1.2 Identify diet and lifestyle factors that contribute to the 15 leading causes of death in North America.

1.3 Define the terms *nutrition, carbohydrate, protein, lipid (fat), alcohol, vitamin, mineral, water, phytochemical, kilocalorie (kcal),* and *fiber.*

1.4 Determine the total calories (kcal) of a food or diet using the weight and calorie content of the energy-yielding nutrients, convert English to metric units, and calculate percentages, such as percent of calories from fat in a diet.

Chapter 1
Nutrition, Food Choices, and Health

What Would You Choose?

We begin each chapter with this activity to get you thinking. We ask you to make a choice that is right for you using the concepts discussed in the chapter. At the end of each chapter, we provide the logic behind what a dietitian would recommend.

You were awake last night until 2:30 A.M. finishing a class project. Unfortunately, your Psychology 101 class meets at 9:00 this morning. When your alarm goes off at 7:30 A.M., you decide to sleep those extra 20 minutes it would take to sit down and enjoy breakfast at the dining hall. What's your best time-saving breakfast option? What factors may hold you back from making the correct choice?

a Skip breakfast but plan to consume a few extra calories at lunch and dinner.

b Eat a low-fat granola bar and iced coffee from the vending machines in your dorm.

c Eat a quick bowl of Wheaties™ with a banana and low-fat milk along with a yogurt, all from your dorm room "pantry."

d Pick up a ham, egg, and cheese bagel.

Think about your choice as you read Chapter 1, then see What the Dietitian Chose at the end of the chapter.

Research has clearly shown that a lifestyle that includes a diet rich in fruits, vegetables, and whole grains, coupled with regular exercise, can enhance our quality of life in the short term and keep us healthy for many years to come. Unfortunately, this healthy lifestyle is not always easy to follow. When it comes to "nutrition," it is clear that some of our diets are out of balance with our metabolism, physiology, and physical activity level.

We begin this chapter with some questions. What influences your daily food choices? How important are factors such as taste, appearance, convenience, or cost? Is nutrition one of the factors you consider? Are your food choices influencing your quality of life and long-term health? By making optimal dietary choices, we can bring the goal of a long, healthy life within reach. This is the primary theme of this chapter and throughout this book.

The ultimate goal of this book is to help you find the best path to good nutrition. The information presented is based on emerging science that is translated into everyday actions that improve health. After completion of your nutrition course, you should understand the knowledge behind the food choices you make and recommend to others. We call this achievement of making food choices that are right for you "nutrition literacy."

1.5 Understand the scientific method as it is used in forming hypotheses and theories in the field of nutrition, including the determination of nutrient needs.

1.6 List the major characteristics of the North American diet, the food habits that often need improvement, and the key "Nutrition and Weight Status" objectives of the *Healthy People 2020* report.

1.7 Describe a basic plan for health promotion and disease prevention and what to expect from good nutrition and a healthy lifestyle.

1.8 Identify food and nutrition issues relevant to college students.

1.1 Why Do You Choose the Food You Eat?

In your lifetime, you will eat about 70,000 meals and 60 tons of food. Many factors—some internal, some external—influence our food choices. This chapter begins with a discussion of these factors and ends with a conversation specifically about eating well as a college student. In between, we examine the powerful effect of dietary habits in determining overall health and take a close look at the general classes of nutrients—as well as the calories—supplied by the food we eat. We also discuss the major characteristics of the North American diet, the food habits that often need improvement, and the key "Nutrition and Weight Status" objectives in the *Healthy People 2020* report. A review of the scientific process behind nutrition recommendations is also included, along with an introduction to our "Newsworthy Nutrition" feature that you will see throughout the book.

Understanding what drives us to eat and what affects food choice will help you understand the complexity of factors that influence eating, especially the effects of our routines and food advertising (Fig. 1-1). You can then appreciate why foods may have different meanings to different people and thus why food habits and preferences of others may differ from yours.

WHAT INFLUENCES YOUR FOOD CHOICES?

Food means so much more to us than nourishment—it reflects much of what we think about ourselves. The Bureau of Labor Statistics estimated that in 2013, Americans spent the equivalent of 19 days eating and drinking. If we live to be 80 years old, that will add up to 4.1 years of eating and drinking. Overall, our daily food choices stem from a complicated mix of biological and social influences (see Fig. 1-1). Let's examine some of the key reasons we choose what we eat.

FIGURE 1-1 ▶ Food choices are affected by many factors. Which have the greatest impact on your food choices?
© BananaStock/PunchStock

© Ingram Publishing

▲ Cereal and milk are two of the most commonly purchased foods in America largely because they are eaten together for breakfast every day by many. © Stockbyte/PunchStock

Flavor, texture, and appearance are the most important factors determining our food choices. Creating more flavorful foods that are both healthy and profitable is a major focus of the food industry. The challenge is to match the "taste" of the foods we prefer with the best nutrition and health characteristics. The good news is that chefs and "food bloggers" are dedicating themselves to promoting nutritious food that is also delicious, resulting in food that is good for us starting to taste better.

Early influences related to various people, places, and events have a continuing impact on our food choices. Many food customs, including ethnic diet patterns, begin as we are introduced to foods during childhood. Parents can lay a strong foundation knowing that early exposure to food choices during infancy, toddler, and preschool years is important in influencing later health behaviors. Developing healthy patterns during childhood will go a long way to ensure healthy preferences and choices when we are teenagers and adults.

Routines and habits are tied to some food choices. Food habits, food availability, and convenience strongly influence choices. Most of us eat from a core group of foods with about 100 basic items accounting for 75% of our total food intake. Recent surveys indicate that the most commonly purchased foods in America are milk (about 23 gallons per person yearly), ready-to-eat cereal, bottled water (about 34 gallons per year), soft drinks (nearly 41 gallons per year), and bread (about 53 pounds per year). It is no surprise that milk and cereal are both on the top-five list because many Americans eat them together as their daily breakfast. Bread is also on the list because it is typically consumed at every meal in America, making it one of the most common forms of grain eaten. Bottled water has become the drink of choice for most events, especially outdoor activities. The popularity of carbonated soft drinks remains a concern because studies have found an association between consumption of sugar-sweetened drinks and obesity in children (see Chapter 19).

Marketing and advertising is a major media tool for capturing the food interest of the consumer. Consumers have more food choices than ever and these choices are well advertised in newspapers and magazines, on billboards, radio, television, and online. The food industry in the United States spends billions on advertising. Some of this advertising is helpful, as it promotes the importance of food components such as calcium and fiber in our diets. However, the food industry also advertises highly sweetened cereals, cookies, cakes, and soft drinks because they bring in the greatest profits. Researchers at Yale University found that in 2012, fast-food restaurant chains spent $4.6 billion on advertising, primarily television ads. In recent years, most fast-food restaurants increased their advertising to children (Fig. 1-2), resulting in preschoolers viewing an average of 2.8 fast-food television ads, older children viewing 3.2 ads, and teens viewing 4.8 ads every day. This is of concern because food advertising has been shown to have a definite

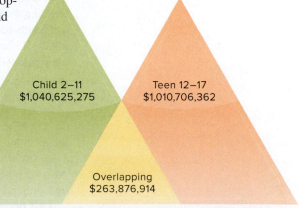

Child 2–11
$1,040,625,275

Teen 12–17
$1,010,706,362

Overlapping
$263,876,914

Total Youth-Directed Marketing: $1,787,454,723

FIGURE 1-2 ▲ This chart shows the marketing expenditures used to promote food and beverages to children and teens in the United States in 2009.

Source: Reading 9: Federal Trade Commission: A Review of Food Marketing to Children and Adolescents, Follow-Up Report, December 2012. www.ftc.gov/os/2012/12/121221food marketingreport.pdf

CRITICAL THINKING

Can healthy choices be legislated? Public health authorities would like to influence health behaviors by banning or taxing unhealthy foods or ingredients; however, industries and many concerned citizens oppose the expanding reach of the government. This struggle gained national attention in the summer of 2014. Mounting evidence for the link between consumption of sugar-sweetened beverages and obesity had prompted the proposal of a ban on the sale of sugary drinks in containers larger than 16 ounces in some establishments. With the backing of then-mayor Michael Bloomberg, this ban was approved by the New York City Board of Health and would have taken effect in 2013. However, the beverage industry staunchly opposed the ban and the New York Supreme Court invalidated the law. In June 2014, the New York Court of Appeals ruled that this ban overreached the health department's regulatory authority. Whose responsibility is it to determine which foods are good for you?

effect on weight gain in children and adolescents. In addition, marketing of fast food via mobile devices and social media has increased exponentially (see Further Reading 9). Recent studies indicate that the association between TV advertising of foods and drinks, and childhood obesity is especially prevalent in the United States (see Further Readings 3 and 10). Concern for the negative effect of advertising and marketing on the diets and health of children led the Council of Better Business Bureaus to establish the Children's Food and Beverage Advertising Initiative, a self-regulatory program. Participants are 17 of the largest food and beverage companies that represent about 80% of child-directed television food advertising. The Initiative is designed to shift the mix of foods advertised to children to encourage healthier dietary choices and healthy lifestyles (see Further Reading 11). Research also indicates that mass media influences the onset of eating disorders through its depiction of extremely thin models as stereotypes of attractive bodies. Eating disorders will be introduced in Eating Well in College (Section 1.8) and discussed at length in Chapter 15.

Restaurant dining plays a significant role in our food choices. Restaurant food is often calorie dense, in large portions, and of poorer nutritional quality compared to foods made at home. Fast-food and pizza restaurant menus typically emphasize meat, cheese, fried foods, and carbonated beverages. In response to recent consumer demands, restaurants have placed healthier options on their menus and many are listing nutritional content there, as well. Mandatory posting of the calorie content of restaurant items will go into effect soon as a result of the Affordable Care Act. The law requires chain restaurants with 20 or more locations to post the calorie content of their offerings on menus or menu boards with other nutritional information available upon request. The intent of the law is to provide consumers with clear and consistent nutrition information so that they can make informed and healthful choices. Although many restaurants have already placed calorie information on their menus, the Food and Drug Administration (FDA) extended the date for which establishments must be compliant with the menu labeling rule to December 1, 2016.

Time and convenience have become significant influences affecting food choices. These stem from a lifestyle that limits the amount of time spent in food preparation (see Further Reading 4). In the 2011 Academy of Nutrition and Dietetics Trends Survey, 62% of American adults indicated that it took too much time to keep track of their diet (see Further Reading 2). Restaurants and supermarkets have responded to our demanding work schedules and long hours away from home by supplying prepared meals, microwavable entrees, and various quick-prep frozen products.

Cost and economics play a role in our food choices. The 2015 Food and Health Survey indicates that after taste, cost is the number two reason why people choose the food they do. While the average American now spends less on food than in the past, young adults and those with higher incomes spend the most on food. As income increases, so do meals eaten away from home and preferences for foods such as cookies, chocolate, cheese, and meat. Also keep in mind that as calorie intake increases, so does the food bill. Tips for eating well on a college student's budget are discussed in Section 1.8.

Last but not least, *nutrition*—or what we think of as "healthy foods"—also directs our food purchases. North Americans who tend to make health-related food choices are often well-educated, middle-class professionals. These same people are generally health oriented, have active lifestyles, and focus on weight control. The recent National Health Interview Survey showed that 74% of women in the study habitually or always read nutrition labels, whereas only 58% of men read labels on food products. Label reading was associated with a lower body mass index (BMI, body weight relative to height), especially in women. Women who read labels had a BMI of 1.48 points lower than women who did not read nutrition labels. This translates to a difference of 8.6 pounds for a woman of average height (see Further Reading 14).

WHY ARE YOU SO HUNGRY?

Two drives, **hunger** and **appetite,** influence our desire to eat. These drives differ dramatically. Hunger is primarily our physical, biological drive to eat and is controlled by internal body mechanisms. For example, as foods are digested and absorbed by the stomach and small intestine, these organs send signals to the liver and brain telling us to reduce further food intake.

Appetite, our primarily psychological drive to eat, is affected by many of the external food choice mechanisms we discussed in the last section, such as environmental and psychological factors and social cues and customs (see Fig. 1-1). Appetite can be triggered simply by seeing a tempting dessert or smelling popcorn at the movie theater. Fulfilling either or both drives by eating sufficient food normally brings a state of **satiety,** a feeling of satisfaction that temporarily halts our desire to continue eating.

A region of the brain helps regulate satiety. The *feeding center* and the *satiety center* work in opposite ways, like a tug-of-war, to promote adequate availability of nutrients at all times. For example, when we haven't eaten for a while, stimulation of the feeding center signals us to eat. As we eat, the nutrient content in the blood rises, and the satiety center is stimulated. This is why we no longer have a strong desire to seek food after a meal. Admittedly, this concept of a tug-of-war between the feeding and satiety centers is an oversimplification of a complex process. The various feeding and satiety messages from body cells to the brain do not single-handedly determine what we eat. We often eat because food comforts us (see Further Reading 20). Almost everyone has encountered a mouthwatering dessert and devoured it, even on a full stomach. It smells, tastes, and looks good. We might eat because it is the right time of day, we are celebrating, or we are seeking emotional comfort to overcome the blues. After a meal, memories of pleasant tastes and feelings reinforce appetite. If stress or depression sends you to the refrigerator, you are mostly seeking comfort, not food calories. Appetite may not be a physical process, but it does influence food intake. We will discuss more about this mechanism, including the effect of meal size and composition on satiety, in Chapter 7 on energy balance and weight control.

PUTTING OUR FOOD CHOICES INTO PERSPECTIVE

The next time you pick up a candy bar or reach for a second helping at a meal, remember the internal and external influences on eating behavior. You should now understand that daily food consumption is a complicated mix of biological and social influences. Body cells, nutrients in the blood, hormones, brain chemicals, and our social and family customs all influence food choices. When food is abundant, appetite—not hunger—most likely triggers eating. Satiety associated with consuming a meal may reside primarily in our psychological frame of mind. Also, because satiety regulation is not perfect, body weight can fluctuate. We become accustomed to a certain amount of food at a meal. Providing less than that amount leaves us wanting more. One way to use this observation for weight-loss purposes is to train your eye to expect less food by slowly decreasing serving sizes to more appropriate amounts. Your appetite then readjusts as you expect less food. Keep track of what triggers your eating for a few days. Is it primarily hunger or appetite? The Rate Your Plate activity in this chapter also asks you to keep track of what influences your food intake on a daily basis.

hunger The primarily physiological (internal) drive to find and eat food.

appetite The primarily psychological (external) influences that encourage us to find and eat food, often in the absence of obvious hunger.

satiety A state in which there is no longer a desire to eat; a feeling of satisfaction.

✔ CONCEPT CHECK 1.1

1. What are the factors that influence our food choices?
2. How do hunger and appetite differ in the way they influence our desire to eat?
3. What factors influence satiety?

▲ Major health problems can be avoided by a healthy diet and adequate physical activity.
© Mike Kemp/Getty Images

▲ Many foods are rich sources of nutrients.
© Pixtal/AGE Fotostock

nutrients Chemical substances in food that contribute to health, many of which are essential parts of a diet. Nutrients nourish us by providing calories to fulfill energy needs, materials for building body parts, and factors to regulate necessary chemical processes in the body.

essential nutrient In nutritional terms, a substance that, when left out of a diet, leads to signs of poor health. The body either cannot produce this nutrient or cannot produce enough of it to meet its needs. If added back to a diet before permanent damage occurs, the affected aspects of health are restored.

risk factors A term used frequently when discussing the factors contributing to the development of a disease. A risk factor is an aspect of our lives, such as heredity, lifestyle choices (e.g., smoking), or nutritional habits.

chronic Long-standing, developing over time. When referring to disease, this term indicates that the disease process, once developed, is slow and lasting. A good example is cardiovascular disease.

cardiovascular disease A general term that refers to any disease of the heart and circulatory system. This disease is generally characterized by the deposition of fatty material in the blood vessels (hardening of the arteries), which in turn can lead to organ damage and death. Also termed coronary heart disease (CHD), as the vessels of the heart are the primary sites of the disease.

1.2 How Is Nutrition Connected to Good Health?

Fortunately, the foods we eat can support good health in many ways depending on their components. You just learned, however, that lifestyle habits and other factors may have a bigger impact on our food choices than the food components themselves. Unfortunately, many North Americans suffer from diseases that could have been prevented if they had known more about the foods and, more importantly, had applied this knowledge to plan meals and design their eating pattern. We will now look at the effect these choices are having on our health both today and in the future.

WHAT IS NUTRITION?

Nutrition is the science that links foods to health and disease. It includes the processes by which the human organism ingests, digests, absorbs, transports, and excretes food substances.

NUTRIENTS COME FROM FOOD

What is the difference between food and **nutrients?** Food provides the energy (in the form of calories) as well as the materials needed to build and maintain all body cells. Nutrients are the substances obtained from food that are vital for growth and maintenance of a healthy body throughout life. For a substance to be considered an **essential nutrient,** three characteristics are needed:

- First, at least one specific biological function of the nutrient must be identified in the body.
- Second, omission of the nutrient from the diet must lead to a decline in certain biological functions, such as production of blood cells.
- Third, replacing the omitted nutrient in the diet before permanent damage occurs will restore those normal biological functions.

WHY STUDY NUTRITION?

We all may feel like nutrition experts because we all eat several times a day. Nutrition knowledge can be confusing, however, and seem like a moving target. Recommendations may seem to differ depending on their source, and there are so many choices when shopping for food or eating out. We just learned that nutrition is only one of many factors that influence our eating habits. There is a lot to learn, and we know that you are interested in what you should be eating and how the food you eat affects you. Studying nutrition will help you erase any misconceptions you have about food and nutrition and make informed choices about the foods you eat and their relationship to health.

Nutrition is a lifestyle factor that is a key to developing and maintaining an optimal state of health for you. A poor diet and a sedentary lifestyle are known to be **risk factors** for life-threatening **chronic** diseases such as **cardiovascular (heart) disease, hypertension, diabetes,** and some forms of **cancer** (Table 1-1). Together, these and related disorders account for two-thirds of all deaths in North America (Fig. 1-3) (see Further Reading 15). Not meeting nutrient needs in younger years makes us more likely to suffer health consequences, such as bone fractures from the disease **osteoporosis,** in later years. At the same time, taking too much of a nutrient—such as a vitamin A supplement—can be harmful. Another dietary problem, drinking too much alcohol, is associated with many health problems.

U.S. government scientists have calculated that a poor diet combined with a lack of sufficient physical activity contributes to hundreds of thousands of fatal cases of cardiovascular

TABLE 1-1 ■ Glossary Terms to Aid Your Introduction to Nutrition*

Cancer	A condition characterized by uncontrolled growth of abnormal cells.
Cardiovascular (heart) disease	A general term that refers to any disease of the heart and circulatory system. This disease is generally characterized by the deposition of fatty material in the blood vessels (hardening of the arteries), which in turn can lead to organ damage and death. Also termed coronary heart disease (CHD), as the vessels of the heart are the primary sites of the disease.
Cholesterol	A waxy lipid found in all body cells; it has a structure containing multiple chemical rings. Cholesterol is found only in foods of animal origin.
Chronic	Long-standing, developing over time. When referring to disease, this term indicates that the disease process, once developed, is slow and lasting. A good example is cardiovascular disease.
Diabetes	A group of diseases characterized by high blood **glucose.** Type 1 diabetes involves insufficient or no release of the hormone insulin by the pancreas and therefore requires daily insulin therapy. Type 2 diabetes results from either insufficient release of insulin or general inability of insulin to act on certain body cells, such as muscle cells. Persons with type 2 diabetes may or may not require insulin therapy.
Hypertension	A condition in which blood pressure remains persistently elevated. Obesity, inactivity, alcohol intake, excess salt intake, and genetics may each contribute to the problem.
Kilocalorie (kcal)	Unit that describes the energy content of food. Specifically, a kilocalorie (kcal) is the heat energy needed to raise the temperature of 1000 grams (1 liter) of water 1 degree Celsius. Although kcal refers to a 1000-calorie unit of measurement, it is commonly referred to as calories on food labels. *Kilocalories* is the technically correct term for the energy content of a food, so we will use it in this book.
Obesity	A condition characterized by excess body fat.
Osteoporosis	Decreased bone mass related to the effects of aging (including estrogen loss during menopause in women), genetic background, and poor diet.
Risk factor	A term used frequently when discussing the factors contributing to the development of a disease. A risk factor is an aspect of our lives, such as heredity, lifestyle choices (e.g., smoking), or nutritional habits.

*Many bold terms are also defined in the page margins within each chapter and in the glossary at the end of this book.

hypertension A condition in which blood pressure remains persistently elevated. Obesity, inactivity, alcohol intake, excess salt intake, and genetics may each contribute to the problem.

diabetes A group of diseases characterized by high blood glucose. Type 1 diabetes involves insufficient or no release of the hormone insulin by the pancreas and therefore requires daily insulin therapy. Type 2 diabetes results from either insufficient release of insulin or general inability of insulin to act on certain body cells, such as muscle cells. Persons with type 2 diabetes may or may not require insulin therapy.

cancer A condition characterized by uncontrolled growth of abnormal cells.

osteoporosis The presence of a stress-induced fracture or a T-score of −2.5 or lower. The bones are porous and fragile due to low mineral density.

glucose A six-carbon sugar that exists in a ring form; found as such in blood, and in table sugar bound to fructose; also known as *dextrose,* it is one of the simple sugars.

Percent of All Deaths

Cause	Percent
Heart disease*	23.6%
Cancer*	22.9%
Chronic lower respiratory disease	5.6%
Stroke*	5.1%
Accidents	5.0%
Alzheimer's disease*	3.3%
Diabetes mellitus*	2.9%
Pneumonia/Influenza	2.0%
Kidney disease*	1.8%
Suicide	1.6%

FIGURE 1-3 ▲ Ten leading causes of death in the United States

Source: Centers for Disease Control and Prevention, National Vital Statistics Report, Deaths: Leading Causes for 2012, August 31, 2015 (see Further Reading 15). Canadian statistics are quite similar.

*Causes of death in which diet plays a part.

obesity Disorder involving excessive body fat that increases the risk of health problems.

stroke A decrease or loss in blood flow to the brain that results from a blood clot or other change in arteries in the brain. This in turn causes the death of brain tissue. Also called a *cerebrovascular accident.*

carbohydrates A compound containing carbon, hydrogen, and oxygen atoms. Most are known as *sugars, starches,* and *fibers.*

lipids A compound containing much carbon and hydrogen, little oxygen, and sometimes other atoms. Lipids do not dissolve in water and include fats, oils, and cholesterol.

proteins Food and body compounds made of more than 100 amino acids; proteins contain carbon, hydrogen, oxygen, nitrogen, and sometimes other atoms in a specific configuration. Proteins contain the form of nitrogen most easily used by the human body.

vitamins An essential organic (carbon-containing) compound needed in small amounts in the diet to help regulate and support chemical reactions and processes in the body.

minerals Element used in the body to promote chemical reactions and to form body structures.

water The universal solvent; chemically, H_2O. The body is composed of about 60% water. Water (fluid) needs are about 9 (women) or 13 (men) cups per day; needs are greater if one exercises heavily.

kilocalorie (kcal) Heat energy needed to raise the temperature of 1000 grams (1 L) of water 1 degree Celsius .

disease, cancer, and diabetes each year among adults in the United States. Thus, the combination of poor diet and too little physical activity may be the second leading cause of death in the United States. In addition, **obesity,** which the American Medical Association recently declared as a disease, is considered the second leading cause of preventable death in North America (smoking is the first). When they occur together, obesity and smoking cause even more health problems. Obesity and chronic diseases are often preventable. An important key to good health and more health care savings is to realize that the cost of prevention, usually when we are children and young adults, is a small fraction of the cost of treating these diseases when we are older.

The good news is that the increased interest in health, fitness, and nutrition shown by Americans has been associated with long-term decreasing trends for heart disease, cancer, and **stroke** (three of the leading causes of death). Mortality from heart disease, the leading cause of death, has been declining steadily since 1980. As you gain understanding about your nutritional habits and increase your knowledge about optimal nutrition, you will have the opportunity to dramatically reduce your risk for many common health problems. Recent research has shown that a healthy diet along with other healthy lifestyle factors can protect women from sudden cardiac death. A healthy diet was defined as one with a high proportion of vegetables, fruits, nuts, omega-3 fats, and fish (see Further Reading 6). For additional help, the U.S. federal government provides two websites that contain links to many sources of health and nutrition information (www.healthfinder.gov and www.nutrition.gov). Other useful sites are www.webmd.com and www.eatright.org.

☑ **CONCEPT CHECK 1.2**

1. How do we define nutrition?
2. What are the three leading causes of death in which diet plays a part?

1.3 What Are the Classes and Sources of Nutrients?

To begin the study of nutrition, let's start with an overview of the six classes of nutrients. You are probably already familiar with the terms **carbohydrates, lipids** (fats and oils), **proteins, vitamins,** and **minerals.** These nutrients, plus **water,** make up the six classes of nutrients found in food.

Nutrients can then be assigned to three functional categories: (1) those that primarily provide us with calories to meet energy needs (expressed in **kilocalories [kcal]**); (2) those important for growth, development, and maintenance; and (3) those that act to keep body functions running smoothly. Some function overlap exists among these categories (Table 1-2). The

TABLE 1-2 ■ **Major Functions of the Various Classes of Nutrients**

Nutrient Classes That Provide Energy	Nutrient Classes That Promote Growth, Development, and Maintenance	Nutrient Classes That Regulate Body Processes
Most carbohydrates	Proteins	Proteins
Proteins	Lipids	Some lipids
Most lipids	Some vitamins	Some vitamins
	Some minerals	Some minerals
	Water	Water

energy-yielding nutrients (carbohydrates, lipids, and protein) along with water are needed in relatively large amounts, so they are called **macronutrients.** Vitamins and minerals are needed in such small amounts in the diet that they are called **micronutrients.**

CARBOHYDRATES

Chemically, carbohydrates can exist in foods as simple sugars and complex carbohydrates. **Simple sugars,** frequently referred to as *sugars,* are relatively small molecules. These sugars are found naturally in fruits, vegetables, and dairy products. Table sugar, known as sucrose, is an example of a simple sugar that is added to many foods we eat. Glucose, also known as blood sugar or dextrose, is an example of a simple sugar in your blood. **Complex carbohydrates** are formed when many simple sugars are joined together. For example, plants store carbohydrates in the form of **starch,** a complex carbohydrate made up of hundreds of glucose units. Breads, cereals, grains, and starchy vegetables are the main sources of complex carbohydrates.

During digestion, complex carbohydrates are broken down into single sugar molecules (such as glucose) and absorbed via **cells** lining the small intestine into the bloodstream (see Chapter 3 for more on digestion and absorption). However, the **bonds** between the sugar molecules in certain complex carbohydrates, called **fiber,** cannot be broken down by human digestive processes. Fiber passes through the small intestine undigested to provide bulk for the stool (feces) formed in the large intestine (colon).

Aside from enjoying their taste, we need sugars and other carbohydrates in our diets primarily to help satisfy the calorie needs of our body cells. Carbohydrates provide a major source of calories for the body, on average 4 kcal per gram. Glucose, a simple sugar that the body can derive from most carbohydrates, is a major source of calories for most cells. When insufficient carbohydrate is consumed, the body is forced to make glucose from proteins—not a healthy change. Chapter 4 focuses on carbohydrates.

LIPIDS

Lipids (mostly fats and oils) in the foods we eat also provide energy. Lipids yield more calories per gram than do carbohydrates—on the average, 9 kcal per gram—because of differences in their chemical composition. They are also the main form for energy storage in the body.

Lipids dissolve in certain chemical solvents (e.g., ether and benzene) but not in water. In this book, the more familiar terms *fats* and *oils* will generally be used, rather than lipids. Generally, fats are lipids that are solid at room temperature, and oils are lipids that are liquid at room temperature. We obtain fats and oils from animal and plant sources. Animal fats, such as butter or lard, are solid at room temperature. Plant oils, such as corn or olive oil, tend to be liquid at room temperature. To promote heart health, most people would benefit from using more plant oils in place of solid fats (see Chapter 5).

Certain fats are essential nutrients that must come from our diet. These key fats that the body cannot produce, called essential fatty acids, perform several important functions in the body: they help regulate blood pressure and play a role in the synthesis and repair of vital cell parts. However, we need only about 4 tablespoons of a common plant oil (such as canola or soybean oil) each day to supply these essential fatty acids. A serving of fatty fish, such as salmon or tuna, at least twice a week is another healthy source of fats. The unique fatty acids in these fish complement the healthy aspects of common vegetable oils. This will be explained in greater detail in Chapter 5, which focuses on lipids.

PROTEINS

Proteins are the main structural material in the body. For example, proteins constitute a major part of bone and muscle; they are also important components in blood, body cells, **enzymes,** and immune factors. Proteins can also provide calories for the body—on average, 4 kcal per gram. Typically, however, the body uses little protein for the purpose of meeting

macronutrient A nutrient needed in gram quantities in a diet.

micronutrient A nutrient needed in milligram or microgram quantities in a diet.

simple sugar Monosaccharide or disaccharide in the diet.

complex carbohydrate Carbohydrate composed of many monosaccharide molecules. Examples include glycogen, starch, and fiber.

starch A carbohydrate made of multiple units of glucose attached together in a form the body can digest; also known as *complex carbohydrate.*

cells The structural basis of plant and animal organization. In animals it is bounded by a cell membrane. Cells have the ability to take up compounds from and excrete compounds into their surroundings.

bonds A linkage between two atoms formed by the sharing of electrons, or attractions.

fiber Substances in plant foods not digested in the human stomach or small intestine. These add bulk to feces. Fiber naturally found in foods is also called *dietary fiber.*

enzymes A compound that speeds up the rate of a chemical reaction but is not altered by the reaction. Almost all enzymes are proteins (some are made of genetic material).

▲ Salmon is a fatty fish that is a healthy source of essential fatty acids. © FoodCollection

amino acid The building block for proteins containing a central carbon atom with nitrogen and other atoms attached.

daily calorie needs. Proteins are formed when **amino acids** are bonded together. Some of these are essential nutrients.

Protein in our diet comes from animal and plant sources. The animal products meat, poultry, fish, dairy products, and eggs are significant sources of protein in most diets. Beans, grains, and some vegetables are good plant protein sources and are important to include in vegetarian diets.

Most North Americans eat up to two times as much protein as the body needs to maintain health. This amount of extra protein in the diet reflects the standard of living and the dietary habits of most North Americans. It is generally not harmful for healthy persons with no evidence of heart or kidney disease, diabetes, or family history of colon cancer or kidney stones. The excess is used for calorie needs and carbohydrate production but ultimately can be converted to and stored as fat. Chapter 6 focuses on proteins.

VITAMINS

chemical reaction An interaction between two chemicals that changes both chemicals.

fat-soluble Soluble in fats, oils, or fat solvents.

water-soluble Capable of dissolving in water.

The main function of vitamins is to enable many **chemical reactions** to occur in the body. Some of these reactions help release the energy trapped in carbohydrates, lipids, and proteins. Remember, however, that vitamins themselves contain no usable calories for the body.

The 13 vitamins are divided into two groups: four are **fat-soluble** because they dissolve in fat (vitamins A, D, E, and K); nine are **water-soluble** because they dissolve in water (the B vitamins and vitamin C). The two groups of vitamins have different sources, functions, and characteristics. Water-soluble vitamins are found mainly in fruits and vegetables, whereas dairy products, nuts, seeds, oils, and breakfast cereals are good sources of fat-soluble vitamins. Cooking destroys water-soluble vitamins much more readily than it does fat-soluble vitamins. Water-soluble vitamins are also excreted from the body much more readily than are fat-soluble vitamins. Thus, the fat-soluble vitamins, especially vitamin A, have the ability to accumulate in excessive amounts in the body, which then can lead to toxicity. Vitamins are discussed in Chapters 8 through 13.

MINERALS

inorganic Any substance lacking carbon atoms bonded to hydrogen atoms in the chemical structure.

atom Smallest combining unit of an element, such as iron or calcium. Atoms consist of protons, neutrons, and electrons.

major mineral Vital to health, a mineral that is required in the diet in amounts greater than 100 milligrams per day.

trace mineral Vital to health, a mineral that is required in the diet in amounts less than 100 milligrams per day.

electrolyte A mineral that separates into positively or negatively charged ions in water. They are able to transmit an electrical current.

Minerals are structurally simple, **inorganic** substances that do not contain carbon **atoms**. Minerals such as sodium and potassium typically function independently in the body, whereas minerals such as calcium and phosphorus combine to function in tissue, such as bone. Because of their simple structure, minerals are not destroyed during cooking, but they can still be lost if they dissolve in the water used for cooking and that water is then discarded. Minerals are critical players in nervous system functioning, water balance, structural (e.g., skeletal) systems, and many other cellular processes but produce no calories as such for the body.

The 16 or more essential minerals required in the diet for good health are divided into two groups: **major minerals** and **trace minerals** because dietary needs and concentrations in the body vary enormously. If daily needs are less than 100 milligrams, the mineral is classified as a trace mineral; otherwise, it is a major mineral. Minerals that function based on their electrical charge when dissolved in water are also called **electrolytes;** these include sodium, potassium, and chloride. Many major minerals are found naturally in dairy products and fruits, whereas many trace minerals are found in meats, poultry, fish, and nuts. Minerals are covered in Chapters 8 through 13.

WATER

solvent A liquid substance in which other substances dissolve.

Water makes up the sixth class of nutrients. Although sometimes overlooked as a nutrient, water (chemically, H_2O) has numerous vital functions in the body. It acts as a **solvent** and lubricant, as a vehicle for transporting nutrients and waste, and as a medium for temperature regulation and chemical processes. For these reasons, and because the human body is approximately 60% water, the average man should consume about 3 liters—equivalent to 3000 grams or about 13 cups—of water and/or other fluids every day. Women need closer to 2200 grams or about 9 cups per day. Fluid needs vary widely, however, based on differences in body mass and environmental conditions. Because thirst is a late sign of dehydration, urine color can be used as another measure of hydration status. Urine color should be no more yellow than lemonade.

Water is not only available from the obvious sources, but it is also the major component in some foods, such as many fruits and vegetables (e.g., lettuce, grapes, and melons). The body even makes some water as a by-product of **metabolism.** Water is examined in detail in Chapter 9.

metabolism Chemical processes in the body by which energy is provided in useful forms and vital activities are sustained.

OTHER IMPORTANT COMPONENTS IN FOOD

Another group of compounds in foods from plant sources, especially within the fruit and vegetable groups, is what scientists call **phytochemicals.** Although these plant components are not considered essential nutrients in the diet, many of these substances provide significant health benefits. Considerable research attention is focused on various phytochemicals in reducing the risk for certain diseases. For example, evidence from animal and laboratory studies indicates that compounds in blueberries and strawberries prevent the growth of certain cancer cells. Although certain phytochemicals are now available as dietary supplements, research suggests that their health benefits are best obtained through the consumption of whole foods. Foods with high phytochemical content are sometimes called "superfoods" because of the health benefits they are thought to confer. There is no legal definition of the term *superfood,* however, and there is concern that it is being overused in marketing certain foods. Table 1-3 lists some noteworthy phytochemicals with their common food sources. Tips for boosting the phytochemical content of your diet will be discussed in Chapter 2.

phytochemical A chemical found in plants. Some phytochemicals may contribute to a reduced risk of cancer or cardiovascular disease in people who consume them regularly.

TABLE 1-3 **Food Sources of Some Phytochemical Compounds Under Study**

Food Sources	Phytochemical
Garlic, onions, leeks	Allyl sulfides/organosulfurs
Garlic, onions, licorice, legumes	Saponins
Orange, red, and yellow fruits and vegetables (egg yolks are a source as well)	Carotenoids (e.g., lycopene)
Oranges, lemons, grapefruit	Monoterpenes
Chili peppers	Capsaicin
Flaxseed, berries, whole grains	Lignans
Cruciferous vegetables (broccoli, cabbage, kale)	Indoles
Cruciferous vegetables, especially broccoli	Isothiocyanates
Soybeans, other legumes, cucumbers, other fruits and vegetables	Phytosterols
Citrus fruit, onions, apples, grapes, red wine, tea, chocolate, tomatoes	Flavonoids
Soybeans, other legumes	Isoflavones
Tea	Catechins
Blueberries, strawberries, raspberries, grapes, apples, bananas, nuts	Polyphenols
Red, blue, and purple plants (blueberries, eggplant)	Anthocyanosides
Onions, bananas, oranges (small amounts)	Fructooligosaccharides
Grapes, peanuts, red wine	Resveratrol

▲ Blueberries are sometimes considered "superfoods" because they are rich in health-promoting phytochemicals. © Lifesize/Getty Images

Some related compounds under study are also found in animal products, such as sphingolipids (meat and dairy products) and conjugated linoleic acid (meat and cheese). These are not phytochemicals per se because they are not from plant sources, but they have been shown to have health benefits.

SOURCES OF NUTRIENTS

Now that we know the six classes of nutrients, it is important to understand that the quantities of the various nutrients that people consume in different foods vary widely. On a daily basis, we consume about 500 grams, or about 1 pound, of protein, fat, and carbohydrate. In contrast, the typical daily mineral intake totals about 20 grams (about 4 teaspoons), and the daily vitamin intake totals less than 300 milligrams (1/15 of a teaspoon). Although we require a gram or so of some minerals, such as calcium and phosphorus, we need only a few milligrams or less of other minerals each day. For example, we need about 10 milligrams of zinc per day, which is just a few specks of the mineral.

The nutrient content of the foods we eat also differs from the nutrient composition of the human body. This is because growth, development, and later maintenance of the human body are directed by the genetic material (DNA) inside body cells. This genetic blueprint determines how each cell uses the essential nutrients to perform body functions. These nutrients can come from a variety of sources. Cells are not concerned about whether available amino acids come from animal or plant sources. The carbohydrate glucose can come from sugars or starches. The food that you eat provides cells with basic materials to function according to the directions supplied by the genetic material (**genes**) housed in body cells. Genetics and nutrition will be discussed in Chapter 3.

genes A specific segment on a chromosome. Genes provide the blueprint for the production of all body proteins.

✓ CONCEPT CHECK 1.3

1. What are the six classes of nutrients?
2. What are the three general functions of nutrients in the body?

1.4 What Math Concepts Will Aid Your Study of Nutrition?

alcohol Ethyl alcohol or ethanol (CH_3CH_2OH) is the compound in alcoholic beverages.

CALORIES

We obtain the energy we need for involuntary body functions and voluntary physical activity from various calorie sources: carbohydrates (4 kcal per gram), fats (9 kcal per gram), and proteins (4 kcal per gram). Foods generally provide more than one calorie source. Plant oils, such as soybean or canola oil, are one exception; these are 100% fat at 9 kcal per gram.

Alcohol is also a potential source of calories, supplying about 7 kcal per gram. It is not considered an essential nutrient, however, because it is not required for human function. Still, alcoholic beverages, such as beer—also rich in carbohydrate—are a contributor of calories to the diets of many adults.

The body releases the energy from the chemical bonds in carbohydrate, protein, and fat (and alcohol) in order to

- build new compounds.
- perform muscular movements.
- promote nerve transmission.
- maintain electrolyte balance within cells.

Chapter 7 describes how that energy is released from the chemical bonds in energy-yielding nutrients and then used by body cells to support the processes just described.

Carbohydrate
4 kcal per gram

Fat
9 kcal per gram

Protein
4 kcal per gram

Alcohol
7 kcal per gram

▲ Calorie content of energy nutrients and alcohol. The weights illustrate their relative energy potential per gram.

WHOLE WHEAT BREAD

Nutrition Facts		% Daily Value*		% Daily Value*		* The % Daily Value
19 servings per container	**Total Fat** 1g	2%	**Total Carbohydrate** 15g	5%		(DV) tells you how much a nutrient in a serving of food contributes to a daily diet. 2,000 calories a day is used for general nutrition advice.
Serving size 1 slice (36g)	Saturated Fat 0g	0%	Dietary Fiber 2g	8%		
	Trans Fat less than 1g	**	Total Sugars 3g			
Amount per serving	**Cholesterol** 0mg	0%	Includes 2g Added Sugars	4%		
Calories 80	**Sodium** 200mg	8%	**Protein** 3g			
	Vitamin D 0mcg 0% • Calcium 30mg 3% • Iron 1mg 5% • Potassium 70mg 2%					

FIGURE 1-4 ▲ Use the nutrient values on the Nutrition Facts panel to calculate calorie content of a food. Based on carbohydrate, fat, and protein content, a serving of this food (whole wheat bread) contains 81 kcal ([15 × 4] + [1 × 9] + [3 × 4] = 81). The label lists 80, suggesting that the calorie value was rounded down.

The energy in food is often expressed using the term *calories* on food labels. As defined earlier, a calorie is the amount of heat energy it takes to raise the temperature of 1 gram of water 1 degree Celsius (1°C, centigrade scale). (Chapter 7 has a diagram of the bomb calorimeter that can be used to measure calories in foods.) A calorie is a tiny measure of heat relative to the amount of calories we eat and use. Food energy is more conveniently expressed in terms of the kilocalorie (kcal), which equals 1000 calories. (If the "c" in calories is capitalized, this also signifies kilocalories.) A kilocalorie is the amount of heat energy it takes to raise the temperature of 1000 grams (1 liter) of water 1°C. The abbreviation *kcal* is used throughout this book. On food labels, the word *calorie* (without a capital "C") is also used loosely to mean *kilocalorie*. Any values given on food labels in calories are actually in kilocalories (Fig. 1-4). A suggested intake of 2000 calories per day on a food label is technically 2000 kcal.

CALCULATING CALORIES

Use the 4-9-4 estimates for the calorie content of carbohydrate, fat, and protein introduced over the last few pages to determine calorie content of a food. Consider these foods:

© Burke/Triolo/Brand X Pictures

1 Grilled Chicken Sandwich

Carbohydrate	46 grams × 4 =	184 kcal
Fat	14 grams × 9 =	126 kcal
Protein	45 grams × 4 =	180 kcal
Alcohol	0 gram × 7 =	0 kcal
Total		**490 kcal**

© C Squared Studios/Getty Images

8-ounce Piña Colada

Carbohydrate	57 grams × 4 =	228 kcal
Fat	5 grams × 9 =	45 kcal
Protein	1 gram × 4 =	4 kcal
Alcohol	23 grams × 7 =	161 kcal
Total		**438 kcal**

You can also use the 4-9-4 estimates to determine what portion of total kilocalorie intake is contributed by the various calorie-yielding nutrients. Assume that one day you consume 290 grams of carbohydrates, 60 grams of fat, and 70 grams of protein. This consumption yields a total of 1980 kcal ([290 × 4] + [60 × 9] + [70 × 4] = 1980). The percentage of your total kilocalorie intake derived from each nutrient can then be determined:

$$
\begin{aligned}
\text{\% of kcal as carbohydrate} &= (290 \times 4) \div 1980 = 0.59\ (\times 100 = 59\%) \\
\text{\% of kcal as fat} &= (60 \times 9) \div 1980 = 0.27\ (\times 100 = 27\%) \\
\text{\% of kcal as protein} &= (70 \times 4) \div 1980 = 0.14\ (\times 100 = 14\%)
\end{aligned}
$$

Check your calculations by adding the percentages together. Do they total 100%?

PERCENTAGES

You will use a few mathematical concepts in studying nutrition. Besides performing addition, subtraction, multiplication, and division, you need to know how to calculate percentages and convert English units of measurement to metric units.

The term *percent* (%) refers to a part of the total when the total represents 100 parts. For example, if you earn 80% on your first nutrition examination, you will have answered the equivalent of 80 out of 100 questions correctly. This equivalent also could be 8 correct answers out of 10; 80% also describes 16 of 20 (16/20 = 0.80 or 80%). The decimal form of percents is based on 100% being equal to 1.00. It is difficult to succeed in a nutrition course unless you know what a percentage means and how to calculate one. Percentages are used frequently when referring to menus and nutrient composition. The best way to master this concept is to calculate some percentages. Some examples follow:

Question	Answer
What is 6% of 45?	6% = 0.06, so 0.06 × 45 = 2.7
What percent of 99 is 3?	3/99 = 0.03 or 3% (0.03 × 100)

Joe ate 15% of the adult Recommended Dietary Allowance for iron (RDA = 8 milligrams) at lunch. How many milligrams did he eat?

0.15 × 8 milligrams = 1.2 milligrams

THE METRIC SYSTEM

The basic units of the metric system are the meter, which indicates length; the gram, which indicates weight; and the liter, which indicates volume. Appendix F in this textbook lists conversions from the metric system to the English system (pounds, feet, and cups) and vice versa. Here is a brief summary:

A gram (g) is about 1/30 of an ounce (an ounce weighs 28 grams).

5 grams of sugar or salt is about 1 teaspoon.

A pound (lb) weighs 454 grams.

A kilogram (kg) is 1000 grams, equivalent to 2.2 pounds.

To convert your weight to kilograms, divide it by 2.2.

A 154-pound man weighs 70 kilograms (154/2.2 = 70).

A gram can be divided into 1000 milligrams (mg) or 1,000,000 micrograms (μg or mcg).

10 milligrams of zinc (approximate adult need) would be a few grains of zinc.

Liters are divided into 1000 units called milliliters (ml); 100 milliliters is a deciliter (dl).

One teaspoon equals about 5 milliliters (ml), 1 cup is about 240 milliliters, and 1 quart (4 cups) equals almost 1 liter (L) (0.946 liter to be exact).

A centimeter is 1/100 of a meter; 2.54 centimeters equals 1 inch.

If you plan to work in any scientific field, you will need to learn the metric system. *For now, remember that a kilogram equals 2.2 pounds, an ounce weighs 28 grams, 2.54 centimeters equals 1 inch, and a liter is almost the same as a quart.* In addition, know the fractions that the following prefixes represent: *micro* (1/1,000,000), *milli* (1/1000), *centi* (1/100), and *kilo* (1000).

✓ CONCEPT CHECK 1.4

1. What are the energy (kilocalorie) values for each of the "energy nutrients"?

1.5 How Do We Know What We Know About Nutrition?

How do we know what we know about nutrient needs? In a word, research. Like other sciences, the research that sets the foundation for nutrition knowledge has developed using the *scientific method,* a testing procedure designed to detect and eliminate error.

THE SCIENTIFIC METHOD

The first step of the scientific method is the observation of a natural phenomenon (Fig. 1-5). Scientists then suggest possible explanations, called **hypotheses,** about its cause. At times, historical events have provided clues to important relationships in nutrition science, such as the link between the need for vitamin C and the development of the disease **scurvy** (see Chapter 8). Another approach is for scientists to study diet and disease patterns among various populations, a research method called **epidemiology.**

Thus, hypotheses about the role of diet in various health problems can be suggested by historical and epidemiological findings. *Proving* the role of particular dietary components, however, requires controlled experiments. The data gathered from experiments may either support or refute each hypothesis. If the results of many experiments support a hypothesis, scientists accept the hypothesis as a **theory.** Often, the results from one experiment suggest a new set of questions.

The most rigorous type of controlled experiment follows a randomized, **double-blind,** placebo-controlled study design. In this type of study, a group of participants—the experimental group—follows a specific protocol (e.g., consuming a certain food or nutrient), and participants in a corresponding **control group** follow their normal habits or

hypotheses Tentative explanations by a scientist to explain a phenomenon.

scurvy The vitamin C deficiency disease characterized by weakness, fatigue, slow wound healing, opening of previously healed wounds, bone pain, fractures, sore and bleeding gums, diarrhea, and pinpoint hemorrhages on the skin.

epidemiology The study of how disease rates vary among different population groups.

theory An explanation for a phenomenon that has numerous lines of evidence to support it.

double-blind study An experimental design in which neither the participants nor the researchers are aware of each participant's assignment (test or placebo) or the outcome of the study until it is completed. An independent third party holds the code and the data until the study has been completed.

control group Participants in an experiment who are not given the treatment being tested.

FIGURE 1-5 ▲ The scientific method. Scientists consistently follow these steps when testing all types of hypotheses. Scientists do not accept a nutrition or other scientific hypothesis until it has been thoroughly tested using the scientific method.

placebo Generally, an inactive medicine or treatment used to disguise the treatments given to the participants in an experiment.

case-control study A study in which individuals who have a disease or condition, such as lung cancer, are compared with individuals who do not have the condition.

consume a **placebo.** People are randomly assigned to each group. Scientists then observe the experimental group over time to see if there is any effect not found in the control group. A **case-control study** compares individuals who have a disease or condition, such as lung cancer, to individuals who do not have the condition.

TESTING A HYPOTHESIS: CAN A HIGH-FAT DIET CAUSE WEIGHT LOSS?

The following example shows how the scientific method (see Fig. 1-5) was used to test a hypothesis about the effects of low-calorie, high-fat diets on weight loss.

Step 1. Observations Made and Questions Asked. In the mid-1950s, physicians note that in short-term experiments, people eating a low-calorie, high-fat diet lost weight more quickly than people eating a low-calorie, high-carbohydrate diet.

Step 2. Hypothesis Generated. Low-calorie, high-fat diets (e.g., Atkins diet) lead to more weight loss over time than low-calorie, high-carbohydrate diets.

Step 3. Research Experiments Conducted. For 1 year, researchers followed 63 people assigned to either a low-calorie, high-fat diet or a low-calorie, high-carbohydrate diet. At the end of the study, weight loss did not differ significantly between the two groups.

Step 4. Results Evaluated by Other Scientists and Published. A peer review indicated that the study was conducted in an unbiased, scientific manner and the results appeared valid. The study was published in *The New England Journal of Medicine* (348:2082, 2003).

Step 5. Follow-up Experiments Conducted to Confirm or Extend the Findings. A study published in 2005 described what happened when 160 people were assigned to a specific diet for a year. One diet was a low-calorie, high-fat diet; the other was a low-calorie, high-carbohydrate diet. Again, at the end of 1 year, weight loss in these two groups did not differ significantly. Peer reviewers indicated that the study was conducted scientifically. It was published in the *Journal of the American Medical Association* (293:43, 2005). A more recent 2-year study compared people who ate one of four reduced-calorie diets that was either low or high in fat, average or high in protein, or low or high in carbohydrates. After 2 years, the amount of weight loss was similar among participants. This study was published in *The New England Journal of Medicine* (360:859, 2009).

Step 6. Accept or Reject Hypothesis? Based on the currently available research studies, the hypothesis is not accepted. Reduced-calorie diets result in weight loss regardless of whether they emphasize fat, protein, or carbohydrate.

TYPES OF EXPERIMENTS

Human experiments provide the most convincing evidence about relationships between nutrients and health, but they are often not practical or ethical. Thus, much of what we know about human nutritional needs and functions has been gleaned from animal experiments. The use of animal experiments to study the role of nutrition in certain human diseases depends on the availability of an **animal model** in which a disease in laboratory animals closely mimics a particular human disease. Often, if no animal model is available and human experiments are ruled out, scientific knowledge cannot advance beyond what can be learned from epidemiological studies.

animal model Use of animals to study disease to understand more about human disease.

Once an experiment is complete, scientists summarize the findings and seek to publish the results in scientific journals. Generally, before articles are published in scientific journals, they are critically reviewed by other scientists familiar with the subject, which helps to ensure that only high-quality, objective research findings are published.

Keep in mind that one experiment is never enough to prove a particular hypothesis or provide a basis for nutritional recommendations. Rather, through follow-up studies, the results obtained in one laboratory must be confirmed by similar experiments conducted in other laboratories and, possibly, under varying circumstances. Only then can we really trust and use the results. As shown in Figure 1-6, the more lines of evidence available to support an idea, the more likely it is to be true.

Case-control studies show that obese patients are much more likely to have type 2 diabetes than the leaner comparison group that is matched for other characteristics.

Observations by physicians indicate that type 2 diabetes is much more common in their obese patients than in leaner patients.

Laboratory animal studies show that overfeeding animals that leads to obesity also often leads to the development of type 2 diabetes.

Growing confidence in the research hypothesis that obesity leads to the development of type 2 diabetes

Epidemiological studies show that type 2 diabetes is more commonly found in obese populations than leaner populations.

Human studies show that weight loss can correct type 2 diabetes in many people. Laboratory researchers also show that enlarged fat cells associated with obesity are much less responsive to the normal hormonal signals involved in blood glucose regulation.

FIGURE 1-6 ▲ Data from a variety of sources can come together to support a research hypothesis. This diagram shows how various types of research data support the hypothesis that obesity leads to the development of type 2 diabetes.

Epidemiological studies may suggest hypotheses, but controlled experiments are needed to rigorously test hypotheses before nutrition recommendations can be made. For example, epidemiologists found that smokers who regularly consumed fruits and vegetables had a lower risk for lung cancer than smokers who ate few fruits and vegetables. Some scientists proposed that beta-carotene, a pigment present in many fruits and vegetables, may be responsible for reducing the damage that tobacco smoke creates in the lungs. However, in double-blind studies involving heavy smokers, the risk of lung cancer was found to be *higher* for those who took beta-carotene supplements than for those who did not (this is not true for the small amount of beta-carotene found naturally in foods). Soon after these results were reported, two other large studies using beta-carotene supplements were stopped by the federal funding agency on the basis that these supplements are ineffective in preventing both lung cancer and cardiovascular disease.

✓ CONCEPT CHECK 1.5

1. What are the six steps used in the scientific method?

1.6 What Is the Current State of the North American Diet and Health?

DOES OBESITY THREATEN OUR FUTURE?

There is no doubt that the obesity epidemic threatens the future health of Americans. It is estimated that more than 35% of adults are currently obese, with *obesity* defined as having an excessive amount of body fat relative to lean tissue. Considered more broadly, two-thirds of adults and one-third of children are overweight or obese. According to the Centers for Disease Control and Prevention (CDC), the average American adult man weighs 195.5 pounds, and the average American adult woman weighs 166.2 pounds. Where you live is also a factor, with obesity rates varying by state. State by state, self-reported obesity data from the CDC (Fig. 1-7) indicates that in 2013, obesity rates were between 20% and 25% in 7 states,

Newsworthy Nutrition

Throughout the textbook, we have highlighted the use of the scientific method in research studies in a feature we call "Newsworthy Nutrition." These are recently published studies that relate to chapter topics and that have made a significant impact on our nutrition knowledge. You will find the first "Newsworthy Nutrition" study in Section 1.6 on the current state of the North American diet and health.

FIGURE 1-7 ▶ Percentage of adults who are obese,* by state, 2013.

Source: CDC, Prevalence of Self-Reported Obesity Among U.S. Adults by State and Territory, BRFSS, 2013.

*Body mass index (BMI) > 30, or about 30 pounds overweight for a 5′9″ person, based on self-reported weight and height.

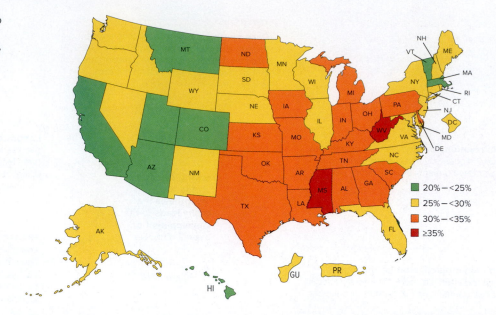

Legend:
- 20%–<25%
- 25%–<30%
- 30%–<35%
- ≥35%

above 30% in 18 states, and above 35% in 2 states (Mississippi and West Virginia; see Further Reading 5). In 2006, only one state was above 30%.

The report, *F as in Fat: How Obesity Threatens America's Future 2013* (see Further Reading 19), shares evidence that since 2005 the rate of increase in obesity has been slowing. This is good news. If the incidence of obesity continued to grow at recent rates, the effects on the health and wealth of our nation would be catastrophic by the year 2030.

Newsworthy Nutrition

No Change in Obesity Prevalence in Youth or Adults Between 2003 and 2012

The prevalence of obesity in the United States is high, with 30% of adults and 17% of children estimated to be obese. Despite its high occurrence, an earlier study found that the prevalence of obesity remained stable between 2003 and 2010. Because of this leveling off rate, scientists at the National Center for Health Statistics developed a hypothesis that the prevalence of obesity in youth and adults would also have remained stable between 2003 and 2012. The purpose of this study was to analyze trends in childhood and adult obesity between 2003 and 2012. The analyses were based on measurements of weight and height in 9120 participants from the 2011–2012 National Health and Nutrition Examination Survey (NHANES). Childhood obesity was defined as a body mass index (BMI) at or above the 95th percentile of the CDC BMI-for-age growth charts in children and adolescents aged 2 to 19 years. In adults, obesity was defined as a BMI greater than or equal to 30. Trends in obesity prevalence were analyzed across five periods (2003–2004, 2005–2006, 2007–2008, 2009–2010, and 2011–2012). Overall, the results of this study indicate no significant change for obesity from 2003–2004 through 2011–2012 in 2- to 19-year-olds or adults. Results for prevalence of obesity in 2011–2012 were 16.9% in youth and 34.9% in adults. There was a significant decrease in obesity from 13.9% to 8.4% among 2- to 5-year-olds and a significant increase in obesity from 31.5% to 38.1% among women aged 60 years and older. Based on these results, the authors of this study conclude that, while not increasing overall, the prevalence of obesity remains high in youth and adults, and thus should continue to be under surveillance.

Source: Ogden CL and others: Prevalence of childhood and adult obesity in the United States, 2011-2012. *Journal of the American Medical Association* 311:806, 2014 (see Further Reading 16).

The report calls for a national commitment to the prevention of obesity and outlines a scenario by which a 9% to 14% (depending on the state) reduction of the states' obesity rates by 2030 could greatly decrease obesity-related diseases and health care costs. There is additional evidence that the prevalence of obesity is leveling off from the National Health and Nutrition Examination Survey (NHANES) conducted over the last decade. Read more about these encouraging results in the Newsworthy Nutrition feature in this section.

It is well documented that this extra weight will continue to have dangerous consequences. In Section 1.2, we pointed out that obesity plays a role in chronic illness, including heart disease, stroke, high blood pressure, high cholesterol, diabetes, arthritis, and certain cancers. It is estimated that obesity kills more than 200,000 Americans a year. Because of its role in so many chronic disorders, obesity is an expensive condition with more than $190 billion spent annually on health care related to obesity. Because of numerous medical conditions, obese individuals are absent from work more often than those of healthy weight. Health economists estimate that obesity-related absenteeism costs employers as much as $6.4 billion a year, whereas loss of on-the-job productivity due to pain, shortness of breath, or other obstacles costs another $30 billion. It has become obvious that the answers to the obesity crisis are not simple. From a nutrition perspective, however, the problem can be clearly stated. Most of us continue to eat too much, especially foods with a high number of calories and a low number of nutrients, and we do not engage in enough physical activity.

ASSESSING THE CURRENT NORTH AMERICAN DIET

With the aim of finding out what North Americans eat, federal agencies conduct surveys to collect data about food and nutrient consumption, as well as connections between diet and health. In the United States, the U.S. Department of Health and Human Services monitors food consumption with the National Health and Nutrition Examination Survey (NHANES). The NHANES was used in the study highlighted in the Newsworthy Nutrition. In Canada, this information is gathered by Health Canada in conjunction with Agriculture and Agrifood Canada. Survey data from 2009-2010 indicate that North American adults consume about 15% of their calorie intake as proteins, 52% as carbohydrates, and 33% as fats. These percentages, which do not consider alcohol, fall within the ranges recommended by the Food and Nutrition Board (FNB) of the National Academy of Sciences. The FNB advocates that 10% to 35% of calories come from protein, 45% to 65% from carbohydrate, and 20% to 35% from fat. These standards apply to people in both the United States and Canada.

Food-consumption data also indicate that animal sources supply about two-thirds of protein intake for most North Americans, whereas plant sources supply only about one-third. In many other parts of the world, it is just the opposite: plant proteins—from rice, beans, corn, and other grains and vegetables—dominate protein intake. About half the carbohydrate in North American diets comes from simple sugars; the other half comes from starches (such as in pastas, breads, and potatoes). About 60% of dietary fat comes from animal sources and 40% from plant sources.

Evidence of positive changes in dietary habits have begun to appear. Results from the 2011—2012 NHANES show that calories consumed daily by the typical U.S. adult are declining for the first time in over 40 years. The fact that the decline in calories has occurred while obesity rates have stopped rising, suggests that the calorie reductions are making a difference. One of the most significant declines has been in the amount of full-calorie soda consumed, which has dropped 25% since the late 1990s. Keep in mind that while these changes in calories consumed are a step in the right direction and appear to stem from our growing awareness of the dangers of eating and drinking too much, we often do not choose the foods that will meet all our nutrient needs.

In the next section, we discuss recommendations to consume a variety of nutrient-dense foods within and across the food groups, especially whole grains, fruits, vegetables, low-fat or fat-free milk or milk products, and lean meats and other protein sources. These foods will provide nutrients that are often overlooked, including various B vitamins, vitamin C, vitamin D, vitamin E, calcium, potassium, magnesium, iron, fiber, and many phytochemicals. Daily intake of a balanced multivitamin and mineral supplement is another strategy to

▲ African-Americans and Hispanics have a greater chance of developing hypertension than do other ethnic groups and therefore should replace salty snack foods with healthier low-sodium options. © Ingram Publishing

help meet nutrient needs but does not make up for a poor diet. Also keep in mind that use of nutrient supplements should be discussed with your health professional to avoid potentially harmful side effects (dietary supplements are discussed in Chapter 8).

Experts also recommend that we pay more attention to balancing calorie intake with needs. An excess intake of calories is usually tied to overindulgence in sugar, fat, and alcoholic beverages. Many North Americans would benefit from a healthier balance of food in their diets. Moderation is the key for some foods that are high in calories from sugar and fat. For other foods, such as fruits and vegetables, increased quantity and variety are warranted. Few adults currently meet the new recommendation to "fill half your plate with fruits and vegetables" promoted in the U.S. Department of Agriculture (USDA) MyPlate guidelines for total servings of vegetables and fruits.

HEALTH OBJECTIVES FOR THE UNITED STATES FOR THE YEAR 2020

Health promotion and disease prevention have been public health strategies in North America for the past 3 decades. One part of this strategy is *Healthy People 2020,* a report issued in December 2010 by the U.S. Department of Health and Human Services' (DHHS) Public Health Service. Every 10 years, DHHS issues a collection of health objectives for the nation. These objectives are developed by experts in federal agencies and target major public health concerns, setting goals for the coming decade. *Healthy People 2020* sets forth more than 600 health objectives across 42 topic areas and outlines national standards to eliminate health disparities, improve access to health education and quality health care, and strengthen public health services. The vision for 2020 is a society in which all people live long, healthy lives. Important features of *Healthy People 2020* include a focus on health equity and social determinants of health, and an interactive, personalized website at www.HealthyPeople.gov.

The overarching goals of *Healthy People 2020* are to:

- Attain high-quality, longer lives free of preventable disease, disability, injury, and premature death.
- Achieve health equity, eliminate disparities, and improve health of all groups.
- Create social and physical environments that promote good health for all.
- Promote quality of life, healthy development, and healthy behaviors across all life stages.

Healthy People 2020, like earlier versions, includes a topic area specific to nutrition. This topic is called Nutrition and Weight Status, and its objectives target individual behaviors, as well as the policies and environments that support these behaviors. Nutrition and weight status are important because a healthful diet helps us reduce our risks for numerous health conditions that burden the public health system, including heart disease, high blood pressure, diabetes, osteoporosis, and some cancers. Good nutrition for children is also emphasized in this report because of its importance for growth and development. The goal of this topic is to promote health and reduce chronic disease risk through the consumption of healthful diets and achievement and maintenance of healthy body weights. This goal also includes increasing household food security and eliminating hunger.

The Nutrition and Weight Status objectives are based on strong science that supports the health benefits of eating a healthful diet and maintaining a healthy body weight. A healthful diet is described as one that includes:

- Consuming a variety of nutrient-dense foods within and across the food groups, especially whole grains, fruits, vegetables, low-fat or fat-free milk or milk products, and lean meats and other protein sources.
- Limiting intake of solid fats, cholesterol, added sugars, sodium (salt), and alcohol.
- Limiting caloric intake to meet caloric needs.

The objectives also emphasize that individual behaviors should be addressed in any efforts to change diet and weight, as well as the policies and environments that support these behaviors in settings such as schools, worksites, health care organizations, and communities.

▲ Many nutrition-related objectives are part of the *Healthy People 2020* report. The report outlines health promotion and disease prevention objectives for the United States for the year 2020.

Source: www.healthypeople.gov

TABLE 1-4 ■ *Healthy People 2020:* **Nutrition and Weight Status Categories and Objectives**

Category 1: Healthier Food Access

1. Increase the number of states with nutrition standards for child care.
2. Increase the proportion of schools that offer nutritious foods and beverages outside of school meals.
3. Increase the number of states that have incentive policies for food retail outlets to provide foods that are encouraged by the 2015—2020 Dietary Guidelines for Americans.
4. Increase the proportion of Americans who have retail access to foods recommended by the 2010 Dietary Guidelines for Americans.

Category 2: Health Care and Worksite Settings

5. Increase the proportion of primary care physicians who measure patients' body mass index (BMI).
6. Increase the proportion of physician office visits that include nutrition or weight counseling or education.
7. Increase the proportion of worksites that offer nutrition and weight-management classes and counseling.

Category 3: Weight Status

8. Increase the proportion of adults who are at a healthy weight.
9. Reduce the proportion of adults who are obese.
10. Reduce the proportion of children and adolescents who are considered obese.
11. Prevent inappropriate weight gain in youth and adults.

Category 4: Food Insecurity

12. Eliminate very low food security among children.
13. Reduce household food insecurity and, in so doing, reduce hunger.

Category 5: Food and Nutrient Consumption

14. Increase the contribution of fruits to the diets of the population ages 2 years and older.
15. Increase the variety and contribution of vegetables to the diets of the population ages 2 years and older.
16. Increase the contribution of whole grains to the diets of the population ages 2 years and older.
17. Reduce consumption of calories from solid fats and added sugars in the population ages 2 years and older.
18. Reduce consumption of saturated fat in the population ages 2 years and older.
19. Reduce consumption of sodium in the population ages 2 years and older.
20. Increase consumption of calcium in the population ages 2 years and older.

Category 6: Iron Deficiency

21. Reduce iron deficiency among young children and females of childbearing age.
22. Reduce iron deficiency among pregnant females.

Table 1-4 lists the six categories of objectives for the Nutrition and Weight Status topic, along with the 22 specific objectives. Table 1-5 provides a more detailed sample of nine specific Nutrition and Weight Status objectives along with the current status of these objectives and their targets for 2020.

Other new topic areas highlight changes in the health needs of specific segments of the population: early and middle childhood, adolescence, and older adults. Because young people develop habits, including eating and physical activity behaviors, that are likely to persist throughout life, new objectives promote strengthened health education in schools and communities, and fostering an environment in which young people can develop healthy habits. Older adults are the fastest-growing segment of the American population and are at high risk for experiencing the chronic health problems that so severely impact our health care system. The objectives for older adults include improving access to health care, helping older adults to manage their own health conditions, and ensuring proper training and support of professionals and nonprofessionals who care for this population.

▲ An increase in the consumption of some foods, such as fruits and vegetables, can lead to a healthier balance of food in the North American diet. © xefstock/Getty Images

TABLE 1-5 ■ A Sample of Nutrition and Weight Status Objectives from *Healthy People 2020* Along with Details About the Current Status and Targets for 2020

	Target	Current Estimate
Increase the proportion of adults at a healthy weight.	33.9%	30.8%
Reduce the proportion of overweight or obese children and adolescents.	14.6%	16.2%
Increase the contribution of the following to the diets of the population ages 2 years and older (per 1000 calories).		
• Fruits	0.9 cup	0.5 cup
• Total vegetables	1.1 cups	0.8 cup
• Whole grains	0.6 ounce	0.3 ounce
Reduce consumption of calories from solid fats (% total calorie intake).	16.7%	18.9%
Reduce consumption of calories from added sugars (% total calorie intake).	10.8%	15.7%
Increase consumption of calcium in the population ages 2 years and older.	1300 mg	1118 mg
Reduce iron deficiency among females of childbearing age.	9.4%	10.4%

Note: In later chapters, we will explore additional nutrition-related objectives, such as those addressing osteoporosis, various forms of cancer, diabetes prevention and treatment, food allergies, cardiovascular disease, low birth weight, nutrition during pregnancy, breastfeeding, eating disorders, physical activity, and alcohol use.

genomics The study of the function and structure of the complete set of DNA within a single cell of an organism, known as the genome.

A scientifically exciting new topic area in the *Healthy People 2020* report is **genomics.** Nine of the 10 leading causes of death have a strong genetic component. Genetic testing is becoming a valuable tool for improving diagnosis and treatment of chronic diseases, especially for cancers of the breast and colon. In combination with family history, genetic testing can help health care professionals guide patients in treatment options, including lifestyle changes. The relationship between genetics and nutrition will be discussed in Chapter 3.

✓ CONCEPT CHECK 1.6

1. Surveys indicate that we could improve our diets by focusing on which types of food sources?

2. The consumption of which types of foods should be reduced to attain and maintain good health?

1.7 What Can You Expect from Good Nutrition and a Healthy Lifestyle?

The obesity epidemic and prevalence of chronic diseases in the United States show that something is not right with many of our dietary patterns and/or lifestyles. The strong association between obesity and poor health is clear. The reverse is also well documented: when an obese or overweight person loses just 5% to 10% of body weight, that person's risks of many chronic diseases are greatly reduced.

HEALTHY WEIGHT

Because weight gain is one of the greatest lifelong nutrition challenges, we encourage you to seek a lifestyle that will make gaining weight more difficult and maintaining a healthy weight easier. Preventing obesity in the first place is the easiest approach. Unfortunately, many aspects of our society make it hard not to gain weight. The earlier (preferably in childhood) we develop lifestyle habits of good nutrition, regular physical activity, and the avoidance of addictions to salt, fat, sweets, high-calorie foods, and sedentary lifestyles, the better. As you enter the workforce, seek out employers who offer wellness programs that encourage weight management and weight loss among their employees. Aim to live in a city or town that has opportunities for physical activity such as bike paths, walking trails, and parks, as well as access to fresh fruits and vegetables through farmers' markets and community gardens. Seek out and join running or walking clubs. Shop at grocery stores that offer a good selection of fruits, vegetables, and other healthy foods. When dining out, choose restaurants that have tasty but healthy options on their menu.

Fortunately, many dietary habits have improved during the past decade. Today, we can choose from a wide variety of food products as a result of continual innovation by food manufacturers. We are eating more breakfast cereals, pizza, pasta entrees, stir-fried meats and vegetables served on rice, salads, tacos, burritos, and fajitas than ever before. Sales of whole milk are down, and sales of fat-free and 1% low-fat milk have increased. Consumption of frozen vegetables rather than canned vegetables is also on the rise. Despite the alarming problem of overweight and obesity, our cultural diversity, varied cuisines, and general lack of nutrient deficiencies should be points of pride for North Americans.

LONGER, HEALTHIER LIVES

Today, North Americans live longer than ever and enjoy better general health. Deaths from cardiovascular disease, for example, have dropped dramatically since the late 1960s, partly because of better medical care and dietary patterns. Affluence, however, has also led to sedentary lifestyles and high intakes of animal fat, salt, and alcohol. This lifestyle pattern has led to problems such as cardiovascular disease, hypertension, diabetes, and, of course, obesity. Greater efforts are needed by the general public to lower intake of animal fats and to improve variety in our diets, especially from fruits, vegetables, and whole grains. With better technology and greater choices, we can have a much better diet today than ever before—if we know what choices to make.

THE TOTAL DIET

Nutrition experts generally agree that there are no "good" or "bad" foods, but some foods provide relatively few nutrients in comparison to calorie content. In Chapter 2, you will learn that an individual's total diet is the proper focus in a nutritional evaluation. It is the position of the Academy of Nutrition and Dietetics that "the total diet or overall pattern of food eaten is the most important focus of healthy eating" (see Further Reading 1). Health experts have prepared many reports and outlined numerous objectives to get us closer to being a "Healthy People" as soon as 2020. In Chapter 2, we will discuss the "Dietary Guidelines" that are published every 5 years and the interactive programs available on **ChooseMyPlate.gov.** As you reexamine your nutritional habits, remember your health is largely your responsibility. Your body has a natural ability to heal itself. Offer it what it needs, and it will serve you well. Confusing and conflicting health messages hinder change in our eating patterns.

Prevention of disease is an important investment of one's time, even during the college years. The following recommendations will help promote your health and prevent chronic diseases: (1) consuming enough essential nutrients, including fiber, while moderating energy, solid fat, added sugar, and alcohol intake; (2) doing adequate, regular physical activity (at least 30 to 60 minutes on most or all days); (3) minimizing alcohol intake (no more than two drinks per day for men and one drink for women and all adults age 65 years and older); and (4) not smoking cigarettes or cigars. In addition to these recommendations, you can optimize your health by getting adequate sleep (7 to 9 hours per night), consuming sufficient water (9 to 13 cups per day from foods and beverages), reducing stress, using medications prudently, and, of course, abstaining from use of illicit drugs. Having close relationships with others and maintaining a positive outlook on life are also linked to lower risk for disease. Finally, consultation with health care professionals on a regular basis is important. This is because early diagnosis is especially useful for controlling the damaging effects of many diseases. In total, these contribute to maximal health and prevention of the

▲ Access to fresh fruits and vegetables through farmers' markets and community gardens is important to a healthy lifestyle.

© Image Source/Getty Images

▼ Regular physical activity complements a healthy diet. Whether it is all at once or in segments throughout the day, incorporate 30 to 60 minutes or more of such activity into your daily routine. © Monkey Business Image/AGE fotostock

registered dietitian (RD) A person who has completed a baccalaureate degree program approved by the Accreditation Council for Education in Nutrition and Dietetics (ACEND), performed at least 1200 hours of supervised professional practice, passed a registration examination, and complies with continuing education requirements.

registered dietitian nutritionist (RDN) The RDN is the updated credential formerly abbreviated RD. The credential was updated to better reflect the scope of practice of the dietitian and to align with the new name of the professional organization for dietitians, the Academy of Nutrition and Dietetics.

diseases listed. Section 1.8 gives you a "sneak peek" of several nutrition issues relevant to most college students. These issues, including the "freshman 15," vegetarianism, fuel for athletes, eating disorders, and alcohol and binge drinking, also will be covered more fully in later chapters of the book.

ASK THE RDN: Who's the Expert?

Dear RDN: I am interested in making positive changes to my eating pattern to reach a healthy weight and feel better. How can I find a qualified nutrition expert who will give me personalized nutrition advice?

You have already made a big step toward better nutrition by taking this nutrition course! The information in this textbook is written by authors who are all qualified nutrition experts, namely *registered dietitian nutritionists* (RDN). The textbook and your instructor will provide a solid foundation in nutrition, but be aware that some people call themselves "nutritionists" without qualified training in nutrition. The best approach to finding answers about your personal nutritional state is to consult your primary care provider, **registered dietitian (RD),** or **registered dietitian nutritionist (RDN).** The RD/RDN has been certified by the Commission on Dietetic Registration of the Academy of Nutrition and Dietetics (AND) after completing rigorous classroom and clinical training in nutrition. The RD/RDN must also complete continuing education. The RD credential was recently updated to RDN to better reflect the scope of practice of dietitians. While both titles signify the same credential, we will use RDN when referring to dietitians in this book.

You can begin your search for a local RDN by asking your primary care provider or calling your health insurance company for a referral. You can also find an RDN by using the AND national referral service, called *Find a Registered Dietitian Nutritionist.* This service links consumers with qualified nutrition practitioners who provide reliable, objective nutrition information. Visit the website, www.eatright.org, and click on "Find an Expert." (In Canada, visit the Dietitians of Canada website, www.dietitians.ca, and click on "Find a Dietitian.") Enter your ZIP code or state to display the providers in your area. Select additional specialties that may apply to your specific needs. The website will display a list of providers. A professional with the RD or RDN credential after his or her name is a qualified nutrition expert who is trained to help you separate facts from fads, and optimize your health with better food choices. You can trust an RDN to translate the latest scientific findings into easy-to-understand nutrition information that you can sink your teeth into.

I hope this answer was helpful. We will use this feature, "Ask the RDN," in every chapter to answer questions about topics that may seem to have conflicting viewpoints.

Your nutrition expert,

Anne M. Smith, PhD, RDN, LD (author)

✓ CONCEPT CHECK 1.7

1. What are some dietary patterns, physical activities, and lifestyle recommendations for health promotion and disease prevention?

1.8 Nutrition and Your Health

Eating Well in College

© BananaStock/PunchStock

The college years are a time for freedom and a chance to make personal lifestyle decisions. Studies show that the diets of college students are not optimal. Typically, students fall short of diet recommendations for whole grains, vegetables, fruits, milk, and meat, opting instead to max out on fats, sweets, and alcohol. This information is disturbing because young adulthood is the time when many health behaviors are formed that will persist throughout life.

What is it about the college lifestyle that makes it so difficult to build healthy habits? In this section, we will discuss several topics and provide possible solutions.

Food Choices

College students face changes in academic requirements, interpersonal relationships, and living environments. These stressful situations contribute to poor health behaviors. For example, when you are writing papers and cramming for exams, balanced meals are all too easily replaced by high-fat and high-calorie fast foods, convenience items, and sugary, caffeinated beverages. Physical activity is sacrificed in favor of study time. In a recent study of college students living on and off campus, two-thirds of the students reported skipping meals, with "no time to prepare" the major reason (see Further Reading 7).

Also consider that on campus, you are faced with a wide variety of dining choices. Dining halls, fast-food establishments, bars, and vending machines combine to offer food 24 hours per day. While it is certainly possible to make wise food choices at each of these outlets, the temptations of convenience, taste, and value (i.e., inexpensive, oversized portions) may persuade the college student to select unhealthy options.

Meals and snacks are also times to socialize. You may unintentionally eat a big lunch at noon without regard to hunger if your peers are meeting in the dining hall to catch up. While chatting, it is easy to lose track of portions and to overeat. In addition, food may be a source of familiarity and comfort in a new and stressful place.

Weight Control and the "Freshman 15"

Studies show that most college students gain weight during their first year (see Further Reading 8). The "freshman 15" is a term used to describe the weight gained by students during their first year of college. Although it is becoming evident that most freshmen do not gain the 15 pounds, a recent study of over 7000 U.S. college students found that students pack on 2.4 to 3.5 pounds on average during their first year away from home (see Further Reading 21). Very few (just under 10%) of freshmen gained 15 pounds or more, and 25% of freshmen actually lost weight. The research also determined cumulative weight gain over the entire years at college and found that women gained approximately 9 pounds and men, 13 pounds, on average. The two lifestyle factors that made a difference in weight gain among the students were heavy drinking and working during college.

There are several reasons to maintain a healthy weight. Over the long term, risk of chronic diseases goes up as weight increases. In the short term, losing excess weight can improve how you feel and perform. Detecting "flab" around your midsection or feeling that your clothes are getting tighter are two good indicators that you are carrying excess weight. If weight loss is necessary, with some knowledge and perseverance, you can safely lose excess pounds.

Behavioral research clearly demonstrates that setting several small, achievable goals will spur motivation. As you will learn in Chapter 7, body weight is a balancing act between calories in and calories burned. Try keeping track of your calorie consumption for several days and comparing that to your energy needs, based on your age, gender, and activity level. You can use one of the equations presented in Chapter 7 or take advantage of the Super-Tracker interactive tools on www.ChooseMyPlate.gov to estimate your energy needs.

A healthy rate of weight loss is 1 to 2 pounds per week. Greater rates of weight loss will not likely be sustained over time. Remember that the numbers on the scale are not as important as your body composition—the amount of fat in relation to lean mass. In order to lose weight, you must create an energy deficit, either by restricting energy intake below what you need to maintain your

CASE STUDY Typical College Student

Andy is like many other college students. He grew up on a quick bowl of cereal and milk for breakfast and a hamburger, French fries, and cola for lunch, either in the school cafeteria or at a local fast-food restaurant. At dinner, he generally avoided eating any of his salad or vegetables, and by 9:00 P.M. he was deep into bags of chips and cookies. Andy has taken most of these habits to college. He prefers coffee for breakfast and possibly a chocolate bar. Lunch is still mainly a hamburger, French fries, and cola, but pizza and tacos now alternate more frequently than when he was in high school. One thing Andy really likes about the restaurants surrounding campus is that, for a few cents more, he can make his hamburger a double or get extra cheese and pepperoni on his pizza. This helps him stretch his food dollar; searching out large-portion value meals for lunch and dinner now has become part of a typical day.

© Image 100/Corbis

Provide some dietary advice for Andy. Start with his positive habits and then provide some constructive criticism, based on what you now know.

Answer the following questions, and check your responses at the end of this chapter. As you make suggestions for Andy, think about your favorite food choices, why they are your favorites, and whether these are positive choices.

1. **Start with Andy's positive habits:** What healthy choices are being made when Andy eats at local restaurants?
2. **Now provide some constructive criticism:**
   a. What are some of the negative aspects of items available at fast-food restaurants?
   b. Why is ordering the "value meals" a dangerous habit?
   c. What healthier substitutions could he make at each meal?
   d. List some healthier choices he could make at fast-food restaurants on campus.

current weight or by increasing your physical activity. For an adult with excess weight, an energy deficit of 500 kcal per day will result in weight loss of about 25 pounds over a year's time. As weight is lost, energy needs gradually decrease, such that further deficits will be required to lose additional weight.

Although many students skip it, breakfast is the *most* important meal of the day. Starting the day off with a serving of lean protein (e.g., an egg, Canadian bacon, or protein shake), a fortified whole-grain breakfast cereal, skim milk, and a serving of fruit puts you on the right path for meeting recommendations for fiber, calcium, and fruit intake. Even though it may seem that coffee gets your brain going in the morning, your brain is fueled best by carbohydrates, not caffeine. Studies also show that eating breakfast prevents overeating later in the day. Read more about breakfast choices in the *What the Dietitian Chose* recommendations at the end of this chapter.

One of the biggest contributors to weight gain for college students is consuming several hundred calories per day in the form of sugary or alcoholic beverages. One 12-ounce can of regular cola contains about 140 kcal. A 12-ounce can of regular beer has 150 kcal. Consuming gourmet coffee beverages, such as lattes and

▲ Research (see Further Reading 18) has shown that gourmet coffee beverages, such as lattes and cappuccinos, can increase calorie consumption by about 200 kcal per day. © BananaStock/PunchStock

▶ Five Simple Tips to Avert Weight Gain

- **Eat breakfast.** Rev up your metabolism with a protein source such as an egg or low-fat yogurt, at least one serving of whole grains such as a breakfast cereal, and a fruit such as a banana.
- **Plan ahead.** Eat a balanced meal or snack every 3 to 4 hours.
- **Limit liquid calories.** Drink water instead of high-calorie soft drinks, fruit juice, alcohol, or coffee; if you drink alcohol, limit it to 1 or 2 drinks per day.
- **Stock the fridge.** Keep a stash of low-calorie, nutritious snacks such as pretzels, light microwave popcorn, and fruit (fresh, canned, or dried).
- **Exercise regularly.** Find a friend to work out with you. Experts recommend 30 minutes of moderate exercise at least 5 days a week.

cappuccinos, can increase average calorie consumption by about 200 kcal per day (see Further Reading 18). Even fruit juices have at least 100 kcal per 8-ounce glass. Furthermore, a 24-ounce mug of a soft drink makes you feel no fuller than an equal volume of water, yet the soft drink adds 300 kcal more. A convenient stash of water is the best way to quench your thirst.

Exercise is very important to any weight loss and weight maintenance plan, but sticking with it is hard to do. When you find yourself short on time, exercise is often the first thing that goes. To ensure your success at boosting daily activity, choose activities you enjoy such as working out with friends at the campus recreation center, participating in intramural sports, or taking an activity class such as dancing. Don't forget the brisk walking to and from classes. For more information on planning an exercise program, see Chapter 14.

Alcohol and Binge Drinking

Excessive alcohol consumption is a big problem on college campuses. Many college students consider drinking alcohol, legally or not, to be a "rite of passage" into adulthood. On campuses, binge drinking—consuming five or more drinks in a row for men or four drinks or more for women—has become an epidemic. A new level of "extreme drinking" goes far beyond binge drinking. For example, recent studies indicate that college students celebrate twenty-first birthdays with an average of about eight drinks more during the week of that birthday compared to a typical week (see Further Reading 12).

The statistics on the impact of binge drinking on college campuses are sobering. An estimated two of every five students on college campuses participate in binge drinking. Each year, 1400 college students between the ages of 18 and 24 die from alcohol-related unintentional injuries, including motor vehicle crashes. In addition to deaths and injuries, other problems stemming from binge drinking include unsafe sex and its consequences, long-term health problems, suicides, academic problems, legal troubles, and alcohol abuse or dependence. Thirty-one percent of college students meet the criteria for alcohol use disorders.

In addition, alcohol consumption definitely contributes to weight gain—by virtue of its own calories and the increased food consumption at events where drinking occurs. If you choose to drink alcohol, do so in moderation—no more than two drinks per day for men and one drink per day for women. Be aware of the warning signs and dangers of alcohol poisoning shown here. Special issues related to alcohol use by adolescents are covered in Chapter 19.

▶ **The warning signs and symptoms of alcohol poisoning:**

- Semiconsciousness or unconsciousness
- Slow respiration of 8 or fewer breaths per minute or lapses between breaths of more than 8 second
- Cold, clammy, pale, or bluish skin
- Strong odor of alcohol, which usually accompanies these symptoms

▲ Late-night pizza can add extra calories to the college student's daily intake. © Stockbyte/PunchStock

Eating Disorders

As many as 30% of college students are at risk of developing an eating disorder. As you will learn in Chapter 15, disordered eating is a mild and short-term change in eating patterns that typically occurs in response to life stress, a desire to change appearance, or a bad habit. Sometimes, disordered eating habits may lead to an eating disorder, such as anorexia nervosa, bulimia nervosa, or binge-eating disorder. Chapter 15 includes advice on what to do if you suspect that your roommate or friend is suffering from an eating disorder.

Starving the body also starves the brain, which limits performance in academics and beyond. The negative consequences of disordered eating may last a lifetime. Ultimately, eating disorders do not arise from problems with food but rather from problems with self-esteem, control, and abusive relationships. Frequently, what begins as a diet spirals into a much larger problem. Eating disorders are not just diets gone bad: they require professional intervention. Left unchecked, eating disorders lead to serious adverse effects, such as loss of menstrual periods, thinning of bones, gastrointestinal problems, kidney problems, heart abnormalities, and eventually death.

Choosing a Vegetarian Lifestyle

Many college students experiment with or adopt a vegetarian eating pattern. Plant-based diets can meet nutrition needs and decrease risk of many chronic diseases, but they require appropriate planning at all life stages.

Protein is not typically deficient, even with a vegan diet, which contains no animal products. However, vegetarians, and especially vegans, may be at risk for deficiencies of several vitamins and minerals. Consuming a ready-to-eat breakfast cereal is an easy and inexpensive way to obtain these nutrients. See Chapter 6 for more information on vegetarian food planning.

▲ Many students adopt a vegetarian diet during college. Guidelines for planning a nutritious vegetarian diet, with items such as this veggie lasagna and spinach salad, are presented in Chapter 6. © Blue Moon Stock/PunchStock

Restaurants and campus dining services have responded to the growing interest in vegetarian meals by offering a variety of vegetarian options. For optimal health benefits, choose foods that are baked, steamed, or stir-fried rather than deep-fried; select whole grains rather than refined carbohydrates; and consume food fortified with vitamins and minerals. Even if you do not follow a plant-based diet all the time, choosing several plant-based meals each week can help with weight control and boost intake of fiber and healthy phytochemicals. You will learn in Chapter 2 that the ChooseMyPlate program recommends that the largest portion of your plate be filled with plant foods, including whole grains, fruits, and vegetables.

Fuel for Competition: Student Athletes

Students who compete in sports such as intramural and intercollegiate athletics need to consume more calories and nutrients. Despite an emphasis on a lean physique, athletes at all levels must take care not to severely restrict calories, as this could impact performance and health. Muscles require adequate carbohydrates for fuel, and protein for growth and repair. Fat, as well, is an important source of stored energy for use during exercise. Low energy availability in women may lead to a loss of menstruation (amenorrhea), a condition costly to long-term bone health.

In addition to the calories needed to fuel the body, fluids are essential for health and performance. Water is adequate for events lasting less than 60 minutes; sports drinks are ideal for longer events, because they supply carbohydrates to fuel fatigued muscles as well as electrolytes to replenish those lost in perspiration. Intentional fluid losses to "cut weight" for a competition are detrimental to health and performance.

Athletes also should take care not to be wooed by the supplement industry. Increasing food intake to meet the energy demands of athletic training is also sufficient to meet most vitamin and mineral needs. As an exception, athletes may be at risk for iron-deficiency anemia. Consuming a balanced multivitamin and mineral supplement is adequate for most people. Individual vitamin, mineral, amino acid, or herbal supplements are not advised, in spite of the hype of supplement makers.

Tips for Eating Well on a College Student's Budget

Because higher education can be hard on the wallet, it is good to know that it is possible to eat well on campus on a budget. If you live on campus, participate in a prepaid campus meal plan. These plans are generally designed to offer great food value with a variety of healthy foods. If you live off campus or have your own kitchen, plan ahead. Packing a lunch from home rather than grabbing lunch on the run will save you money and put you in control of healthy choices. For example, preparing a sandwich at home costs half as much as purchasing one at a fast-food restaurant or deli.

Never go grocery shopping on an empty stomach: everything will look good and you'll buy more. Also, go to the store with a list in hand and stick to it, because impulse buys tend to drain your wallet. Buy store-brand rather than name-brand items. Make use of canned and frozen fruits and vegetables; they are just as nutritious as fresh varieties, particularly if you choose low-sodium and low-sugar options. Rather than buying cartons of fruit juice, select cans of fruit juice concentrate and mix with water at home. Likewise, preparing other drinks, such as iced tea, from store-brand powder (look for sugar-free types) will save over gallon jugs or vending machine containers of drinks. Canned (fruits, tuna) and dry (oatmeal) foods can be nutritious and last a long time, so you can avoid throwing out spoiled items. Finally, eggs and peanut butter are inexpensive and simple sources of protein.

In conclusion, *The College Student's Guide to Eating Well on Campus* (see Further Reading 13) and *The Dorm Room Diet* (see Further Reading 17) are excellent books with more details on ways college students can plan a healthy diet and stay fit.

Some Calorie Traps for College Students

	Number of Calories
Two handfuls of almonds	500
Two handfuls of granola	330
Personal-size pizza	500 to 600
1 cup of ice cream	300
Two handfuls of frosted cereal	250
Six-pack of regular beer	900

Source: Ann Litt, *The College Student's Guide to Eating Well on Campus*

Summary (Numbers refer to numbered sections in the chapter.)

1.1 The flavor, texture, and appearance of foods primarily influence our food choices. Several other factors also help determine food habits and choices: food availability and convenience, early childhood experiences and ethnic customs, nutrition and health concerns, advertising, restaurants, social changes, and economics. A variety of external (appetite-related) forces affect satiety (feeling of satisfaction that halts our desire to continue eating). Hunger cues combine with appetite cues, such as easy availability of food, to promote food intake.

1.2 Nutrition is a lifestyle factor that is a key to developing and maintaining an optimal state of health. A poor diet and a sedentary lifestyle are known to be risk factors for life-threatening chronic diseases such as heart disease, hypertension, diabetes, and cancer. Not meeting nutrient needs in younger years makes us more likely to suffer health consequences in later years. Too much of a nutrient also can be harmful. Drinking too much alcohol is another dietary problem associated with many health problems.

1.3 Nutrition is the study of how the body uses food substances to promote and support growth, maintenance, and reproduction of cells. Nutrients in foods fall into six classes: (1) carbohydrates, (2) lipids (mostly fats and oils), (3) proteins, (4) vitamins, (5) minerals, and (6) water. The first three, along with alcohol, provide calories for the body to use. Phytochemicals are plant chemicals that may contribute to a reduced risk of disease in people who consume them.

1.4 The body transforms the energy contained in carbohydrate, protein, and fat into other forms of energy that in turn allow the body to function. Fat provides, on average, 9 kcal per gram, whereas both protein and carbohydrate provide, on average, 4 kcal per gram. Calculating percentages and converting English units to metric units are important skills needed for the study of nutrition.

1.5 The scientific method is the procedure for testing the validity of possible explanations of a phenomenon, called hypotheses. Experiments are conducted to either support or refute a specific hypothesis. Once we have enough experimental information to support a specific hypothesis, it then can be called a theory. All of us need to be skeptical of new ideas in the nutrition field, waiting until many lines of experimental evidence support a concept before adopting any suggested dietary practice.

1.6 The obesity problem has worsened with 35% of people in the United States reported to be overweight or obese in 2013. This increase is a result of eating too much, especially foods with a high number of calories and a low number of nutrients, and not engaging in enough physical activity. Results from large nutrition surveys in the United States and Canada suggest that some of us need to concentrate on consuming foods that supply more of certain vitamins, minerals, and fiber. *Healthy People 2020* is a national initiative that includes Nutrition and Weight Status objectives related to eating a healthful diet and maintaining a healthy body weight. A healthful diet includes consuming a variety of nutrient-dense foods within and across the food groups, especially whole grains, fruits, vegetables, low-fat or fat-free milk or milk products, and lean meats and other protein sources; limiting intake of solid fats, cholesterol, added sugars, sodium (salt), and alcohol; and limiting intake of calories to meet energy needs.

1.7 A basic plan for health promotion and disease prevention includes eating a varied diet, performing regular physical activity, not smoking, not abusing nutrient supplements (if used), consuming adequate water and other fluids, getting enough sleep, limiting alcohol intake (if consumed), and limiting or appropriately coping with stress. The primary focus of nutrition planning should be on food, not on dietary supplements. The focus on foods to supply nutrient needs avoids the possibility of severe nutrient imbalances.

1.8 Studies show that the diets and other health habits of college students are not optimal. Students fall short of recommendations for servings of grains, vegetables, fruits, milk, and meat, opting instead for fats, sweets, and alcohol. This information is disturbing from a public health standpoint, because young adulthood is the time when many health behaviors are formed and will likely persist throughout life. Issues of particular importance on college campuses are weight control, making healthy meal choices, alcohol and binge drinking, and eating disorders.

Check Your Knowledge (Answers are available at the end of this question set.)

1. Our primary psychological drive to eat that is affected by many external food-choice mechanisms is called
   a. hunger.   b. appetite.   c. satiety.   d. feeding.

2. Energy-yielding nutrients include
   a. vitamins, minerals, and water.
   b. carbohydrates, proteins, and fats.
   c. trace minerals and fat-soluble vitamins.
   d. iron, vitamin C, and potassium.

3. The *essential* nutrients
   a. must be consumed at every meal.
   b. are required for infants but not adults.
   c. can be made in the body when they are needed.
   d. cannot be made by the body and therefore must be consumed to maintain health.

4. Sugars, starches, and dietary fibers are examples of
   a. proteins.   c. carbohydrates.
   b. vitamins.   d. minerals.

5. Which nutrient classes are most important in the regulation of body processes?
   a. vitamins   c. minerals
   b. carbohydrates   d. both a and c

6. A kcal is a
   a. measure of heat energy.
   b. measure of fat in food.
   c. heating device.
   d. term used to describe the amount of sugar and fat in foods.

7. A food that contains 10 grams of fat would yield _____ kcal.
   a. 40   b. 70   c. 90   d. 120

8. If you consume 300 grams of carbohydrate in a day that you consume 2400 kcal, the carbohydrates will provide _____% of your total energy intake.
   a. 12.5   b. 30   c. 50   d. 60

9. Which of the following is true about the North American diet?
   a. Most of our protein comes from plant sources.
   b. About half of the carbohydrates come from simple sugars.
   c. Most of our fats come from plant sources.
   d. Most of our carbohydrates come from starches.

10. A behavior that will decrease the risk of weight gain in college is to
    a. skip breakfast.
    b. drink more liquid calories.
    c. stock your fridge with nutritious snacks.
    d. exercise infrequently.

Study Questions (Numbers refer to Learning Outcomes)

1. Describe the process that controls hunger and satiety in the body. List other factors that influence our food choices. **(LO 1.1)**

2. Describe how your food preferences have been shaped by the following factors:
   a. Exposure to foods at an early age
   b. Advertising (What is the newest food you have tried?)
   c. Eating out
   d. Peer pressure
   e. Economic factors **(LO 1.1)**

3. What products in your supermarket reflect the consumer demand for healthier foods? For convenience? **(LO 1.1)**

4. Name one chronic disease associated with poor nutrition habits. Now list a few corresponding risk factors. **(LO 1.2)**

5. Describe two sources of fat and explain why the differences are important in terms of overall health. **(LO 1.3)**

6. Identify three ways that water is used in the body. **(LO 1.3)**

7. Explain the concept of calories as it relates to foods. What are the values used to calculate kilocalories from grams of carbohydrate, fat, protein, and alcohol? **(LO 1.4)**

8. A bowl of Panera's broccoli cheddar soup contains 21 grams carbohydrate, 13 grams fat, and 12 grams protein. Calculate the percentage of kilocalories derived from fat. **(LO 1.4)**

9. According to national nutrition surveys, which nutrients tend to be underconsumed by many North Americans? Why do you think this is the case? **(LO 1.5)**

10. List four *Healthy People 2020* objectives for the United States. How would you rate yourself in each area? Why? **(LO 1.5 & 1.6)**

11. List five strategies to avoid weight gain during college. **(LO 1.7)**

What the Dietitian Chose

Even bleary-eyed procrastinators can fuel their bodies for a new day of higher education! *Skipping breakfast is not a smart plan.* After a period of fasting (i.e., overnight), the body and the brain need fuel to operate at peak efficiency. In addition, many research studies demonstrate that eating a sensible breakfast is a good way to control weight. Compared to those who eat breakfast, people who skip breakfast tend to crave higher calorie foods, snack more throughout the day, and eat more at subsequent meals. Consider eating breakfast each day as part of your plan to fend off the "freshman 15."

Grab-and-go food options, such as those available in vending machines or from fast-food establishments, are often high in calories but low in nutrients. For example, a low-fat granola bar has only 100 kcal and 3 grams of fat but offers little else in terms of nutrition. Also, a granola bar is not likely to stave off hunger for very long.

On the other hand, a fast-food breakfast sandwich will probably promote satiety, but its calorie, fat, and sodium contents are too high. This type of sandwich provides 550 kcal, 23 grams of fat (38% of a day's total kilocalories in the sandwich and 35% of the whole day's limit for fat), and 1490 mg sodium (just under the 1500 mg Adequate Intake for this nutrient). A fast-food breakfast sandwich can fit into an otherwise healthy diet on occasion but should not be part of your normal routine.

Keeping nutritious but convenient breakfast options accessible is a good strategy for any time-pressed college student. Whole-grain,

fortified, ready-to-eat breakfast cereal with fat-free milk is a great choice: it is quick, provides a wide variety of vitamins and minerals, and boosts fiber intake. Adding a source of protein will help to support body processes and maintain fullness for a longer time. Hard-boiled eggs or a handful of dry-roasted nuts provide protein in ready-to-eat form. A cup of low-fat Greek yogurt offers protein with the added benefit of calcium. Fresh and dried fruit are portable and nutritious options for breakfast. Many fruit choices are loaded with potassium and vitamin C, plus they provide fiber.
A 1.5-ounce box of raisins, which can be stored for months without a refrigerator, provides about 130 kcal, no fat or cholesterol, very little sodium, 2 grams of fiber, and 320 milligrams of potassium.

So, the bowl of Wheaties with a banana and low-fat milk along with a yogurt, all from your dorm room "pantry," would be the healthiest choice for most.

▲ With a little bit of planning, breakfast can be both quick and healthy.
© Stockbyte/Getty Images

CASE STUDY SOLUTION | Typical College Student

1. The most positive aspect of Andy's diet is that it contains good sources of protein from animal products also rich in zinc and iron. Alternating his hamburger and fries for lunch with pizza or tacos is a move in the right direction.

2a. On the downside, Andy's diet is low in dairy products, fruits, and vegetables. This will result in a low intake of calcium, several of the vitamins, and the phytochemical (plant-based) substances discussed in this chapter. His diet is also low in fiber because fast-food restaurants primarily use refined-grain products rather than whole-grain products and have few fruit and vegetable choices on the menu. Most of the beverages are soft drinks loaded with sugar. Many menu items, especially fries and chicken nuggets, are high in fat.

2b. Most value menu options apply to foods rich in fat (French fries) and sugar (soft drinks), resulting in excessive amounts of these two components.

2c. He could choose a low-fat fruit and granola bar instead of the candy bar for breakfast, or he could take the time to eat a bowl of whole-grain breakfast cereal with fruit and low-fat or fat-free milk to increase fiber and calcium (in the latter case) intake. Juices such as orange juice for breakfast are beverage options that will add fruits or vegetables to his diet. Overall, Andy could improve his intake of fruits, vegetables, and dairy products by focusing on variety in food choice and balance among the food groups.

2d. Andy could alternate between tacos and bean burritos to gain the benefits of plant proteins in a diet. To incorporate more veggies and fruits in the diet, Andy could add lettuce, tomato, and onion to his tacos and hamburgers. When choosing pizza, he can replace high-fat toppings (e.g., pepperoni) and extra cheese with veggies (e.g., green peppers and onions). Many sub shops and delis offer several low-fat sandwiches, emphasizing lean meats such as turkey and vegetable toppings. For his beverages, Andy could order milk at least half of the time at his restaurant visits and substitute diet soft drinks for the regular variety. This would help moderate his sugar intake.

Further Readings

1. Academy of Nutrition and Dietetics: Position of the Academy of Nutrition and Dietetics: Total diet approach to healthy eating. *Journal of the Academy of Nutrition and Dietetics* 113:307, 2013.

2. Academy of Nutrition and Dietetics: Nutrition and you: Trends 2011. http://www.eatrightpro.org/resource/media/press-releases/new-in-food-nutrition-and-health/ada-releases-findings-of-nutrition-and-you-trends-2011-survey. Accessed September 14, 2015.

3. Andreyeva T and others: Exposure to food advertising on television: Associations with children's fast food and soft drink consumption and obesity. *Economics and Human Biology* 9:221, 2011.

4. Blake CE and others: Behavioral contexts, food-choice coping strategies, and dietary quality of a multiethnic sample of employed parents. *Journal of American Dietetic Association* 111:401, 2011.

5. Centers for Disease Control and Prevention: Overweight and obesity 2013. www.cdc.gov/obesity/data/adult.html. Accessed March 6, 2013.

6. Chiuve SE and others: Adherence to a low-risk, healthy lifestyle and risk of sudden cardiac death among women. *Journal of the American Medical Association* 306:62, 2011.

7. Choi S and Lee Y: Relationship of college students' residence to frequency of meal skipping and snacking pattern. *Journal of the Academy of Nutrition and Dietetics* 112:A24, 2012.

8. Edmonds MJ and others: Body weight and percent body fat increase during the transition from high school to university in females. *Journal of the American Dietetic Association* 108:1033, 2008.

9. Federal Trade Commission: A review of food marketing to children and adolescents, follow-up report, December 2012. www.ftc.gov/os/2012/12/121221foodmarketingreport.pdf. Accessed September 2, 2015.

10. Goris JM and others: Television food advertising and the prevalence of childhood overweight and obesity: A multicountry comparison. *Public Health Nutrition* 13:1003, 2010.

11. Kolish ED and Hernandez M: The Children's Food and Beverage Advertising Initiative, A Report on Compliance and Progress During 2012, December 2013.

12. Lewis MA and others: Examining the relationship between typical drinking behavior and 21st birthday drinking behavior among college students: Implications for event-specific prevention. *Addiction* 104:760, 2009.

13. Litt AS: *The college student's guide to eating well on campus.* Glen Echo, MD: Tulip Hill Press, 2005.

14. Loureiro ML and others: The effects of nutritional labels on obesity. *Agricultural Economics* 43:333, 2012.

15. Murphy SL and others: Death: Final data for 2012. *National Vital Statistics Reports* 63, 2015.

16. Ogden CL and others: Prevalence of childhood and adult obesity in the United States, 2011-2012. *Journal of the American Medical Association* 311:806, 2014.

17. Oz D: *The dorm room diet: The 10-step program for creating a healthy lifestyle plan that really works.* New York: Newmarket Press, 2010.

18. Shields DH and others: Gourmet coffee beverage consumption among college women. *Journal of the American Dietetic Association* 104:650, 2004.

19. Trust for America's Health: *F as in fat: How obesity threatens America's future, 2013.* Robert Wood Johnson Foundation, August 2013. healthyamericans.org/report/100/ Accessed September 10, 2015.

20. Yanover T and Sacco WP: Eating beyond satiety and body mass index. *Eating and Weight Disorders* 13:119, 2008.

21. Zagorsky JL and Smith PK: The freshman 15: A critical time for obesity intervention or media myth? *Social Science Quarterly* 92:1389, 2011.

 connect To get the most out of your study of nutrition, go to McGraw-Hill's online resources: Connect www.mcgrawhillconnect.com, where you will find NutritionCalc Plus, LearnSmart, and many other dynamic tools.

I. Examine Your Eating Habits More Closely

Choose a day of the week that is typical of your eating pattern. Using the first table found in Appendix C, list all foods and drinks you consumed for 24 hours. In addition, write down the approximate amounts of food you ate in units, such as cups, ounces, teaspoons, and tablespoons. Place the corresponding abbreviation from the list below in the *Reason for Choice* column to indicate why you picked that food or drink. There can be more than one reason for choosing a particular food or drink.

FLVR	Flavor/texture	ADV	Advertisement	PEER	Peers
CONV	Convenience	WTCL	Weight control	NUTR	Nutritive value
EMO	Emotions	HUNG	Hunger	$	Cost
AVA	Availability	FAM	Family/cultural	HLTH	Health

Application

Ask yourself what your most frequent reason is for eating or drinking. To what degree is health or nutritive value a reason for your food choices? Should you make these higher priorities?

II. Observe the Supermarket Explosion

Today's supermarkets carry up to 60,000 items. Think about your last grocery shopping trip and the items you purchased to eat. Following is a list of 20 newer food products added to supermarket shelves. For those items you have tried, use the key from Part I to identify why you chose these products.

_____ Prepackaged salad greens (variety packs other than iceberg lettuce)

_____ Gourmet or sprayable salad oils (e.g., walnut, almond, olive, or sesame oil)

_____ Precooked frozen turkey patties, precooked bacon

_____ Microwavable sandwiches (e.g., Hot Pockets® or frozen sandwiches)

_____ Microwavable meals in a bowl (e.g., mac and cheese, or soup)

_____ Refrigerated, precooked pasta (e.g., tortellini or fettucini) and accompanying sauces (e.g., pesto or tomato basil)

_____ Imported grain products (e.g., risotto, farfalline, gnocchi, or fusilli)

_____ Whole-grain pasta or rice

_____ Frozen dinners (list your favorite of any of the wide variety)

_____ Bottled waters (flavored or unflavored)

_____ Trendy juices (e.g., draft apple cider, acai, or pomegranate)

_____ Roasted and/or flavored coffees (e.g., beans, ground, instant, or K-Cups®)

_____ Instant hot cereal in a bowl (add water and go!)

_____ "Fast-shake" pancake mix (add water, shake, and ready to cook)

_____ Breakfast bars or cookies (e.g., granola or fruit-flavored bars)

_____ Dried fruit and nut mixes

_____ Meal replacement/fitness products (e.g., "energy" bars, high-protein bars, or sports drinks)

_____ Low-calorie muffin tops or bagel thins

_____ Packaged yogurt smoothies

_____ Milk substitutes (e.g., rice milk or soy milk)

Finally, identify three new food products not on this list that you have seen in the past year. Discuss the appeal of these products to the North American consumer.

© BloomImage RF/Getty Images

Student Learning Outcomes

Chapter 2 is designed to allow you to:

2.1 Use variety, proportionality, and moderation, as well as nutrient and energy density, to develop a healthy eating plan.

2.2 List the purpose and key recommendations of the Dietary Guidelines and the 2008 Physical Activity Guidelines for Americans.

2.3 Design a meal that conforms to the MyPlate recommendations as well as the Mediterranean diet and/or other diet planning guides.

2.4 Describe the three states of nutritional health.

2.5 Outline the measurements used (ABCDEs) in nutritional assessment: *A*nthropometric, *B*iochemical, *C*linical, *D*ietary, and *E*nvironmental status.

Designing a Healthy Dietary Pattern

What Would You Choose?

In between classes, you stop at a nearby convenience store to pick up a cold drink that will quench your thirst and fill your growling stomach. Immediately, you reach for your favorite cola, but the Jones Soda Co.® display with its personalized labels catches your eye. You notice that these sodas are made with no high-fructose corn syrup but instead contain pure cane sugar. Is there a nutritional difference between the added sugars in these two types of sodas? Which of the following beverages provides the best of calories, nutrients, and energy for an afternoon snack?

a 20-ounce bottle of regular cola (e.g., Coca-Cola®) containing high-fructose corn syrup

b 20-ounce bottle of diet cola (e.g., Coke Zero®) containing an artificial sweetener

c 12-ounce bottle of Jones Soda Co.® Pure Cane Cola Soda

d ½ pint (8 fluid ounces) of low-fat (1%) chocolate milk

e 16-ounce bottle of water

Think about your choice as you read Chapter 2, then see What the Dietitian Chose at the end of the chapter.

How many times have you heard wild claims about how healthful certain foods are for you? As consumers focus more on diet and disease, food manufacturers are asserting that their products have all sorts of health benefits. "Eat more olive oil and oat bran to lower blood cholesterol." "Drink pomegranate juice to guard your body against free radicals." Hearing these claims, you would think that food manufacturers have all the answers.

Advertising aside, nutrient intakes that are out of balance with our needs—such as excess calories, saturated fat, cholesterol, *trans* fat, salt, alcohol, and sugar intakes—are linked to many leading causes of death in North America, including obesity, hypertension, cardiovascular disease, cancer, liver disease, and type 2 diabetes. Physical inactivity is also too common. In this chapter, you will explore the components of a healthy diet and lifestyle—an approach that will minimize your risks of developing nutrition-related diseases. The goal is to provide you with a firm understanding of these concepts before you study the nutrients in detail.

2.6 Describe the specific nutrient recommendations categories within the Dietary Reference Intakes.

2.7 Identify reliable sources of nutrition information.

2.8 Describe the components of the Nutrition Facts panel and the various health claims and label descriptors that are allowed.

▲ A menu full of fruits, vegetables, and whole-grain breads and cereals will help ward off disease and control body weight. © McGraw-Hill Education/Ken Karp, photographer

2.1 A Food Philosophy That Works

You may be surprised that what you should eat to minimize the risk of developing the nutrition-related diseases seen in North America is exactly what you have heard many times before: *Consume a variety of foods balanced by a moderate intake of each food.* Health professionals have recommended the same basic dietary and lifestyle pattern for many years:

- Control *how much* you eat.
- Pay attention to *what* you eat: choose whole grains, fruits, and vegetables.
- Stay physically active.

A healthy dietary pattern does not have to mean deprivation and misery; it simply requires some basic nutrition know-how and planning. Besides, eliminating favorite foods typically does not work for "dieters" in the long run. The best plan consists of learning the basics of a healthful dietary pattern: variety, moderation, and proportionality. Monitoring total calorie intake is also important for many of us, especially if unwanted weight gain is taking place.

Many nutrition experts agree that there are no exclusively "good" or "bad" foods. Even so, many North Americans have dietary patterns that miss the mark when it comes to the foundations of healthy eating. Eating patterns overloaded with fatty meats, fried foods, sugared soft drinks, and refined starches can result in substantial risk for nutrition-related chronic diseases.

We are more likely to maintain a healthy dietary pattern and lifestyle when we emphasize a total diet pattern that is balanced and moderate. Let's now define *variety, moderation,* and *proportionality.* We will also introduce two very important concepts that will help us to make healthy food choices: nutrient density and energy density.

phytochemical A chemical found in plants. Some phytochemicals may contribute to a reduced risk of cancer or cardiovascular disease in people who consume them regularly.

VARIETY MEANS EATING MANY DIFFERENT FOODS

Variety in your dietary pattern means choosing foods from all the food groups and sub-groups, rather than eating the "same old thing" day after day. Variety makes meals more interesting and helps ensure that they contain sufficient nutrients. A variety of foods is best because no one food meets all your nutrient needs. For example, meat provides protein and iron but little calcium and no vitamin C. Eggs are a source of protein, but they provide little calcium because the calcium is mostly in the shell. Cow's milk contains calcium but very little iron. None of these foods contains fiber.

One way to balance your dietary pattern as you consume a variety of foods is to select foods from each of these five major food groups every day:

- Grains
- Fruits
- Vegetables
- Dairy
- Protein

MyPlate, a food guide plan discussed in Section 2.3, offers a visual reminder and advice to help you make smart choices from each of these food groups. A dinner consisting of a bean burrito, lettuce and tomato salad with oil-and-vinegar dressing, a glass of milk, and an apple covers all groups.

Carrots—a source of fiber and a pigment that forms vitamin A—may be your favorite vegetable. However, if you choose carrots every day as your only vegetable source, you may miss out on the vitamin folate. Other vegetables, such as broccoli and asparagus, are rich sources of this nutrient. Hopefully, you're beginning to get a sense of how different foods and food groups vary in the nutrients they contain. For now, just recognize that you need a variety of foods in your dietary pattern because the required nutrients are scattered among many foods.

An added bonus of dietary variety, especially within the fruit and vegetable groups, is the inclusion of a rich supply of **phytochemicals.** Many of these substances provide significant health benefits. Considerable research attention is focused on various phytochemicals in reducing the risk for certain diseases (e.g., cancer). You can't just buy a bottle of

▲ Tomatoes are considered functional foods because they contain phytochemicals such as lycopene that are important for health.
© Sawayasu Tsuji/Getty Images

phytochemicals: they are generally available only within whole foods. Current multivitamin and mineral supplements contain few or none of these beneficial plant chemicals.

Numerous population studies show reduced cancer risk among people who regularly consume fruits and vegetables (see Further Reading 8). Researchers suspect that some phytochemicals present in fruits and vegetables block the cancer process. Links between cancer and nutrition are described more thoroughly in Chapter 8. Some phytochemicals have also been linked to a reduced risk of cardiovascular disease (see Further Readings 2 and 8). Because humans evolved eating a wide variety of plant-based foods, the body may have developed a need for these phytochemicals, along with the various nutrients present, to maintain optimal health.

Foods rich in phytochemicals are now part of a family of foods referred to as **functional foods.** A functional food provides health benefits beyond those supplied by the traditional nutrients it contains. For example, a tomato contains the phytochemical lycopene, so it can be called a functional food.

It will likely take many years for scientists to unravel all of the important effects of the myriad of phytochemicals in foods, and it is unlikely that all will ever be available or effective in supplement form. For this reason, leading nutrition and medical experts suggest that a dietary pattern rich in fruits, vegetables, and whole-grain breads and cereals is the most reliable way to obtain the potential benefits of phytochemicals.

Table 2-1 provides a number of suggestions for including more phytochemicals from fruits, vegetables, and whole grains in your eating pattern, as does the website www.fruitsandveggiesmorematters.org. A note of caution: Some research suggests that increasing

▲ Vegetables such as sliced cucumbers can be added to salads, sandwiches, pizza, tacos, soups, and much more to increase your phytochemical intake. © Jupiterimages

functional foods Foods that have health benefits beyond basic nutrition.

TABLE 2-1 ■ Tips for Boosting the Phytochemical Content of Your Dietary Pattern

- Include vegetables in main and side dishes. Add these to rice, omelets, potato salad, and pastas. Try broccoli or cauliflower florets, mushrooms, peas, carrots, corn, or peppers.

- Look for quick-to-fix grain side dishes in the supermarket. Pilafs, couscous, rice mixes, and tabbouleh are just a few that you'll find.

- Choose fruit-filled cookies, such as fig bars, instead of sugar-rich cookies. Use fresh or canned fruit as a topping for pudding, hot or cold cereal, pancakes, and frozen desserts.

- Put raisins, grapes, apple chunks, pineapples, grated carrots, zucchini, or cucumber into coleslaw, chicken salad, or tuna salad.

- Be creative at the salad bar: Try fresh spinach, leaf lettuce, red cabbage, zucchini, yellow squash, cauliflower, peas, mushrooms, or red or yellow peppers.

- Pack fresh or dried fruit for snacks away from home instead of grabbing a candy bar or going hungry.

- Add slices of cucumber or zucchini, spinach, or carrot slivers to the lettuce and tomato on your sandwiches.

- Each week try one or two vegetarian meals such as beans and rice, vegetable stir-fry, or pasta with tomato sauce.

- If your daily protein intake exceeds the recommended amounts, reduce the meat, fish, or poultry in casseroles, stews, and soups by one-third to one-half and add more vegetables and legumes.

- Keep a container of fresh vegetables in the refrigerator for snacks.

- Choose fruit or vegetable juices (preferably 100% juice varieties) instead of soft drinks.

- Substitute tea for coffee or soft drinks on a regular basis.

- Have a bowl of fresh fruit on hand.

- Switch from crisp head lettuce to leaf lettuce, such as romaine.

- Use salsa as a dip for chips in place of creamy dips.

- Choose whole-grain breakfast cereals, breads, and crackers.

- Add flavor to your plate with ginger, rosemary, basil, thyme, garlic, onions, parsley, and chives in place of salt.

- Incorporate soy products, such as tofu, soy milk, soy protein isolate, and roasted soybeans, into your meals (see Chapter 6).

CRITICAL THINKING

Andy usually eats the same foods every day: corn flakes for breakfast, a peanut butter and jelly sandwich for lunch, and meat with potatoes for dinner. What are some practical tips he can use to increase his fruit and vegetable intake?

nutrient density The ratio derived by dividing a food's nutrient content by its calorie content. When the food's contribution to our nutrient need for that nutrient exceeds its contribution to our calorie need, the food is considered to have a favorable nutrient density.

dietary variety can lead to overeating. Thus, as you incorporate a wide variety of foods in your eating pattern, be mindful of your total calorie intake.

PROPORTIONALITY MEANS EATING MORE NUTRIENT-DENSE FOODS

Proportionality, also referred to as balance, is eating more of nutrient-dense foods and beverages such as fruits, vegetables, whole grains, and fat-free or low-fat milk products, and less of foods high in certain types of fat, sugars, cholesterol, salt, and alcohol. Balance also refers to matching your energy intake (how many total calories you consume) with energy expenditure (calories burned by metabolism and physical activity) over time. A prolonged imbalance between energy intake and energy expenditure leads to fluctuations in body weight.

The **nutrient density** of a food is a characteristic used to determine its nutritional quality. Nutrient density of a food is determined by comparing its protein, vitamin, or mineral content with the amount of calories it provides. A food is deemed nutrient dense if it provides a large amount of a nutrient for a relatively small amount of calories when compared with other food sources. The higher a food's nutrient density is, the better it is as a nutrient source. Comparing the nutrient density of different foods is an easy way to estimate their relative nutritional quality.

Generally, nutrient density is determined with respect to individual nutrients. For example, many fruits and vegetables have a high content of vitamin C compared with their modest calorie content; that is, they are nutrient-dense foods for vitamin C. Figure 2-1 shows that fat-free milk is much more nutrient dense than sugared soft drinks for many nutrients, especially protein, vitamin A, riboflavin, and calcium.

As noted previously, menu planning should focus mainly on the total dietary pattern, not on the selection of one critical food as the key to an adequate eating pattern. Many low-cost, nutrient-dense foods—such as fat-free and low-fat milk, lean meats, legumes (beans),

FIGURE 2-1 ▶ Comparison of the nutrient contributions of a sugared soft drink with that of fat-free (i.e., nonfat or skim) milk. Choosing a glass of fat-free milk makes a significantly greater contribution to nutrient intake than does a sugared soft drink. An easy way to determine nutrient density from this chart is to compare the lengths of the bars indicating vitamin or mineral contribution with the bar that represents calorie contribution. For the soft drink, there are no nutrients to surpass the calorie content. Fat-free milk, in contrast, has longer nutrient bars for protein, vitamin A, the vitamins thiamin and riboflavin, and the mineral calcium than it does for calories. Including many nutrient-dense foods in your diet is a good way to meet nutrient needs without exceeding calorie needs.

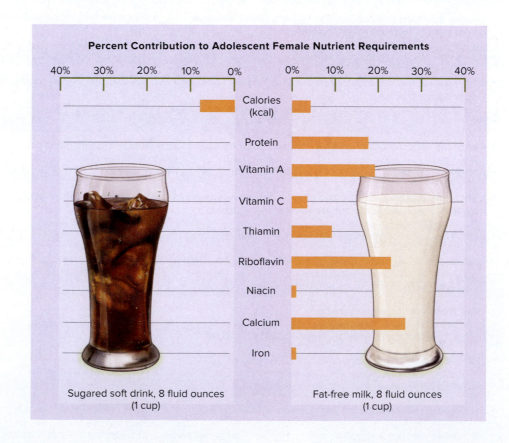

Percent Contribution to Adolescent Female Nutrient Requirements

40% 30% 20% 10% 0%		0% 10% 20% 30% 40%
	Calories (kcal)	
	Protein	
	Vitamin A	
	Vitamin C	
	Thiamin	
	Riboflavin	
	Niacin	
	Calcium	
	Iron	

Sugared soft drink, 8 fluid ounces (1 cup)   Fat-free milk, 8 fluid ounces (1 cup)

oranges, carrots, broccoli, whole-wheat bread, and whole-grain breakfast cereals—do help balance less nutrient-dense foods such as cookies and potato chips, which many people like to eat. The latter are often called empty-calorie foods because they tend to be high in sugar and/or fat but provide few other nutrients.

Eating nutrient-dense foods is especially important for people who have dietary patterns relatively low in calories. This includes some older people and those following weight-loss diets. This is because nutrient needs remain high even though calorie needs may be diminished.

MODERATION REFERS MOSTLY TO PORTION SIZE

Eating in moderation requires paying attention to portion sizes and planning your daily eating pattern so that you do not overconsume any nutrients. It is especially important to choose foods that help you limit intake of animal fat, added sugars, salt, and alcohol. Americans typically consume too much of these food components—and too many calories overall. For example, if you plan to eat a bacon cheeseburger (relatively high in fat, salt, and calories) at lunch, you should eat foods such as fruits and salad greens (less concentrated sources of these nutrients) at other meals that same day. If you prefer whole milk to low-fat or fat-free milk, reduce the fat elsewhere in your meals. Try low-fat salad dressings or use jam rather than butter or margarine on toast. Overall, it is more feasible to consume moderate portions of foods that supply lots of fat, salt, and sugar than to try to eliminate these foods altogether.

Let's be clear that moderation is important for all food components. For example, many North Americans do not consume enough vitamin E, which is found in plant oils, nuts, and some fruits and vegetables. However, taking large doses of vitamin E (e.g., from supplements) can lead to excessive bleeding because of its effects on blood clotting. You *can* get too much of a good thing!

Energy density is a measurement that best describes the calorie content of a food. Energy density of a food is determined by comparing the calorie (kcal) content with the weight of food. A food that is rich in calories but weighs relatively little is considered energy dense. Examples include nuts, cookies, fried foods in general, and even fat-free snacks such as fat-free pretzels. Foods with low energy density include fruits, vegetables, and any food that incorporates lots of water during cooking, such as oatmeal (Table 2-2).

Researchers have shown that eating a meal with many foods of low energy density promotes satiety without contributing many calories (see Further Readings 5 and 6). This is probably because we typically consume a constant weight of food at a meal rather than a constant number of calories. How this constant weight of food is regulated is not known, but careful laboratory studies show that people consume fewer calories in a meal if most of the food choices are low in energy density, compared with foods high in energy density. An eating pattern low in energy density can aid in losing (or maintaining) weight.

Overall, foods with lots of water and fiber (i.e., low-energy-density foods) contribute few calories even though they help one feel full. Alternatively, foods with high energy density must be eaten in greater amounts to promote fullness. This is one more reason to fill your plate with a variety of fruits, vegetables, and whole-grain breads and cereals—a pattern that is typical of many ethnic diets throughout rural areas of the world. Unfortunately, low-energy-density foods, such as fresh fruits and vegetables, are often more expensive than those that have high energy density. Read more about this situation in Further Reading 3, which is summarized in the Newsworthy Nutrition feature in this section.

Many foods such as peanut butter are both energy and nutrient dense. Even energy-dense foods can have a place in your dietary pattern, but you will have to plan for them. For example, chocolate is a very energy-dense food, but a small portion at the end of a meal can supply a satisfying finale. In addition, foods with high energy density can help individuals with poor appetites, such as some older people, to maintain or gain weight.

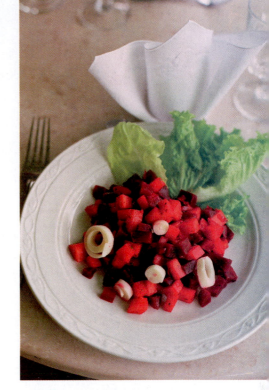

▲ Focus on nutrient-rich foods as you strive to meet your nutrient needs. The more colorful the food on your plate, the greater the content of nutrients and phytochemicals.
© Stockbyte/Getty Images

energy density A comparison of the calorie (kcal) content of a food with the weight of the food. An energy-dense food is high in calories but weighs very little (e.g., potato chips), whereas a food low in energy density has few calories but weighs a lot (e.g., an orange).

▲ Salsa is full of phytochemicals and a great, very low-energy-density alternative to higher calorie chip dips. It helps to balance out the high-energy-density tortilla chips. © C Squared Studios/Getty Images

TABLE 2-2 ■ Energy Density of Common Foods (Listed in Relative Order)

Very Low Energy Density (less than 0.6 kcal per gram)	Low Energy Density (0.6–1.5 kcal per gram)	Medium Energy Density (1.5–4 kcal per gram)	High Energy Density (greater than 4 kcal per gram)
Lettuce	Whole milk	Eggs	Graham crackers
Tomatoes	Oatmeal	Ham	Fat-free sandwich cookies
Strawberries	Cottage cheese	Pumpkin pie	Chocolate
Broccoli	Beans	Whole-wheat bread	Chocolate chip cookies
Salsa	Bananas	Bagels	Tortilla chips
Grapefruit	Broiled fish	White bread	Bacon
Fat-free milk	Fat-free yogurt	Raisins	Potato chips
Carrots	Ready-to-eat breakfast cereals with 1% low-fat milk	Cream cheese	Peanuts
Vegetable soup		Cake with frosting	Peanut butter
		Pretzels	Mayonnaise
Celery	Plain baked potato	Rice cakes	Butter or margarine
Cabbage	Cooked rice		Vegetable oils
Melon	Spaghetti noodles		

Source: Data adapted from Rolls B, *The ultimate volumetrics diet.* New York: HarperCollins, 2012.

Newsworthy Nutrition

Energy density impacts waistlines and wallets

Dietary patterns with low energy density are associated not only with higher intakes of nutrients but also with higher food costs. Researchers used food-frequency question-naires to assess dietary intake and food costs among 164 men and women in Seattle, Washington. Dietary data were compared with components of socioeconomic status. Household income and especially education were strong predictors of dietary energy density. The association between food spending and energy density was particularly strong for women. Nutrition advice to consume foods with lower energy density may be difficult to follow for people with limited financial resources. The increasing cost of consuming foods with low energy density and high nutrient density may play a role in the correlations between socioeconomic status (e.g., income and education) and rates of obesity and diet-related chronic diseases.

Source: Monsivais P., Drewnowski A. Lower-energy-density diets are associated with higher monetary costs per kilocalorie and are consumed by women of higher socioeconomic status. *Journal of the American Dietetic Association* 109:804, 2009. Further Reading 3.

✓ CONCEPT CHECK 2.1

1. What do variety, proportionality, and moderation mean, and how do they work together to result in a healthy dietary pattern?

2. How do the concepts of nutrient density and energy density differ?

2.2 Dietary and Physical Activity Guidelines

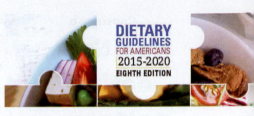

▲ U.S. Department of Health and Human Services and U.S. Department of Agriculture. *2015–2020 Dietary Guidelines for Americans.* 8th Edition. December 2015.

Since the early twentieth century, researchers have worked to translate the science of nutrition into practical terms so that people with no special training could estimate whether their nutritional needs were being met. Early food guidance systems aimed to reduce risk for nutrient deficiencies, but severe deficiency diseases are no longer common. Marginal deficiencies of calcium, iron, folate and other B vitamins, vitamin C, vitamin D, vitamin E, potassium, magnesium, and fiber are still a problem; but for many North Americans, major health problems stem from overconsumption of one or more of the following: calories, added sugars, saturated fat, *trans* fat, alcohol, and sodium.

The following sections of this chapter describe guidelines and tools for planning healthy lifestyles. You will notice how those core concepts of variety, proportionality, and moderation keep showing up throughout our discussions of the Dietary Guidelines, the Physical Activity Guidelines, and MyPlate.

DIETARY GUIDELINES—THE BASIS FOR MENU PLANNING

The USDA and U.S. Department of Health and Human Services (DHHS) have published Dietary Guidelines since 1980 (see Further Reading 12). The Dietary Guidelines are designed to inform the development of food, nutrition, and health policies and programs. Although not intended for direct use by the general public, the Dietary Guidelines are an important tool for health professionals to use in helping Americans design healthy eating and activity patterns (see Further Reading 7). The federal government uses them to develop nutrition education materials for the public, such as MyPlate.

The 2015–2020 Dietary Guidelines were derived from the *Scientific Report of the 2015 Dietary Guidelines Advisory Committee,* written by scientific experts and submitted to the USDA and DHHS in February 2015. The *Scientific Report* was based on the most current evidence from nutrition research. The Dietary Guidelines were published in January 2016 after congressional hearings and feedback from federal agencies, industry groups, and the general public. The full 2015–2020 Dietary Guidelines report contains background on the Dietary Guidelines, tables and charts to support the recommendations, and a list of consumer behaviors and key strategies for achieving its recommendations (see Further Reading 10). The aim of the Dietary Guidelines is to translate nutrition science into food-based guidelines that will help Americans meet nutrient needs and reduce risk for many chronic diseases. They are not intended for treating disease.

Following are the five foundational guidelines of the 2015–2020 Dietary Guidelines:

1. **Follow a healthy eating pattern across the lifespan.** All food and beverage choices matter. Choose a healthy eating pattern at an appropriate calorie level to help achieve and maintain a healthy body weight, support nutrient adequacy, and reduce the risk of chronic disease.
2. **Focus on variety, nutrient density, and amount.** To meet nutrient needs within calorie limits, choose a variety of nutrient-dense foods across and within all food groups in recommended amounts.
3. **Limit calories from added sugars and saturated fats and reduce sodium intake.** Consume an eating pattern low in added sugars, saturated fats, and sodium. Cut back on foods and beverages higher in these components to amounts that fit within healthy eating patterns.
4. **Shift to healthier food and beverage choices.** Choose nutrient-dense foods and beverages across and within all food groups in place of less healthy choices. Consider cultural and personal preferences to make these shifts easier to accomplish and maintain.
5. **Support healthy eating patterns for all.** Everyone has a role in helping to create and support healthy eating patterns in multiple settings nationwide, from home to school to work to communities.

The Dietary Guidelines are accompanied by Key Recommendations (Fig. 2-2) that provide detail on the elements of healthy eating patterns.

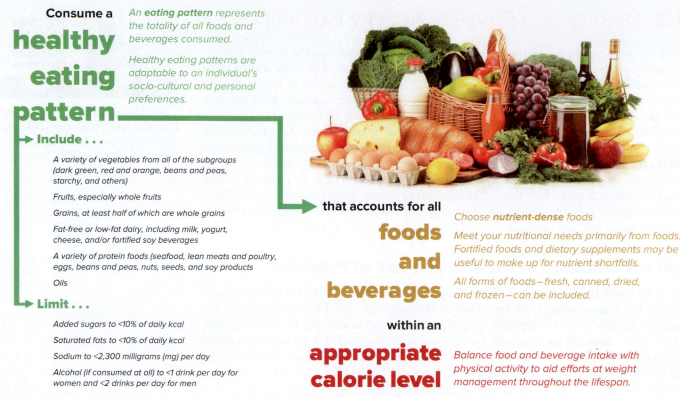

Consume a

healthy eating pattern

*An **eating pattern** represents the totality of all foods and beverages consumed.*

Healthy eating patterns are adaptable to an individual's socio-cultural and personal preferences.

→ Include . . .

A variety of vegetables from all of the subgroups (dark green, red and orange, beans and peas, starchy, and others)

Fruits, especially whole fruits

Grains, at least half of which are whole grains

Fat-free or low-fat dairy, including milk, yogurt, cheese, and/or fortified soy beverages

A variety of protein foods (seafood, lean meats and poultry, eggs, beans and peas, nuts, seeds, and soy products)

Oils

→ Limit . . .

Added sugars to <10% of daily kcal

Saturated fats to <10% of daily kcal

Sodium to <2,300 milligrams (mg) per day

Alcohol (if consumed at all) to <1 drink per day for women and <2 drinks per day for men

that accounts for all

foods and beverages

*Choose **nutrient-dense** foods*

Meet your nutritional needs primarily from foods. Fortified foods and dietary supplements may be useful to make up for nutrient shortfalls.

All forms of foods—fresh, canned, dried, and frozen—can be included.

within an

appropriate calorie level

Balance food and beverage intake with physical activity to aid efforts at weight management throughout the lifespan.

FIGURE 2-2 ▲ Key Recommendations from the 2015–2020 Dietary Guidelines for Americans.
© Getty Images/iStockphoto

Shifting to Healthy Eating Patterns Healthy eating patterns are the hallmark of the 2015–2020 Dietary Guidelines and are designed to help people meet the five foundational guidelines and Key Recommendations. The ultimate goal of a healthy eating pattern is to support a healthy body weight and help reduce the risk of chronic disease. The Dietary Guidelines use the Healthy U.S.-Style Eating Pattern (see Table 2-5 in Section 2.3) to exemplify the specific amounts of food groups and other dietary components that make up healthy eating patterns. It is based on foods Americans typically consume, but in nutrient-dense forms and appropriate amounts. The Dietary Guidelines also include the Healthy Mediterranean-Style Eating Pattern and the Healthy Vegetarian Eating Pattern as alternative plans.

Shifts are needed to align current dietary intakes with healthy eating patterns. As seen in Figure 2-3, certain aspects of our eating patterns are close to recommendations, whereas others will require significant improvement. Many Americans have eating patterns that are low in vegetables, fruits, whole grains, dairy, seafood, and oil; and high in refined grains, added sugars, saturated fats, and sodium.

Importance of Calorie Balance Within Healthy Eating Patterns The balance between calories consumed (from foods and beverages) and calories expended (through physical activity and metabolic processes) determines body weight. Consuming too many calories without increasing physical activity will inevitably lead to weight gain, which exacts an enormous toll on individuals and communities. Meeting nutrient needs within calorie limits could alleviate many chronic diseases, especially cardiovascular disease, type 2 diabetes, and osteoporosis. In light of the current epidemic of overweight and obesity, the message of calorie balance within a healthy eating pattern continues to be woven throughout the Dietary Guidelines, which encourage all Americans to achieve and maintain a healthy body weight. Knowing how many calories you need each day is a good place to start (Fig. 2-4). Use an online calculator such as Supertracker (www.choosemyplate.gov/tools-supertracker) to calculate your estimated calorie needs. Next, become familiar with the calorie content of foods and beverages. Finally, monitoring weight over time will allow you to see how your food and physical activity choices are balancing out.

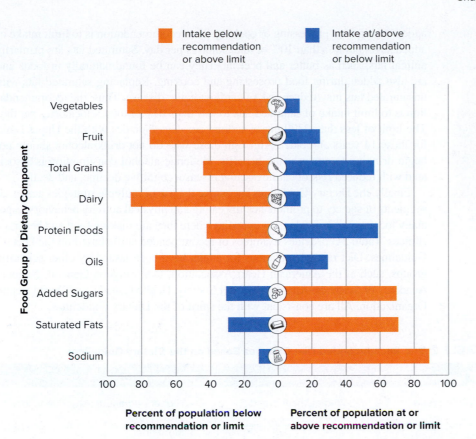

FIGURE 2-3 ◄ Comparing current eating patterns in the United States to the Dietary Guidelines.

Source: 2015–2020 Dietary Guidelines for Americans. Based on data from U.S. Department of Agriculture, Agricultural Research Service and U.S. Department of Health and Human Services, Centers for Disease Control and Prevention. *What we eat in America, NHANES 2007–2010 for average intakes by age-sex group. Healthy U.S.-Style Food Patterns, which vary based on age, sex, and activity level, for recommended intakes and limits.*

Food Components to Include in Your Healthy Eating Pattern To improve nutritional status and overall health, the Dietary Guidelines promote the consumption of vegetables, fruits, whole grains, fat-free or low-fat dairy, seafood, lean meats and poultry, eggs, beans and peas, nuts and seeds, and oils, without exceeding calorie needs. This type of dietary pattern will (1) contribute to nutrient adequacy; (2) lower intake of problem nutrients; (3) improve gastrointestinal function; (4) aid in weight management; and (5) decrease risk for chronic diseases.

A basic premise of the Dietary Guidelines is that nutritional needs should be met primarily from foods. Each of the food groups provides an array of nutrients, and the recommended amounts reflect eating patterns that have been associated with positive health outcomes (see Table 2-5 in Section 2.3). For vegetables, eating a variety from all five vegetable subgroups—dark green, red and orange, legumes (beans and peas), starchy, and other—are recommended, because each subgroup contributes different combinations of nutrients. For fruits, at least half of the recommended amount should come from whole fruits. At least half of grains should be whole grains. Dairy, including milk, yogurt, cheese, or fortified soy beverages, should be fat free or low fat. Protein foods should include several subgroups: seafood, meats, poultry, eggs, nuts, seeds, and soy products, as well as legumes and dairy. Oils are part of healthy eating patterns because they contribute essential fatty acids and vitamin E. In certain cases, fortified foods and dietary supplements may be useful sources of one or more nutrients that otherwise might be consumed in less than recommended amounts.

Food Components to Limit in Your Healthy Eating Pattern Because typical American dietary patterns contain too much added sugars, saturated and *trans* fats, and sodium, the Dietary Guidelines emphasize the need to limit these components (see Fig. 2-3). Added sugars and saturated fats are energy dense (high in calories), but provide few essential nutrients. Dietary patterns predominated by these food components especially increase risk for obesity, type 2 diabetes, hypertension, cardiovascular disease, and cancer. Added sugars include sugars and other sweeteners that are

	Calorie Range (kcal)		
Children	Sedentary	→	Active
2–3 years	1000	→	1400
Females			
4–8 years	1200	→	1800
9–13	1400	→	2200
14–18	1800	→	2400
19–30	1800	→	2400
31–50	1800	→	2200
51+	1600	→	2200
Males			
4–8 years	1200	→	2000
9–13	1600	→	2600
14–18	2000	→	3200
19–30	2400	→	3000
31–50	2200	→	3000
51+	2000	→	2800

FIGURE 2-4 ▲ Estimates of calorie (kcal) needs.

Source: 2015–2020 Dietary Guidelines for Americans.

▲ Choose low-sugar, high-fiber cereal with fresh fruit instead of sugary breakfast cereal.
© Peter Cade/Getty Images

added during food processing or cooking. The recommendation is to limit intake of added sugars to less than 10% of total calories per day. Saturated fats are primarily animal fats, such as butter and beef fat. They can be found naturally in foods and are also added during food processing and cooking. Replacing saturated fats with unsaturated fats may reduce risk of cardiovascular disease. Thus, the recommendation is to limit intake of saturated fats to less than 10% of total kilocalories per day. The limit of less than 2300 mg of sodium per day coincides with the Upper Limit for those 14 years and older. Although those who do not drink alcohol should not begin drinking to attain health benefits, moderate alcohol consumption is associated with reduced risk of cardiovascular disease, cognitive decline, and death.

Finally, the Dietary Guidelines encourage the use of multiple strategies across all segments of society to promote healthy eating and physical activity behaviors, especially focusing on individuals at the point where they are making food and beverage choices. Table 2-3 provides examples of recommended shifts based on the Dietary Guidelines. Diet recommendations for adults have been issued by other scientific groups, such as the American Heart Association, U.S. Surgeon General, National Academy of Sciences, American Cancer Society, Health Canada, and World Health Organization. All are consistent with the spirit of the Dietary Guidelines.

TABLE 2-3 ■ Recommended Diet Changes Based on the Dietary Guidelines

If You Usually Eat This,	Try This Instead	Benefits
White bread	Whole-wheat bread	• Higher nutrient density, due to less processing • More fiber
Sugary breakfast cereal	Low-sugar, high-fiber cereal with fresh fruit	• Higher nutrient density • More fiber • More phytochemicals
Cheeseburger with French fries	Hamburger and baked beans	• Less saturated fat and *trans* fat • Less cholesterol • More fiber • More phytochemicals
Potato salad	Three-bean salad	• More fiber • More phytochemicals
Doughnut	Bran muffin or bagel with light cream cheese	• More fiber • Less fat
Regular soft drinks	Diet soft drinks	• Fewer calories
Boiled vegetables	Steamed vegetables	• Higher nutrient density, due to reduced loss of water-soluble vitamins
Canned vegetables	Fresh or frozen vegetables	• Higher nutrient density, due to reduced loss of heat-sensitive vitamins • Lower in sodium
Fried meats	Broiled meats	• Less saturated fat
Fatty meats, such as ribs or bacon	Lean meats, such as ground round, chicken, or fish	• Less saturated fat
Whole milk	Low-fat or fat-free milk	• Less saturated fat • Fewer calories • More calcium

(continued)

TABLE 2-3 ■ (continued)

If You Usually Eat This,	Try This Instead	Benefits
Ice cream	Sherbet or frozen yogurt	• Less saturated fat • Fewer calories
Mayonnaise or sour cream salad dressing	Oil-and-vinegar dressings or light creamy dressings	• Less saturated fat • Less cholesterol • Fewer calories
Cookies	Popcorn (air popped with minimal margarine or butter)	• Fewer calories and *trans* fat
Heavily salted foods	Foods flavored primarily with herbs, spices, lemon juice	• Lower in sodium
Chips	Pretzels	• Less fat

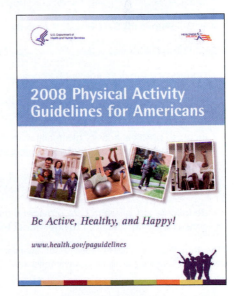

▲ Active means a lifestyle that includes physical activity equivalent to walking more than 3 miles per day at 3 to 4 miles per hour, in addition to the light physical activity associated with typical day-to-day life.
© Don Hammond/Design Pics/Corbis

PHYSICAL ACTIVITY GUIDELINES FOR AMERICANS

In line with its goal for all Americans to live healthier, more prosperous, and more productive lives, the U.S. Department of Health and Human Services issued its first Physical Activity Guidelines for Americans in 2008 as a complement to the Dietary Guidelines (see Further Reading 9). The overarching idea is that regular physical activity—for people of all ages, races, ethnicities, and physical abilities—produces long-term health benefits. The guidelines are truly meant to inform the work of health professionals and policy makers, but consumer materials are available. *Be Active Your Way: A Guide for Adults,* available at www.health.gov, translates the guidelines into consumer-friendly, practical advice.

The key guidelines, listed in Table 2-4, provide measurable physical activity standards for Americans age 6 and older. Specific recommendations (not listed in Table 2-4) also apply to special population groups, including pregnant women, adults with disabilities, and people with chronic medical conditions. For adults, the guidelines emphasize that health benefits occur with at least 150 minutes per week of moderate-intensity physical activity. Adults may accumulate activity throughout the week in a variety of ways: extended sessions (e.g., 50 minutes on 3 days a week) or in short bursts throughout the week that amount to at least 150 minutes. Children and adolescents should strive to include 60 minutes of physical activity per day. For optimum benefits, include both aerobic and muscle-strengthening activities. Overall, physical activity should be enjoyable and safe for each individual. In 2012, a follow-up report, *Physical Activity Guidelines for Americans Midcourse Report: Strategies to Increase Physical Activity Among Youth,* was published, identifying interventions that can help increase physical activity in youth across a variety of settings.

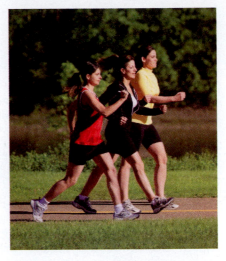

2008 Physical Activity Guidelines for Americans

Be Active, Healthy, and Happy!

www.health.gov/paguidelines

▲ www.health.gov/PAGuidelines/

TABLE 2-4 ■ Selected Recommendations of the 2008 Physical Activity Guidelines for Americans*

Key Guidelines for Children and Adolescents
• Children and adolescents should do 60 minutes or more of physical activity daily.
• Aerobic: Most of the 60 or more minutes a day should be either moderate- or vigorous-intensity aerobic physical activity and should include vigorous-intensity activity at least 3 days a week.
• Muscle strengthening: As part of their 60 or more minutes of daily physical activity, children and adolescents should include muscle-strengthening physical activity on at least 3 days of the week.
• Bone strengthening: As part of their 60 or more minutes of daily physical activity, children and adolescents should include bone-strengthening physical activity on at least 3 days of the week.
• It is important to encourage young people to participate in physical activities that are appropriate for their age, are enjoyable, and offer variety.

(continued)

TABLE 2-4 ■ *(continued)*

Key Guidelines for Adults

- All adults should avoid inactivity. Some physical activity is better than none, and adults who participate in any amount of physical activity gain some health benefits.

- For substantial health benefits, adults should do at least 150 minutes a week of moderate-intensity or 75 minutes a week of vigorous-intensity aerobic physical activity, or an equivalent combination of moderate- and vigorous-intensity aerobic activity. Aerobic activity should be performed in episodes of at least 10 minutes, and preferably, it should be spread throughout the week.

- For additional and more extensive health benefits, adults should increase their aerobic physical activity to 300 minutes a week of moderate-intensity or 150 minutes a week of vigorous-intensity aerobic physical activity, or an equivalent combination of moderate- and vigorous-intensity activity. Additional health benefits are gained by engaging in physical activity beyond this amount.

- Adults should also do muscle-strengthening activities that are moderate or high intensity and involve all major muscle groups on 2 or more days a week, as these activities provide additional health benefits.

Key Guidelines for Older Adults

- When older adults cannot do 150 minutes of moderate-intensity aerobic activity a week because of chronic conditions, they should be as physically active as their abilities and conditions allow.

- Older adults should do exercises that maintain or improve balance if they are at risk of falling.

- Older adults should determine their level of effort for physical activity relative to their level of fitness.

- Older adults with chronic conditions should understand whether and how their conditions affect their ability to do regular physical activity safely.

Key Guidelines for Safe Physical Activity

To do physical activity safely and reduce the risk of injuries and other adverse events, people should:

- Understand the risks and yet be confident that physical activity is safe for almost everyone.

- Choose to do types of physical activity that are appropriate for their current fitness level and health goals because some activities are safer than others.

- Increase physical activity gradually over time whenever more activity is necessary to meet guidelines or health goals. Inactive people should "start low and go slow" by gradually increasing how often and how long activities are done.

- Protect themselves by using appropriate gear and sports equipment; looking for safe environments; following rules and policies; and making sensible choices about when, where, and how to be active.

- Be followed by a health care provider if they have chronic conditions or symptoms. People with chronic conditions and symptoms should consult their health care provider about the appropriate types and amounts of activity.

*The 2008 Physical Activity Guidelines for Americans also include recommendations for pregnant women, adults with disabilities, and people with chronic medical conditions. These are available at www.health.gov.

✓ **CONCEPT CHECK 2.2**

1. What are three of the major guidelines of the 2015–2020 Dietary Guidelines for Americans?

2. How many minutes of moderate-intensity physical activity are advised per week in the 2008 Physical Activity Guidelines for Americans?

2.3 MyPlate—A Menu-Planning Tool

The titles, food groupings, and shapes of food guides have evolved since the first edition published by the U.S. Department of Agriculture (USDA) a century ago. The most recent food-guidance systems have provided a means for individualization of dietary advice via interactive technology available on the Internet.

To keep pace with updated nutrition advice presented by the 2015–2020 Dietary Guidelines for Americans and *Healthy People 2020* (see Section 1.6), MyPlate was released in 2011 as the leading depiction of healthy eating for Americans (Fig. 2-5). MyPlate, which replaced the familiar MyPyramid, shapes the key recommendations from the Dietary Guidelines into an easily recognizable and extremely applicable visual: a place setting.

DISHING UP MYPLATE

Although it is not intended to stand alone as a source of dietary advice, MyPlate serves as a reminder of how to build a healthy plate at mealtimes (see Further Reading 11). It emphasizes important areas of the American diet that are in need of improvement. Recall from the discussion of the Dietary Guidelines that Americans need to increase the relative proportions of fruits, vegetables, whole grains, and fat-free or low-fat dairy products while simultaneously decreasing consumption of refined grains and high-fat meats.

The MyPlate icon includes five food groups:

FIGURE 2-5 ▲ MyPlate is a visual representation of the advice contained in the 2015–2020 Dietary Guidelines for Americans.
Source: ChooseMyPlate.gov.

- *Fruits* and *vegetables* cover half of the plate. These foods are dense sources of nutrients and health-promoting phytochemicals despite their low calorie contents.
- *Grains* occupy slightly more than one-fourth of the plate. The message to make half your grains whole is stressed throughout accompanying consumer-education materials.
- The remaining space on the plate is reserved for sources of **protein.** Specifically, the 2015–2020 Dietary Guidelines recommend a variety of protein foods, including seafood, lean meats and poultry, eggs, legumes (beans and peas), nuts, seeds, and soy products.
- A cup of *dairy* appears next to the plate. Depending on personalized calorie recommendations, users should have 2 to 3 cups per day of low-fat or fat-free dairy products or other rich sources of calcium.

MyPlate does not display a separate group for fats and oils, as they are mostly incorporated into other foods. MyPlate food guide recommends limiting solid fats and focusing instead on plant oils, which are sources of essential fatty acids and vitamin E.

CONSUMER HEALTH MESSAGES

Consumer research points to the need for simple, actionable health messages to capture the attention of the public and achieve successful behavior change. Accordingly, ChooseMyPlate.gov provides a series of succinct recommendations to help Americans make healthier food choices. Consumer messages include:

Balancing Calories

- Enjoy your food, but eat less.
- Avoid oversized portions.

Food Components to Increase

- Make half your plate fruits and vegetables.
- Make at least half your grains whole.
- Switch to skim or 1% milk.

Food Components to Limit

- Compare sodium in foods such as soup, bread, and frozen meals—and choose the foods with lower numbers.
- Drink water instead of sugary drinks.

DAILY FOOD PLANS

On ChooseMyPlate.gov, you will find an interactive tool that estimates your calorie needs and suggests a food pattern based on your age, gender, height, and weight (Table 2-5). These daily food plans provide useful information for each food group, including recommended daily amounts in common household measures. Modified daily food plans are also available for preschoolers, pregnant or breastfeeding mothers, and those interested in losing weight. Be sure to visit the site to generate your own daily food plan.

▲ In 1942, Canada released its first set of Official Food Rules. Since then, food guidance has evolved based on nutrition research and the changing needs of the population. Now, Health Canada publishes Canada's Food Guide to Healthy Eating, available at http://www.hc-sc.gc.ca/fn-an/food-guide-aliment/index-eng.php © All rights reserved. Eating Well with Canada's Food Guide. Health Canada, 2011. Adapted and reproduced with permission from the Minister of Health, 2016.

TABLE 2-5 ■ Healthy U.S.-Style Eating Pattern: Recommended Amounts of Food From Each MyPlate Food Group at 12 Kilocalorie Levels

Daily Amount of Food from Each Group Based on Kilocalorie Level												
Kilocalories	1000	1200	1400	1600	1800	2000	2200	2400	2600	2800	3000	3200
Fruits	1 cup	1 cup	1.5 cups	1.5 cups	1.5 cups	2 cups	2 cups	2 cups	2 cups	2.5 cups	2.5 cups	2.5 cups
Vegetables[1,2]	1 cup	1.5 cups	1.5 cups	2 cups	2.5 cups	2.5 cups	3 cups	3 cups	3.5 cups	3.5 cups	4 cups	4 cups
Grains[3]	3 oz-eq	4 oz-eq	5 oz-eq	5 oz-eq	6 oz-eq	6 oz-eq	7 oz-eq	8 oz-eq	9 oz-eq	10 oz-eq	10 oz-eq	10 oz-eq
Protein Foods	2 oz-eq	3 oz-eq	4 oz-eq	5 oz-eq	5 oz-eq	5.5 oz-eq	6 oz-eq	6.5 oz-eq	6.5 oz-eq	7 oz-eq	7 oz-eq	7 oz-eq
Dairy[4]	2 cups	2 cups	2 cups	3 cups	3 cups	3 cups	3 cups	3 cups	3 cups	3 cups	3 cups	3 cups

Note: oz-eq stands for ounce equivalent; tsp stands for teaspoon.

[1]Vegetables are divided into five subgroups (dark green, orange, legumes, starchy, and other). Over a week's time, a variety of vegetables should be eaten, especially green and orange vegetables.

[2]Dry beans and peas can be counted either as vegetables (dry beans and peas subgroup) or in the protein foods group. Generally, individuals who regularly eat meat, poultry, and fish would count dry beans and peas in the vegetable group. Individuals who seldom eat meat, poultry, or fish (vegetarians) would consume more dry beans and peas, and count some of them in the protein foods group until enough servings from that group are chosen for the day.

[3]At least half of the grain servings should be whole-grain varieties.

[4]Most of the dairy servings should be fat free or low fat.

FIGURE 2-6 ▲ MyPlate: What counts as a serving?

The recommended numbers of servings are given in cups for vegetables, fruits, and dairy foods. Grains and protein foods are listed in ounces. See Figure 2-6 for a description of what counts as a MyPlate serving. Pay close attention to the stated serving size for each choice when following your daily food plan to help control calorie intake.

Portion sizes

2 tbsp salad dressing, peanut butter, margarine, etc.	**= 2 tbsp measure**
Baked potato Small/medium fruit Ground or chopped food Bagel English muffin	**= ½ to ⅔ cup measure**
3 ounce meat, poultry, or fish	**= ½ to ¾ cup**
Large apple or orange 1 cup ready-to-eat breakfast cereal	**= 1 cup**

FIGURE 2-7 ▲ A golf ball, tennis ball, deck of cards, and baseball are standard-size objects that make convenient guides for judging serving sizes.

(golf ball): © Ryan McVay/Getty Images; (tennis ball): © C Squared Studios/Getty Images; (cards): © Photodisc Collection/Getty Images; (baseball): © C Squared Studios/Getty Images

How familiar are you with serving-size measurements? Figure 2-7 shows a convenient guide to estimate common serving-size measurements. Common household units are listed in Appendix F with their metric equivalents. Ounces and fluid ounces differ: ounces are a measure of weight, whereas fluid ounces are a measure of volume.

MyPlate sets limits for empty calories, which come from solid fats and/or added sugars (SoFAS) (Fig. 2-8). SoFAS add calories to the diet but contribute few nutrients. Solid fats are solid at room temperature and include butter, beef fat, and shortening. Some solid fats, such as the marbling in a ribeye steak, are naturally present in foods. Others, such as the shortening used to make a flaky croissant, are added during food processing or preparation. Added sugars include sugars and syrups that are added to foods during processing or preparation. Examples of foods that are major contributors of empty calories in the American diet are cakes, cookies, pastries, soft drinks, energy drinks, cheese, pizza, ice cream, and processed meats. The daily food plans available on ChooseMyPlate.gov make some allowance for empty calories throughout the day; depending on total energy needs, allowances range from 120 to 600 kcal per day.

ADDITIONAL MyPLATE RESOURCES

ChooseMyPlate.gov also offers in-depth information regarding the Dietary Guidelines, as well as the following additional interactive tools for consumers.

- USDA's 10 Tips Nutrition Education series provides access to one-page printable documents for consumers and health educators. The materials cover over two dozen topics,

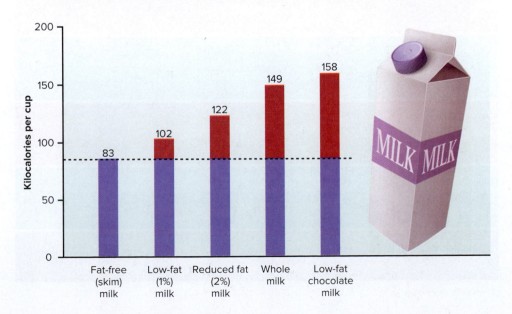

FIGURE 2-8 ◄ Empty calories come from solid fats and/or added sugars (SoFAS). This bar graph compares the amounts of empty kilocalories, shown by the red bars, in various types of milk.

such as "Kid-friendly veggies and fruits," "Healthy eating for vegetarians," and "Got your dairy today?" The printouts are perfect for posting on a refrigerator, and the suggestions can help you get started toward a healthy dietary pattern.

- Sample menus and recipes are available online for consumers who are ready to make a change and need a place to start.
- Food-A-Pedia allows users to locate calorie and food group information for specific food entries.
- The SuperTracker enables users to self-monitor food and activity.

MENU PLANNING WITH MyPLATE

Overall, MyPlate exemplifies the foundations of a healthy dietary pattern you have already learned: variety, proportionality, and moderation. To achieve optimal nutrition, remember the following points when using MyPlate to plan your daily menus:

- The guide does not apply to infants or children under 2 years of age. Daily food plans for children from ages 2 to 8 are based on average height and weight for age and gender.
- Variety is a key to successful implementation of MyPlate. There is no single, perfect food that is absolutely essential to good nutrition. Each food is rich in some nutrients but deficient in at least one essential nutrient. Likewise, no food group is more important than another; each food group makes an important, distinctive contribution to nutritional intake (Table 2-6). Choose foods from each food group and also choose different foods within each food group. For a sample meal plan, see Table 2-7.
- The foods within a group may vary widely with respect to nutrients and calories. For example, the calorie content of 3 ounces of baked potato is 98 kcal, whereas that of 3 ounces of potato chips is 470 kcal. With respect to vitamin C, an orange has 70 mg and an apple has 10 mg.
- Choose primarily low-fat and fat-free items from the dairy group. By reducing calorie intake in this way, you can select more items from other food groups. If milk causes intestinal gas and bloating, emphasize yogurt and cheese (see Chapter 4 for details on the problem of lactose intolerance).

> Solid fats contribute almost 20% of total calories in the typical American's dietary pattern, but they have little to offer in terms of essential nutrients and dietary fiber. Instead of solid fats, choose foods containing plant oils.

TABLE 2-6 ■ Nutrient Contributions of MyPlate Food Groups

Food Category	Major Nutrient Contributions
Grains	Carbohydrate Vitamins such as thiamin Minerals such as iron Fiber*
Vegetables	Carbohydrate Vitamins such as plant pigments that form vitamin A Minerals such as magnesium Fiber
Fruits	Carbohydrate Vitamins such as folate and vitamin C Minerals such as potassium Fiber
Dairy	Carbohydrate Protein Vitamins such as vitamin D Minerals such as calcium and phosphorus
Protein Foods	Protein Vitamins such as vitamin B-6 Minerals such as iron and zinc

*In whole-grain varieties

© Mitch Hrdlicka/Getty Images

© Masterfile

© C Squared Studios/Getty Images

TABLE 2-7 ■ Putting MyPlate into Practice

Meal	Food Group
Breakfast	
1 small orange	Fruits
¾ cup Healthy Choice Low-fat Granola	Grains
with ½ cup fat-free milk	Dairy
½ toasted, small raisin bagel	Grains
with 1 tsp soft margarine	Oils
Lunch	
Turkey sandwich	
2 slices whole-wheat bread	Grains
2 oz turkey	Protein
2 tsp mustard	
1 small apple	Fruits
2 oatmeal-raisin cookies (small)	Empty Calories
3 P.M. Study Break	
6 whole-wheat crackers	Grains
1 tbsp peanut butter	Protein
½ cup fat-free milk	Dairy
Dinner	
Tossed salad	
1 cup romaine lettuce	Vegetables
½ cup sliced tomatoes	Vegetables
1½ tbsp Italian dressing	Oils
½ carrot, grated	Vegetables
3 oz broiled salmon	Protein
½ cup rice	Grains
½ cup green beans	Vegetables
with 1 tsp soft margarine	Oils
Late-Night Snack	Dairy
1 cup "light" fruit yogurt	
Nutrient Breakdown	56% of kcal
1800 kcal	18% of kcal
Carbohydrate	26% of kcal
Protein	
Fat	

This menu meets nutrient needs for all vitamins and minerals for an average adult who needs 1800 kcal.
For adolescents, teenagers, and older adults, add one additional serving of milk or other calcium-rich sources.

- Include plant foods that are good sources of proteins, such as beans and nuts, at least several times a week because many are rich in vitamins (such as vitamin E), minerals (such as magnesium), and fiber.
- For vegetables and fruits, try to include a dark-green or orange vegetable for vitamin A, and a vitamin-C-rich fruit, such as an orange, every day. Do not focus primarily on

potatoes (e.g., French fries) for your vegetable choices. Surveys show that fewer than 5% of adults eat a full serving of a dark-green vegetable on any given day. Increased consumption of these foods is important because they contribute vitamins, minerals, fiber, and phytochemicals.

- Choose whole-grain varieties of breads, cereals, rice, and pasta because they contribute vitamin E and fiber. A daily serving of a whole-grain, ready-to-eat breakfast cereal is an excellent choice because the vitamins (such as vitamin B-6) and minerals (such as zinc) typically added to it, along with fiber, help fill in common nutritional gaps.
- Include some plant oils on a daily basis, such as those in salad dressing, and eat fish at least twice a week. This supplies you with health-promoting essential fatty acids.

LIMITATIONS OF MyPLATE

Although MyPlate will promote important changes in American dietary patterns, it has certain limitations. Some critics say that the icon is too simple. For example, it does not immediately provide information about overall calories, serving sizes, or number of servings to choose from each food group. However, many of these details will vary by person. Users will need to access the accompanying materials available on ChooseMyPlate.gov to obtain a personally tailored daily food plan.

The MyPlate icon does not address the types of foods to choose within each food group. Making appropriate food choices for weight management and prevention of diet-related chronic diseases requires consumers to have some nutrition knowledge. Fortunately, public health messages and online content related to MyPlate are available to educate Americans.

MyPlate shows how to build a healthy plate at mealtimes, but it does not adequately address the total diet, which in reality includes many snacks between meals. Consumer messages about healthy snacking will be part of the consumer communications initiative over the next few years.

As with any public health campaign, it is possible that the people who need it most will overlook the MyPlate message. Educated consumers with access to interactive MyPlate tools likely already comply with many of the Dietary Guidelines. Populations with poor diets may be unlikely or unable to click through to find a personalized daily food plan.

Overall, the MyPlate icon is an attractive and relevant tool that immediately shows us how to build a healthy plate at mealtimes. The strength of MyPlate lies in its simplicity. It conveys the major messages that are needed when shopping, cooking, and eating and can be enhanced with the details provided on ChooseMyPlate.gov.

HOW DOES YOUR PLATE RATE?

Regularly comparing your daily food intake with your personalized daily food plan recommendations is a relatively simple way to evaluate the quality of your overall dietary pattern. Identify the nutrients that are low in your eating pattern based on the nutrients found in each food group. For example, if you do not consume enough servings from the milk group, your calcium intake is most likely too low. Look for foods that you enjoy that supply calcium, such as calcium-fortified orange juice.

For a more detailed analysis of your current dietary pattern, use the SuperTracker tool on ChooseMyPlate.gov. Your NutritionCalc software also helps you compare your food choices to MyPlate. With a detailed dietary analysis, you can compare your intakes of individual nutrients to standards set by the Food and Nutrition Board and clearly see the areas that need improvement. Even small dietary and exercise changes can have positive results.

THE MEDITERRANEAN DIET PYRAMID

Updated in 2009, the Mediterranean Diet Pyramid (Fig. 2-9) is a useful alternative to MyPlate. It is based on the dietary patterns of the southern Mediterranean region, which has enjoyed the lowest recorded rates of chronic diseases and the highest adult life expectancy. An abundance of research supports the health benefits of following the Mediterranean Diet (see Further Reading 8). The 2015–2020 Dietary Guidelines include the Healthy

Choose Your Foods booklets from the American Diabetes Association offer alternative menu-planning tools. These food lists organize foods based on calorie, protein, carbohydrate, and fat content. The result is a manageable framework for designing diets, especially for treatment of diabetes. For more information on the food lists, see Appendix B.

▲ Typical restaurant meals contain oversized portions that do not align with MyPlate.
© Burke/Triolo/Brand X Pictures

Food *quality* is just as important as food *quantity* when it comes to good nutrition. Consider the difference in calorie contents of the following two meals, both of which fit the proportions suggested by MyPlate:

Fried chicken fillet sandwich with mayonnaise on a white sandwich roll, 1 each

French fries, 1 medium order

Apple-filled pastry, 1 each

Whole milk, 1 cup

1293 kcal

Skinless grilled chicken breast, 3 ounces

Brown rice, prepared with reduced-fat tub margarine, 1 cup

Steamed green beans, 1 cup

Cubed watermelon, 1 cup

Skim milk, 1 cup

513 kcal

Mediterranean Diet Pyramid

A contemporary approach to delicious, healthy eating

Meats and Sweets
Less often

Wine
In moderation

Poultry and Eggs
Moderate portions, every two days or weekly

Cheese and Yogurt
Moderate portions, daily to weekly

Drink Water

Fish and Seafood
Often, at least two times per week

Fruits, Vegetables, Grains (mostly whole), Olive oil, Beans, Nuts, Legumes and Seeds, Herbs and Spices
Base every meal on these foods

Be Physically Active; Enjoy Meals with Others

Illustration by George Middleton   © 2009 Oldways Preservation and Exchange Trust   www.oldwayspt.org

Mediterranean-Style Eating Pattern, which contains more fruits and seafood and less dairy than the Healthy U.S.-Style Eating Pattern.

Oldways—a respected, international, nonprofit culinary think tank—also publishes the Latin-American Diet Pyramid and was the force behind development of the Whole Grain stamp seen on food packages.

ASK THE RDN   The Mediterranean Diet

Dear RDN: I know that olives, olive oil, Greek yogurt, and feta cheese are Mediterranean foods but could you share some more specific tips on how to follow the Mediterranean Diet eating plan?

The Mediterranean dietary pattern is not limited to Greek and Italian food. As shown on the pyramid in Figure 2-9, foods from plant sources form the foundation of every meal. A variety of fruits and vegetables (other than potatoes) is a big part of this plan. Eat 5 to 10 servings a day, especially of seasonally fresh and locally grown foods. For most produce, each serving is ½ cup cooked or 1 cup raw.

You are right about including olives and olive oil. These and avocados are considered healthy sources of fat, compared to many other plant oils and animal fats. Choose 4 to 6 servings a day–a serving is equal to 1 teaspoon of olive oil, 5 olives, or 1/8 of an avocado. Also include a handful of nuts or seeds daily as good sources of healthy fats, fiber, and protein.

Legumes (beans) are also plant sources of fiber and protein. Eat ½ cup of cooked legumes, including hummus, at least twice a week. You can have bread, but only four small (1-ounce) portions of whole-grain bread, pasta, or quinoa each day. A serving of grains is 1 slice of bread or ½ cup of cooked pasta, rice, or cereal. Plenty of herbs and spices, such as basil and oregano, are also used in the Mediterranean eating plan and have antioxidant and anti-inflammatory properties.

As you make your way up the pyramid, eat a 4-ounce serving of fish two to three times a week. Moderate portions (3 to 4 ounces) of lean meat and poultry or 2 eggs are recommended once a week or every few days. Choose low-fat dairy (up to three 1-cup servings a day) from cultured sources such as yogurt or kefir. These are easier to digest and supply beneficial bacteria. Water is the beverage of choice. Moderate drinking of wine (one to two 5-ounce glasses of red wine per day) also has proven health benefits. Finally, remember that regular physical activity that promotes a healthy weight is an important aspect of the Mediterranean lifestyle as well as eating meals with family and friends.

Buon appetito!

Anne M. Smith, PhD, RDN, LD (author)

✓ **CONCEPT CHECK 2.3**

1. What is the website where you can find all of the tools associated with MyPlate?
2. What are the five major food groups represented on MyPlate?

2.4 States of Nutritional Health

The ultimate intent of the sound nutrition advice found in the Dietary Guidelines and the MyPlate food guide is to promote optimal nutritional status for individuals. The amount of each nutrient needed to maintain a state of desirable nutrition is the basis for published dietary intake recommendations. We have already discussed general dietary guidelines and cover more specific nutrient recommendations in Section 2.6. The body's nutritional health is determined by considering the **nutritional state** of each needed nutrient. Three general categories of nutritional status are recognized: desirable nutrition, undernutrition, and overnutrition. The common term **malnutrition** can refer to either **overnutrition** or **undernutrition.** Neither state is conducive to good health. Furthermore, it is possible to be both overnourished (e.g., consume excess calories) and undernourished (e.g., consume too few essential vitamins and minerals) at the same time.

The amount of each nutrient needed to maintain a state of desirable nutrition is the basis for published dietary intake recommendations.

DESIRABLE NUTRITION

The nutritional state for a particular nutrient is desirable when body tissues have enough of the nutrient to support normal metabolic functions and surplus stores that can be used in times of increased need. A desirable nutritional state can be achieved by obtaining essential nutrients from a variety of foods.

UNDERNUTRITION

Undernutrition occurs when nutrient intake does not meet nutrient needs. At first, any surpluses are put to use; then, as stores are exhausted, health begins to decline. Many nutrients are in high demand due to constant cell loss and regeneration in the body, such as in the gastrointestinal tract. For this reason, the stores of certain nutrients, including many of the

nutritional state The nutritional health of a person as determined by anthropometric measurements (height, weight, circumferences, and so on), biochemical measurements of nutrients or their by-products in blood and urine, a clinical (physical) examination, a dietary analysis, and economic evaluation; also called nutritional status.

malnutrition Failing health that results from longstanding dietary practices that do not coincide with nutritional needs.

overnutrition A state in which nutritional intake greatly exceeds the body's needs.

undernutrition Failing health that results from a longstanding dietary intake that is not enough to meet nutritional needs.

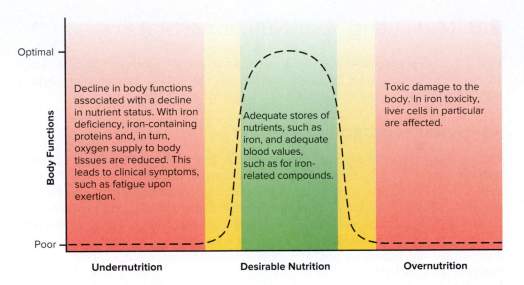

Optimal

Body Functions

Decline in body functions associated with a decline in nutrient status. With iron deficiency, iron-containing proteins and, in turn, oxygen supply to body tissues are reduced. This leads to clinical symptoms, such as fatigue upon exertion.

Adequate stores of nutrients, such as iron, and adequate blood values, such as for iron-related compounds.

Toxic damage to the body. In iron toxicity, liver cells in particular are affected.

Poor

Undernutrition   **Desirable Nutrition**   **Overnutrition**

FIGURE 2-10 ◄ The general scheme of nutritional status. Green reflects good status, yellow marginal status, and red poor status (undernutrition or overnutrition). This general concept can be applied to all nutrients. Iron was chosen as an example because iron deficiency is the most common nutrient deficiency worldwide.

B vitamins, are exhausted rapidly and therefore require a regular intake. In addition, some women in North America do not consume sufficient iron to compensate for monthly losses and eventually deplete their iron stores (Fig. 2-10).

Once availability of a nutrient falls sufficiently low, biochemical evidence indicates that the body's metabolic processes have slowed or stopped. At this state of deficiency, there are no outward **symptoms;** thus, it is termed a **subclinical** deficiency. A subclinical deficiency can go on for some time before clinicians are able to detect its effects.

Eventually, clinical symptoms will develop. Clinical evidence of a nutritional deficiency—perhaps in the skin, hair, nails, tongue, or eyes—can occur within months but may take years to develop. Often, clinicians do not detect a problem until a deficiency produces outward symptoms, such as small areas of bruising on the skin from a vitamin C deficiency.

symptom A change in health status noted by the person with the problem, such as stomach pain.

subclinical Stage of a disease or disorder not severe enough to produce symptoms that can be detected or diagnosed.

OVERNUTRITION

Prolonged consumption of more nutrients than the body needs can lead to overnutrition. In the short run (e.g., 1 to 2 weeks), overnutrition may cause only a few symptoms, such as stomach distress from excess iron intake. If an excess intake continues, however, some nutrients may accumulate to toxic amounts, which can lead to serious disease. For example, too much vitamin A during pregnancy can cause birth defects.

The most common form of overnutrition in developed nations is an excess intake of calories that leads to obesity. In the long run, outcomes of obesity include other serious diseases, such as type 2 diabetes and certain forms of cancer. Use the website www.shapeup.org to learn more about the importance of lifelong weight control.

For most vitamins and minerals, the gap between desirable intake and overnutrition is wide. Therefore, even if people take a typical balanced multivitamin and mineral supplement daily, they probably will not receive a harmful dose of any nutrient. The gap between desirable intake and overnutrition is the smallest for vitamin A and the minerals calcium, iron, and copper. Thus, if you take nutrient supplements, keep a close eye on your total vitamin and mineral intake from both food and supplements to avoid toxicity (see Section 8.5) for further advice on use of nutrient supplements).

▲ The most common type of overnutrition in North America is the excess intake of calories, which often leads to obesity. © 2007 Getty Images, Inc.

✓ **CONCEPT CHECK 2.4**

1. What are the main differences between the undernutrition, desirable nutrition, and overnutrition states of nutritional health?

2.5 Measuring Your Nutritional State

To find out how nutritionally fit *you* are, a nutritional assessment—either whole or in part—needs to be performed (Table 2-8). Generally, this is performed by a primary care provider, often with the aid of a registered dietitian nutritionist (RDN).

ANALYZING BACKGROUND FACTORS

Because family health history plays an important role in determining nutritional and health status, it must be carefully recorded and critically analyzed as part of a nutritional assessment. Other related background information includes (1) a medical history, especially for any disease states or treatments that could decrease nutrient absorption or ultimate use; (2) a list of medications taken; (3) a social history (e.g., marital status and living conditions); (4) level of education to determine the degree of complexity that can be used in written materials and oral discussions; and (5) economic status to determine the ability to purchase, transport, and cook food.

ASSESSING NUTRITIONAL STATUS USING THE ABCDEs

In addition to background factors, four nutritional-assessment categories complete the picture of nutritional status. **Anthropometric assessment** of height, weight (and weight changes), skinfold thicknesses, and body circumferences provide information about the current state of nutrition. Most measures of body composition are easy to obtain and are generally reliable. However, an in-depth examination of nutritional health is impossible without the more expensive process of **biochemical assessment.** This involves the measurement of the concentrations of nutrients and nutrient by-products in the blood, urine, and feces and the activities of specific blood enzymes.

A **clinical assessment** would follow, during which a health professional would search for any physical evidence (e.g., high blood pressure) of diet-related diseases or deficiencies. Then, a close look at the person's dietary pattern (**dietary assessment**), including a record of at least the previous few days' food intake, would help to determine any possible problem areas.

Finally, adding the **environmental assessment** (from the background analysis) provides further details about the living conditions, education level, and ability to purchase and prepare foods needed to maintain health. Now the true nutritional state of a person emerges. Taken together, these five assessments form the ABCDEs of nutritional assessment: anthropometric, biochemical, clinical, dietary, and environmental (Fig. 2-11).

anthropometric assessment Measurement of body weight and the lengths, circumferences, and thicknesses of parts of the body.

biochemical assessment Measurement of biochemical functions (e.g., concentrations of nutrient by-products or enzyme activities in the blood or urine) related to a nutrient's function.

clinical assessment Examination of general appearance of skin, eyes, and tongue; evidence of rapid hair loss; sense of touch; and ability to cough and walk.

dietary assessment Estimation of typical food choices relying mostly on the recounting of one's usual intake or a record of one's previous days' intake.

environmental assessment Includes details about living conditions, education level, and the ability of the person to purchase, transport, and cook food. The person's weekly budget for food purchases is also a key factor to consider.

TABLE 2-8 ■ Conducting an Evaluation of Nutritional Health

Parameters	Example
Background	Medical history (e.g., current diseases, past surgeries, current weight, weight history, and current medications)
	Social history (e.g., marital status and living conditions)
	Family health history
	Education level
	Economic status
Nutritional	Anthropometric assessment: height, weight, skinfold thickness, arm muscle circumference, and other parameters
	Biochemical (laboratory) assessment of blood and urine: enzyme activities, concentrations of nutrients or their by-products
	Clinical assessment (physical examination): general appearance of skin, eyes, and tongue; rapid hair loss; sense of touch; and ability to walk
	Dietary assessment: usual intake or record of previous days' meals

Anthropometric

Biochemical

Clinical

Dietary

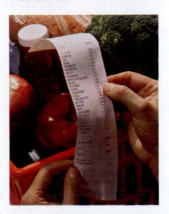
Environmental

FIGURE 2-11 ◄ A complete nutritional assessment includes anthropometric, biochemical, clinical, and dietary information. Environmental status adds further information, rounding out the ABCDEs of nutritional assessment.

(anthropometric): © Royalty-Free/Corbis; (biochemical): © C. Borland/PhotoLink/Getty Images; (clinical): © Fuse/Getty Images; (dietary): © Mike Kemp/Rubberball/Getty Images; (environmental): © Comstock/PunchStock

A practical example using the ABCDEs for evaluating nutritional status can be illustrated in a person who chronically abuses alcohol. Upon evaluation, the physician notes that this person needs medical attention, including nutrient repletion based on the following nutritional assessment results:

(A) Low weight for height, recent 10-pound weight loss, muscle wasting in the upper body
(B) Low amounts of the vitamins thiamin and folate in the blood
(C) Psychological confusion, facial sores, and uncoordinated movement
(D) Dietary intake of mostly wine and hamburgers for the last week
(E) Currently residing in a homeless shelter; $35 in wallet; unemployed

RECOGNIZING THE LIMITATIONS OF NUTRITIONAL ASSESSMENT

A long time may elapse between the initial development of poor nutritional health and the first clinical evidence of a problem. A dietary pattern high in animal and other solid fat often increases blood cholesterol but without producing any clinical evidence for years. However, when the blood vessels become sufficiently blocked by cholesterol and other materials, chest pain during physical activity or a **heart attack** may occur. An active area of nutrition research is the development of better methods for early detection of nutrition-related problems such as heart attack risk.

Another example of a serious health condition with delayed symptoms is low bone density resulting from a calcium deficiency—a particularly relevant issue for adolescent and young adult females. Many young women do not consume the needed amount of calcium but suffer no obvious effects in their younger years; however, the bone structures of these women with low calcium intakes do not reach full potential during the years of growth, making osteoporosis more likely later in life.

Furthermore, clinical symptoms of some nutritional deficiencies (e.g., diarrhea, inability to walk normally, and facial sores) are not very specific. These may have causes other than

heart attack Rapid fall in heart function caused by reduced blood flow through the heart's blood vessels. Often part of the heart dies in the process. Technically called a myocardial infarction.

poor nutrition. The long time it takes for symptoms to develop and their potential to be vague often make it difficult to establish a link between an individual's current dietary pattern and nutritional state.

CONCERN ABOUT THE STATE OF YOUR NUTRITIONAL HEALTH IS IMPORTANT

The good news is that people who focus on maintaining nutritional health are apt to enjoy a long, vigorous life. For example, a recent study found that women with a healthy lifestyle had a decreased risk for heart attacks (80% reduction) compared to women without such healthy practices (see the Newsworthy Nutrition). The healthy habits included:

- Maintained a healthy dietary pattern:
  - Varied
  - Included some fish
  - Rich in fiber
  - Low in animal fat and *trans* fat
- Maintained a healthy weight
- Occasionally consumed alcohol in small amounts
- Exercised for at least 30 minutes daily
- Avoided use of tobacco

Should all adults follow this example (with optional use of alcohol)?

Newsworthy Nutrition

Healthy dietary pattern lowers women's risk of sudden cardiac death

Sudden cardiac death (death occurring within 1 hour after symptom onset) is the cause of more than half of all heart-related deaths and usually occurs as the first sign of heart disease, especially in women. Lifestyle information from the Nurses' Health Study (81,722 women) was used to determine if adherence to a healthy lifestyle lowers the risk of sudden cardiac death among women. Low-risk lifestyle was considered as not smoking, not overweight, exercising 30 minutes per day or longer, and following the Mediterranean Diet. Risk of sudden cardiac death dropped by 92% with a combination of the four healthy lifestyles; and women who ate a diet most similar to the Mediterranean Diet with a high proportion of vegetables, fruits, nuts, omega-3 fats, and fish, along with moderate amounts of alcohol and small amounts of red meat, had a 40% less risk than women whose diets least resembled this diet. The conclusion is that a healthy dietary pattern along with other healthy lifestyle factors can protect women from sudden cardiac death.

Source: Chiuve SE and others: Adherence to a low risk, healthy lifestyle and risk of sudden cardiac death among women. *Journal of the American Medical Association* 306:62, 2011 (see Further Reading 2).

Although nutrition recommendations are often made for the entire healthy population, each of us has individual needs based on our particular health status and genetic background. It would be more appropriate, but also more expensive, if recommendations were made on an individual basis once a person's health status is known.

✓ CONCEPT CHECK 2.5

1. What are the ABCDE steps used in assessing nutritional status?

2.6 Specific Nutrient Standards and Recommendations

The overarching goal of any healthy dietary plan is to meet nutrient needs. To begin, we must determine what amount of each essential nutrient is necessary to maintain health. Most

TABLE 2-9 ■ Dietary Reference Intakes and Daily Value

RDA	Recommended Dietary Allowance. Use to evaluate your current intake for a specific nutrient. The further you stray above or below this value, the greater your chances of developing nutritional problems.
AI	Adequate Intake. Use to evaluate your current intake of nutrients but realize that an AI designation implies that further research is required before scientists can establish a more definitive recommendation.
EER	Estimated Energy Requirement. Use to estimate kilocalorie needs of the average person within a specific height, weight, gender, age, and physical activity pattern.
UL	Upper Level. Use to evaluate the highest amount of daily nutrient intake unlikely to cause adverse health effects in the long run in almost all people (97% to 98%) in a population. This number applies to chronic use and is set to protect even very susceptible people in the healthy general population. As intake increases above the Upper Level, the potential for adverse effects generally increases.
DV	Daily Value. Use as a rough guide for comparing the nutrient content of a food to approximate human needs. Typically, the Daily Value used on food labels refers to ages 4 years through adulthood. It is based on a 2000-kcal diet. Some Daily Values also increase slightly with higher kilocalorie intakes (see Fig. 2-13 in Section 2.8 on food labeling).

of the terms that describe nutrient needs fall under one umbrella term: **Dietary Reference Intakes (DRIs).** The development of DRIs is an ongoing, collaborative effort between the Food and Nutrition Board of the Institute of Medicine in the United States and Health Canada (see Further Reading 12). Included under the DRI umbrella are **Recommended Dietary Allowances (RDAs), Adequate Intakes (AIs), Estimated Energy Requirements (EERs),** and **Tolerable Upper Intake Levels (Upper Levels or ULs).**

As you begin your study of nutrition, all these acronyms can seem like an alphabet soup of abbreviations! To help you more easily sift through these nutrient standards, some basic knowledge about their use is summarized in Table 2-9.

RECOMMENDED DIETARY ALLOWANCE

A Recommended Dietary Allowance (RDA) is the daily amount of a nutrient that will meet the needs of nearly all individuals (about 97%) in a particular age and gender group. A person can compare his or her daily intake of specific nutrients to the RDA. Although an intake slightly above or below the RDA for a particular nutrient on any given day is no reason for concern, a significant deviation below (about 70%) or above (about three times or more for some nutrients) the RDA for an extended time can eventually result in a deficiency or toxicity of that nutrient, respectively.

ADEQUATE INTAKE

An RDA can be set for a nutrient only if there is sufficient information on the human needs for that particular nutrient. Today, there is not enough information on some nutrients, such as chromium, to set such a precise standard as an RDA. For this and other nutrients, the DRIs include a category called an Adequate Intake (AI). This standard is based on the dietary intakes of people who appear to be maintaining nutritional health. That amount of intake is assumed to be adequate, as no evidence of a nutritional deficiency is apparent.

ESTIMATED ENERGY REQUIREMENT

For kilocalorie needs, we use the Estimated Energy Requirement (EER) instead of an RDA or AI. In contrast to the RDAs, which are set somewhat higher than the average needs for nutrients, the EER is set for the average person. While a slight excess of vitamins and minerals is

Dietary Reference Intakes (DRIs) Term used to encompass nutrient recommendations made by the Food and Nutrition Board of the Institute of Medicine. These include RDAs, AIs, EERs, and ULs.

Recommended Dietary Allowance (RDA) Nutrient intake amount sufficient to meet the needs of 97% to 98% of the individuals in a specific life stage.

Adequate Intake (AI) Nutrient intake amount set for any nutrient for which insufficient research is available to establish an RDA. AIs are based on estimates of intakes that appear to maintain a defined nutritional state in a specific life stage.

Estimated Energy Requirement (EER) Estimate of the energy (kcal) intake needed to match the energy use of an average person in a specific life stage.

Tolerable Upper Intake Level (UL) Maximum chronic daily intake level of a nutrient that is unlikely to cause adverse health effects in almost all people in a specific life stage.

Nutrition Facts

12 servings per container

Serving size	1 donut (about 52g)

Amount per serving

Calories 200

	% Daily Value*
Total Fat 12g	**18**%
Saturated Fat 3g	**15**%
Trans Fat 4g	
Cholesterol 5mg	**1**%
Sodium 95mg	**4**%
Total Carbohydrate 22g	**7**%
Dietary Fiber <1g	**1**%
Total Sugars 12g	
Includes 10g Added Sugars	**20**%
Protein 2g	

Vitamin D 0mcg	0%
Calcium 60mg	6%
Iron 1mg	6%
Potassium 39mg	1%

* The % Daily Value (DV) tells you how much a nutrient in a serving of food contributes to a daily diet. 2,000 calories a day is used for general nutrition advice.

▲ The Daily Value is the nutrient standard used on the Nutrition Facts portion of the food label. The percent Daily Value for each nutrient is based on consuming a 2000-kcal diet.
© David A. Tietz/Editorial Image, LLC

not harmful, a long-term excess of even a small amount of kilocalories will lead to weight gain. Therefore, the calculation of EER needs to be more specific, taking into account age, gender, height, weight, and physical activity (e.g., sedentary or moderately active). In some cases, the additional kilocalorie needs for growth and lactation are also included (see Chapters 7, 14, and 15 for the specific formulas used). Note that the EER is based on the "average" person. Thus, it can only serve as a starting point for estimating kilocalorie needs.

TOLERABLE UPPER INTAKE LEVEL

A Tolerable Upper Intake Level (Upper Level or UL) has been set for some vitamins and minerals (see Appendix G). The UL is the highest amount of a nutrient unlikely to cause adverse health effects in the long run. As intake exceeds the UL, the risk of ill effects increases. These amounts generally should not be exceeded day after day, as toxicity could develop. For people eating a variety of foods and/or using a balanced multivitamin and mineral supplement, exceeding the UL is unusual. Problems are more likely to arise with dietary patterns that promote excessive intakes of a limited variety of foods, with the use of many fortified foods, or with excessive doses of individual vitamins or minerals.

DAILY VALUE

A nutrition standard more relevant to everyday life is the Daily Value (DV). This is a generic standard used on food labels. It is applicable to both genders from 4 years of age through adulthood and is based on consuming a 2000-kcal diet. DVs are mostly set at or close to the highest RDA value or related nutrient standard seen in the various age and gender categories for a specific nutrient (see Appendix A). DVs have been set for vitamins, minerals, protein, and other dietary components. For fat and cholesterol, the DVs represent a maximum level, not a goal one should strive to reach. DVs allow consumers to compare their intake from a specific food to desirable (or maximum) intakes.

HOW SHOULD THESE NUTRIENT STANDARDS BE USED?

As nutrient intake increases, the RDA for the nutrient, if set, is eventually met and a deficient state is no longer present (Fig. 2-12). An individual's needs most likely will be met

FIGURE 2-12 ▶ This figure shows the relationship of the Dietary Reference Intakes (DRIs) to each other and the percentage of the population covered by each. At intakes between the RDA and the UL, the risk of either an inadequate diet or adverse effects from the nutrient in question is close to zero. The UL is then the highest level of nutrient intake likely to pose no risks of adverse health effects to almost all individuals in the general population. At intakes above the UL, the margin of safety to protect against adverse effects is reduced. The AI is set for some nutrients instead of an RDA. The Food and Nutrition Board states that there is no established benefit for healthy individuals if they consume nutrient intakes above the RDA or AI.

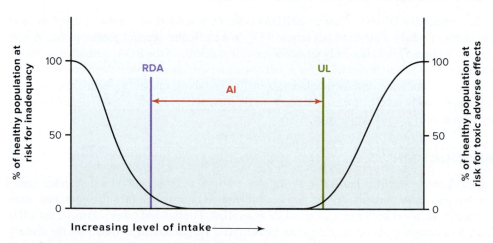

Recommended Dietary Allowance (RDA): The dietary intake level that is sufficient to meet the nutrient requirement of nearly all (97% to 98%) healthy individuals in a particular life stage and gender group. When set for a nutrient, aim for this intake.

Adequate Intake (AI): A recommended intake value based on observed or experimentally determined approximations or estimates of nutrient intake by a group (or groups) of healthy people that is assumed to be adequate; used when an RDA cannot be determined. When set for a nutrient, aim for this intake.

Tolerable Upper Intake Level (Upper Level or UL): The highest level of nutrient intake that is likely to pose no risk of adverse health effects for almost all individuals in the general population. As intake increases above the Upper Level, the risk of adverse effects increases.

since RDAs are set high to include almost all people. Related to the RDA concept of meeting an individual's needs are the standards of AI and the EER. These can be used to estimate an individual's needs for some nutrients and kilocalories, respectively. Still, keep in mind that these standards do not share the same degree of accuracy as the RDA. For example, EER may have to be adjusted upward if the individual is very physically active. Finally, as nutrient intake increases above the UL, poor nutritional health is again likely. However, this poor health is due now to the toxic effects of a nutrient, rather than those of a deficiency.

The type of standard set for nutrients depends on the quality of available evidence. A nutrient recommendation backed by lots of experimental research will be expressed as an RDA. For a nutrient that still requires more research, only an AI is presented. We use the EER as a starting point for determining calorie needs. Some nutrients also have a UL if information on toxicity or adverse health effects is available. Periodically, new DRIs become available as expert committees review and interpret the available research.

RDAs and related standards are intended mainly for diet planning. Specifically, a dietary plan should aim to meet the RDA or AI as appropriate and not to exceed the UL over the long term (see Fig. 2-12). Specific RDA, AI, EER, and UL standards are found in Appendix G. To learn more about these nutrient standards, visit the link for Dietary Guidance at the Food and Nutrition Information Center's website (https://fnic.nal.usda.gov/dietary-guidance/dietary-reference-intakes).

✓ CONCEPT CHECK 2.6

1. How do the definitions of RDA and AI differ?
2. Which DRI category includes the highest amounts of a nutrient unlikely to cause adverse health effects?

2.7 Evaluating Nutrition Information

The following suggestions should help you make healthful and logical nutrition decisions:

1. Apply the basic principles of nutrition along with the Dietary Guidelines for Americans and related resources to any nutrition claim, including those on websites. Do you note any inconsistencies? Do reliable references support the claims? Beware of the following:
   - Testimonials about personal experience
   - Disreputable publication sources
   - Promises of dramatic results (rarely true)
   - Lack of evidence from other scientific studies
2. Examine the background and scientific credentials of the individual, organization, or publication making the nutritional claim. Usually, a reputable author is one whose educational background or present affiliation is with a nationally recognized university or medical center that offers programs or courses in the field of nutrition, medicine, or a closely allied specialty.
3. Be wary if the answer is "Yes" to any of the following questions about a health-related nutrition claim:
   - Are only advantages discussed and possible disadvantages ignored?
   - Are claims made about "curing" disease? Do they sound too good to be true?
   - Is extreme bias against the medical community or traditional medical treatments evident? Health professionals as a group strive to cure diseases in their patients, using what proven techniques are available. They do not ignore reliable cures.
   - Is the claim touted as a new or secret scientific breakthrough?

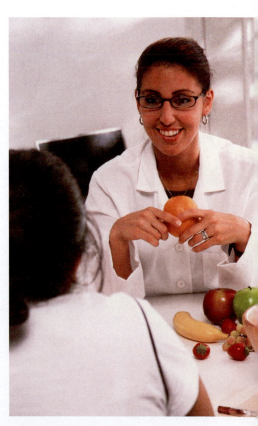

▲ Registered dietitian nutritionists are a reliable source of nutrition advice. © liquidlibrary/PictureQuest

4. Note the size and duration of any study cited in support of a nutrition claim. The larger it is and the longer it went on, the more dependable its findings. Also consider the type of study: epidemiology versus case-control versus double-blind study. Check out the group studied; a study of men or women in Sweden may be less relevant than one of men or women of Southern European, African, or Hispanic descent, for example. Keep in mind that "contributes to," "is linked to," or "is associated with" does not mean "causes."

5. Beware of news conferences and other hype regarding the latest findings. Much of this will not survive more detailed scientific evaluation.

6. When you meet with a nutrition professional, you should expect that he or she will do the following:
   - Ask questions about your medical history, lifestyle, and current eating habits.
   - Formulate a dietary plan tailored to your needs, as opposed to simply tearing a form from a tablet that could apply to almost anyone.
   - Schedule follow-up visits to track your progress, answer any questions, and help keep you motivated.
   - Involve family members in the dietary plan, when appropriate.
   - Consult directly with your physician and readily refer you back to your physician for those health problems a nutrition professional is not trained to treat.

7. Avoid practitioners who prescribe **megadoses** of vitamin and mineral supplements for everyone.

8. Examine product labels carefully. Be skeptical of any promotional information about a product that is not clearly stated on the label. A product is not likely to do something not specifically claimed on its label or package insert (legally part of the label).

Remember from the Ask the RDN in Chapter 1 that the best approach to finding answers about your nutritional state is to consult your primary care provider or registered dietitian nutritionist first (see Further Reading 1). Appendix E also lists many reputable sources of nutrition advice for your use. Overall, nutrition is a rapidly advancing field, and there are always new findings. Finally, the following websites can help you evaluate ongoing nutrition and health claims:

acsh.org
American Council on Science and Health

www.quackwatch.org
Quackwatch: Your Guide to Quackery, Health Fraud, and Intelligent Decisions

www.ncahf.org
National Council Against Health Fraud

http://ods.od.nih.gov
National Institutes of Health, Office of Dietary Supplements

www.fda.gov
U.S. Food and Drug Administration

megadose Large intake of a nutrient beyond estimates of needs or what would be found in a balanced diet; 2 to 10 times human needs is a starting point.

Diet and Nutrition Apps

Science-based reviews of the most popular diet and nutrition apps for phones and tablets are available from the Academy of Nutrition and Dietetics. Food and nutrition experts—registered dietitian nutritionists—have written these reviews of top-rated, free smartphone apps for those looking to lose weight, manage their diabetes, or eat gluten-free foods. Ratings are based on a scale of 1 to 5 stars. The reviews are available at http://www.eatrightpro.org/resources/media/trends-and-reviews/app-reviews.

2.8 Nutrition and Your Health
Food Labels and Diet Planning

© Photodisc/Getty Images

Today, nearly all foods sold in stores must be in a package that has a label containing the following information: the product name, name and address of the manufacturer, amount of product in the package, and ingredients listed in descending order by weight. This food and beverage labeling is monitored in North America by government agencies such as the Food and Drug Administration (FDA) in the United States. The listing of certain food constituents is also required—specifically, on a Nutrition Facts panel (Fig. 2-13). Consumers can use the information in the Nutrition Facts panel to learn more about what they eat. The following components must be listed:

- Total calories (kcal)
- Calories from fat
- Total fat
- Saturated fat
- *Trans* fat
- Cholesterol
- Sodium
- Total carbohydrate

- Fiber
- Sugars
- Protein
- Vitamin A
- Vitamin C
- Calcium
- Iron

In addition to these required components, manufacturers can choose to list polyunsaturated and monounsaturated fat, potassium, and others. Listing these components becomes *required* if the food is fortified with that nutrient or if a claim is made about the health benefits of the specific nutrient.

Remember that the Daily Value is a generic standard used on the food label. The percentage of the Daily Value (% Daily Value or % DV) is usually given for each nutrient per serving. These percentages are based on a 2000-kcal diet and must be adjusted for people who require considerably more or less than 2000 kcal per day with respect to fat and carbohydrate intake. DVs are mostly set at or close to the highest RDA value or related nutrient standard seen in the various age and gender categories for a specific nutrient.

Serving sizes on the Nutrition Facts panel must be consistent among similar foods. This means that all brands of ice cream, for example, must use the same serving size on their label. These serving sizes may differ from those of MyPlate because those on food labels are based on more typical portion sizes. In addition, food claims made on packages must follow legal definitions. A long list of definitions for nutrient claims allowed on food labels is given in Table 2-10. For example, if a product claims to be "low sodium," it must have 140 milligrams of sodium or less per serving.

Many manufacturers list the Daily Values set for dietary components such as fat, cholesterol, and carbohydrate on the Nutrition Facts panel. This can be useful as a reference point. As noted, they are based on 2000 kcal; if the label is large enough, amounts based on 2500 kcal are listed as well. As mentioned, DVs allow consumers to compare their intake from a specific food to desirable (or maximum) daily intakes.

Changes to Nutrition Labels Approved

For the first time in 20 years, the FDA finalized new rules for the Nutrition Facts panel in May 2016. The changes are designed to promote healthier eating and combat obesity, aiming to help consumers make informed decisions about the foods they eat (Fig. 2-14). Several changes, such as increasing the type size for "Calories," "servings per container," and the "Serving size" declaration, and bolding the number of calories and the "Serving size" declaration, are aimed at making it easier for Americans to know how many calories they are consuming. The Daily Value information for nutrients is being updated and will include the actual amount, in addition to percent Daily Value of vitamin D, calcium, iron and potassium. The Daily Value footnote is changing to better explain the meaning of percent Daily Value. Along with potassium and vitamin D, "Added Sugars," is an addition to the label, whereas calories from fat is being eliminated. These changes to sugar and fat are based on scientific data showing that it is difficult to meet nutrient needs and stay within calorie limits if added sugar is more than 10 percent of total daily calories, and that the type of fat is more important than the amount. One of the most significant changes is that serving size information will now more accurately reflect how much is consumed in one sitting. For example, the serving sizes for a soda will go from 8 ounces to 12 ounces, and ice cream will increase from ½ cup to ⅔ cup. To eliminate confusion about the number of servings in a container and calories in a serving, larger packages, such as a pint of ice cream, would have two columns on

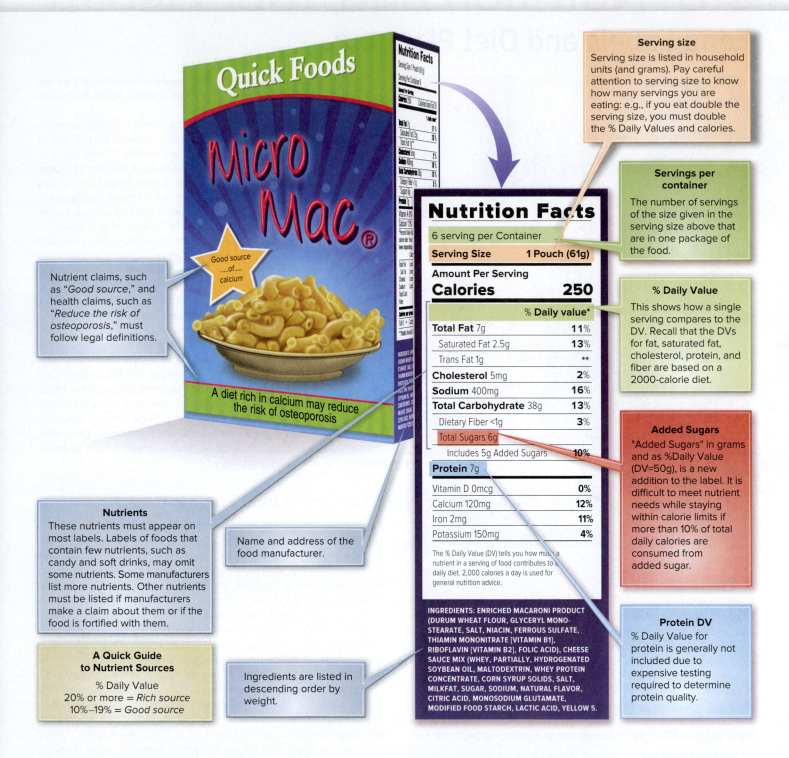

Serving size

Serving size is listed in household units (and grams). Pay careful attention to serving size to know how many servings you are eating: e.g., if you eat double the serving size, you must double the % Daily Values and calories.

Servings per container

The number of servings of the size given in the serving size above that are in one package of the food.

% Daily Value

This shows how a single serving compares to the DV. Recall that the DVs for fat, saturated fat, cholesterol, protein, and fiber are based on a 2000-calorie diet.

Added Sugars

"Added Sugars" in grams and as %Daily Value (DV=50g), is a new addition to the label. It is difficult to meet nutrient needs while staying within calorie limits if more than 10% of total daily calories are consumed from added sugar.

Protein DV

% Daily Value for protein is generally not included due to expensive testing required to determine protein quality.

Nutrient claims, such as "Good source," and health claims, such as "Reduce the risk of osteoporosis," must follow legal definitions.

Nutrients

These nutrients must appear on most labels. Labels of foods that contain few nutrients, such as candy and soft drinks, may omit some nutrients. Some manufacturers list more nutrients. Other nutrients must be listed if manufacturers make a claim about them or if the food is fortified with them.

Name and address of the food manufacturer.

A Quick Guide to Nutrient Sources

% Daily Value
20% or more = *Rich source*
10%–19% = *Good source*

Ingredients are listed in descending order by weight.

Nutrition Facts

6 serving per Container

| Serving Size | 1 Pouch (61g) |

Amount Per Serving

Calories 250

	% Daily value*
Total Fat 7g	11%
Saturated Fat 2.5g	13%
Trans Fat 1g	**
Cholesterol 5mg	2%
Sodium 400mg	16%
Total Carbohydrate 38g	13%
Dietary Fiber <1g	3%
Total Sugars 6g	
Includes 5g Added Sugars	10%
Protein 7g	
Vitamin D 0mcg	0%
Calcium 120mg	12%
Iron 2mg	11%
Potassium 150mg	4%

The % Daily Value (DV) tells you how much a nutrient in a serving of food contributes to a daily diet. 2,000 calories a day is used for general nutrition advice.

INGREDIENTS: ENRICHED MACARONI PRODUCT (DURUM WHEAT FLOUR, GLYCERYL MONO-STEARATE, SALT, NIACIN, FERROUS SULFATE, THIAMIN MONONITRATE [VITAMIN B1], RIBOFLAVIN [VITAMIN B2], FOLIC ACID), CHEESE SAUCE MIX (WHEY, PARTIALLY, HYDROGENATED SOYBEAN OIL, MALTODEXTRIN, WHEY PROTEIN CONCENTRATE, CORN SYRUP SOLIDS, SALT, MILKFAT, SUGAR, SODIUM, NATURAL FLAVOR, CITRIC ACID, MONOSODIUM GLUTAMATE, MODIFIED FOOD STARCH, LACTIC ACID, YELLOW 5.

FIGURE 2-13 ▲ Food packages must list product name, name and address of the manufacturer, amount of product in the package, and ingredients. The Nutrition Facts panel is required on virtually all packaged food products. The % Daily Value listed on the label is the percent of the amount of a nutrient needed daily that is provided by a single serving of the product. Canadian food labels use a slightly different group of health claims and label descriptors.

the labels, "per serving" and "per package." Manufacturers with more than $10 million in annual food sales must begin using the new label by July 26, 2018, while others will have an additional year to comply. More information can be found at http://www.fda.gov/Food/GuidanceRegulation/GuidanceDocumentsRegulatory Information/LabelingNutrition/ucm385663.htm.

TABLE 2-10 ■ Definitions for Nutrient Claims Allowed on Food Labels

Sugar

- **Sugar free:** less than 0.5 gram (g) per serving

- **No added sugar; without added sugar; no sugar added:**
  - No sugars were added during processing or packing, including ingredients that contain sugars (e.g., fruit juices, applesauce, or jam).
  - Processing does not increase the sugar content above the amount naturally present in the ingredients. (A functionally insignificant increase in sugars is acceptable for processes used for purposes other than increasing sugar content.)
  - The food that it resembles and for which it substitutes normally contains added sugars.
  - If the food doesn't meet the requirements for a low- or reduced-calorie food, the product bears a statement that the food is not low calorie or calorie reduced and directs consumers' attention to the Nutrition Facts panel for further information on sugars and calorie content.

- **Reduced sugar:** at least 25% less sugar per serving than reference food

Calories

- **Calorie free:** fewer than 5 kcal per serving

- **Low calorie:** 40 kcal or less per serving and, if the serving is 30 grams or less or 2 tablespoons or less, per 50 grams of the food

- **Reduced or fewer calories:** at least 25% fewer kcal per serving than reference food

Fiber

- **High fiber:** 5 grams or more per serving (Foods making high-fiber claims must meet the definition for low fat, or the level of total fat must appear next to the high-fiber claim.)

- **Good source of fiber:** 2.5 to 4.9 grams per serving

- **More or added fiber:** at least 2.5 grams more per serving than reference food

Fat

- **Fat free:** less than 0.5 gram of fat per serving

- **Saturated fat free:** less than 0.5 gram per serving, and the level of *trans* fatty acids does not exceed 0.5 gram per serving

- **Low fat:** 3 grams or less per serving and, if the serving is 30 grams or less or 2 tablespoons or less, per 50 grams of the food; 2% milk can no longer be labeled low fat, as it exceeds 3 grams per serving; *reduced fat* will be the term used instead.

- **Low saturated fat:** 1 gram or less per serving and not more than 15% of kcal from saturated fatty acids

- **Reduced or less fat:** at least 25% less per serving than reference food

- **Reduced or less saturated fat:** at least 25% less per serving than reference food

Cholesterol

- **Cholesterol free:** less than 2 milligrams (mg) of cholesterol and 2 grams or less of saturated fat per serving

- **Low cholesterol:** 20 milligrams or less of cholesterol and 2 grams or less of saturated fat per serving or, if the serving is 30 grams or less or 2 tablespoons or less, per 50 grams of the food

- **Reduced or less cholesterol:** at least 25% less cholesterol than reference food and 2 grams or less of saturated fat per serving

Sodium

- **Sodium free:** less than 5 milligrams per serving

- **Very low sodium:** 35 milligrams or less per serving and, if the serving is 30 grams or less or 2 tablespoons or less, per 50 grams of the food

- **Low sodium:** 140 milligrams or less per serving or, if the serving is 30 grams or less or 2 tablespoons or less, per 50 grams of the food

- **Light in sodium:** at least 50% less per serving than reference food

- **Reduced or less sodium:** at least 25% less per serving than reference food

Other Terms

- **Fortified or enriched:** Vitamins and/or minerals have been added to the product in amounts in excess of at least 10% of that normally present in the usual product. *Enriched* generally refers to replacing nutrients lost in processing, whereas *fortified* refers to adding nutrients not originally present in the specific food.

- **Healthy:** An individual food that is low fat and low saturated fat and has no more than 360 to 480 milligrams of sodium or 60 milligrams of cholesterol per serving can be labeled "healthy" if it provides at least 10% of the Daily Value for vitamin A, vitamin C, protein, calcium, iron, or fiber.

- **Light or lite:** The descriptor *light* or *lite* can mean two things: first, that a nutritionally altered product contains one-third fewer kcal or half the fat of reference food (if the food derives 50% or more of its kcal from fat, the reduction must be 50% of the fat) and, second, that the sodium content of a low-calorie, low-fat food has been reduced by 50%. In addition, "light in sodium" may be used for foods in which the sodium content has been reduced by at least 50%. The term *light* may still be used to describe such properties as texture and color, as long as the label explains the intent; for example, "light brown sugar" and "light and fluffy."

- **Diet:** A food may be labeled with terms such as *diet, dietetic, artificially sweetened,* or *sweetened with nonnutritive sweetener* only if the claim is not false or misleading. The food can also be labeled *low calorie* or *reduced calorie.*

- **Good source:** *Good source* means that a serving of the food contains 10% to 19% of the Daily Value for a particular nutrient. If 5% or less, it is a *low source.*

(continued)

TABLE 2-10 ■ (continued)

- **High:** *High* means that a serving of the food contains 20% or more of the Daily Value for a particular nutrient.

- **Organic:** Federal standards for organic foods allow claims when much of the ingredients do not use chemical fertilizers or pesticides, genetic engineering, sewage sludge, antibiotics, or irradiation in their production. At least 95% of ingredients (by weight) must meet these guidelines to be labeled "organic" on the front of the package. If the front label instead says "made with organic ingredients," only 70% of the ingredients must be organic. For animal products, the animals must graze outdoors, be fed organic feed, and cannot be exposed to large amounts of antibiotics or growth hormones.

- **Natural:** The food must be free of food colors, synthetic flavors, or any other synthetic substance.

The following terms apply only to meat and poultry products regulated by USDA.

- **Extra lean:** less than 5 grams of fat, 2 grams of saturated fat, and 95 milligrams of cholesterol per serving (or 100 grams of an individual food)

- **Lean:** less than 10 grams of fat, 4.5 grams of saturated fat, and 95 milligrams of cholesterol per serving (or 100 grams of an individual food)

Many definitions are from FDA's *Dictionary of Terms,* as established in conjunction with the 1990 Nutrition Labeling and Education Act (NLEA).

USDA Organic label: Source: www.usda.gov/

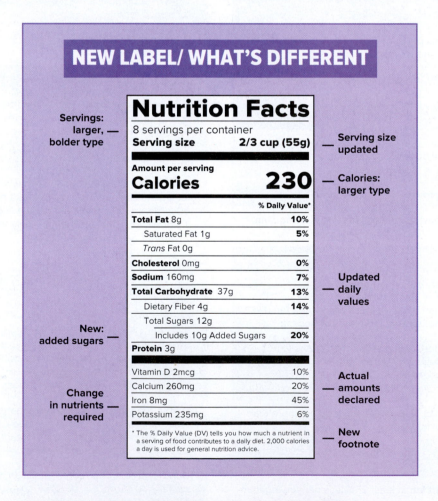

FIGURE 2-14 ▲ New Nutrition Facts Label with changes noted.

Source: FDA: Changes to the Nutrition Facts Label, http://www.fda.gov/Food/GuidanceRegulation/ GuidanceDocumentsRegulatoryInformation/LabelingNutrition/ucm385663.htm

The Nutrition Facts label uses the term *calorie* to express energy content in some cases, but kilocalorie (kcal) values are actually listed.

▲ Use the Nutrition Facts label to learn more about the nutrient content of the foods you eat. Nutrient content is expressed as a percent of Daily Value. Canadian food laws and related food labels have a slightly different format.
© Ryan McVay/Getty Images

Menu Planning with Labels

All of the tools discussed in this chapter greatly aid in menu planning. Menu planning can start with MyPlate. The totality of choices made within the groups can then be evaluated using the Dietary Guidelines. Individual foods that make up a dietary pattern can be examined more closely using the Daily Values listed on the Nutrition Facts panel of the product. For the most part, these Daily Values are in line with the Recommended Dietary Allowances and related nutrient standards. The Nutrition Facts panel is especially useful in identifying nutrient-dense foods (foods high in a specific nutrient, such as the vitamin folate, but low in the relative amount of kilocalories provided) and the energy-dense foods (foods that fill you up without providing a lot of kilocalories). Generally speaking, the more you learn about and use these tools together, the more they will benefit your diet. Research has shown that individuals who read the Nutrition Facts when shopping for food report healthier nutrient consumption compared to nonusers (see Further Reading 4).

Exceptions to Food Labeling

Foods such as fresh fruits, vegetables, and fish currently are not required to have Nutrition Facts labels. However, many grocers have voluntarily chosen to provide their customers with information about these products on posters or pamphlets that may contain recipes that can assist you in your endeavor to improve your dietary pattern.

The % Daily Value for protein is not mandatory on foods because protein deficiency is not a public health concern in the United States. If the % Daily Value for protein is given on a label, FDA requires that the product be analyzed for protein quality. This procedure is expensive and time consuming, so many companies opt not to list a % Daily Value for protein. However, labels on food for infants and children under 4 years of age must include the % Daily Value for protein, as must the labels on any food carrying a claim about protein content.

Health Claims on Food Labels

As a marketing tool directed toward the health-conscious consumer, food manufacturers like to claim that their products have all sorts of health benefits. FDA has legal oversight over most food products and permits some health claims with certain restrictions. Overall, claims on foods fall into one of four categories:

- Health claims—closely regulated by FDA
- Preliminary health claims—regulated by FDA, but evidence may be scant for the claim
- Nutrient claims—closely regulated by FDA (review Table 2-10)
- Structure/function claims—these are not FDA approved, or necessarily valid

Table 2-10 lists the definitions for nutrient claims on food labels. Currently, FDA limits the use of health messages to specific instances in which there is significant scientific agreement that a relationship exists between a nutrient, food, or food constituent and the disease. The claims allowed at this time may show a link (a "may" or "might" qualifier must be used in the statement) between a dietary pattern

- with enough calcium and vitamin D and a reduced risk of osteoporosis.
- low in total fat and a reduced risk of some cancers.
- low in saturated fat and cholesterol and a reduced risk of cardiovascular disease (typically referred to as heart disease on the label).
- rich in fiber—containing grain products, fruits, and vegetables—and a reduced risk of some cancers.
- low in sodium and high in potassium and a reduced risk of hypertension and stroke.
- rich in fruits and vegetables and a reduced risk of some cancers.
- adequate in the synthetic form of the vitamin folate (called folic acid) and a reduced risk of neural tube defects (a type of birth defect).
- with sugarless gum and a reduced risk of tooth decay, especially when compared with foods high in sugars and starches.
- rich in fruits, vegetables, and grain products that contain fiber and a reduced risk of cardiovascular disease. Oats (oatmeal, oat bran, and oat flour) and psyllium are two fiber-rich ingredients that can be singled out in reducing the risk of cardiovascular disease, as long as the statement also says that the diet should be low in saturated fat and cholesterol.
- a diet rich in whole-grain foods and other plant foods, as well as low in total fat, saturated fat, and cholesterol, and a reduced risk of cardiovascular disease and certain cancers.
- low in saturated fat and cholesterol that also includes 25 grams of soy protein and a reduced risk of cardiovascular disease. The statement "one serving of the (name of food) provides _____ grams of soy protein" must also appear as part of the health claim.
- that includes fatty acids from oils present in fish and a reduced risk of cardiovascular disease.
- that includes margarines containing plant stanols and sterols and a reduced risk of cardiovascular disease.

▲ Specific health claims can be made on food labels for whole-grain cereals. Cheerios® are made from oats, which can be singled out in reducing the risk of cardiovascular disease as long as the statement also says that the diet should be low in saturated fat and cholesterol. © McGraw-Hill Education/Jill Braaten, photographer

In addition, before a health claim can be made for a food product, it must meet two general requirements. First, the food must be a "good source" (before any fortification) of fiber, protein, vitamin A, vitamin C, calcium, or iron. (The legal definition of "good source" appears in Table 2-10.) Second, a single serving of the food product cannot contain more than 13 grams of fat, 4 grams of saturated fat, 60 milligrams of cholesterol, or 480 milligrams of sodium. If a food exceeds any one of these requirements, no health claim can be made for it, despite its other nutritional qualities. For example, even though whole milk is high in calcium, its label can't make the health claim about calcium and osteoporosis because whole milk contains 5 grams of saturated fat per serving. In another example, a health claim regarding fat and cancer can be made only if the product contains 3 grams or less of fat per serving, the standard for low-fat foods.

The FDA's 2003 Consumer Health Information for Better Nutrition Initiative also allows the use of qualified health claims when there is emerging evidence for a relationship between a food, food component, or dietary supplement and reduced risk of a disease or health-related condition. In this case, the evidence is not well enough established to meet the significant scientific agreement standard required for an FDA-authorized health claim. The following are examples of "Qualified Health Claims Subject to Enforcement Discretion." More information can be found at http://www.fda.gov/Food/IngredientsPackagingLabeling/LabelingNutrition/ucm073992.htm.

Qualified claims about cancer risk:
- Tomatoes and/or tomato sauce and prostate, ovarian, gastric, and pancreatic cancers
- Calcium and colon/rectal cancer and calcium and recurrent colon/rectal polyps

Qualified claims about cardiovascular disease risk:
- Nuts and heart disease
- Omega-3 fatty acids and coronary heart disease
- Monounsaturated fatty acids from olive oil and coronary heart disease

CASE STUDY Using the Nutrition Facts Label to Make Food Choices

On her way home from her afternoon nutrition class, Laura stops at the supermarket to pick up a few items she needs for the rest of the week. After picking up bananas, yogurt, bagels, and milk, she heads to the frozen food section to find a quick meal before a busy evening. She is in the mood for pasta and finds two brands of frozen cheese manicotti. Laura remembers to check out the Nutrition Facts panel for the two products to help her choose the healthiest option. Help Laura make the best choice by studying the Nutrition Facts labels for the two brands (Luigi's and Mario's) and answering the following questions.

1. Given that a serving of each product of manicotti weighs the same, which product has the highest energy density?
2. Compare the calories from fat for each manicotti product. Divide the calories from fat by the total calories for each product. What is the percent calories from fat for Luigi's and Mario's?
3. Compare the saturated fat content to the total kilocalorie content of each manicotti product. For each, what is the percent of the total kilocalories that is saturated fat?
4. Laura sees that the total calories for Mario's manicotti are much lower than the calories for Luigi's. If she ate two packages of Mario's manicotti, how many calories would she consume?
5. How many servings of Luigi's manicotti would Laura need to consume to get 100% of her Daily Value of sodium?
6. The Daily Value for vitamin C is 60 milligrams. What is the percent Daily Value for vitamin C in each manicotti product?
7. Which product has the higher nutrient density for vitamin C?

8. The Daily Value for calcium is 1000 milligrams. What is the percent Daily Value in each manicotti product?
9. Which product has the higher nutrient density for calcium?
10. Which of the two brands would you choose? What information on the Nutrition Facts label in the figure contributed to this decision?

(a) Luigi's Manicotti

Nutrition Facts

1 servings per container

Serving size   1 Package (260g)

Amount per serving

Calories   390

	% Daily Value*
Total Fat 18g	**27%**
Saturated Fat 9g	**45%**
Trans Fat 2g	
Cholesterol 45mg	**14%**
Sodium 880mg	**36%**
Total Carbohydrate 38g	**13%**
Dietary Fiber	**15%**
Total Sugars 12g	
Includes 10g Added Sugars	**20%**
Protein 17g	
Vitamin D 0mcg	0%
Calcium 400mg	40%
Iron 2mg	11%
Potassium 470mg	13%

* The % Daily Value (DV) tells you how much a nutrient in a serving of food contributes to a daily diet. 2,000 calories a day is used for general nutrition advice.

(b) Mario's Manicotti

Nutrition Facts

1 servings per container

Serving size   1 Package (260g)

Amount per serving

Calories   230

	% Daily Value*
Total Fat 4g	**6%**
Saturated Fat 2g	**10%**
Trans Fat 1g	
Cholesterol 15mg	**4%**
Sodium 590mg	**24%**
Total Carbohydrate 28g	**9%**
Dietary Fiber 3g	**12%**
Total Sugars 10g	
Includes 8g Added Sugars	**16%**
Protein 19g	
Vitamin D 0mcg	0%
Calcium 350mg	35%
Iron 1mg	6%
Potassium 280mg	8%

* The % Daily Value (DV) tells you how much a nutrient in a serving of food contributes to a daily diet. 2,000 calories a day is used for general nutrition advice.

Summary (Numbers refer to numbered sections in the chapter.)

2.1 A healthy eating plan is based on consuming a *variety* of foods balanced by a *moderate* intake of each food and will minimize the risk of developing nutrition-related diseases.

Proportionality is eating foods with greater nutrient density and reflects the nutrient content of a food in relation to its calorie content. Nutrient-dense foods are relatively rich in nutrients, in comparison with kilocalorie content.

Energy density of a food is determined by comparing kilocalorie content with the weight of food. A food rich in kilocalories but weighing relatively very little, such as nuts, cookies, fried foods in general, and most snack foods (including fat-free brands), is considered energy dense. Foods with low energy density include fruits, vegetables, and any food that incorporates lots of water during cooking, such as oatmeal.

2.2 Dietary Guidelines for Americans have been issued to help improve the health of all Americans ages 2 and older. The guidelines emphasize a healthy eating pattern that includes a variety of vegetables from all of the subgroups, whole fruits, whole grains, fat-free or low-fat dairy, a variety of protein foods, and oils; and limits saturated fats and *trans* fats, added sugars, and sodium.

2.3 MyPlate and accompanying online tools are designed to translate nutrient recommendations into a food plan that exhibits variety, proportionality, and moderation. The best results are obtained by using low-fat or fat-free dairy products, incorporating some vegetable proteins in the dietary pattern in addition to animal-protein foods, including citrus fruits and dark-green vegetables, and emphasizing whole-grain breads and cereals.

2.4 A person's nutritional state can be categorized as *desirable nutrition,* in which the body has adequate stores for times of increased needs; *undernutrition,* which may be present with or without clinical symptoms; and *overnutrition,* which can lead to vitamin and mineral toxicities and various chronic diseases.

2.5 Evaluation of nutritional state involves analyzing background factors, as well as anthropometric, biochemical, clinical, dietary, and environmental assessments. It is not always possible to detect nutritional inadequacies via nutritional assessment because symptoms of deficiencies are often nonspecific and may not appear for many years.

2.6 Recommended Dietary Allowances (RDAs) are set for many nutrients. These amounts yield enough of each nutrient to meet the needs of healthy individuals within specific gender and age categories. Adequate Intake (AI) is the standard used when not enough information is available to set a more specific RDA. Estimated Energy Requirements (EERs) set calorie needs for both genders at various ages and physical activity patterns. Tolerable Upper Intake Levels (Upper Levels or ULs) for nutrient intake have been set for some vitamins and minerals. All of these dietary standards fall under the term *Dietary Reference Intakes (DRIs).*

Daily Values are used as a basis for expressing the nutrient content of foods on the Nutrition Facts panel and are based for the most part on the RDAs.

2.7 Apply the basic principles of nutrition to evaluate any nutrition claim. Several indicators of nutrition misinformation include insufficient scientific evidence to support a product claim, lack of credible sources, promises of unbelievable results, or distrust of the medical community. To sort nutrition fact from fiction, seek the advice of a registered dietitian nutritionist.

2.8 Food labels, especially the Nutrition Facts panels, are a useful tool to track your nutrient intake and learn more about the nutritional characteristics of the foods you eat. Any health claims listed must follow FDA-set criteria.

Check Your Knowledge (Answers are available at the end of this question set.)

1. Anthropometric measurements include
   a. height, weight, skinfolds, and body circumferences.
   b. blood concentrations of nutrients.
   c. a diet history of the previous days' intake.
   d. blood levels of enzyme activities.

2. Foods with *high* nutrient density offer the_____nutrients for the_____kilocalories.
   a. least, lowest
   b. least, most
   c. most, lowest
   d. most, most

3. A meal of a bean burrito, tossed salad, and glass of milk represents foods from all MyPlate food groups except
   a. dairy.
   b. protein.
   c. vegetables.
   d. fruits.

4. The Dietary Guidelines for Americans provide advice for Americans
   a. from birth and older.
   b. from age 2 and older.
   c. from age 6 and older.
   d. from age 18 and older.

5. The 2015–2020 Dietary Guidelines recommend that we increase which of the following foods?
   a. refined grains
   b. whole milk products
   c. seafood
   d. added sugars

6. How many minutes of moderate-intensity physical activity are recommended for adults in the 2008 Physical Activity Guidelines for Americans?
   a. 150 minutes per week
   b. 60 minutes every day
   c. 50 minutes every day
   d. 30 minutes three days a week

7. The term Daily Value is used on
   a. restaurant menus.
   b. food labels.
   c. medical charts.
   d. none of the above.

8. The Tolerable Upper Intake Level, or UL, is used to
   a. estimate calorie needs of the average person.
   b. evaluate the highest amount of daily nutrient intake unlikely to cause adverse health effects.
   c. evaluate your current intake for a specific nutrient.
   d. compare the nutrient content of a food to approximate human needs.

9. The current food label must list
   a. a picture of the product.
   b. a uniform and realistic serving size.
   c. the RDA for each age group.
   d. ingredients alphabetically.

10. The most common type of undernutrition in industrialized nations, such as the United States, is
    a. anorexia.
    b. protein deficiency.
    c. obesity.
    d. iron deficiency.

Answer Key: 1. a (LO 2.5), 2. c (LO 2.1), 3. d (LO 2.3), 4. b (LO 2.2), 5. c (LO 2.2), 6. a (LO 2.2), 7. b (LO 2.8), 8. b (LO 2.6), 9. b (LO 2.8), 10. d (LO 2.4)

Study Questions (Numbers refer to Learning Outcomes)

1. How would you explain the concepts of nutrient density and energy density to a fourth-grade class? **(LO 2.1)**

2. Describe the intent of the Dietary Guidelines for Americans. Based on the discussion of the Dietary Guidelines for Americans, suggest two key dietary changes the typical North American adult should consider making. **(LO 2.2)**

3. What dietary changes would you need to make to comply with the healthy eating guidelines exemplified by MyPlate on a regular basis? **(LO 2.3)**

4. Describe what would happen to the status of a nutrient in the body for a person who transitions from an overnourished to an undernourished state. **(LO 2.4)**

5. What steps would you follow to evaluate the nutritional state of an undernourished person? **(LO 2.5)**

6. How do RDAs and AIs differ from Daily Values in intention and application? **(LO 2.6)**

7. What would you list as the top five sources of reliable nutrition information? What makes these sources reliable? **(LO 2.7)**

8. Dietitians encourage all people to read labels on food packages to learn more about what they eat. What four nutrients could easily be tracked in your diet if you read the Nutrition Facts panels regularly on food products? **(LO 2.8)**

9. Define the USDA definition for the term "organic." **(LO 2.8)**

10. List some specific health claims that can be made on food labels. **(LO 2.8)**

What the Dietitian Chose

It is smart to reach for a carbohydrate-containing beverage when you need quick energy. Some of us also rely on caffeine in drinks to give us a boost. Many beverages on the market contain high concentrations of carbohydrate as "added sugar." This added sugar has recently been the subject of many debates because the consumption of added sugars has been on the rise since 1970, and excessive sugar intake has been linked to several adverse health conditions. The major sources of added sugars are sodas, energy drinks, and sports drinks.

The main issue here is the abundance of empty calories supplied by soft drinks. Studies show that liquid calories do not promote satiety in the same way as food calories do. In other words, consuming 250 kcal of cola does not mean that you will feel full enough to eat one less slice of pizza to compensate for those extra kilocalories. Excess calories from any source will lead to weight gain over time.

For these empty calories, portion size is a concern. A 20-ounce bottle of regular cola contains about 68 grams (about 15 teaspoons) of sweeteners. Both types of soft drink provide about 250 kcal. In terms of a soft drink, a 12-ounce soda, such as the Jones Root Beer Soda®, will have proportionally less sugar (48 grams) due to its smaller volume. If you consume one soft drink per day or less, the type of sweetener is not likely to make a big difference. If you consume several soft drinks per day, you would be better off choosing a beverage that does not contain calories, such as diet cola or water. Beverages with artificial sweeteners, such as Coke Zero®, typically are calorie free and therefore provide you with no energy when you need a boost. You may feel a temporary lift from the caffeine in some of these products. Water is the perfect drink to restore fluid losses and prevent dehydration, but it contains no calories for energy.

Your best choice when needing a quick energy boost in this case is low-fat chocolate milk. The nutrient-dense chocolate milk not only provides less sugar than the sodas on our list, but it is also the best source of total nutrition. Most convenience stores sell chocolate milk in pint bottles or half-pint (8-ounce) cartons (similar to those served in school cafeterias). The 8-ounce carton of chocolate milk provides a good amount of kilocalories (150 kcal) as well as 8 grams of protein, 2.5 grams of fat, and 25 grams of sugar. It also provides calcium (290 milligrams), vitamin A (490 IU), and vitamin D (2.8 micrograms), as well as other vitamins and minerals. A pint bottle (16 ounces) would provide twice the amount of kilocalories and other nutrients. In addition, the chocolate provides a source of caffeine that you may be looking for.

▲ Chocolate milk is a very nutritious beverage that provides protein, vitamins, and minerals, along with calories. © Real Food by Warren Diggles/ Alamy

CASE STUDY SOLUTION — Using the Nutrition Facts Label to Make Food Choices

1. Luigi's has the highest energy density because it has the highest kilocalories per weight **(390 per 260 grams)**.

2. The percent kilocalories from fat for Luigi's is **41%**, and the percent kilocalories from fat for Mario's is **15%**.

3. The percent of the total fat that is saturated fat is **50%** for Luigi's and **50%** for Mario's. They both have the same ratio of saturated fat to total fat, even though Luigi's has more grams of saturated fat per serving.

4. If she ate two packages of Mario's manicotti, she would consume 460 kilocalories because **230 × 2 = 460.**

5. Laura would need to consume a little less than three servings of Luigi's manicotti to get 100% of her Daily Value of sodium because **100%/36% = 2.78.**

6. The percent Daily Value for vitamin C is **4%** for Luigi's manicotti and **10%** for Mario's manicotti.

7. Mario's manicotti has a higher nutrient density for vitamin C.

8. The percent Daily Value for calcium is **40%** for Luigi's manicotti and **35%** for Mario's manicotti.

9. Mario's manicotti has a higher nutrient density for calcium (**35%** DV per 230 kcal) than that of Luigi's (**40%** DV per 390 kcal) because Mario's has significantly fewer kilocalories, even though the DV is lower.

10. Mario's manicotti would be the best choice because it has greater nutrient density and lower energy density. This means that Laura will get more nutrients and fewer kilocalories. If she wants to increase her kilocalorie intake, it would be healthier to eat two servings of Mario's manicotti rather than one serving of Luigi's. This will increase her protein, vitamin, mineral, and fiber intake but will keep her total fat and saturated fat intake below that in just one serving of Luigi's.

Further Readings

1. Academy of Nutrition and Dietetics: Practice Paper of the Academy of Nutrition and Dietetics: Communicating accurate food and nutrition information. *Journal of the Academy of Nutrition and Dietetics* 112:759, 2012.

2. Chiuve SE and others: Adherence to a low risk, healthy lifestyle and risk of sudden cardiac death among women. *Journal of the American Medical Association* 306:62, 2011.

3. Monsivais P, Drewnowski A: Lower-energy-density diets are associated with higher monetary costs per kilocalorie and are consumed by women of higher socioeconomic status. *Journal of the American Dietetic Association* 109:804, 2009.

4. Ollberding NJ and others: Food label use and its relation to dietary intake among U.S. adults. *Journal of the American Dietetic Association* 110:1233, 2010.

5. Perez-Escamilla R and others: Dietary energy density and body weight in adults and children: A systematic review. *Journal of the Academy of Nutrition and Dietetics* 112:671, 2012.

6. Rolls B, Hermann M: *The ultimate volumetrics diet: Smart, simple, science-based strategies for losing weight and keeping it off.* New York: HarperCollins, 2012.

7. Rowe S and others: Translating the Dietary Guidelines for Americans 2010 to bring about real behavior change. *Journal of the American Dietetic Association* 111:28, 2011.

8. Sofi F and others: Adherence to Mediterranean Diet and health status: Meta-analysis. *British Medical Journal* 337:a1344, 2008.

9. U.S. Department of Health and Human Services: *2008 Physical Activity Guidelines for Americans.* 2008. www.health.gov/PAGuidelines/. Updated/accessed September 25, 2015.

10. U.S. Department of Health and Human Services: *Dietary Guidelines for Americans, 2015–2020.* 2016. http://health.gov/dietaryguidelines/2015/guidelines/ Accessed 2/1/2016.

11. United States Department of Agriculture: *USDA's MyPlate.* July 2015. www.choosemyplate.gov. Accessed September 25, 2015.

12. Watts ML and others: The art of translating nutritional science into dietary guidance: History and evolution of the Dietary Guidelines for Americans. *Nutrition Reviews* 69:404, 2011.

 connect To get the most out of your study of nutrition, go to McGraw-Hill's online resources: Connect www.mcgrawhillconnect.com, where you will find NutritionCalc Plus, LearnSmart, and many other dynamic tools.

Does Your Diet Compare to MyPlate?

Using your food-intake record from Chapter 1, place each food item in the appropriate group of the accompanying MyPlate chart. That is, for each food item, indicate how many servings it contributes to each group based on the amount you ate (see Food Composition Table Supplement for serving sizes). Many of your food choices may contribute to more than one group. For example, spaghetti with meat sauce contributes to three categories: grains, vegetables, and proteins. After entering all the values, add the number of servings consumed in each group. Finally, compare your total in each food group with the recommended number of servings shown in Table 2-5 or obtained from the ChooseMyPlate.gov website. Enter a minus sign (−) if your total falls below the recommendation or a plus sign (+) if it equals or exceeds the recommendation.

Indicate the number of servings from MyPlate that each food yields:

Food or Beverage	Amount Eaten	Grains	Vegetables	Fruits	Dairy	Protein
Group totals						
Recommended servings						
Shortages/overages in numbers of servings						

© Getty Images/Jonelle Weaver

Student Learning Outcomes

Chapter 3 is designed to allow you to:

3.1 Understand some basic roles of nutrients in human physiology.

3.2 Identify the functions of the common cellular components.

3.3 Define tissue, organ, and organ system.

3.4 Identify the role of the cardiovascular and lymphatic systems in nutrition.

3.5 List basic characteristics of the nervous system and its role in nutrition.

3.6 List basic characteristics of the endocrine system, especially the pancreas, and its role in nutrition.

3.7 List basic characteristics of the immune system and its role in nutrition.

3.8 Outline the overall processes of digestion and absorption in the mouth, stomach, small intestine, and large intestine, as well as the roles played by the liver, gallbladder, and pancreas.

3.9 List basic characteristics of the urinary system and its role in nutrition.

Merely eating food won't nourish you. You must first digest the food by breaking it down into usable forms of the essential nutrients that can be absorbed into the bloodstream. Once nutrients are taken up by the bloodstream, they can be distributed to and used by body cells.

We rarely think about digesting and absorbing foods. Except for a few voluntary responses—such as deciding what and when to eat, how well to chew food, and when to eliminate the remains—most digestion and absorption processes control themselves. We don't consciously decide when the pancreas will secrete digestive substances into the small intestine or how quickly foodstuffs will be propelled down the intestinal tract. Hormones and nerve impulses control these functions. Your only awareness of these involuntary responses may be a hunger pang right before lunch or a "full" feeling after eating that last slice of pizza.

You've learned about cells, tissues, and organs before, but now let's look at the human body from a nutrition perspective. Refresh your memory of the basic anatomy (structure) and physiology (function) of the circulatory system, nervous system, endocrine system, immune system, and urinary system. In particular, as you focus on the digestive system, you will gain an in-depth understanding of how the food you eat nourishes your body.

3.10 Understand the importance of the body storage areas for nutrients.

3.11 Understand the emerging field of nutritional genomics.

3.12 Identify the major nutrition-related gastrointestinal health problems and approaches to treatment.

3.1 Nutrition's Role in Human Physiology

tissues Collections of cells adapted to perform a specific function.

organ A group of tissues designed to perform a specific function; for example, the heart, which contains muscle tissue, nerve tissue, and so on.

organ system A collection of organs that work together to perform an overall function.

The everyday function of the human body relies on the coordination of many highly structured organ systems. Together, these systems are composed of trillions of cells. Each cell is a self-contained, living entity. Cells of the same type normally join together, using intercellular substances to form **tissues,** such as muscle tissue. One, two, or more tissues then combine in a particular way to form more complex structures called **organs.** All organs contribute to nutritional health, and a person's overall nutritional state determines how well each organ functions. At a still higher level of coordination, several organs that work together form an **organ system,** such as the digestive system.

Chemical processes (reactions) occur constantly in every living cell; the production of new substances is balanced by the breakdown of older ones. An example is the constant formation and degradation of bone. For this turnover of substances to occur, cells require a continuous supply of energy derived from dietary carbohydrate, protein, and/or fat. Cells also need water; building supplies, especially protein and minerals; and chemical regulators, such as the vitamins. Almost all cells also need a steady supply of oxygen. These substances enable the tissues, made of individual cells, to function properly.

Getting an adequate supply of all nutrients to the body's cells begins with a healthy diet. To ensure optimal use of nutrients, the body's cells, tissues, organs, and organ systems also must work efficiently.

This chapter covers the anatomy and physiology of the cell and major organ systems, especially as they relate to human nutrition. In later chapters, you will examine the intricacies of each of the essential nutrients, but let us start out by admiring the "big picture" of the human body.

✓ CONCEPT CHECK 3.1

1. Discuss the levels of organization of the human body.
2. Describe three ways essential nutrients support cell functions.

3.2 The Cell: Structure, Function, and Metabolism

organelles Compartments, particles, or filaments that perform specialized functions within a cell.

The cell is the basic structural and functional component of life. Living organisms are made of many different kinds of cells specialized to perform particular functions, and all cells are derived from preexisting cells. In the human body, all cells have certain common features. These cells have membranes and **organelles** that perform specialized functions (Fig. 3-1). There are at least 15 different organelles, but the nutritional relevance of just six of the organelles will be examined here. Metabolism, the chemical processes that take place in body cells, is also discussed.

CELL (PLASMA) MEMBRANE

phospholipid Any of a class of fat-related substances that contain phosphorus, fatty acids, and a nitrogen-containing component. Phospholipids are an essential part of every cell.

There is an outside and inside to every cell, separated by the cell (plasma) membrane. (Please note that animal cells do not have cell walls.) The cell membrane itself is not an organelle, but it holds the cellular contents (cytoplasm and organelles) together and regulates the flow of substances into and out of the cell. Cell-to-cell communication also occurs by way of this membrane.

The cell membrane, illustrated in Figure 3-1(b), is a lipid bilayer (or double membrane) of **phospholipids** with their water-soluble heads facing both the interior and the exterior of the cell. Their water-insoluble tails are tucked into the interior of the cell membrane.

FIGURE 3-1 ▶ (a) An animal cell. Almost all human cells contain these various organelles. Shown here, but not discussed in the text, are the nucleolus, nuclear envelope, and centrioles. The nucleolus participates in genetic-related functions. The nuclear envelope encloses the nucleus. The centrioles participate in cell division. (b) A detailed view of the cell membrane.

Cholesterol is another component of the cell membrane. It is fat soluble, so it is embedded within the bilayer. This cholesterol provides rigidity and thus stability to the membrane.

There are also various proteins embedded in the cell membrane. Proteins provide structural support, act as transport vehicles, and function as **enzymes** that affect chemical processes within the membrane (see Section 3.9 on digestion for more about enzymes). Some proteins form open channels that allow water-soluble substances to pass into and out of the cell. Proteins on the outside surface of the membrane act as receptors, snagging essential substances that the cell needs and drawing them into the cell. Other proteins act as gates that open and close to control the flow of various particles into and out of the cell.

In addition to lipids and proteins, the membrane also contains carbohydrates that mark the exterior of the cell. These carbohydrates are combined with either protein or fat, and they help send messages to the cell's organelles and act as identification markers for the cell.

cholesterol A waxy lipid found in all body cells. It has a structure containing multiple chemical rings that is found only in foods that contain animal products.

enzymes A compound that speeds the rate of a chemical reaction but is not altered by the reaction. Almost all enzymes are proteins.

In addition, they detect invaders and initiate defensive actions. In sum, these carbohydrates provide tags that are important to cellular identity and interaction.

CYTOPLASM

cytoplasm The fluid and organelles (except the nucleus) in a cell.

The **cytoplasm** is the combination of fluid material and organelles within the cell, not including the nucleus. (A handful of these organelles will be described within this section.) A small amount of energy for use by the cell can be produced by chemical processes that occur in the cytoplasm. This contributes to the survival of all cells and is the sole source of energy production in red blood cells. This energy production is called **anaerobic** metabolism because it does not require oxygen.

MITOCHONDRIA

mitochondria Organelles that are the main sites of energy production in a cell. They contain the pathway for oxidizing fat for fuel, among other metabolic pathways.

Mitochondria are sometimes called the "power plants," or the "powerhouse" of the cell. These organelles are capable of converting the food energy in energy-yielding nutrients (carbohydrate, protein, and fat) to a form of energy that cells can use. This is an **aerobic** process that uses the oxygen we inhale, along with water, enzymes, and some vitamins and minerals (see Chapter 12 for details). Except for red blood cells, all cells contain mitochondria; only the size, shape, and quantity vary.

CELL NUCLEUS

cell nucleus An organelle bound by its own double membrane and containing chromosomes, the genetic information for cell protein synthesis and cell replication.

chromosomes A single, large DNA molecule and its associated proteins; contains many genes to store and transmit genetic information.

gene A specific segment on a chromosome. Genes provide the blueprint for the production of cell proteins.

deoxyribonucleic acid (DNA) The site of hereditary information in cells; DNA directs the synthesis of cell proteins.

ribonucleic acid (RNA) The single-stranded nucleic acid involved in the transcription of genetic information and translation of that information into protein structure.

transcription Process by which genetic information stored as DNA within the nucleus is copied to RNA during protein synthesis.

ribosomes Cytoplasmic particles that mediate the linking together of amino acids to form proteins; may exist freely in the cytoplasm or attached to endoplasmic reticulum.

translation Process by which genetic information copied into RNA dictates the amino acid sequence to form a protein.

With the exception of the red blood cell, all cells have one or more nuclei. The **cell nucleus** is bounded by its own double membrane. The nucleus contains the genetic material responsible for controlling actions that occur in the cell. The genetic material includes many **chromosomes,** which contain several **genes** made up of **deoxyribonucleic acid (DNA).** DNA is the "code book" that contains directions for making substances, specifically proteins, the cell needs. This code book remains in the nucleus of the cell but sends its information to other cell organelles by way of a "messenger" molecule called **ribonucleic acid (RNA).** The information stored on the DNA in the nucleus is copied onto RNA through the process of **transcription** and then moves out to the cytoplasm through pores in the nuclear membrane. The RNA carries the transcribed DNA code to protein-synthesizing sites called **ribosomes.** There, the RNA template is used in the process of **translation** to make a specific protein (see Section 6.2 for details on protein synthesis). Altogether, this process is known as **gene expression.**

All of the DNA in a cell is copied during cell replication. DNA is a double-stranded molecule, and when the cell begins to divide, each strand is separated and an identical copy of each is made. Thus, each new DNA contains one new strand of DNA and one strand from the original DNA. In this way, the genetic code is preserved from one cell generation to the next. (The mitochondria contain their own DNA, so they reproduce themselves within a cell independent of action in the cell's nucleus.)

gene expression Use of DNA information on a gene to produce a protein. Thought to be a major determination of cell development.

ENDOPLASMIC RETICULUM

endoplasmic reticulum (ER) An organelle composed of a network of canals running through the cytoplasm. Part of the endoplasmic reticulum contains ribosomes.

The outer membrane of the cell nucleus is continuous with a network of tubes called the **endoplasmic reticulum (ER).** Part of the endoplasmic reticulum (termed the rough [as opposed to smooth] ER) contains the ribosomes, where the RNA code is translated into proteins during protein synthesis. Many of these proteins play a central role in human nutrition. Parts of the endoplasmic reticulum are also involved in lipid synthesis, detoxification of toxic substances, and calcium storage and release in the cell.

GOLGI COMPLEX

Golgi complex The cell organelle near the nucleus that processes newly synthesized protein for secretion or distribution to other organelles.

secretory vesicles Membrane-bound vesicles produced by the Golgi complex; contain protein and other compounds to be secreted by the cell.

The **Golgi complex** is a packaging site for proteins used in the cytoplasm or exported from the cell. It consists of sacs within the cytoplasm in which proteins are "packaged" as **secretory vesicles** for secretion by the cell.

LYSOSOMES

Lysosomes are the cell's digestive system. They are sacs that contain enzymes for the digestion of foreign material. Sometimes known as "suicide bags," they are responsible for digesting worn-out or damaged cell components. Certain cells associated with immune functions contain many lysosomes.

PEROXISOMES

Peroxisomes contain enzymes that detoxify harmful chemicals. Peroxisomes get their name from the fact that hydrogen peroxide (H_2O_2) is formed as a result of such enzyme action. Peroxisomes also contain a protective enzyme called *catalase*, which prevents excessive accumulation of hydrogen peroxide in the cell, which would be very damaging. Peroxisomes also play a minor role in metabolizing one possible source of energy for cells—alcohol.

CELL METABOLISM

Metabolism refers to the entire collection of chemical processes involved in maintaining life. It encompasses all the sequences of chemical reactions that occur in the body's cells. These biochemical reactions take place in the cell cytoplasm and organelles that we have just discussed. They enable us to release and use energy from foods, synthesize one substance from another, and prepare waste products for excretion.

The reactions of metabolism that take place within your body can be categorized into one of two types. One type of reaction, *anabolic*, puts different molecules together and, therefore, requires energy. The other type of reaction, *catabolic*, takes molecules apart and, therefore, releases energy. The metabolism of carbohydrates, proteins, and fats yields energy. Vitamins and minerals contribute to the enzyme activity that supports metabolic reactions in the cell.

The metabolism of energy production begins in the cytoplasm with the initial anaerobic breakdown of glucose. The remaining aerobic steps of energy production take place in the mitochondria. Ultimately, the cells of the body use these interconnected processes to convert the energy found in food to energy stored in the high-energy compound **adenosine triphosphate (ATP).** You will learn more about the metabolism of energy sources in Chapter 12.

lysosome A cellular organelle that contains digestive enzymes for use inside the cell for turnover of cell parts.

peroxisome A cell organelle that destroys toxic products within the cell.

adenosine triphosphate (ATP) The main energy currency for cells. ATP energy is used to promote ion pumping, enzyme activity, and muscular contraction.

▲ The body is made up of numerous organ systems including the endocrine, nervous, and circulatory systems shown here. © M. Freeman/PhotoLink/Getty Images

✓ CONCEPT CHECK 3.2

1. What is an organelle?
2. Choose three organelles and explain their relevance to human nutrition.
3. What is the difference between anabolic and catabolic reactions? How does ATP fit into cellular metabolism?

3.3 Body Systems

As noted earlier, when groups of similar cells work together to accomplish a specialized task, the arrangement is referred to as a tissue. Humans are composed of four primary types of tissue: **epithelial, connective, muscle,** and **nervous** tissue. Epithelial tissue is composed of cells that cover surfaces both inside and outside the body. For example, the lining of the respiratory tract is made up of epithelial cells. Epithelial cells secrete important substances, absorb nutrients, and excrete waste. Connective tissue supports and protects the body, stores fat, and produces blood cells. Muscle tissue is designed for movement. Nervous tissue found in the brain and spinal cord is designed for communication. These four types of tissues then go on to form various organs and, ultimately, organ systems (Fig. 3-2).

epithelial tissue The surface cells that line the outside of the body and all external passages within it.

connective tissue Protein tissue that holds different structures in the body together. Some body structures are made up of connective tissue—notably, tendons and cartilage. Connective tissue also forms part of bone and the nonmuscular structures of arteries and veins.

muscle tissue A type of tissue adapted to contract, to cause movement.

nervous tissue Tissue composed of highly branched, elongated cells that transport nerve impulses from one part of the body to another.

Cardiovascular System

Major components
heart, blood vessels, and blood

Functions
• Carries blood and regulates blood supply

• Transports nutrients, waste products, hormones, and gases (oxygen and carbon dioxide) throughout the body

• Regulates blood pressure

Lymphatic and Immune Systems

Major lymphatic components
lymph, lymphocytes, lymphatic vessels, and lymph nodes

Major immune components
white blood cells, lymph vessels and nodes, spleen, thymus gland, and other lymph tissues

Lymphatic functions
• Removes foreign substances from blood and lymph

• Maintains tissue fluid balance

• Aids fat absorption

Immune functions
• Provides defense against pathogens

• Formation of white blood cells

Urinary System

Major components
kidneys, urinary bladder, and the ducts that carry urine

Functions
• Removes waste products from the blood and forms urine

• Regulates blood acid–base (pH) balance, overall chemical balance, and water balance

Nervous System

Major components
brain, spinal cord, nerves, and sensory receptors

Functions
• Detects and interprets sensation

• Controls movements, physiological, and intellectual functions

Endocrine System

Major components
endocrine glands, such as the pituitary, thyroid, and adrenal glands; hypothalamus; and pancreas

Functions
• Regulates metabolism, growth, reproduction, and many other functions by producing and releasing hormones

Digestive System

Major components
mouth, esophagus, stomach, intestines, and accessory organs (liver, gallbladder, and pancreas)

Functions
• Performs the mechanical and chemical processes of digestion of food, absorption of nutrients, and elimination of wastes

• Assists the immune system by destroying some pathogens and forming a barrier against foreign materials

FIGURE 3-2 ▲ Organ systems of the body. © McGraw-Hill Education

Integumentary System

Major components
skin, hair, nails, and sweat glands

Functions
- Protects the body
- Regulates body temperature
- Prevents water loss
- Produces vitamin D

Skeletal System

Major components
bones, cartilage, ligaments, and joints

Functions
- Protects organs
- Supports body weight
- Allows body movement
- Produces blood cells
- Stores minerals

Muscular System

Major components
smooth, cardiac, and skeletal muscle

Functions
- Produces body movement, heartbeat, and body heat
- Propels food in the digestive tract
- Maintains posture

Respiratory System

Major components
lungs and respiratory passages

Functions
- Exchanges gases (oxygen and carbon dioxide) between the blood and the air
- Regulates blood acid–base (pH) balance

Reproductive System

Major components
gonads (ovaries and testes), genitals, and breasts

Functions
- Performs the processes of sexual maturation and reproduction
- Influences sexual functions and behaviors
- Produces human milk to nourish an infant

FIGURE 3-2 ▲ *(Continued)*

We focus primarily on the digestive system in this chapter. The nutrients we consume in food are unavailable until they have been processed by the digestive system. Chemical and mechanical digestive processes alter food so that the nutrients can be released and absorbed into the body for distribution to body tissues.

Sometimes organs within a system can serve another system. For example, the basic function of the digestive system is to convert the food we eat into absorbable nutrients. At the same time, the digestive system serves the immune system by preventing dangerous pathogens from invading and causing illness in the body. As you study nutrition, you will note the multiple roles played by many organs (see Fig. 3-2).

The main objective of this chapter is to understand the actions of nutrients as they affect different cells, tissues, organs, and organ systems. As we explore several key organ systems—cardiovascular, lymphatic, urinary, nervous, endocrine, immune, and digestive systems—look for the ways each system both *affects* and *is affected by* nutrition.

Also in this chapter, we introduce the study of interactions between genetics and nutrition. Throughout this book, discussions will point out how you can personalize nutrition advice based on your genetic background. In this way, you can identify and avoid some controllable risk factors that would contribute to development of genetically linked diseases present in your family.

> ✓ **CONCEPT CHECK 3.3**
>
> 1. List the four types of tissues and give an example of where you could find each in the body.
> 2. Examine Figure 3-2. Provide three examples of ways the organs of one system support the functions of another system.

3.4 Cardiovascular System and Lymphatic System

cardiovascular system The body system consisting of the heart, blood vessels, and blood. This system transports nutrients, waste products, gases, and hormones throughout the body and plays an important role in immune responses and regulation of body temperature.

lymphatic system A system of vessels and lymph that accepts fluid surrounding cells and large particles, such as products of fat absorption. Lymph eventually passes into the bloodstream from the lymphatic system.

lymph A clear fluid that flows through lymph vessels; carries most forms of fat after their absorption by the small intestine.

plasma The fluid, extracellular portion of blood.

artery A blood vessel that carries blood away from the heart.

capillary A microscopic blood vessel that connects the smallest arteries and veins; site of nutrient, oxygen, and waste exchange between body cells and the blood.

vein A blood vessel that carries blood to the heart.

The body has two separate organ systems that circulate fluids in the body: the **cardiovascular system** and the **lymphatic system.** Some texts group these two systems together as the *circulatory system,* but each system has distinct components and functions. The cardiovascular system consists of the heart and blood vessels. The lymphatic system consists of lymphatic vessels and a number of lymph tissues. Blood flows through the cardiovascular system, while **lymph** flows through the lymphatic system.

CARDIOVASCULAR SYSTEM

The heart is a muscular pump that normally contracts and relaxes 50 to 90 times per minute when the body is at rest. This continual pumping, measured by taking your pulse, keeps blood moving through the blood vessels. The blood that flows through the cardiovascular system is composed of **plasma,** red blood cells, white blood cells, platelets, and many other substances. It travels two basic routes. In the first route, blood circulates from the right side of the heart, through the lungs, and then back to the heart. In the lungs, blood picks up oxygen and releases carbon dioxide. After this exchange of gases has taken place, blood is said to be *oxygenated* and returns to the left side of your heart. In the second route, the oxygenated blood circulates from the left side of the heart to all other body cells, eventually returning back to the right side of the heart (Fig. 3-3). After blood has circulated throughout the body, it is *deoxygenated.* (As you review the cardiovascular system, recall from your previous studies of biology that *left* and *right* designations of the heart refer to the left and right sides of your body, not of the diagram in front of you.)

In the cardiovascular system, blood leaves the heart via **arteries,** which branch into **capillaries,** a network of tiny blood vessels. Exchange of nutrients, oxygen, and waste products between the blood and cells occurs through the minute, weblike pores of the capillaries (Fig. 3-4). Capillaries service every region of the body via individual capillary beds that are only one cell layer thick. The blood then returns to the heart via the **veins.**

The cardiovascular system facilitates the exchange of oxygen, nutrients, and wastes between the body's internal and external environments. Other functions include delivery of hormones to their target cells, maintenance of a constant body temperature, and distribution of white blood cells throughout the body to protect against pathogens as part of the immune system (see Section 3.8).

(b)

1 Right side of the heart accepts oxygen-depleted venous blood that has already circulated to body cells.

2 Blood is pumped out of right side of the heart to lungs.

3 Gas exchange takes place in the lungs. Blood picks up oxygen and releases carbon dioxide.

4 Left side of the heart receives oxygen-rich blood from the lungs.

5 Oxygenated blood from the left side of the heart is destined for body cells.

6 Blood reaching the small intestine supplies oxygen and nutrients to intestinal cells; also picks up nutrients from digestion of food.

7 Nutrient-rich venous blood leaves the small intestine and travels via a portal vein to liver.

8 When blood reaches the kidney, waste products, excess nutrients, and water are removed. The removed substances are excreted via urine. Filtered blood returns back into circulation.

Capillaries
Vein
Artery
Head and arms
CO_2
O_2
Lungs
Heart
Liver
Portal vein
Intestine
Kidneys
Trunk and legs
CO_2
O_2
Capillaries

(a)

FIGURE 3-3 ▲ Blood circulation through the body. (a) The heart and some examples of the major arteries and veins of the cardiovascular system. (b) The paths that blood takes from the heart to the lungs (1–3), back to the heart (4), and through the rest of the body (5–8). The red color indicates blood richer in oxygen; blue is for blood carrying more carbon dioxide. Keep in mind that arteries and veins go to all parts of the body.

Portal Circulation in the Gastrointestinal Tract Water-soluble nutrients are transferred to the circulatory system through capillary beds. Once absorbed through the stomach or intestinal wall, nutrients reach one of two destinations. Some nutrients are taken up by cells in the intestines and portions of the stomach to nourish those organs. Most of these water-soluble nutrients from recently eaten foods, however, are transferred into the **hepatic portal circulation.** (The term *hepatic* refers to the liver. There are other portal systems in physiology, but the simpler terms *portal circulation* or *portal vein* usually refer to hepatic portal circulation.) To enter portal circulation, the nutrients pass from the intestinal capillaries into

hepatic portal circulation The portion of the circulatory system that uses a large vein (portal vein) to carry nutrient-rich blood from capillaries in the intestines and portions of the stomach to the liver.

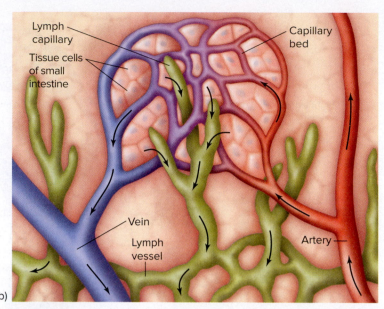

FIGURE 3-4 ▲ Capillary and lymph vessels. (a) Exchange of oxygen (O_2) and nutrients for carbon dioxide (CO_2) and other waste products occurs between the capillaries and the surrounding tissue cells. (b) Lymph vessels are also present in capillary beds, such as in the small intestine. Lymph vessels in the small intestine are also called *lacteals*. The lymph vessels have closed ends and are important for fat absorption.

hepatic portal vein Large vein leaving the intestine and stomach and connecting to the liver.

veins that eventually merge into a very large vein called the **hepatic portal vein.** Unlike most veins in the body—which carry blood back to the heart—this portal vein leads directly to the liver. This enables the liver to process absorbed nutrients before they enter the general circulation of the bloodstream. Overall, hepatic portal circulation represents a special form of circulation in the cardiovascular system.

LYMPHATIC SYSTEM

lymphatic system A system of vessels and lymph that accepts fluid surrounding cells and large particles, such as products of fat absorption. Lymph eventually passes into the bloodstream from the lymphatic system.

The **lymphatic system** consists of a network of lymphatic vessels and the fluid (lymph) that moves through them. The lymph vessels take up excess fluid that collects between cells and return it to the bloodstream. Lymph is similar to blood, consisting largely of blood plasma that has found its way out of capillaries and into the spaces between cells. It contains a full array of the various white blood cells that play an important role in the immune system. However, neither red blood cells nor platelets are present. Lymph is collected in tiny lymph vessels all over the body and moves through even larger vessels until it eventually enters the cardiovascular system through major veins near the heart. The lymphatic system does not have a pump (like the heart); its flow is driven by muscle contractions arising from normal body movements.

lacteal Lymphatic vessels that absorb fats from the small intestine.

Lymphatic Circulation in the Gastrointestinal Tract Besides contributing to the defense of the body against invading pathogens, lymphatic vessels that serve the small intestine, which are also called **lacteals,** play an important role in nutrition. These vessels pick up and transport the majority of products of fat digestion and fat absorption. These fat-related products are too large to enter the bloodstream directly and therefore are generally emptied into the bloodstream only after passing through the lymphatic system.

✓ CONCEPT CHECK 3.4

1. What is hepatic portal circulation?
2. Which nutrients are absorbed into the lymph? Why?
3. Describe how nutrients, oxygen, and wastes are exchanged between the body's internal and external environments.

- **1** Kidneys produce urine
- **2** Ureters transport urine
- **3** Urinary bladder stores urine
- **4** Urethra passes urine to outside

Artery leading to the kidney

Vein exiting the kidney

FIGURE 3-5 ◀ Organs of the urinary system. The kidneys (1), bean-shaped organs located on either side of the spinal column, filter waste from the blood and form urine, which is transported to the bladder by the ureters (2) and stored in the bladder (3) as urine. The urethra (4) transports the urine to outside the body. The urinary system of the female is shown. The male's urinary system is the same, except that the urethra extends through the penis.

3.5 Urinary System

The **urinary system** is composed of two kidneys, one on each side of the spinal column. Each kidney is connected to the bladder by a **ureter.** The bladder is emptied by way of the **urethra** (Fig. 3-5). The main function of the kidneys is to remove waste from the body. The kidneys are constantly filtering blood to control its composition. This results in the formation of urine, which is composed of water, dissolved waste products of metabolism such as **urea,** and excess or unneeded water-soluble vitamins and various minerals.

Together with the lungs, the kidneys also maintain the acid–base balance (**pH**) of the blood. The kidneys contribute to bone health because they convert a form of vitamin D into its active hormone form. The kidneys also produce a hormone that stimulates red blood cell synthesis (**erythropoietin;** see Section 14.6 for information on misuse of this hormone by some athletes). During times of fasting, the kidneys even produce glucose from certain amino acids. Thus, the kidneys perform many important functions related to nutrition and are a vital component of the body.

The proper function of the kidneys is closely tied to the strength of the cardiovascular system, particularly its ability to maintain adequate blood pressure, and the consumption of sufficient fluid. Uncontrolled diabetes, hypertension, and drug abuse are harmful to the kidneys.

✓ CONCEPT CHECK 3.5

1. The kidneys filter wastes from the blood. Trace the path of waste products out of the body.
2. How are the kidneys involved in bone health?

3.6 Nervous System

The **nervous system** is a regulatory system that centrally controls most body functions. The nervous system can detect changes occurring in various organs and the external environment and initiate corrective action when needed to maintain a constant internal body environment. The nervous system also regulates activities that change almost instantly, such as voluntary muscle contractions and the body's response to stress or danger. The body has many receptors that receive information about what is happening within the body and in the

urinary system The body system consisting of the kidneys, urinary bladder, and the ducts that carry urine. This system removes waste products from the circulatory system and regulates blood acid-base balance, overall chemical balance, and water balance in the body.

ureter Tube that transports urine from the kidney to the urinary bladder.

urethra Tube that transports urine from the urinary bladder to the outside of the body.

urea Nitrogenous waste product of protein metabolism; major source of nitrogen in the urine.

pH A measure of relative acidity or alkalinity of a solution. The pH scale is 0 to 14. A pH of 7 is neutral; a pH below 7 is acidic; a pH above 7 is alkaline.

erythropoietin A hormone secreted mostly by the kidneys that enhances red blood cell synthesis and stimulates red blood cell release from bone marrow.

nervous system The body system consisting of the brain, spinal cord, nerves, and sensory receptors. This system detects sensations, directs movements, and controls physiological and intellectual functions.

neuron The structural and functional unit of the nervous system. Consists of a cell body, dendrites, and an axon.

outside environment. For the most part, these receptors are found in our eyes, ears, skin, nose, and stomach. We act on information from these receptors via the nervous system.

The basic structural and functional unit of the nervous system is the **neuron.** Neurons are elongated, highly branched cells. The body contains about 100 billion neurons. Neurons respond to electrical and chemical signals, conduct electrical impulses, and release chemical regulators. Overall, neurons allow us to perceive what is occurring in our environment, engage in learning, store vital information in memory, and control the body's voluntary (and involuntary) actions.

The brain stores information, reacts to incoming information, solves problems, and generates thoughts. In addition, the brain plans a course of action based on the other sensory inputs. Responses to the stimuli are carried out mostly through the rest of the nervous system. Nutrition and brain health will be discussed in Section 13.7.

Simply put, the nervous system receives information through stimulation of various receptors, processes this information, and sends out signals through its various branches for an action that needs to be taken. Actual transmission of the signal occurs through a change in the concentration of two nutrients, sodium and potassium, in the neuron. There is an influx of sodium into the neuron and a loss of potassium as the message is sent. Concentrations of these minerals are then restored to normal amounts in the neuron after the signal passes, making it ready to conduct another message. You will learn more about the role of these electrolyte minerals in nerve transmission in Section 9.4.

synapse The space between one neuron and another neuron (or cell).

neurotransmitter A compound made by a nerve cell that allows for communication between it and other cells.

When the signal must bridge a gap (**synapse**) between the branches of different neurons, the message is generally converted into a chemical signal called a **neurotransmitter.** The neurotransmitter is then released into the gap, and its target may be another neuron or another type of cell, such as a muscle cell (Fig. 3-6). If the signal is sent to another neuron,

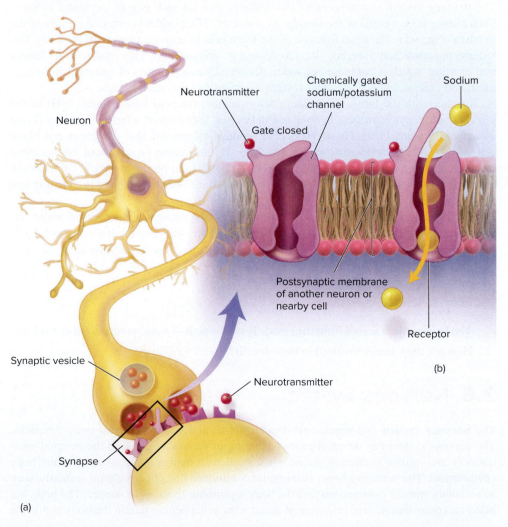

FIGURE 3-6 ▶ Transmission of a message from one neuron to another neuron or to another type of cell that relies on neurotransmitters. Figure (a) shows how vesicles containing neurotransmitters, formed within the neuron, fuse with the membrane of the neuron and the neurotransmitter is released into the synapse. Enlarged in (b), the neurotransmitter then binds to the receptors on the nearby neuron (or cell). In this way, the message is transmitted from one neuron to another or to the cell that ultimately performs the action directed by the message.

this allows it to continue on to its final destination. The neurotransmitters used in this process are often made from common nutrients found in foods, such as amino acids. The amino acid tryptophan is converted to the neurotransmitter serotonin, and the amino acid tyrosine is converted to the neurotransmitters **norepinephrine** and **epinephrine** (also called adrenaline).

Other nutrients also play a role in the nervous system. Calcium is needed for the release of neurotransmitters from neurons. Vitamin B-12 plays a role in the formation of the **myelin** sheath, which provides insulation around specific parts of most neurons. Finally, a regular supply of carbohydrate in the form of glucose is important for supplying fuel for the brain. The brain can use other calorie sources but generally relies on glucose.

norepinephrine A neurotransmitter from nerve endings and a hormone from the adrenal gland. It is released in times of stress and is involved in hunger regulation, blood glucose regulation, and other body processes.

epinephrine A hormone also known as *adrenaline;* it is released by the adrenal glands (located on each kidney) at times of stress. It acts to increase glycogen breakdown in the liver, among other functions.

myelin A lipid and protein combination (lipoprotein) that covers nerve fibers.

✔ CONCEPT CHECK 3.6

1. How are sodium and potassium involved in nerve impulse transmission?

2. How are signals transmitted between one neuron and the next? Why are amino acids important in this process?

3. Which nutrient is the brain's preferred source of fuel?

3.7 Endocrine System

The **endocrine system** plays a major role in the regulation of metabolism, reproduction, water balance, and many other functions by producing hormones in the **endocrine glands** of the body and subsequently releasing them into the blood (Table 3-1). The term *hormone* comes from a Greek word, meaning "to stir or excite." A true hormone is a regulatory compound that has a specific site of synthesis from which it then enters the bloodstream to reach target cells. Hormones are the messengers of the body. They can be permissive (turn on), antagonistic (turn off), or synergistic (work in cooperation with another hormone) in performing a task. Some compounds must undergo chemical changes before they can function as hormones. For example, vitamin D, synthesized in the skin or obtained from food, is converted into an active hormone by chemical changes made in the liver and kidneys.

The hormone **insulin,** synthesized in and released from the pancreas, helps control the amount of glucose in the blood (Fig. 3-7). Insulin is mostly produced when glucose in the blood rises to a certain level, usually after a meal. At this point, insulin is released and travels to the muscle, adipose, and liver cells of the body. Among its many functions, insulin allows for the movement of glucose from the blood into muscle and adipose cells. In the liver cells, insulin causes an increase in stored glycogen by stimulating the synthesis of glycogen from glucose. Once a sufficient amount of glucose has been cleared from the blood, the production of insulin lessens. The hormones epinephrine, norepinephrine, glucagon, and growth hormone have just the opposite effect on blood glucose. They all cause an increase in blood glucose through a variety of actions (see Table 3-1). **Thyroid hormones,** synthesized in and released from the thyroid gland, help to control the body's rate of metabolism. Other hormones are especially important in regulating digestive processes (see Section 3.9).

Hormones are not taken up by all cells in the body but only by those with the correct **receptor** protein. These binding sites, which generally are found on the cell membrane, are highly specific for a certain hormone. The hormone attaches to its receptor on the cell membrane. This binding activates additional compounds called second messengers within the cell to carry out the assigned task. This is true of insulin. A few hormones can penetrate the cell membrane and eventually bind to receptors on the DNA in the nucleus (e.g., thyroid hormone and estrogen).

endocrine system The body system consisting of the various glands and the hormones these glands secrete. This system has major regulatory functions in the body, such as reproduction and cell metabolism.

endocrine gland A hormone-producing gland.

insulin A hormone produced by the pancreas. One of insulin's roles is to increase the synthesis of glycogen in the liver and the movement of glucose from the bloodstream into body cells.

thyroid hormones Hormones produced by the thyroid gland that regulate growth and metabolic rate.

receptor A site in a cell at which compounds (such as hormones) bind. Cells that contain receptors for a specific compound are partially controlled by that compound.

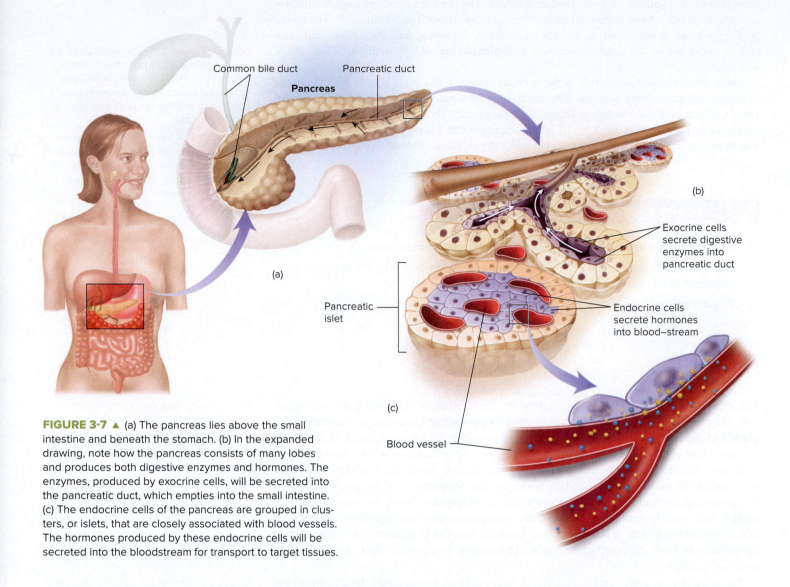

FIGURE 3-7 ▲ (a) The pancreas lies above the small intestine and beneath the stomach. (b) In the expanded drawing, note how the pancreas consists of many lobes and produces both digestive enzymes and hormones. The enzymes, produced by exocrine cells, will be secreted into the pancreatic duct, which empties into the small intestine. (c) The endocrine cells of the pancreas are grouped in clusters, or islets, that are closely associated with blood vessels. The hormones produced by these endocrine cells will be secreted into the bloodstream for transport to target tissues.

TABLE 3-1 ■ **Some Hormones of the Endocrine System with Nutritional Significance**

Hormone	Gland/Organ	Target	Effect	Role in Nutrition
Insulin	Pancreas	Adipose, muscle, and liver cells	Decreased blood glucose	Uptake and storage of glucose, fat, and amino acids by cells
Glucagon	Pancreas	Liver	Increased blood glucose	Release of glucose from liver stores, synthesis of glucose from amino acids, release of fat from adipose tissue
Epinephrine, Norepinephrine	Adrenal glands	Heart, blood vessels, brain, lungs	Increased body metabolism and blood glucose	Release of glucose and fat into the blood
Growth hormone	Pituitary gland	Most cells	Promotion of amino acid uptake by cells, increased blood glucose	Promotion of protein synthesis and growth, increased fat use for energy
Thyroid hormones	Thyroid gland	Most organs	Increased oxygen consumption, overall growth, brain development of the nervous system	Protein synthesis, increased body metabolism

☑ **CONCEPT CHECK 3.7**

1. Examine Figure 3-7. How does the pancreas have both endocrine and exocrine roles?
2. What effect does insulin have on the storage of nutrients?
3. List at least three hormones that tend to increase blood sugar.
4. If a person has hypothyroidism, the thyroid gland produces low levels of thyroid hormone. Will a person with hypothyroidism tend to lose weight or gain weight? Explain your answer.

3.8 Immune System

The immune system provides a very clear example of the interrelationship between nutrition status and organ system function. In developing nations, where food shortages are common, malnutrition increases susceptibility to infectious diseases, such as diarrheal disease. Cells throughout the body—skin and intestinal cells—work in concert with the cells and tissues of the immune system to defend the body against infection.

We are born with some aspects of immune function, such as physical and chemical barriers against infection, the inflammatory response, and the ability of some **white blood cells** to engulf microorganisms by **phagocytosis.** These are termed **nonspecific (innate) immunity,** because they protect the body against invasion by any microorganism. The skin and the intestinal cells support the immune system by forming an important barrier against invading microorganisms. If the integrity of either one of these barriers is compromised, microorganisms can invade the body and cause illness. Substances secreted by the skin and intestinal cells can also destroy pathogens.

If the body's nonspecific immune defenses are unable to block a microorganism's entry into the bloodstream, cells and chemicals involved in **specific (adaptive) immunity** will identify and destroy the invading pathogen. Specific immunity involves the process by which certain white blood cells produce **antibodies** (also called **immunoglobulins**) that target specific microorganisms or foreign proteins (known as **antigens**). After initial exposure to an antigen, a "memory" is created such that a second exposure to the substance will produce a more vigorous and rapid attack.

The turnover of many cells of the immune system is quite rapid—only a few hours or days. The constant resynthesis of cells requires steady nutrient intake. Nutrients that are important for the health of the immune system include protein, essential fatty acids, iron, copper, zinc, vitamins A, C, and D, and some B vitamins (see Chapter 10).

☑ **CONCEPT CHECK 3.8**

1. Contrast nonspecific (innate) and specific (adaptive) immunity.
2. What are the roles of antigens and antibodies in the immune response?
3. List three nutrients that support the immune system.

3.9 Digestive System

The foods and beverages we consume, for the most part, must undergo extensive alteration by the **digestive system** to provide us with usable nutrients. The processes of **digestion** and **absorption** take place in a long tube that is open at both ends and extends from the mouth to the anus. This tube is called the **gastrointestinal (GI) tract** (Fig. 3-8). The open space

white blood cells One of the formed elements of the circulating blood system; also called *leukocytes*. White blood cells are able to squeeze through intracellular spaces and migrate. They phagocytize bacteria, fungi, and viruses, as well as detoxify proteins that may result from allergic reactions, cellular injury, and other immune system cells.

phagocytosis A process in which a cell forms an indentation, and solid particles enter the indentation and are engulfed by the cell.

nonspecific immunity Defenses that stop the invasion of pathogens; requires no previous encounter with a pathogen; also called *innate immunity*.

specific immunity Function of white blood cells directed at specific antigens; also called *adaptive immunity*.

antibody Blood protein that binds foreign proteins found in the body.

antigen Any substance that induces a state of sensitivity and/or resistance to microorganisms or toxic substances after a lag period; a foreign substance that stimulates a specific aspect of the immune system.

digestive system System consisting of the gastrointestinal tract and accessory structures (liver, gallbladder, and pancreas). This system performs the mechanical and chemical processes of digestion, absorption of nutrients, and elimination of wastes.

digestion Process by which large ingested molecules are mechanically and chemically broken down to produce basic nutrients that can be absorbed across the wall of the GI tract.

absorption The process by which substances are taken up from the GI tract and enter the bloodstream or the lymph.

gastrointestinal (GI) tract The main sites in the body used for digestion and absorption of nutrients. It consists of the mouth, esophagus, stomach, small intestine, large intestine, rectum, and anus. Also called the *digestive tract*.

Organ	Digestive Functions
1 Mouth and salivary glands	Chew food Perceive taste Moisten food with saliva Lubricate food with mucus Release small amount of starch-digesting (amylase) and fat-digesting (lipase) enzymes Initiate swallowing reflex
2 Esophagus	Lubricate with mucus Move food to stomach by peristaltic waves (swallowing)
3 Stomach	Store, mix, dissolve, and continue digestion of food Dissolve food particles with secretions Kill microorganisms with acid Release protein-digesting (pepsin) and fat-digesting (lipase) enzymes Lubricate and protect stomach surface with mucus Regulate emptying of dissolved food into small intestine Produce intrinsic factor for vitamin B-12 absorption
4 Liver	Produce bile to aid fat digestion and absorption
5 Gallbladder	Store, concentrate, and later release bile into the small intestine
6 Pancreas	Secrete sodium bicarbonate and enzymes for digesting carbohydrate (amylase), fat (lipase), and protein (trypsin and chymotrypsin)
7 Small intestine	Mix and propel contents Lubricate with mucus Digest and absorb most substances using enzymes made by the pancreas (see above) and small intestinal cells (lactase, sucrase, maltase, and peptidases)
8 Large intestine	Mix and propel contents Absorb sodium, potassium, and water House bacteria Lubricate with mucus Synthesize some vitamins and short-chain fatty acids Form feces
9 Rectum	Hold feces and expel via the anus, which is the opening to the outside of the body

FIGURE 3-8 ▲ Physiology of the GI tract. Many organs cooperate in a regulated fashion to allow the digestion and absorption of nutrients in foods. Partially digested food spends about 2 to 3 hours in the stomach (longer for large meals). Passage through the small intestine takes 3 to 10 hours, followed by up to 72 hours in the large intestine. On average, digestion and absorption of a meal takes about 2 days. Food matter tends to pass more quickly through the GI tract of men than women.

lumen The hollow opening inside a tube, such as the GI tract.

motility Generally, the ability to move spontaneously. It also refers to movement of food through the GI tract.

inside the GI tract is called the **lumen.** Nutrients from the food we eat must pass through the walls of the GI tract—from the lumen through the cells lining the GI tract—to be absorbed into the bloodstream. The organs that make up the GI tract, as well as some additional accessory organs located nearby, are collectively known as the digestive system.

In the digestive system, food is broken down mechanically and chemically. Mechanical digestion takes place as soon as you begin chewing your food and continues as muscular contractions simultaneously mix and move food through the length of the GI tract (as part of a process known as **motility**).

Chemical digestion refers to the chemical breakdown of foods by acid and enzymes secreted into the GI tract. Enzymes are a key part of digestion. Each enzyme is specific to one type of chemical process. For example, the enzyme that recognizes and digests table sugar (sucrose) ignores milk sugar (lactose). Besides working on only specific types of chemicals, enzymes are sensitive to acidic and alkaline conditions, temperature, and the types of vitamins and minerals they require to function. Digestive enzymes that work in the

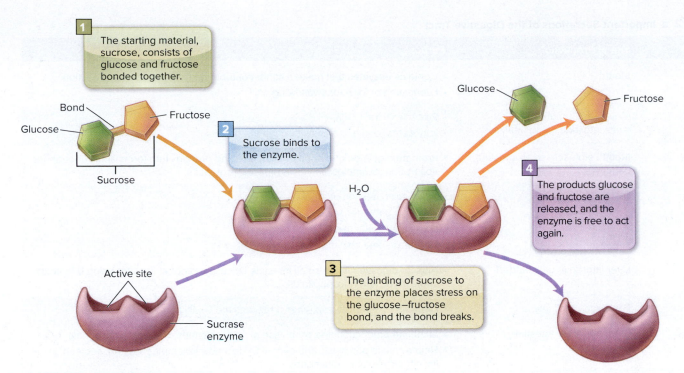

1. The starting material, sucrose, consists of glucose and fructose bonded together.

Bond

Glucose

Fructose

Sucrose

Active site

Sucrase enzyme

2. Sucrose binds to the enzyme.

H_2O

3. The binding of sucrose to the enzyme places stress on the glucose–fructose bond, and the bond breaks.

Glucose

Fructose

4. The products glucose and fructose are released, and the enzyme is free to act again.

FIGURE 3-9 ▲ A model of enzyme action. The enzyme sucrase splits the sugar sucrose into two simpler sugars, glucose and fructose. [Note that sometimes energy input is needed to make reactions occur.]

acidic environment of the stomach do not work well in the alkaline environment of the small intestine. The pancreas and small intestine produce most of the digestive enzymes; however, the mouth and the stomach also contribute their own enzymes to the process of digestion. The organs of the digestive system are able to fine-tune the production of each type of digestive enzyme in response to the nutritional makeup and amount of food consumed. Overall, the enzymes of the digestive system work together to hasten the breakdown of ingested food into absorbable nutrients (Fig. 3-9).

As food moves along the GI tract, nutrients are absorbed and the waste products reach the large intestine. In addition to nutrients from the food we eat, the bacteria that live in the large intestine produce some vitamins (vitamin K and biotin) that can be absorbed. The final role of the digestive system is elimination of wastes.

Most of the processes of digestion and absorption are under autonomic control; that is, they are involuntary. Almost all of the functions involved in digestion and absorption are controlled by signals from the nervous system, hormones from the endocrine system, and hormonelike compounds. Many common ailments arise from problems with the digestive system. Several of these digestive problems are discussed in Section 3.12.

The digestive system is composed of six separate organs; each organ performs one (or more) specific job(s). Let's look briefly at the role of each organ. These organs are shown in Figure 3-8. More detailed descriptions of digestive processes will be provided in later chapters as each nutrient is introduced.

MOUTH

The mouth performs many functions in the digestion of food. Besides chewing food to reduce it to smaller particles, the mouth also senses the taste of the foods we consume. The tongue, through the use of its taste buds, identifies foods on the basis of their specific flavor(s). Sweet, sour, salty, bitter, and **umami** comprise the primary taste sensations we experience. Recently, researchers have also proposed a sixth taste sensation—a taste for fat. Surprisingly, the nose and our sense of smell greatly contribute to our ability to sense the taste of food. When we chew a food, chemicals are released that stimulate the nasal passages. Thus, it makes perfect sense that when we have a cold and our nose is stuffed up and congested, even our favorite foods will not taste as good as they normally do.

umami A brothy, meaty, savory flavor in some foods. Monosodium glutamate enhances this flavor when added to foods.

TABLE 3-2 ■ **Important Secretions of the Digestive Tract**

Secretion	Site of Production	Purpose
Saliva	Mouth	• Contains enzymes that make a minor contribution to starch and fat digestion • Lubrication of food for swallowing
Mucus	Mouth, esophagus, stomach, small intestine, large intestine	• Protects GI tract cells • Lubricates food as it travels through the GI tract
Enzymes	Mouth, stomach, small intestine, pancreas	• Promote digestion of carbohydrates, fats, and proteins into forms small enough for absorption (examples: amylases, lipases, proteases)
Acid	Stomach	• Promotes digestion of protein • Destroys pathogens • Solubilizes some minerals • Activates some enzymes
Bile	Liver (stored in gallbladder)	• Aids fat digestion in the small intestine by suspending fat in water using **bile acids**, cholesterol, and phospholipids.
Bicarbonate	Pancreas, small intestine	• Neutralizes stomach acid when it reaches the small intestine
Hormones	Stomach, small intestine, pancreas	• Stimulate production and/or release of acid, enzymes, bile, and bicarbonate • Help regulate peristalsis and overall GI tract flow (examples: gastrin, secretin, insulin, cholecystokinin, glucagon)
Intrinsic factor	Stomach	• Facilitates absorption of vitamin B-12 in the small intestine

bile acid A compound produced by the liver. Bile acids are the main component of bile, which aids in emulsification of fat during digestion in the small intestine.

amylase Starch-digesting enzyme produced by the salivary glands and the pancreas.

lipase Fat-digesting enzyme produced by the salivary glands, stomach, and pancreas.

esophagus A tube in the GI tract that connects the pharynx with the stomach.

pharynx The organ of the digestive tract and respiratory tract located at the back of the oral and nasal cavities, commonly known as the throat.

epiglottis The flap that folds down over the trachea during swallowing.

bolus A moistened mass of food swallowed from the oral cavity into the pharynx.

peristalsis A coordinated muscular contraction used to propel food down the gastrointestinal tract.

lower esophageal sphincter A circular muscle that constricts the opening of the esophagus to the stomach. Also called the *gastroesophageal sphincter* or the *cardiac sphincter.*

The taste of food, or the anticipation of it, signals the rest of the GI tract to prepare for the digestion of food. Once in the mouth, mechanical and chemical digestion begins. Salivary glands produce **saliva,** which functions as a solvent so that food particles can be further separated and tasted. In addition, saliva contains a starch-digesting enzyme, salivary **amylase** (see Section 4.4 for more on starch-digesting enzymes) and a fat-digesting enzyme, **lipase** (see Section 5.4). **Mucus,** another component of saliva, makes it easy to swallow a mouthful of food. The food then travels to the esophagus. The important secretions and products of digestion are listed in Table 3-2.

ESOPHAGUS

The **esophagus** is a long tube that connects the **pharynx** with the stomach. Near the pharynx is a flap of tissue (called the **epiglottis**) that prevents the **bolus** of swallowed food from entering the trachea (wind pipe) (Fig. 3-10). During swallowing, food lands on the epiglottis, folding it down to cover the opening of the trachea. Breathing also stops automatically. These responses ensure that swallowed food will only travel down the esophagus. If food instead travels down the trachea, choking may occur (the victim will not be able to speak, cough, or breathe). A group of techniques to treat such a person is called the Heimlich maneuver (see www.heimlichinstitute.org for details).

At the top of the esophagus, nerve fibers release signals to tell the GI tract that food has been consumed. This results in an increase in GI muscle action, called **peristalsis.** These continual waves of muscle contractions, followed by muscle relaxation, force the food along the digestive tract from the esophagus onward (Fig. 3-11).

At the end of the esophagus is the **lower esophageal sphincter,** a muscle that constricts (closes) after food enters the stomach. The main function of sphincters is to prevent the backflow of GI tract contents. Sphincters respond to various stimuli, such as signals from the nervous system, hormones, acidic versus alkaline conditions, and pressure that builds up around the sphincter. The primary function of the lower esophageal sphincter is to prevent the acidic contents of the stomach from flowing back up into the esophagus. Dysfunction of this sphincter can cause some of the health problems we will discuss in Section 3.12.

FIGURE 3-10 ▲ The process of swallowing. (a) During swallowing, food does not normally enter the trachea because the epiglottis closes over the larynx. (b) The closed epiglottis allows food to proceed down the esophagus. When a person chokes, food becomes lodged in the trachea, blocking airflow to the lungs. (c) The food moves down the esophagus and the airway reopens.

No digestion or absorption occurs in the esophagus; it serves merely to transport food from the mouth to the stomach. The cells of the esophagus secrete mucus to lubricate the passage of food, but no digestive enzymes are produced.

STOMACH

The stomach is a large sac that can hold up to 4 cups (or 1 quart) of food for several hours until all of the food is able to enter the small intestine. Stomach size varies individually and can be reduced surgically as a radical treatment for obesity (more on this in Section 7.9). While in the stomach, the food is mixed with gastric juice, which contains water, hydrochloric acid, and enzymes. (*Gastric* is a term pertaining to the stomach.) The acid in the gastric juice destroys the biological activity of proteins, converts inactive digestive enzymes to their active form, partially digests food protein, and makes dietary minerals soluble so that they can be absorbed. The mixing that takes place in the stomach produces a watery food mixture, called **chyme,** which slowly leaves the stomach a teaspoon (5 milliliters) at a time and enters the small intestine. Following a meal, the stomach contents are emptied into the small intestine over the course of 1 to 4 hours. The **pyloric sphincter,** located at the base of the stomach, controls the rate at which the chyme is released into the small intestine (Fig. 3-12). There is very little absorption of nutrients from the stomach, except for some water and alcohol.

You might wonder how the stomach prevents itself from being digested by the acid and enzymes it produces. First, the stomach has a thick layer of mucus that lines and protects it. The production of acid and enzymes also requires the release of a specific hormone (gastrin). This release happens primarily when we are eating or thinking about eating. Last, as the concentration of acid in the stomach increases, hormonal control causes acid production to taper off.

One other important function of the stomach is the production of a substance called **intrinsic factor.** This vital proteinlike compound is essential for the absorption of vitamin B-12.

SMALL INTESTINE

The small intestine is considered "small" because its diameter is only 1 inch (2.5 centimeters). It is actually quite long—about 10 feet (3 meters), beginning at the stomach and extending to the large intestine (Fig. 3-13). The three parts of the small intestine are the **duodenum** (first 10 inches), the **jejunum** (second 4 feet), and the **ileum** (last 5 feet). Most of the digestion and absorption of food occurs in the small intestine. As chyme moves from the stomach into the first part of the small intestine, it is still very acidic. You just learned that the stomach secretes a thick layer of mucus to protect itself from the strong acid. However, if the small intestine were coated with mucus, digestion and absorption would be very limited.

FIGURE 3-11 ▲ Peristalsis. Peristalsis is a progressive type of movement, propelling material from point to point along the GI tract. To begin this, a ring of contraction occurs where the GI wall is stretched, passing the food mass forward. The moving food mass triggers a ring of contraction in the next region, which pushes the food mass even farther along. The result is a ring of contraction that moves like a wave along the GI tract, pushing the food mass down the tract.

chyme A mixture of stomach secretions and partially digested food.

pyloric sphincter Ring of smooth muscle between the stomach and the small intestine.

intrinsic factor A proteinlike compound produced by the stomach that enhances vitamin B-12 absorption.

duodenum First segment of the small intestine that receives chyme from the stomach and digestive juices from the pancreas and gallbladder. This is the site of most chemical digestion of nutrients; approximately 10 inches in length.

jejunum Middle segment of the small intestine; approximately 4 feet in length.

ileum Last segment of the small intestine; approximately 5 feet in length.

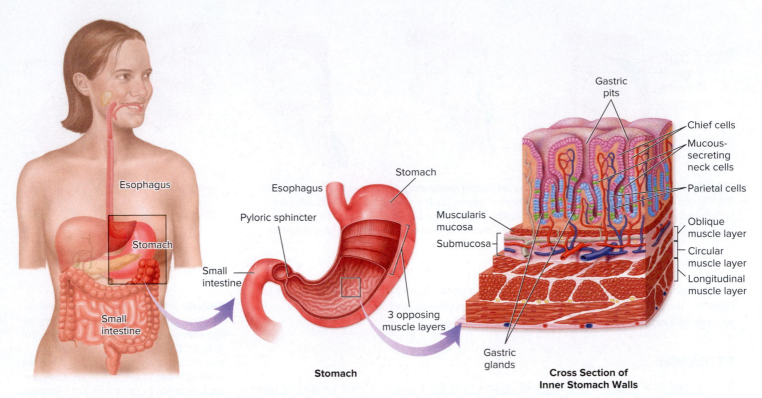

FIGURE 3-12 ▲ Physiology of the stomach. The interior surface mucous cells produce mucus for protection from stomach acid and enzymes. Parietal cells produce the hydrochloric acid (HCl), and chief cells produce the enzymes. Mucous neck cells, scattered among the cells in the gastric pits, also produce mucus. The exterior surface is made up of three layers of muscle that facilitate mechanical digestion.

villi (singular, villus) The fingerlike protrusions into the small intestine that participate in digestion and absorption of food.

absorptive cells Also known as *enterocytes;* the intestinal cells that line the villi and participate in nutrient absorption.

microvilli Extensive folds on the muscosal surface of the absorptive cells.

passive diffusion Movement of a substance across a semipermeable membrane from an area of higher solute concentration to an area of lower solute concentration. This type of transport does not require a carrier and does not require energy.

Therefore, the pancreas and intestinal cells secrete bicarbonate to neutralize the acid. The neutral pH also optimizes the activity of the digestive enzymes that work in the small intestine. Muscular contractions move the chyme through the small intestine and thoroughly mix food particles with digestive juices (review Fig. 3-11). These juices contain many enzymes that break down carbohydrates, protein, fat, and some vitamins into absorbable units.

The physical structure of the small intestine is very important to the body's ability to digest and absorb the nutrients it needs. The lining of the small intestine is called the mucosa and is folded many times; within these folds are fingerlike projections called **villi.** These "fingers" are constantly moving, which helps them trap food to enhance absorption. Each individual villus (singular) is made up of many **absorptive cells** (also called enterocytes), and the mucosal surface of each of these cells is folded even further into **microvilli.** The combined folds, villi, and microvilli in the small intestine increase its surface area 600 times beyond that of a simple tube (see Fig. 3-13).

The absorptive cells have a short life. New intestinal absorptive cells are constantly produced in the crypts of the small intestinal lining (see Fig. 3-13) and appear daily along the surface of each villus "finger." This is probably because absorptive cells are subjected to a harsh environment, so renewal of the intestinal cell lining is necessary. This rapid cell turnover leads to high nutrient needs for the small intestine. Fortunately, many of the old cells can be broken down and have their component parts reused. The health of the cells is further enhanced by various hormones and other substances that participate in or are produced as part of the digestive process.

The small intestine absorbs nutrients through the intestinal wall through various means and processes, as illustrated in Figure 3-14.

- **Passive diffusion:** When the nutrient concentration is higher in the lumen of the small intestine than in the absorptive cells, the difference in nutrient concentration drives the nutrient into the absorptive cells by diffusion. Fats, water, and some minerals are examples of nutrients that move down a concentration gradient to be absorbed by passive diffusion.

(a)

(b)

(c)

(d)

(e)

FIGURE 3-13 ▲ Organization of the small intestine. (a) The three parts of the small intestine are the duodenum (10 in), jejunum (4 ft), and ileum (5 ft). (b) Several layers of muscle work together to mix and propel chyme through the small intestine. (c) The highly folded lining of the small intestine increases the surface area for absorption up to 600 times that of a simple tube. (d) The villi are covered with absorptive cells. Capillaries and lacteals inside each villus transport nutrients from the absorptive cells of the small intestine through the blood and lymph. (e) The mucosal side of the absorptive cells is covered with microvilli, which maximize nutrient absorption.

FIGURE 3-14 ◄ Nutrient absorption relies on four major absorptive processes. (1) Passive diffusion (in blue) is diffusion of nutrients across the absorptive cell membranes. (2) Facilitated diffusion (in green) uses a carrier protein to move nutrients down a concentration gradient. (3) Active absorption (in purple) involves a carrier protein as well as energy to move nutrients (against a concentration gradient) into absorptive cells. (4) Phagocytosis and pinocytosis (in green and brown) are forms of active transport in which the absorptive cell membrane forms an indentation that engulfs a nutrient to bring it into the cell.

facilitated diffusion Movement of a substance across a semipermeable membrane from an area of higher solute concentration to an area of lower solute concentration. This type of transport does not require energy, but it does require a carrier.

active absorption Movement of a substance across a semipermeable membrane from an area of lower solute concentration to an area of higher solute concentration. This type of transport requires energy and a carrier.

phagocytosis A process in which a cell forms an indentation, and solid particles enter the indentation and are engulfed by the cell.

pinocytosis A process in which a cell forms an indentation, and fluid enters the indentation and is engulfed by the cell.

ileocecal sphincter The ring of smooth muscle between the end of the small intestine and the beginning of the large intestine.

- **Facilitated diffusion:** Some compounds require a carrier protein to follow a concentration gradient into absorptive cells. This type of absorption is called faciliated diffusion. Fructose is one example of a compound that makes use of such a carrier to allow for facilitated diffusion.
- **Active absorption:** In addition to the need for a carrier protein, some nutrients also require energy input to move from the lumen of the small intestine into the absorptive cells. This mechanism makes it possible for cells to take up nutrients even when they are consumed in low concentrations (i.e., against a concentration gradient). Some sugars, such as glucose, are actively absorbed, as are amino acids.
- **Phagocytosis** and **pinocytosis:** In a further means of active absorption, absorptive cells literally engulf compounds (phagocytosis) or liquids (pinocytosis). A cell membrane can form an indentation of itself so that when particles or fluids move into the indentation, the cell membrane surrounds and engulfs them. This process is used when an infant absorbs immune substances from human milk (see Section 18.7).

Once absorbed, water-soluble compounds such as glucose and amino acids are transported by the capillaries to the portal vein. Recall that the liver is the end of this process. Most fats are absorbed into the lymph vessels, which eventually empty into the bloodstream (review Figs. 3-3 and 3-4).

Undigested food cannot be absorbed into cells of the small intestine. Any undigested food that reaches the end of the small intestine must pass through the **ileocecal sphincter** on the way to the large intestine (Fig. 3-15). This sphincter prevents the contents of the large intestine from reentering the small intestine.

CRITICAL THINKING

The authors of some popular (fad) diet books contend that eating certain combinations of foods, such as meats and fruits together, hinders the digestive processes. Based on what you have learned so far about the enzymes and digestion, does this sound accurate?

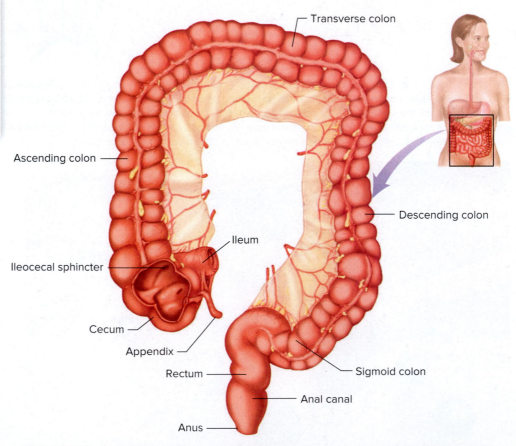

FIGURE 3-15 ▲ The parts of the large intestine include the cecum, ascending colon, transverse colon, descending colon, and sigmoid colon. Overall, the large intestine is about 3 ½ feet (1.1 meters) long.

LARGE INTESTINE

When the contents of the small intestine enter the large intestine, the material left bears little resemblance to the food originally eaten. Under normal circumstances, only a minor amount (5%) of carbohydrate, protein, and fat escapes absorption to reach the large intestine (Table 3-3).

The large intestine (sometimes called the *colon*) can be subdivided into five main segments: the **cecum, ascending colon, transverse colon, descending colon,** and **sigmoid colon** (see Fig. 3-15). Physiologically, the large intestine differs from the small intestine in that there are no villi or digestive enzymes. The absence of villi means that little absorption takes place in the large intestine in comparison to the small intestine. Nutrients absorbed from the large intestine include water, some vitamins, some fatty acids, and the minerals sodium and potassium. Unlike the small intestine, the large intestine has a number of mucus-producing cells. The mucus secreted by these cells functions to hold the feces together and protect the large intestine from the bacterial activity within it.

The large intestine is home to a large population of bacteria (over 500 different species). While the stomach and small intestine have some bacterial activity, the large intestine is the organ most heavily colonized with bacteria. Starting at infancy, the diet plays a major part in determining the type of bacteria in our digestive tracts. The number and type of bacteria in the human colon recently has become of great interest. Research has shown that intestinal bacteria play a significant role in the maintenance of health, especially health of the colon. It is speculated that higher levels of beneficial organisms can reduce the activity of disease-causing bacteria. This is another illustration of the GI tract working as an important immune organ. The strains *bifidobacteria* and *lactobacilli* are typically associated with health, whereas *clostridia* are considered problematic. Bacteria in the large intestine are able to break down some of the remaining food products that enter the large intestine, such as the milk sugar lactose (in lactose-intolerant people), and some components of fiber. Some of the products of bacterial metabolism in the large intestine, which include various fatty acids and gases, can then be absorbed.

cecum A pouch at the first part of the large intestine that houses many bacteria.

ascending colon Segment of the large intestine that carries feces from the cecum, up the right side of the abdomen, to the transverse colon.

transverse colon Segment of the large intestine that carries feces from the ascending colon, from right to left across the top of the abdomen, to the descending colon.

descending colon Segment of the large intestine that carries feces from the transverse colon, down the left side of the abdomen, to the sigmoid colon.

sigmoid colon Last segment of the large intestine that carries feces from the descending colon to the rectum.

TABLE 3-3 ■ Major Sites of Absorption Along the GI Tract

Organ	Primary Nutrients Absorbed
Stomach	Alcohol (20% of total)
	Water (minor amount)
Small intestine	Calcium, magnesium, iron, and other minerals
	Glucose
	Amino acids
	Fats
	Vitamins
	Water (70% to 90% of total)
	Alcohol (80% of total)
	Bile acids
Large intestine	Sodium
	Potassium
	Some fatty acids
	Gases
	Water (10% to 30% of total)

Newsworthy Nutrition

Probiotics Provide Relief from Constipation

Up to 25% of adults suffer from functional constipation, a problem characterized by infrequent or difficult bowel movements not due to a physical cause. Typically, functional constipation is treated with medications that can have side effects or lead to dependence. In this study, 40 adults with functional constipation were randomly assigned to receive a daily probiotic supplement containing *Lactobacillus reuteri* or placebo for 4 weeks. By the end of the study period, subjects who received the probiotics reported increased frequency of bowel movements (5.3 per week) compared with subjects who received placebo (2.7 per week). No adverse effects were reported. This study demonstrated that taking a probiotic supplement can significantly increase the frequency of bowel movements among adults with functional constipation.

Source: Ojetti V and others: The effect of *Lactobacillus reuteri* supplementation in adults with chronic functional constipation: A randomized, double-blind, placebo-controlled trial. *Journal of Gastrointestinal and Liver Diseases* 23(4):387, 2014 (see Further Reading 16).

probiotic Live microorganisms that, when administered in adequate amounts, confer health benefits on the host.

prebiotic Selectively fermented ingredient that results in specific changes in the composition and/or activity of the gastrointestinal microbiota, thus conferring benefits upon the host.

feces Mass of water, fiber, tough connective tissues, bacterial cells, and sloughed intestinal cells that passes through the large intestine and is excreted through the anus; also called *stool*.

rectum Terminal portion of the large intestine.

anus Last portion of the GI tract; serves as an outlet for the digestive system.

anal sphincters A group of two sphincters (inner and outer) that help control expulsion of feces from the body.

gallbladder An organ attached to the underside of the liver; site of bile storage, concentration, and eventual secretion.

bile A liver secretion stored in the gallbladder and released through the common bile duct into the first segment of the small intestine. It is essential for the digestion and absorption of fat.

Foods containing certain live microorganisms such as *lactobacilli* have been linked to some health benefits, such as improving intestinal tract health. These microorganisms are called **probiotics** because once consumed, they take up residence in the large intestine and confer health benefits. You can find these probiotic microorganisms in certain forms of fluid milk, fermented milk, and yogurt, and in pill form (see Further Reading 16). A related term is **prebiotic.** These are substances that increase growth of probiotic microorganisms. One example is fructooligosaccharides (see Table 1-3 in Chapter 1 for dietary sources). The beneficial organisms of the large intestine and their use as probiotics are highlighted in Newsworthy Nutrition.

Some water remains in the material that enters the large intestine because the small intestine absorbs only 70% to 90% of the fluid it receives, which includes large amounts of GI-tract secretions produced during digestion. The remnants of a meal also contain some minerals and some fiber. Because water is removed from the large intestine, its contents become semisolid by the time they have passed through the first two-thirds of it. What remains in the **feces,** besides water and undigested fiber, is tough connective tissues (from animal foods); bacteria from the large intestine; and some body wastes, such as parts of dead intestinal cells.

RECTUM

The feces or stool remains in the last portion of the large intestine, the **rectum,** until muscular movements push it into the **anus** to be eliminated. The presence of feces in the rectum stimulates elimination. The anus contains two **anal sphincters** (internal and external), one of which is under voluntary control (external sphincter). Relaxation of this sphincter allows for elimination.

ACCESSORY ORGANS

The liver, **gallbladder,** and pancreas work with the GI tract and are considered accessory organs to the process of digestion (review Fig. 3-8). These accessory organs are not part of the GI tract through which food passes, but they play necessary roles in the process of digestion. These organs secrete digestive fluids into the GI tract and enable the process of converting food into absorbable nutrients.

The liver produces a substance called **bile.** The bile is stored and concentrated in the gallbladder until the gallbladder receives a hormonal signal to release the bile. This signal is induced by the presence of fat in the small intestine. Bile is released and delivered to the duodenum via a tube called the bile duct (Fig. 3-16).

In action, bile is like soap. Components of the bile enable large portions of fat to break into smaller bits so that they can be suspended in water (Chapter 5 will cover this process in detail). Interestingly, some of the bile constituents can be "recycled" in a process known as **enterohepatic circulation.** These components of bile are reabsorbed from the small intestine, returned to the liver via the portal vein, and reused.

In addition to bile, the liver releases a number of other unwanted substances that travel with the bile to the gallbladder and end up in the small intestine and eventually in the large intestine for excretion. The liver functions in this manner to remove unwanted substances from the blood. (Other by-products are excreted via the urine; see Section 3.5.)

The pancreas has both endocrine and digestive functions. As a gland of the endocrine system, the pancreas manufactures hormones—insulin and glucagon—that are secreted into the blood to regulate blood glucose levels (review Fig. 3-7). As an organ of the digestive system, it produces "pancreatic juice," a mixture of water, bicarbonate, and a variety of digestive enzymes capable of breaking apart carbohydrates, proteins, and fats into small fragments. Bicarbonate is a base that neutralizes the acidic chyme as it moves from the stomach into the duodenum. As noted earlier, the small intestine does not have a protective layer of mucus because mucus would impede nutrient absorption. Instead, the neutralizing capacity of bicarbonate from the pancreas protects the walls of the small intestine from erosion by acid, which would otherwise lead to the formation of an ulcer (see Section 3.12).

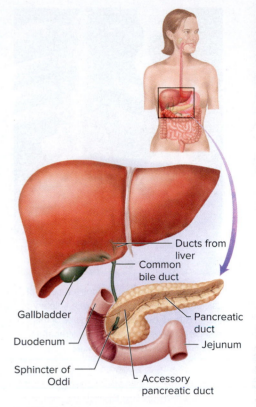

FIGURE 3-16 ▲ Bile is produced by the liver and stored in the gallbladder. The pancreas produces pancreatic juice, which contains water, bicarbonate, and digestive enzymes. When chyme reaches the small intestine, bile is released from the gallbladder through the common bile duct. In addition, pancreatic juices flow through the pancreatic duct, which joins the common bile duct at the sphincter of Oddi. Relaxation of this sphincter releases both bile and pancreatic juice into the duodenum to facilitate digestion.

enterohepatic circulation A continual recycling of compounds such as bile acids between the small intestine and the liver.

adipose tissue Connective tissue made up of cells that store fat and also cushions and insulates the body.

✅ **CONCEPT CHECK 3.9**

1. Choose three secretions of the digestive system. Where is each secreted? What is the role of each in the process of digestion?

2. What are enzymes? Is bile an enzyme?

3. How do mucus and surface area affect absorption?

4. Which absorptive processes use energy? How does *concentration gradient* factor into this?

5. What did you have for lunch today? Trace the path of your meal through the digestive system. Where is each nutrient broken down as it passes through the GI tract? Where is each absorbed?

3.10 Nutrient Storage Capabilities

The human body must maintain reserves of nutrients; otherwise, we would need to eat continuously. Storage capacity varies for each different nutrient. Most fat is stored in **adipose tissue,** made up of cells designed specifically for this. Short-term storage of carbohydrate occurs in muscle and liver in the form of glycogen. The blood maintains a small reserve of glucose and amino acids. Many vitamins and minerals are stored in the liver, whereas other nutrient stores are found in other sites in the body.

When people do not meet their needs for certain nutrients, blood levels of these nutrients can be maintained by breaking down body tissues. For example, calcium is taken from bone and protein is taken from muscle. In cases of long-term deficiency, these nutrient losses weaken and harm these tissues.

Many people believe that if too much of a nutrient is obtained—for example, from a vitamin or mineral supplement—only what is needed is stored and the rest is excreted by the body. Though true for some nutrients, such as vitamin C, the large dosages of other nutrients frequently found in supplements, such as vitamin A and iron, can cause harmful side effects because they are not readily excreted. This is one reason why obtaining your nutrients primarily (or exclusively) from a balanced diet is the safest means to acquire the building blocks you need to maintain the good health of all organ systems.

▲ The skeletal system provides a reserve of calcium for day-to-day needs when dietary intake is inadequate. Long-term use of this reserve, however, reduces bone strength.
© Jason Reed/Ryan McVay/Getty Images

epigenome A network of chemical compounds surrounding DNA that modify the genome without altering the DNA sequences and have a role in determining which genes are active (expressed) or inactive (silenced) in a particular cell.

epigenetics Heritable changes in gene function that are independent of DNA sequence. For example, malnutrition during pregnancy may modify gene expression in the fetus and affect long-term body weight regulation in the offspring.

Nutrition and genetics interact in various ways:
- Genes dictate much of our individual nutrient requirements.
- Genes may make us more susceptible or resistant to certain nutrition-related diseases.
- Nutrients and other dietary components can affect gene expression.

nutritional genomics Study of interactions between nutrition and genetics; includes nutrigenetics and nutrigenomics.

nutrigenetics Study of the effects of genes on nutritional health, such as variations in nutrient requirements and responsiveness to dietary modifications.

nutrigenomics Study of how food impacts health through its interaction with our genes and its subsequent effect on gene expression.

✓ **CONCEPT CHECK 3.10**

1. What is the body's most efficient form of energy storage?
2. Why is it important to consume nutrients daily?
3. When it comes to vitamins and minerals, is consuming more than the RDA or AI a good way to ensure optimal nutrition status? Why or why not?

3.11 Nutrition and Genetics

Once nutrients and other dietary components are taken up by cells, they may interact with our genes and may affect gene expression. The growth, development, and maintenance of cells, and ultimately of the entire organism, are directed by genetic mechanisms present in the cells. Each gene essentially represents instructions for a recipe, noting the ingredients (nucleic acids forming amino acids) and how these ingredients are arranged (to create proteins). The products (proteins) of all the recipes in the cookbook (the human genome) make up the human organism. The genome and the **epigenome** control the expression of genes and determine individual traits such as eye color and susceptibility to many diseases. **Epigenetics** refers to changes in gene expression caused by mechanisms other than changes in the underlying DNA sequence. While our genome contains the code for the proteins that can be made by our bodies, our epigenome is an extra layer of instructions that influences gene activity. In many cases, it is the epigenome that can be altered by environmental and dietary factors, rather than altering the genetic sequence.

The causes of chronic diseases are complex and include both genetic and environmental components. Fortunately, scientific breakthroughs in our understanding of the links between nutrition and genetics are beginning to become clearer. Genetic discoveries are leading to new drugs that target disease processes at the molecular level as well as affordable genetic tests that predict our risk for disease.

THE EMERGING FIELD OF NUTRITIONAL GENOMICS

In the near future, the accessibility of genetic information will enhance the ability of health professionals to personalize nutrition recommendations that can optimize nutritional status and improve the outcomes of nutrition-related diseases. Collectively, the interactions between genetics and nutrition are known as **nutritional genomics.** It is evident that nutritional status can both *affect* and *be affected by* an individual's genetic makeup. **Nutrigenetics** is the branch of nutritional genomics that examines how variations in genes can affect nutritional health. For example, the efficiency of absorption, metabolism, and excretion of a particular nutrient is controlled by genes. On the other hand, **nutrigenomics** refers to the many ways dietary components affect gene expression—particularly as it relates to development and treatment of nutrition-related diseases, such as cardiovascular disease. Let us examine each of these branches of nutritional genomics more closely.

In Section 2.6, you learned how Dietary Reference Intakes are set. Recall that nutrient recommendations, such as RDAs, are not absolute but are actually estimates of a level of intake that is likely to meet the needs of most (97% to 98%) of the population. For example, the RDA for folic acid (a B vitamin) is 400 micrograms per day. For most of the population, consuming 400 micrograms per day of folic acid from foods or supplemental sources will supply enough of the vitamin to optimize its function in body processes, such as the formation of red blood cells and metabolism of amino acids. There are certain subgroups of the population, however, for whom 400 micrograms of folic acid is not sufficient. These people have a genetic variation that alters the production of an enzyme necessary for amino acid metabolism, so their dietary requirements for folic acid may be as much as 10 times higher than the RDA. Nutrigenetics researchers are actively examining how genetic variations like this can affect individual nutrient requirements, how we can identify these people, and how we can personalize nutrition advice based on this knowledge (see Further Readings 1 and 6).

With nutrigenomics, researchers are interested in finding out how nutrients or other dietary components can influence gene expression, particularly as it relates to development of chronic diseases. Traditionally, nutrition and lifestyle recommendations have been based on the results of observational or experimental research that links diet to disease within the population as a whole. Nutrigenomics research now highlights the fallacy of a "one-size-fits-all" approach to nutrition interventions for disease prevention and management. It is becoming clear that generalized nutrition recommendations may not apply to all individuals within a population group. Nutrients or other compounds in the diet can turn certain genes on or off (like a light switch), thus manipulating the production of proteins that can affect—positively or negatively—the development or progression of diseases. Current areas of research include obesity, diabetes, cardiovascular disease, celiac disease, cancer, osteoporosis, and Alzheimer's disease. With a better understanding of the interactions between genes and our diet, it will not be long before dietary recommendations can be tailored to help those with genetically linked diseases.

▲ Studies of twins have provided strong evidence for the interaction between genes and diet and their combined effects on disease risk. © Royalty-Free/Corbis

NUTRITIONAL DISEASES WITH A GENETIC LINK

Studies of families, including those with identical twins and adopted children, provide strong support for the effects of genetics in various disorders. In fact, family history is considered to be an important risk factor in the development of many nutrition-related diseases.

Cardiovascular Disease There is strong evidence that cardiovascular disease is the result of gene–environment interactions. About one of every 500 people in North America has a defective gene that greatly delays cholesterol removal from the bloodstream. Another genetic variation can lead to elevated blood levels of an amino acid, called homocysteine, which increases cardiovascular disease risk. As discussed in Section 1.2, elevated blood cholesterol is one of the risk factors for development of cardiovascular disease. Discoveries of gene–diet interactions related to management of blood lipids will allow for personalized treatment plans for medications and nutrition therapy to reduce disease risk and improve health outcomes. Although dietary modifications are important and can make a difference, medications and even surgery are often warranted to fully address these problems.

Obesity Most obese North Americans have at least one obese parent. This strongly suggests a genetic link. Findings from many human studies suggest that a variety of genes (likely 60 or more) are involved in the regulation of body weight. For example, specific gene variations have been linked to the propensity to overeat and alterations in metabolism.

Still, although some individuals may be genetically predisposed to store body fat, whether they do so depends on how many calories they consume relative to their needs. A common concept in nutrition is that *nurture*—how people live and the environmental factors that influence them—allows *nature*—each person's genetic potential—to be expressed. Although not every person with a genetic tendency toward obesity becomes obese, those genetically predisposed to weight gain have a higher lifetime risk than individuals without a genetic predisposition to obesity.

Diabetes Both of the two common types of diabetes—type 1 and type 2—have genetic links. Evidence for these genetic links comes from studies of families, including twins, and from the high incidence of diabetes among certain population groups (e.g., South Asians or Pima Indians). Diabetes, in fact, is a complex disease with more than 200 genes identified as possible causes. Only sensitive and expensive testing can identify who is at greatest risk. Type 2 diabetes is the most common form of diabetes (90% of all cases) and is linked to obesity. Typically, type 2 diabetes is diagnosed after a person becomes obese, not before. In this case, nurture affects nature.

Cancer Approximately 10% of cancers have a genetic link. Approximately 90% of cancers are related to environmental and lifestyle factors. Body weight and dietary patterns have

▲ Genetic testing for disease susceptibility will be more common in the future as the genes that increase the risk of developing various diseases are isolated and decoded.

© Rob Meinychuk/Getty Images

been estimated to account for approximately 60% of all cancers. Other environmental influences on cancer risk include tobacco, sedentary lifestyles, family history, viruses, radiation, and toxic exposures.

YOUR GENETIC PROFILE

From this discussion, you can see that your genes can greatly influence your risk of developing certain diseases. By recognizing your potential for developing a particular disease, you can avoid behaviors and exposures that further raise your risk. How can you figure out your genetic profile? Genetic testing can be valuable if it confirms that you carry a genetic mutation associated with a disease and might alter the course of treatment. Testing is also of interest when you do not know your family medical history or there are gaps in your family tree. Depending on the gene of interest, it typically costs under $1000 to have your DNA sequenced to reveal potential susceptibility for diseases or disorders. Many genetic tests are now covered by health insurance plans. The Genetic Information Nondiscrimination Act (GINA), which became a law in May 2008, prohibits health insurers from raising premiums or denying coverage based on genetic information. DNA testing includes providing a DNA sample (blood, saliva, hair). Areas of interest in the genome are sequenced and read in a process known as genotyping. If you are considering genetic testing, it is best to consult a Certified Genetic Counselor. You can find one at nsgc.org.

Many of the genes involved in common diseases, such as diabetes, are still unknown. Although there are genetic tests available for some diseases, your family history of certain diseases is still a much better indicator of your genetic profile and risk of disease. Put together a family tree of illnesses and deaths by compiling a few key facts on your primary relatives: siblings, parents, aunts and uncles, and grandparents, as suggested in the Rate Your Plate section. In general, the greater number of your relatives who had a genetically transmitted disease and the closer they are related to you, the greater your risk. If there is a significant family history of a certain disease, lifestyle changes may be appropriate. For example, women with a family history of breast cancer should avoid becoming overweight or obese, minimize alcohol use, and continue regular checkups.

Figure 3-17 shows an example of a medical family tree (also called a *genogram*). Risk is high when two or more first-degree relatives in a family have a specific disease (first-degree relatives include one's biological parents, siblings, and offspring) or when a first-degree relative develops a disease before the age of 50 to 60 years. In the family depicted in Figure 3-17, prostate cancer killed the man's father. Knowing this, the man should be tested regularly for prostate cancer. His sisters should have frequent mammograms and breast exams because their mother died of breast cancer. Because heart attack and stroke are also common in the family, all the children should adopt a lifestyle that minimizes the risk of developing these conditions, such as avoiding excessive animal fat and salt intake. Colon cancer is also evident, so careful screening throughout life is important.

Information about our genetic makeup should increasingly influence our dietary and lifestyle choices. Throughout this text, we will discuss "controllable" risk factors that could contribute to development of genetically linked diseases present in your family. This information will help you personalize nutrition advice based on your genetic background, and identify and avoid the risk factors that could lead to the diseases present in your family.

PERSONALIZING NUTRITION ADVICE

Nutrition professionals already recognize that dietary advice must be tailored to personal and cultural preferences. Research is now paving the way for even more personalized nutrition that incorporates the results of genetic testing to determine which diet will work most effectively for each person. There are genetic tests available for at least 1500 diseases and conditions. Many companies—most of them online—are already offering dietary advice and supplements based on direct-to-consumer genetic tests.

As we discussed in Section 2.7 caution is always needed when evaluating nutrition information and claims. Some DNA-testing companies are responsible organizations, but many

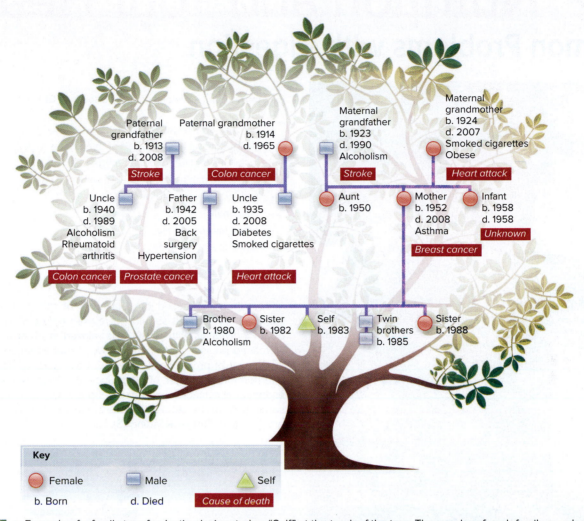

FIGURE 3-17 ▲ Example of a family tree for Justin, designated as "Self" at the trunk of the tree. The gender of each family member is identified by color (blue squares for males and orange circles for females). Dates of birth (b) and death (d) are listed below each family member. If deceased, the cause of death is highlighted using white text against a red background. Other medical conditions the family members experienced are noted beneath each name. Create your own family tree of frequent diseases using the diagram in Rate Your Plate or the interactive tool available at https://familyhistory.hhs.gov/FHH/html/index.html. Then show your family tree to your physician to get a more complete picture of what the information means for your health.

are not. Marketing schemes may belittle the science of genetics to consumers. Even though there have been some great advancements in nutritional genomics in recent years, there is still much to learn. Not only is the science of nutritional genomics in its infancy, but application of this technology will require advanced training for health practitioners. Most health professionals agree that genetic testing complements carefully planned nutrient recommendations and dietary guidelines, but on its own, it is not quite ready for "prime time."

This chapter's review of human anatomy, physiology, and genetics from a nutrition perspective sets the stage for a more in-depth look at the nutrients in Chapters 4 through 13. As you learn about recommendations for specific nutrients or prevention of diseases, keep in mind that individual variations in genetic profiles will prove to be important considerations when tailoring nutrition advice.

✓ **CONCEPT CHECK 3.11**

1. What is the difference between nutrigenetics and nutrigenomics?
2. List two nutrition-related diseases that are strongly affected by genetics.
3. Predict how nutritional genomics will affect nutrition recommendations in the future.

Common Problems with Digestion

© Royalty-Free/Corbis

When suffering from persistent heartburn or GERD, see a doctor if you have

- difficulty swallowing or pain when swallowing.
- heartburn that has persisted for more than 10 years.
- initial onset of heartburn after age 50.
- heartburn that resists treatment with medications.
- sudden, unexplained weight loss.
- chest pain.
- blood loss or anemia.
- blood in stool or vomit.

Heartburn is caused by relaxation of the gastroesophageal sphincter. Typically, it should be relaxed only during swallowing, but in individuals with GERD, it is relaxed at other times as well. Increased pressure against the lower esophageal sphincter (e.g., as a result of pregnancy or obesity) heightens risk for heartburn. The hormonal changes of pregnancy also tend to relax the lower esophageal sphincter. For some people, slow movement of gastric contents from the stomach to the small intestine complicates the problem (see Further Reading 13).

Without fanfare, the digestive system does the important work of extracting nutrients from the food you eat to supply the needs of your body's trillions of cells. It is not until something goes awry that you notice digestion at all. In this section, you learn about nutritional strategies to cope with heartburn, ulcers, constipation, hemorrhoids, irritable bowel syndrome (IBS), diarrhea, gallstones, and celiac disease. Three other digestive disorders—lactose maldigestion, diverticulosis, and cystic fibrosis—will be discussed in Section 4.4 and Section 5.6.

Heartburn

About half of North American adults experience occasional heartburn, also known as acid reflux (Fig. 3-18). This gnawing pain in the upper chest is caused by the movement of acid from the stomach into the esophagus. Unlike the stomach, the esophagus has very little mucus to protect it, so acid quickly erodes the lining of this organ. Acid reflux symptoms may include pain, nausea, gagging, cough, or hoarseness. The recurrent and therefore more serious form of the problem is called **gastroesophageal reflux disease (GERD).** GERD is diagnosed when symptoms occur two or more times per week.

gastroesophageal reflux disease (GERD) Disease that results from stomach acid backing up into the esophagus. The acid irritates the lining of the esophagus, causing pain.

Esophagus

Stomach

Relaxed lower esophageal sphincter

Inflamed esophagus

Acid reflux

FIGURE 3-18 ▲ Heartburn is a sign of reflux of stomach acid into the esophagus.

If left untreated, heartburn can damage the lining of the esophagus, leading to chronic esophageal inflammation and an increased risk of esophageal cancer. Heartburn sufferers should follow the general recommendations given in Table 3-4. For occasional heartburn, quick relief can be found with over-the-counter (OTC) antacids. Taking antacids will reduce the acid in the stomach but will not stop the acid reflux. For more persistent (few days a week or everyday) heartburn or GERD, H$_2$ blockers or **proton pump inhibitors (PPIs)** may be needed (see Medicine Cabinet). PPIs provide long-lasting relief by reducing stomach acid production and should be taken before the first meal of the day because they take longer to work. Medications that improve GI motility may also be useful. If the proper medications are not effective at controlling GERD, surgery may be needed to strengthen the weakened esophageal sphincter (see Further Reading 4).

Ulcers

A peptic **ulcer** occurs when the lining of the esophagus, stomach, or small intestine is eroded by the acid secreted by stomach cells (Fig. 3-19). A disruption of the layer of mucus that usually protects the stomach allows acid and protein-digesting enzymes to damage the stomach lining. Acid can also erode the lining of the esophagus and the first part of the small intestine, the duodenum. This can cause pain, blood loss, and even perforation. At any given time, about 4.5 million people in the United States are affected by peptic ulcers. In young people, most ulcers occur in the small intestine, whereas in older people, they occur primarily in the stomach.

proton pump inhibitor   A medication that inhibits the ability of gastric cells to secrete hydrogen ions. Low doses of this class of medications are also available without prescription (e.g., omeprazole [Prilosec] ^{R}).

ulcer   Erosion of the tissue lining, usually in the stomach or the upper small intestine. As a group these are generally referred to as peptic ulcers.

perforation   A hole made by boring or piercing. With reference to the gastrointestinal tract, the hole is in the wall of the esophagus, stomach, intestine, rectum, or gallbladder. Complications include bleeding and infection.

TABLE 3-4 ■ Nutrition and Lifestyle Recommendations for Care of Heartburn and Peptic Ulcers

	Heartburn	Peptic Ulcers
Avoid smoking.	√	√
Avoid large doses of aspirin, ibuprofen, and other NSAID compounds unless a physician advises otherwise.[a]	√	√
Achieve or maintain a healthy body weight.	√	√
Eat small, low-fat meals.	√	√
Limit alcohol consumption.	√	√
Limit consumption of caffeine (e.g., coffee, some soft drinks).	√	√
Consume a nutritionally complete diet with adequate fiber (see Section 4.3 for sources of fiber).	√	√
Avoid foods that worsen symptoms.[b]		
• Acidic foods (e.g., orange juice, tomato products)	√	√
• Highly spiced foods (e.g., chili, cayenne, and black pepper)	√	√
• Foods that relax the lower esophageal sphincter (e.g., peppermint, spearmint, chocolate)	√	
• Carbonated beverages	√	√
• Onions and garlic	√	
Avoid tight-fitting clothing.	√	
Elevate the head of the bed 6 to 8 inches.	√	
Avoid eating at least 3 to 4 hours before lying down.	√	
Wash hands often and follow food safety guidelines (see Section 17.8).		√

[a]For people who must use these medications, FDA has approved an NSAID combined with a medication to reduce gastric damage. The medication reduces gastric acid production and enhances mucus secretion.

[b]These foods do not cause heartburn or ulcers, but they may irritate sites of existing damage in the esophagus or stomach.

CASE STUDY Gastroesophageal Reflux Disease

Caitlin is a 20-year-old college sophomore. Over the last few months, she has been experiencing regular bouts of heartburn. This usually happens after a large lunch or dinner. Occasionally, she has even bent down after dinner to pick up something and had some stomach contents travel back up her esophagus and into her mouth. This especially frightened Caitlin, so she visited the University Health Center.

The nurse practitioner at the center told Caitlin it was good that she came in for a checkup because she suspects Caitlin has a disease called gastroesophageal reflux disease (GERD). She tells Caitlin that this can lead to serious problems, such as a rare form of cancer, if not controlled. She provides Caitlin with a pamphlet describing GERD and schedules an appointment with a physician for further evaluation.

Answer the following questions, and check your responses at the end of this chapter.

1. What dietary and lifestyle habits may have contributed to Caitlin's symptoms of GERD?
2. What is the dietary and lifestyle management advice that will help Caitlin cope with this health problem?
3. What types of medications have been especially useful for treating this problem?
4. Overall, how will Caitlin cope with this health problem, and will it ever go away?
5. Why is management of GERD so important?

▲ Caitlin was wise to see a health professional about her persistent heartburn. © Stockdisc/PunchStock

Small intestine (duodenal) ulcer

Stomach ulcer

(a)

Healthy gastric mucosa

Ulcer

(b)

FIGURE 3-19 ▲ (a) A peptic ulcer in the stomach or small intestine. *H. pylori* bacteria and NSAIDs (e.g., aspirin) cause ulcers by impairing mucosal defense, especially in the stomach. Smoking, genetics, and stress also can impair mucosal defense or cause an increase in the release of pepsin and stomach acid. (b) Close-up of a stomach ulcer. This needs to be treated or eventual perforation of the stomach is possible.
© J. James/Science Source

How do you know if you have a peptic ulcer? Some people experience no symptoms at all, but most notice stomach pain about 2 hours after eating. Stomach acid acting on a meal irritates the ulcer after most of the meal has moved from the site of the ulcer. Other symptoms may include weight loss, lack of appetite, nausea and vomiting, or bloating. Vomiting blood or what looks like coffee grounds and the appearance of black, tarry stools are signs of bleeding in the GI tract. Any evidence of GI bleeding warrants immediate medical attention.

The two chief culprits of peptic ulcer disease are infection of the stomach by the acid-resistant bacteria, *Helicobacter pylori (H. pylori),* and heavy use of medications that impair mucus production by the stomach. Conditions that cause excessive stomach acid production also play a role. In addition, cigarette smoking is known to cause ulcers, increase ulcer complications such as bleeding, and lead to ulcer treatment failure.

H. pylori bacteria is found in more than 80% of patients with stomach and duodenal ulcers. The bacteria is common but results in ulcer disease in only 10% to 15% of those infected. Although the mechanism by which *H. pylori* causes ulcers is not well understood, treatment of the infection with antibiotics heals the ulcers and prevents their recurrence. Two Australian physicians were awarded the Nobel Prize in 2005 "for their discovery of the bacterium *H. pylori* and its role in gastritis and peptic ulcer disease."

Nonsteroidal anti-inflammatory drugs (NSAIDs) are medications for painful inflammatory conditions such as arthritis. Aspirin, ibuprofen, and naproxen are the most commonly used types. NSAIDs reduce the mucus secreted by the stomach. Newer medications, called "Cox-2 inhibitors" (e.g., celecoxib [Celebrex®]), have been used as a replacement for NSAIDs because they are less likely to cause stomach ulcers. They do offer some advantages over NSAIDs, but they may not be totally safe for some people, especially those with a history of cardiovascular disease or strokes.

The primary risk associated with an ulcer is the possibility that it will erode entirely through the stomach or intestinal wall. The GI contents could then spill into the body cavities, causing a massive infection. In addition, an ulcer may damage a blood vessel, leading to substantial blood loss. For these reasons, it is important to never ignore the early warning signs of ulcer development, which include a persistent gnawing or burning near the stomach that may occur immediately following a meal or awaken you at night.

Today, a combination approach is used for ulcer therapy. People infected with *H. pylori* are given antibiotics and stomach acid-blocking medications (see Medicine Cabinet). There is a 90% cure rate for *H. pylori* infections in the first week of this treatment. Recurrence is unlikely if the infection is cured, but an incomplete cure almost certainly leads to repeated ulcer formation (see Further Reading 14).

Are dietary changes effective for prevention or treatment of peptic ulcers? Many people think that eating spicy or acidic foods can cause ulcers. Contrary to popular belief, these foods do not cause ulcers. However, once an ulcer has developed, these foods may irritate damaged tissues. Thus, for some people, avoidance of spicy or acidic foods may help to relieve symptoms.

In the past, milk and cream were thought to help cure ulcers. Clinicians now know that milk and cream are two of the worst foods for a person with ulcers because the calcium in these foods stimulates acid secretion and actually inhibits ulcer healing.

Medicine Cabinet

Proton pump inhibitors (PPIs) are medications that inhibit the ability of gastric cells to secrete hydrogen ions (i.e., protons). Low doses of this class of medications may be available without a prescription. Because stomach acid is important for the absorption of vitamin B-12, prolonged use of PPIs could impair vitamin B-12 status.

Examples:

- Omeprazole (Prilosec OTC®)
- Lansoprazole (Prevacid®)
- Rabeprazole (Aciphex®)
- Esomeprazole (Nexium®)

H_2 blockers impede the stimulating effect of histamine on acid-producing cells in the stomach.

Examples:

- Cimetidine (Tagamet®)
- Ranitidine (Zantac®)
- Nizatidine (Axid®)
- Famotidine (Pepcid®)

medicine cabinet - pills: © Footage supplied by Goodshoot/Punchstock

Overall, medical treatment of *H. pylori* infection has so revolutionized ulcer therapy that dietary changes are of minor importance. People with ulcers should refrain from smoking and minimize the use of NSAIDs. Current dietary therapy approaches simply recommend avoidance of foods that tend to worsen ulcer symptoms (see Table 3-4).

Constipation

Constipation, difficult or infrequent evacuation of the bowels, is commonly reported by adults. Slow movement of fecal material through the large intestine causes constipation. More fluid is absorbed during the extended time the feces stay in the large intestine, so the feces become dry and hard.

Constipation can result when people regularly ignore their normal bowel reflexes for long periods. People may ignore normal urges when it is inconvenient to interrupt occupational or social activities. Muscle spasms of an irritated large intestine can also slow the movement of feces and contribute to constipation. Calcium or iron supplements, and medications such as antacids, can also cause constipation.

NSAIDs Nonsteroidal anti-inflammatory drugs; include aspirin, ibuprofen (Advil®), and naproxen (Aleve®).

constipation A condition characterized by infrequent bowel movements.

▲ Dried fruits are a natural source of fiber and can help prevent constipation when consumed with an adequate amount of fluid. © C Squared Studios/Getty Images

Fiber and fluid are the best strategies for treating mild cases of constipation (see Further Reading 10). Whole-grain breads and cereals, beans, and dried fruits are excellent sources of fiber. Fiber stimulates peristalsis by drawing water into the large intestine and helping to form a bulky, soft fecal output. Additional fluid should be consumed to facilitate fiber's action in the large intestine. Also, people with constipation may need to develop more regular bowel habits; allowing the same time each day for a bowel movement can help to train the large intestine to respond routinely. Finally, relaxation facilitates regular bowel movements, as does regular physical activity.

Laxatives can lessen constipation. Some laxatives work by irritating the intestinal nerve junctions to stimulate the peristaltic muscles, while others that contain fiber draw water into the intestine to enlarge fecal output. The larger output stretches the peristaltic muscles, making them rebound and then constrict. Regular use of laxatives, however, should be supervised by a physician. Overall, the bulk-forming fiber laxatives are the safest to use.

CRITICAL THINKING

Amelia has heard that taking laxatives after overeating prevents deposition of body fat from excess calorie intake. Laxatives hasten emptying of the large intestine and increase fluid losses. Based on what you have learned about digestion and absorption of nutrients, do you think Amelia can count on laxatives to prevent fat gain from excess calorie intake?

---

laxative A medication or other substance that stimulates evacuation of the intestinal tract.

hemorrhoid A pronounced swelling of a large vein, particularly veins found in the anal region.

FODMAPs Fermentable oligosacchardes, disaccharides, monosaccharides, and polyols. These carbohydrates may be poorly digested and lead to GI symptoms such as bloating, gas, and diarrhea in some people.

Hemorrhoids

Hemorrhoids, also called *piles,* are swollen veins of the rectum and anus. The blood vessels in this area are subject to intense pressure, especially during bowel movements. Added stress to the vessels from pregnancy, obesity, prolonged sitting, violent coughing or sneezing, or straining during bowel movements (particularly with constipation), can lead to a hemorrhoid.

Hemorrhoids can develop unnoticed until a strained bowel movement precipitates symptoms. Itching (caused by moisture in the anal canal), swelling, and irritation are the most common symptoms. Pain, if present, is usually aching and steady. Bleeding may result from a hemorrhoid and appear in the toilet as a bright red streak in the feces. The sensation of a mass in the anal canal after a bowel movement is a symptom of an internal hemorrhoid that protrudes through the anus.

Anyone can develop a hemorrhoid, and about half of adults over age 50 do. Diet, lifestyle, and heredity may contribute to the problem. For example, a low-fiber diet can lead to hemorrhoids as a result of straining during bowel movements. If you think you have a hemorrhoid, you should consult your physician. Rectal bleeding, although usually caused by hemorrhoids, may also indicate other problems, such as cancer.

A physician may suggest a variety of self-care measures for hemorrhoids. Pain can be lessened by applying warm, soft compresses or sitting in a tub of warm water for 15 to 20 minutes. Dietary recommendations are the same as those for treating constipation, emphasizing the need to consume adequate fiber and fluid. OTC remedies, such as Preparation H®, can also offer relief from symptoms.

Irritable Bowel Syndrome

Many adults (25 million or more in the United States) have irritable bowel syndrome (IBS), characterized by a combination of cramps, gassiness, bloating, and irregular bowel function (diarrhea, constipation, or alternating episodes of both). It is about twice as common in women as it is in men. The disease leads to about 3.5 million visits to physicians in the United States each year.

Symptoms associated with IBS include visible abdominal distention, pain relief after a bowel movement, increased stool frequency, loose stools with pain onset, mucus in stool, and a feeling of incomplete elimination after a bowel movement. Although IBS can be uncomfortable and upsetting, it is harmless as it carries no risk for cancer or other serious digestive problems.

It is difficult to pinpoint an exact cause for IBS. Recent studies indicate that alterations in some of the hormones that regulate the movement of food matter through the GI tract may be to blame. Also, inflammatory responses in the GI tract could be involved for some people with IBS. The majority of people who suffer from IBS perceive that their symptoms are food related, but there is little evidence of actual food allergies or intolerances (see Further Reading 5). When it comes to specific foods, poorly digested carbohydrates are a prime suspect (see Further Reading 9 and the discussion of **FODMAPs** in Chapter 4). Fructose, sugar alcohols, and other carbohydrates may lead to diarrhea or excessive gas if they reach the large intestine undigested. Depression and stress are also associated with IBS; up to 50% of sufferers report a history of verbal or sexual abuse.

Given the diversity of symptoms and possible causes, therapy must be individualized. Increasing **viscous fiber** (e.g., oats, apples, legumes) may be helpful for some people with IBS, but **nonfermentable fiber** (e.g., whole grains, vegetables) seems to worsen symptoms (see Section 4.2). Elimination diets that focus on avoiding dairy products and gas-forming foods, such as legumes, certain vegetables (cabbage, beans, and broccoli), and some fruits (grapes, raisins, cherries, and cantaloupe), can alleviate symptoms. Herbal formulations, certain probiotics, and cognitive behavioral therapy have been shown to decrease symptoms of IBS and improve overall quality of life (see Further Readings 3 and 8). The patient should limit or eliminate caffeine-containing foods and beverages. Low-fat and more frequent, small meals may help because large meals can trigger contractions of the large intestine. Other strategies include a reduction in stress, psychological counseling, and certain antidepressant and other medications. Hypnosis has been shown to relieve symptoms in severe cases.

Following a diet that eliminates certain foods or entire food groups can limit nutritional adequacy. Indeed, research indicates that intakes of some nutrients, including calcium and vitamin A, are inadequate among people with IBS. For help with dietary monitoring, identifying problem foods, and planning a nutritionally adequate diet, a registered dietitian can be a valuable resource for a person with IBS.

Diarrhea

Diarrhea is defined as increased fluidity, frequency, or amount of bowel movements compared to a person's usual pattern. Most cases of diarrhea are of short duration and result from viral or bacterial infections. These microorganisms produce substances that cause the intestinal cells to secrete fluid rather than absorb fluid. Another form of diarrhea can be caused by consumption of substances that are not readily absorbed, such as the sugar alcohol sorbitol found in sugarless gum (see Chapter 4, Section 4.3) or large amounts of a high-fiber source such as bran. When consumed in large amounts, the unabsorbed substance draws water into the intestines, in turn leading to diarrhea.

The goal of diet therapy for any form of diarrhea is to prevent dehydration. Increasing intake of water and **electrolytes** is the first line of defense against dehydration. Prompt treatment of dehydration—within 24 to 48 hours—is critical, especially for infants and older adults (see Section 19.2 and Section 20.2). Diarrhea that lasts more than 7 days in adults should be investigated by a physician as it can be a sign of a more serious intestinal disease, especially if there is also blood in the stool.

For diarrhea caused by infection, dietary changes (besides increased fluid intake) are usually not necessary. Some sources recommend temporarily decreasing intake of caffeine, fat, fiber, and poorly absorbed carbohydrates (see Further Reading 11), but other sources show that maintaining a regular diet speeds recovery. Foods containing probiotics may assist recovery. For diarrhea caused by a poorly absorbed substance, such as excess sugar alcohols or lactose, avoidance of the offending substance is the key to relief.

Gallstones

Gallstones are a major cause of illness and surgery, affecting 10% to 20% of U.S. adults. Gallstones are pieces of solid material that develop in the gallbladder when substances in the bile—primarily

FIGURE 3-20 ▲ Gallbladder and gallstones seen after surgical removal from the body. Size and composition of the stones vary from one case to another. © Dr. Gladden Willis/Visuals Unilmited/Corbis

cholesterol (80% of gallstones)—form crystal-like particles. They may be as small as a grain of sand or as large as a golf ball (Fig. 3-20). These stones are caused by a combination of factors, with excess weight being the primary modifiable factor, especially in women 20 to 60 years old. Other factors include genetic background (e.g., Native Americans), advanced age (>60 years for both women and men), pregnancy, reduced activity of the gallbladder (contracts less than normal), altered bile composition (e.g., too much cholesterol or not enough bile salts), diabetes, and diet (e.g., low-fiber diets). In addition, gallstones may develop during rapid weight loss or prolonged fasting (as the liver metabolizes more fat, it secretes more cholesterol into the bile).

Attacks due to gallstones include intermittent pain in the upper right abdomen, gas and bloating, nausea or vomiting, or other health problems. Medications are available to dissolve gallstones, but these take a long time to work, and the recurrence of gallstones after therapy is common. Therefore, surgical removal of the gallbladder is the most common method for treating gallstones (500,000 surgeries per year in the United States).

The best prevention strategy is to avoid becoming overweight, especially for women. Avoiding rapid weight loss (>3 pounds per week), limiting animal protein and focusing more on plant protein intake (especially some nut intake), and following a high-fiber diet can help as well. Regular physical activity is also recommended, as is moderate to no caffeine and alcohol intake (see Further Reading 12).

Celiac Disease and Gluten Sensitivity

Celiac disease (sometimes called celiac sprue) affects about 1% of the U.S. population. Development of celiac disease depends on two factors: a genetic predisposition and dietary exposure to a protein

viscous fiber A fiber that is readily fermented by bacteria in the large intestine; also called *soluble fiber*.

nonfermentable fiber A fiber that is not easily metabolized by intestinal bacteria; also called *insoluble fiber*.

electrolyte A mineral that separates into positively or negatively charged ions in water. They are able to transmit an electrical current.

celiac disease Chronic, immune-mediated disease precipitated by exposure to dietary gluten in genetically predisposed people.

called gluten. Gluten is a type of protein found in certain grains: wheat, rye, and barley. Protein-digesting enzymes in the GI tract break down some of the bonds in gluten, but digestion is incomplete. These partially digested proteins can be absorbed into the cells lining the small intestine. When people with a genetic predisposition for celiac disease are exposed to these small proteins from gluten, they experience an inflammatory reaction. Although many people think celiac disease is a food allergy, it is actually an autoimmune response: the immune system attacks and destroys its own cells. (You will learn more about food allergies in Section 6.3 and Section 19.7.)

The immune response that occurs after exposure to gluten targets the cells of the small intestine, causing a flattening of the villi, which thereby reduces the absorptive surface (Fig. 3-21). The production of some digestive enzymes is decreased and the ability of the small intestine to absorb nutrients is impaired. Malabsorption leads to a variety of GI complaints: diarrhea, bloating, cramps, and flatulence. In fact, it is common for celiac disease to be misdiagnosed as IBS. However, the pathology underlying celiac disease has far worse consequences than IBS. Over time, malabsorption of nutrients can lead to fatigue, weight loss (or poor growth in children), anemia, infertility, and even bone loss (see Further Readings 7 and 15).

If celiac disease is suspected, the first step in making a formal diagnosis is a blood test for the presence of antibodies to gluten. This may be followed by one or more biopsies of the small intestine to confirm the pathological defects. There is also a genetic test for celiac disease, but having the gene does not always predict development of the disease.

Strict dietary avoidance of food products containing wheat, rye, and barley is the only proven way to manage the disease. On food labels, food manufacturers must identify the presence of wheat (one of eight major food allergens). However, rye and barley are not as easy to spot. Therefore, people following a gluten-free diet must learn to carefully interpret the list of ingredients to identify sources of gluten. Within the grains group, rice, potato flour, cornmeal, buckwheat, arrowroot, and soy are gluten free, but ingredients such as wheat, rye, barley, bran, graham flour, semolina, spelt, and malt are sources of gluten and must be avoided. Oats do not traditionally contain gluten, but contamination in the field or during food processing could introduce gluten into this grain as well.

People with celiac disease quickly learn that wheat, barley, and rye can be hidden ingredients in any food group. Wheat and its derivatives are used to thicken sauces and condiments, as flavoring agents in dairy products and many other processed foods, and in breading for deep-fried vegetables and meats. It is helpful that many food manufacturers now voluntarily disclose the presence or absence of gluten in their products. However, not all products clearly identify gluten. Dining out is yet another challenge: even a dusting of wheat flour can have adverse effects for a person with celiac disease.

After several weeks on a gluten-free diet, the small intestinal lining regenerates, GI symptoms subside, and nutrient absorption improves. So far, the gluten-free diet is the only proven way to manage celiac disease, but research on other treatments is underway. Food scientists are working toward developing strains of wheat, barley, and rye that do not contain gluten. From a gastroenterological perspective, other approaches are to supply digestive enzymes that will break down the gluten proteins before they stimulate an autoimmune response and to use polymers that will bind to gluten in the GI tract and prevent it from being absorbed. From an immunological perspective, researchers are looking at medications that could block immune responses that damage the small intestine.

A related issue is **nonceliac gluten sensitivity (NCGS),** or sometimes called gluten intolerance. Some people experience symptoms of celiac disease after ingestion of gluten, but they do not have the small intestinal pathology of celiac disease, nor do they express the antibodies typical of CD. Some reports indicate that for each person who is diagnosed with CD, as many as six others have NCGS. Aside from GI symptoms, patients with NCGS may also report fatigue, headache, muscle and joint pain, and/or sleep disorders. Symptoms subside with a gluten-free diet but reappear when gluten is reintroduced. The medical community recognizes NCGS as a verifiable condition, but the immunological mechanism that causes it is not well understood. There is no diagnostic test for the condition—only the effectiveness of the gluten-free diet in alleviating symptoms (see Further Reading 2). Many questions remain: Is NCGS a permanent condition? Is there a level of gluten intake that would not trigger symptoms? It seems that there are multiple immunological reactions to gluten that are predicted by different genetic traits (see Further Reading 7).

Overall, the prevalence and awareness of celiac disease and NCGS seem to be on the rise. A cause for the increased prevalence has not been pinpointed, but some scientists speculate that changes in wheat production or widespread use of wheat in the food supply may be to blame. Others suspect that an infection or exposure to some environmental toxin could increase gut permeability and lead to gluten sensitization.

(a)

(b)

FIGURE 3-21 ▲ Biopsy findings in patients with and without celiac disease. (a) Normal small intestinal cells. Note the intact villi, which increase the surface area of the small intestine to maximize nutrient absorption. (b) The small intestinal cells of a person with celiac disease. The villi appear flattened. (a): © Cultura Science/Alvin Telser, PhD/Getty Images; (b): © Cultura Science/Michael J. Klein, M.D./Getty Images

nonceliac gluten sensitivity (NCGS) One or more of a variety of immune-related conditions with symptoms similar to celiac disease that are precipitated by the ingestion of gluten in people who do not have celiac disease.

ASK THE RDN   Gluten-Free Diet

Dear RDN: I have heard that a gluten-free diet is a healthier choice. Will a gluten-free diet help me lose weight?

The media is brimming with popular advice to eliminate wheat and other grains from the diet, promising everything from a clear mind to a trim waistline. For individuals with celiac disease and nonceliac gluten sensitivity, avoiding gluten is a health priority. It will likely correct gastrointestinal complications and a range of other symptoms such as fatigue and body pain. Weight loss, however, is not one of the benefits of a gluten-free diet.

The only reason a gluten-free diet might induce weight loss is because it can be restrictive. For the person who regularly overconsumes bread, pasta, pizza, and baked goods, eliminating all sources of gluten could limit these food choices, thus leading to weight loss. Important point: Weight loss is the result of a calorie deficit, not the lack of gluten. Now, with the increased availability of gluten-free options in grocery stores and restaurants, you will soon realize that a gluten-free diet may not be that restrictive after all.

In fact, you may actually *gain* weight on a gluten-free diet. For a person with celiac disease, as the small intestine heals, nutrient absorption will increase and appetite will likely improve. In addition, many gluten-free products contain more calories than their wheat-based counterparts. To compensate for losses of taste and texture, some gluten-free products incorporate extra fat or sugar. For example, a typical slice of whole-grain wheat bread is about 80 kcal; some brands of gluten-free bread provide as many as 140 kcal per slice. Keep in mind that the "Gluten-Free" claim does not make a food healthy!

Lastly, grains are an important part of a balanced diet. They provide calories, of course, but they also supply dietary fiber and essential vitamins and minerals. Wheat flour is fortified with thiamin, niacin, riboflavin, folic acid, and iron. So, if you are planning to try a gluten-free diet, work with a registered dietitian nutritionist to ensure that your diet meets your nutrient needs. Choose whole gluten-free grains and unprocessed fruits and vegetables to replace wheat and balance calories to avoid weight gain.

With a grain of truth,

Angela Collene, MS, RDN, LD (author)

Summary

The conditions discussed here can be very serious, possibly leading to malnutrition, internal bleeding, and life-threatening infections. It is important to seek competent medical advice if you or someone you know suspects a GI disorder. However, you should feel empowered to know that you can control some risks and complement medical treatment with nutrition and other lifestyle changes. Overall, keeping body weight within a healthy range, meeting recommendations for fiber and fluid intake, and avoiding smoking and overuse of NSAID medications are useful strategies that can help you cope with several common disorders of the GI tract.

Summary (Numbers refer to numbered sections in the chapter.)

3.1 Cells join together to make up tissues, tissues unite to form organs, and organs work together as an organ system.

3.2 The basic structural unit of the human body is the cell. Almost all cells contain the same organelles, but cell structure varies according to the type of job cells must perform.

3.3 Epithelial, connective, muscle, and nervous tissues are the four primary types of tissues in the human body. Each type of organ system is affected by nutrient intake.

3.4 From the cells of the GI tract, water-soluble nutrients are absorbed into capillaries and fat-soluble nutrients are absorbed into lymph vessels, which eventually connect to the bloodstream. Blood delivers nutrients and oxygen to cells and picks up waste as it circulates around the body.

3.5 The urinary system, including the kidneys, is responsible for filtering the blood, removing body waste, and maintaining the chemical composition of the blood.

3.6 The nervous system allows for communication and regulation. Vitamin B-12 is part of the insulation that surrounds neurons. Transmission of nerve impulses relies on sodium and potassium. Neurotransmitters are made from amino acids.

3.7 The endocrine system produces hormones—protein-based chemical messengers—to regulate metabolic reactions and the levels of nutrients in the blood.

3.8 With assistance from the skin and the gastrointestinal tract, the immune system protects the body from pathogens. Optimal immune system function relies on protein; essential fatty acids; vitamins A, C, and D; some B vitamins; and the minerals iron, zinc, and copper.

3.9 The GI tract consists of the mouth, esophagus, stomach, small intestine, large intestine (colon), rectum, and anus.

Spaced along the GI tract are sphincters that regulate the flow of food matter. Peristalsis moves food matter along the GI tract. Nerves, hormones, and other substances control the activity of sphincters and peristaltic muscles.

Digestive enzymes are secreted by the mouth, stomach, small intestine, and pancreas. Little digestion and absorption occur in the stomach or large intestine, but some protein is digested in the stomach.

Most absorption occurs through the cells of the villi, which line the small intestine. Absorptive processes include passive diffusion, facilitated diffusion, active transport, phagocytosis, and pinocytosis.

Some water and mineral absorption takes place in the large intestine. Some constituents of undigested carbohydrates are broken down by bacteria in the large intestine. Some of these products are absorbed; remaining undigested materials are eliminated in the feces.

The liver, gallbladder, and pancreas participate in digestion and absorption. Products from these organs, such as enzymes and bile, enter the small intestine and help in digesting protein, fat, and carbohydrate.

3.10 Limited stores of nutrients are present in the blood for immediate use. Some nutrients, such as minerals and fat-soluble vitamins, can be stored extensively in bone, adipose, and liver tissues. Excessive storage of nutrients can be toxic. Conversely, breakdown of vital tissues can supply nutrients in times of need, but continued breakdown eventually leads to ill health.

3.11 Nutritional genomics includes the study of how genes influence nutritional status (nutrigenetics) and how nutrients and other dietary components influence genetic expression (nutrigenomics). Genograms and genetic testing can be useful tools for identifying prevalence for disease. Personalized nutritional prescriptions can then be applied to promote optimal health.

3.12 Common GI tract diseases, such as heartburn, constipation, and irritable bowel syndrome, can be treated with a combination of diet changes and medications.

Check Your Knowledge (Answers are available at the end of this question set.)

1. The stomach is protected from digesting itself by producing
   a. bicarbonate.
   b. a thick layer of mucus.
   c. hydroxyl ions to neutralize acid.
   d. antipepsin that destroys enzymes.

2. The lower esophageal sphincter is located between the
   a. stomach and esophagus.
   b. stomach and duodenum.
   c. ileum and the cecum.
   d. colon and the anus.

3. A muscular contraction that propels food down the GI tract is called
   a. a sphincter.
   b. enterohepatic circulation.
   c. gravitational pull.
   d. peristalsis.

4. Bicarbonate ions (HCO_3^-) from the pancreas
   a. neutralize acid in the stomach.
   b. are synthesized in the pyloric sphincter.
   c. neutralize bile in the duodenum.
   d. neutralize acid in the duodenum.

5. Most digestive processes occur in the
   a. mouth.
   b. stomach.
   c. small intestine.
   d. large intestine.
   e. liver.

6. Bile is formed in the _____ and stored in the _____.
   a. stomach, pancreas
   b. duodenum, kidney
   c. liver, gallbladder
   d. gallbladder, liver

7. Much of the digestion that occurs in the large intestine is caused by
   a. lipase.
   b. pepsin.
   c. saliva.
   d. bacteria.

8. Treatment of ulcers may include
   a. H₂ blockers.
   b. proton pump inhibitors.
   c. antibiotics.
   d. all of these.

9. The study of how food impacts health through interaction with genes is
   a. nutrigenomics.
   b. epidemiology.
   c. immunology.
   d. nutrigenetics.

10. Energy production that takes place in the cytoplasm is anaerobic metabolism because it does not require
    a. water.
    b. oxygen.
    c. anabolic steroids.
    d. anaerobic bacteria.

Answer Key: 1. b (LO 3.8); 2. a (LO 3.8); 3. d (LO 3.8)
4. d (LO 3.8); 5. c (LO 3.8); 6. c (LO 3.8); 7. d (LO 3.8);
8. d (LO 3.12); 9. a (LO 3.11); 10. b (LO 3.2)

Study Questions (Numbers refer to Learning Outcomes)

1. Identify at least one function of the 12 organ systems related to nutrition. **(LO 3.3)**

2. Draw and label parts of the cell and explain the function of each organelle as it relates to human nutrition. **(LO 3.2)**

3. Trace the flow of blood from the right side of the heart and back to the same site. How is blood routed through the small intestine? Which class of nutrients enters the body via the blood? Via the lymph? **(LO 3.4)**

4. Explain why the small intestine is better suited than the other GI tract organs to carry out the absorptive process. **(LO 3.8)**

5. Identify the five basic tastes. Give an example of one food that exemplifies each of these basic taste sensations. **(LO 3.8)**

6. What is one role of acid in the process of digestion? Where is it secreted? **(LO 3.8)**

7. Contrast the processes of active absorption and passive diffusion of nutrients. **(LO 3.8)**

8. Identify two accessory organs that empty their contents into the small intestine. How do the digestive substances secreted by these organs contribute to the digestion of food? **(LO 3.8)**

9. In which organ systems would the following substances be found? chyme **(LO 3.8)**, plasma **(LO 3.4)**, lymph **(LO 3.4)**, urine **(LO 3.9)**

10. Describe the nutrition-related diseases for which genetics or family history is considered to be an important risk factor. **(LO 3.11)**

CASE STUDY SOLUTION — Gastroesophageal Reflux Disease

1. Overeating at mealtimes appears to bring on Caitlin's regular bouts of heartburn.

2. Typical dietary advice includes consuming smaller, more frequent meals low in fat, not overeating at mealtimes, waiting about 2 hours after meals before lying down, and elevating the head of the bed about 6 inches (review Table 3-4). These recommendations reduce the risk of stomach contents forcing their way back up the esophagus. In addition, losing excess weight (if overweight) can alleviate GERD.

3. If dietary advice does not control symptoms, the primary medication used to control GERD inhibits acid production in the stomach (see the discussion in Section 3.12 on the proton pump inhibitors such as omeprazole [Prilosec®]). If this and other medical therapy fail to control the problem, surgery to strengthen the lower esophageal sphincter is possible.

4. Caitlin's GERD can be treated but most likely will be a lifelong condition. Even surgery will generally not cure the problem. Lifetime diet and lifestyle management, and most likely medications, will still be needed to manage the problem.

5. Lifelong management of GERD is important because long-standing GERD increases the risk of esophageal cancer.

What the Dietitian Chose

Constipation results from slow movement of fecal material through the large intestine. Increasing fiber and water in your diet can often relieve constipation without the aid of an over-the-counter laxative. To boost your fiber intake, choose whole grains, fruits, vegetables, and legumes (beans). This can be a tough task when most of the menu options you will find in fast-food restaurants and convenience stores are low in fiber.

As you select your pizza, look for slices with extra vegetables or fruit. This will increase the fiber content by about 1 gram per slice. Pizza with whole-grain crust would add another 1 gram of fiber per slice. These are small improvements, so you will probably still need to look for additional fiber sources.

What about your side dish? Unless they are made with whole grains, the pasta and breadsticks will not add much fiber to your meal. A breadstick and a cup of pasta with Alfredo sauce provide about 1 and 2 grams of fiber, respectively. These carbohydrate-rich add-ons are supplying extra calories and would be better off skipped. The salad provides about 1 to 3 grams of fiber, depending on its size and ingredients. The core ingredients of tossed salad—lettuce, cucumbers, tomato—are mostly water and not particularly high in fiber. Toppings such as cheese, egg, or diced meat will not help relieve constipation. Instead, dried fruit (e.g., dried cranberries or raisins) and nuts supply some additional fiber.

◄ Whole-grain pasta and beans used in salads and soups are good sources of fiber that can prevent intestinal issues such as constipation. (salad): © Getty Images/Jonelle Weaver; (soup): © Royalty-Free/Corbis

An even better choice, however, is the soup! A cup of bean and pasta soup is just what the doctor ordered to help relieve constipation. It provides about 6 grams of fiber and some extra water, as well.

Lastly, be sure to drink plenty of water. Dehydration is an often overlooked cause of constipation. Water helps lubricate the digestive tract and adds bulk to the feces when absorbed by fiber in the large intestine.

Further Readings

1. Baumler, MD: Nutrigenetics—building a platform for dietitians to offer personalized nutrition. *Today's Dietitian* 14:48, 2012.

2. Bizzaro N and others: Cutting-edge issues in celiac disease and in gluten intolerance. *Clinical Reviews in Allergy and Immunology* 42:279, 2012.

3. Camilleri M: Probiotics and irritable bowel syndrome: Rationale, putative mechanisms, and evidence of clinical efficacy. *Journal of Clinical Gastroenterology* 40:264, 2006.

4. DeVault KR, Castell DO: Updated guidelines for the diagnosis and treatment of gastroesophageal reflux disease. *American Journal of Gastroenterology* 100:190, 2005.

5. El-Salhy M and others: The role of diet in the pathogenesis and management of irritable bowel syndrome (review). *International Journal of Molecular Medicine* 29:723, 2012.

6. Fenech M and others: Nutrigenetics and nutrigenomics: Viewpoints on the current status and applications in nutrition research and practice. *Journal of Nutrigenetics and Nutrigenomics* 4:69, 2011.

7. Ferretti GF and others: Celiac disease, inflammation, and oxidative damage: A nutrigenetic approach. *Nutrients* 4:243, 2012.

8. Lynch A, Webb C: What are the most effective nonpharmacologic therapies for irritable bowel syndrome? *Journal of Family Practice* 57:57, 2008.

9. Marcason W: What is the FODMAP diet? *Journal of the Academy of Nutrition and Dietetics* 112:12, 2012.

10. Muller-Lisser SA and others: Myths and misconceptions about constipation. *American Journal of Gastroenterology* 100:232, 2005.

11. National Digestive Diseases Information Clearinghouse: Diarrhea. 2013. Available at http://digestive.niddk.nih.gov/ddiseases/pubs/diarrhea/index. aspx. Accessed September 24, 2015.

12. National Digestive Diseases Information Clearinghouse: Gallstones. 2013. Available at http://digestive.niddk.nih.gov/ddiseases/pubs/gallstones/index. aspx. Accessed September 24, 2015.

13. National Digestive Diseases Information Clearinghouse: Gastroesophageal reflux (GER) and gastroesophageal reflux disease (GERD) in adults. 2013. Available at http://www.niddk.nih.gov/health-information/health-topics/ digestive-diseases/ger-and-gerd-in-adults/Documents/gerd_508.pdf Accessed September 25, 2015.

14. National Digestive Diseases Information Clearinghouse: Peptic ulcer disease and *H. pylori*. 2014. Available at http://www.niddk.nih.gov/health-information/health-topics/digestive-diseases/peptic-ulcer/Documents/ hpylori_508.pdf. Accessed September 25, 2015.

15. Presutti RJ and others: Celiac disease. *American Family Physician* 76:1795, 2007.

16. Wallace TC and others: Human gut microbiota and its relationship to health and disease. *Nutrition Reviews* 69:392, 2011.

Rate Your Plate

I. Are You Taking Care of Your Digestive Tract?

People need to think about the health of their own digestive tract. There are symptoms we need to notice, as well as habits we need to practice to protect it. The following assessment is designed to help you examine your habits and symptoms associated with the health of your digestive tract. Put a *Y* in the blank to the left of the question to indicate yes and an *N* to indicate no.

_____ 1. Are you currently experiencing greater than normal stress and tension?

_____ 2. Do you have a family history of digestive tract problems (e.g., ulcers, hemorrhoids, recurrent heartburn, and constipation)?

_____ 3. Do you experience pain in your stomach region about 2 hours after you eat?

_____ 4. Do you smoke cigarettes?

_____ 5. Do you take aspirin frequently?

_____ 6. Do you have heartburn at least once per week?

_____ 7. Do you commonly lie down after eating a large meal?

_____ 8. Do you drink alcoholic beverages more than 2 or 3 times per day?

_____ 9. Do you experience abdominal pain, bloating, or gas 1 ½ to 2 hours after consuming milk products?

_____ 10. Do you often have to strain while having a bowel movement?

_____ 11. Do you consume less than 9 (women) or 13 (men) cups of a combination of water and other fluids per day?

_____ 12. Do you perform physical activity for less than 60 minutes on most or all days of the week (e.g., jog, swim, walk briskly, row, and stair climb)?

_____ 13. Do you eat a diet relatively low in fiber? (Recall that significant fiber is found in whole fruits, vegetables, legumes, nuts and seeds, whole-grain breads, and whole-grain cereals.)

_____ 14. Do you frequently have diarrhea?

_____ 15. Do you frequently use laxatives or antacids?

Add up the number of yes answers and record the total. If your score is from 8 to 15, your habits and symptoms put you at risk for experiencing future digestive tract problems. Take particular note of the habits to which you answered yes. Consider trying to cooperate more with your digestive tract.

II. Create Your Family Tree for Health-Related Concerns

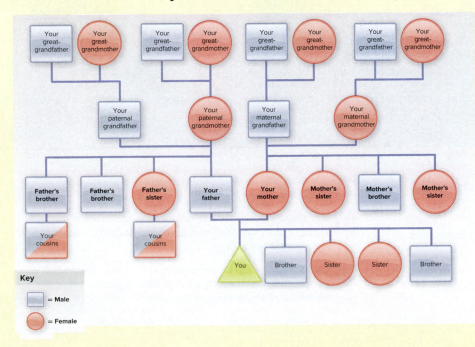

Adapt this diagram to your family tree. Under each heading, list year born, year died (if applicable), major diseases that developed during the person's lifetime, and cause of death (if applicable). Figure 3-17 shows one such example. You may also use the interactive tool available at https://familyhistory.hhs.gov/FHH/html/index.html to generate a medical family tree.

You are likely to be at risk for any diseases listed. Creating a plan for preventing such diseases when possible, especially those that developed in your family members before age 50 to 60 years, is advised. Speak with your physician about any concerns arising from this exercise.

Student Learning Outcomes

Chapter 4 is designed to allow you to:

4.1 Explain the most important nutritional role of carbohydrates and how they are created.

4.2 Identify the basic structures of the major carbohydrates: monosaccharides, disaccharides, polysaccharides (e.g., starches), and fiber.

4.3 Describe food sources of carbohydrates and list some alternative sweeteners.

4.4 Explain how carbohydrates are taken in and used by the body, including the processes of digestion, absorption, metabolism, and glucose regulation.

4.5 List the functions of carbohydrates in the body, the problems that result from not eating enough carbohydrates, and the beneficial effects of fiber on the body.

Chapter 4
Carbohydrates

What Would You Choose?

It is lunchtime and you have a 30-minute break between classes. You stop at Doug's Deli for a quick sandwich. In making a sandwich choice, you remember that meals should resemble the MyPlate food pattern and that several of the food groups provide sources of carbohydrates. All of the sandwiches provide about 350 kcal. The fiber content ranges from about 1 gram to about 7.5 grams. Which sandwich would you choose to maximize the number of servings from a variety of healthy carbohydrate sources?

a Turkey and Swiss on rye, with tomato slices, sliced cucumbers, romaine lettuce, and mustard

b Ham and Swiss on sourdough, made with extra-lean ham and mayonnaise

c Tuna salad on whole wheat, made with tuna, grated carrots, onions, and mayonnaise and served with alfalfa sprouts, romaine lettuce, and cucumber slices

d Hotdog on a white bun, with relish, mustard, and ketchup

e Soy burger on whole-wheat English muffin, with tomato, pickle slices, romaine lettuce, and mayonnaise

f Peanut butter and jelly on soft white bread, made with strawberry jelly and smooth peanut butter

Think about your choice as you read Chapter 4, then see What the Dietitian Chose at the end of the chapter.

What did you eat to obtain the energy you are using right now? Chapters 4 through 6 will examine this question by focusing on the main nutrients the human body uses for fuel. These nutrients are carbohydrates (on average, 4 kcal per gram) and fats and oils (on average, 9 kcal per gram). Although protein (on average, 4 kcal per gram) *can* be used for energy needs, the body typically reserves this nutrient for other processes.

It is likely that you have recently consumed fruits, vegetables, dairy products, cereal, breads, and pasta. These foods supply carbohydrates. Although some carbohydrate sources are more beneficial than others, carbohydrates should be a major part of our dietary patterns. Many people think carbohydrate-rich foods cause weight gain, but they do not any more so than fat or protein. In fact, pound for pound, carbohydrates are much less fattening than fats and oils. Furthermore, high-carbohydrate foods, especially fiber-rich foods such as fruits, vegetables, whole-grain breads and cereals, and legumes, provide many important health benefits in addition to the calories they contain. Almost all carbohydrate-rich foods, except pure sugars, provide several essential nutrients and should generally constitute 45% to 65% of our daily calorie intake. Let's take a closer look at carbohydrates.

4.6 State the RDA for carbohydrate and various guidelines for carbohydrate intake.

4.7 Identify the consequences of diabetes and explain appropriate dietary measures that will reduce the adverse effects of this health problem.

4.1 Carbohydrates—Our Most Important Energy Source

Carbohydrates are a main fuel source for some cells, especially those in the brain, nervous system, and red blood cells. Muscles also rely on a dependable supply of carbohydrates to fuel intense physical activity. Carbohydrates provide on average 4 kcal per gram and are a readily available fuel for all cells, in the form of both blood glucose and **glycogen** stored in the liver and muscles. The glycogen stored in the liver can be used to maintain blood glucose concentrations in times when you have not eaten for several hours or the food you eat does not supply enough carbohydrates. Regular intake of carbohydrates is important because liver glycogen stores are depleted in about 18 hours if no carbohydrates are consumed. After that point, the body is forced to produce carbohydrates, mostly from breakdown of proteins in the body. This eventually leads to health problems, including the loss of muscle tissue. To obtain adequate energy, the Food and Nutrition Board of the Institute of Medicine recommends that 45% to 65% of the calories we consume each day be from carbohydrates. (See the Acceptable Macronutrient Distribution Range table in the DRI charts in Appendix G.)

Despite their important role as a calorie source, some forms of carbohydrate promote health more than others. As you will see in this chapter, whole-grain breads and cereals have greater health benefits than refined and processed forms of carbohydrate. Choosing the healthiest carbohydrate sources most often, while moderating intake of less healthful sources, contributes to a healthy dietary pattern. It is difficult to eat so little carbohydrate that body fuel needs are not met, but it is easy to overconsume the simple carbohydrates, namely sugars, that can contribute to health problems. Let's explore this concept further as we look at carbohydrates in detail.

Green plants synthesize most of the carbohydrates in our foods. Leaves capture the sun's solar energy in their cells and transform it into chemical energy. This energy is then stored in the chemical bonds of the carbohydrate glucose as it is produced from carbon dioxide in the air and water in the soil. This complex process is called **photosynthesis** (Fig. 4-1).

glycogen A carbohydrate made of multiple units of glucose with a highly branched structure. It is the storage form of glucose in humans and is synthesized (and stored) in the liver and muscles.

▲ Fruits such as oranges and pears are an excellent source of carbohydrates, especially simple sugars and fiber. © Imagestate Media (John Foxx)/Imagestat

photosynthesis Process by which plants use energy from the sun to synthesize energy-yielding compounds, such as glucose.

$$6 \text{ carbon dioxide} + 6 \text{ water} + \text{solar energy} \rightarrow \text{glucose} + 6 \text{ oxygen}$$
$$(CO_2) \qquad (H_2O) \qquad (C_6H_{12}O_6) \qquad (O_2)$$

6 carbon dioxide (CO_2) + 6 water (H_2O)

Sun   Energy →

Glucose ($C_6H_{12}O_6$) + 6 oxygen (O_2)

FIGURE 4-1 ▲ A summary of photosynthesis. Plants use carbon dioxide, water, and the sun's energy to produce glucose. Glucose is then stored in the leaf and can also undergo further metabolism to form starch and fiber in the plant. With the addition of nitrogen from soil or air, glucose can also be transformed into protein.

Translated into English, this reads: 6 molecules of carbon dioxide combine with 6 molecules of water to form 1 molecule of **glucose.** Converting solar energy into chemical bonds in the sugar is a key part of the process. Six molecules of oxygen are then released into the air.

glucose A six-carbon sugar that exists in a ring form; found as such in blood, and in table sugar bound to fructose; also known as *dextrose,* it is one of the simple sugars.

✓ CONCEPT CHECK 4.1

1. Why are carbohydrates considered our most valuable energy source?

4.2 Forms of Carbohydrates

As the name suggests, most carbohydrate molecules are composed of carbon, hydrogen, and oxygen atoms. Simple forms of carbohydrates are called **sugars.** Larger, more complex forms are primarily called either **starches** or **fibers,** depending on their digestibility by human GI-tract enzymes. Starches are digestible, whereas fibers are not. The Concept Map at the end of this section summarizes the forms and characteristics of carbohydrates.

The simple carbohydrates contain only one or two sugar units and are called monosaccharides and disaccharides, respectively. Food labels lump all of these sugars under one category, listing them as "sugars."

MONOSACCHARIDES—GLUCOSE, FRUCTOSE, AND GALACTOSE

Monosaccharides are the **simple sugar** units (*mono* means "one") that serve as the basic unit of all carbohydrate structures. The most common monosaccharides in foods are glucose, fructose, and galactose (Fig. 4-2).

Glucose is the major monosaccharide found in the body. Glucose is also known as *dextrose,* and glucose in the bloodstream may be called blood sugar. Glucose is an important source of energy for human cells, although foods contain very little carbohydrate as this single sugar. Most glucose comes from the digestion of starches and **sucrose** (common table sugar) from our food. Sucrose is made up of the monosaccharides glucose and fructose. For the most part, sugars and other carbohydrates in foods are eventually converted into glucose in the liver. This glucose then goes on to serve as a source of fuel for cells.

Fructose, also called *fruit sugar,* is another monosaccharide. Fructose is found naturally in fruits and forms half of each sucrose molecule. After it is consumed, fructose is absorbed by the small intestine and then transported to the liver, where it is quickly metabolized. Much is converted to glucose, but the rest goes on to form other compounds, such as fat, if fructose is consumed in very high amounts. Most of the free fructose in the food we eat comes from the use of **high-fructose corn syrup (HFCS)** in soft drinks, candies, jams, jellies, and many other fruit products and desserts (see the discussion on nutritive sweeteners in Section 4.3). Fructose is also found naturally in fruits and forms half of each sucrose molecule.

The sugar **galactose** has nearly the same structure as glucose. Large quantities of pure galactose do not exist in nature. Instead, galactose is usually found bonded to glucose in **lactose,** a sugar found in milk and other milk products. After lactose is digested and absorbed, galactose arrives in the liver. There it is either transformed

sugar A simple carbohydrate with the chemical composition (CH_2O) *n.* The basic unit of all sugars is glucose, a six-carbon ring structure. The primary sugar in the diet is sucrose, which is made up of glucose and fructose.

starch A carbohydrate made of multiple units of glucose attached together in a form the body can digest; also known as *complex carbohydrate.*

fiber Substances in plant foods not digested in the human stomach or small intestine. These add bulk to feces. Fiber naturally found in foods is also called *dietary fiber.*

monosaccharide Simple sugar, such as glucose, that is not broken down further during digestion.

simple sugar Monosaccharide or disaccharide in the diet.

sucrose Fructose bonded to glucose; table sugar.

fructose A six-carbon monosaccharide that usually exists in a ring form; found in fruits and honey; also known as *fruit sugar.*

high-fructose corn syrup (HFCS) Corn syrup that has been manufactured to contain between 42% and 90% fructose.

galactose A six-carbon monosaccharide that usually exists in a ring form; closely related to glucose.

lactose Glucose bonded to galactose; also known as *milk sugar.*

Monosaccharides

Glucose   Fructose   Galactose

FIGURE 4-2 ▲ Chemical forms of the important monosaccharides.

Disaccharides

Sucrose: glucose + fructose
Lactose: glucose + galactose
Maltose: glucose + glucose

Sucrose

FIGURE 4-3 ▲ Chemical form of the disaccharide sucrose.

disaccharide Class of sugars formed by the chemical bonding of two monosaccharides.

maltose Glucose bonded to glucose.

fermentation The conversion of carbohydrates to alcohols, acids, and carbon dioxide without the use of oxygen.

polysaccharides Carbohydrates containing many glucose units, from 10 to 1000 or more.

amylose A digestible straight-chain type of starch composed of glucose units.

amylopectin A digestible branched-chain type of starch composed of glucose units.

▲ Root vegetables such as potatoes, yams, and tapioca are high in amylopectin starch.
© C Squared Studios/Getty Images

into glucose or further metabolized into glycogen. This is a good example of the body not using all nutrients in their original states. Some of these substances are broken down and later reassembled into the same or a different substance when and where they are needed.

Much of the galactose in the diet is metabolized to glucose. When later required for milk production in the mammary gland of a lactating woman, galactose is resynthesized from glucose to help form the milk sugar lactose. Therefore, it is not necessary for the lactating woman to drink milk in order to make milk!

DISACCHARIDES: SUCROSE, LACTOSE, AND MALTOSE

Disaccharides are formed when two monosaccharides combine (*di* means "two"). The disaccharides in food are sucrose, lactose, and **maltose.** All contain glucose.

Sucrose forms when the two sugars glucose and fructose bond together (Fig. 4-3). Sucrose is found naturally in sugarcane, sugar beets, honey, and maple sugar. These products are processed to varying degrees to make brown, white, and powdered sugars. Animals do not produce sucrose or much of any carbohydrate except glycogen.

Lactose forms when glucose bonds with galactose during the synthesis of milk. Therefore, our major food source for lactose is milk products. The discussion in Section 4.4 on lactose maldigestion and lactose intolerance looks at the problems that result when a person can't readily digest lactose.

Maltose results when starch is broken down to just two glucose molecules bonded together. Maltose plays an important role in the beer and liquor industry. In the production of these alcoholic beverages, starches in various cereal grains are first converted to simpler carbohydrates by enzymes present in the grains. The products of this step—maltose, glucose, and other sugars—are then mixed with yeast cells in the absence of oxygen. The yeast cells convert most of the sugars to alcohol (ethanol) and carbon dioxide through a process called **fermentation.** Little maltose remains in the final product. Few other food products or beverages contain maltose. In fact, most maltose that we ultimately digest in the small intestine is produced during our own digestion of starch.

COMPLEX CARBOHYDRATES

In many foods, numerous single-sugar units are bonded together to form a chain, known as a polysaccharide (*poly* means "many"). **Polysaccharides,** also called *complex carbohydrates* or *starch,* may contain 1000 or more glucose units and are found chiefly in grains, vegetables, and fruits. When the Nutrition Facts panel on food labels lists "Other Carbohydrates," this primarily refers to starch content.

Plants store carbohydrates in two forms of starch digestible by humans: **amylose** and **amylopectin.** Amylose, a long, straight chain of glucose units, comprises about 20% of the digestible starch found in vegetables, beans, breads, pasta, and rice. Amylopectin is a highly branched chain and makes up the remaining 80% of digestible starches in the diet (Fig. 4-4). Cellulose (a fiber) is another complex carbohydrate in plants. Although similar to amylose, it cannot be digested by humans, as discussed in Section 4.3.

The enzymes that break down starches to glucose and other related sugars act only at the end of a glucose chain. Amylopectin, because it is branched, provides many more sites (ends) for enzyme action. Therefore, amylopectin is digested more rapidly and raises blood glucose much more readily than amylose (see the discussion of glycemic index in Section 4.5).

As noted earlier, animals—including humans—store glucose in the form of glycogen. Glycogen consists of a chain of glucose units with many branches, providing even more sites for enzyme action than amylopectin (review Fig. 4-4). Because of its branched structure that can be broken down quickly, glycogen is an ideal storage form of carbohydrate in the body.

FIGURE 4-4 ▼ Some common starches, amylose and amylopectin, and glycogen. We consume essentially no glycogen. All glycogen found in the body is made by our cells, primarily in the liver and muscles.

Glucose

Glucose

Glucose

Amylose   **Amylopectin**   **Glycogen**

The liver and muscles are the major storage sites for glycogen. Because the amount of glucose immediately available in body fluids can provide only about 120 kcal, the carbohydrate energy stored as glycogen—amounting to about 1800 kcal—is extremely important. Of this 1800 kcal, liver glycogen (about 400 kcal) can readily contribute to blood glucose. Muscle glycogen stores (about 1400 kcal) cannot raise blood glucose but instead supply glucose for muscle use, especially during high-intensity and endurance exercise. Although animals store glycogen in their muscles, animal products such as meats, fish, and poultry are not good sources of carbohydrates because glycogen stores quickly degrade after the animal dies.

FIBER

Fiber as a class is mostly made up of polysaccharides, but fibers differ from starches insofar as the chemical bonds that join the individual sugar units cannot be digested by human enzymes in the GI tract. This prevents the small intestine from absorbing the sugars because they cannot be released from the various fibers. Fiber is not a single substance but a group of substances with similar characteristics. The group is composed of the carbohydrates **cellulose, hemicelluloses, pectins, gums,** and **mucilages,** as well as the noncarbohydrate **lignin.** In total, these constitute all the nonstarch polysaccharides in foods. Nutrition Facts labels generally do not list these individual forms of fiber but instead lump them together under the term **dietary fiber.**

Cellulose, hemicelluloses, and lignin form the structural parts of plants. Bran layers form the outer covering of all grains and are rich in hemicelluloses and lignin. (The woody fibers in broccoli are partly lignin.) **Whole grains** (i.e., unrefined) are good sources of bran fiber (Fig. 4-5). Because the majority of these fibers neither readily dissolve in water nor are easily metabolized by intestinal bacteria, they are called **nonfermentable** or insoluble fibers. Insoluble fiber is found in wheat bran, nuts, fruit skins, and some vegetables. Insoluble fiber acts as a natural laxative because it speeds up the transit time of food through the GI tract.

Pectins, gums, and mucilages are contained around and inside plant cells. These fibers either dissolve or swell when put into water and are therefore called **viscous** or soluble fibers. They also are readily fermented by bacteria in the large intestine. These fibers are found in beans, oats, oat bran, and some fruits and vegetables, as well as salad dressings, some frozen desserts, jams, and jellies as gum arabic, guar gum, locust bean gum, and various pectin forms. Soluble fiber slows the rate of absorption by attracting water into the GI tract, reduces blood cholesterol, and controls blood glucose.

Most foods contain mixtures of soluble and insoluble fibers. Food labels do not generally distinguish between the two types, but manufacturers have the option to do so. Often, if food is listed as a good source of one type of fiber, it usually contains some of the other type of fiber as well. The definition of fiber has recently been expanded to include (1) *dietary fiber,* which describes the nondigestible carbohydrates and lignin that are naturally occurring and

cellulose An undigestible, nonfermentable, straight-chain polysaccharide made of glucose molecules.

hemicellulose A nonfermentable fiber containing xylose, galactose, glucose, and other monosaccharides bonded together.

pectin A viscous fiber containing chains of galacturonic acid and other monosaccharides; characteristically found between plant cell walls.

gums Polysaccharides occurring naturally that cause an increase in viscosity; used as thickeners, gels, emulsifiers, and stabilizers.

mucilage A viscous fiber consisting of chains of galactose, mannose, and other monosaccharides; characteristically found in seaweed.

lignin A nonfermentable fiber made up of a multiringed alcohol (noncarbohydrate) structure.

dietary fiber Fiber found in food.

whole grains Grains containing the entire seed of the plant, including the bran, germ, and endosperm (starchy interior). Examples are whole wheat and brown rice.

nonfermentable fiber A fiber that is not easily metabolized by intestinal bacteria; also called *insoluble fiber.*

viscous fiber A fiber that is readily fermented by bacteria in the large intestine; also called *soluble fiber.*

FIGURE 4-5 ▶ Viscous (soluble) and nonfermentable (insoluble) fiber. (a) The skin of an apple consists of the nonfermentable fiber cellulose, which provides structure for the fruit. The viscous fiber pectin "glues" the fruit cells together. (b) The outside layer of a wheat kernel is made of layers of bran—primarily hemicellulose, a nonfermentable fiber—making this whole grain a good source of fiber. Overall, fruits, vegetables, whole-grain breads and cereals, and beans are rich in fiber.

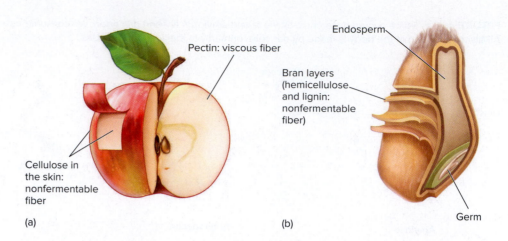

Pectin: viscous fiber

Cellulose in the skin: nonfermentable fiber

(a)

Endosperm

Bran layers (hemicellulose and lignin: nonfermentable fiber)

Germ

(b)

▶ This Concept Map summarizes the various forms and characteristics of the simple and complex carbohydrates.

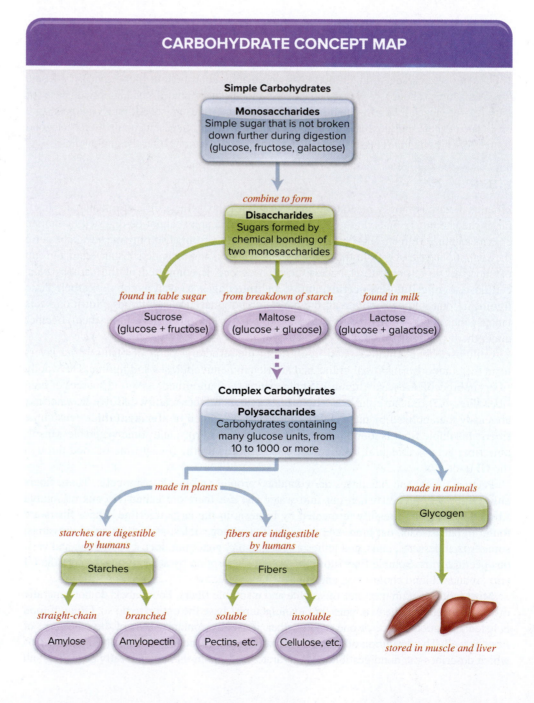

CARBOHYDRATE CONCEPT MAP

Simple Carbohydrates

Monosaccharides
Simple sugar that is not broken down further during digestion (glucose, fructose, galactose)

combine to form

Disaccharides
Sugars formed by chemical bonding of two monosaccharides

found in table sugar

Sucrose (glucose + fructose)

from breakdown of starch

Maltose (glucose + glucose)

found in milk

Lactose (glucose + galactose)

Complex Carbohydrates

Polysaccharides
Carbohydrates containing many glucose units, from 10 to 1000 or more

made in plants

made in animals

Glycogen

starches are digestible by humans

Starches

fibers are indigestible by humans

Fibers

straight-chain

Amylose

branched

Amylopectin

soluble

Pectins, etc.

insoluble

Cellulose, etc.

stored in muscle and liver

intact in plants; and (2) **functional fiber,** which consists of the isolated nondigestible carbohydrates that are added to food because they have beneficial physiological effects in human
beings. The commercially produced functional or isolated fibers include resistant starch,
polydextrose, indigestible dextrins, and inulin, which is one of the most popular varieties
currently added to products. The health benefits of many of these fibers are still unclear and
are therefore a hot discussion topic (see Further Readings 7 and 10).

Many of these fibers fall into a category of functional fiber called the **prebiotics.**
Prebiotics include a group of short-chain carbohydrates or oligosaccharides, resistant
to digestion but fermented by bacteria in the colon. They are thought to stimulate the
growth or activity of beneficial bacteria in the large intestine and therefore promote the
host's health.

functional fiber Fiber added to foods
that has been shown to provide health
benefits.

prebiotic Selectively fermented ingredient that results in specific changes in the
composition and/or activity of the gastrointestinal microbiota, thus conferring
benefits upon the host.

✓ CONCEPT CHECK 4.2

1. What are the names and definitions of the monosaccharides and disaccharides, and
   what happens to them when they are digested and absorbed?
2. What is a polysaccharide and what are the differences between the plant
   polysaccharides?
3. What is the name of the storage form of glucose and its locations in the body?
4. What makes fiber a very different kind of carbohydrate, and what is the difference
   between nonfermentable, viscous, and functional fiber?

4.3 Carbohydrates in Foods

Four of the groups on MyPlate—grains, vegetables, fruits, and dairy—contain the most
nutrient-dense sources of carbohydrates (Fig. 4-6). A healthy, carbohydrate-rich dietary
pattern emphasizes foods from these groups that do not contain too much sugar or fat.
Most dietary carbohydrate comes from starches. Because plants store glucose in the
form of starches, plant-based foods (beans, potatoes, and the grains used to make breads,
cereals, and pasta) are the best sources of starch. A dietary pattern rich in these starches
also provides many micronutrients and phytochemicals along with the carbohydrates. A
dietary pattern rich in whole grains, beans, and potatoes also provides significant amounts
of dietary fiber along with starch. Soluble fibers (pectin, gums, and mucilages) are found
in the skins and flesh of many fruits and berries; as thickeners and stabilizers in jams,
yogurts, sauces, and fillings; and in products that contain psyllium and seaweed. Fiber is
also available as a supplement or as an additive to certain foods (functional fiber) such
that individuals with relatively low intakes of natural dietary fiber can still obtain the
health benefits of fiber.

Unfortunately, the top five carbohydrate sources for U.S. adults in recent years have been:
white bread; soft drinks; cookies and cakes (including doughnuts); sugars, syrups, and jams;
and potatoes. Remember that these foods are on the Dietary Guidelines list of foods and
food components to reduce. Many North Americans are starting to take a closer look at their
carbohydrate sources and improve them from a nutritional standpoint by including more
whole-grain versions of breads, pasta, rice, and cereals, as well as fruits and vegetables. The
decline in soft drink consumption in the United States over the past 8 years is particularly
encouraging, with shoppers turning to water, energy drinks, and coffee instead. Although
data from *Beverage Digest* indicates that Americans still drink an average of 44 gallons of
soda a year, this is an 18.5% drop from the peak in 1998.

It is important to understand the percentage of calories from carbohydrates when
planning a healthy dietary pattern. The food components that yield the highest percentage of calories from carbohydrates are table sugar, honey, jam, jelly, fruit, and plain baked

MyPlate:
Sources of Carbohydrates

Grains	Vegetables	Fruits	Dairy	Protein
• All varieties	• All varieties	• All varieties	• Milk • Yogurt	• Beans • Nuts
15 grams per serving	5 grams per serving	18 grams per serving	12 grams per serving	4–10 grams per serving

FIGURE 4-6 ▲ Sources of carbohydrates from MyPlate. The fill of the background color (none, 1/3, 2/3, or completely covered) within each group in the plate indicates the average nutrient density for carbohydrates in that group. Overall, the grain group, vegetable group, fruit group, and dairy group contain many foods that are nutrient-dense sources of carbohydrate. (breads): Keith Weller/USDA; (vegetables): © Mitch Hrdlicka/Getty Images; (fruits): © Ingram Publishing/SuperStock

▲ How does this lunch of a turkey, cheese, lettuce, and tomato sandwich on whole-grain bread with an apple and a glass of low-fat milk compare to MyPlate? © McGraw-Hill Education/Ken Karp

potatoes (Fig. 4-7). Cornflakes, rice, bread, and noodles are next, all containing at least 75% of calories as carbohydrates. Foods with moderate amounts of carbohydrate calories are peas, broccoli, oatmeal, dry beans and other legumes, cream pies, French fries, and fat-free milk. In these foods, the carbohydrate content is diluted either by protein, as in the case of fat-free milk, or by fat, as in the case of cream pies. Foods with essentially no carbohydrates include beef, eggs, chicken, fish, vegetable oils, butter, and margarine.

WHOLE GRAINS

The 2015–2020 Dietary Guidelines recommend that we consume at least half of all grains as whole grains; increase whole-grain intake by replacing refined grains with whole grains; and limit the consumption of foods that contain refined grains, especially refined grain foods that contain solid fats, added sugars, and sodium. The Dietary Guidelines define whole grain as the entire grain seed or kernel made of three components: bran, germ, and endosperm. When the term *whole grain* is used on a food package, it also means that the product contains a minimum of 51% whole-grain ingredients by weight per serving. In contrast, refined grains typically contain only the starchy endosperm portion of the seed or kernel. These highly processed grains are low in fiber because much of the fiber in whole grains is found in the outer layers, which are removed in processing.

Although more fiber is one of the primary advantages of whole grains, many benefits of whole grains are thought to be due to the combined effects of several compounds. These compounds include fiber, minerals, trace minerals, vitamins, carotenoids, and other phytochemicals and are mainly contained in the bran and germ parts of the grains. The Dietary Guidelines recommend consuming two to three servings of whole grains per day. Several studies have

Food Sources of Carbohydrates

Food Item	Carbohydrate (grams)	% RDA
RDA	130	100%
Baked potato, 1 each	51	39%
Cola drink, 12 fluid oz	39	30%
Plain M&Ms, ½ oz	30	23%
Banana, 1 each	28	22%
Cooked rice, ½ cup	22	17%
Cooked corn, ½ cup	21	16%
Light yogurt, 1 cup	19	15%
Kidney beans, ½ cup	19	15%
Spaghetti noodles, ½ cup	19	15%
Orange, 1 each	16	12%
Seven-grain bread, 1 slice	12	9%
Fat-free milk, 1 cup	12	9%
Pineapple chunks, ½ cup	10	8%
Cooked carrots, ½ cup	8	6%
Peanuts, 1 oz	6	5%

Key:
- Grains
- Vegetables
- Fruits
- Dairy
- Protein
- Empty calories

FIGURE 4-7 ◀ Food sources of carbohydrate compared to the RDA of 130 grams for carbohydrate.

Is White Whole Wheat Really Whole Grain?

White whole wheat is a whole grain. It has the nutritional benefits of whole wheat but a milder taste, softer texture, and the lighter color of white bread. Traditional whole wheat is made from red wheat, which has a darker color and strongly flavored phenolic compounds. Switching to white whole wheat may be an acceptable option for those who prefer the taste and texture of white bread.

▲ The Whole Grains Council developed the Whole Grain stamp for use on grain products to help us identify whole-grain foods. There are two versions of the stamp. The 100% stamp is used if all grain ingredients are whole grains and there is a minimum of 16 grams (a full serving) of whole grain per serving. The basic stamp is used if a product contains at least 8 grams (a half serving) of whole grain, but it may also contain some refined grain.

Whole Grains Council, An Oldways Program. Used by permission.

shown that this is enough to impart numerous health benefits, including reducing risks of cardiovascular disease, diabetes, metabolic syndrome, some cancers, and obesity.

It is estimated that 9 in 10 people don't meet the whole-grain recommendation of three servings per day. Although Americans like grains and consume an average of 6.4 ounces of them daily, only 0.6 ounce is whole grain. This average consumption of less than one serving of whole grains per day falls far short of the recommendation. The reasons Americans are reluctant to consume whole grains include differences in the taste, texture, cost, and availability of whole grains, compared to products made with refined flour.

In addition to our preference for refined grains, many consumers who are trying to choose a whole-grain product are very confused by the deceptive marketing messages on the labels of grain products. For example, a label that says a cereal is "made with whole grains" does not guarantee that the cereal is 100% whole grain. Terms such as *cracked wheat bread, stoneground wheat, enriched wheat flour, 12-grain bread,* and *multigrain* are confusing because these products may contain little to no whole grain. Multigrain cereals may contain multiple grains, but many of them may be refined with just a small amount of whole grains added to a substantial amount of refined grains. Some "whole-grain breads" are white bread in disguise because brown coloring is added to enriched white flour (see Further Reading 6).

With all of the confusing buzzwords, it is crucial to look beyond the front-of-the-package claims and examine the list of ingredients. To confirm that products contain 100% whole grain, look for *whole* as the first word on the ingredient list. Sugary breakfast cereals that claim to be whole grain may list the first ingredient as a whole grain such as corn, rice, oat, or wheat, but then the next several ingredients may be various forms of sugar that together weigh more than the whole grain (see Further Readings 13 and 15).

Although whole grains make up only about 10% to 15% of grains on the grocery shelves, it is getting easier to find whole-wheat products and other whole-grain pastas. See Table 4-1 for information on several whole grains that are available, including their potential health benefits. To help simplify the process of finding whole-grain foods, the Whole Grains Council developed the Whole Grain stamp for food manufacturers to use on grain products. There are two versions of the stamp. The 100% Whole Grain stamp is used on a product if all of its grain ingredients are whole grains. It must also have a minimum of 16 grams (a full serving) of whole grain per serving. The basic Whole Grain stamp may be used if a product contains at least 8 grams (a half serving) of whole grain, but it may also contain some refined grain. The basic stamp is also used even if a product contains large amounts

TABLE 4-1 ■ Know Your Whole Grains

Grain	Characteristics	How to Spot Whole Grain	Health Benefits
Barley	Highest in fiber with a tough hull, which is difficult to remove without losing some of the bran; very slow cooking	Look for whole barley, hulled barley, or hull-less barley. Pearled barley is not technically a whole grain because small amounts of the bran are missing.	Barley fiber may lower cholesterol even more effectively than oat fiber.
Buckwheat	High levels of the antioxidant rutin and a high level of protein; cousin of rhubarb, not technically a grain at all—and certainly not a kind of wheat	If buckwheat is on ingredient list, it is almost always whole buckwheat.	Rutin improves circulation and prevents LDL cholesterol from blocking blood vessels.
Corn	Known for its sweet flavor	Avoid labels that say "degerminated" and look for the words *whole corn.*	Corn has highest level of antioxidants of any grain or vegetable.
Oats	High in protein and almost never have their bran and germ removed in processing; sweet flavor makes them popular for breakfast cereals	*Oats, oatmeal,* or *oat groats* on an ingredient list are almost always whole oats. Steel-cut oats are the entire oat kernel sliced into smaller pieces to help water penetrate and cook the grain. In the United States, most oats are steamed and flattened to produce "old-fashioned" or regular oats, quick oats, and instant oats, which cook more quickly.	Oat fiber is especially effective in lowering cholesterol.
Quinoa	Rich in high-quality protein, this small, light-colored round grain is similar in appearance to sesame seeds.	*Quinoa* on ingredient list almost always means whole quinoa.	Complete protein that contains all the essential amino acids.
Rice	Many whole-grain varieties, including brown, black, purple, or red. Brown rice is lower in fiber than most other whole grains but rich in many nutrients. White rice is refined, with the germ and bran removed.	Brown rice is always whole grain, as are most other colored rices, such as black rice or red rice.	One of the most easily digested grains; ideal for those on a restricted diet or who are gluten intolerant.
Rye	Unusual among grains for the high level of fiber in its endosperm—not just in its bran	Look for whole rye or rye berries in the ingredient list.	Rye fiber promotes a rapid feeling of fullness, making rye a good choice for people trying to lose weight. Rye products generally have a lower glycemic index than products made from wheat and most other grains, making them a good choice for diabetics.
Wheat	Dominates the grains we eat because it contains large amounts of gluten, a stretchy protein that enables bakers to create satisfying risen breads	Look for the term *whole wheat* (in Canada, for the term *whole-grain whole wheat*).	Since wheat is the most common grain eaten in the United States, most U.S. studies of "whole grains" can attest to the benefits of whole wheat. These benefits include reduced risk of stroke, type 2 diabetes, heart disease, inflammatory disease, and asthma; and better weight maintenance and healthier blood pressure levels.

Source: Adapted from the Whole Grains Council, Whole grains A to Z, at http://wholegrainscouncil.org/whole-grains-101/whole-grains-a-to-z.

of whole grain (23 grams, 37 grams, 41 grams, etc.) but also contains extra bran, germ, or refined flour. This reminds us that even if a product has whole grains, it can also contain a lot of sugar or solid fats. As of September 2015, the Whole Grain stamp is on over 10,500 different products and in over 44 countries. Choosing products with the 100% stamp will help us reach the minimum goal to get three servings of whole grains per day (see Further Reading 6). Schools are doing their part to increase whole-grain consumption by children, by meeting requirements of the Healthy, Hunger-Free Kids Act of 2010. Foods must contain at least 50% whole grains to meet the whole-grain–rich criteria for the federal school meal and child nutrition.

VEGETABLES

Vegetables are a valuable source of carbohydrates in the form of starch and fiber. They are naturally low in fat and calories and come packed with many other nutrients vital for health, including potassium, folate, vitamin A, and vitamin C. Eating the recommended amount of vegetables has been shown to reduce the risk of several chronic diseases. As we discussed with whole grains, the fiber in vegetables may reduce the risk of heart disease, obesity, and type 2 diabetes. Within the MyPlate guidelines, any vegetable or 100% vegetable juice counts as a member of the vegetables group. Vegetables are organized into five subgroups (dark-green vegetables, starchy vegetables, red and orange vegetables, beans and peas, and other vegetables) based on their nutrient content. Vegetable choices should be selected from among the vegetable subgroups but may be raw or cooked; fresh, frozen, canned, or dried/dehydrated; and whole, cut up, or mashed. Although it is not necessary to eat vegetables from each subgroup daily, the amounts listed from each subgroup should be eaten over a week as a way to reach your daily intake recommendation.

The amount of vegetables you need depends on your age, sex, and level of physical activity. For example, recommended total daily amounts for women age 19 to 50 years are 2 ½ cups. In general, 1 cup of raw or cooked vegetables or vegetable juice or 2 cups of raw leafy greens can be considered as "1 cup" from the vegetables group. Recommended weekly amounts from each vegetable subgroup are given as amounts to eat weekly. For example, the recommendations for women age 19 to 50 years are 1 ½ cups of dark-green vegetables, 5 ½ cups of red and orange vegetables, 1 ½ cups of beans and peas, 5 cups of starchy vegetables, and 4 cups of other vegetables such as cauliflower or mushrooms.

FRUITS

Fruits provide carbohydrates primarily in the form of natural sugar and fiber. Eating fruits provides health benefits similar to those discussed for vegetables; people who eat more fruits as part of an overall healthy diet are more likely to have a reduced risk of several chronic diseases. Dietary fiber from fruits helps reduce blood cholesterol levels, may lower risk of heart disease, and is important for proper bowel function. The fiber in fruits helps with weight maintenance by providing a feeling of fullness with fewer calories. Remember that whole or cut-up fruits are a great source of dietary fiber, compared to fruit juices that contain little or no fiber.

DAIRY

Foods in the dairy group provide carbohydrates in the form of lactose. Dairy products also provide other key nutrients, including calcium, potassium, vitamin D, and protein, which are responsible for many health benefits, especially improved bone health. While calcium-fortified soymilk (soy beverage) is part of the dairy group, foods made from milk that are primarily fat, such as cream cheese, cream, and butter, are not part of this group. The lactose content of dairy products varies somewhat. There are approximately 5 to 8 grams of lactose in the following high-lactose foods: ½ cup of fluid milk (whole, reduced fat, fat free, and buttermilk), half-and-half, plain yogurt, sour cream, and heavy cream; and ¾ cup of cottage cheese, ricotta cheese, ice cream, and ice milk. The following low-lactose foods

Dear RDN: *Is juicing healthier than eating whole fruits or vegetables?*

Juicing has become a popular way to consume fruits and vegetables and can be a fun way to drink the fruits and vegetables you do not enjoy eating. It is also a smart way to get your vitamins and minerals if you have gas or cramping when you eat fiber-rich produce. The good news is that most of the vitamins, minerals, and phytochemicals remain in the juice that is extracted from the fruits and vegetables during the juicing process. Also, you control the amount of added sugars and preservatives in the end product. The downside of the juicing process is that the natural fiber found in whole fruits and vegetables is typically lost. Thus, the juice is not healthier than whole fruit. In fact, there is no scientific evidence to support claims that juice extracts provide any health benefits or that nutrients are better absorbed from juice. Remember that juices from both fruits and vegetables contain a significant amount of natural sugar and juicing concentrates the sugar and calories. If consumed in excess, those calories can quickly add up! For example, juicing three apples will result in 40 grams of sugar and 200 calories. To make your juice healthier, add some of the pulp back to obtain valuable fiber that can help you feel full. Even better, instead of a juicer, you can use an extractor (e.g., NutriBullet®), which pulverizes fruits, vegetables, and nuts into the consistency of juice. Finally, keep sugar, calories, and fiber content in mind when buying ready-made juices at trendy juice bars.

To your health,

Anne M. Smith, PhD, RDN, LD (author)

▲ There are many forms of sugar on the market. Together they contribute to our daily intake of approximately 100 grams (20 teaspoons) of sugar in our diets.
(honey jar): © Burke/Triolo Productions/Getty Images; (measuring spoons): © C Squared Studios/ Getty Images

contain about 0 to 2 grams of lactose: ½ cup milk treated with lactase enzyme and sherbet; and 1 ounce aged cheese (blue, brick, cheddar, Colby, Swiss, and Parmesan) and processed cheese. Some individuals experience the condition of lactose intolerance and maldigestion when they consume high-lactose foods. (This situation is discussed in Section 4.4.) The amount of food you need to eat from the dairy group depends on your age, with the recommended daily amounts being 3 cups for all males and females 9 years and older. Typically, 1 cup of milk, yogurt, or soymilk (soy beverage), 1 ½ ounces of natural cheese, or 2 ounces of processed cheese is considered as "1 cup" from the dairy group.

NUTRITIVE SWEETENERS

The various substances that impart sweetness to foods fall into two broad classes: nutritive sweeteners, which can provide calories for the body, and alternative sweeteners, which for the most part provide no calories. As given in Table 4-2, the alternative sweeteners are much sweeter on a per-gram basis than the nutritive sweeteners. The taste and sweetness of sucrose make it the benchmark against which all other sweeteners are measured. Sucrose is obtained from sugarcane and sugar beet plants. Both sugars and sugar alcohols provide calories along with sweetness. Sugars are found in many different food products, whereas sugar alcohols have rather limited uses.

Sugars. All of the monosaccharides (glucose, fructose, and galactose) and disaccharides (sucrose, lactose, and maltose) discussed earlier are designated *nutritive sweeteners* because they provide calories. Many forms of sugar, including those naturally present in food and those added during processing or preparation, add up to an average intake of about 30 teaspoons of total sugar per day. The 2015–2020 Dietary Guidelines recommend that we reduce the intake of calories from added sugars. Added sugars are defined as caloric sweeteners added to foods during processing or preparation or before consumption. It is estimated that Americans consume an average of 20 teaspoons of added sugar per day, far exceeding the recommendation of no more than 8 teaspoons daily for adults. Data from a recent

TABLE 4-2 ■ The Sweetness of Sugars (Nutritive) and Alternative Sweeteners

Type of Sweetener	Relative Sweetness* (Sucrose = 1)	Typical Sources
Sugars		
Lactose	0.2	Dairy products
Maltose	0.4	Sprouted seeds
Glucose	0.7	Corn syrup
Sucrose	1.0	Table sugar, most sweets
Invert sugar†	1.3	Some candies, honey
Fructose	1.2–1.8	Fruit, honey, some soft drinks
Sugar Alcohols		
Sorbitol	0.6	Dietetic candies, sugarless gum
Mannitol	0.7	Dietetic candies
Xylitol	0.9	Sugarless gum
Maltitol	0.9	Baked goods, chocolate, candies
Alternative Sweeteners		
Stevia (Truvia®)	100–300	Tabletop sweetener, food ingredient
Luo han guo (Nectresse®)	150–300	Intended for use as a tabletop sweetener, a food ingredient, and a component of other sweetener blends
Aspartame (Equal®)	180	Diet soft drinks, diet fruit drinks, sugarless gum, tabletop sweetener
Acesulfame-K (Sunette®)	200	Sugarless gum, diet drink mixes, tabletop sweetener, puddings, gelatin desserts
Saccharin (Sweet'N Low®)	300	Diet soft drinks, tabletop sweetener
Sucralose (Splenda®)	600	Diet soft drinks, tabletop sweetener, sugarless gum, jams, frozen desserts
Neotame	7000–13,000	Tabletop sweetener, baked goods, frozen desserts, jams
Advantame	20,000	Tabletop sweetener, soft drinks, baked goods, frozen desserts, syrups, jams

*On a per gram basis.

†Sucrose broken down into glucose and fructose.

Source: From the Academy of Nutrition and Dietetics, 2012, and other sources (see Further Reading 11).

▲ Soft drinks are typical sources of either sugars or alternative sweeteners, depending on the type of soft drink chosen.
© BananaStock/PunchStock

National Health and Nutrition Examination Survey (NHANES) indicate that 14.6% of our total energy intake is from added sugar and that 60% of it comes from sugar-sweetened beverages, grain-based desserts, and fruit drinks.

HFCS is a sweetener now used in all kinds of foods, from soft drinks to barbecue sauce. It is called "high-fructose" corn syrup because it contains 55% fructose, compared to sucrose, which contains only 50% fructose. HFCS is made by an enzymatic process that converts some of the glucose in cornstarch into fructose, which tastes sweeter than glucose. In the United States, corn is abundant and inexpensive compared to sugarcane or sugar beets, much of which is imported. Food manufacturers prefer HFCS because of its low cost and broad range of food-processing applications, and because it is easy to transport, has better shelf stability, and improves food properties. An average American consumes about 60 pounds of HFCS each year. There has been much confusion and controversy surrounding the use and possible health effects of HFCS. Much of the controversy stemmed from a scientific commentary that was published in 2004 and suggested a link between HFCS consumption and obesity. Since then, the scientific community has examined this issue and concluded that there are no metabolic or endocrine response differences between HFCS and sucrose related to obesity or any other adverse health outcome (see Further Reading 12).

In addition to sucrose and HFCS, brown sugar, turbinado sugar (sold as raw sugar), honey, maple syrup, agave nectar, and other sugars are also added to foods. Brown sugar is essentially sucrose containing some molasses that is not totally removed from the sucrose during processing or is added to the sucrose crystals. Turbinado sugar is a partially refined version of raw sucrose. Maple syrup is made by boiling down and concentrating the sap that runs in sugar maple trees during the late winter. Because pure maple syrup is expensive, most pancake syrup is primarily corn syrup and HFCS with maple flavor added.

Honey is a product of plant nectar that has been altered by bee enzymes. The enzymes break down much of the nectar's sucrose into fructose and glucose. Honey offers essentially the same nutritional value as other simple sugars—a source of energy and little else. However, honey is not safe to feed to infants because it can contain spores of the bacterium *Clostridium botulinum* that causes fatal foodborne illness. Unlike the acidic environment of an adult's stomach, which inhibits the growth of the bacteria, an infant's stomach does not produce much acid, making infants susceptible to the threat that this bacterium poses.

Sugar Alcohols. Food manufacturers and consumers have numerous options for obtaining sweetness while using less sugar and calories. A primary purpose of sugar alcohols and alternative sweeteners is to enable people with diabetes to enjoy the flavor of sweetness while controlling sugars; they also provide noncaloric or very-low-calorie sugar substitutes for persons trying to lose (or control) body weight.

sorbitol Alcohol derivative of glucose that yields about 3 kcal/g but is slowly absorbed from the small intestine; used in some sugarless gums and dietetic foods.

xylitol Alcohol derivative of the five-carbon monosaccharide xylose.

Sugar alcohols, or polyols, such as **sorbitol** and **xylitol** are used as nutritive sweeteners but contribute fewer calories (about 2.6 kcal per gram) than sugars. They are also absorbed and metabolized to glucose more slowly than are simple sugars. Because of this, they remain in the intestinal tract for a longer time and in large quantities can cause diarrhea. In fact, any products that may be consumed in amounts that result in a daily ingestion of 50 grams or more of sugar alcohols must bear the statement, "Excess consumption may have a laxative effect," on the label.

Sugar alcohols must be listed on labels. If only one sugar alcohol is used in a product, its name must be listed; however, if two or more are used in one product, they are grouped together under the heading "sugar alcohols." The caloric value of each sugar alcohol used in a food product is calculated so that when one reads the total amount of calories a product provides, it includes the sugar alcohols in the overall amount.

Sugar alcohols are used in sugarless gum, breath mints, and candy. Unlike sucrose, sugar alcohols are not readily metabolized by bacteria to acids in the mouth and thus do not promote tooth decay.

ALTERNATIVE SWEETENERS

Alternative sweeteners yield little or no calories when consumed in amounts typically used in food products. They also are not metabolized by bacteria in the mouth, so they do not promote dental caries. Eight alternative sweeteners (see Table 4-2) are currently available in the United States, resulting in a $1.2 billion industry.

Acceptable Daily Intake (ADI) Estimate of the amount of a sweetener that an individual can safely consume daily over a lifetime. ADIs are given as milligrams per kilogram of body weight per day.

For each sweetener, FDA determines an **Acceptable Daily Intake (ADI)** guideline. ADIs are set at a level 100 times less than the level at which no harmful effects were noted in animal studies. Alternative sweeteners can be used safely by adults and children, and are considered safe during pregnancy.

saccharin Alternative sweetener that yields no energy to the body; 300 times sweeter than sucrose.

Saccharin The oldest alternative sweetener, **saccharin** represents about half of the alternative sweetener market in North America (typically packaged in pink packets, including Sweet 'N Low®). Based on laboratory animal studies, saccharin was once thought to increase the risk of bladder cancer, but it is no longer listed as a potential cause of cancer.

The FDA lists the ADI for saccharin at 5 milligrams per kilogram, or the equivalent of 9 to 12 packets of the sweetener.

Aspartame. Aspartame is in widespread use throughout the world (typically packaged in blue packets, including Equal®). It has been approved for use in more than 90 countries, and its use has been endorsed by the World Health Organization, the American Medical Association, the American Diabetes Association, among other groups.

The components of aspartame are the amino acids phenylalanine and aspartic acid, along with methanol. Recall that amino acids are the building blocks of proteins, so aspartame is more like a protein than a carbohydrate. Like protein, aspartame yields about 4 kcal per gram, but because it is about 200 times sweeter than sucrose, only a small amount is needed to obtain the desired sweetness. Like other proteins, however, aspartame is damaged when heated for a long time and thus would lose its sweetness if used in products that require cooking. Aspartame is used in beverages, gelatin desserts, chewing gum, and toppings.

The ADI of aspartame is 50 milligrams per kilogram of body weight. This is equivalent to about 18 cans of aspartame-containing diet soft drink or 8 packets of Equal. Aspartame appears to be safe for pregnant women and children, but some scientists suggest cautious use by these groups, especially young children, who need ample calories to grow. Although questions have been raised about a connection between aspartame and brain tumors, the National Cancer Institute conducted an extensive review of its data and declared, in 2009, that there is no link between aspartame and brain tumor development.

Persons with an uncommon disease called **phenylketonuria (PKU),** which interferes with the metabolism of phenylalanine, should avoid aspartame because of its high phenylalanine content. People with PKU will find a mandatory warning label on products containing aspartame (see label for sugarless gum).

Sucralose. Sucralose (Splenda®) is made by adding three chlorines to sucrose. It cannot be broken down or absorbed, so it yields no calories, and it is about 600 times sweeter than sucrose. It can be used in cooking and baking because it does not break down under high heat conditions. Sucralose is approved as an additive to foods such as soft drinks, gum, baked goods, syrups, gelatins, frozen dairy desserts such as ice cream, jams, processed fruits, and fruit juices, and for tabletop use. The ADI for sucralose is 5 milligrams per kilogram (about 30 packets of Splenda or 6 cans of diet soda for an adult).

Neotame. Neotame was recently approved by FDA for use as a general-purpose sweetener but is used in very few foods. Depending on its food application, Neotame is approximately 7000 to 13,000 times sweeter than table sugar. Neotame is heat stable and can be used as a tabletop sweetener as well as in cooking applications. Neotame is safe for use by the general population, including children, pregnant and lactating women, and people with diabetes. Although similar to aspartame, neotame does not require labeling for people with PKU because it is not broken down in the body to its amino acid components.

Acesulfame-K. Acesulfame-K is an organic acid linked to potassium (K) and is 200 times sweeter than sucrose. It was originally approved by FDA in 1988 and is sold as Sunette®. Acesulfame-K can be used in baking because it does not lose its sweetness when heated. In the United States, it is currently approved for use as a general-purpose sweetener. The ADI for acesulfame-K is 15 milligrams per kilogram, or the equivalent of 6 cans of diet soda.

Stevia. Stevia, sold as Truvia® and Sweet Leaf®, is an alternative sweetener derived from a South American shrub. Stevia extracts are 100 to 300 times sweeter than sucrose but provide no energy. It has been used in teas and as a sweetener in Japan since the 1970s, and FDA stated in December 2008 that stevia is considered generally recognized as safe (GRAS) for use in foods.

Luo Han Guo. Luo han guo is the extract of the monk fruit. It was approved by FDA in 2009 and is sold as the sweeteners Nectresse™ and Monk Fruit in the Raw™. Luo han guo is between 150 and 300 times sweeter than sucrose.

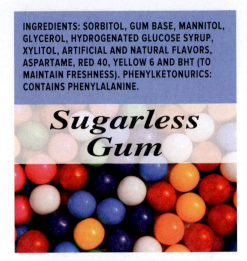

INGREDIENTS: SORBITOL, GUM BASE, MANNITOL, GLYCEROL, HYDROGENATED GLUCOSE SYRUP, XYLITOL, ARTIFICIAL AND NATURAL FLAVORS, ASPARTAME, RED 40, YELLOW 6 AND BHT (TO MAINTAIN FRESHNESS). PHENYLKETONURICS: CONTAINS PHENYLALANINE.

Sugarless Gum

▲ Sugar alcohols and the alternative sweetener aspartame are used to sweeten this product. Note the warning for people with phenylketonuria (PKU) that this product is made with aspartame and, thus, contains phenylalanine. © Nancy R. Cohen/Getty Images

aspartame Alternative sweetener made of two amino acids and methanol; about 200 times sweeter than sucrose.

phenylketonuria (PKU) Disease caused by a defect in the liver's ability to metabolize the amino acid phenylalanine into the amino acid tyrosine; untreated, toxic by-products of phenylalanine build up in the body and lead to mental retardation.

sucralose Alternative sweetener that has chlorines in place of 3 hydroxyl (—OH) groups on sucrose; 600 times sweeter than sucrose.

neotame General-purpose, nonnutritive sweetener that is approximately 7000 to 13,000 times sweeter than table sugar. It has a chemical structure similar to aspartame.

acesulfame-K Alternative sweetener that yields no energy to the body; 200 times sweeter than sucrose.

stevia Alternative sweetener derived from South American shrub; 100 to 300 times sweeter than sucrose.

▲ A variety of alternative sweeteners are available. © McGraw-Hill Education/Jill Braaten, photographer

Advantame. In May 2014, the FDA announced that a new food additive, advantame, is safe for use as a general-purpose sweetener and flavor enhancer in food. Advantame is stable at higher temperatures and can be used as a tabletop sweetener as well as in cooking applications. Chemically, advantame is similar to aspartame but is much sweeter. Because only a small amount is needed to achieve the same level of sweetness (it is 20,000 times sweeter than sucrose), foods that contain advantame do not need to include alerts for people with PKU.

> ✔ **CONCEPT CHECK 4.3**
>
> 1. Which food groups are the primary sources of carbohydrate in our diets?
> 2. What specific foods contain the highest percentage of calories from carbohydrates?
> 3. What are the common nutritive sweeteners?
> 4. Which alternative sweeteners are approved for use in food?

4.4 Making Carbohydrates Available for Body Use

As discussed in Chapter 3, simply eating a food does not supply nutrients to body cells. Digestion and absorption must occur first.

STARCH AND SUGAR DIGESTION

Food preparation can be viewed as the start of carbohydrate digestion because cooking softens tough connective structures in the fibrous parts of plants, such as broccoli stalks. When starches are heated, the starch granules swell as they soak up water, making them much easier to digest. All of these effects of cooking generally make carbohydrate-containing foods easier to chew, swallow, and break down during digestion.

The enzymatic digestion of starch begins in the mouth, when the saliva, which contains an enzyme called salivary **amylase,** mixes with the starchy products during the chewing of food. This amylase breaks down starch into many smaller units, primarily disaccharides, such as maltose (Fig. 4-8). You can taste this conversion while chewing a saltine cracker. Prolonged chewing of the cracker causes it to taste sweeter as some starch breaks down into the sweeter disaccharides, such as maltose. Usually, food is in the mouth for such a short amount of time that this phase of digestion is negligible. In addition, once the food moves down the esophagus and reaches the stomach, the acidic environment inactivates salivary amylase.

When the carbohydrates reach the small intestine, the more alkaline environment of the intestine is better suited for further carbohydrate digestion. The pancreas releases enzymes, such as pancreatic amylase, to aid the last stage of starch digestion. After amylase action, the original carbohydrates in a food are now present in the small intestine as the monosaccharides glucose and fructose, originally present as such in food, and disaccharides (maltose from starch breakdown, lactose mainly from dairy products, and sucrose from food and that added at the table).

The disaccharides are digested to their monosaccharide units once they reach the wall of the small intestine, where the specialized enzymes on the absorptive cells digest each disaccharide into monosaccharides. The enzyme **maltase** acts on maltose to produce two glucose molecules. **Sucrase** acts on sucrose to produce glucose and fructose. **Lactase** acts on lactose to produce glucose and galactose.

LACTOSE MALDIGESTION AND LACTOSE INTOLERANCE

Deficient production of the enzyme lactase will impair the digestion of lactose. The most common form of this condition is **primary lactose maldigestion,** a normal pattern of

amylase Starch-digesting enzyme produced by the salivary glands and the pancreas.

maltase An enzyme made by absorptive cells of the small intestine; this enzyme digests maltose to two glucoses.

sucrase An enzyme made by absorptive cells of the small intestine; this enzyme digests sucrose to glucose and fructose.

lactase An enzyme made by absorptive cells of the small intestine; this enzyme digests lactose to glucose and galactose.

primary lactose maldigestion Develops after early childhood, at about age 3 to 5 years, when the production of the enzyme lactase decreases.

Carbohydrate Digestion and Absorption

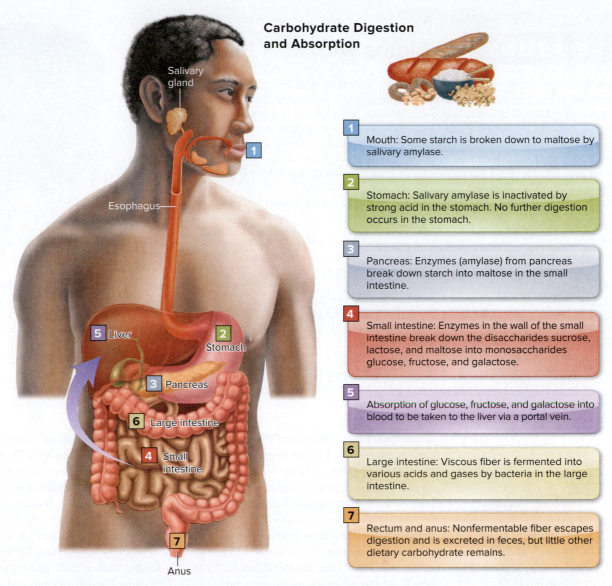

Salivary gland

Esophagus

5 Liver

2 Stomach

3 Pancreas

6 Large intestine

4 Small intestine

7

Anus

1 Mouth: Some starch is broken down to maltose by salivary amylase.

2 Stomach: Salivary amylase is inactivated by strong acid in the stomach. No further digestion occurs in the stomach.

3 Pancreas: Enzymes (amylase) from pancreas break down starch into maltose in the small intestine.

4 Small intestine: Enzymes in the wall of the small intestine break down the disaccharides sucrose, lactose, and maltose into monosaccharides glucose, fructose, and galactose.

5 Absorption of glucose, fructose, and galactose into blood to be taken to the liver via a portal vein.

6 Large intestine: Viscous fiber is fermented into various acids and gases by bacteria in the large intestine.

7 Rectum and anus: Nonfermentable fiber escapes digestion and is excreted in feces, but little other dietary carbohydrate remains.

FIGURE 4-8 ▲ Carbohydrate digestion and absorption. Enzymes made by the mouth, pancreas, and small intestine participate in the process of digestion. Most carbohydrate digestion and absorption take place in the small intestine. Chapter 3 covered the physiology of digestion and absorption in detail.

physiology that often begins to develop after early childhood, at about age 3 to 5 years. This primary form of lactose maldigestion is estimated to be present in about 75% of the world's population, although not all of these individuals experience symptoms. **Secondary lactose maldigestion** is a temporary condition in which lactase production is decreased in response to another condition, such as intestinal diarrhea. Rarely, lactase production is absent from birth, a condition known as **congenital lactase deficiency.** Any of these types of lactose maldigestion can lead to symptoms of gas, abdominal bloating, cramps, and diarrhea when lactose is consumed. The bloating and gas are caused by bacterial fermentation of lactose in the large intestine. The diarrhea is caused by undigested lactose in the large intestine as it draws water from the circulatory system into the large intestine. When significant symptoms develop after lactose intake, it is then called **lactose intolerance.** It is important to note that lactose maldigestion and resultant lactose intolerance are not equivalent to a milk allergy.

It is hypothesized that approximately 3000 to 5000 years ago, a genetic mutation occurred in regions that relied on milk and dairy foods as a main food source, allowing those individuals (mostly in northern Europe, pastoral tribes in Africa, and the Middle East) to retain the ability to maintain high lactase output for their entire lifetime. In North America, only about 25% of

secondary lactose maldigestion Occurs when production of the enzyme lactase declines for no apparent reason. When significant symptoms develop after lactose intake, it is then called *lactose intolerance.*

congenital lactase deficiency Birth defect resulting in the inability to produce lactase, such that a lactose-free diet is required from birth.

lactose intolerance A condition in which symptoms such as abdominal gas and bloating appear as a result of severe lactose maldigestion.

© Photodisc/Getty Images

CASE STUDY Problems with Milk Intake

Myeshia is a 19-year-old African-American female who recently read about the health benefits of calcium and decided to increase her intake of dairy products. To start, she drank a cup of 1% milk at lunch. Not long afterward, she experienced bloating, cramping, and increased gas production. She suspected that the culprit of this pain was the milk she consumed, especially because her parents and her sister complain of the same problem. She wanted to determine if other milk products were, in fact, the cause of her discomfort, so the next day she substituted a cup of yogurt for the glass of milk at lunch. Consuming the yogurt did not cause any pain.

Answer the following questions and check your response at the end of this chapter.

1. Why did Myeshia believe that she was sensitive to milk?
2. What component of milk is likely causing the problems that Myeshia experiences after drinking milk?
3. Why does this component cause intestinal discomfort in some individuals?
4. What is the name of this condition?
5. What groups of people are most likely to experience this condition?
6. Why did consuming yogurt not cause the same effects for Myeshia?
7. Are there any other products on the market that can replace regular milk or otherwise alleviate symptoms for individuals with this problem?
8. Can people with this condition ever drink regular milk?
9. What nutrients may be inadequate in the diet if dairy products are not consumed?
10. Why do some individuals have trouble tolerating milk products during or immediately after an intestinal viral infection?

▲ Use of yogurt helps lactose maldigesters meet calcium needs. © Ingram Publishing/ SuperStock

adults show signs of decreased lactose digestion in the small intestine. Asian Americans, African Americans, and Latino/Hispanic Americans are the population groups most likely to suffer lactose maldigestion, and the occurrence increases as people age. Many of these individuals can consume moderate amounts of lactose with minimal or no gastrointestinal discomfort because of eventual lactose breakdown by bacteria in the large intestine. Studies have shown that nearly all individuals with decreased lactase production can tolerate ½ to 1 cup of milk with meals and that most individuals adapt to intestinal gas production resulting from the fermentation of lactose by bacteria in the large intestine. Thus, it is unnecessary for these people to totally restrict their intake of lactose-containing foods, such as milk and milk products, which are important for maintaining bone health. Obtaining enough calcium and vitamin D from the diet is much easier if milk and milk products are included in a diet.

Combining lactose-containing foods with other foods also helps because certain properties of foods can have positive effects on rates of digestion. For example, fat in a meal slows digestion, leaving more time for lactase action. Hard cheese and yogurt are also more easily tolerated than milk. Much of the lactose is lost during the production of cheese, and the active bacteria cultures in yogurt digest the lactose with their lactase. In addition, products such as lactose-free or lactose-reduced milk (Lactaid® and Dairy Ease®) are made by treating regular milk with the lactase enzyme. Lactase supplements are also available to assist lactose maldigesters when they decide to consume products containing lactose. Many plant-based "milks," including soy milk, almond milk, and rice milk, are naturally lactose free and can be used as an alternative to regular milk.

CARBOHYDRATE ABSORPTION

Monosaccharides found naturally in foods and those formed as by-products of starch and disaccharide digestion in the mouth and small intestine generally follow an active absorption process. Recall from Chapter 3 that this is a process that requires a specific carrier and energy input for the substance to be taken up by the absorptive cells in the small intestine. Glucose and its close relative, galactose, undergo active absorption. They are pumped into the absorptive cells along with sodium.

Fructose is taken up by the absorptive cells via facilitated diffusion. In this case, a carrier is used, but no energy input is needed. This absorptive process is thus slower than that seen with glucose or galactose. So, large doses of fructose are not readily absorbed and can contribute to diarrhea as the monosaccharide remains in the small intestine and attracts water.

Once glucose, galactose, and fructose enter the absorptive cells, some fructose is metabolized into glucose. The single sugars in the absorptive cells are then transferred to the portal vein that goes directly to the liver. The liver then metabolizes those sugars by transforming the monosaccharides galactose and fructose into glucose and

- releasing it directly into the bloodstream for transport to organs such as the brain, muscles, kidneys, and adipose tissues.
- producing glycogen for storage of carbohydrate.
- producing fat (minor amount, if any).

Of these three options, producing fat occurs when carbohydrates are consumed in high amounts and overall calorie needs are exceeded.

Unless an individual has a disease that causes malabsorption or an intolerance to a carbohydrate such as lactose (or fructose), only a minor amount of some sugars (about 10%) escapes digestion. Any undigested carbohydrate travels to the large intestine and is fermented there by bacteria. The acids and gases produced by bacterial metabolism of the undigested carbohydrate are absorbed into the bloodstream. Scientists suspect that some of these products of bacterial metabolism promote the health of the large intestine by providing it with a source of calories.

FIBER AND INTESTINAL HEALTH

Bacteria in the large intestine ferment soluble fibers into such products as acids and gases. The acids, once absorbed, also provide calories for the body. In this way, soluble fibers provide about 1.5 to 2.5 kcal per gram. Although the intestinal gas (flatulence) produced by this bacterial fermentation is not harmful, it can be painful and sometimes embarrassing. Over time, however, the body tends to adapt to a high-fiber intake, eventually producing less gas. You may notice that some potentially gas-forming foods are good sources of soluble fiber.

Because insoluble fiber is an indigestible carbohydrate, it remains in the intestinal tract and supplies mass to the feces, making elimination much easier. When enough fiber is consumed, the stool is large and soft because many types of plant fibers attract water. The larger size stimulates the intestinal muscles to contract, which aids elimination. Consequently, less pressure is necessary to expel the stool. When too little fiber is eaten, the opposite can occur: very little water is present in the feces, making it small and hard. Constipation may result, which forces one to exert excessive pressure in the large intestine during defecation. This high pressure can force parts of the large intestine (colon) wall out from between the surrounding bands of muscle, forming many small pouches called **diverticula** (Fig. 4-9). **Hemorrhoids** (discussed in Section 3.12) may also result from excessive straining during defecation. Diverticula are asymptomatic in about 80% of affected people; that is, they go unnoticed. The asymptomatic form of this disease is called **diverticulosis.** If feces (and bacteria) become trapped within diverticuli, they may become inflamed or infected, a painful condition known as **diverticulitis.** In the short term, intake of fiber then should be reduced to limit further bacterial activity. Once the inflammation subsides, a high-fiber diet is resumed to ease stool elimination and reduce the risk of a future attack.

Very high intakes of fiber—for example, 60 grams per day—can also pose some health risks and therefore should be followed only under the guidance of a primary care provider. Increased fluid intake is extremely important with a high-fiber diet. Inadequate fluid intake can leave the stool very hard and painful to eliminate. In more severe cases, the combination of excess fiber and insufficient fluid may contribute to blockages in the intestine, which may require surgery. Aside from problems with the passage of materials through the GI tract, a high-fiber diet may also decrease the availability of nutrients. Certain components of fiber

What Are FODMAPs?

You learned in Section 3.12, that a group of carbohydrates known as FODMAPs (fermentable oligo-, di-, and monosaccharides and polyols) may cause gastrointestinal symptoms such as gas, bloating, and diarrhea in some people. The FODMAPs include fructose, lactose, fructans (in wheat, onions, and garlic), galactans (in legumes), and polyols (sugar alcohols, see Section 4.3). Some individuals are poor digesters of FODMAPs. These carbohydrates reach the large intestine without being digested. They draw water into the digestive tract and undergo fermentation by the bacteria that reside in the large intestine, leading to bloating and gas. Following a low-FODMAP dietary pattern may be the key to relief for many people with irritable bowel syndrome (IBS). It is important to work with a gastroenterologist and RDN when limiting FODMAPs. Ideally, you should eliminate only those foods that trigger digestive problems; overly restrictive dietary patterns can lead to nutrient inadequacies. The following websites provide practical information on foods to avoid and foods to include when restricting FODMAPs: http://www.gidoctor.net/fodmap.php; http://www.stefaniemendez.com/ibs-low-fodmap-diet/.

diverticula Pouches that protrude through the exterior wall of the large intestine.

hemorrhoid A pronounced swelling of a large vein, particularly veins found in the anal region.

Large intestine (colon)   Diverticula

FIGURE 4-9 ▲ Diverticula in the large intestine. A low-fiber dietary pattern increases the risk of developing diverticula. About one-third of people over age 45 and two-thirds over age 85 have diverticulosis.

diverticulosis The condition of having many diverticula in the large intestine.

diverticulitis An inflammation of the diverticula caused by acids produced by bacterial metabolism inside the diverticula.

▲ Beano® is a dietary supplement that contains natural digestive enzymes. Such products can be used to reduce intestinal gas produced by bacterial metabolism of undigested sugars in beans and some vegetables in the large intestine. © McGraw-Hill Education/Mark Dierker, photographer

ketone bodies Partial breakdown products of fat that contain three or four carbons.

may bind to essential minerals, keeping them from being absorbed. For example, when fiber is consumed in large amounts, zinc and iron absorption may be hindered.

Many population studies have shown a link between increased fiber intake and a decrease in colon cancer development. Most research on diet and colon cancer focuses on the potential preventive effects of fruits, vegetables, whole-grain breads and cereals, and beans (rather than just fiber). It is more advisable to increase fiber intake using fiber-rich foods than mostly relying on fiber supplements. Overall, the health benefits to the colon that stem from a high-fiber dietary pattern are partially due to the nutrients that are commonly present in most high-fiber foods, such as vitamins, minerals, phytochemicals, and, in some cases, essential fatty acids.

✓ **CONCEPT CHECK 4.4**

1. In what form are carbohydrates absorbed, and what happens to these compounds after absorption?

2. What are the names and locations of the enzymes that digest carbohydrates?

3. Why do some individuals feel discomfort after they consume large amounts of lactose? How can they avoid these symptoms?

4. What are the beneficial effects of fiber in the intestinal tract?

4.5 Putting Carbohydrates to Work in the Body

As just discussed, all of the digestible carbohydrate that we eat is eventually converted into glucose. Glucose is then the form of carbohydrate that goes on to function in body metabolism. The other sugars can generally be converted into glucose, and the starches are broken down to yield glucose, so the functions described here apply to most carbohydrates. The functions of glucose in the body start with supplying calories to fuel the body.

PROVIDING ENERGY

The main function of glucose is to supply calories for use by the body. Certain tissues in the body, such as red blood cells, can use only glucose and other simple carbohydrate forms for fuel. Most parts of the brain and central nervous system also derive energy only from glucose, unless the diet contains almost none. In that case, much of the brain can use partial breakdown products of fat—called **ketone bodies**—for energy needs. Other body cells, including muscle cells, can use simple carbohydrates as fuel, but many of these cells can also use fat or protein for energy needs.

A dietary pattern that supplies enough digestible carbohydrates to prevent breakdown of proteins for energy needs is considered *protein sparing*. Under normal circumstances, digestible carbohydrates in the diet mostly end up as blood glucose, and protein is reserved for functions such as building and maintaining muscles and vital organs. However, if you don't eat enough carbohydrates, your body is forced to make glucose from body proteins, draining the pool of amino acids available in cells for other critical functions. During long-term starvation, the continuous withdrawal of proteins from the muscles, heart, liver, kidneys, and other vital organs can result in weakness, poor function, and even failure of body systems.

The wasting of protein that occurs during long-term fasting can be life threatening. This has prompted companies that make formulas for rapid weight loss to include sufficient carbohydrates in the products to decrease protein breakdown and thereby protect vital tissues and organs, including the heart. Most of these very-low-calorie products are powders that can be mixed with different types of fluids and are consumed five or six times per day. When considering any weight-loss products, be sure that your total diet provides at least the RDA for carbohydrate.

In addition to the loss of protein, when you don't eat enough carbohydrates, the metabolism of fats is inefficient. In the absence of adequate carbohydrates, fats are not broken down completely in metabolism and instead form ketone bodies. This condition, known as **ketosis,** should be avoided because it disturbs the body's normal acid–base balance and leads to other health problems. This is a good reason to question the long-term safety of the low-carbohydrate diets that have been popular.

ketosis The condition of having a high concentration of ketone bodies and related breakdown products in the bloodstream and tissues.

REGULATING BLOOD GLUCOSE

Under normal circumstances, a person's blood glucose concentration is regulated within a narrow range. When carbohydrates are digested and taken up by the absorptive cells of the small intestine, the resulting monosaccharides are transported directly to the liver. One of the liver's roles, then, is to guard against excess glucose entering the bloodstream after a meal. The liver works together with the pancreas to regulate blood glucose.

When the concentration of glucose in the blood is high, such as during and immediately after a meal, the pancreas releases the hormone **insulin** into the bloodstream. Insulin delivers two different messages to various body cells to cause the level of glucose in the blood to fall. First, insulin directs the liver to store glucose as glycogen. Second, insulin directs muscle, adipose, and other cells to remove glucose from the bloodstream by taking it into those cells. By triggering both glycogen synthesis in the liver and glucose movement out of the bloodstream into certain cells, insulin keeps the concentration of glucose from rising too high in the blood (Fig. 4-10).

insulin A hormone produced by the pancreas. One of insulin's roles is to increase the synthesis of glycogen in the liver and the movement of glucose from the bloodstream into body cells.

On the other hand, when a person has not eaten for a few hours and blood glucose begins to fall, the pancreas releases the hormone **glucagon.** This hormone has the opposite effect of insulin. It prompts the breakdown of liver glycogen into glucose and the generation of glucose from noncarbohydrate substances, which is then released into the bloodstream to keep blood glucose from falling too low.

A different mechanism increases blood glucose during times of stress. **Epinephrine** (adrenaline) is the hormone responsible for the "flight or fight" reaction. Epinephrine and a related compound are released in large amounts from the adrenal glands (located on each kidney) and various nerve endings in response to a perceived threat, such as a car approaching head-on. These hormones cause glycogen in the liver to be quickly broken down into glucose. The resulting rapid flood of glucose from the liver into the bloodstream helps fuel quick mental and physical reactions.

glucagon A hormone made by the pancreas that stimulates the breakdown of glycogen in the liver into glucose; this ends up increasing blood glucose. Glucagon also increases the generation of glucose from non-carbohydrate substances.

epinephrine A hormone also known as *adrenaline;* it is released by the adrenal glands (located on each kidney) at times of stress. It acts to increase glycogen breakdown in the liver, among other functions.

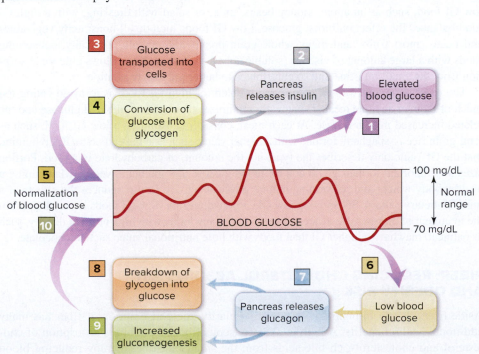

FIGURE 4-10 ◄ Regulation of blood glucose. Insulin and glucagon are key factors in controlling blood glucose. When blood glucose rises above the normal range of 70 to 100 milligrams per deciliter (mg/dl) (1), insulin is released (2) to lower it (3), and (4) blood glucose then falls back into the normal range (5). When blood glucose falls below the normal range (6), glucagon is released (7), which has the opposite effect of insulin (8), and (9) this then restores blood glucose to the normal range (10). Other hormones, such as epinephrine, norepinephrine, cortisol, and growth hormone, also contribute to blood glucose regulation.

hyperglycemia High blood glucose, above 125 milligrams per 100 milliliters of blood.

hypoglycemia Low blood glucose, below 40 to 50 milligrams per 100 milliliters of blood for nondiabetics.

This complex regulatory system is responsible for maintaining blood glucose within an acceptable range. It provides a safeguard against extremely high blood glucose (**hyperglycemia**) or low blood glucose (**hypoglycemia**). In essence, the actions of insulin on blood glucose are balanced by the actions of glucagon, epinephrine, and other hormones. If hormonal balance is not maintained, such as during over- or underproduction of insulin or glucagon, major changes in blood glucose concentrations occur. The disease type 1 diabetes is an example of the underproduction of insulin. The failure of blood glucose regulation will be discussed in Section 4.7.

The Glycemic Index and Blood Glucose. Our bodies react uniquely to different sources of carbohydrates. For example, a serving of a high-fiber food, such as baked beans, results in lower blood glucose levels compared to the same size serving of mashed potatoes. The effects of various foods on blood glucose are important to know because foods that result in a high blood glucose cause a large release of insulin from the pancreas. When this type of high insulin output occurs frequently, it leads to many deleterious effects on the body. Some of these undesirable effects are high blood triglycerides, increased fat deposition in the adipose tissue, increased tendency for blood to clot, increased fat synthesis in the liver, and a more rapid return of hunger after a meal (insulin rapidly lowers the macronutrients in the blood as it stimulates their storage, signaling hunger). Over time, this increase in insulin output may also cause the muscles to become resistant to the action of insulin and eventually lead to type 2 diabetes in some people.

glycemic index (GI) The blood glucose response of a given food, compared to a standard (typically, glucose or white bread). Glycemic index is influenced by starch structure, fiber content, food processing, physical structure, and macronutrients in the meal such as fat.

The **glycemic index (GI)** is a measurement of how the carbohydrate in a food raises blood glucose and, therefore, is helpful for planning a diet to avoid hyperglycemia (high blood glucose) and high insulin output. Glycemic index is a ratio of the blood glucose response to a given food compared to the response to a reference such as glucose or white bread (Table 4-3). Foods are ranked based on this comparison with a high GI food raising blood glucose more than a medium or low GI food.

The GI of a food is influenced by starch structure, fiber content, food processing, physical structure, and other macronutrients in the meal, such as fat. Thus, the GI of a food is different when the food is eaten alone compared to when it is combined with other foods. In general, the more highly processed foods have a higher GI. For example, juice has a higher GI than whole fruit. Foods with particularly high glycemic index values are baking potatoes (due to higher amylopectin content compared to red potatoes), mashed potatoes (due to greater surface area exposed), short-grain white rice, honey, and jelly beans. Combining a low GI food, such as an apple, kidney beans, milk, or salad with dressing, with a high GI food balances the effect on blood glucose. Low GI foods include all nonstarchy vegetables and beans, most fruits, and many whole-grain breads and cereals. Typically, consuming foods with a large amount of viscous (soluble) fiber, such as oat fiber, slows glucose absorption from the small intestine and so contributes to better glucose regulation.

The most important way to address the problem of high GI foods is to avoid eating too much of them at any one meal. This greatly minimizes their effects on blood glucose and the related increased insulin release. At each meal, consider substituting a low GI food, such as long-grain rice or spaghetti, for one with a higher value, such as a baked potato. Keep in mind that the GI value only describes the type, not the amount, of carbohydrate in a food. Portion sizes are important to manage, to control blood glucose and maintain weight. Maintaining a healthy body weight and performing regular physical activity further reduces the effects of a high GI dietary pattern. Substituting low GI carbohydrates for high GI foods is very helpful in the treatment of diabetes. Be aware, however, that many foods with high nutrient density, such as oatmeal, may have a higher GI than foods with little nutritional value such as chocolate.

You might wonder why the glycemic index of white bread and whole-wheat bread are similar. This is because whole-wheat flour is typically so finely ground that it is quickly digested. Thus, the effect of fiber in slowing digestion and related absorption of glucose is no longer present. Some experts suggest we focus more on minimally processed varieties of grains, such as coarsely ground whole-wheat flour and steel-cut or rolled oatmeal, to get the full benefits of these fiber sources in reducing blood glucose levels.

FIBER: REDUCING CHOLESTEROL ABSORPTION AND OBESITY RISK

Aside from its role in maintaining bowel regularity, the consumption of fiber has many additional health benefits. A high intake of viscous fiber also inhibits absorption of cholesterol and cholesterol-rich bile acids from the small intestine, thereby reducing blood

TABLE 4-3 ■ Glycemic Index (GI) of Common Foods*

Reference food glucose = 100			
Low GI foods—below 55			
Intermediate GI foods—between 55 and 70			
High GI foods—more than 70			

	Glycemic Index (GI)		Glycemic Index (GI)
Pastas/Grains		**Breads and Muffins**	72
White rice, long grain	56	Bagel	69
White rice, short grain	72	Whole-wheat bread	70
Spaghetti	41	White bread	
Vegetables		**Fruits**	
Carrots, boiled	49	Apple	38
Sweet corn	55	Banana	55
Potato, baked	85	Orange	44
Dairy Foods		**Beverages**	
Milk, skim	32	Orange juice	46
Yogurt, low fat	33	Gatorade	78
Ice cream	61	Coca-Cola	63
Legumes		**Snack Foods**	
Baked beans	48	Potato chips	54
Kidney beans	27	Vanilla wafers	77
Navy beans	38	Jelly beans	80
Sugars	73		
Honey	65		
Sucrose	23		
Fructose			

*Based on a serving of food that supplies 50 grams of CHO

Source: Foster-Powell K and others: International table of glycemic index and glycemic load. *American Journal of Clinical Nutrition* 76:5, 2002.

▲ The glycemic index of a food is not always a clear indicator of its nutritional value. For example, potato chips have a low glycemic index, but they are not very nutrient dense. © BananaStock/PunchStock

cholesterol and possibly reducing the risk of cardiovascular disease and gallstones. Recall that good sources of viscous fiber are apples, bananas, oranges, carrots, barley, oats, and kidney beans. The beneficial bacteria in the large intestine degrade soluble fiber and produce certain fatty acids that probably also reduce cholesterol synthesis in the liver. In addition, the slower glucose absorption that occurs with diets high in viscous fiber is linked to a decrease in insulin release. One of the effects of insulin is to stimulate cholesterol synthesis in the liver, so this reduction in insulin may contribute to the ability of viscous fiber to lower blood cholesterol. Overall, a fiber-rich diet containing fruits, vegetables, beans, and whole-grain breads and cereals (including whole-grain breakfast cereals) is advocated as part of a strategy to reduce risk of cardiovascular disease (i.e., coronary heart disease and stroke). Again, this is something that a low-carbohydrate dietary pattern cannot promise.

A diet high in fiber likely controls weight and reduces the risk of developing obesity (see Further Reading 14). Due to their bulky nature, high-fiber foods require more time to chew and thus fill us up without yielding many calories. Increasing intake of foods rich in fiber is one strategy for feeling satisfied or full after a meal (review the discussion of energy density in Section 2.1).

▲ Oatmeal is a rich source of viscous fiber. The FDA allows a health claim for the benefits of oatmeal to lower blood cholesterol because of the effects of this viscous fiber. © John A. Rizzo/Getty Images

▲ Whole grain as the entire grain seed or kernel made of three components: bran, germ, and endosperm. © Nancy R. Cohen/Getty Images

1. What is the primary role of carbohydrates in the body?
2. How does the body respond when too little carbohydrate is consumed?
3. What are the mechanisms by which blood glucose levels are maintained within a narrow range?
4. How can the glycemic index be applied in meal planning?
5. What are some of the important functions of fiber?

4.6 Carbohydrate Needs

The RDA for carbohydrates is 130 grams per day for adults. This is based on the amount needed to supply adequate glucose for the brain and nervous system, without having to rely on ketone bodies from incomplete fat breakdown as a calorie source. Somewhat exceeding this amount is fine; the Food and Nutrition Board recommends that carbohydrate intake should range from 45% to 65% of total calorie intake. The Nutrition Facts panel on food labels uses 60% of calorie intake as the standard for recommended carbohydrate intake. This would be 300 grams of carbohydrate when consuming a 2000-calorie diet.

Survey data from the USDA indicate that carbohydrates are available for the average American in greater amounts (474 grams per day in 2010) than any other components in the food system. Recommendations for carbohydrate consumption, however, emphasize the type of carbohydrates we should consume rather than just the total amount. Experts agree that one's carbohydrate intake should be based primarily on fruits, vegetables, whole-grain breads and cereals, and beans, rather than on refined grains, potatoes, and sugars.

The 2015–2020 Dietary Guidelines for Americans recommend that we choose fiber-rich fruits, vegetables, and whole grains often. More specifically, 3 or more ounces of grains—roughly one-half of one's grains—should be whole. Whole grain is defined as the entire grain seed or kernel made of three components: the bran, germ, and endosperm, which must be in nearly the same relative proportions as the original grain if cracked, crushed, or flaked (see Further Readings 13 and 15).

HOW MUCH FIBER DO WE NEED?

An Adequate Intake for fiber has been set based on the ability of fiber to reduce risk of cardiovascular disease (and likely many cases of diabetes). The Adequate Intake for fiber for adults is 25 grams per day for women and 38 grams per day for men. The goal is to provide at least 14 grams per 1000 kcal in a diet. After age 50, the Adequate Intake falls to 21 grams per day and 30 grams per day, respectively. The Daily Value used for fiber on food and supplement labels is 25 grams for a 2000-kcal diet. In North America, fiber intake averaged 17 grams per day between 2007 and 2010, and the average whole-grain intake was 0.8 ounce, less than one serving per day. This low intake is attributed to the lack of knowledge on the benefits of whole grains and the inability to recognize whole-grain products at the time of purchase. Thus, most of us should increase our fiber intake. At least three servings of whole grains per day are recommended. Eating a high-fiber cereal (at least 3 grams of fiber per serving) for breakfast is one easy way to increase fiber intake (Fig. 4-11; see Further Readings 7 and 10).

The Rate Your Plate exercise shows a diet containing 25 or 38 grams of fiber within moderate calorie intakes. Diets to meet the fiber recommendations are possible and enjoyable if you incorporate plenty of whole-wheat bread, fruits, vegetables, and beans. Use the Rate Your Plate exercise to estimate the fiber content of your diet and determine *your* fiber score.

Remember that very high intakes of fiber can be unhealthy and that fluid intake must be increased with a high-fiber diet. A high-fiber diet may also decrease the absorption of essential minerals, especially zinc and iron.

In the final analysis, keep in mind that any nutrient can lead to health problems when consumed in excess. High carbohydrate, high fiber, and low fat do not mean zero calories.

▲ When buying a bread labeled as "wheat bread," most people think they are buying a whole-wheat product. Because the flour is from the wheat plant, manufacturers can correctly list enriched white (refined) flour as wheat flour on food labels; however, if "whole-wheat flour" is not listed first on the ingredient list, then the product is not primarily a whole-wheat bread and thus does not contain as much fiber as it could. Careful reading of labels is important in the search for more fiber. Look for the term *whole-grain* or *whole-wheat* flour on the label for breads that are an excellent source of fiber. © Getty Images

Nutrition Facts

10 servings per container
Serving size   1 cup (55g/2.0 oz.)

Amount per serving	Cereal	Cereal with ½ Cup Vitamins A & D Skim Milk
Calories	**170**	**210**

	% Daily Value**	
Total Fat 1.0g*	2%	2%
Sat. Fat 0g	0%	0%
Trans Fat 0g		*
Cholesterol 0mg	0%	0%
Sodium 300mg	13%	15%
Potassium 340mg	10%	16%
Total Carbohydrate 43g	14%	16%
Dietary Fiber 7g	28%	28%
Total Sugars 16g		
Includes 10g Added Sugars	20%	20%
Protein 4g		
Vitamin D 1mcg, 2.5mcg	10%	25%
Calcium 20mg, 120mg	2%	12%
Iron 12mg, 12mg	65%	65%
Potassium 225mg, 402 mg	6%	11%
Vitamin A 225mcg, 300mcg	15%	20%
Vitamin C 12mg, 13mg	20%	22%
Thiamin 0.3mg, 0.5mg	25%	30%
Riboflavin 0.4mg, 0.6mg	25%	35%
Niacin 5mg, 5mg	25%	25%
Vitamin B6 0.5mg, 0.5mg	25%	25%
Folic acid 120mcg, 120mcg	30%	30%
Vitamin B12 1.5mcg, 2.1mcg	25%	35%
Phosphorus 200mg, 300mg	20%	30%
Magnesium 80mg, 100mg	20%	25%
Zinc 3.7mg, 3.7mg	25%	25%
Copper 0.2mg, 0.2mg	10%	10%

* Amount in cereal. One half cup skim milk contributes an additional 40 calories, 65mg sodium, 6g total car-bohydrate (6g sugars), and 4g protein.

** The % Daily Value (DV) tells you how much a nutrient in a serving of food contributes to a daily diet. 2,000 calories a day is used for general nutrition advice.

Nutrition Facts

17 servings per container
Serving size   ¾ cup (30g)

Amount per serving	Cereal	Cereal with ½ Cup Skim Milk
Calories	**170**	**210**

	% Daily Value**	
Total Fat 0g*	0%	1%
Saturated Fat 0g	0%	1%
Trans Fat 0g		*
Cholesterol 0mg	0%	1%
Sodium 60mg	2%	4%
Potassium 80mg	2%	8%
Total Carbohydrate 35g	9%	11%
Dietary Fiber 1g	4%	4%
Total Sugars 20g		
Includes 15g Added Sugars	30%	30%
Protein 3g		
Vitamin D 1mcg, 2mcg	10%	20%
Calcium 0mg, 150mg	0%	15%
Iron 1.8mg, 1.8mg	10%	10%
Potassium 95mg, 272 mg	3%	8%
Vitamin A 375mcg, 450mcg	25%	30%
Vitamin C 0mg, 1.2mg	0%	2%
Thiamin 0.3mg, 0.3mg	25%	25%
Riboflavin 0.4mg, 0.6mg	25%	35%
Niacin 5mg, 5mg	25%	25%
Vitamin B6 0.5mg, 0.5mg	25%	25%
Folic acid 100mcg, 100mcg	25%	25%
Vitamin B12 1.5mcg, 1.8mcg	25%	30%
Phosphorus 40mg, 150mg	4%	15%
Magnesium 16mg, 32mg	4%	8%
Zinc 1.5mg, 1.5mg	10%	10%
Copper 0.04mg, 0.04mg	2%	2%

* Amount in Cereal. One-half cup skim milk contributes an additional 65mg sodium, 6g total carbohydrate (6g sugars), and 4g protein.

** The % Daily Value (DV) tells you how much a nutrient in a serving of food contributes to a daily diet. 2,000 calories a day is used for general nutrition advice.

FIGURE 4-11 ◄ Reading the Nutrition Facts on food labels helps us choose more nutritious foods. Based on the information from these nutrition labels, which cereal is the better choice for breakfast? Consider the amount of fiber in each cereal. Did the ingredients lists give you any clues? (Note: Ingredients are always listed in descending order by weight on a label.) When choosing a breakfast cereal, it is generally wise to focus on those that are rich sources of fiber. Sugar content can also be used for evaluation; however, sometimes this number does not reflect added sugar but simply the addition of fruit, such as raisins, thus complicating the evaluation.

▲ Whole-grain foods, such as granola, are excellent sources of fiber. © Brand X Pictures/ PunchStock

Carbohydrates help moderate calorie intake in comparison with fats, but high-carbohydrate foods also contribute to total calorie intake.

HOW MUCH SUGAR IS TOO MUCH?

The main problems with consuming an excess amount of sugar are that it provides empty calories and increases the risk for dental decay.

The 2015–2020 Dietary Guidelines for Americans provide the following recommendations regarding carbohydrate intake as part of a healthy eating pattern while staying within calorie needs:

- Include a variety of vegetables from all of the subgroups—dark green, red and orange, legumes (beans and peas), starchy, and other.
- Include fruits, especially whole fruits.
- Include grains, at least half of which are whole grains.
- Limit intake of calories from added sugars to less than 10% per day.

Diet Quality Declines When Sugar Intake Is Excessive. Overcrowding the diet with sweet treats can leave little room for important, nutrient-dense foods, such as fruits and vegetables. Children and teenagers are at the highest risk for consuming too many empty calories in place of nutrients essential for growth. Many children and teenagers are drinking an excess of sugared soft drinks and other sugar-containing beverages and much less milk than ever before. This exchange of soft drinks for milk can compromise bone health, because milk contains calcium and vitamin D, which are both essential for bone health.

With regard to sugar intake, an upper limit of 25% of total calorie intake from "added sugars" has been set by the Food and Nutrition Board. Remember that "added sugars" are sugars added to foods during processing and preparation. Diets that go beyond this upper limit are likely to be deficient in vitamins and minerals. The World Health Organization (WHO) continues to reiterate a "strong recommendation" that added sugars provide no more than 10% of total daily calorie intake. A moderate intake of about 10% of calorie intake corresponds to a maximum of approximately 50 grams (or 12 teaspoons) of sugars per day, based on a 2000-kcal diet. Because of the association between excessive consumption of sugars and several metabolic abnormalities and adverse health conditions, the American Heart Association recommends reductions in the intake of added sugars such that the upper limit of intake for most American women is no more than 100 kcal (25 grams) per day from added sugars and no more than 150 kcal (37.5 grams) per day for most American men (see Further Reading 9). In March 2014, the WHO proposed a similar "conditional recommendation" that a sugar intake of less than 5% of daily kilocalories (25 grams for an adult of normal BMI) should be the target in order to avoid health risks such as weight gain and tooth decay.

Most of the sugars we eat come from foods and beverages to which sugar has been added during processing and/or manufacture. The Food Consumption Survey data from 2007–2010 indicates that the average daily intake of added sugars for American adults was 73 grams and for children was 77 grams, amounting to about 15% of calorie intake. Major sources of added sugars include soft drinks, cakes, cookies, fruit drinks, and dairy desserts such as ice cream (Fig. 4-12). Table 4-4 lists suggestions to limit sources of added sugars, including sweet desserts such as cakes, cookies, and ice cream (full and reduced fat). Also limit low-fat and fat-free snack products which typically contain lots of added sugar to produce an acceptable taste but resulting in a high-calorie food with as much or more calories than the high-fat food product it was designed to replace.

Supersizing sugar-rich beverages has also become common and has led to more sugar consumption; for example, in the 1950s, a typical serving size of a soft drink was a 6.5-ounce bottle, and now a 20-ounce plastic bottle is a typical serving. This one change in serving size contributes an extra 170 kcal to the diet—all from added sugars. Most convenience stores now offer

FIGURE 4-12 ▶ Sources of added sugars in the diets of the U.S. population age 2 years and older.

Sources: Dietary Guidelines for Americans; Chapter 3; National Cancer Institute, Sources of added sugars in the diets of the U.S. population ages 2 years and older, NHANES 2005–2006. Risk factor monitoring and methods. Cancer Control and Population Sciences. http://riskfactor.cancer.gov/diet/foodsources/added_sugars/table5a.html

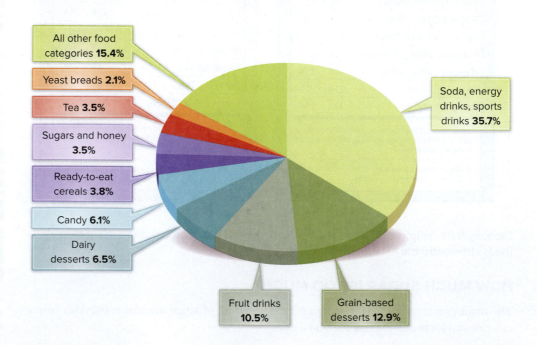

All other food categories **15.4%**

Yeast breads **2.1%**

Tea **3.5%**

Sugars and honey **3.5%**

Ready-to-eat cereals **3.8%**

Candy **6.1%**

Dairy desserts **6.5%**

Soda, energy drinks, sports drinks **35.7%**

Fruit drinks **10.5%**

Grain-based desserts **12.9%**

TABLE 4-4 ■ Suggestions for Reducing Added Sugar Intake

At the Grocery Store

- Read the ingredients list on food labels. Look for all forms of added sugars including as corn syrup. Select items lower in total sugar.
- Buy unsweetened versions of foods typically high in sugar such as cereals, oatmeal, applesauce, yogurt, and canned fruit (buy fresh fruits or fruits packed in water, juice, or light syrup rather than in heavy syrup).
- Buy nuts and dried fruits to replace candy for snacks.

© Photodisc/Getty Images

In the Kitchen

- Reduce the sugar in foods prepared at home. Make more foods from "scratch" to lower the sugar typically found in processed foods. Try low-sugar recipes or adjust your own. The amount of sugar can be decreased in recipes for foods such as pancakes, waffles, cookies, and cakes that will still taste great. Start by reducing the sugar gradually until you've decreased it by one-third or more.
- Add sweetness to foods with flavors and spices such as vanilla, citrus zest, cinnamon, cardamom, coriander, nutmeg, ginger, and mace.

© CMCD/Getty Images

At the Table

- Choose fewer foods high in sugar, such as prepared baked goods and sweet desserts. Reach for fresh fruit instead of cookies or candy for dessert and between-meal snacks.
- Include more protein such as eggs and turkey, and healthy fats such as nuts, seeds, and olive oil to decrease the desire for sugar.
- Add less sugar to foods such as coffee, tea, cereal, and fruit. Reduce the use of white and brown sugars, honey, molasses, syrups, jams, and jellies. Cut back gradually to a quarter or half the amount. Resist using sugar alternatives, which can confuse the body's taste for sweets.
- Substitute water for sugared soft drinks, sweet tea, coffee drinks, energy drinks, punches, and fruit juices.

©McGraw-Hill Education/ Jack Holtel photographer

▲ Cookies and cakes are one of the top five carbohydrate sources for U.S. adults. © Brand X Pictures/PunchStock

An excess intake of sugared soft drinks has recently been linked to a risk for both weight gain and type 2 diabetes in adults.

cups that will hold 64 ounces of soft drink. In 2012, the New York City Board of Health tried to ban the sale of sugary drinks in containers larger than 16 ounces in restaurants and other establishments in an effort to lower the intake of excess calories from sugar. Controversy over the authority of the health board to limit or ban a legal item led to a New York appeals court ruling in July 2013 that the city Board of Health exceeded its legal authority and acted unconstitutionally by trying to put a size limit on soft drinks served in city restaurants. Health messages about the sugary beverages appear to be having some positive effects, resulting in a decrease in soft drink sales over the past 8 years. Market research indicates that youth are choosing more water, energy drinks, and coffee in place of soft drinks. Read more about trends in added sugar consumption and the decline in soda consumption in the Newsworthy Nutrition and Further Reading 16.

Sugar and Hyperactivity. There is a widespread notion that high sugar intake causes hyperactivity in children, typically part of the syndrome called *attention deficit hyperactivity disorder (ADHD)*. In the 1990s, however, several well-controlled studies found that sugar in the diet did not affect children's behavior. Some researchers suggest that expecting sugar to affect a child can influence parents' interpretation of what they see. A study of parents' perceptions showed that parents who believe a child's behavior is affected by sugar are more likely to perceive their child as hyperactive when they believe the child just had a sugary drink. Experts recommend that other factors associated with hyperactivity, including temperament, emotional disturbances, learning disorders (e.g., ADHD), and sleep problems, be considered.

Sugar and Oral Health. Sugars in the diet (and starches readily fermented in the mouth, such as crackers and white bread) also increase the risk of developing **dental caries.** Recall that caries, also known as cavities, are formed when sugars and other carbohydrates are metabolized

▲ Many foods we enjoy are sweet. These should be eaten in moderation. © BananaStock/ PunchStock

dental caries Erosions in the surface of a tooth caused by acids made by bacteria as they metabolize sugars.

Newsworthy Nutrition

Americans are decreasing Consumption of sugar-sweetened beverages

Sugar-sweetened beverages (SSBs) are high in added sugars and calories, and have few, if any, nutrients. Consumption of SSBs has been associated with dental caries and risk factors of cardiovascular disease, and calories from SSBs contribute to obesity. Reducing SSB consumption, therefore, has been recommended to promote optimal health. The objective of this study was to examine trends in SSB consumption among youth and adults in the United States. This design was a large cross-sectional study of the energy intake from SSBs of 22,367 youth aged 2–19 years and 29,133 adults aged ≥20 years using dietary data from NHANES between 1999 and 2010. SSBs included soda, fruit drinks, sports and energy drinks, sweetened coffee and tea, and other sweetened beverages. The location and meal occasion of SSB consumption was also examined. The results of this study indicate that between 1999–2000 and 2009–2010, the intake of kilocalories from SSBs decreased from 223 to 155 kcal per day for youth and from 196 to 151 kcal per day for adults. During the 12-year study, SSB consumption decreased both in the home and away from home and with both meals and snacks. The percentage of total energy from SSBs also decreased to 8% among youth and 7% among adults in 2009–2010. The authors conclude from their analysis that there is a declining trend in SSB consumption among youth and adults in the United States.

Source: Kit BK and others: Trends in sugar-sweetened beverage consumption among youth and adults in the United States: 1999–2010. *American Journal of Clinical Nutrition* 98:180, 2013.

CRITICAL THINKING

John and Mike are identical twins who like the same games, sports, and foods. However, John likes to chew sugar-free gum and Mike doesn't. At their last dental visit, John had no cavities but Mike had two. Mike wants to know why John, who chews gum after eating, doesn't have cavities and he does. How would you explain this to him?

into acids by bacteria that live in the mouth. These acids dissolve the tooth enamel and underlying structure. Bacteria also use the sugars to make plaque, a sticky substance that both adheres acid-producing bacteria to teeth and diminishes the acid-neutralizing effect of saliva.

The worst offenders in terms of promoting dental caries are sticky and gummy foods high in sugars, such as caramel, because they stick to the teeth and supply the bacteria with a long-lived carbohydrate source. For this reason, snacking regularly on sugary foods is likely to cause caries because it gives the bacteria on the teeth a steady source of carbohydrates from which to continually make acid. Frequent consumption of liquid sugar sources (e.g., fruit juices) can also cause dental caries. Sugared gum chewed between meals is a prime example of a poor dental habit. Still, sugar-containing foods are not the only foods that promote acid production by bacteria in the mouth. As mentioned, if starch-containing foods (e.g., crackers and bread) are held in the mouth for a long time, the starch will be broken down to sugars by enzymes in the mouth; bacteria can then produce acid from these sugars. Overall, the sugar and starch contents of a food and its ability to remain in the mouth largely determine its potential to cause caries.

Fluoridated water and toothpaste are major factors in the prevention of dental caries in North American children due to fluoride's tooth-strengthening effect (see Chapter 9). Research has also indicated that certain foods—such as cheese, peanuts, and sugar-free chewing gum—can help reduce the amount of acid on teeth. In addition, rinsing the mouth after meals and snacks reduces the acidity in the mouth. Certainly, good nutrition, habits that do not present an overwhelming challenge to oral health (e.g., chewing sugar-free gum), and routine visits to the dentist all contribute to improved dental health.

✔ CONCEPT CHECK 4.6

1. What is the recommended intake of total carbohydrate per day, and how do typical dietary intakes compare?
2. How much fiber is recommended each day?
3. How can we reduce our consumption of added sugars?
4. What is the link between sugar and oral health?

Diabetes—When Blood Glucose Regulation Fails

© BananaStock/Photolibrary

Improper regulation of blood glucose results in either hyperglycemia (high blood glucose) or hypoglycemia (low blood glucose). High blood glucose is most commonly associated with diabetes (technically, *diabetes mellitus*), a disease that affects 28.9 million adults, or 12.3% of the North American population 20 years or older (see Further Reading 4). It is estimated that over 38% of these people do not know that they have the disease. Diabetes contributed to 234,051 deaths in 2010 in North America. Diabetes is currently increasing in epidemic proportions in the United States, with 1.7 million new cases diagnosed in people 20 years or older in 2012. The American Diabetes Association (ADA) recommends testing fasting blood glucose in adults over age 45 every 3 years to screen for diabetes. Diabetes was diagnosed for decades using a fasting blood glucose of 126 milligrams per 100 milliliters of blood or greater. In 2010, the ADA along with several international diabetes organizations recommended use of the hemoglobin A1c (HbA1c) test to diagnose diabetes with a threshold of greater than 6.5%. The HbA1c is a more sensitive, long-term indicator of poor blood glucose control than the fasting blood glucose level. When blood glucose is too high, the glucose builds up in the blood and combines with hemoglobin (protein in red blood cells), making it glycated. The amount of glycated hemoglobin, or HbA1c, reflects the last several weeks of blood glucose levels (see Further Reading 3).

Diabetes

There are two major forms of diabetes: **type 1** (formerly called insulin-dependent or juvenile-onset diabetes) and **type 2 diabetes** (formerly called noninsulin-dependent or adult-onset diabetes) (Table 4-5). The change in names to type 1 and type 2 diabetes stems from the fact that many type 2 diabetics eventually must also rely on insulin injections as a part of their treatment. In addition, many children today have type 2 diabetes. A third form, called gestational diabetes, occurs in some pregnant women (see Chapter 18). It is usually treated with an insulin regimen and diet, and resolves after delivery of the baby. However, women who have gestational diabetes during pregnancy are at high risk for developing type 2 diabetes later in life.

Traditional symptoms of diabetes are excessive urination, excessive thirst, and excessive hunger. No one symptom is diagnostic of diabetes, and other symptoms—such as unexplained weight loss, exhaustion, blurred vision, tingling in hands and feet, frequent infections, poor wound healing, and impotence—often accompany traditional symptoms.

Type 1 Diabetes

Type 1 diabetes often begins in late childhood, around age 10 to 14 years, but can occur at any age. The occurrence of the disease rose 3% from 2002 to 2009 in children and teens. Children usually are admitted to the hospital with abnormally high blood glucose after eating, as well as evidence of ketosis.

The onset of type 1 diabetes is generally associated with decreased release of insulin from the pancreas. As insulin in the blood declines, blood glucose increases, especially after eating. Figure 4-13 shows a typical glucose response observed in a patient with this form of diabetes after consuming about 75 grams of glucose. When blood glucose levels are high, the kidneys let excess glucose spill into the urine, resulting in frequent urination this is high in sugar.

Most cases of type 1 diabetes begin with an immune system disorder, which causes destruction of the insulin-producing cells in the pancreas. The disease may stem from genetic, autoimmune, or environmental factors. Most likely, a virus or protein foreign to the body sets off the destruction. In response to their damage, the affected pancreatic cells release other proteins, which stimulate a more aggressive attack. Eventually, the pancreas loses its ability to synthesize insulin, and the clinical stage of the disease begins. Hyperglycemia and other symptoms develop slowly and only after

type 1 diabetes A form of diabetes characterized by total insulin deficiency due to destruction of insulin-producing cells of the pancreas. Insulin therapy is required.

type 2 diabetes A form of diabetes characterized by insulin resistance and often associated with obesity. Insulin therapy can be used but is often not required.

TABLE 4-5 ■ Comparison of Type 1 and Type 2 Diabetes

	Type 1 Diabetes	Type 2 Diabetes
Occurrence	5% to 10% of cases of diabetes	90% to 95% of cases of diabetes
Cause	Autoimmune destruction of the pancreas	Insulin resistance
Risk factors	Moderate genetic predisposition	Strong genetic predisposition Obesity and physical inactivity Ethnicity Metabolic syndrome Prediabetes
Characteristics	Distinct symptoms (frequent thirst, hunger, and urination) Ketosis Weight loss	Mild symptoms, especially in early phases of the disease (fatigue and nighttime urination) No ketosis generally
Treatment	Insulin Diet Exercise	Diet Exercise Oral medications to lower blood glucose Insulin (in advanced cases)
Complications	Cardiovascular disease Kidney disease Nerve disease Blindness Infections	Cardiovascular disease Kidney disease Nerve damage Blindness Infections
Monitoring	Blood glucose Urine ketones HbA1c*	Blood glucose HbA1c

*Hemoglobin A1c.

90% or more of the insulin-secreting cells have been destroyed. HbA1c, fasting blood glucose, or an oral glucose tolerance test can be used to diagnose diabetes. Remember that HbA1c is the recommended measure because over time, blood glucose attaches to hemoglobin in red blood cells, especially when blood glucose remains elevated. A HbA1c value of over 7% indicates poor blood glucose control.

Type 1 diabetes is treated primarily by insulin therapy, either with injections or with an insulin infusion pump. The pump dispenses insulin at a steady rate into the body, with greater amounts delivered after each meal. Dietary therapy includes balancing carbohydrate intake with the insulin regimen and physical activity schedule to manage blood glucose levels. The amount and timing of carbohydrates eaten should be consistent from day to day to maintain blood glucose control. Insulin should be adjusted to match carbohydrate intake in persons who adjust their mealtime insulin doses or who are using an insulin pump. There are several methods available to estimate carbohydrate content of foods, including carbohydrate counting, exchange lists, and the glycemic index of foods (see Further Readings 2 and 5). For more information on nutrition treatment of diabetes, see Further Readings 1, 2, and 3. If one does not eat often enough, the injected insulin can cause a severe drop in blood glucose or hypoglycemia because it acts

Symptoms of Diabetes

The symptoms of diabetes may occur suddenly and include one or more of the following:

- Extreme thirst
- Frequent urination
- Drowsiness, lethargy
- Sudden vision changes
- Increased appetite
- Sudden weight loss
- Sugar in urine
- Fruity, sweet, or winelike odor on breath
- Heavy, labored breathing
- Stupor, unconsciousness

on whatever glucose is available. The diet should be moderate in simple carbohydrates, include ample fiber and polyunsaturated fat but be low in both animal and *trans* fats, and supply an amount of calories in balance with needs. Providing adequate calories and nutrients to promote growth and development in children is crucial for young diabetics.

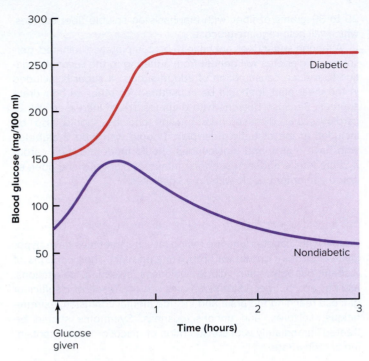

FIGURE 4-13 ▲ Glucose tolerance test. A comparison of blood glucose concentrations in untreated diabetic and healthy nondiabetic persons after consuming a 75-gram test load of glucose.

The hormone imbalances that occur in people with untreated type 1 diabetes—primarily, not enough insulin—lead to mobilization of body fat, taken up by liver cells. Ketosis is the result because the fat is partially broken down to ketone bodies. Ketone bodies can rise excessively in the blood, and eventually spill into the urine. These pull sodium and potassium ions as well as water into the urine. This series of events also causes frequent urination and can contribute to a chain reaction that eventually leads to dehydration,

▲ Insulin pumps alleviate the discomfort of injecting insulin under the skin multiple times per day. © Realistic Reflections

ion imbalance, coma, and even death, especially in patients with poorly controlled type 1 diabetes. Treatment includes provision of insulin, fluids, and minerals such as sodium and potassium.

Several degenerative complications, including cardiovascular disease, blindness, kidney disease, and nerve damage result from poor blood glucose regulation, specifically long-term hyperglycemia. The high blood sugar concentration physically deteriorates small blood vessels (capillaries) and nerves. When improper nerve stimulation occurs in the intestinal tract, intermittent diarrhea and constipation result. Because of nerve deterioration in the extremities, many people with diabetes lose the sensation of pain associated with injuries or infections. They do not have as much pain, so they often delay treatment of hand or foot problems. This delay, combined with a rich environment for bacterial growth (bacteria thrive on glucose), sets the stage for damage and death of tissues in the extremities, sometimes leading to the need for amputation of feet and legs. Elevated blood glucose also leads to glucose binding (known as glycation) to proteins and fats in the body, forming what are called *advanced glycation endproducts (AGEs)*. These have been shown to be toxic to cells, especially those of the immune system and kidneys.

Current research has shown that aggressive treatment directed at keeping blood glucose within the normal range can slow the development of blood vessel and nerve complications of diabetes. Maintaining near-normal HbA1c (6% or less) greatly reduces the risk of death and developing other diseases in people with diabetes. A person with diabetes generally must work closely with a physician and registered dietitian nutritionist to make the correct alterations in diet and medications and to perform physical activity safely. Physical activity enhances glucose uptake by muscles independent of insulin action, which in turn can lower blood glucose. This outcome is beneficial, but people with type 1 diabetes need to be aware of their blood glucose response to physical activity and compensate appropriately to avoid hypoglycemia.

Type 2 Diabetes

Type 2 diabetes usually begins after age 30. This is the most common type of diabetes, accounting for about 90% to 95% of the cases diagnosed in North America. The disease is progressive and is present, in many cases, long before it is diagnosed. Hyperglycemia develops slowly such that the classic symptoms are not noticed in the early stages of the disease, even though the risk for complications is rising. Risk factors for type 2 diabetes are both genetic and environmental and include a family history of diabetes; older age; obesity, especially intra-abdominal obesity; physical inactivity; prior history of gestational diabetes; prediabetes; and race or ethnicity. Latino/Hispanic Americans, African Americans, Asian Americans, Native Americans, and Pacific Islanders are at particular risk. The overall number of people affected is also on the rise, primarily because of widespread inactivity and obesity in our population. There has been a substantial increase in type 2 diabetes in children, due mostly to an increase in overweight in this population (coupled with limited physical activity).

Type 2 diabetes arises when the insulin receptors on the cell surfaces of certain body tissues, especially muscle and fat tissue, become insulin resistant. During the onset of the disease there is an abundance of insulin, but it is not used properly and blood glucose is not readily transferred into cells. The person develops high blood glucose as a result of the glucose remaining in the bloodstream. As the pancreas attempts to increase insulin output to compensate, the beta cells in the pancreas lose the ability to produce sufficient quantities of the hormone. As the disease develops, pancreatic function can fail, leading to reduced insulin output. Because of the genetic link for type 2 diabetes, those who have a family history should schedule regular blood glucose tests and be careful to avoid risk factors such as obesity and inactivity.

Many cases of type 2 diabetes (about 90%) are associated with overweight and obesity (especially with fat located in the abdominal region), but high blood glucose is not directly caused by the obesity. In fact, some lean people also develop this type of diabetes. Obesity associated with oversized adipose cells increases the risk for insulin resistance by the body as more fat is added to these cells during weight gain.

Because type 2 diabetes is linked to obesity, achieving a healthy weight should be a primary goal of treatment, with even limited weight loss leading to better blood glucose regulation. Although many cases of type 2 diabetes can be relieved by reducing excess adipose tissue stores, many people are not able to lose weight. They remain affected with diabetes and may experience the degenerative complications seen in the type 1 form of the disease. Ketosis, however, is not usually seen in type 2 diabetes. Glucose-lowering medications and insulin are used as needed in patients with type 2 diabetes. New classes of drugs that mimic gut hormones are helping diabetic patients overcome the chronic problems that conventional treatments alone have been unable to control. (See the Medicine Cabinet for information about drugs used to manage diabetes.)

Regular patterns of meals and physical activity are important elements of therapy for type 2 diabetes. Physical activity helps the muscles take up more glucose. Dietary therapy should emphasize overall calorie control, increased intakes of fiber-rich foods and fish, and reduced intakes of added sugars and solid fats. Distributing carbohydrates throughout the day helps minimize the high and low swings in blood glucose concentrations. As in type 1 diabetes, carbohydrate counting, exchange lists, and glycemic index of foods are excellent tools to manage carbohydrate intake. Using the glycemic index of foods combined with carbohydrate counting is an excellent way for motivated individuals to achieve blood glucose goals. It is also important to consume the recommended

25 to 30 grams of fiber, with emphasis on soluble fiber sources, which will help regulate glucose.

Although sugar does not have to be completely eliminated, persons with diabetes will benefit from adhering to the recommendation to reduce consumption of added sugars. If sugar is included in the meal plan, it should be substituted for other carbohydrate sources. Because persons with diabetes are at increased risk of cardiovascular disease, heart-healthy choices should also be included in the diabetic meal plan. People with type 2 diabetes who have high blood triglycerides should moderate their carbohydrate intake and increase their intake of plant oils and fiber, as noted earlier for people with type 1 diabetes.

Hypoglycemia

People with diabetes who are taking insulin sometimes have hypoglycemia if they do not eat frequently enough. The first signs of diabetic hypoglycemia include shakiness, sweating, palpitations, anxiety, and hunger. Later symptoms are the result of insufficient glucose reaching the brain and include mental confusion, extreme fatigue, seizures, and unconsciousness. Symptoms should be treated immediately with consumption of glucose or food containing carbohydrate.

Metabolic Syndrome

Metabolic syndrome is characterized by the presence of several risk factors for diabetes and cardiovascular disease. A person with metabolic syndrome must have at least three of the following

For more information on diabetes, consult the following websites: www.diabetes.org and www.ndep.nih.gov.

▲ Regular exercise is a key part of a plan to prevent (and control) type 2 diabetes (see Further Reading 8). © Ariel Skelley/Blend Images LLC

metabolic syndrome A condition in which a person has poor blood glucose regulation, hypertension, increased blood triglycerides, and other health problems. This condition is usually accompanied by obesity, lack of physical activity, and a diet high in refined carbohydrates. Also called Syndrome X.

metabolic risk factors (or be on medication to treat these risk factors) to be diagnosed with metabolic syndrome: a large waistline from abdominal obesity (accumulation of fat around and within the midsection), high blood triglycerides, low HDL or "good" cholesterol, hypertension, and high fasting blood glucose (Fig. 4-14). Each aspect of metabolic syndrome is a unique health problem with its own treatment. In metabolic syndrome, however, these risk factors are clustered together, making a person twice as likely to develop cardiovascular disease and five times more likely to develop diabetes.

It is generally accepted that one key element unifies all the aspects of metabolic syndrome: *insulin resistance.* As you learned in this chapter, insulin is a hormone that directs tissues to pull glucose out of the blood and into cells for storage or fuel. With insulin resistance, the pancreas produces plenty of insulin, but the cells of the body do not respond to it effectively. Instead, excess glucose stays in the bloodstream. For a while, the pancreas may be able to compensate for the resistance of cells to insulin by overproducing insulin. Over time, however, the pancreas is unable to keep up the accelerated insulin production, and blood glucose levels remain elevated. With metabolic syndrome, blood glucose is not high enough to be classified as diabetes (≥126 mg/dl), but without intervention, it is likely to get worse and eventually lead to diabetes.

Genetics and aging contribute to the development of insulin resistance and the other elements of metabolic syndrome, but

▲ Decreasing body weight and increasing physical activity are interventions to help prevent metabolic syndrome. © Dynamic Graphics/JupiterImages

environmental factors such as diet and activity play an important role. Obesity, particularly abdominal obesity, is highly related to insulin resistance. More than half of adults in the United States are overweight, 30% are obese, and these numbers continue to climb year after year. Increases in body weight among children and adolescents are of great concern because childhood obesity places them at high risk for these health problems. This increase in body weight has precipitated a dramatic surge in cardiovascular disease and diabetes risk: an estimated 50 million Americans now have metabolic syndrome.

The insulin resistance that precedes and causes type 2 diabetes also leads to several other components of the metabolic syndrome. The chief culprits contributing to the high blood triglycerides of metabolic syndrome are excessively large meals full of foods rich in simple sugars and refined starches and low in fiber, coupled with little physical activity. Nutrition and lifestyle changes are key strategies in addressing all of the unhealthy conditions of metabolic syndrome as a whole. Suggested interventions include:

- Decrease body weight. Even small improvements (e.g., 5% weight loss) for overweight and obese individuals can lessen disease risk. The most successful weight-loss and weight-maintenance programs include moderate dietary restriction combined with physical activity.
- Increase physical activity. To alleviate risks for chronic diseases, the 2008 Physical Activity Guidelines for Americans include a recommendation to do the equivalent of at least 150 minutes of moderate-intensity physical activity each week.
- Limit total fat consumption, especially animal and *trans* fat sources. Omega-3 fats, however, such as those found in fish and nuts, are considered healthy fats and should be included in your meal plan because they help combat several chronic diseases. We will explore the different types and sources of fats and their effects in Chapter 5.
- For those with particularly high risk for cardiovascular disease, medications to lower blood pressure, total cholesterol, and triglycerides may be warranted.

Metabolic Syndrome Risk Indicators

For a patient to be diagnosed with metabolic syndrome, he or she must have **three** of the five risk factors listed below.

- *High blood pressure*
  130/85 mmHg or higher

- *Low HDL cholesterol*
  - Men with HDL level less than 40 mg/dL

  - Women with HDL level less than 50 mg/dL

- *Elevated glucose*
  Fasting level of 100 mg/dL or higher

- *Elevated triglycerides (blood fat)*
  150 mg/dL or higher

- *Abdominal obesity*
  - Men with waist circumference greater than 40 inches

  - Women with waist circumference greater than 35 inches

FIGURE 4-14 ▲ Metabolic syndrome is characterized by the presence of several risk factors for diabetes and cardiovascular disease.

Medicine Cabinet

Insulin. Synthetic "human" insulin or their analogs used to treat diabetes are classified by how fast they start to work and how long their effects last.

- Rapid-acting insulin starts working within a few minutes and lasts for a couple of hours. *Examples:* Humalog®, NovoLog®, and Apidra®.

- Regular- or short-acting insulin takes about 30 minutes to work and lasts for 3 to 6 hours. *Examples:* Humulin R and Novolin R.

- Intermediate-acting insulin takes 2 to 4 hours to work, and its effects can last for up to 18 hours. *Examples:* Humulin N® and Novolin N®.

- Long-acting insulin takes 6 to 10 hours to reach the bloodstream, but it can keep working for an entire day. *Examples:* Lantus® and Levemir®.

Injectable diabetes medications are used to stimulate the release of insulin. These drugs mimic the gut hormones amylin and incretin and are used with injectable insulin (Symlin®) or with metformin and sulfonylurea. *Examples:* Byetta® and Victoza®.

Oral diabetes medications are usually prescribed to people with type 2 diabetes because they help control blood sugar levels when the body still produces some insulin. Each category of these drugs works differently.

- **Sulfonylureas.** Lower blood sugar by stimulating the pancreas to release more insulin. *Examples:* Glucotrol®, DiaBeta®, Micronase®, Glynase PresTab®, and Amaryl®.

- **Biguanides.** Improve insulin's ability to move sugar into cells, especially muscle cells, and prevent the liver from releasing stored sugar. *Example:* metformin (Glucophage®, Riomet®, Fortamet®, and Glumetza®).

- **Thiazolidinediones.** Improve insulin's effectiveness (decreasing insulin resistance) in muscle and in fat tissue, and lower the amount of sugar released by the liver. These drugs have been linked to adverse cardiovascular events. *Examples:* Actos® and Avandia®.

- **Alpha-glucosidase inhibitors.** Block enzymes that help digest starches to slow the rise in blood sugar. These diabetes pills may cause diarrhea or gas. *Examples:* Precose® and Glyset®.

- **Meglitinides.** Lower blood sugar by stimulating the pancreas to release more insulin when blood sugar is high. *Examples:* Prandin® and Starlix®.

- **Dipeptidyl peptidase IV (DPP-IV) inhibitors.** Lower blood sugar in patients with type 2 diabetes by increasing insulin secretion from the pancreas when blood sugars are high and reducing sugar production by the liver. *Examples:* Januvia®, Nesina®, Onglyza®, and Tradjenta®.

- **Combination therapy.** Combine two medications into one pill. *Example:* Glucovance® combines glyburide, a sulfonylurea, and metformin.

© McGraw-Hill Education/Jill Braaten, photographer

medicine cabinet - pills: © Footage supplied by Goodshoot/Punchstock

Summary (Numbers refer to numbered sections in the chapter.)

4.1 Carbohydrates are created in plants through photosynthesis. They are our main fuel source for body cells. Refined and processed products lack many of the health benefits provided by unprocessed sources of carbohydrates (e.g., whole grains, beans, fruits, and vegetables).

4.2 The common monosaccharides in food are glucose, fructose, and galactose. Once these are absorbed from the small intestine and delivered to the liver, much of the fructose and galactose is converted into glucose.

The major disaccharides are sucrose (glucose + fructose), maltose (glucose + glucose), and lactose (glucose + galactose). When digested, these yield their component monosaccharides.

One major group of polysaccharides consists of storage forms of glucose: starches in plants and glycogen in humans. These can be broken down by human digestive enzymes, releasing the glucose units. The main plant starches—straight-chain amylose and branched-chain amylopectin—are digested by enzymes in the mouth and small intestine.

In humans, glycogen is synthesized in the liver and muscle tissue from glucose. Under the influence of hormones, liver glycogen is readily broken down to glucose, which can enter the bloodstream.

Fiber is composed primarily of the polysaccharides cellulose, hemicellulose, pectin, gum, and mucilage, as well as the noncarbohydrate lignins. These substances are not broken down by human digestive enzymes. Soluble (also called viscous) fiber, however, is fermented by bacteria in the large intestine.

4.3 Table sugar, honey, jelly, fruit, and plain baked potatoes are some of the most concentrated sources of carbohydrates. Other high-carbohydrate foods, such as pie and fat-free milk, are diluted by either fat or protein. Nutritive sweeteners in food include sucrose, high-fructose corn syrup, brown sugar, and maple syrup. Several alternative sweeteners are approved for use by FDA: saccharin, aspartame, sucralose, neotame, and acesulfame-K.

4.4 Some starch digestion occurs in the mouth. Carbohydrate digestion is completed in the small intestine. Some plant fibers are digested by the bacteria present in the large intestine; undigested plant fibers become part of the feces. Monosaccharides in the intestinal contents mostly follow an active absorption process. They are then transported via the portal vein that leads directly to the liver.

The ability to digest lactose often diminishes with age. Lactose maldigestion also can develop early in childhood and is most common among people of African, Asian, or Hispanic descent. Undigested lactose travels to the large intestine, resulting in such symptoms as abdominal gas, pain, and diarrhea. The occurrence of severe symptoms after consuming lactose is called lactose intolerance. Most people with lactose maldigestion can tolerate cheese, yogurt, and moderate amounts of milk.

4.5 Carbohydrates provide calories (on average, 4 kcal per gram), protect against wasteful use of food and body protein for energy,

and prevent ketosis. The RDA for carbohydrate is 130 grams per day. If carbohydrate intake is inadequate for the body's needs, protein is metabolized to provide glucose for energy needs. However, the price is loss of body protein, ketosis, and eventually a general body weakening. For this reason, low-carbohydrate diets are not recommended for extended periods.

Blood glucose concentration is regulated within a narrow range of 70 to 99 milligrams per deciliter. Insulin and glucagon are hormones that control blood glucose concentration. When we eat a meal, insulin promotes glucose uptake by cells. When fasting, glucagon promotes glucose release from glycogen stores in the liver.

Insoluble (also called nonfermentable) fiber provides mass to the feces, thus easing elimination. In high doses, soluble fiber can help control blood glucose in diabetic people and lower blood cholesterol.

4.6 Diets high in complex carbohydrates are encouraged as a replacement for high-fat diets. A goal of about half of calories as complex carbohydrates is a good one, with about 45% to 65% of total calories coming from carbohydrates in general. Foods to consume are whole-grain cereal products, pasta, legumes, fruits, and vegetables. Many of these foods are rich in fiber.

Moderating sugar intake, especially between meals, reduces the risk of dental caries. Alternative sweeteners, such as aspartame, aid in reducing intake of sugars.

4.7 Diabetes is characterized by a persistent high blood glucose concentration. Regular physical activity and a balanced meal plan that emphasizes fiber and limits added sugars and solid fats are helpful in treating both type 1 and type 2 diabetes. Insulin is the main medication employed: it is required in type 1 diabetes and may be used in type 2 diabetes.

Check Your Knowledge (Answers are available at the end of this question set.)

1. Dietary fiber
   a. raises blood cholesterol levels.
   b. speeds up transit time for food through the digestive tract.
   c. causes diverticulosis.
   d. causes constipation.

2. When the pancreas detects excess glucose, it releases the
   a. enzyme amylase.
   b. monosaccharide glucose.
   c. hormone insulin.
   d. hormone glucagon.

3. Cellulose is a(n)
   a. indigestible fiber.
   b. simple carbohydrate.
   c. energy-yielding nutrient.
   d. animal polysaccharide.

4. Digested white sugar is broken into _____ and _____.
   a. glucose, lactose
   b. glucose, fructose
   c. sucrose, maltose
   d. fructose, sucrose

5. Starch is a
   a. complex carbohydrate.
   b. fiber.
   c. simple carbohydrate.
   d. gluten.

6. Fiber content of the diet can be increased by adding
   a. fresh fruits.
   b. fish and poultry.
   c. eggs.
   d. whole grains and cereals.
   e. both a and d.

7. Which form of diabetes is most common?
   a. type 1   b. type 2   c. type 3   d. gestational

8. The recommended daily intake for fiber is approximately _____ grams.
   a. 5   b. 30   c. 100   d. 450

9. Lactose intolerance is the result of
   a. drinking high-fat milk.
   b. eating a large amount of yogurt.
   c. low lactase activity.
   d. a high-fiber diet.

10. One of the components of metabolic syndrome is
    a. high body weight.
    b. high waist circumference.
    c. low blood sugar.
    d. low blood pressure.

Answer Key: 1. b (LO 4.5), 2. c (LO 4.5), 3. a (LO 4.2), 4. b (LO 4.2), 5. a (LO 4.2), 6. e (LO 4.3), 7. b (LO 4.7), 8. b (LO 4.6), 9. c (LO 4.4), 10. b (LO 4.7)

Study Questions (Numbers refer to Learning Outcomes)

1. Why do we need carbohydrates in the diet? **(LO 4.3)**

2. What are the three major monosaccharides and the three major disaccharides? Describe how each plays a part in the human diet. **(LO 4.2)**

3. Why are some foods that are high in carbohydrates, such as cookies and fat-free milk, not considered to be concentrated sources of carbohydrates? **(LO 4.3)**

4. Describe the digestion of the various types of carbohydrates in the body. **(LO 4.4)**

5. Describe the reason why some people are unable to tolerate high intakes of milk. **(LO 4.4)**

6. List three alternatives to simple sugars for adding sweetness to the diet. **(LO 4.3)**

7. Outline the basic steps in blood glucose regulation, including the roles of insulin and glucagon. **(LO 4.5)**

8. What are the important roles that fiber plays in the diet? **(LO 4.5)**

9. Summarize current carbohydrate intake recommendations. **(LO 4.6)**

10. What, if any, are the proven ill effects of sugar in the diet? **(LO 4.6)**

What the Dietitian Chose

Sandwiches can be a great option for a quick lunch that includes several, if not all, of the food groups on MyPlate. Most of us define a sandwich as meat and perhaps cheese between two slices of bread. This idea will guarantee plenty of grains, protein, and even dairy. All of the sandwiches on this menu provide 1 ½ to 2 ½ ounces of protein. The hotdog and the peanut butter sandwich are the lowest, at 1 ½ ounces, and the soy burger is the highest with 2 ½ ounces of protein. All the others provide 2 ounces of protein, and all of the sandwiches are equal in terms of their grain servings, at 2 ounces.

The challenge arises in filling the other half of the plate—that is, getting some vegetables and perhaps fruit onto a sandwich. Additionally, we want to consider the nutritional quality of the grains, protein, and dairy items. If we evaluate the sandwiches at Doug's Deli based on their carbohydrate sources, we see that only three of the sandwiches offer servings of vegetables. The addition of two tomato slices, four slices of cucumber or pickles, and two lettuce leaves to the turkey sandwich and the soy burger provides ¾ cup of vegetables to each. The tuna salad sandwich provides the most vegetables, 1 ¼ cups, from the carrots and onions in the tuna salad and the ½ cup of sprouts, two leaves of lettuce, and four cucumber slices added to the sandwich.

We typically do not find fruits on a sandwich and that is true of the menu at Doug's Deli. Although we see strawberry jelly on the peanut butter sandwich, jelly does not count as a fruit serving and instead provides 32 kcal (~10% of total kilocalories in the sandwich) from added sugars.

As we move to the grains aspect of MyPlate, we want to examine the whole-grain content of the breads offered. Fortunately, two of the options we already highlighted for their vegetable content are served on whole-grain breads. The tuna salad on whole wheat and the soy burger on a whole-wheat English muffin both offer 2 ounces of whole grain for this quick lunch. The combination of vegetables and whole grain provides a significant amount of dietary fiber. The

tuna salad sandwich has 7 grams and the soy burger has 7.5 grams of dietary fiber, which is close to 30% of the daily recommendation of 25 to 38 grams per day. The soy burger on whole wheat also has the benefit of having both soluble fiber from the soybean and insoluble fiber from the whole wheat. The

© BananaStock/PunchStock

peanut butter sandwich also provides 3 grams of primarily soluble fiber from the peanut butter.

The turkey and Swiss sandwich is also a good choice with 4 grams of fiber, and it provides a ¾-cup serving of dairy. Unfortunately, the rye is not necessarily a whole-grain bread. The ham and Swiss provides 2 ounces of lean protein and ¾ cup of dairy but provides only 1.5 grams of fiber because it is on sourdough bread made from refined white flour. It is also low on the list of choices because of its high sodium content (about 1100 milligrams).

Although it is sometimes described as America's favorite, the hotdog on a white bun has the least to offer nutritionally. It provides the lowest amount of grain at 1 ½ ounces, and the grain is refined rather than whole. It also has the lowest protein content at 1 ½ ounces and offers only 1 gram of fiber. It is high in sodium at over 700 milligrams and contains 6 grams of animal fat.

In summary, the dietitian would choose either the meatless soy burger or the tuna salad sandwich at Doug's Deli to maximize the number of servings from a variety of healthy carbohydrate sources including vegetables and whole grains.

CASE STUDY SOLUTION Problems with Milk Intake

1. Myeshia suspected that she was sensitive to milk because she developed bloating and gas when she consumed milk during one meal.

2. The disaccharide lactose is the most likely cause of Myeshia's symptoms.

3. When the enzyme lactase is missing or in short supply in the small intestine, undigested lactose travels to the large intestine and is fermented by bacteria there. The fermentation of lactose by bacteria produces abdominal gas, bloating, and pain. Diarrhea can also occur because the presence of lactose in the colon draws water from the blood vessels into the large intestine.

4. Lactose maldigestion is a normal pattern of physiology that often begins to develop at about age 3 to 5 years in populations that do not rely on milk and other dairy foods as a main food source. When significant symptoms develop after lactose intake, it is then called lactose intolerance.

5. The primary form of lactose maldigestion is estimated to occur in about 75% of the world's population. In the United States, most lactose maldigesters are African-Americans (like Myeshia), Asian-Americans, and Latino/Hispanic Americans. The occurrence of lactose maldigestion also increases as people age.

6. The active bacteria cultures in yogurt digest the lactose when these bacteria are broken apart in the small intestine and release their lactase.

7. Many products, such as low-lactose milk and lactase pills, are available to enable lactose maldigesters to tolerate milk.

8. Many lactose maldigesters can consume moderate amounts of lactose with minimal or no intestinal discomfort because of the eventual lactose breakdown by bacteria in the large intestine.

9. In North America and Western Europe, milk and other dairy products are important sources of calcium and vitamin D. These are important for maintaining bone health.

10. Secondary lactose maldigestion occurs when a condition (e.g., long-standing diarrhea from a viral infection) results in a significant decline in lactase production.

Further Readings

1. American Diabetes Association: Nutrition recommendations and interventions for diabetes: A position statement of the American Diabetes Association. *Diabetes Care* 31 (suppl 1):S61, 2008.

2. American Diabetes Association and Academy of Nutrition and Dietetics: *Choose your foods: Food lists for diabetes.* 2014.

3. American Diabetes Association: Standards of Medical Care in Diabetes-2014: *Diabetes Care* 37:S14, 2014.

4. Centers for Disease Control and Prevention: *National Diabetes Statistics Report, 2014.* Atlanta, GA: U.S. Department of Health and Human Services, Centers for Disease Control and Prevention, 2014.

5. Franz MJ and others: The evidence for medical nutrition therapy for type 1 and type 2 diabetes in adults. *Journal of the American Dietetic Association* 110:1852, 2010.

6. Getz L: Deciphering whole grain food labels: Separating fact from fiction. *Today's Dietitian* 14(6):44, 2012.

7. Hall M: Fiber facts about cereal. *Today's Dietitian* 14(12):30, 2012.

8. Hayes C, Kriska A: Role of physical activity in diabetes management and prevention. *Journal of the American Dietetic Association* 108:S19, 2008.

9. Johnson RK and others: Dietary sugars intake and cardiovascular health: A scientific statement from the American Heart Association. *Circulation* 120(11):1011, 2009.

10. Position of the Academy of Nutrition and Dietetics: Health implications of dietary fiber. *Journal of the Academy of Nutrition and Dietetics* 115:1861, 2015.

11. Position of the Academy of Nutrition and Dietetics: Use of nutritive and nonnutritive sweeteners. *Journal of the Academy of Nutrition and Dietetics* 112:739, 2012.

12. Rippe JM, Angelopoulos TJ: Sucrose, high-fructose corn syrup, and fructose, their metabolism and potential health effects: What do we really know? *Advances in Nutrition* 4:236, 2013.

13. Schaeffer J: Boosting whole grain consumption. *Today's Dietitian* 15(2):33, 2013.

14. Slavin J and others: How fiber affects weight regulation. *Food Technology,* p. 34, February 2008.

15. Webb D: Whole grain goodness. *Today's Dietitian* 14(9):56, 2012.

16. Welsh JA and others: Consumption of added sugars is decreasing in the United States. *American Journal of Clinical Nutrition* 94:726, 2011.

 To get the most out of your study of nutrition, go to McGraw-Hill's online resources: Connect www.mcgrawhillconnect.com, where you will find NutritionCalc Plus, LearnSmart, and many other dynamic tools.

Rate Your Plate

Estimate Your Fiber Intake

Review the sample menus shown in Table 4-6. The first menu contains 1600 kcal and 25 grams of fiber (AI for women); the second menu contains 2100 kcal and 38 grams of fiber (AI for men).

TABLE 4-6 ■ Sample Menus Containing 1600 kcal with 25 grams of Fiber and 2000 kcal with 38 Grams of Fiber*

Menu	25 Grams of Fiber			38 grams of Fiber		
	Serving Size	Carbohydrate Content (g)	Fiber Content (g)	Serving Size	Carbohydrate Content (g)	Fiber Content (g)
Breakfast						
Muesli cereal	1 cup	60	6	1 cup	60	6
Raspberries	½ cup	11	2	½ cup	11	2
Whole-wheat toast	1 slice	13	2	2 slices	26	4
Margarine	1 tsp	0	0	1 tsp	0	0
Orange juice	1 cup	28	0	1 cup	28	0
1% milk	1 cup	24	0	1 cup	24	0
Coffee	1 cup	0	0	1 cup	0	0
Lunch						
Bean and vegetable burrito	2 small	50	4.5	3 small	75	7
Guacamole	¼ cup	5	4	¼ cup	5	4
Monterey Jack cheese	1 oz	0	0	1 oz	0	0
Pear (with skin)	1	25	4	1	25	4
Carrot sticks	—	—	—	¾ cup	6	3
Sparkling water	2 cups	0	0	2 cups	0	0
Dinner						
Grilled chicken (no skin)	3 oz	0	0	3 oz	0	0
Salad		7	3	½ cup	19	6
Red cabbage	½ cup					
Romaine	½ cup			½ cup		
Peach slices	¼ cup			1 cup		
Toasted almonds	—	—	—	½ oz	3	2
Fat-free salad dressing	2 tbsp	0	0	2 tbsp	0	0
1% milk	1 cup	24	0	1 cup	24	0
Total		247	25		306	38

© Image Source/Corbis

© BananaStock/PunchStock

© Getty Images/Jonelle Weaver

*The overall diet is based on MyPlate breakdown of approximate energy content: carbohydrate, 58%; protein, 12%; and fat, 30%.

To roughly estimate your daily fiber consumption, determine the number of servings that you ate yesterday from each food category listed here. If you are not meeting your needs, how could you do so? Multiply the serving amount by the value listed and then add up the total amount of fiber.

Food	Servings	Grams
Vegetables		
(serving size: 1 cup raw leafy greens or 1/2 cup other vegetables)	_____ × 2	_____
Fruits		
(serving size: 1 whole fruit, 1/2 grapefruit, 1/2 cup berries or cubed fruit, and 1/4 cup dried fruit)	_____ × 2.5	_____
Beans, lentils, split peas		
(serving size: 1/2 cup cooked)	_____ × 7	_____
Nuts, seeds		
(serving size: 1/4 cup; 2 tbsp peanut butter)	_____ × 2.5	_____
Whole grains		
(serving size: 1 slice whole-wheat bread; 1/2 cup whole-wheat pasta, brown rice, or other whole grain; and 1/2 each bran or whole-grain muffin)	_____ × 2.5	_____
Refined grains		
(serving size: 1 slice bread, 1/2 cup pasta, rice, or other processed grains; and 1/2 each refined bagels or muffins)	_____ × 1	_____
Breakfast cereals		
(serving size: check package for serving size and amount of fiber per serving)	_____ × grams of fiber per serving	_____
Total Grams of Fiber =		_____

Source: Adapted from Fiber: Strands of protection. *Consumer Reports on Health,* p. 1, August 1999.

How does your total fiber intake for yesterday compare with the general recommendation of 25 to 38 grams of fiber per day for women and men, respectively?

If you are not meeting your needs, how could you do so?

▲ This dessert is an excellent source of fiber from 2 slices of whole-wheat banana bread (7 grams) with ½ cup of berries (1.8 grams) and 2 ounces of yogurt for a total of 8.8 grams of fiber. © Kevin Sanchez/Cole Group/Getty Images

© Ingram Publishing/SuperStock

Student Learning Outcomes

Chapter 5 is designed to allow you to:

5.1 Understand the common properties of lipids.

5.2 List three structural forms of lipids (fats) and the role of each in our food supply. Distinguish between fatty acids and triglycerides. Discuss the importance of the essential fatty acids, as well as the balance between omega-3 and omega-6 fatty acids, with respect to health.

5.3 Differentiate among food sources of saturated, monounsaturated, and polyunsaturated fatty acids and cholesterol.

5.4 Explain how lipids are digested and absorbed.

5.5 Name the classes of lipoproteins and classify them according to their functions.

5.6 List the function of lipids, including the roles of phospholipids and the functions of cholesterol in the body.

Chapter 5
Lipids

Lipids are energy dense: fatty acids from triglycerides contain more than twice the calories per gram (on average, 9 kcal) as proteins and carbohydrates (on average, 4 kcal each). Consumption of common solid fats also contributes to the risk of cardiovascular disease. For these reasons, some concern about excessive consumption of certain lipids is warranted. Lipids do play vital roles, however, both in the body and in foods. Their presence in the diet is essential to good health. In fact, lipids found in seafood, such as the salmon pictured here, have been linked to *lower* risk for several chronic diseases. In general, lipids should comprise 20% to 35% of an adult's total calorie intake.

Humans need very little fat in their diet to maintain health. In fact, the body's need for the essential fatty acids can be met by daily consumption of only about 2 to 4 tablespoons of plant oil incorporated into foods and consumption of fatty fish such as salmon or tuna at least twice weekly. The Food and Nutrition Board suggests that fat intake can be as high as 35% of calories consumed for an adult. Some experts suggest that an intake as high as 40% of calories is appropriate as long as the predominant type of fat is a healthy one, such as olive oil. After learning more about lipids—fats, oils, and related compounds—in this chapter, you can decide for yourself how much fat you want to consume.

Let us look at lipids in detail—their forms, functions, metabolism, and food sources. This chapter will also discuss the link between various lipids and the major "killer" disease in North America: cardiovascular disease, which involves the heart, including the coronary arteries (coronary heart disease) and other arteries in the body.

5.7 Explain the recommendations for fat intake.

5.8 Characterize the symptoms of cardiovascular disease and highlight some known risk factors.

5.1 Lipids: Common Properties

Lipids are composed primarily of the elements carbon and hydrogen; they contain fewer oxygen atoms than do carbohydrates. Chemical energy can be derived from breakdown of all those carbon-hydrogen bonds, so lipids yield more than twice as much energy (9 kcal per gram) as carbohydrates or proteins (4 kcal per gram).

Lipid is a generic term that includes **triglycerides, phospholipids,** and **sterols.** Food experts, such as chefs, call lipids that are solid at room temperature *fats,* and call lipids that are liquid at room temperature *oils.* Most people use the word *fat* to refer to all lipids because they do not realize that there is a difference. To simplify our discussion, this chapter primarily uses the term *fat.* When necessary for clarity, the name of a specific lipid, such as cholesterol, will be used. This word use is consistent with the way many people use these terms.

As a class of nutrients, lipids share one main characteristic: they do not readily dissolve in water. Think of an oil-and-vinegar salad dressing. The oil is not soluble in the water-based vinegar; on standing, the two separate into distinct layers, with oil on the top and vinegar on the bottom.

As you will learn in Section 5.2, the chemical structures of lipids are diverse. Triglycerides are the most common type of lipid found in the body and in foods. Each triglyceride molecule consists of three fatty acids bonded to **glycerol.** Phospholipids and sterols (including **cholesterol**) are also classified as lipids, although their structures can be quite different from the structure of triglycerides. All of these lipid compounds are described in this chapter.

> ✔ **CONCEPT CHECK 5.1**

1. What is the common property that all lipid compounds share?

5.2 Lipids: Triglycerides, Phospholipids, and Sterols

FATTY ACIDS AND TRIGLYCERIDES

Fatty Acids: The Simplest Form of Lipids Triglycerides are the primary form of lipids in the body and in foods. Fatty acids are found in triglycerides. A fatty acid is basically a long chain of carbons bonded together and flanked by hydrogens. At one end of the molecule (the alpha end) is an **acid group.** At the other end (the omega end) is a **methyl group** (Fig. 5-1).

Fats in foods are not composed of a single type of fatty acid. Rather, each dietary fat, or triglyceride, is a complex mixture of many different fatty acids, the combination of which provides each food its unique taste and smell.

Fatty acids can be saturated or unsaturated with hydrogen. Chemically speaking, a carbon atom can form four bonds. Within the carbon chain of a fatty acid, each carbon bonds to two other carbons and to hydrogens. The carbons that make up the chain of a **saturated fatty acid** are all connected to each other by single bonds. This allows the maximum number of hydrogens to be bound. Just as a sponge can be saturated (full) with water, a saturated fatty acid, such as stearic acid, is saturated with hydrogen [see Fig. 5-1(a)]. The saturated fatty acids are very straight and linear and therefore can pack very close together. This close packing or stacking of saturated fat molecules makes them solidify at room temperature.

Animal fats are high in saturated fatty acids and remain solid at room temperature. A good example is the solid fat surrounding a piece of uncooked steak. Chicken fat, semi-solid at room temperature, contains less saturated fat than beef fat. However, in some foods,

triglyceride The major form of lipid in the body and in food. It is composed of three fatty acids bonded to glycerol.

phospholipid Any of a class of fat-related substances that contain phosphorus, fatty acids, and a nitrogen-containing component. Phospholipids are an essential part of every cell.

sterol A compound containing a multi-ring (steroid) structure and a hydroxyl group (—OH). Cholesterol is a typical example.

glycerol A three-carbon alcohol used to form triglycerides.

cholesterol A waxy lipid found in all body cells. It has a structure containing multiple chemical rings that is found only in foods that contain animal products.

acid group In chemistry, a functional group that consists of a carbon atom that shares bonds with two oxygen atoms. This is the site where fatty acids are linked to glycerol to form triglycerides.

methyl group In chemistry, a carbon atom that shares bonds with three hydrogen atoms. The methyl group is the omega end of a fatty acid.

saturated fatty acid A fatty acid containing no carbon-carbon double bonds.

▲ Saturated fats, such as butter, are solid at room temperature, whereas unsaturated fats, such as olive and corn oil, are liquid at room temperature. © Tetra Images/Getty Images

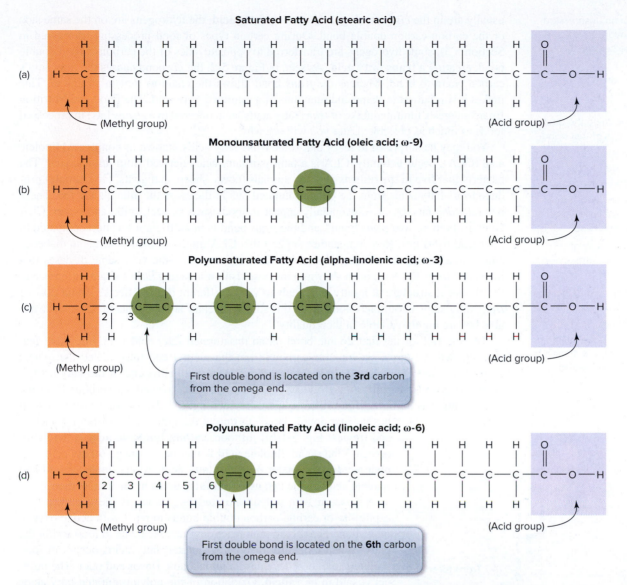

FIGURE 5-1 ▲ (a-d) Chemical forms of saturated, monounsaturated, and polyunsaturated fatty acids. Each of the depicted fatty acids contains 18 carbons, but they differ from each other in the number and location of double bonds. The double bonds are shaded. The linear shape of saturated fatty acids, as shown in (a), allows them to pack tightly together and so form a solid at room temperature. In contrast, unsaturated fatty acids (b-d) have "kinks" where double bonds interrupt the carbon chain (see Fig. 5-2). Thus, unsaturated fatty acids pack together only loosely and are usually liquid at room temperature.

monounsaturated fatty acid A fatty acid containing one carbon-carbon double bond.

polyunsaturated fatty acid A fatty acid containing two or more carbon-carbon double bonds.

saturated fats are suspended in liquid, such as the butterfat in whole milk, so the solid nature of these fats at room temperature is less apparent.

If the carbon chain of a fatty acid contains a double bond, those carbons in the chain have fewer bonds to share with hydrogen, and the chain is said to be *unsaturated*. A fatty acid with only one double bond is **monounsaturated** [see Fig. 5-1(b)]. Canola oil, olive oil, and avocados contain a high percentage of monounsaturated fatty acids.

If two or more of the bonds between the carbons are double bonds, the fatty acid is even less saturated with hydrogens, and so it is **polyunsaturated** [see Fig. 5-1(c), (d)]. The double bonds in unsaturated fatty acids create kinks in their structure that keep them from packing closely together, so they are liquid at room temperature. Corn, soybean, sunflower, and safflower oils are rich in polyunsaturated fatty acids.

Unsaturated fatty acids, with their double bonds, can exist in two different structural forms: the *cis* and *trans* forms. In nature, monounsaturated and polyunsaturated fatty acids

▲ Avocados are a rich source of monounsaturated fat. © McGraw-Hill Education/Ken Cavanagh, photographer

cis fatty acid A form of an unsaturated fatty acid that has the hydrogens lying on the same side of the carbon-carbon double bond.

trans fatty acid A form of an unsaturated fatty acid, usually a monounsaturated one when found in food, in which the hydrogens on both carbons forming the double bond lie on opposite sides of that bond.

omega-3 (ω-3) fatty acid An unsaturated fatty acid with the first double bond on the third carbon from the methyl end ($-CH_3$).

omega-6 (ω-6) fatty acid An unsaturated fatty acid with the first double bond on the sixth carbon from the methyl end ($-CH_3$).

alpha-linolenic acid An essential omega-3 fatty acid with 18 carbons and three double bonds.

linoleic acid An essential omega-6 fatty acid with 18 carbons and two double bonds.

essential fatty acids Fatty acids that must be supplied by the diet to maintain health. Currently, only linoleic acid and alpha-linolenic acid are classified as essential.

usually are in the *cis* form (Fig. 5-2). In a **cis fatty acid,** the hydrogens are on the same side of the carbon-carbon double bond. During certain types of food processing (discussed in Section 5.3), some hydrogens are transferred to opposite sides of the carbon-carbon double bond, creating a **trans fatty acid.** As seen in Figure 5-2, the *cis* bond causes the fatty acid's carbon chain to bend, whereas the *trans* bond allows the chain to remain straighter. This makes it similar to the shape and functions of a saturated fatty acid. The Food and Nutrition Board suggests limiting intake of *trans* fatty acids (also referred to as *trans* fats) in processed foods as much as possible. Later you will see why.

You may be surprised to learn that some *trans* fatty acids, known as conjugated linoleic acid (CLA), occur naturally. CLA is a family of fatty acids derived from linoleic acid. The bacteria that live in the rumens of some animals (cows, sheep, and goats, for example) produce *trans* fatty acids from the polyunsaturated fats in the grass the animals are fed. These natural *trans* fats, or CLA, eventually appear in foods such as beef, milk, and butter. CLA contains both *cis* and *trans* bonds, and the *trans* bond is in a different location compared to industrial *trans* fats. Research studies suggest that CLA improves insulin levels in diabetics and decreases the risk of heart disease, cancer, and obesity—the very same diseases that industrial *trans* fats have been shown to increase. Isn't it amazing how a slight difference in the chemical structure of a fatty acid leads to vastly different health effects? About 20% of *trans* fatty acids in our diets come from this source. Dietary supplements of CLA are available but are highly variable in their quality.

The location of the first double bond on an unsaturated fatty acid is an important feature and will be three, six, or nine carbons from the methyl end (also called the *omega* end). If the first double bond starts three carbons from the methyl end of the fatty acid, it is an **omega-3 (ω-3) fatty acid** [review Fig. 5-1(c)]. If it is located six carbons from the methyl end, it is an **omega-6 (ω-6) fatty acid** [review Fig. 5-1(d)]. An omega-9 fatty acid has its first double bond starting at the ninth carbon from the methyl end [review Fig. 5-1(b)]. In foods, **alpha-linolenic acid** is the major omega-3 fatty acid, **linoleic acid** is the major omega-6 fatty acid, and **oleic acid** is the major omega-9 fatty acid. Alpha-linolenic acid and linoleic acid are the two **essential fatty acids** in the human diet.

A concern with polyunsaturated fatty acids is the chemical susceptibility of carbon-carbon double bonds to react with active oxygen molecules. These oxidation reactions can take place in food and in the body. When oxidation of polyunsaturated fatty acids occurs in food products, the food develops an unpalatable flavor and odor. The product is said to be **rancid.** Oxidation of the polyunsaturated fatty acids in the body can cause inflammation and tissue damage. This process is thought to contribute to aging, atherosclerosis, and cancer. Fortunately, antioxidants such as vitamin E halt the process of oxidation. Many of the dietary recommendations for fat intake aim to decrease the likelihood of these harmful oxidation reactions.

Essential Fatty Acids The various classes of lipids have diverse functions in the body and are necessary for health. Of all the types of lipids found in foods, however, only two polyunsaturated fatty acids are essential in the human diet. Linoleic acid (an omega-6 fatty acid) and alpha-linolenic acid (an omega-3 fatty acid) are called *essential* fatty acids because we must obtain them from foods to maintain health. The essential fatty acids form parts of vital body structures, perform important roles in immune system function and vision, help form cell membranes, and produce **eicosanoids,** which are involved in practically all important functions in the body.

Many fatty acids that serve important functions in the body are derived from the essential dietary omega-3 and omega-6 parents, alpha-linolenic acid and linoleic acid (Fig. 5.3). Human enzymes convert the

Cis form
(Causes carbon chain to bend)

Trans form

Oleic acid

Elaidic acid

FIGURE 5-2 ▲ *Cis* and *trans* fatty acids. In the *cis* form, the hydrogens (in white) that flank the carbon-carbon double bond lie on the same side of the double bond. This causes a "kink" at that point in the fatty acid, typical of unsaturated fatty acids in foods. In contrast, in the *trans* form, the hydrogens that flank a double bond lie on opposite sides of the double bond. This causes the fatty acid to exist in a linear form, like a saturated fatty acid. *Cis* fatty acids are much more common in foods than *trans* fatty acids. The latter are primarily found in foods containing partially hydrogenated fats, notably stick margarine, shortening, and deep-fat fried foods.

two essential fatty acids to other long-chain polyunsaturated fatty acids, such as **eicosapentaenoic acid (EPA)** and **docosahexaenoic acid (DHA),** which are particularly important for proper function of the brain and nervous system. EPA is needed for concentration and vision and is converted into a powerful anti-inflammatory agent. Because of its role in brain structure, DHA is especially important during pregnancy for fetal brain and nervous system development.

If humans fail to consume enough essential fatty acids, their skin becomes flaky and itchy, and diarrhea and other symptoms such as infections often are seen. Growth and wound healing may be restricted. These signs of deficiency have been seen in people fed intravenously by **total parenteral nutrition** containing little or no fat for 2 to 3 weeks, as well as in infants receiving formulas low in fat.

FIGURE 5-3 ▲ The essential fatty acid (EFA) family. Linoleic acid (the essential omega-6 fatty acid) and alpha-linolenic acid (the essential omega-3 fatty acid) must be consumed as part of the diet because the body lacks the enzymes required to make them. When these two essential fatty acids are obtained from the diet, the body can then make other fatty acids, which eventually give rise to a variety of eicosanoids that regulate body functions.

Triglycerides The lipids in foods and in body structures are mostly in the form of triglycerides. Although some fatty acids are transported in the bloodstream attached to proteins, most fatty acids are formed into triglycerides by cells in the body.

Triglycerides contain a simple three-carbon alcohol, called glycerol, which serves as a backbone for the three attached fatty acids [Fig. 5-4(a)]. Removing one fatty acid from a triglyceride forms a **diglyceride.** Removing two fatty acids from a triglyceride forms a **monoglyceride.** Later you will see that before most dietary fats are absorbed, the two outer fatty acids are typically removed from the triglyceride during digestion in the small intestine. This produces a mixture of fatty acids and monoglycerides that can be absorbed into the intestinal cells. After absorption, the fatty acids and monoglycerides are mostly reformed into triglycerides inside body cells.

PHOSPHOLIPIDS

Phospholipids are another class of lipids. Like triglycerides, they are built on a backbone of glycerol. However, at least one fatty acid is replaced with a compound containing phosphorus (and often other elements, such as nitrogen) [see Fig. 5-4(b)]. Many types of phospholipids exist in the body, especially in the brain. They are an important part of cell membranes. **Lecithin** is a common example of a phospholipid. Various forms of phospholipids are found in body cells, and they participate in fat digestion, absorption, and transport. The body is able to produce all the phospholipids it needs. Even though lecithin is sold as a dietary supplement and is used as an additive in many foods, phospholipids are not essential components of the diet.

STEROLS

Sterols are a class of lipids characterized by a multi-ringed structure that makes them structurally and functionally different from the other lipids already discussed [see Fig. 5-4(c)]. The most common example of a sterol is cholesterol. This waxy substance does not look like a triglyceride; it does not have a glycerol backbone or any fatty acids. Still, because it does not readily dissolve in water, it is a lipid. Among other functions, cholesterol is used to form certain hormones and bile acids, and is incorporated into cell structures. The body can make all the cholesterol it needs, so sterols are not essential components of the diet.

The following Concept Map summarizes the various forms of lipids.

eicosanoids A class of hormone compounds, including the prostaglandins, derived from the essential polyunsaturated fatty acids. These signaling compounds are involved in cellular activity that affects practically all important functions in the body.

eicosapentaenoic acid (EPA) An omega-3 fatty acid with 20 carbons and five carbon-carbon double bonds. It is present in large amounts in fatty fish and is slowly synthesized in the body from alpha-linolenic acid.

docosahexaenoic acid (DHA) An omega-3 fatty acid with 22 carbons and six carbon-carbon double bonds. It is present in large amounts in fatty fish and is slowly synthesized in the body from alpha-linolenic acid. DHA is especially present in the retina and brain.

total parenteral nutrition The intravenous feeding of all necessary nutrients, including the most basic forms of protein, carbohydrates, lipids, vitamins, minerals, and electrolytes.

diglyceride A breakdown product of a triglyceride consisting of two fatty acids bonded to a glycerol backbone.

monoglyceride A breakdown product of a triglyceride consisting of one fatty acid attached to a glycerol backbone.

lecithin A group of phospholipid compounds that are major components of cell membranes.

(a)

(b)

(c)

FIGURE 5-4 ▲ Chemical forms of common lipids: (a) triglyceride, (b) phospholipid (in this case, lecithin), and (c) sterol (in this case, cholesterol).

✓ **CONCEPT CHECK 5.2**

1. What are the four possible structural forms of lipids?
2. What is the difference between saturated and unsaturated fatty acids?
3. What is the difference between omega-3 and omega-6 fatty acids?
4. Which two fatty acids are essential?
5. How do triglycerides differ from phospholipids?
6. What are the main functions of cholesterol in the body?

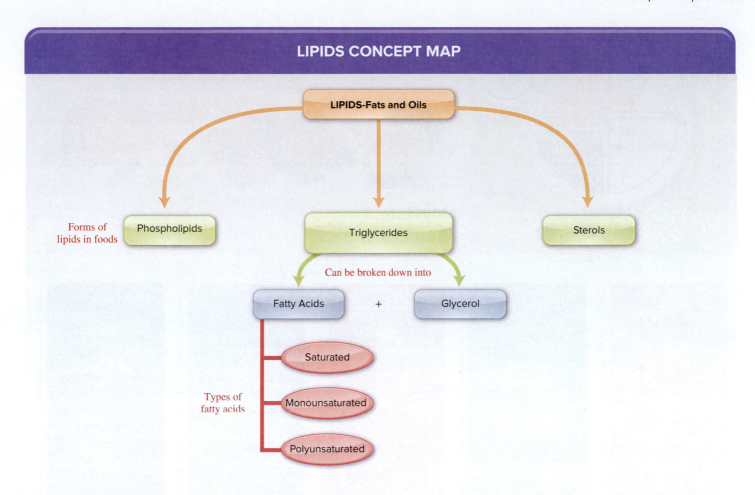

LIPIDS CONCEPT MAP

LIPIDS-Fats and Oils

Forms of lipids in foods

Phospholipids

Triglycerides

Sterols

Can be broken down into

Fatty Acids + Glycerol

Types of fatty acids

Saturated

Monounsaturated

Polyunsaturated

5.3 Fats and Oils in Foods

FATTY ACIDS AND TRIGLYCERIDES IN FOODS

Lipids (in the form of triglycerides) are abundant in the North American diet. The foods highest in fat (and therefore energy density) include salad oils and spreads such as butter, margarine, and mayonnaise. All of these foods contain close to 100% of calories as fat.

Other high-fat foods include nuts, bologna, avocados, and bacon, which have about 80% of calories as fat (Fig. 5-5). Next, peanut butter and cheddar cheese have about 75% of calories from fat. Marbled steak and hamburgers (ground chuck) have about 60% of calories from fat, and chocolate bars, ice cream, doughnuts, and whole milk have about 50% of calories as fat. Eggs, pumpkin pie, and cupcakes have 35%, as do lean cuts of meat such as top round, ground round, and sirloin. Bread contains about 15% of calories as fat. Foods such as cornflakes, sugar, and fat-free milk have essentially no fat. Figure 5-6 shows examples of food sources of fat.

While you certainly should monitor the *total amount* of fat, the *type* of fat in foods is another important consideration when it comes to selecting a dietary pattern that promotes optimal health. Remember that triglycerides are composed of a mixture of fatty acids of various lengths and degrees of saturation. Overall, a fat or an oil is classified as saturated, monounsaturated, or polyunsaturated based on the type of fatty acids present in the greatest concentration (Fig. 5-7). Fats in foods that contain primarily saturated fatty acids are solid at room temperature, especially if the fatty acids have long carbon chains (i.e., a **long-chain fatty acid**), as opposed to shorter versions. In contrast, fats containing primarily polyunsaturated or monounsaturated fatty acids (regardless of the length of the carbon chain) are usually liquid at room temperature. Almost all fatty acids in the body and in foods are long-chain fatty acids.

long-chain fatty acid A fatty acid that contains 12 or more carbons.

▲ This peanut butter (protein) and jelly sandwich on whole-grain bread (grain) with low-fat milk (dairy) provides a healthy source of plant fat from the peanut butter. Which sections of MyPlate are we missing? © McGraw-Hill Education/ Elite Images

ChooseMyPlate.gov

MyPlate: Sources of Fats

Grains	Vegetables	Fruits	Dairy	Protein
• Crackers • Pasta dishes with added fat	• French fried potatoes • Deep-fried vegetables • Vegetables roasted with oil	• Fruit pies • Avocados	• Whole milk • Low-fat milk (1%, 2%) • Some yogurts • Many cheeses • Premium ice cream	• Marbled meat • Bacon • Poultry (skin) • Deep-fat-fried meat • Nuts
0–18 grams per serving	0–27 grams per serving	0–11 grams per serving	0–10 grams per serving	7–17 grams per serving

FIGURE 5-5 ▲ Sources of fats from MyPlate. The fill of the background color (none, 1/3, 2/3, or completely covered) within each group in the plate indicates the average nutrient density for fat in that group. The fruit group and vegetable group are generally low in fat. In the other groups, both high-fat and low-fat choices are available. Careful reading of food labels can help you choose lower fat versions of some foods. In general, any type of frying adds significant amounts of fat to a product, as with French fries and fried chicken.

(avocado): © Ingram Publishing/SuperStock; (chicken): © Ingram Publishing/Alamy; (cheese): © Pixtal/age fotostock

▲ Dairy products are a primary contributor of saturated fat to our diets. © D. Hurst/Alamy

Animal fats are the chief contributors of saturated fatty acids to the North American diet. About 40% to 60% of total fat in dairy and meat products is in the form of saturated fatty acids. Palm oil and coconut oil are two plant oils that are rich sources of saturated fatty acids.

Aside from palm oil and coconut oil, most plant oils are rich in unsaturated fatty acids, ranging from 73% to 94% of total fat. The major sources of monounsaturated fatty acids in the diet are canola oil, olive oil, and peanut oil. Corn, cottonseed, sunflower, soybean, and safflower oils contain mostly polyunsaturated fatty acids (54% to 77%).

Food Sources of Essential Fatty Acids Rich food sources of linoleic acid—the essential omega-6 fatty acid—include safflower, sunflower, corn, and cottonseed oils, as well as nuts and seeds. In the North American diet, chicken is the leading source of linoleic acid, simply because it is so frequently consumed.

Two nutrient-dense food sources of alpha-linolenic acid (the essential omega-3 fatty acid) are flax seeds and walnuts (see Further Reading 6). Flax seeds can be purchased in many natural food stores rather inexpensively. These need to be chewed thoroughly, or they will pass through the GI tract undigested. Many people find it easier to grind them in a coffee grinder before eating them. Flax seed oil is also available, but it turns rancid very quickly, especially if not refrigerated. Compared to other nuts and seeds, walnuts are one

Food Sources of Fat

Food Item	Fat (grams)	% AHA Recommendation
Daily value	65	███████████ 100%
T-bone steak, 3 ounces	17	██ 26%
Mixed nuts, 1 ounce	16	██ 25%
Canola oil, 1 tablespoon	14	██ 22%
Hamburger with bun, 1 each	12	██ 18%
Stick margarine, 1 tablespoon	12	██ 18%
Avocado, 1/2 cup	11	██ 17%
Cheddar cheese, 1 ounce	10	█ 15%
Salmon, 3 ounces	10	█ 15%
Whole milk, 1 cup	8	█ 12%
Chicken breast with skin, 3 ounces	7	█ 11%
Whole-milk yogurt, 8 ounces	7	█ 11%
Snack crackers, 1 ounce	7	█ 11%
Baked beans, 1/2 cup	7	█ 11%
M&M chocolate candies, 1 ounce	6	█ 9%
Flax seeds, 1 tablespoon	3	█ 5%
Fig Newton cookies, 2	3	█ 5%

Key:
- Grains
- Vegetables
- Fruits
- Dairy
- Protein
- Empty calories
- Oils

FIGURE 5-6 ◄ Food sources of fat compared to the American Heart Association (AHA) recommendation of 70 grams per day, or 30% of calories from fat for a 2100-kcal diet.

▲ Walnuts are one of the richest plant sources of the omega-3 fatty acid, alpha-linolenic acid, and are a good source of plant sterols. © Jack Star/PhotoLink/Getty Images

Omega-3 Fatty Acids in Fish (grams per 3-ounce serving):

Atlantic salmon	1.8
Anchovy	1.7
Sardines	1.4
Rainbow trout	1.0
Coho salmon	0.9
Bluefish	0.8
Striped bass	0.8
Tuna, white, canned	0.7
Halibut	0.4
Catfish, channel	0.2

Recommended omega-3 fatty acid (alpha-linolenic acid) intake per day:

Men	1.6 grams
Women	1.1 grams

of the richest sources of alpha-linolenic acid (2.6 grams per 1-ounce serving or 14 walnut halves). In addition, walnuts are a rich source of plant sterols known to inhibit intestinal absorption of cholesterol. Other rich food sources of alpha-linolenic acid include oils from perilla seeds, chia seeds, canola, and soybeans.

Omega-3 Fatty Acids in Fish Looking at Figure 5-3, you can see that eicosapentaenoic acid (EPA) and docosahexaenoic acid (DHA) can be made in the body, so they are not essential fatty acids. However, by consuming food sources of EPA and DHA, you effectively skip a few rather slow and inefficient steps in the conversion of alpha-linolenic acid to EPA and DHA. These two omega-3 fatty acids are naturally high in fatty fish such as salmon, tuna, sardines, anchovies, striped bass, catfish, herring, mackerel, trout, and halibut. The Dietary Guidelines for Americans and recommendations from the American Heart Association encourage us to consume two servings of fatty fish per week for optimal cardiovascular health (see Section 5.7). An EPA/DHA supplement is useful for people who do not regularly consume fatty fish.

A word of caution: some types of fish can be a source of mercury, which is toxic in high amounts (see Section 17.6). Fish species that are highest in mercury include shark, swordfish, king mackerel, tilefish, marlin, orange roughy, and bigeye, or ahi, tuna. Salmon, sardines, herring, and albacore or yellowfin tuna are better choices because they are lower

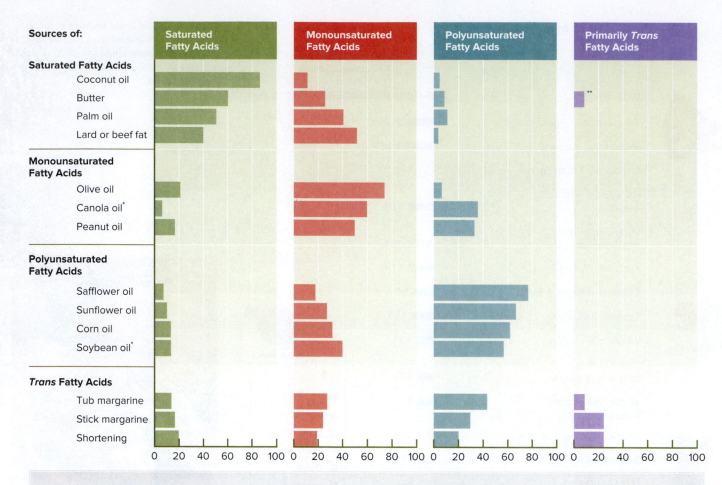

Sources of:	Saturated Fatty Acids	Monounsaturated Fatty Acids	Polyunsaturated Fatty Acids	Primarily *Trans* Fatty Acids
Saturated Fatty Acids				
Coconut oil				
Butter				**
Palm oil				
Lard or beef fat				
Monounsaturated Fatty Acids				
Olive oil				
Canola oil*				
Peanut oil				
Polyunsaturated Fatty Acids				
Safflower oil				
Sunflower oil				
Corn oil				
Soybean oil*				
***Trans* Fatty Acids**				
Tub margarine				
Stick margarine				
Shortening				

*Rich source of the omega-3 fatty acid alpha-linolenic acid (7% and 12% of total fatty acid content for soybean oil and canola oil, respectively).

**The natural *trans* fatty acids in butter are not harmful and may even have health-promoting properties, such as preventing certain forms of cancer.

FIGURE 5-7 ▲ Saturated, monounsaturated, polyunsaturated, and *trans* fatty acid composition of common fats and oils (expressed as percent of all fatty acids in the product).

emulsifier A compound that can suspend fat in water by isolating individual fat droplets, using a shell of water molecules or other substances to prevent the fat from coalescing.

in mercury, yet still provide heart-healthy omega-3 fatty acids. Varying your choices rather than always eating the same species of fish and limiting overall intake to 12 ounces per week (on average two to three meals of fish or shellfish per week) is recommended to reduce mercury exposure, especially for pregnant women and children. Overall, research indicates that the benefits of fish intake, especially in reducing the risk of cardiovascular disease, outweigh the possible risks of mercury contamination.

FOOD SOURCES OF PHOSPHOLIPIDS

Wheat germ, peanuts, egg yolk, soy beans, and organ meats are rich sources of phospholipids. Phospholipids such as lecithin, a component of egg yolks, are often added to salad dressing. Lecithin is used as an **emulsifier** in these and other products because of its ability to keep mixtures of lipids and water from separating (Fig. 5-8). Emulsifiers are added to salad dressings to keep the vegetable oil suspended in water. Eggs added to cake batters likewise emulsify the fat with the milk.

▲ Peanuts are a source of lecithins, as are wheat germ and egg yolks. © C Squared Studios/ Getty Images

Emulsifiers and Agitation in Salad Dressing

Oil

Water

Water

Emulsified fat

Oil droplet attracted
to fatty acid core

Water attracted
to shell

Phospholipid
acting as an
emulsifier

FIGURE 5-8 ◄ Emulsifiers in action. Emulsifiers prevent many brands of salad dressings and other condiments from separating into layers of water and fat. Emulsifiers attract fatty acids inside and have a water-attracting group on the outside. Add them to salad dressing, shake well, and they hold the oil in the dressing away from the water. Emulsification is important in both food production and fat digestion/absorption.

FOOD SOURCES OF STEROLS

Cholesterol is found only in animal foods (Table 5-1). An egg yolk contains about 210 milligrams of cholesterol. Eggs are our main dietary source of cholesterol, along with meats and whole milk. Manufacturers who advertise their brand of peanut butter, vegetable shortening, margarines, and vegetable oils as "cholesterol free" are taking advantage of uninformed consumers: all of these products are naturally cholesterol free! Some plants contain other sterols similar to cholesterol, but they do not pose the heart-health risks associated with cholesterol. In fact, some plant sterols have blood cholesterol-lowering properties (refer to the discussion in Section 5.8 on medical interventions to lower blood lipids).

TABLE 5-1 ■ **Cholesterol Content of Foods**

3 oz beef brains	2635 mg
3 oz beef liver	337 mg
1 large egg yolk*	209 mg
3 oz shrimp	166 mg
3 oz beef*	75 mg
3 oz pork	75 mg
3 oz chicken or turkey (white meat)*	75 mg
1 cup ice cream	63 mg
3 oz trout	60 mg
3 oz tuna	45 mg
3 oz hot dog	38 mg
1 oz cheddar cheese*	30 mg
1 cup whole milk*	24 mg
1 cup 1% milk	12 mg
1 cup fat-free milk	5 mg
1 large egg white	0 mg

*Leading dietary sources of cholesterol in American diets.

▲ The North American diet contains many high-fat foods, such as pastries. To limit calorie intake from such energy-dense foods, control portion sizes and choose these foods only in moderation. © Allan Rosenberg/Cole Group/Getty Images

USING FOOD LABELS TO IDENTIFY FAT

Some fat discussed so far is obvious: butter on bread, mayonnaise in potato salad, and marbling in raw meat. Fat is harder to detect in other foods that also contribute significant amounts of fat to our diets. Foods that contain hidden fat include whole milk, pastries, cookies, cake, cheese, hot dogs, crackers, French fries, and ice cream. When we try to cut down on fat intake, hidden fats need to be considered, along with the more obvious sources.

A place to begin searching for hidden fat and learn more about the fat content of the foods you eat is on the Nutrition Facts labels of foods you buy (Fig. 5-9). The label lists calories from fat right next to total calories for easy comparison. Pay attention to the type of fat in the product, as well. Foods that are high in saturated fat should be chosen less frequently.

Also, check out the list of ingredients on the food label. Some signals from the ingredients list that can alert you to the presence of fat are animal fats (e.g., bacon, beef, ham, lamb, pork, chicken, and turkey fats), lard, dairy fats (e.g., butter and cream), egg and egg-yolk solids, nuts, vegetable oils, and partially hydrogenated shortening or vegetable oil. Conveniently, the label lists ingredients by order of weight in the product. If fat is one of the first ingredients listed, you are probably looking at a high-fat product.

FAT IN FOOD PROVIDES SOME SATIETY, FLAVOR, AND TEXTURE

Controversy exists about whether high-fat foods increase satiety. Fats tend to slow the process of digestion, which could help you to feel full after a meal; however, fats also improve the flavor and texture of foods, so they may stimulate increased food intake. Fat's effect on satiety may depend on the size and saturation of the fatty acids in foods. What everyone knows for sure is that fats contain more than twice the calories of carbohydrates and proteins. Therefore, a high-fat meal is likely to be a high-calorie meal.

Fat provides important textures and carries flavors in foods. If you have ever eaten a high-fat yellow cheese or cream cheese, you probably agree that the feel of fat melting on the tongue is good. The fat in reduced-fat and whole milk also gives body, which fat-free milk lacks. The most tender cuts of meat are high in fat, visible as the marbling of meat. In addition, many flavorings dissolve in fat. Heating spices in oil intensifies the flavors of an Indian

FIGURE 5-9 ▲ Reading labels helps locate hidden fat. Who would think that wieners (hot dogs) can contain about 85% of food calories as fat? Looking at the hot dog does not suggest that almost all of its food calories come from fat, but the label shows otherwise. Let us do the math: 13 grams total fat × 9 kcal per gram of fat = 120 kcal from fat; 120 kcal/140 kcal per link = 0.86 or 86% kcal from fat.

curry or a Mexican dish. Because fat contributes to our enjoyment of eating, reducing the fat content of foods (or the overall diet) takes some ingenuity.

FAT-REPLACEMENT STRATEGIES FOR REDUCED-FAT FOODS

Manufacturers have introduced reduced-fat versions of numerous food products. The fat content of these alternatives ranges from 0% in fat-free Fig Newtons to about 75% of the original fat content in other products. However, the total calorie content of most fat-reduced products is not substantially lower than that of the regular products. Generally, when fat is removed from a product, something must be added—commonly, sugars—in its place. It is difficult to reduce both the fat and sugar contents of a product at the same time and maintain flavor and texture. For this reason, many reduced-fat products (e.g., cakes and cookies) are still energy dense. Use the Nutrition Facts panel on the food label to choose the portion size that fits into your daily calorie needs.

To lower the fat in foods, manufacturers may replace some of the fat with water, protein (Simplesse®, Dairy-Lo®), or forms of carbohydrates such as starch derivatives (Z-trim®), fiber (Maltrin®, Stellar™, Oatrim), and gums. In reduced-fat margarines, water replaces some of the fat. While regular margarines are 80% fat by weight (11 grams per tablespoon), some reduced-fat margarines are as low as 30% fat by weight (4 grams per tablespoon). When used in recipes, the extra water added to these margarines can cause texture and volume changes in the finished product. Cookbooks can suggest alterations in recipes to compensate for the increased water content of these products.

Manufacturers also may use engineered fats, such as olestra (Olean®) and salatrim (Benefat®), that are made with fat and sucrose (table sugar) but that provide few or no calories because they cannot be digested and/or absorbed well. The main problem with the fat replacer olestra is that it can bind the fat-soluble vitamins and reduce their absorption.

To date, fat replacements have had little impact on our diets. This is partly because currently approved fat replacements lack versatility and are not used extensively by manufacturers. In addition, fat replacements are not practical for use in the foods that provide the most fat in our diets: beef, cheese, whole milk, and pastries.

FAT RANCIDITY LIMITS SHELF LIFE OF FOODS

Decomposing oils emit a disagreeable odor and taste sour and stale. Stale potato chips are a good example. The double bonds in unsaturated fatty acids break down, producing rancid by-products. Ultraviolet light, oxygen, and heat (as in deep-fat frying) can break double bonds and, in turn, destroy the structure of polyunsaturated fatty acids. Saturated fats and *trans* fats can more readily resist these effects because they contain fewer carbon-carbon double bonds.

Rancidity is not a major problem for consumers because the odor and taste generally discourage us from eating enough to become sick. However, rancidity is a problem for the food industry and restaurant business because it reduces a product's shelf life. To increase shelf life, manufacturers often add partially hydrogenated plant oils to products. Foods most likely to become rancid are deep-fried foods and those with a large amount of exposed surface. Polyunsaturated oils are a good choice for products such as salad dressings, whereas more saturated fats are best for high-heat cooking. The fat in fish is also susceptible to rancidity because it is highly polyunsaturated.

Antioxidants such as vitamin E help protect foods against rancidity by guarding against fat breakdown. The vitamin E naturally occurring in plant oils reduces the breakdown of double bonds in fatty acids. When food manufacturers want to prevent rancidity in polyunsaturated fats, they often add the synthetic antioxidants **BHA** and **BHT** or vitamin C to products that contain fat, such as salad dressings and cake mixes. Manufacturers also tightly seal products and use other methods to reduce oxygen levels inside packages.

HYDROGENATION OF FATTY ACIDS IN FOOD PRODUCTION INCREASES *TRANS* FATTY ACID CONTENT

As mentioned previously, most fats with long-chain saturated fatty acids are solid at room temperature, and those with unsaturated fatty acids are liquid at room temperature. In the production of some foods, solid fats work better than liquid oils. In pie crust,

▲ Fat replacements such as gum fiber are typically seen in soft serve ice cream. © Ingram Publishing/Alamy

Canada has not approved the use of olestra in food products; the United States is the sole country that permits the use of this fat substitute in foods.

BHA, BHT Butylated hydroxyanisole and butylated hydroxytoluene: two common synthetic antioxidants added to foods.

Hydrogen source

Unsaturated vegetable oil (liquid)	Adding hydrogen under pressure	Partially hydrogenated fat (semisolid)
(a)	(b)	(c)

FIGURE 5-10 ▲ How liquid oils are made into solid fats. (a) Unsaturated fatty acids are present in liquid form in large metal tanks. (b) Hydrogens are added (hydrogenation), changing some carbon-carbon double bonds to single bonds and producing some *trans* fatty acids. (c) The partially hydrogenated product is likely to be used in margarine, shortening, or for deep-fat frying.

hydrogenation The addition of hydrogen to a carbon-carbon double bond, producing a single carbon-carbon bond with two hydrogens attached to each carbon.

for example, solid fats yield a flaky product, whereas crusts made with liquid oils tend to be greasy and more crumbly. If oils with unsaturated fatty acids are used to replace solid fats, they often must be made more saturated (with hydrogen), as this solidifies the vegetable oils into shortenings and margarines. Hydrogen is added by bubbling hydrogen gas under pressure into liquid vegetable oils in a process called **hydrogenation** (Fig. 5-10). The fatty acids are not fully hydrogenated to the saturated fatty acid form, as this would make the product too hard and brittle. Partial hydrogenation—leaving some monounsaturated fatty acids—creates a semisolid product.

The process of hydrogenation produces *trans* fatty acids, which were described in Section 5.2. Most natural monounsaturated and polyunsaturated fatty acids exist in the *cis* form, causing a bend in the carbon chain, whereas the straighter carbon forms of *trans* fat more closely resemble saturated fatty acids. This may be the mechanism whereby *trans* fat increases the risk for heart disease. Studies also indicate that *trans* fats increase overall inflammation in the body, which is not healthful. Thus, the Dietary Guidelines for Americans, the American Heart Association, and the Food and Nutrition Board each recommend minimal *trans* fat intake.

Partially hydrogenated soybean oil—rich in *trans* fat—became the major fat in food processing when manufacturers eliminated the tropical oils rich in saturated fat (palm, palm olein, and coconut). While foods made with partially hydrogenated oil were becoming popular, there was very little known about the *trans* fats they contained and their harmful effects. It was not until the 1990s that scientists began identifying the adverse health effects of *trans* fats. Currently, *trans* fat intake in North America amounts to 3 to 4 grams per day. Table 5-2 includes typical sources of *trans* fat.

▲ Fried foods are a rich source of fat and *trans* fats. Reducing the intake of these foods can help lower blood lipid levels. © Getty Images/Digital Vision

TABLE 5-2 ■ Main Sources of Fatty Acids and Their State at Room Temperature

Type and Health Effects	Main Sources	State at Room Temperature
Saturated Fatty Acids Increase blood levels of cholesterol		
Long chain	Lard; fat in beef, pork, and lamb	Solid
Medium and short chain	Milk fat (butter), coconut oil, palm oil, palm kernel oil	Soft or liquid
Monounsaturated Fatty Acids Decrease blood levels of cholesterol	Olive oil, canola oil, peanut oil	Liquid
Polyunsaturated Fatty Acids Decrease blood levels of cholesterol	Sunflower oil, corn oil, safflower oil, fish oil	Liquid
Essential Fatty Acids Omega-3: alpha-linolenic acid Reduces inflammation responses, blood clotting, and plasma triglycerides	Cold-water fish (salmon, tuna, sardines, mackerel), walnuts, flaxseed, hemp oil, canola oil, soybean oil, chia seeds, and perilla oil	Liquid
Omega-6: linoleic acid Regulates blood pressure and increases blood clotting	Beef, poultry, safflower oil, sunflower oil, corn oil	Solid to liquid
***Trans* Fatty Acids** Increase blood cholesterol more than saturated fat	Margarine (squeeze, tub, stick), shortening	Soft to very solid

The American Heart Association strongly advises that we limit *trans* fat intake to less than 1% of total daily calories. This means only 2 grams of *trans* fats a day, or 20 kcal, if you need 2000 kcal per day. FDA has taken action to make consumers more aware of the amounts of *trans* fat in foods. Since 2006, federal regulations have required the disclosure of *trans* fat content on food packages (review Fig. 5-9). Food labels in Canada also must list *trans* fat content. In 2015, FDA determined that partially hydrogenated oils—the main sources of *trans* fats in the diet—are no longer "generally recognized as safe" for use in human food products (see Further Reading 4). North American companies have already been responding to consumer demands by creating products that are free of *trans* fat. For example, Promise®, Smart Balance®, and Fleischmann's® margarines are free of *trans* fat (less than 0.5 gram per serving) compared to typical margarines. By 2018, most *trans* fats will be eliminated from food products.

To minimize *trans* fat intake, a general guideline is to limit consumption of fried (especially deep-fat fried) food items, any pastries or flaky bread products (such as pie crusts, crackers, croissants, and biscuits), and cookies. Most importantly, use little or no stick margarine or shortening. Instead, substitute vegetable oils and softer tub margarines (whose labels list vegetable oil or water as the first ingredient). Avoid deep-fat frying any food in shortening. Substitute baking, panfrying, broiling, steaming, grilling, or deep-fat frying in unhydrogenated oils with high "smoke points," meaning they do not break down at deep-frying temperatures. Peanut, safflower, sunflower, and canola oils are good choices. Replace nondairy creamers with reduced-fat or fat-free milk, as most nondairy creamers are rich in partially hydrogenated vegetable oils. Finally, read the ingredients on food labels, using the previous tips to estimate *trans* fat content. If partially hydrogenated vegetable oil is one of the first three ingredients on the label, you can assume that there is a significant amount of *trans* fat in the product.

✓ CONCEPT CHECK 5.3

1. Which foods are the most fat dense (>60% total calories as fat)?
2. Where is cholesterol found in the food supply?
3. Which types of fat are used as emulsifiers, and what is their function in food?
4. What are some strategies used to produce reduced-fat foods?
5. How do fats become rancid, and how can this be prevented?
6. What happens to unsaturated fats during the process of hydrogenation?
7. What regulations are in place to educate and protect the public from *trans* fats in foods?

5.4 Making Lipids Available for Body Use

It is no secret that fats and oils make foods more appealing. Their presence in foods adds flavor, moistness, and texture. What happens to lipids once they are eaten? Let us take a closer look at the digestion, absorption, and physiological roles of lipids in the body.

DIGESTION

In the first phase of fat digestion, the stomach (and salivary glands to some extent) secretes the enzyme **lipase.** Lipase acts primarily on triglycerides that have fatty acids with short chain lengths, such as those found in butterfat. The action of these lipase enzymes, however, is dwarfed by that of the lipase enzyme that is released from the pancreas to digest fats in the small intestine. Most of the triglycerides in the diet contain fatty acids with longer chain lengths and are generally not digested until they reach the small intestine (Fig. 5-11).

Nut Butters: Are They "Good" Fat?

Nut butters are plant products, so they are naturally cholesterol free and provide 2 or 3 grams of fiber, which can lower blood cholesterol. Nuts are also a good source of unsaturated fats. Two tablespoons of peanut butter provide about 12 grams of unsaturated fats and only 3 grams of saturated fat. As you've learned, monounsaturated and polyunsaturated fats tend to lower blood cholesterol levels. To steer clear of *trans* fats, be on the lookout for partially hydrogenated oils in the list of ingredients. These have been used in some products to increase shelf life, although food manufacturers are gradually phasing them out. Lastly, check the sugar content. Nut butters naturally contain 1 or 2 grams of sugar, but processed varieties (e.g., cinnamon swirl) may contain up to 9 grams of sugar. Reap the most heart-health benefits by choosing natural nut butters and controlling the size of your portion.

© McGraw-Hill Education/Elite Images

lipase Fat-digesting enzyme produced by the salivary glands, stomach, and pancreas.

FIGURE 5-11 ▶ A summary of fat digestion and absorption. Section 3.9 covered general aspects of this process.

Fat Digestion and Absorption

1 Stomach: Only minor digestion of fat takes place in the stomach through the action of lipase enzymes.

2 Liver: The liver produces bile, stored in the gallbladder and released through the bile duct into the small intestine. Bile aids in fat digestion and absorption by emulsifying lipids in the digestive juices.

3 Pancreas: The pancreas secretes a mixture of enzymes, including lipase, into the small intestine.

4 Small intestine: The small intestine is the primary site for digestion and absorption of lipids. Once absorbed, long-chain fatty acids are packaged for transport through the lymph and bloodstream. (Shorter-chain fatty acids are absorbed directly into portal circulation.)

5 Large intestine: Less than 5% of ingested fat is normally excreted in the feces.

In the small intestine, triglycerides are broken down by lipase into smaller products, namely monoglycerides (glycerol backbones with a single fatty acid attached) and fatty acids. Under the right circumstances, digestion is rapid and thorough. The "right" circumstances include the presence of bile from the gallbladder. Bile acids (components of bile) act to emulsify fats in the watery digestive juices. Emulsification improves digestion and absorption because it separates large fat globules into smaller ones, thereby increasing the total surface area for lipase action (Fig. 5-12). After participating in fat digestion, most bile acids are absorbed in the last segment of the small intestine and transported back to the liver. Through this process, approximately 98% of bile acids are recycled. Only 1% to 2% of bile acids end up in the large intestine to be eliminated in the feces.

With regard to phospholipid digestion, certain enzymes from the pancreas and cells in the wall of the small intestine digest phospholipids. The eventual products are glycerol, fatty acids, and the remaining phosphorus-containing parts. With regard to cholesterol digestion, any cholesterol with a fatty acid attached is broken down to free cholesterol and fatty acids by certain enzymes released from the pancreas. Any fatty acids that are part of these structures could be broken down to yield energy, but contribution to overall calorie intake is miniscule compared to the energy stored in triglycerides.

If the gallbladder is surgically removed (e.g., in cases of gallstone formation), bile will enter the small intestine directly from the liver. Moderate intakes of fat can still be digested adequately, but some people experience loose stools after eating high-fat meals because some fat reaches the large intestine unabsorbed.

1 Large fat droplets enter small intestine after meal.

2 Bile acids (mostly) and lecithin emulsify fats into smaller particles.

3 Lipase breaks down fat into fatty acids and monoglycerides.

4 Monoglycerides and fatty acids are absorbed as micelles through the brush border and then re-formed into triglycerides.

5 Short- and medium-chain fatty acids enter the bloodstream (cardiovascular system).

6 Triglycerides combine with cholesterol, protein, and phospholipids to form chylomicrons, which enter the lymphatic system.

FIGURE 5-12 ▲ Bile acids facilitate the digestion of triglycerides by emulsifying fat droplets in the chyme in the small intestine. This allows for efficient action of pancreatic lipase and subsequent absorption of monoglycerides and fatty acids into the mucosal cells of the small intestine.

ABSORPTION

The products of fat digestion in the small intestine are fatty acids and monoglycerides. These products diffuse into the absorptive cells of the small intestine. About 95% of dietary fat is absorbed in this way. The chain length of fatty acids affects the ultimate fate of fatty acids and monoglycerides after absorption. If the chain length of a fatty acid is less than 12 carbon atoms, it is water soluble and will therefore probably travel as such through the portal vein that connects directly to the liver. Longer chain fatty acids are too large to be absorbed directly into portal circulation. These larger products of fat digestion are reformed into triglycerides within the absorptive cells of the small intestine and eventually enter circulation via the lymphatic system.

> ✓ **CONCEPT CHECK 5.4**
>
> 1. What enzyme is responsible for digestion of triglycerides?
> 2. What are the end products of fat digestion?
> 3. What are the differences between the absorption of long- versus short-chain fatty acids?

5.5 Carrying Lipids in the Bloodstream

lipoprotein A compound found in the bloodstream containing a core of lipids with a shell composed of protein, phospholipid, and cholesterol.

As noted earlier, fat and water do not mix easily. This incompatibility presents a challenge for the transport of fats through the watery media of the blood and lymph. **Lipoproteins** serve as vehicles for transport of lipids from the small intestine and liver to the body tissues (Table 5-3). They are found in the bloodstream and contain a core of lipids with a shell composed of protein, phospholipid, and cholesterol (Fig. 5-13).

Lipoproteins are classified into four groups—chylomicrons, VLDL, LDL, and HDL—based on their densities. Lipids are less dense than proteins. Therefore, lipoproteins that contain a large percentage of lipids in comparison to protein are less dense than those depleted of lipids (Fig. 5-14).

DIETARY FATS ARE CARRIED BY CHYLOMICRONS

chylomicron Lipoprotein made of dietary fats surrounded by a shell of cholesterol, phospholipids, and protein. Chylomicrons are formed in the absorptive cells of the small intestine after fat absorption and travel through the lymphatic system to the bloodstream.

lipoprotein lipase An enzyme attached to the cells that form the inner lining of blood vessels; it breaks down triglycerides into free fatty acids and glycerol.

As you learned in Section 5.4, digestion of dietary fats results in a mixture of glycerol, monoglycerides, and fatty acids. Once these products are absorbed by the cells of the small intestine, they are reassembled into triglycerides. Then, the intestinal cells package the triglycerides into **chylomicrons,** which enter the lymphatic system and eventually the bloodstream. Chylomicrons are the largest of the lipoproteins; they are loaded with dietary fat and originate only from the intestinal cells. Like the other lipoproteins, chylomicrons are composed of large droplets of lipid surrounded by a thin, water-soluble shell of phospholipids, cholesterol, and protein (see Fig. 5-14). The water-soluble shell around a chylomicron allows the lipid to float freely in the lymph and blood, which are both water based. Some of the proteins present may also help other cells identify the lipoprotein as a chylomicron.

Once a chylomicron enters the bloodstream, the triglycerides in its core are broken down into fatty acids and glycerol by an enzyme called **lipoprotein lipase,** attached to the inside

TABLE 5-3 ■ **Composition and Roles of the Major Lipoproteins in the Blood**

Lipoprotein	Primary Component	Key Role
Chylomicron	Triglyceride	Carries dietary fat from the small intestine to cells
VLDL	Triglyceride	Carries lipids made and taken up by the liver to cells
LDL	Cholesterol	Carries cholesterol made by the liver and from other sources to cells
HDL	Protein	Contributes to cholesterol removal from cells and, in turn, excretion of it from the body

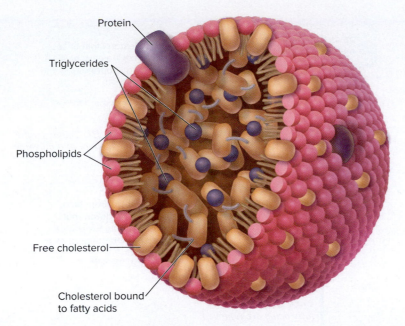

FIGURE 5-13 ▲ The structure of a lipoprotein (specifically, LDL). This structure allows fats to circulate in the water-based bloodstream. Various lipoproteins are found in the bloodstream. The primary component of LDL is cholesterol.

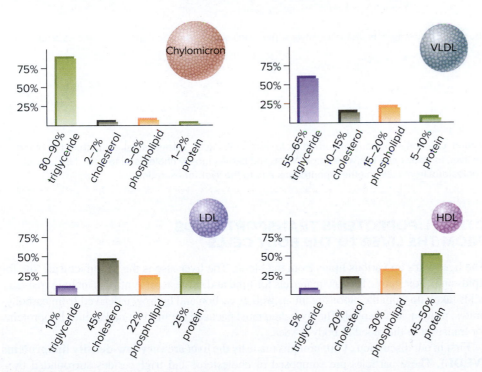

FIGURE 5-14 ▲ Composition of lipoproteins.

walls of the blood vessels (Fig. 5-15). As soon as the fatty acids are released to the bloodstream, they are absorbed by nearby cells. The remaining glycerol backbone circulates back to the liver. Muscle cells can immediately use the absorbed fatty acids for fuel. Adipose cells, on the other hand, tend to reform the fatty acids into triglycerides for storage. After triglycerides have been removed, a chylomicron remnant remains. Chylomicron remnants are removed from circulation by the liver, and their components are recycled to make other lipoproteins and bile acids.

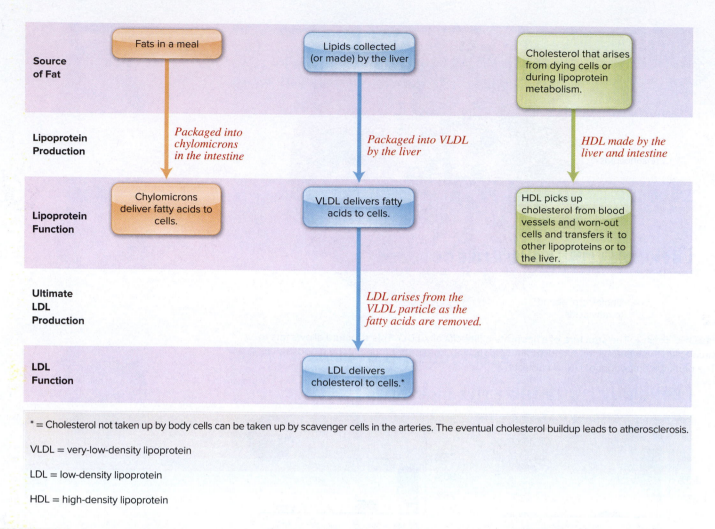

Source of Fat	Fats in a meal	Lipids collected (or made) by the liver	Cholesterol that arises from dying cells or during lipoprotein metabolism.
Lipoprotein Production	*Packaged into chylomicrons in the intestine*	*Packaged into VLDL by the liver*	*HDL made by the liver and intestine*
Lipoprotein Function	Chylomicrons deliver fatty acids to cells.	VLDL delivers fatty acids to cells.	HDL picks up cholesterol from blood vessels and worn-out cells and transfers it to other lipoproteins or to the liver.
Ultimate LDL Production		*LDL arises from the VLDL particle as the fatty acids are removed.*	
LDL Function		LDL delivers cholesterol to cells.*	

* = Cholesterol not taken up by body cells can be taken up by scavenger cells in the arteries. The eventual cholesterol buildup leads to atherosclerosis.

VLDL = very-low-density lipoprotein

LDL = low-density lipoprotein

HDL = high-density lipoprotein

FIGURE 5-15 ▲ Lipoprotein production and function. Chylomicrons carry absorbed fat to body cells. VLDL carries fat taken up from the bloodstream by the liver, as well as any fat made by the liver, to body cells. LDL arises from VLDL and carries mostly cholesterol to cells. HDL arises mostly from the liver and intestine. HDL carries cholesterol from cells to other lipoproteins and to the liver for excretion.

OTHER LIPOPROTEINS TRANSPORT LIPIDS FROM THE LIVER TO THE BODY CELLS

The liver takes up various lipids from the blood. The liver also is the manufacturing site for lipids and cholesterol. The raw materials for lipid and cholesterol synthesis include free fatty acids taken up from the bloodstream, as well as carbon and hydrogen derived from carbohydrates, protein, and alcohol. The liver then must package the lipids it makes into lipoproteins for transport in the blood to body tissues.

First in our discussion of lipoproteins made by the liver are **very-low-density lipoproteins (VLDL).** These particles are composed of cholesterol and triglycerides surrounded by a water-soluble shell. VLDLs are rich in triglycerides and thus are very low in density. Once in the bloodstream, lipoprotein lipase on the inner surface of the blood vessels breaks down the triglyceride in the VLDL into fatty acids and glycerol. Fatty acids and glycerol are released into the bloodstream and taken up by the body cells.

As its triglycerides are released, the VLDL becomes proportionately more dense. Much of what eventually remains of the VLDL fraction is then called **low-density lipoprotein (LDL);** this is composed primarily of the remaining cholesterol. The primary function of LDL is to transport cholesterol to tissues. LDL particles are taken up from the bloodstream by specific receptors on cells, especially liver cells, and are then broken down. The cholesterol and protein components of LDL provide some of the building blocks

very-low-density lipoprotein (VLDL) The lipoprotein created in the liver that carries cholesterol and lipids that have been taken up or newly synthesized by the liver.

low-density lipoprotein (LDL) The lipoprotein in the blood containing primarily cholesterol; elevated LDL is strongly linked to cardiovascular disease risk.

necessary for cell growth and development, such as synthesis of cell membranes and hormones.

The final group of lipoproteins, **high-density lipoproteins (HDL),** is a critical and beneficial participant in this process of lipid transport. Its high proportion of protein makes it the densest lipoprotein. The liver and intestine produce most of the HDL in the blood. It roams the bloodstream, picking up cholesterol from dying cells and other sources. HDL donates the cholesterol primarily to other lipoproteins for transport back to the liver to be excreted. Some HDL travels directly back to the liver.

"GOOD" AND "BAD" CHOLESTEROL IN THE BLOODSTREAM

HDL and LDL are often described as "good" and "bad" cholesterol, respectively. Many studies demonstrate that the amount of HDL in the bloodstream can closely predict the risk for cardiovascular disease. Risk increases with low HDL because little cholesterol is transported back to the liver and excreted. Women tend to have high amounts of HDL, especially before **menopause,** compared to men. High amounts of HDL slow the development of cardiovascular disease, so any cholesterol carried by HDL can be considered "good" cholesterol.

On the other hand, LDL is sometimes considered "bad" cholesterol. In our discussion of LDL, you learned that it is taken up by receptors on various cells. If LDL is not readily cleared from the bloodstream, **scavenger cells** in the arteries take up the lipoprotein, leading to a buildup of cholesterol in the blood vessels. This buildup, known as **atherosclerosis,** greatly increases the risk for cardiovascular disease. Scientists believe that atherosclerosis starts because the innermost layer of the artery becomes damaged. Because of the damage, over time, fats, cholesterol, platelets, cellular debris, and calcium are deposited in the artery wall. The longer LDL cholesterol is in the bloodstream, the more likely it is to be oxidized and cleared by scavenger cells, which "swallow" the cholesterol to become **"foam cells"** that embed in the artery wall (see Section 5.8). Low amounts of LDL are needed as part of routine body functions, but a high level of LDL cholesterol is a risk factor for cardiovascular disease.

Here is an important point: the cholesterol in foods is not designated as "good" or "bad." It is only after cholesterol has been made or processed by the liver that it shows up in the bloodstream as LDL or HDL. Dietary patterns can affect the metabolism of cholesterol, however. Diets low in saturated fat, *trans* fat, and cholesterol encourage the uptake of LDL by the liver, thereby removing LDL from the bloodstream and decreasing the ability of scavenger cells to form atherosclerotic plaque in blood vessels. Likewise, diets high in saturated fat, *trans* fat, and cholesterol reduce the uptake of LDL by the liver, increasing cholesterol in the blood and the risk for cardiovascular disease. Consider what foods in your diet are high in saturated fat, *trans* fat, or cholesterol.

✔ CONCEPT CHECK 5.5

1. How do lipids move through the watery environment of the lymph and blood?
2. How are dietary fats packaged in the small intestine and transported?
3. Where are VLDLs made and what do they contain?
4. Where do the LDLs originate and what is their destination?
5. Why are HDLs considered "good" cholesterol?

5.6 Roles of Lipids in the Body

Many key functions of fat in the body require the use of fatty acids in the form of triglycerides. Triglycerides are used for energy storage, insulation, and transportation of fat-soluble vitamins.

high-density lipoprotein (HDL) The lipoprotein in the blood that picks up cholesterol from dying cells and other sources and transfers it to the other lipoproteins in the bloodstream, as well as directly to the liver; low HDL increases the risk for cardiovascular disease.

menopause The cessation of the menstrual cycle in women, usually beginning at about 50 years of age.

scavenger cells Specific form of white blood cells that can bury themselves in the artery wall and accumulate LDL. As these cells take up LDL, they contribute to the development of atherosclerosis.

atherosclerosis A buildup of fatty material (plaque) in the arteries, including those surrounding the heart.

foam cells Lipid-loaded white blood cells that have surrounded large amounts of a fatty substance, usually cholesterol, on the blood vessel walls.

It appears that saturated fatty acids promote an increase in the amount of free cholesterol (not attached to fatty acids) in the liver, whereas unsaturated fatty acids do the opposite. As free cholesterol in the liver increases, it causes the liver to reduce cholesterol uptake from the bloodstream, contributing to elevated LDL in the blood. (*Trans* fatty acids are thought to act in the same ways as saturated fatty acids.)

▲ When at rest or during light activity, the body uses mostly fatty acids for fuel.
© SW Productions/Getty Images

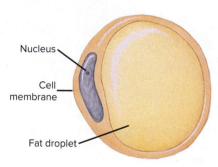

Nucleus

Cell membrane

Fat droplet

Adipose cell

PROVIDING ENERGY

Triglycerides contained in the diet and stored in adipose tissue provide the fatty acids that are the main fuel for muscles while at rest and during light activity. A mix of fat and carbohydrates is burned for fuel during endurance exercise, but muscles rely mainly on carbohydrates during short, intense exercise. As the duration of exercise increases, the percent of fatty acids used for exercise rises as the percent of carbohydrates falls. Other body tissues also use fatty acids for energy needs. Overall, about half of the energy used by the entire body at rest and during light activity comes from fatty acids. When considering the whole body, the use of fatty acids by skeletal and heart muscle is balanced by the use of glucose by the nervous system and red blood cells. Recall from Section 4.5 that cells need a supply of carbohydrate to efficiently process fatty acids for fuel. The details about how we burn fat as a fuel will be discussed throughout Chapter 12 and in Section 14.3.

STORING ENERGY FOR LATER USE

We store energy mainly in the form of triglycerides. The body's ability to store fat is essentially limitless. Its fat storage sites, adipose cells, can increase about 50 times in weight. If the amount of fat to be stored exceeds the ability of the existing cells to expand, the body can form new adipose cells.

An important advantage of using triglycerides to store energy in the body is that they are energy dense. Recall that these yield, on average, 9 kcal per gram, whereas proteins and carbohydrates yield only about 4 kcal per gram. In addition, triglycerides are chemically stable, so they are not likely to react with other cell constituents, making them a safe form for storing energy. Finally, when it comes to storage, triglycerides are space savers. Adipose cells contain about 80% lipid and only 20% water and protein. When we store triglycerides in adipose cells, we store little else. In contrast, muscle tissue is about 73% water. What if we had to store energy as muscle tissue? Body weight linked to energy storage would increase dramatically. The same would be true if we stored energy primarily as glycogen, as about 3 grams of water are stored for every gram of glycogen.

INSULATING AND PROTECTING THE BODY

The insulating layer of fat just beneath the skin is made mostly of triglycerides. Fat tissue also surrounds and protects some organs—kidneys, for example—from injury. We usually do not notice the important insulating function of fat tissue, because we wear clothes and add more as needed. A layer of insulating fat is important in animals living in cold climates. Polar bears, walruses, and whales all build a thick layer of fat tissue around themselves to insulate against cold-weather environments. The extra fat also provides energy storage for times when food is scarce.

TRANSPORTING FAT-SOLUBLE VITAMINS

Triglycerides and other fats in food carry fat-soluble vitamins to the small intestine and aid their absorption. People who absorb fat poorly, such as those with the disease cystic fibrosis, are at risk for deficiencies of fat-soluble vitamins, especially vitamin K. A similar risk comes from taking mineral oil as a laxative at mealtimes. The body cannot digest or absorb mineral oil, so the undigested oil carries the fat-soluble vitamins from the meal into the feces, where they are eliminated. Unabsorbed fatty acids can bind minerals, such as calcium and magnesium, and draw them into the stool for elimination. This can harm mineral status. Recall that the main problem with the fat replacer olestra is that it can bind the fat-soluble vitamins and reduce their absorption.

REGULATING BODY PROCESSES

The lipids are potent regulators of chemical processes within the body. Sterols are important in the synthesis of hormones, including estrogen, testosterone, and the active form of vitamin D. Individual fatty acids also orchestrate many aspects of human metabolism. As you learned in Section 5.2, the essential omega-3 and omega-6 fatty acids can be converted in the body into other fatty acids, which give rise to eicosanoids. Eicosanoids act as chemical messengers that direct growth and development, immune function, and the work of the central nervous system. The essential omega-3 fatty acid, alpha-linolenic acid, can be converted into EPA and DHA in the body. Eicosanoids made from these omega-3 fatty acids tend to decrease blood clotting and inflammatory processes in the body. This is in contrast to the pro-inflammatory effects of omega-6 fatty acids. The omega-6 parent fat, linoleic acid, is converted by the body into the long-chain fatty acid **arachidonic acid (AA).** Arachidonic acid has some important functions in the body, but when omega-6 fatty acids are consumed in excess, arachidonic acid can contribute to inflammatory conditions such as arthritis, blood clotting, and other cardiovascular problems.

arachidonic acid (AA) An omega-6 fatty acid made from linoleic acid with 20 carbon atoms and four carbon-carbon double bonds.

Some studies show that people who eat fish at least twice a week (total weekly intake of 8 ounces) run lower risks for heart attack than do people who rarely eat fish. In these cases, the omega-3 fatty acids in fish oil are probably acting to reduce blood clotting. As will be covered in detail in Section 5.8, blood clots are part of the heart attack process. In addition, omega-3 fatty acids have a favorable effect on heart rhythm. Consequently, the risk of heart attack decreases with the consumption of omega-3 fatty acids from fish, especially for people already at high risk.

Recognize that excessive intakes of omega-3 fatty acids can be unhealthy, too! Certain groups of people, such as the Greenlandic Inuit, eat so much seafood that their normal blood-clotting ability can be impaired. An excess of omega-3 fatty acid intake can allow uncontrolled bleeding and may cause **hemorrhagic stroke.** An excessive intake of long-chain fatty acids in seafood can also depress immune function, resulting in more infections.

hemorrhagic stroke Damage to part of the brain resulting from rupture of a blood vessel and subsequent bleeding within or over the internal surface of the brain.

PHOSPHOLIPIDS IN THE BODY

Many types of phospholipids exist in the body, especially in the brain. They form important parts of cell membranes. Phospholipids are found in body cells, and they participate in fat digestion in the intestine. Recall that the various forms of lecithin (discussed in Section 5.5) are common examples of phospholipids [review Fig. 5-4(b)].

Cell membranes are composed primarily of phospholipids. A cell membrane looks much like a sea of phospholipids with protein "islands" (Fig. 5-16). The proteins form receptors for hormones, function as enzymes, and act as transporters for nutrients. The fatty acids on the phospholipids serve as a source of essential fatty acids for the cell. Some cholesterol is also present in the membrane.

By breaking fat globules into small droplets, emulsifiers enable a fat to be suspended in water. They act as bridges between the oil and water that in turn lead to the formation of tiny oil droplets surrounded by thin shells of water. Phospholipids in the shells of lipoproteins suspend fats in blood in much the same way lecithin suspends vinegar in oil in salad dressing. Sphingomyelin is a phospholipid that protects nerve cells.

The body's main emulsifiers are the lecithins and bile acids, produced by the liver and released into the small intestine via the gallbladder during digestion.

CHOLESTEROL IN THE BODY

Cholesterol plays many vital roles in the body. It forms part of some important hormones, such as estrogen, testosterone, and a precursor of the active vitamin D hormone. Cholesterol is an essential structural component of cells and the outer layer of the lipoprotein particles that transport lipids in the blood. The cholesterol content of the heart, liver, kidney, and brain is high, reflecting its critical role in these organs. Cholesterol is also the building block of bile acids, needed for fat digestion. As discussed earlier, about 98% of the bile acids are absorbed and end up back at the liver after participating in fat digestion. Using medicines that block some of this reabsorption of bile acids is one way to treat high blood cholesterol. The liver takes cholesterol from the bloodstream to form replacement bile acids. Viscous fiber in the diet can also bind to bile acids to produce the same effect

Cell (plasma) membrane

Carbohydrate chains

Protein chain

Phospholipid bilayer

Globular protein

Cholesterol

FIGURE 5-16 ▲ Phospholipids are the main components of cell membranes, forming a double layer (bilayer) of lipid.

▲ Trimming the fat off meats can help reduce saturated fat intake, but you cannot remove the marbling (streaks of fat running through the meat). Limit portion size to 3 ounces and choose fatty cuts of meat less often to help keep your blood cholesterol levels in check.
© Royalty-Free/Corbis

(see the discussion in Section 5.8 on medical interventions related to cardiovascular disease for details).

About two-thirds of the cholesterol circulating through your body is made by body cells; the remaining one-third is consumed in the diet. Except in cases of genetically related high blood cholesterol, cholesterol synthesis by the body is well regulated: a higher intake of dietary cholesterol leads to an overall decrease in body production, whereas a lower intake from food results in more cholesterol made in the body. Generally, each day, your body's cells produce approximately 875 milligrams of cholesterol. Of these, about 400 milligrams are used to make new bile acids to replenish those lost in the feces, and about 50 milligrams are used to make hormones. In addition to all the cholesterol cells make, we consume about 180 to 325 milligrams of cholesterol per day from animal-derived food products, with men consuming the higher amount compared to women. Absorption of cholesterol from food ranges from about 40% to 65%. The effect of blood cholesterol, especially LDL cholesterol, on cardiovascular disease risk will be discussed in Section 5.8.

✔ **CONCEPT CHECK 5.6**

1. What are the functions of triglycerides in the body?

2. Where are phospholipids found in the body?

3. What are some compounds that are made from cholesterol in the body?

5.7 Recommendations for Fat Intake

There is no RDA for total fat intake for adults, although there is an Adequate Intake set for total fat for infants (see Section 19.2). The Dietary Guidelines for Americans and the Food and Nutrition Board recommend that total fat intake should be 20% to 35% of total calories, which equates to 44 to 78 grams per day for a person who consumes 2000 kcal daily.

Regarding essential fatty acids, the Food and Nutrition Board has issued recommendations for linoleic acid and alpha-linolenic acid. Table 5-4 lists the AIs for adults. To meet our dietary requirements for essential fatty acids, we only need to consume 2 to 4 tablespoons of plant oil each day, which equates to roughly 5% of our total calories. We can easily get that much from cooking oils, salad dressings, nuts and seeds, vegetables, and whole-grain breads. Even a low-fat diet will provide enough essential fatty acids if it follows a balanced plan such as MyPlate.

The advice to consume 20% to 35% of calories as fat does not apply to infants and toddlers below the age of 2 years. These youngsters are forming new tissue that requires fat, especially in the brain, so their intake of fat and cholesterol should not be greatly restricted.

EATING FOR HEART HEALTH

The most specific recommendations for fat intake come from the American Heart Association (AHA) (see Further Reading 2). Many North Americans are at risk for developing cardiovascular disease, so AHA promotes dietary and lifestyle goals aimed at reducing this risk. The AHA diet and lifestyle goals for cardiovascular disease risk reduction for the general public include aiming for an overall healthy eating pattern; appropriate body weight; and a desirable blood cholesterol profile, blood pressure, and blood glucose level. In Table 5-5, a more detailed list of recommendations is provided for those who currently are at high risk or have cardiovascular disease.

To reduce risk for cardiovascular disease, the AHA recommends reducing *trans* fat and limiting saturated fat to no more than 5% to 6% of total calories. These are the primary fatty acids that raise LDL. Table 5-6 is an example of a diet that adheres to 20% or 30% of calories as fat. Compare these recommendations to the actual dietary intake patterns of these fats by North Americans: 33% of calories from total fat, with about 13% of calories from saturated fat each day.

▲ Whole grains (shredded wheat, whole-wheat bread, oatmeal cookies, popcorn), fruits (orange juice, apple, banana, raisins), vegetables (carrots, lettuce, tomato), lean meats (roast beef, turkey, chicken), and fat-free milk are the primary components of the dietary patterns described in Table 5-5. © Digital Vision/Getty Images

TABLE 5-4 ■ **Food and Nutrition Board Recommendations for Essential Omega-6 and Omega-3 Fatty Acids**

	Men (grams per day)	Women (grams per day)
Linoleic acid (omega-6)	17 (3.6 tsp)	12 (2.6 tsp)
Alpha-linolenic acid (omega-3)	1.6 (0.35 tsp)	1.1 (0.24 tsp)

TABLE 5-5 ■ **American Heart Association's Diet and Lifestyle Recommendations**

Use up at least as many calories as you take in.

Eat a variety of nutritious foods from all the food groups, including:
- A variety of fruits and vegetables
- Whole grains
- Low-fat dairy products
- Skinless poultry and fish
- Nuts and legumes
- Nontropical vegetable oils

Eat less of the nutrient-poor foods:
- Limit foods and beverages that are high in calories but low in nutrients.
- Limit the amount of saturated fat, *trans* fat, and sodium you eat.

(continued)

TABLE 5-5 ■ American Heart Association's Diet and Lifestyle Recommendations—*Continued*

As you make daily food choices, base your eating pattern on these recommendations:

• Eat a variety of fresh, frozen, and canned fruits and vegetables without high-calorie sauces or added salt and sugars.
• Choose fiber-rich whole grains for most grain servings.
• Choose poultry and fish without the skin and prepare them in healthy ways.
• Eat a variety of fish (especially those rich in omega-3 fatty acids) at least twice a week.
• Select fat-free and low-fat dairy products.
• Avoid foods containing partially hydrogenated vegetable oils to reduce *trans* fat in your diet.
• Limit saturated fat and *trans* fat and replace them with monounsaturated and polyunsaturated fats. If you need to lower blood cholesterol, reduce saturated fats to no more than 5% to 6% of total calories.
• Cut back on beverages and foods with added sugars.
• Choose foods with less sodium and prepare foods with little or no salt.
• If you drink alcohol, drink in moderation (no more than 1 drink per day for women and no more than 2 drinks per day for men).
• Follow the AHA recommendations when you eat out and keep an eye on portion sizes.

Source: Eckel RH and others: 2013 AHA/ACC guideline on lifestyle management to reduce cardiovascular risk. a report of the American College of Cardiology/ American Heart Association Task Force on Practice Guidelines. *Circulation* 129:S76, 2013.

TABLE 5-6 ■ Daily Menu Examples Containing 2000 kcal and 30% or 20% of Calories as Fat

30% of Calories as Fat		20% of Calories as Fat	
Food	Fat (grams)	Food	Fat (grams)
Breakfast			
Orange juice, 1 cup	0.5	Same	0.5
Shredded wheat, ¾ cup	0.5	Shredded wheat, 1 cup	0.7
Toasted whole-grain bagel	1.1	Same	1.1
Peanut butter, 3 teaspoons	8.0	Same	8.0
1% low-fat milk, 1 cup	2.5	Fat-free milk, 1 cup	0.6
Lunch			
Whole-wheat bread, 2 slices	2.4	Same	2.4
Roast beef, 2 ounces	4.9	Light turkey roll, 2 ounces	0.9
Mustard, 3 teaspoons	0.6	Same	0.6
Swiss cheese, 2 slices	15.6	Swiss cheese, 1 slice	7.8
Lettuce	—	Same	—
Tomato	—	Same	—
Oatmeal cookie, 1	3.3	Oatmeal cookie, 2	6.6
Snack			
Apple	—	Same	—
Dinner			
Chicken tenders frozen meal	18.0	Fat-free chicken tenders	—
Carrots, ½ cup	—	Same	—
Dinner roll, 1	2.0	Same	2.0
Olive oil, 1.5 teaspoon	6.8	Same	6.8
Banana	0.6	Same	0.6
1% low-fat milk, 1 cup	2.5	Fat-free milk, 1 cup	0.6
Snack			
Raisins, 2 teaspoons	—	Raisins, ½ cup	—
Air-popped popcorn, 3 cups	1.0	Air-popped popcorn, 6 cups	2.0
Parmesan cheese, 2 tablespoons	2.8	Same	2.8
Totals	**73.1**		**44.0**

ASK THE RDN | Coconut Oil

Dear RDN: My friend at the health food store said I should start using coconut oil in my cooking because it has all kinds of health benefits. Is coconut oil a good choice?

Recently, coconut oil has been promoted for weight loss, heart health, cancer protection, and brain health. Indeed, there is some interesting research on the health effects of the particular fatty acids in coconut oil. At this point, however, there is little evidence to back up the claims that coconut oil is a miracle cure for anything.

Coconut oil is highly saturated. In fact, nearly 90% of the fatty acids in coconut oil are saturated, which is even more than butter or beef fat. This makes for a desirable product: it has that "melt in your mouth" quality and it is very shelf stable, which is attractive for food manufacturers and consumers alike. How do saturated fats impact your health? In this chapter, you have seen the recommendations from all the major health authorities urging Americans to limit their intakes of saturated fat. This is because saturated fatty acids have been shown to increase blood levels of LDL cholesterol, which are linked to atherosclerosis. Proponents of coconut oil point to research showing that the fatty acids in coconut oil, while they do raise LDL, also raise HDL levels. It remains to be seen how these alterations ultimately affect risk for cardiovascular disease.

When it comes to weight loss, the producers of coconut oil focus on the size of the fatty acids in their product. Most dietary fats are long-chain fatty acids. About 60% of the fatty acids in coconut oil, however, are medium-chain fatty acids, which are more likely to be burned as fuel and less likely to be stored in adipose tissue. Does coconut oil help you lose weight? There are two small human studies that show a decrease in waist circumference with coconut oil, but there is not yet enough evidence to promote coconut oil as a weight-loss aid.

If you like coconut oil, *use it in moderation.* Like any dietary fat, coconut oil is a dense source of calories. Simply adding coconut oil to your dietary pattern is not a wise choice because those extra fat calories can quickly add up. Extra calories from any source inevitably lead to weight gain. Use it instead of butter or margarine, aiming to keep your total intake of saturated fat less than 10% of total calories. Most of the time, though, choose unsaturated plant oils, which have proven benefits for heart health. Coconut oil is not a cure-all, but it can be included as part of an overall healthy dietary pattern that meets your calorie needs.

Yours in health,

Angela Collene, MS, RDN, LD (author)

Please note that the latest guidelines set no specific limits on dietary cholesterol. This is because dietary cholesterol intake has little impact on blood cholesterol levels. Instead, evidence shows that saturated fat and *trans* fat have the greatest impact on blood lipids. That doesn't mean you should eat limitless quantities of cholesterol-rich foods! As it turns out, rich food sources of cholesterol are usually sources of saturated fat, as well. Thus, as you reduce the saturated fat in your diet, you will likely reduce your cholesterol intake, too.

RECOMMENDATIONS FOR FISH CONSUMPTION

The Dietary Guidelines and the American Heart Association's Diet and Lifestyle Recommendations encourage Americans to eat 2 or more servings of fatty fish each week. Fish is not only a rich source of omega-3 fatty acids, but also a valuable source of protein and trace elements that may provide protective effects for the cardiovascular system. Broiled or baked fish is recommended rather than fried fish because frying may increase the ratio of omega-6 to omega-3 fatty acids and may produce *trans* fatty acids and oxidized lipid products that may increase cardiovascular disease risk.

Although consuming fish is thought to have greater benefits than using fish oil supplements, in some instances, fish oil capsules can be safely substituted for fish if a person does not like fish. Generally, about 1 gram of omega-3 fatty acids (about three capsules)

▲ The American Heart Association recommends eating fatty fish such as salmon at least twice a week. As a source of omega-3 fatty acids, fish is a heart-healthy alternative to other animal sources of protein, which can be high in saturated fat and cholesterol.

© Purestock/SuperStock

Do those fish oil capsules leave a nasty taste in your mouth? Freezing fish oil capsules before consumption, using enteric-coated capsules, and using capsules with vitamin E will reduce the fishy aftertaste.

from fish oil per day is recommended, especially for people with evidence of cardiovascular disease. The American Heart Association also recently suggested that fish oil supplements (providing 2 to 4 grams of omega-3 fatty acids per day) could be employed to treat elevated blood triglycerides. However, fish oil capsules should be limited for individuals who have bleeding disorders, take anticoagulant medications, or anticipate surgery, because they may increase risk of uncontrollable bleeding and hemorrhagic stroke. Thus, for fish oil capsules, as well as other dietary supplements, it is important to follow a physician's recommendations. Remember that fish oil supplements are not regulated by FDA. The quality of these supplements, therefore, is not standardized, and contaminants naturally present in the fish oil may not have been removed.

DIETARY PATTERNS THAT PROMOTE CARDIOVASCULAR HEALTH

In recent years, the Mediterranean diet (see Further Readings 3 and 12, and Newsworthy Nutrition) has attracted a lot of attention because of the lower rates of chronic diseases seen among people following such a diet plan. Reduction of cardiovascular disease has been one of the most consistent results of the Mediterranean diet. The major sources of fat in the Mediterranean diet include liberal amounts of olive oil compared to a small amount of animal fat (from animal flesh, eggs, and dairy products). In contrast, major sources of fat in the typical North American diet include animal flesh, whole milk, pastries, cheese, margarine, and mayonnaise. While dietary fat sources definitely play a role in prevention of chronic disease, it is important to remember that other aspects of one's lifestyle also contribute to disease risk. People who follow a Mediterranean diet also tend to consume moderate alcohol (usually in the form of red wine, which contains many antioxidants), eat plenty of whole grains and few refined carbohydrates, and are also more physically active than typical North Americans (see Further Reading 10).

An alternative plan for reduction of cardiovascular disease is Dr. Dean Ornish's purely vegetarian (**vegan**) diet plan (see Further Reading 9). This diet is very low in fat, including only a scant quantity of vegetable oil used in cooking and the small amount of oils present

vegan A person who eats only plant foods.

Newsworthy Nutrition

Mediterranean diet decreases risk of cardiovascular disease

Based on earlier observations of an inverse relationship between adherence to the Mediterranean diet and risk of cardiovascular disease, the effect of the Mediterranean diet pattern on the primary prevention of cardiovascular disease events was studied in Spain, using a randomized multicenter trial design. Participants (7447 persons, 55 to 80 years, 57% women) were at high cardiovascular risk but had no cardiovascular disease at the beginning of the study and were randomly assigned to either a Mediterranean diet supplemented with extra-virgin olive oil; a Mediterranean diet supplemented with mixed nuts; or a control diet with advice to reduce dietary fat. Participants were followed for a median of 4.8 years and assessed for the occurrence of the following major cardiovascular events: myocardial infarction, stroke, or death from cardiovascular causes. There was good adherence to the interventions for the two Mediterranean-diet groups. At least one major cardiovascular event occurred in 288 participants. This included 96 events for the group assigned to a Mediterranean diet with extra-virgin olive oil and 83 events for the group assigned to a Mediterranean diet with nuts versus 109 events for the control group. The authors concluded that a Mediterranean diet, unrestricted in calories but supplemented with extra-virgin olive oil or nuts, resulted in a substantial reduction in the incidence of major cardiovascular events among persons at high cardiovascular risk. These results, therefore, support the benefits of the Mediterranean diet for the prevention of cardiovascular disease.

Source: Estruch R and others: Primary prevention of cardiovascular disease with a Mediterranean diet. *New England Journal of Medicine* 368:1279–1290, 2013.

in plant foods. Individuals restricting fat intake to 20% of calories should be monitored by a physician, as the resulting increase in carbohydrate intake can increase blood triglycerides in some people, which is not a healthful change. Over time, however, the initial problem of high blood triglycerides on a low-fat diet may self-correct. Among people following the Ornish plan, blood triglycerides initially increased but within a year fell to normal values as long as the individuals emphasized high-fiber carbohydrate sources, controlled (or improved) body weight, and followed a regular exercise program.

FAT *QUALITY* VERSUS FAT *QUANTITY*

Weight control is a vitally important way to minimize risk for a variety of chronic diseases. Because it is a dense source of calories, many people seek to limit fat intake as a way to manage body weight. However, it is important to recognize that excess calories from any source–fat, carbohydrates, or protein–contribute to weight gain. If weight loss is needed, understand that your overall calorie intake is more important than the specific ratio of carbohydrates, fats, and protein in your diet.

As you have learned, the general consensus among nutrition experts is that fat should comprise 20% to 35% of total calories. When it comes to improving your dietary pattern, it is usually not necessary to drastically lower the *quantity* of fat in your diet. However, we should aim to choose more foods that provide omega-3 fatty acids, while choosing fewer sources of saturated and *trans* fats (see Further Reading 13). In short, most Americans need to improve their fat *quality*.

Simply selecting the reduced-fat versions of pastries, cookies, and cakes will not improve the quality of your diet. Often, extra sugar or salt has been added to these foods to compensate for losses of taste and texture. Instead, focus your efforts on choosing plant sources of fat more often than animal sources (Table 5-7). Fruits, vegetables, and whole grains are usually low in total fat and saturated fat; the (mostly unsaturated) fats they do provide are accompanied by vitamin E, vitamin K, and a variety of health-promoting phytochemicals.

TABLE 5-7 ■ Tips for Cutting Back on Saturated Fats and *Trans* Fats

	Eat Less of These Foods	Eat More of These Foods
Grains	• Pasta dishes with cheese or cream sauces • Croissants • Pastries • Doughnuts • Pie crust	• Whole-grain breads • Whole-grain pasta • Brown rice • Air-popped popcorn
Vegetables	• French fries • Potato chips • Vegetables cooked in butter, cheese, or cream sauces	• Fresh, frozen, baked, or steamed vegetables
Fruit	• Fruit pies	• Fresh, frozen, or canned fruits
Dairy	• Whole milk • Ice cream • High-fat cheese • Cheesecake	• Fat-free and reduced-fat milk • Low-fat frozen desserts (e.g., yogurt, sherbet, and ice milk) • Reduced-fat/part-skim cheese
Protein	• Bacon • Sausage • Organ meats (e.g., liver) • Egg yolks	• Fish • Skinless poultry • Lean cuts of meat (with fat trimmed away) • Soy products • Egg whites/egg substitutes

CASE STUDY   Planning a Heart-Healthy Diet

Jackie is a 21-year-old health-conscious individual majoring in business. She recently learned that a diet high in saturated fat can contribute to high blood cholesterol and that exercise is beneficial for the heart. Jackie now takes a brisk 30-minute walk each morning before going to class, and she has started to cut as much fat out of her diet as she can, replacing it mostly with carbohydrates. A typical day for Jackie now begins with a 2-cup bowl of Fruity Pebbles™ with 1 cup of skim milk and ½ cup of apple juice. For lunch, she might pack a turkey sandwich on white bread with lettuce, tomato, and mustard; a 1-ounce package of fat-free pretzels; and five reduced-fat vanilla wafers. Dinner could be a 2-cup portion of pasta with some olive oil and garlic mixed in, and a small iceberg lettuce salad with lemon juice squeezed over it. Her snacks are usually baked chips, low-fat cookies, fat-free frozen yogurt, or fat-free pretzels. She drinks five diet soft drinks throughout the day as her main beverage.

Answer the following questions, and check your response at the end of this chapter.

▲ Are there important food groups missing from Jackie's new diet plan? © trbfoto/Brand X Pictures/ Jupiterimages

1. Has Jackie made the best diet changes with regard to lowering blood cholesterol and maintaining heart health?
2. Is there much fat left in Jackie's new diet plan? Is it necessary for her to drastically lower her fat intake?
3. What types of fat should Jackie try to consume? Why are these types of fat the most desirable?
4. What types of foods has Jackie used to replace the fat in her diet?
5. What food groups are missing from her new diet plan? How many servings should she be including from these food groups?
6. Is Jackie's new exercise routine appropriate?

✓ CONCEPT CHECK 5.7

1. How does the percent of calories as fat in the North American diet compare to recommendations?
2. What are the recommendations for saturated fat and *trans* fat intake?
3. What are the characteristics of the Mediterranean diet?

5.8 Nutrition and Your Health
Lipids and Cardiovascular Disease

© Foodcollection

The typical forms of cardiovascular disease—coronary heart disease and strokes—are associated with inadequate blood circulation in the heart and brain related to buildup of this plaque. Blood supplies the heart muscle, brain, and other body organs with oxygen and nutrients. When blood flow via the coronary arteries surrounding the heart is interrupted, the heart muscle can be damaged. A heart attack, or **myocardial infarction,** may result (review Fig. 5-17). This may cause the heart to beat irregularly or to stop. About 25% of people do not survive their first heart attack. If blood flow to parts of the brain is interrupted long enough, part of the brain dies, causing a **cerebrovascular accident,** or stroke.

A heart attack can strike with the sudden force of a sledgehammer, with pain radiating up the neck or down the arm. It can sneak up at night, masquerading as indigestion, with slight pain or pressure in the chest. Crushing chest pain is a more common symptom in men (see Further Reading 11). Many times, the symptoms are so subtle in women that death occurs before she or the health professional realizes that a heart attack is taking place. If there is any suspicion that a heart attack is taking place, the person should first

▲ Cardiovascular disease kills more women than any other disease. © image100/PunchStock

Cardiovascular disease is the major killer of North Americans. It typically involves the coronary arteries and, thus, frequently the term *coronary heart disease (CHD)* or *coronary artery disease (CAD)* is used. Each year, about 610,000 people die of coronary heart disease in the United States. About 735,000 people in the United States have a heart attack each year. Women generally lag about 10 years behind men in developing the disease. Still, it eventually kills more women than any other disease. The cost of coronary heart disease alone is $108.9 billion each year, which includes the costs of health care services, medications, and lost productivity.

Development of Cardiovascular Disease

The symptoms of cardiovascular disease develop over many years and often do not become obvious until old age. Nonetheless, autopsies of young adults under 20 years of age have shown that many of them had atherosclerotic **plaque** in their arteries (Fig. 5-17). This finding indicates that plaque buildup can begin in childhood and continue throughout life, although it usually goes undetected for some time (see Further Reading 11).

plaque A cholesterol-rich substance deposited in the blood vessels; it contains various white blood cells, smooth muscle cells, various proteins, cholesterol and other lipids, and eventually calcium.

myocardial infarction Death of part of the heart muscle. Also termed a *heart attack.*

cerebrovascular accident (CVA) Death of part of the brain tissue due typically to a blood clot. Also termed a *stroke.*

FIGURE 5-17 ▶ The road to a heart attack. Injury to an artery wall begins the process. This is followed by a progressive buildup of plaque in the artery walls. The heart attack represents the terminal phase of the process. Blockage of the left coronary artery by a blood clot is evident. The heart muscle served by the portion of the coronary artery beyond the point of blockage lacks oxygen and nutrients, leading to cell damage and death of the cardiac tissue. This damage can lead to a significant drop in heart function and often total heart failure.

call 911 and then chew an aspirin (325 milligrams) thoroughly. Aspirin helps to reduce the blood clotting that leads to a heart attack.

Continuous formation and breakdown of blood clots in the blood vessels is a normal process. However, in areas where plaques build up, blood clots are more likely to remain intact and then lead to a blockage, cutting off or diminishing the supply of blood to the heart (via the coronary arteries) or brain (via the carotid arteries). More than 95% of heart attacks are caused by total blockage of the coronary arteries due to a blood clot forming in an area of the artery already partially blocked by plaque. Disruption of the plaque may even lead to eventual clot formation.

Atherosclerosis probably first develops to repair damage in a vessel lining. Ongoing inflammation in the blood vessel is suspected of causing blood vessel damage. (A laboratory test for C-reactive protein in the blood is used to detect inflammation; see Further Reading 8). The damage that starts this process can also be caused by smoking, diabetes, hypertension, viral and bacterial infection, and LDL. In addition to causing damage to arteries, LDL then enters the damaged areas of the artery walls and begins to accumulate. Atherosclerosis can be seen in arteries throughout the

body. The damage develops especially at points where an artery branches into two smaller vessels. A great deal of stress is placed on the vessel walls at these points due to changes in blood flow.

Once blood vessel damage has occurred, the next step in the development of atherosclerosis is the progression phase. This step is characterized by deposition of plaque at the site of initial damage. The rate of plaque buildup during the progression phase is directly related to the amount of LDL in the blood. The form of LDL that contributes to atherosclerosis has been changed by free radicals into **oxidized** LDL. This form is preferentially taken up by scavenger cells in the arterial wall. Nutrients and phytochemicals that have **antioxidant** properties may reduce LDL oxidation.

oxidize In the most basic sense, the loss of an electron or gain of an oxygen by a chemical substance. This change typically alters the shape and/or function of the substance.

antioxidant A substance that has the ability to prevent or repair the damage caused by oxidation.

Fruits and vegetables are particularly rich in these compounds. Eating fruits and vegetables regularly is one positive step we can make to reduce plaque buildup and slow the progression of cardiovascular disease. Some fruits and vegetables particularly helpful in this regard include legumes (beans), nuts, dried plums (prunes), raisins, berries, plums, apples, cherries, oranges, grapes, spinach, broccoli, red bell peppers, and onions. Tea, coffee, and dark chocolate are also sources of antioxidants. The American Heart Association does not support use of antioxidant supplements (such as vitamin E) to reduce cardiovascular disease risk. This is because large-scale studies have shown no decrease in cardiovascular disease risk with use of antioxidant supplements.

The body also sends white blood cells called macrophages to the location of the cholesterol accumulation on the blood vessel wall. In an attempt to destroy it, the macrophage surrounds the fatty deposit and produces lipid-loaded foam cells. Over years, as cholesterol plaques form and grow inside arteries, they eventually can begin to block off blood flow. The LDL-rich center of the plaque grows in a slow, controlled way and seldom causes heart attacks but arteries harden, narrow, and lose their elasticity. Affected arteries become further damaged as blood pumps through them and pressure increases. Some plaques can become unstable and tear away from the artery. If they rupture, a blood clot will form inside the artery, and within minutes, blood flow is cut off, resulting in a heart attack or stroke.

Factors that typically bring on a heart attack in a person already at risk include dehydration; acute emotional stress (such as firing an employee); strenuous physical activity when not otherwise physically fit (shoveling snow, for example); waking during the night or getting up in the morning (linked to an abrupt increase in stress); and consuming large, high-fat meals (increases blood clotting).

Risk Factors for Cardiovascular Disease

For a person at low risk of cardiovascular disease, the advice of health experts is to consume a balanced diet, perform regular physical activity, have a complete fasting lipoprotein analysis performed at age 20 or beyond, and reevaluate risk factors every 5 years.

How do you know if you are at risk? The most likely risk factors are:

- **Total blood cholesterol over 200 milligrams per 1 deciliter of blood** (200 mg/dl; 1 deciliter equals 100 milliliters). Risk is especially high when total cholesterol is at or over 240 mg/dl and

LDL-cholesterol readings are over 130 to 160 mg/dl. (The terms *LDL cholesterol* and *HDL cholesterol* are used when expressing the blood concentration because it is the cholesterol content of these lipoproteins that is measured.)

- **Smoking.** Smoking is the main cause of about 20% of cardiovascular disease deaths and generally negates the female advantage of later occurrence of the disease. A combination of smoking and oral contraceptive use increases the risk of cardiovascular disease in women even more. Smoking greatly increases the expression of a person's genetically linked risk for cardiovascular disease, even if one's blood lipids are low. Smoking also makes blood more likely to clot. Even second-hand smoke has been implicated as a risk factor.
- **Hypertension.** **Systolic blood pressure** over 139 (millimeters of mercury) and **diastolic blood pressure** over 89 indicate hypertension. Healthy blood pressure values are less than 120 and 80, respectively. (Treatment of hypertension is reviewed in Section 9.9.)
- **Diabetes.** Diabetes virtually guarantees development of cardiovascular disease and so puts a person with diabetes in the high-risk group. Insulin increases cholesterol synthesis in the liver, in turn increasing LDL in the bloodstream. This disease negates any female advantage (see Further Reading 5).

Together, the previous four risk factors explain most cases of cardiovascular disease.

Other risk factors to consider are:

- **HDL cholesterol** under 40 mg/dl, especially when the ratio of total cholesterol to HDL cholesterol is greater than 4:1 (3.5:1 or less is optimal). Women often have high values for HDL cholesterol; therefore, it is important for this to be measured in women to establish cardiovascular disease risk. A value of 60 mg/dl or more is especially protective. Exercising for at least 45 minutes four times a week can increase HDL by about 5 mg/dl. Losing excess weight (especially around the waist) and avoiding smoking and overeating also help maintain or raise HDL, as does moderate alcohol consumption.
- **Age.** Men over 45 years and women over 55 years.
- **Family history** of cardiovascular disease, especially before age 50.
- **Blood triglycerides** 200 mg/dl or greater in the fasting state (less than 100 mg/dl is optimal).
- **Obesity** (especially fat accumulation in the waist). Typical weight gain seen in adults is a chief contributor to the increase in LDL seen with aging. Obesity also typically leads to insulin resistance, creating a diabetes-like state, and ultimately the disease itself. It also increases overall inflammation throughout the body.
- **Inactivity.** Exercise conditions the arteries to adapt to physical stress. Regular exercise also improves insulin action in the body.

systolic blood pressure The pressure in the arterial blood vessels associated with the pumping of blood from the heart.

diastolic blood pressure The pressure in the arterial blood vessels when the heart is between beats.

▲ The buildup of plaque within artery walls is called atherosclerosis. The body sends white blood cells called macrophages to the location of the plaque in an attempt to destroy it. The macrophage surrounds the fatty deposit and produces lipid-loaded foam cells, seen here as a foamy appearance on the artery wall. © MedicalRF.com

The corresponding reduction in insulin output leads to a reduction in lipoprotein synthesis in the liver. Both regular aerobic exercise and resistance exercise are recommended. A person with existing cardiovascular disease should seek physician approval before starting such a program, as should older adults.

The term *risk factor* is not equivalent to cause of disease; nevertheless, the more of these risk factors one has, the greater the chances of ultimately developing cardiovascular disease. A good example is the **metabolic syndrome,** discussed in Section 4.7. A person with the metabolic syndrome would have abdominal obesity, high blood triglycerides, low HDL cholesterol, hypertension, poor blood glucose regulation (i.e., high fasting blood glucose), and increased blood clotting. This profile raises the risk for cardiovascular disease considerably. On a positive note, cardiovascular disease is rare in populations that have low LDL cholesterol, normal blood pressure, and do not smoke or have diabetes. By minimizing these risk factors, as well as following the dietary recommendations of the American Heart Association in Section 5.7 and staying physically active, one will most likely reduce many of the other controllable risk factors listed. In other words, develop and follow a total lifestyle plan. Medications may also be added to lower blood lipids, as discussed next. Finally, if a person has a family history of cardiovascular disease but the usual risk factors are not present, a rarer defect may be the cause. In this case, having a detailed physical examination for other potential causes is advised.

Medications to Lower Blood Lipids

For some people, diet and lifestyle changes are simply not enough to lower blood cholesterol. Fortunately, medications offer a more

Healthy People 2020 has set a goal of reducing total blood cholesterol among adults from the average of 198 mg/dl to 178 mg/dl, as well as reducing the percentage of adults with high blood cholesterol from 15% to 13.5%.

metabolic syndrome A condition in which a person has poor blood glucose regulation, hypertension, increased blood triglycerides, and other health problems. This condition is usually accompanied by obesity, lack of physical activity, and a diet high in refined carbohydrates. Also called Syndrome X.

aggressive approach to treating high cholesterol. Populations that may need cholesterol-lowering medications include individuals who

- have clinical evidence of atherosclerotic cardiovascular disease (see Fig. 5-17),
- have LDL levels of 190 mg/dl or higher,
- are ages 40 to 75 and have LDL levels 70 to 189 mg/dl *and* diabetes, or
- are ages 40 to 75 and have LDL levels 70 to 189 mg/dl *and* greater than 7.5% risk for atherosclerotic cardiovascular disease within the next 10 years (determined by a global risk assessment tool; Table 5-8).

The global risk assessment tool is based on data from several large observational studies of the development and progression of cardiovascular disease. It is meant to assess non-Hispanic black and non-Hispanic white men and women between the ages of 40 and 79 who do not have existing cardiovascular disease. Alternative calculators are available for individuals of other ages and races.

Medications work to lower blood cholesterol in several ways. The statins are a group of medications that reduce cholesterol synthesis in the liver. Examples are listed in the Medicine Cabinet feature in this section. These medications may lead to adverse effects, especially on liver function, so physician monitoring is required. The cost of treatment with one of these drugs can vary widely, from as little as $12 per month to more than $500 (see Further Reading 1).

TABLE 5-8 ■ **Factors Used in Interpreting Risk for Atherosclerotic Cardiovascular Disease***

Risk Factors	Interpretation
Gender	Compared to women, men are at higher risk of developing atherosclerotic cardiovascular disease.
Age	As age increases, risk also increases.
Race	African-Americans are at higher risk than whites.
Total cholesterol	Risk progressively increases as total cholesterol rises above 170 mg/dl.
HDL cholesterol	Risk progressively increases as HDL cholesterol decreases below 50 mg/dl.
Systolic blood pressure	Risk progressively increases as systolic blood pressure rises above 110 mmHg.
Taking medications to treat hypertension	Risk is higher for a person with a history of hypertension.
Diabetes	Risk is higher for a person with a history of diabetes.
Smoking	Compared to nonsmokers, risk is higher for smokers.

*Goff DC and others: 2013 ACC/AHA guideline on the assessment of cardiovascular risk: A report of the American College of Cardiology/American Heart Association Task Force on Practice Guidelines. *Journal of the American College of Cardiology* 63:2935, 2014.

A second group of medications works to lower cholesterol by binding to bile acids in the small intestine, thus preventing their reabsorption and allowing them to be excreted as part of the feces. Recall from Section 3.9 that bile (which contains cholesterol) is secreted from the liver (via the gallbladder) into the small intestine to help digest fats. Usually, about 98% of bile acids is reabsorbed and recycled. When these medications bind to bile acids, they cannot be reabsorbed and recycled, so the liver must synthesize new bile acids. The liver removes LDL from the blood to do this. Medications that block cholesterol absorption are not as effective at lowering cholesterol as statins. Also, some of these medications taste gritty and therefore are not popular.

A third group of drugs can be used to lower blood triglycerides by decreasing the triglyceride production of the liver. These include gemfibrozil (Lopid®) and megadoses of the vitamin nicotinic acid. The use of nicotinic acid results in side effects, however, but these are typically manageable.

Some pharmaceutical companies combine medications with different mechanisms of action. A statin drug (simvastatin) has been combined with another drug (ezetimibe) and is marketed as Vytorin®, a drug that will treat the two sources of cholesterol, "food and family." While the statin reduces the cholesterol made by the liver, the ezetimibe helps to block the absorption of cholesterol from food.

The intensity of therapy depends on the severity of the patient's condition and his or her tolerance of the medication. For example, a patient who has already suffered a heart attack would be treated with a high-dose statin, with the aim of reducing LDL cholesterol by 50%. However, if that patient suffered adverse effects from the high-dose medication (e.g., impaired liver function), the physician would either lower the dose or try a different medication.

Plant Sterols for Cardiovascular Disease

CoroWise® is a leading brand of natural cholesterol reducers called plant sterols. Plant sterols have been clinically shown to reduce LDL (bad) cholesterol, and products that contain these natural cholesterol reducers are backed by the following FDA-approved health claim: *Foods containing at least 0.4 gram per serving of plant sterols, eaten twice a day with meals for a daily total intake of at least 0.8 gram, as part of a diet low in saturated fat and cholesterol, may reduce the risk of heart disease.* Products such as Smart Balance® margarines and Minute Maid Heart Wise® orange juice contain these plant sterols. The plant stanols/sterols, also called phytosterols, work by reducing cholesterol absorption in the small intestine and lowering its return to the liver. The liver responds by taking up more cholesterol from the blood so it can continue to make bile acids. The studies done on the cholesterol-lowering effect of these plant compounds have found that 2 to 5 grams of plant stanols/sterols per day reduces total blood cholesterol by 8%

Two approaches have been shown to cause reversal of atherosclerosis in the body. One employs a vegan diet and other lifestyle changes that are part of the Dr. Dean Ornish program. The other employs aggressive LDL lowering with medications.

Medicine Cabinet

Aspirin. Most common medication recommended to prevent heart attacks in people with coronary artery disease by helping to maintain blood flow to the heart.

Statins. Most frequently prescribed cholesterol-lowering drugs that block a liver enzyme involved in cholesterol synthesis and thus reduce the amount of cholesterol in the blood.

Examples:

- Atorvastatin (Lipitor®)
- Fluvastatin (Lescol, Lescol XL®)
- Lovastatin (Altoprev, Mevacor®)
- Pravastatin (Pravachol®)
- Simvastatin (Zocor®)
- Rosuvastatin (Crestor®)
- Simvastatin + ezetimibe (Vytorin®)

Bile acid sequestering agents (resins). These resins bind to bile acids in the intestine and are excreted in the feces, reducing their supply. This stimulates the liver to produce more bile acids, which uses more cholesterol and causes a decrease in blood cholesterol levels.

Examples:

- Cholestyramine (Questran®)
- Colestipol (Colestid®)
- Colesevelam (Welchol®)

◄ At the first sign of a possible heart attack, the person should call 911 and then thoroughly chew an aspirin. Aspirin in small doses reduces blood clotting. It is often used under a physician's guidance to treat people at risk for heart attack or stroke, especially if one has already occurred. About 80 to 160 milligrams per day is needed to experience benefits. Individuals who may especially benefit from aspirin therapy are men over 40, smokers, postmenopausal women, and people with diabetes, hypertension, or a family history of cardiovascular disease. © McGraw-Hill Education/Photo by Eric Misko, Elite Images Photography

medicine cabinet - pills: © Footage supplied by Goodshoot/Punchstock

▲ Dark chocolate has a high percentage of cocoa solids that contain phytonutrients called flavonols known to have antioxidant and anti-inflammatory properties. Eating dark chocolate has been found to decrease LDL cholesterol and increase HDL cholesterol. © Foodcollection

to 10% and LDL-cholesterol by 9% to 14% (similar to what is seen with some cholesterol-lowering drugs; see Further Reading 7).

In people who have borderline high total blood cholesterol (between 200 and 239 mg/dl), these plant compounds can be helpful in avoiding future drug therapy. Plant stanols/sterols have been made available in pill form as well. Remember that plant sterols are naturally present in nuts in high concentrations. Wheat germ, sesame seeds, pistachios, and sunflower seeds are some of the richest sources.

Surgical Treatment for Cardiovascular Disease

The two most common surgical treatments for coronary artery blockage are percutaneous transluminal coronary angioplasty (PTCA) and coronary artery bypass graft (CABG). PTCA involves the insertion of a balloon catheter into an artery. Once it is advanced to the area of the lesion, the balloon is expanded to crush the lesion. This method works best when only one vessel is blocked, and it may be held open with metal mesh, called a stent. CABG involves the removal and use of a saphenous vein (a large vein in the leg) or use of a mammary artery. The relocated vein is sewn to the main heart vessel (aorta) and then used to bypass the blocked artery. The procedure can be performed on one or more blockages.

For more information on cardiovascular disease, see the website of the American Heart Association at www.heart.org or the heart disease section of Healthfinder at healthfinder.gov. This is a site created by the U.S. government for consumers. In addition, visit the website www.nhlbi.nih.gov/.

Summary (Numbers refer to numbered sections in the chapter.)

5.1 Lipids are a group of compounds that do not dissolve in water. Fatty acids are the simplest form of lipid. There are three fatty acids on every triglyceride, the most common type of lipid found in the body and foods. Phospholipids and sterols are two other classes of lipids in food and our bodies.

5.2 Saturated fatty acids contain no carbon-carbon double bonds, monounsaturated fatty acids contain one carbon-carbon double bond, and polyunsaturated fatty acids contain two or more carbon-carbon double bonds in the carbon chain. In omega-3 polyunsaturated fatty acids, the first of the carbon-carbon double bonds is located three carbons from the methyl end of the carbon chain. In omega-6 polyunsaturated fatty acids, the first carbon-carbon double bond counting from the methyl end occurs at the sixth carbon. The essential fatty acids are linoleic acid (an omega-6 fatty acid) and alpha-linolenic acid (an omega-3 fatty acid). These must be included in the diet to maintain health. The hormonelike compounds produced from omega-3 fatty acids tend to reduce blood clotting, blood pressure, and inflammatory responses in the body. Those produced from omega-6 fatty acids tend to increase blood clotting.

Triglycerides are formed from a glycerol backbone with three fatty acids. Triglycerides rich in long-chain saturated fatty acids tend to be solid at room temperature, whereas those rich in monounsaturated and polyunsaturated fatty acids are liquid at room temperature. Triglycerides are the major form of fat in both food and the body. They allow for efficient energy storage, protect certain organs, transport fat-soluble vitamins, and help insulate the body.

5.3 Foods rich in fat include salad oils, butter, margarine, and mayonnaise. Nuts, bologna, avocados, and bacon are also high in fat, as are peanut butter and cheddar cheese. Steak and hamburger are moderate in fat content, as is whole milk. Many grain products and fruits and vegetables in general are low in fat.

Fats and oils have several functions as components of foods. Fats add flavor and texture to foods and provide some satiety after meals. Some phospholipids are used in foods as emulsifiers, which suspend fat in water.

When fatty acids break down, food becomes rancid, resulting in a foul odor and unpleasant flavor. Hydrogenation is the process of converting carbon-carbon double bonds into single bonds by adding hydrogen at the point of unsaturation. The partial hydrogenation of fatty acids in vegetable oils changes the oils to semisolid fats and helps in food formulation and reduces rancidity. Hydrogenation also increases *trans* fatty acid content. High amounts of *trans* fat in the diet are discouraged, as these increase LDL and reduce HDL.

5.4 Fat digestion takes place primarily in the small intestine. Lipase enzyme released from the pancreas digests long-chain triglycerides into monoglycerides (glycerol backbones with single fatty acids attached) and fatty acids. The breakdown products are then taken up by the absorptive cells of the small intestine. These products are mostly remade into triglycerides inside intestinal cells and eventually enter the lymphatic system, in turn passing into the bloodstream.

5.5 Lipids are carried in the bloodstream by various lipoproteins, which consist of a lipid core encased in a shell of protein, cholesterol, and phospholipid. Chylomicrons are released from intestinal cells and carry lipids arising from dietary intake. Very-low-density lipoprotein (VLDL) and low-density lipoprotein (LDL) carry lipids both taken up by and synthesized in the liver. High-density lipoprotein (HDL) picks up cholesterol from cells and facilitates its transport back to the liver.

5.6 Triglycerides are used for energy storage, insulation, and transportation of fat-soluble vitamins. Phospholipids are derivatives of triglycerides in which one or two of the fatty acids are replaced by phosphorus-containing compounds. Phospholipids are important parts of cell membranes, and some act as efficient emulsifiers.

Cholesterol forms vital biological compounds, such as hormones, components of cell membranes, and bile acids. Cells in the body make cholesterol whether we eat it or not. It is not a necessary part of an adult's diet.

5.7 There is currently no RDA for fat for adults. Plant oils should contribute at least 5% of total calories to achieve the Adequate Intakes proposed for essential fatty acids (linoleic acid and alpha-linolenic acid). Fatty fish are a rich source of omega-3 fatty acids and should be consumed at least twice a week.

Many health agencies and scientific groups suggest a fat intake of no more than 30% to 35% of total calories. Some health experts advocate an even further reduction to 20% of calorie intake for some people to maintain a normal LDL value, but such a diet requires professional guidance. Medications such as "statins" may be added also to lower LDL. If fat intake exceeds 30% of total calories, the diet should emphasize monounsaturated fat. The typical North American diet contains about 33% of total calories as fat.

5.8 In the blood, elevated amounts of LDL and low amounts of HDL are strong predictors of risk for cardiovascular disease. Additional risk factors for the disease are smoking, hypertension, diabetes, obesity, and inactivity.

Check Your Knowledge (Answers are available at the end of this question set.)

1. Margarine usually is made by a process called _____, in which hydrogen atoms are added to carbon-carbon double bonds in the polyunsaturated fatty acids found in vegetable oils.
   a. saturation
   b. esterification
   c. isomerization
   d. hydrogenation

2. Fatty acids that cause a decrease in blood clotting are
   a. omega-3 fatty acids.
   b. omega-6 fatty acids.
   c. omega-9 fatty acids.
   d. prostacyclins.

3. Cholesterol is
   a. a dietary essential; the human body cannot synthesize it.
   b. found in foods of plant origin.
   c. an important part of human cell membranes and necessary to make some hormones.
   d. all of the above.

4. Which of the following groups of foods would be important sources of saturated fatty acids?
   a. olive oil, peanut oil, canola oil
   b. palm oil, palm kernel oil, coconut oil
   c. safflower oil, corn oil, soybean oil
   d. all of the above

5. Lipoproteins are important for
   a. transport of fats in the blood and lymphatic system.
   b. synthesis of triglycerides.
   c. synthesis of adipose tissue.
   d. enzyme production.

6. Which of the following foods is the best source of omega-3 fatty acids?
   a. fatty fish
   b. peanut butter and jelly
   c. lard and shortenings
   d. beef and other red meats

7. Immediately after a meal, newly digested and absorbed dietary fats appear in the lymph and then the blood as part of which of the following?
   a. LDL
   b. HDL
   c. chylomicrons
   d. cholesterol

8. High blood concentrations of _____ decrease the risk for cardiovascular disease.
   a. low-density lipoproteins
   b. chylomicrons
   c. high-density lipoproteins
   d. cholesterol

9. Phospholipids such as lecithin are used extensively in food preparation because they
   a. provide the agreeable feel of fat melting on the tongue.
   b. are excellent emulsifiers.
   c. provide important textural features.
   d. impart delicate flavors.

10. The main form of lipid found in the food we eat is
    a. cholesterol.
    b. phospholipids.
    c. triglycerides.
    d. plant sterols.

Answer Key: 1. d (LO 5.3), 2. a (LO 5.2), 3. c (LO 5.6), 4. b (LO 5.3), 5. a (LO 5.5), 6. a (LO 5.3), 7. c (LO 5.5), 8. c (LO 5.5), 9. b (LO 5.6), 10. c (LO 5.2)

Study Questions (Numbers refer to Learning Outcomes)

1. Describe the chemical structures of saturated and polyunsaturated fatty acids and their different effects in both food and the human body. **(LO 5.2)**

2. Relate the need for omega-3 fatty acids in the diet to the recommendation to consume fatty fish at least twice a week. **(LO 5.7)**

3. Describe the structures, origins, and roles of the four major blood lipoproteins. **(LO 5.5)**

4. What are the recommendations from various health care organizations regarding fat intake? What does this mean in terms of food choices? **(LO 5.7)**

5. What are two important attributes of fat in food? How are these different from the general functions of lipids in the human body? **(LO 5.3)**

6. Describe the significance of and possible uses for reduced-fat foods. **(LO 5.6)**

7. Does the total cholesterol concentration in the bloodstream tell the whole story with respect to cardiovascular disease risk? **(LO 5.8)**

8. List the four main risk factors for the development of cardiovascular disease. **(LO 5.8)**

9. What three lifestyle factors decrease the risk of cardiovascular disease development? **(LO 5.8)**

10. When are medications most needed in cardiovascular disease therapy, and how in general do the various classes of medications operate to reduce risk? **(LO 5.8)**

What the Dietitian Chose

With heart health in mind, you will want to choose the ground meat with the lowest fat, saturated fat, and cholesterol. Check the Nutrition Facts panel, if available, to compare the lipid content of various products. Look for cuts of meat with "round " or "loin" in the name for lowest fat content.

USDA allows up to 30% fat (by weight) in raw ground beef, so the cut of beef makes a difference. Regular ground beef typically contains the most fat (about 20% to 30% fat). Next comes ground chuck (about 15% fat), followed by ground round (about 10% fat), and ground sirloin (about 3% fat). Table 5-9 shows a further breakdown of the fat content of varieties of ground beef. Based on this information, you can see that the ground sirloin will give you the leanest burgers.

The ground sirloin, however, will also be the most expensive variety of ground beef. You may, therefore, want to take advantage of the fact that ground beef loses a lot of fat during cooking—as much as 50% for the highest fat products. Typically, regular ground beef is the least expensive product. As the percent lean increases, so does price.

For foods in which the ground beef will be shaped, then cooked (e.g., hamburger patties, meatballs, or meatloaf), bake, grill, or broil the ground meat on a rack so that fat will drain from the product as it cooks, then let the cooked product rest on paper towels for 1 minute after cooking. For recipes that incorporate browned ground beef into a mixed dish (e.g., casseroles or spaghetti sauce), brown ground beef, crumbling as you cook, then blot with paper towels or rinse under warm water to achieve a final cooked product with nearly the same fat content

▲ Whereas the more expensive ground round and ground sirloin will give you lowest-fat burgers to start, the less expensive regular ground beef or ground chuck burgers will lose fat while cooking. You will therefore want to consider both fat content and cost when making your choice. © Comstock/PunchStock

as the ground round. Using the rinsing method, 100 grams (about 3.5 ounces) of ground beef yields a final product with just 4 grams of fat. Because a greater percentage of the starting product is lost during cooking, you will end up with less meat in the final product. However, this is not such a big deal because most Americans consume two to three times as much protein as they need. To further enhance the heart healthiness of mixed dishes, replace some of that lost product with beans. Chili or tacos would be excellent recipes to try with this method.

TABLE 5-9 ■ Calorie, Fat, and Cholesterol Content of Types of Ground Beef

	Energy (kcal)	Total Fat (g)	Saturated Fat (g)	Cholesterol (mg)
Regular ground beef, 3.5 ounces cooked	273	18	7	82
Ground chuck, 3.5 ounces cooked	232	14	5	86
Ground round, 3.5 ounces cooked	204	11	4	82
Ground sirloin, 3.5 ounces cooked	164	6	3	76

CASE STUDY SOLUTION Planning a Heart-Healthy Diet

1. Jackie's approach to lowering blood cholesterol does not incorporate the best choices. She has excluded a great deal of fat in her diet, perhaps more than necessary, and has failed to include some key food groups that have cholesterol-lowering components.

2. Lowering fat as drastically as she has is not really necessary, especially for a physically active 21-year-old female.

3. Jackie could allow a more liberal amount of fat in her diet by including more monounsaturated fats. Canola oil and olive oil, as well as fats found in nuts and avocados, are rich sources of monounsaturated fats. These fats do not increase blood cholesterol. In addition, she should include good sources of omega-3 fatty acids such as fatty fish, walnuts, flaxseeds, or soybean oil. One option is to use a canola oil-and-vinegar dressing on her salad, rather than lemon juice.

4. She has excluded a great deal of fat in her diet by merely replacing it with refined carbohydrates.

5. To make a shift to a more heart-healthy diet, Jackie would need to include at least 2 cups of fruit and 3 cups of vegetables a day, along with more whole-grain products. She should use whole-wheat bread instead of white bread for her sandwiches and eat a breakfast cereal that has at least 3 grams of fiber per serving.

6. Taking a brisk walk each morning is an excellent way to guarantee at least 30 minutes of activity on most days of the week. Exercise has been shown to increase concentration of HDL cholesterol in the blood and decrease risk of cardiovascular disease.

Further Readings

1. Consumers Union: Evaluating statin drugs to treat high cholesterol and heart disease: Comparing effectiveness, safety, and price. *Consumer Reports Health Best Buy Drugs.* Consumers Union of United States, Inc. 2012. http://www.consumerreports.org/health/resources/pdf/best-buy-drugs/StatinsUpdate-FINAL.pdf. Accessed March 10, 2013.

2. Eckel RH and others: 2013 AHA/ACC guideline on lifestyle management to reduce cardiovascular risk: A report of the American College of Cardiology/American Heart Association Task Force on Practice Guidelines. *Circulation* 129:S76, 2013.

3. Estruch R and others: Primary prevention of cardiovascular disease with a Mediterranean diet. *New England Journal of Medicine* 368:1279–1290, 2013.

4. Food and Drug Administration: Talking about *trans* fat: What you need to know. *Food Facts.* June 2015. http://www.fda.gov/downloads/Food/IngredientsPackagingLabeling/UCM239579.pdf. Accessed October 19, 2015.

5. Fox CS and others: Update on prevention of cardiovascular disease in adults with type 2 diabetes mellitus in light of recent evidence: A scientific statement from the American Heart Association and the American Diabetes Association. *Diabetes Care* 38:1777, 2015.

6. Kris-Etherton PM, Hill AM: omega-3 fatty acids: Food or supplements? *Journal of the American Dietetic Association* 108:1125, 2008.

7. Micallef MA, Garg ML: The lipid-lowering effects of phytosterols and (omega-3) polyunsaturated fatty acids are synergistic and complementary in hyperlipidemic men and women. *Journal of Nutrition* 138:1086, 2008.

8. Myers GL and others: National Academy of Clinical Biochemistry laboratory medicine practice guidelines: Emerging biomarkers for primary prevention of cardiovascular disease. *Clinical Chemistry* 55:378, 2009.

9. Palmer S: Fighting heart disease the Dean Ornish way. *Today's Dietitian* 2:48, 2009.

10. Palmer S: The Mediterranean diet: A practical guide to shopping, menu ideas, and recipes. *Today's Dietitian* 14(5):30, 2012.

11. Schaeffer J: Prevent heart disease: How to dispel the five common heart-health myths with clients and set the record straight. *Today's Dietitian* 15(2):20, 2013.

12. Shai I and others: Weight loss with a low-carbohydrate, Mediterranean, or low-fat diet. *New England Journal of Medicine* 359:229, 2008.

13. Vannice G and others: Position of the Academy of Nutrition and Dietetics: Dietary fatty acids for healthy adults. *Journal of the Academy of Nutrition and Dietetics* 114:136, 2014.

 To get the most out of your study of nutrition, go to McGraw-Hill's online resources: Connect www.mcgrawhillconnect.com, where you will find NutritionCalc Plus, LearnSmart, and many other dynamic tools.

Rate Your Plate

I. Choosing Foods for Heart Health

Instructions: The foods listed in column A tend to be high in saturated fat, *trans* fatty acids, cholesterol, and total fat. Fill in column B with alternative foods that are generally low in these dietary components. After filling in your ideas, see our suggestions for column B for foods that will reduce your risk of cardiovascular disease.

Column A		Column B
Bacon and eggs	or	
Doughnut or sweet roll	or	
Breakfast sausage	or	
Whole milk	or	
Cheeseburger	or	
French fries	or	
Ground chuck	or	
Soup with cream base	or	
Macaroni and cheese	or	
Cream/fruit pie	or	
Cream-filled cookies	or	
Ice cream	or	
Butter or stick margarine	or	

Ready-to-eat whole-grain breakfast cereal
Whole-wheat roll, bagel, or bread
Fruit
Reduced-fat, low-fat, or fat-free milk
Turkey sandwich, no cheese
Plain baked potato with salsa
Ground round
Soup with broth base
Macaroni with marinara sauce
Graham crackers
Granola bar
Frozen yogurt, sherbet, or reduced-fat ice cream
Vegetable oils or soft margarine in a tub

II. Applying the Nutrition Facts Label to Your Daily Food Choices

Imagine that you are at the supermarket looking for a quick snack to help you keep your energy up during afternoons. In the snack section, you settle on two choices [see labels (a) and (b)]. Evaluate the products using the accompanying table.

Compare the nutrients in each product by completing this list. For each serving, which product is lower in each of the following?

	(a)	(b)	no difference
Calories	(a)	(b)	no difference
Calories from Fat	(a)	(b)	no difference
Total Fat	(a)	(b)	no difference
Saturated Fat	(a)	(b)	no difference
Trans Fat	(a)	(b)	no difference
Cholesterol	(a)	(b)	no difference
Sodium	(a)	(b)	no difference
Total Carbohydrates	(a)	(b)	no difference
Dietary Fiber	(a)	(b)	no difference
Sugars	(a)	(b)	no difference
Protein	(a)	(b)	no difference
Iron	(a)	(b)	no difference

Which package has more servings per container?

        (a)   (b)   no difference

Nutrition Facts

6 servings per container

Serving size   **2 bars (42g)**

Amount per serving

Calories   **180**

	% Daily Value*
Total Fat 6g	9%
Saturated Fat 0.5g	3%
Trans Fat 0g	
Cholesterol 0mg	0%
Sodium 160mg	7%
Total Carbohydrate 29g	10%
Dietary Fiber 2g	8%
Total Sugars 11g	
Includes 8g Added Sugars	16%
Protein 4g	
Iron 1mg	6%
Potassium 100mg	3%

Not a significant source of vitamin D and calcium.

The % Daily Value (DV) tells you how much a nutrient in a serving of food contributes to a daily diet. 2,000 calories a day is used for general nutrition advice.

INGREDIENTS: WHOLE GRAIN ROLLED OATS, SUGAR, CANOLA OIL, CRISP RICE WITH SOY PROTEIN (RICE FLOUR, SOY PROTEIN CONCENTRATE, SUGAR, MALT, SALT), HONEY, BROWN SUGAR SYRUP, HIGH FRUCTOSE CORN SYRUP, SALT, SOY LECITHIN, BAKING SODA, NATURAL FLAVOR, PEANUT FLOUR, ALMOND FLOUR, HAZELNUT FLOUR, WALNUT FLOUR, PECAN FLOUR.

(a)

Nutrition Facts

12 servings per container

Serving size   **2 cookies (38g)**

Amount per serving

Calories   **180**

	% Daily Value*
Total Fat 7g	11%
Saturated Fat 2g	10%
Trans Fat 2g	
Cholesterol 0mg	0%
Sodium 100mg	4%
Total Carbohydrate 26g	9%
Dietary Fiber 1g	4%
Total Sugars 12g	4%
Includes 10g Added Sugars	20%
Protein 2g	
Iron 0.4mg	2%
Potassium 75mg	2%

Not a significant source of vitamin D and calcium.

The % Daily Value (DV) tells you how much a nutrient in a serving of food contributes to a daily diet. 2,000 calories a day is used for general nutrition advice.

INGREDIENTS: ENRICHED FLOUR (WHEAT FLOUR, NIACIN, REDUCED IRON, THIAMINE MONONITRATE, RIBOFLAVIN, FOLIC ACID), SUGAR, VEGETABLE OIL SHORTENING (PARTIALLY HYDROGENATED SOYBEAN, COCONUT, COTTONSEED, CORN AND/OR SAFFLOWER AND/OR CANOLA OIL), CORN SYRUP, HIGH FRUCTOSE CORN SYRUP, WHEY (A MILK INGREDIENT), CORN STARCH, SALT, SKIM MILK, LEAVENING (BAKING SODA, AMMONIUM BICARBONATE), ARTIFICIAL FLAVOR, SOYBEAN LECITHIN, COLOR (CONTAINING FD&C YELLOW #5 LAKE).

(b)

1. Which of the two brands would you choose?

_____

_____

2. What information on the Nutrition Facts labels contributed to your decision?

_____

_____

© Digital Vision/age fotostock

Student Learning Outcomes

Chapter 6 is designed to allow you to:

6.1 Distinguish between essential and nonessential amino acids and explain why adequate amounts of each of the essential amino acids are required for protein synthesis.

6.2 Describe how amino acids form proteins.

6.3 Identify food sources of protein, distinguish between high-quality and low-quality proteins, and describe the concept of complementary proteins.

6.4 Describe how protein is digested, absorbed, and metabolized in the body.

6.5 List the primary functions of protein in the body.

Chapter 6
Proteins

Consuming enough protein is vital for maintaining health. Proteins form important structures in the body, make up a key part of the blood, help regulate many body functions, and can fuel body cells.

North Americans generally eat more protein than is needed to maintain health. Our daily protein intake comes mostly from animal sources, such as meat, poultry, fish, eggs, milk, and cheese. In contrast, in the developing world, diets can be deficient in protein.

Diets that are mostly vegetarian still predominate in much of Asia and areas of Africa, and many North Americans practice some form of vegetarianism. North Americans are encouraged to consume a greater portion of their food, including protein, from plant sources. Over the years, plant sources of protein such as nuts, seeds, and legumes have been sidelined by meats. Some popular misconceptions have been that (1) nuts were only high-fat foods, and (2) beans were "the poor man's meat." Sources of plant proteins, however, offer a wealth of nutritional benefits—from lowering blood cholesterol to preventing certain forms of cancer.

We can benefit from eating more plant sources of proteins, but it takes some knowledge to get the right quantity and quality of protein at each meal to meet protein needs. This chapter takes a close look at protein, including the benefits of plant proteins in a diet. It will also examine the benefits and potential risks of vegetarian diets. Let's see why a detailed study of protein is worth your attention.

6.6 Apply current recommendations for protein intake to determine protein needs for healthy adults.

6.7 Describe the harmful effects of a high-protein diet and describe what is meant by positive protein balance, negative protein balance, and protein equilibrium.

6.8 Describe how protein-calorie malnutrition eventually can lead to disease in the body.

6.9 Develop vegetarian diet plans that meet the body's nutritional needs.

6.1 Amino Acids—Building Blocks of Proteins

protein Food and body compounds made of more than 100 amino acids; proteins contain carbon, hydrogen, oxygen, nitrogen, and sometimes other atoms in a specific configuration. Proteins contain the form of nitrogen most easily used by the human body.

amino acid The building block for proteins containing a central carbon atom with nitrogen and other atoms attached.

TABLE 6-1 ■ Classification of Amino Acids

Essential Amino Acids	Nonessential Amino Acids
Histidine	Alanine
Isoleucine*	Arginine
Leucine*	Asparagine
Lysine	Aspartic acid
Methionine	Cysteine
Phenylalanine	Glutamic acid
Threonine	Glutamine
Tryptophan	Glycine
Valine*	Proline
	Serine
	Tyrosine

*A branched-chain amino acid.

branched-chain amino acids Amino acids with a branching carbon backbone; these are leucine, isoleucine, and valine. All are essential amino acids.

nonessential amino acids Amino acids that can be synthesized by a healthy body in sufficient amounts; there are 11 nonessential amino acids. These are also called *dispensable amino acids.*

People in the developed parts of the world, such as the United States and Canada, typically eat enough **protein.** In the developing world, however, it is important to focus on protein in diet planning because dietary patterns in those areas of the world can be deficient in protein.

Thousands of substances in the body are made of proteins. Aside from water, proteins form the major part of lean body tissue, totaling about 17% of body weight. **Amino acids** are compounds that serve as the building blocks for proteins. They are chemically unique in that they contain nitrogen along with carbon, oxygen, and hydrogen. Plants combine nitrogen from the soil with carbon and other elements to form amino acids. They then link these amino acids together to make proteins. Proteins are thus an essential part of a dietary pattern because they supply nitrogen in a form we can readily use, namely, amino acids. Using simpler forms of nitrogen is, for the most part, impossible for humans.

Proteins are crucial to the *regulation* and *maintenance* of the body. Body functions such as blood clotting, fluid balance, hormone and enzyme production, visual processes, transport of many substances in the bloodstream, and cell repair require specific proteins. The body makes proteins in many configurations and sizes so that they can serve these greatly varied functions. Formation of these body proteins begins with amino acids from both the protein-containing foods we eat and those synthesized from other compounds within the body. Proteins can also be broken down to *supply energy* for the body—on average, 4 kcal per gram.

If you fail to consume an adequate amount of protein for weeks at a time, many metabolic processes slow down. This is because the body does not have enough amino acids available to build the proteins it needs. For example, the immune system no longer functions efficiently when it lacks key proteins, thereby increasing the risk of infections, disease, and death.

Amino acids are formed mostly of carbon, hydrogen, oxygen, and nitrogen. Figure 6-1 shows the structure of a generic amino acid and two examples of specific amino acids. The amino acids are slight variations of the generic amino acid pictured but all have different chemical makeups (see Appendix D). Each amino acid has an "acid" group, an "amino" group, and a "side" or R group specific to the amino acid.

The R group on some amino acids has a branched shape, like a tree. These so-called **branched-chain amino acids** are leucine, isoleucine, and valine. The branched-chain amino acids are the primary amino acids used by muscles for energy needs. Whey protein (from milk) is popular among strength-training athletes because it is particularly rich in branched-chain amino acids (see Section 14.4).

Your body uses 20 different amino acids to function (Table 6-1). Although all these commonly found amino acids are important, 11 (alanine, arginine, asparagine, aspartic acid, cysteine, glutamic acid, glutamine, glycine, proline, serine, and tyrosine) are considered **nonessential** with respect to our diets. All tissues have some ability for synthesis of the nonessential amino acids as long as the right ingredients are present—the key factor being

FIGURE 6-1 ▲ Amino acid structure. The side chain (R) differentiates glycine (H) and alanine (CH₃).

nitrogen that is already part of another amino acid. Therefore, it is not essential that these amino acids be consumed.

ESSENTIAL AMINO ACIDS

The nine amino acids (histidine, isoleucine, leucine, lysine, methionine, phenylalanine, threonine, tryptophan, and valine) the body cannot make in sufficient amounts or at all are known as **essential.** The essential amino acids must be obtained from foods, because body cells cannot make the needed carbon-based foundation of the amino acid, cannot put a nitrogen group on the needed carbon-based foundation, or just cannot do the whole process fast enough to meet body needs. If you do not eat enough essential amino acids, your body first struggles to conserve what essential amino acids it can. However, eventually your body slows production of new proteins until at some point, you will break protein down faster than you can make it. When that happens, health deteriorates.

Animal sources of protein, such as meat and dairy products, and plant sources of protein, such as soy, can supply us with an adequate amount of both the essential and nonessential amino-acid building blocks needed to maintain good health. Both nonessential and essential amino acids are present in foods that contain protein.

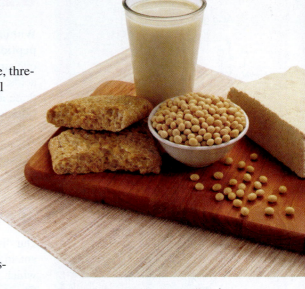

▲ Soy products such as soy milk, tofu, soy bread, and soybeans themselves provide a plant source of all the essential amino acids.
© Mitch Hrdlicka/Getty Images

The essential amino acid in smallest supply in a food or meal in relation to body needs becomes the limiting factor (called the **limiting amino acid**) because it limits the amount of protein the body can synthesize. Fortunately, adults need only about 11% of their total protein requirement to be supplied by essential amino acids. Typically, 50% of the amino acids in dietary proteins are essential.

The estimated requirements for essential amino acids for infants and preschool children are greater (40% of total protein intake) because of the needs of rapid growth and development; however, in later childhood, the need drops to 20%. Dietary plans designed for infants and young children need to take this into account to make sure enough high-quality proteins are present. Providing animal products, such as human milk or cow's milk-based formula for infants, or cow's milk for children, helps ensure this. A major health risk for infants and children occurs in famine situations in which only one type of cereal grain, such as rice, is available, increasing the probability that one or more of the nine essential amino acids are lacking in the total diet. This is discussed further in Section 6.8 on protein-calorie malnutrition (PCM).

essential amino acids The amino acids that cannot be synthesized by humans in sufficient amounts or at all and therefore must be included in the diet; there are nine essential amino acids. These are also called *indispensable amino acids.*

limiting amino acid The essential amino acid in lowest concentration in a food or diet relative to body needs.

conditionally essential amino acids Amino acids that must be made from essential amino acids if insufficient amounts are eaten.

Conditionally Essential Amino Acids Some of the nonessential amino acids, which are usually synthesized in the body, can become essential during times of rapid growth, disease, or metabolic stress. For example, patients recovering from surgery or burns have very high needs for amino acids to heal their injuries, so the activity of enzymes that synthesize nonessential amino acids cannot keep up with demands. Arginine and glutamine are two examples of **conditionally essential amino acids.**

The disease phenylketonuria (PKU) illustrates how a nonessential amino acid can become conditionally essential as a result of a genetic disease. A person with PKU has a limited ability to metabolize the essential amino acid phenylalanine. Normally, the body uses an enzyme to convert much of our dietary phenylalanine intake into tyrosine. In PKU-diagnosed persons, the activity of the enzyme used in processing phenylalanine to tyrosine is insufficient. The results are that (1) tyrosine becomes essential (it must be obtained from the diet); whereas (2) phenylalanine builds up to toxic levels in the blood. Elevated phenylalanine disrupts brain function, leading to mental retardation. PKU is treated with a special diet that limits phenylalanine.

▲ Within the first few days of life, all newborns are tested for phenylketonuria.
© Corbis/PictureQuest

✓ CONCEPT CHECK 6.1

1. What is the basic structure of an amino acid?
2. What is the difference between the essential and nonessestial amino acids?

FIGURE 6-2 ▲ Peptide bonds link amino acids. The synthesis of a peptide bond is a dehydration reaction in which a molecule of water is removed. When peptide bonds are broken (as in digestion), a molecule is added (hydrolysis).

peptide bond A chemical bond formed between amino acids in a protein.

▲ Genes are present on DNA—a double-stranded helix. The cell nucleus contains most of the DNA in the body. DNA can be compared to a "cookbook" that contains the "recipes" (genes) for the synthesis of all proteins that cells need to make. Because the cookbook cannot leave the nucleus to get to the "cooks" (the ribosomes), the recipes for proteins must be transcribed into a form (mRNA) that can leave the nucleus. The amino acids that form a protein can be equated to the "ingredients" required for the recipe.© Andrey Prokhorov/Getty Images

6.2 Protein Synthesis and Organization

Within body cells, amino acids are linked together by chemical bonds—technically called **peptide bonds**—to form proteins (Fig. 6-2). Peptide bonds form between the amino group of one amino acid and the acid (carboxyl) group of another. Through peptide bonding of amino acids, cells can synthesize dipeptides (joining of two amino acids), tripeptides (joining of three amino acids), oligopeptides (joining of four to nine amino acids), and **polypeptides** (joining of 10 or more amino acids). Most proteins are polypeptides ranging from about 50 to 2000 amino acids. These bonds are difficult to break, but heat, acids, enzymes, and other agents are able to do so during cooking and chemical digestion.

The body can synthesize many different proteins by linking together the 20 common types of amino acids with peptide bonds.

PROTEIN SYNTHESIS

Our discussion of protein synthesis begins with deoxyribonucleic acid (DNA). DNA is present in the nucleus of the cell and contains coded instructions for protein synthesis (i.e., which specific amino acids are to be placed in a protein and in which order). Recall from Chapter 3 that DNA is a double-stranded molecule.

Protein synthesis in a cell, however, takes place in the cytoplasm, not in the nucleus. Thus, the DNA code used for synthesis of a specific protein must be transferred from the nucleus to the cytoplasm to allow for protein synthesis. This transfer is the job of messenger RNA (mRNA). Enzymes in the nucleus first read the code (a gene) on a DNA base sequence that encodes one or more proteins and then *transcribe* that information into a single-stranded mRNA molecule (Fig. 6-3) that is ready to leave the nucleus.

Once in the cytoplasm, mRNA travels to the ribosomes. The ribosomes read the mRNA code and *translate* those instructions to produce a specific protein. Amino acids are added one at a time to the growing polypeptide chain according to the instructions on the mRNA. Another key participant in protein synthesis, transfer RNA (tRNA), is responsible for bringing the specific amino acids to the ribosomes as needed during protein synthesis (review Fig. 6-3). Energy input is required to add each amino acid to the chain, making protein synthesis "costly" in terms of calorie use.

Once synthesis of a polypeptide is complete, it twists and folds into the appropriate three-dimensional shape of the intended protein. These structural changes occur based on specific interactions among the amino acids on the polypeptide chain. Some polypeptides, such as the hormone insulin, also undergo further changes in the cell before they are functional.

PROTEIN ORGANIZATION

Through the bonding together of the 20 common types of amino acids into various combinations, the body synthesizes thousands of different proteins. The sequential order of the amino acids then ultimately determines the protein's shape. An important point is that only correctly positioned amino acids can interact and fold properly to form the intended shape for the protein. The resulting unique, three-dimensional form, such as that shown for the protein hemoglobin in Figure 6-4, goes on to dictate the function of each particular protein. If it lacks the proper structure, a protein cannot function.

The relationship between DNA and the proteins eventually produced by a cell is very important. If the DNA code contains errors, an incorrect mRNA will be produced. The ribosomes will then read this incorrect message and an incorrect amino acid will be added and an incorrect polypeptide chain will be produced. Genetic engineering may ultimately be able to correct many gene defects in humans by placing the correct DNA code in the nucleus, so that the correct protein can be made by the ribosomes.

Sickle cell disease (also called **sickle cell anemia**) is one example of what happens when amino acids are out of order on a protein (Fig. 6-5). In North America, people of African descent are especially prone to this genetic disease. Sickle cell anemia is not a nutritional

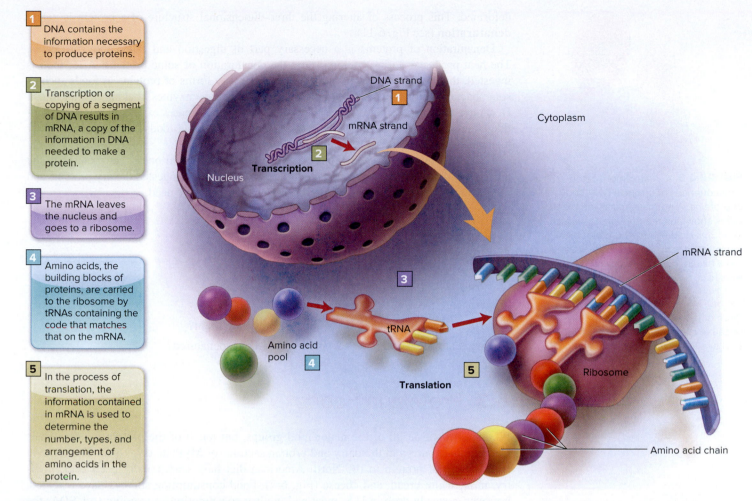

1. DNA contains the information necessary to produce proteins.

2. Transcription or copying of a segment of DNA results in mRNA, a copy of the information in DNA needed to make a protein.

3. The mRNA leaves the nucleus and goes to a ribosome.

4. Amino acids, the building blocks of proteins, are carried to the ribosome by tRNAs containing the code that matches that on the mRNA.

5. In the process of translation, the information contained in mRNA is used to determine the number, types, and arrangement of amino acids in the protein.

DNA strand

mRNA strand

Cytoplasm

Nucleus

Transcription

tRNA

Amino acid pool

Translation

mRNA strand

Ribosome

Amino acid chain

FIGURE 6-3 ▲ Protein synthesis (simplified). Once the mRNA is fully read, the amino acids have been connected into the polypeptide, which is released into the cytoplasm. It generally is then processed further to become a functioning cell protein.

polypeptide A group of 10 to 2000 or more amino acids bonded together to form proteins.

sickle cell disease (sickle cell anemia) An illness that results from a malformation of the red blood cell because of an incorrect structure in part of its hemoglobin protein chains.

disease but is caused by a mutation in the genetic code for hemoglobin, the protein depicted in Figure 6-4 that carries oxygen in red blood cells. The mutation causes the amino acid glutamic acid to be replaced with the amino acid valine. This error produces a profound change in hemoglobin structure. It can no longer form the shape needed to carry oxygen efficiently inside the red blood cell. Instead of forming normal circular disks, the red blood cells collapse into crescent (or sickle) shapes (see Fig. 6-5). Sickle red blood cells become hard and sticky, which causes them to clog blood flow and break apart. This can cause severe bone and joint pain, abdominal pain, headache, convulsions, paralysis, and even death due to the lack of oxygen.

These life-threatening symptoms are caused by a minute, but critical, error in amino-acid order. Why does this error happen? It results from a defect in a person's genetic blueprint, DNA, inherited from one's parents. A defect in the DNA can dictate that a wrong amino acid will be built into the sequence of the body proteins. Many diseases, including cancer, stem from errors in the DNA code.

DENATURATION OF PROTEINS

Changing the shape of a protein often destroys its ability to function normally, such that it loses its biological activity. Exposure to acid or alkaline substances, heat, or agitation (e.g., whipping egg whites) can alter a protein's structure, leaving it uncoiled or otherwise

FIGURE 6-4 ▲ Protein organization. Proteins often form a coiled shape, as shown by this drawing of the blood protein hemoglobin. This shape is dictated by the order of the amino acids in the protein chain. To get an idea of its size, consider that each teaspoon (5 milliliters) of blood contains about 10^{18} hemoglobin molecules. (One billion is 10^{9}.)

FIGURE 6-5 ▲ An example of the consequences of errors in DNA coding of proteins. A normal circular red blood cell is shown on the right along with an abnormal sickle-shaped red blood cell on the left. CDC/Sickle Cell Foundation of Georgia: Jackie George, Beverly Sinclair/photo by Janice Haney Carr

denaturation Alteration of a protein's three-dimensional structure, usually because of treatment by heat, enzymes, acid or alkaline solutions, or agitation.

deformed. This process of altering the three-dimensional structure of a protein is called **denaturation** (see Fig. 6-11).

Denaturation of proteins is a necessary part of digestion and other body processes. The heat produced during cooking starts the denaturation of some proteins. After food is ingested, the secretion of stomach acid denatures many forms of proteins in foods such as some bacterial proteins, plant hormones, and many active enzymes, making it safer to eat. Denaturation enhances digestion because the unraveling increases exposure of the polypeptide chain to digestive enzymes. Denaturing proteins in some foods can also reduce their tendencies to cause allergic reactions.

Recognize that we need the amino acids. especially essential ones, that proteins in the diet supply—not the intact proteins themselves. We dismantle ingested dietary proteins and use the amino-acid building blocks to assemble the proteins we need.

✓ **CONCEPT CHECK 6.2**

1. What is the role of DNA in protein synthesis?
2. What are the steps of protein synthesis?
3. Why is the amino-acid order within a protein important?
4. What are some of the ways a protein can become denatured?

6.3 Protein in Foods

Protein is found in all of the major food groups, but much of the protein we eat comes from animal sources in the dairy and protein sections of MyPlate (Fig. 6-6). The top five contributors of protein to the North American diet have traditionally been beef, poultry, milk, white bread, and cheese (Fig. 6-7). Food consumption surveys have revealed, however, a steady drop in U.S. meat and poultry consumption. According to USDA, the average American consumed 202 pounds of red meat and poultry in 2014, 8% less than in 2004. This decrease was primarily related to a sharp drop in beef consumption. In 2014, the U.S. beef consumption per person of 54.2 pounds, was down 18% from 10 years ago and down about 30% from 1980. The downward trend seems to be a result of the rising cost of beef as well as conscious decisions to eat less red meat for health, environmental, and social reasons.

While the consumption of animal products has declined in the United States, world meat and dairy consumption doubled between 1950 and 2009, and is set to increase by an additional factor of four over the next 40 years (see Further Reading 7). It is particularly interesting that the demand for meat, eggs, and dairy products has increased in developing nations at a dramatic rate. The United Nations Food and Agriculture Organization (FAO) reports that in developing countries, milk consumption per person has almost doubled between 1980 and 2005, meat consumption more than tripled, and egg consumption increased fivefold. The greatest increases in consumption are occurring in East and Southeast Asia. For example, China's dairy production and consumption has soared, averaging a 12.8% increase annually since 2000, while per capita meat consumption has quadrupled since 1980. India has also boosted its milk production and consumption and is now the largest milk producer in the world. Overall, these increases in demand and consumption have had a substantial impact on agriculture, because of the significant increase (23%) in the farm animal population over the past three decades. The "factory farms" that have developed have a significant environmental impact because of the large amount of land and water used, and the high level of waste produced. These negative effects are in addition to the adverse health implications of consuming a diet high in animal products (see Further Reading 8). It is predicted that the increasing intake of meat and dairy will have profound impacts on our agricultural and ecological resources, and our ability to provide

▲ This grilled chicken (protein) sandwich with lettuce and tomato (vegetables) on foccacia bread (grains) completes three sections of MyPlate. Which sections are missing?© Ingram Publishing/SuperStock

MyPlate: Sources of Protein

Grains	Vegetables	Fruits	Dairy	Protein
• Bread • Breakfast cereals • Rice • Noodles	• Carrots • Corn • Broccoli	• Apples • Oranges • Bananas	• Milk • Yogurt • Cheese	• Meat • Eggs • Fish • Dry beans • Nuts
2–3 grams per serving	2–3 grams per serving	<1 gram per serving	8–10 grams per serving	7 grams per serving

FIGURE 6-6 ▲ Sources of protein from MyPlate. The fill of the background color (none, 1/3, 2/3, or completely covered) within each group on the plate indicates the average nutrient density for protein in that group. Overall, the dairy group and the protein group contain many foods that are nutrient-dense sources of protein. Based on serving sizes listed for MyPlate, the fruits group provides little or no protein (less than 1 gram per serving). Food choices from the vegetables group and grains group provide moderate amounts of protein (2 to 3 grams per serving). The dairy group provides much protein (8 to 10 grams per serving), as does the protein group (7 grams per serving). © IT Stock/PunchStock; © Pixtal/AGE Fotostock; © IT Stock/PunchStock

food in the future. Because the Mediterranean diet is recognized as being low in meat, rich in fresh fruit and vegetables, and low in added sugar and saturated fatty acids, it is recommended as a sustainable alternative dietary pattern. It has been advocated by the FAO and could be a starting point for discussing the creation of policies to support sustainable food production (see Further Reading 2).

PROTEIN QUALITY OF FOODS

Animal and plant proteins can differ greatly in their proportions of essential and nonessential amino acids. Animal proteins contain ample amounts of all nine essential amino acids. (Gelatin—made from the animal protein collagen—is an exception because it is low in essential amino acids.) With the exceptions of soy protein and quinoa seed, plant proteins do not match our need for essential amino acids as precisely as animal proteins. Many plant proteins, especially those found in grains, are low in one or more of the nine essential amino acids.

As you might expect, humans are able to use proteins from any single animal source more efficiently to support growth and maintenance than from any single plant source.

▲ Small amounts of animal protein in a meal easily add up to meet daily protein needs when mixed with grains and vegetables.© Creatas/PunchStock

FIGURE 6-7 ▶ Food sources of protein compared to the RDA of 56 grams for a 70-kilogram man.

Food Sources of Protein

Food Item and Amount	Protein (grams)	% RDA
RDA	56*	100%
Canned tuna, 3 ounces	21.6	38.6%
Broiled chicken, 3 ounces	21.3	38%
Roast beef, 3 ounces	15.3	27%
Yogurt, 1 cup	10.6	19%
Kidney beans, ½ cup	8.1	14.5%
1% low-fat milk, 1 cup	8.0	14%
Peanuts, 1 ounce	7.3	13%
Cheddar cheese, 1 ounce	7.0	12.5%
Egg, 1	5.5	10%
Cooked corn, ½ cup	2.7	5%
Seven-grain bread, 1 slice	2.6	4.6%
White rice, ½ cup	2.1	4%
Pasta, 1 ounce	1.2	2%
Banana, 1	1.2	2%

* for 70 kilogram man

Key:
- Grains
- Vegetables
- Fruits
- Dairy
- Protein

high-quality (complete) proteins Dietary proteins that contain ample amounts of all nine essential amino acids.

lower quality (incomplete) proteins Dietary proteins that are low in or lack one or more essential amino acids.

complementary proteins Two food protein sources that make up for each other's inadequate supply of specific essential amino acids; together, they yield a sufficient amount of all nine and so provide high-quality (complete) protein for the diet.

For this reason, animal proteins (except gelatin) are considered **high-quality (also called complete) proteins,** which contain sufficient amounts of the nine essential amino acids. Individual plant sources of proteins (except for soy beans and quinoa seed) are considered **lower quality (also called incomplete) proteins** because their amino-acid patterns can be quite different from ours. Thus, a single plant protein source, such as corn alone, cannot easily support body growth and maintenance. To obtain a sufficient amount of essential amino acids, a variety of plant proteins needs to be consumed because each plant protein lacks adequate amounts of one or more essential amino acids.

When only lower quality protein foods are consumed, an adequate amount of the essential amino acids needed for protein synthesis may not be obtained. Therefore, a greater amount of lower quality protein is needed to meet the demands of protein synthesis, compared to high-quality proteins. Once any of the nine essential amino acids in the plant protein we have eaten is used up, further protein synthesis becomes impossible. Because the depletion of just one of the essential amino acids prevents protein synthesis, the process illustrates the *all-or-none principle:* either all essential amino acids are available, or none can be used. The remaining amino acids would then be used for energy needs or converted into carbohydrate or fat.

When two or more protein sources are combined to compensate for deficiencies in their essential amino-acid contents, the proteins are called **complementary proteins.** Meals with a variety of high-quality protein sources generally result in a complementary protein pattern. Many legumes, for example, are deficient in the essential amino acid methionine, whereas grains are limited in lysine. Eating a combination of legumes and grains, such as beans and rice, will supply the body with adequate amounts of all essential amino acids (Fig. 6-8). Likewise vegetables, which are limited in methionine, can be combined with nuts, which are limited in lysine. With these combinations, healthy adults should have little concern about obtaining enough of all nine essential amino acids. Even when following a plant-based dietary pattern, complementary proteins need not be consumed at the same meal. Meeting amino-acid needs over the course of a day is a reasonable goal because there is a ready supply of amino acids present in body cells and in the blood (see Fig. 6-14).

In general, many North Americans should consume a higher proportion of plant sources of protein than they currently do. Plant foods contribute fewer calories than most animal products, but supply an ample amount of protein (Fig. 6-9). Vegetable sources of proteins, especially legumes and nuts, are a heart-healthy alternative to animal proteins because they contain very little saturated fat, aside from that added during processing or cooking.

A CLOSER LOOK AT PLANT SOURCES OF PROTEINS

Per gram of protein, plant foods provide more magnesium, fiber, folate, vitamin E, iron (absorption is increased by the vitamin C also present), zinc, and some calcium than animal sources of protein. Also, phytochemicals from these foods are implicated in prevention of a wide variety of chronic diseases.

Legumes are a plant family with pods that contain a single row of seeds. Examples include garden and black-eyed peas, kidney beans, great northern beans, lentils, soy beans, and peanuts. Dried varieties of the mature legume seeds—what we know as beans—also make an impressive contribution to the protein, vitamin, mineral, and fiber content of a meal. A ½-cup serving of legumes provides 100 to 150 kcal, 5 to 10 grams of protein, less than 1 gram of fat, and about 5 grams of fiber. Recall from Chapter 4 that consumption of beans can lead to intestinal gas because our bodies lack the enzymes to break down certain carbohydrates in beans. Gas production can be decreased by soaking dry beans in water to leach the indigestible carbohydrates into the water, which then can be disposed.

Nuts and seeds are also excellent sources of plant protein. Commonly consumed nuts include almonds, pistachios, walnuts, and pecans. The defining characteristic of a nut is that it grows on a tree. Remember that peanuts, because they grow underground, are legumes. Seeds, including pumpkin, sesame, and sunflower seeds, are similar to nuts in nutrient composition. A 1-ounce serving of nuts or seeds generally supplies 160 to 190 kcal, 6 to 10 grams of protein, and 14 to 19 grams of fat. Although they are a dense source of calories, nuts and seeds make a powerful contribution to health when consumed in moderation.

In summary, plant proteins are a nutritious alternative to animal proteins. They are inexpensive, versatile, tasty, a colorful addition to your plate, and beneficial to health beyond their contribution of protein to the diet. Learning to substitute plant proteins in place of less healthy foods is one way to reduce your risk for many diseases. The impact of plant proteins on health will be discussed in Section 6.9.

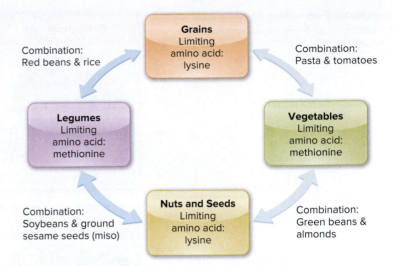

FIGURE 6-8 ▲ Plant group combinations in which the proteins complement each other in a meal based on their limiting amino acids.

FIGURE 6-9 ▲ Legumes are rich sources of protein. These kidney beans provide a significant amount of protein per serving: 7 grams per 1/2 cup.
© McGraw-Hill Education/Mark Dierker, photographer

FOOD PROTEIN ALLERGIES

Allergies occur when the immune system reacts to what it thinks is a foreign protein. In the case of food allergies, the immune system mistakes a food protein for a harmful invader. For some of us, food allergies to soy, peanuts and tree nuts (e.g., almonds and walnuts), and wheat are a concern. Overall, food allergies occur in up to 8% of children 4 years of age or younger and in up to 2% of adults. Eight foods account for 90% of food-related allergies (soy, peanuts, tree nuts, wheat, milk, eggs, fish, and shellfish; Fig. 6-10). The allergic reactions

FIGURE 6-10 ▶ Most common food allergens. (all) Photos courtesy of Dennis Gottlieb

FIGURE 6-10 ▶ Most common food allergens. (all) Photos courtesy of Dennis Gottlieb

Peanut/tree nuts | Milk products | Soy | Wheat | Eggs | Fish/shellfish

can range from a mild intolerance to fatal allergic reactions. Introducing allergenic foods such as peanut butter and eggs to infants as young as 4 to 6 months old is a new approach to combating food allergies that will be discussed further in Section 19.7.

✓ CONCEPT CHECK 6.3

1. What types of foods contain high-quality proteins?
2. Why are complementary proteins important when pairing plant food sources?

pepsin A protein-digesting enzyme produced by the stomach.

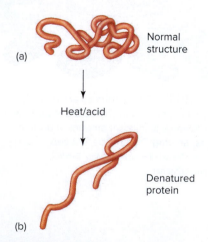

(a) Normal structure

Heat/acid

(b) Denatured protein

FIGURE 6-11 ▲ Denaturation. (a) Protein showing typical coiled state. (b) Protein is partly uncoiled by heat or acid. This uncoiling can reduce biological activity and allow digestive enzymes to act on peptide bonds.

6.4 Protein Digestion and Absorption

As with carbohydrate digestion, protein digestion begins with the cooking of food. Cooking unfolds (denatures) proteins (Fig. 6-11) and softens tough connective tissue in meat. Cooking also makes many protein-rich foods easier to chew and swallow, and facilitates their breakdown during later digestion and absorption. Cooking also makes many protein-rich foods, such as meats, eggs, fish, and poultry, much safer to eat.

DIGESTION

The enzymatic digestion of protein begins in the stomach (Fig. 6-12). Proteins are first denatured by stomach acid. **Pepsin,** a major stomach enzyme for digesting proteins, then goes to work on the unraveled polypeptide chains. Pepsin only breaks the polypeptide into shorter chains of amino acids because it can break only a few of the many peptide bonds found in these large molecules. The release of pepsin is controlled by the hormone gastrin. Thinking about food or chewing food stimulates gastrin release in the stomach. Gastrin then stimulates the stomach to release pepsin and produce acid.

FIGURE 6-12 ▶ A summary of protein digestion and absorption. Enzymatic protein digestion begins in the stomach and ends in the absorptive cells of the small intestine, where any remaining short groupings of amino acids are broken down into single amino acids. Stomach acid and enzymes contribute to protein digestion. Absorption from the intestinal lumen into the absorptive cells requires energy input.

Protein Digestion and Absorption

1 Partial protein digestion by the enzyme pepsin and stomach acid.

2 Pancreas releases enzymes that will further digest polypeptides in the small intestine.

3 Final digestion of peptides into single amino acids takes place mostly inside cells of the small intestine. Once in the small intestine, the partially digested proteins (and fats) trigger the release of the hormone cholecystokinin (CCK) from the walls of the small intestine. CCK causes the pancreas to release protein-splitting enzymes, such as trypsin.

4 Amino acids absorbed into the portal vein and transported to the liver. From there, they enter the general bloodstream.

5 Little dietary protein is present in feces.

4 Liver
1 Stomach
2 Pancreas
3 Small intestine
5 Anus

The partially digested proteins move from the stomach into the small intestine along with the rest of the nutrients and other substances in a meal (chyme). Once in the small intestine, the partially digested proteins (and any fats accompanying them) trigger the release of the hormone cholecystokinin (CCK) from the walls of the small intestine. CCK, in turn, travels through the bloodstream to the pancreas where it causes the pancreas to release protein-splitting enzymes, such as **trypsin.** These digestive enzymes further divide the chains of amino acids into segments of two to three amino acids and some individual amino acids. Eventually, this mixture is digested into amino acids, using other enzymes from the lining of the small intestine and enzymes present in the absorptive cells themselves.

trypsin A protein-digesting enzyme secreted by the pancreas to act in the small intestine.

ABSORPTION

The short chains of amino acids and any individual amino acids in the small intestine are taken up by active transport into the absorptive cells lining the small intestine. Any remaining peptide bonds are broken inside intestinal cells to yield individual amino acids. They are water soluble, so the amino acids travel to the liver via the portal vein, which drains absorbed nutrients from the intestinal tract (see Fig. 6-12). In the liver, individual amino acids can undergo several modifications, depending on the needs of various body tissues. Individual amino acids may be (1) combined into the proteins needed by specific cells; (2) broken down for energy needs; (3) released into the bloodstream; or (4) converted into

Gluten Sensitivity

Recall from the discussion of celiac disease and the gluten-free diet in Chapter 3 that gluten is a type of protein found in wheat, rye, and barley. Small peptides that arise from partial gluten digestion can be absorbed into the cells lining the small intestine and cause an inflammatory reaction in people with a genetic predisposition for celiac disease. Celiac disease is not a food allergy, but an autoimmune response. Strict dietary avoidance of food products containing wheat, rye, and barley is the only proven way to manage the disease. (See Further Reading 3. You will learn more about food allergies in Section 19.7.)

nonessential amino acids, glucose, or fat. With excess protein intake, amino acids are converted into fat as a last resort.

Except during infancy, it is uncommon for intact proteins to be absorbed from the digestive tract. In infants up to 4 to 5 months of age, the gastrointestinal tract is somewhat permeable to small proteins, so some whole proteins can be absorbed. Because proteins from some foods (e.g., cow's milk and egg whites) may predispose an infant to food allergies, experts recommend waiting until an infant reaches 4 to 6 months of age to introduce solid foods (see Further Reading 5 and Chapter 19 for details).

✓ **CONCEPT CHECK 6.4**

1. Where and how does protein digestion begin?
2. What digestion steps take place in the stomach and small intestine?
3. What are the final products of protein digestion, and where do they go after absorption?

6.5 Putting Proteins to Work in the Body

Proteins function in many crucial ways in human metabolism and in the formation of body structures (see Protein Concept Map). We rely on foods to supply the amino acids needed to form these proteins; however, only when we also eat enough carbohydrate and fat can food proteins be used most efficiently. If we do not consume enough calories to meet needs, proteins are broken down to supply energy to cells. This renders the amino acids unavailable for growth and repair of body tissues.

protein turnover The process by which cells break down old proteins and resynthesize new proteins. In this way, the cell will have the proteins it needs to function at that time.

PRODUCING VITAL BODY STRUCTURES

The amino-acid pool in a cell can be used to form body proteins, as well as a variety of other possible compounds. Every cell contains protein. Muscles, connective tissue, mucus, blood-clotting factors, transport proteins in the bloodstream, lipoproteins, enzymes, immune antibodies, some hormones, visual pigments, and the support structure inside bones are made of protein. Excess protein in the diet does not enhance the synthesis of these body components, but eating too little protein can prevent it.

Most vital body proteins are in a constant state of breakdown, rebuilding, and repair. For example, the cells of the intestinal tract lining are constantly sloughed off. The digestive tract treats sloughed cells just like food particles, digesting them and absorbing their amino acids. In fact, most of the amino acids released throughout the body can be recycled to become part of the pool of amino acids available for the synthesis of future proteins. Overall, **protein turnover** is a process by which a cell can respond to its changing environment by making proteins that are needed and disassembling proteins that are not needed.

During any day, an adult makes and degrades about 250 grams of protein, recycling many of the amino acids. Relative to the 65 to 100 grams of protein typically consumed by adults in North America, recycled amino acids make an important contribution to total protein metabolism.

If a person's diet is low in protein for a long period, the processes of rebuilding and repairing body proteins will slow down. Over time, skeletal muscles, blood proteins, and vital organs such as the heart and liver will decrease in size or volume. Only the brain resists protein breakdown.

▲ Protein contributes to the structure and function of muscle. © Dynamic Graphics/JupiterImages

Arterial end of a capillary bed

Venous end of a capillary bed

Blood cells

Fluid forced into tissue spaces by blood pressure generated by pumping action of heart

(a)

Proteins

Fluid drawn into bloodstream by the proteins as blood pressure declines in the capillary bed

Normal tissue

Swollen tissue (edema)

Blood pressure is balanced by counteracting force of protein.

Blood pressure exceeds counteracting force of protein, so fluid remains in the tissues.

(b)

FIGURE 6-13 ◄ Proteins help to maintain fluid balance. (a) As blood is pumped through the circulatory system, some fluid leaks out of the vessels. Normally, proteins in the blood draw water back into the blood vessels. (b) Without sufficient protein in the bloodstream, fluid remains in the tissues and edema develops.

MAINTAINING FLUID BALANCE

Blood proteins help maintain body fluid balance. Normal blood pressure in the arteries forces blood into capillary beds. The blood fluid then moves from the **capillary beds** into the spaces between nearby cells (**extracellular spaces**) to provide nutrients to those cells (Fig. 6-13). Proteins in the bloodstream are too large, however, to move out of the capillary beds into the tissues. The presence of these proteins in the capillary beds attracts the proper amount of fluid back to the bloodstream, partially counteracting the force of blood pressure.

With an inadequate consumption of protein, the concentration of proteins in the bloodstream drops below normal. Excessive fluid then builds up in the surrounding tissues because the counteracting force produced by the smaller amount of blood proteins is too weak to pull enough of the fluid back from the tissues into the bloodstream. As fluids accumulate in the tissues, the tissues swell, causing **edema.** Because edema may be a symptom of other medical problems, an important step in diagnosing the cause is to measure the concentration of blood proteins.

capillary bed Network of one-cell-thick vessels that create a junction between arterial and venous circulation. It is here that gas and nutrient exchange occurs between body cells and the blood.

extracellular space The space outside cells; represents one-third of body fluid.

edema The buildup of excess fluid in extracellular spaces.

CONTRIBUTING TO ACID–BASE BALANCE

Proteins help regulate acid-base balance in the blood. Proteins located in cell membranes pump chemical ions in and out of cells. The ion concentration that results from the pumping action, among other factors, keeps the blood slightly alkaline. In addition, some blood proteins are especially good **buffers** in the bloodstream. Buffers are compounds that maintain acid-base conditions within a narrow range.

buffer Compounds that cause a solution to resist changes in acid-base conditions.

FORMING HORMONES AND ENZYMES

Many hormones, our internal body messengers, are proteins, and therefore require amino acids for synthesis. Some hormones, such as the thyroid hormones, are made from only one type of amino acid, tyrosine. Insulin, on the other hand, is a hormone composed of 51 amino acids. Almost all enzymes are proteins or have a protein component.

Neurotransmitters, released by nerve endings, are often derivatives of amino acids. This is true for dopamine and norepinephrine (both synthesized from the amino acid tyrosine) and serotonin (synthesized from the amino acid tryptophan).

PROTEIN CONCEPT MAP

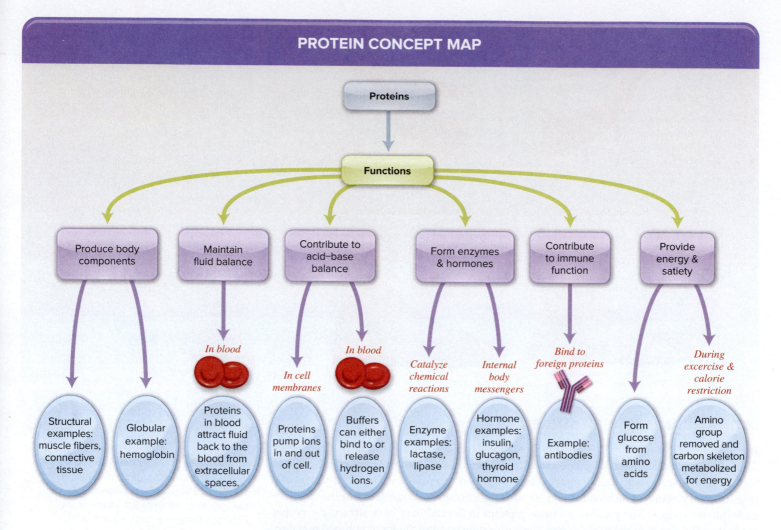

CONTRIBUTING TO IMMUNE FUNCTION

Proteins are a key component of cells within the immune system. Consider, for example, antibodies, which are proteins produced by one type of white blood cell. These antibodies can bind to foreign proteins in the bloodstream—an important step in removing invaders from the body. Without sufficient dietary protein, the immune system lacks the materials needed to function properly. For example, a low-protein status can turn measles into a fatal disease for a malnourished child.

FORMING GLUCOSE

In Chapter 4, you learned that a fairly constant concentration of glucose must be maintained in the blood to supply energy for the brain, red blood cells, and nervous tissue. At rest, the brain uses about 19% of the body's energy requirements, and it gets most of that energy from glucose. If you do not consume enough carbohydrate to supply the glucose, your liver (and kidneys, to a lesser extent) will be forced to make glucose from amino acids present in body tissues (Fig. 6-14).

Making some glucose from amino acids is normal. For example, when you skip breakfast and have not eaten since 7:00 P.M. the preceding evening, glucose must be manufactured. In an extreme situation, however, such as in starvation, amino acids from muscle tissue start to be converted into glucose, which wastes muscle tissue and can produce edema.

The vitamin niacin can be made from the amino acid tryptophan, illustrating another role of proteins.

PROVIDING ENERGY

Proteins supply little energy for a person at a healthy weight. Two situations in which a person does use protein to meet energy needs are during prolonged exercise and during calorie

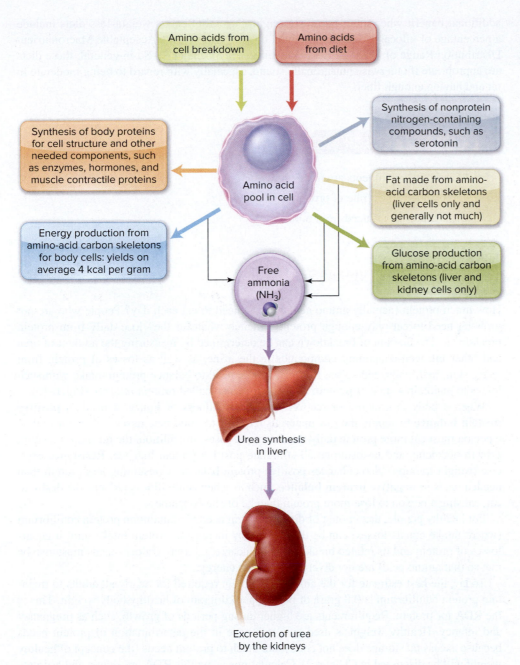

FIGURE 6-14 ◄ Amino-acid metabolism. The amino-acid **pool** in a cell can be used to form body proteins, as well as a variety of other possible products. When the **carbon skeletons** of amino acids are metabolized to produce glucose or fat, ammonia (NH_3) is a resulting waste product. The ammonia is converted into urea and excreted in the urine.

pool The amount of a nutrient stored within the body that can be mobilized when needed.

carbon skeleton Amino-acid structure that remains after the amino group ($⌘NH_2$) has been removed.

restriction, as with a weight-loss diet. In these cases, the amino group ($-NH_2$) from the amino acid is removed, and the remaining carbon skeleton is metabolized for energy needs (see Fig. 6-14). When the carbon skeletons of amino acids are metabolized to produce glucose or fat, ammonia (NH_3) is a resulting waste product. The ammonia is converted into **urea** and excreted in the urine. Under most conditions, cells primarily use fats and carbohydrates for energy needs. Although proteins contain the same amount of kilocalories (on average, 4 kcal per gram) as carbohydrates, proteins are a costly source of kilocalories, considering the amount of processing the liver and kidneys must perform to use this kilocalorie source.

urea Nitrogenous waste product of protein metabolism; major source of nitrogen in the urine,

$$\begin{array}{c} O \\ \| \\ \text{chemically} \quad NH_2-C-NH_2 \end{array}$$

CONTRIBUTING TO SATIETY

Compared to the other macronutrients, proteins provide the highest feeling of **satiety** after a meal. Thus, including some protein with each meal helps control overall food intake. Many experts warn against skimping on protein when trying to reduce energy intake to lose weight. Meeting protein needs is still important, and exceeding needs somewhat may provide an

satiety A state in which there is no longer a desire to eat; a feeling of satisfaction.

additional benefit when dieting to lose weight. Several effective weight-loss diets include a percentage of kilocalories from protein at the upper end of the Acceptable Macronutrient Distribution Range of 10% to 35% for protein (see Appendix G). So in general, these diets are appropriate if otherwise nutritionally sound, especially with regard to being moderate in fat and having enough fiber.

✓ CONCEPT CHECK 6.5

1. Which body constituents are mainly proteins?
2. What is the turnover rate of protein each day?
3. How is glucose produced from protein?

6.6 Protein Needs

How much protein (actually amino acids) do we need to eat each day? People who are not growing need to eat only enough protein to match whatever they lose daily from protein breakdown. The amount of breakdown can be determined by measuring the amount of urea and other nitrogen-containing compounds in the urine, as well as losses of protein from feces, skin, hair, nails, and so on. In short, people need to balance protein intake with such losses to maintain a state of **protein equilibrium,** also called *protein balance* (Fig. 6-15).

When a body is growing or recovering from an illness or injury, it needs a **positive protein balance** to supply the raw materials required to build new tissues. To achieve this, a person must eat more protein daily than he or she loses. In addition, the hormones insulin, growth hormone, and testosterone all stimulate positive protein balance. Resistance exercise (weight training) also enhances positive protein balance. Consuming less protein than needed leads to **negative protein balance,** such as when acute illness reduces the desire to eat, causing a person to lose more protein than he or she consumes.

For healthy people, the amount of dietary protein needed to maintain protein equilibrium (where intake equals losses) can be determined by increasing protein intake until it equals losses of protein and its related breakdown products (e.g., urea). Calorie needs must also be met so that amino acids are not diverted for use as energy.

Today, the best estimate for the amount of protein required for nearly all adults to maintain protein equilibrium is 0.8 gram of protein per kilogram of healthy body weight. This is the RDA for protein. Requirements are higher during periods of growth, such as pregnancy and infancy. Healthy weight is used as a reference in the determination of protein needs because excess fat storage does not contribute much to protein needs (the concept of healthy weight will be discussed in Chapter 7). Calculations using this RDA are shown and estimate a requirement of about 56 grams of protein daily for a typical 70-kilogram (154-pound) man and about 46 grams of protein daily for a typical 57-kilogram (125-pound) woman.

---

protein equilibrium A state in which protein intake is equal to related protein losses; the person is said to be in protein balance.

positive protein balance A state in which protein intake exceeds related protein losses, as is needed during times of growth.

negative protein balance A state in which protein intake is less than related protein losses, such as often seen during acute illness.

The 2015–2020 Dietary Guidelines for Americans recommend a variety of protein foods, including seafood, lean meats and poultry, eggs, legumes (beans and peas), nuts, seeds, and soy products. The following shifts are also recommended to increase variety in protein food choices and to make more nutrient-dense choices:

- Increase the amount and variety of seafood consumed by choosing seafood in place of some meat and poultry.
- Increase seafood intake, but the foods to be replaced depend on the individual's current intake from the other protein subgroups.
- Incorporate seafood as the protein foods choice in meals twice per week in place of meat, poultry, or eggs.
- Use legumes or nuts and seeds in mixed dishes instead of some meat or poultry.
- Shift to nutrient-dense options, including lean and lower sodium options, to improve the nutritional quality of protein food choices and support healthy eating patterns.
- Some individuals, especially teen boys and adult men, also need to reduce overall intake of protein foods by decreasing intakes of meats, poultry, and eggs and increasing amounts of vegetables or other underconsumed food groups.

Convert weight from pounds to kilograms:

$$\frac{154 \text{ pounds}}{2.2 \text{ pounds/kilogram}} = 70 \text{ kilograms}$$

$$\frac{125 \text{ pounds}}{2.2 \text{ pounds/kilogram}} = 57 \text{ kilograms}$$

Calculate protein RDA:

$$70 \text{ kilograms} \times \frac{0.8 \text{ gram protein}}{\text{kilogram body weight}} = 56 \text{ grams}$$

$$57 \text{ kilograms} \times \frac{0.8 \text{ gram protein}}{\text{kilogram body weight}} = 46 \text{ grams}$$

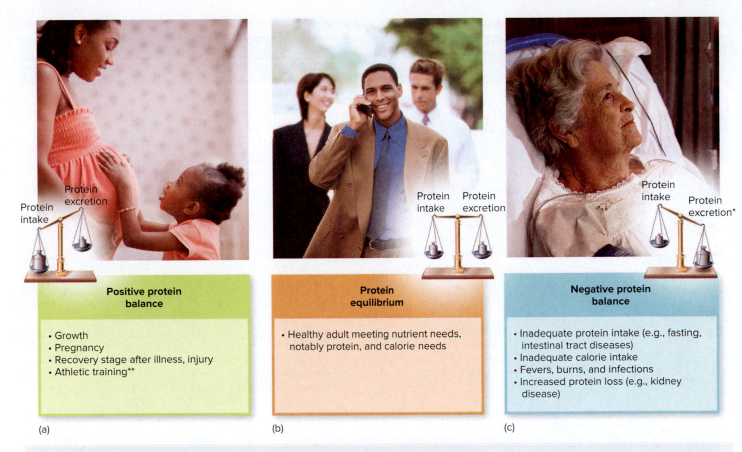

Protein
intake

Protein
excretion

**Positive protein
balance**

- Growth
- Pregnancy
- Recovery stage after illness, injury
- Athletic training**

(a)

Protein
intake

Protein
excretion

**Protein
equilibrium**

- Healthy adult meeting nutrient needs, notably protein, and calorie needs

(b)

Protein
intake

Protein
excretion*

**Negative protein
balance**

- Inadequate protein intake (e.g., fasting, intestinal tract diseases)
- Inadequate calorie intake
- Fevers, burns, and infections
- Increased protein loss (e.g., kidney disease)

(c)

*Based on losses of urea and other nitrogen-containing compounds in the urine, as well as protein lost from feces, skin, hair, nails, and other minor routes.
**Only when additional lean body mass is being gained. Nevertheless, the athlete is probably already eating enough protein to support this extra protein synthesis; protein supplements are not needed.

FIGURE 6-15 ▲ Protein balance in practical terms: (a) positive protein balance, (b) protein equilibrium, and (c) negative protein balance.
© Jose Luis Pelaez Inc/Blend Images LLC; © Stockbyte/Punchstock Images; © Dynamic Graphics/JupiterImages

The RDA for protein translates into about 10% of total calories. Many experts recommend up to 15% of total calories to provide more flexibility in diet planning and to allow for the variety of protein-rich foods North Americans typically consume. The Dietary Guidelines encourage the consumption of protein-rich foods such as beans, nuts, seeds, fat-free milk, and seafood. The Food and Nutrition Board has set an upper range for protein intake at 35% of calories consumed. It is easy to meet currently suggested daily protein needs, as given in Table 6-2. On a daily basis in North America, the typical man and woman consume about 100 and 65 grams of protein, respectively. Thus, most of us consume much more protein than the RDA recommends because we like many high-protein foods and can afford to buy them. Our bodies cannot store excess protein once it is consumed, so the excess amino acids are stripped of the nitrogen-containing amino group and may be turned into glucose or fat and then stored as fat or metabolized for energy needs (review Fig. 6-14).

Current research shows that a goal for a more equal distribution of protein at each meal is important in maintaining body composition and bone health and in regulating glucose. Researchers recommend that adults consume at least 30 grams of protein at more than one meal in order to maintain healthy muscles and bones. Protein at breakfast is especially critical to regulate appetite and daily food intake and to replenish body proteins after an overnight fast.

Mental stress, physical labor, and recreational weekend sports activities do not require an increase in the protein RDA. For some highly trained athletes, such as those participating in endurance or strength training, protein consumption may need to exceed the RDA. Many North Americans, especially men, already consume that much protein.

TABLE 6-2 ■ **Protein Content of Sample Menus Containing 1600 and 2000 kcal**

Menu		1600 kcal		2000 kcal	
		Serving Size	Protein (g)	Serving Size	Protein (g)
Breakfast					
	Low-fat granola	⅔ cup	5	⅔ cup	5
	Blueberries	1 cup	1	1 cup	1
	Fat-free (skim) milk	1 cup	8.5	1 cup	8.5
	Coffee	1 cup	0	1 cup	0
© Image Source/Corbis					
Lunch					
	Broiled chicken breast	3 ounces	25	4 ounces	33
	Salad greens	3 cups	5	3 cups	5
	Baked taco shell strips	½ cup	2	½ cup	2
	Low-fat salad dressing	2 tbsp	0	2 tbsp	0
© John A. Rizzo/Getty Images					
Dinner					
	Fat-free (skim) milk	1 cup	8.5	1 cup	8.5
	Yellow rice	1 ¼ cups	5	2 ½ cups	10 small
	Shrimp	4 large	5	6 large	7
	Mussels	4 medium	8	6 medium	12
	Clams	5 small	12	10 small	24
	Peas	½ cup	2	¼ cup	4
	Sweet red pepper	½ cup	0	½ cup	0
© Kevin Sanchez/Cole Group/Getty Images					
Snack					
	Muffin	1 small	4	1 small	4
	Swiss cheese	1 ounce	7.5	1 ounce	7.5
	Banana	½ small	0.5	½ small	0.5
© John A. Rizzo/Getty Images					
	Total		101		132

✔ **CONCEPT CHECK 6.6**

1. During what situations is the body in positive protein balance?

2. What is the RDA for protein for a 70-kilogram person?

3. How much protein does the average American consume?

6.7 Does Eating a High-Protein Diet Harm You?

Problems with dietary patterns that include excessive protein intakes primarily stem from their typical reliance on animal sources of protein. A high animal-protein diet is unlikely to follow the recommendations of the Dietary Guidelines for Americans or the American Heart Association in terms of reducing risk for cardiovascular disease. Eating patterns rich in animal products are most likely low in beneficial substances found in plant sources, including fiber, some vitamins (e.g., folate), some minerals (e.g., magnesium), and phytochemicals, and are high in substances such as saturated fat.

Newsworthy Nutrition

Red meat consumption linked to deaths

Red meat is a major source of protein and fat in most diets and has been associated with an increased risk of several chronic diseases, leading researchers to hypothesize that red meat consumption would be associated with an increase in early deaths. This study assessed meat consumption and causes of death from two prospective studies that included 37,698 men from the Health Professionals Follow-up Study (1986–2008) and 83,644 women from the Nurses' Health Study (1980–2008) who were free of cardiovascular disease (CVD) and cancer when the study began. During the study, there were 23,926 deaths, including 5910 caused by CVD and 9,464 caused by cancer. Consumption of both unprocessed and processed red meat was associated with an increased risk of total, CVD, and cancer deaths in men and women. Substituting one serving per day of other healthy protein sources (including fish, poultry, nuts, legumes, low-fat dairy, and whole grains) for one serving per day of red meat was associated with a 7% to 19% lower mortality risk. They also estimated that 9.3% of deaths in men and 7.6% in women could be prevented at the end of the study if all the individuals consumed less than one-half serving per day (approximately 42 grams per day) of red meat. These results support the hypothesis that red meat consumption is associated with an increased risk of total and early deaths from CVD and cancer.

Source: Pan A and others: Red meat consumption and mortality: Results from two prospective cohort studies. *Archives of Internal Medicine* 172:555, 2012 (see Further Reading 10).

▲ Animal-protein foods, such as roast beef (2 ounces) and Swiss cheese (1 ounce) on a bagel (3.5 inches), are typically our main sources of protein in the North American diet. This sandwich provides 332 kcal and 31 grams of protein. © Ingram Publishing/SuperStock

Although meat is one of the richest sources of protein, excessive intake of red meat, especially processed forms, has been linked to colon cancer. A 2015 report of the World Health Organization confirmed that consumption of high levels of red and processed meat is associated with an increased risk of colorectal cancer. The report, based on the review of more than 800 studies, indicated that reducing consumption of processed meats can reduce the risk of colorectal cancer. Experts concluded that each 50-gram portion of processed meat eaten daily increases the risk of colorectal cancer by 18%.

An association also has been found between red meat consumption and deaths caused by cardiovascular disease and cancer (see Further Readings 6 and 10, and Newsworthy Nutrition in this section). This connection could be caused by the curing agents used to process meats such as ham and salami, as well as substances that form during cooking of meats at high temperatures. Any type of meat should be trimmed of all visible fat before cooking, especially grilling. The excessive fat or low-fiber contents of diets high in red meat may also be a contributing factor. Because of these concerns, some nutrition experts suggest we focus more on poultry, fish, nuts, legumes, and seeds to meet protein needs.

Some researchers have expressed concern that a high-protein intake may overburden the kidneys by forcing them to excrete the extra nitrogen as urea. Also, animal proteins may contribute to kidney stone formation in certain individuals. A high-protein diet is not recommended for persons preserving kidney function such as those who have diabetes, early signs of kidney disease, or only one functioning kidney. There is some evidence that low-protein diets are helpful in slowing the decline in kidney function somewhat. High-protein diets increase urine output, which can lead to dehydration, especially in athletes.

AMINO-ACID SUPPLEMENTS

Protein and amino-acid supplements are used primarily by those trying to lose weight and by athletes hoping to build muscle. The branched-chain amino acids are especially popular with athletes looking to enhance their performance. Although the right amount of protein in the diet will aid athletic performance and help in weight control, consuming protein in the form of amino-acid supplements cannot be considered safe. Because the body's gastrointestinal system is adapted to handle whole proteins as a dietary source of amino acids, individual amino-acid supplements can overwhelm the absorptive mechanisms in the small intestine. Amino-acid imbalances occur in the intestinal tract because groups of chemically similar amino acids compete for absorption sites in the absorptive cells. For example, an excess of lysine can impair absorption of arginine because they are absorbed by the same transporter. The amino acids methionine, cysteine, and histidine are most likely to cause toxicity when consumed in large amounts. Due to this potential for imbalances and toxicities, the best advice to ensure adequacy is to stick to whole foods as sources of amino acids rather than supplements. Amino-acid supplements also have a disagreeable odor and flavor and are much more expensive than food protein. In Canada, the sale of individual amino acids to consumers is banned. Read more about this issue in What the Dietitian Chose at the end of this chapter.

ASK THE RDN   Paleo Diet

Dear RDN: Is the Paleo Diet™ a healthy way to include a good amount of high-quality protein into my eating plan?

The Paleo Diet, also called the Stone Age or Caveman Diet, is based on what was eaten during the Paleolithic period. Acceptable foods, therefore, are ones that can be hunted, fished, or gathered. Meats include those that are grass fed and pasture raised or wild game such as venison. Wild-caught fish, poultry, eggs, vegetables, fruits, fungi, roots, and nuts are also part of the diet. Dairy products and grains are excluded based on the assumption that the human body has not adapted genetically to allow for the consumption of grains and dairy, and that these foods contribute to health problems such as overweight/obesity and heart disease. Legumes (beans and peanuts), potatoes, added salt, refined sugar, and processed oils are also excluded.

Desirable aspects of the Paleo Diet are that it is rich in high-quality proteins and produce, yet low in added sugar and sodium—all factors that can help keep blood sugar, blood pressure, and weight under control. This very strict diet, however, has inadequate research to support its proposed benefits; and it is nearly impossible to gather and consume foods in the manner they existed in prehistoric times. Most of the meat we eat today is domesticated rather than wild game. Available fruits and vegetables are also grown on farms rather than harvested from the wild. Paleo followers often modify the plan by eating wild-caught fish, grass-fed meat, and organic fruits and vegetables, but even this becomes a challenge given the expense, lack of variety, and need for extensive planning and supplementation.

In sum, the Paleo Diet typically exceeds recommendations for fat and protein intake yet falls short of carbohydrate needs. The elimination of whole grains, legumes, and dairy—foods that are rich in nutrients and fiber—is more likely to lead to nutrient deficiencies than to weight loss. The lack of dairy jeopardizes calcium and vitamin D status and necessitates the use of supplements. Some good attributes of the diet that you can incorporate into a healthy dietary pattern are to eat more lean protein and less refined carbohydrates (more whole grains) to promote weight loss and satiety; a wide variety of fruits and vegetables to obtain vitamins, minerals, fiber, and phytochemicals; and more foods that are local, seasonal, and minimally processed because they provide more nutrients and fiber than a highly processed version of the food.

Eating for today,

Anne M. Smith, PhD, RDN, LD (author)

✓ CONCEPT CHECK 6.7

1. What are some of the harmful effects of regularly consuming a high-protein diet?

6.8 Protein-Calorie Malnutrition

Protein deficiency is rarely an isolated condition and usually accompanies a deficiency of calories and other nutrients resulting from insufficient food intake. In the developed world, alcoholism can lead to cases of protein deficiency because of the low protein content of alcoholic beverages that make up a high percent of calories. Protein and calorie malnutrition is a significant problem in hospitals worldwide, affecting patients from infancy through older adulthood. Malnutrition can be caused by the illnesses or injuries for which patients are admitted to the hospital and by the hospitalization itself (see Further Reading 4). In developing areas of the world, people often have diets low in calories and protein. This state of undernutrition stunts the growth of children and makes them more susceptible to disease throughout life. (Undernutrition is a main focus of Chapter 16.) People who consume too few of their calories as protein can eventually develop **protein-calorie malnutrition (PCM),** also referred to as *protein-energy malnutrition (PEM).* In its milder form, it is difficult to tell if a person with PCM is consuming too little calories or protein, or both. When an inadequate intake of nutrients, including protein, is combined with an existing disease, especially an infection, a form of malnutrition called **kwashiorkor** can develop. But if the nutrient deficiency—especially for calories—becomes severe, a deficiency disease called **marasmus** can result. Both conditions are seen primarily in children but also may develop in adults, even in those hospitalized in North America. These two conditions form the tip of the iceberg with respect to states of undernutrition, and symptoms of these two conditions can even be present in the same person (Fig. 6-16).

KWASHIORKOR

Kwashiorkor is a word from Ghana that means "the disease that the first child gets when the new child comes." Infants in developing areas of the world are usually breastfed from birth. Often by the time the child reaches 1 to 1.5 years of age, the mother is pregnant or has already given birth again, and the newborn infant gets preference for breastfeeding. The older child's diet then abruptly changes from nutritious human milk to starchy roots and **gruels,** which are low in protein compared to their calorie content. Additionally, the foods are usually high in bulky plant fibers, which are very filling and thus prevent the child from consuming enough food to meet calorie needs. Infections also raise calorie and protein needs. For these reasons, it is a challenge to meet the child's calorie needs, and their protein consumption is grossly inadequate, especially in view of the increased amount needed to combat infections. Many vitamin and mineral needs are also far from being fulfilled. Famine victims face similar problems.

protein-calorie malnutrition (PCM) A condition resulting from regularly consuming insufficient amounts of calories and protein. The deficiency eventually results in body wasting, primarily of lean tissue, and an increased susceptibility to infections. Also known as *protein-energy malnutrition (PEM).*

kwashiorkor A disease occurring primarily in young children who have an existing disease and consume a marginal amount of calories and insufficient protein in relation to needs. The child generally suffers from infections and exhibits edema, poor growth, weakness, and an increased susceptibility to further illness.

marasmus A disease resulting from consuming a grossly insufficient amount of protein and calories; one of the diseases classed as protein-calorie malnutrition. Victims have little or no fat stores, little muscle mass, and poor strength. Death from infections is common.

gruel A thin mixture of grains or legumes in milk or water.

FIGURE 6-16 ◄ Classification of undernutrition in children. (kwashiorkor): © Paul Souders/Worldfoto; (marasmus): © Peter Turnley/Corbis

Severe protein (with moderate energy) deficit; often accompanied by infections or other diseases

Protein Calorie Malnutrition

Severe energy and protein deficit

Characteristics of Kwashiorkor

- Edema
- Mild to moderate weight loss
- Maintenance of some muscle and subcutaneous fat
- Growth impairment (60%–80% of normal weight for age)
- Rapid onset
- Fatty liver

Characteristics of Marasmus

- Severe weight loss
- Wasting of muscle and body fat (skin and bones appearance)
- Severe growth impairment (less than 60% of normal weight for age)
- Develops gradually

▲ Unsafe water supplies in developing countries contribute to the incidence of marasmus, particularly in bottle-fed infants.
© Digital Vision/PunchStock

The major symptoms of kwashiorkor are apathy, diarrhea, listlessness, failure to grow and gain weight, and withdrawal from the environment. These symptoms complicate other diseases present. For example, a condition such as measles, a disease that normally makes a well-nourished child ill for only a week or so, can become severely debilitating and even fatal. Further symptoms of kwashiorkor are changes in hair color, potassium deficiency, flaky skin, fatty liver, reduced muscle mass, and massive edema in the abdomen and legs. The presence of edema in a child who has some subcutaneous fat (i.e., directly under the skin) is the hallmark of kwashiorkor (review Fig. 6-16). In addition, these children seldom move or cry. When you hold them, you feel the plumpness of edema, not muscle and fat tissue.

Many symptoms of kwashiorkor can be explained based on what we know about proteins. Proteins play important roles in fluid balance, lipoprotein transport, immune function, production of tissues such as skin, cells lining the GI tract, and hair. Children with an insufficient protein intake do not grow and mature normally. If children with kwashiorkor are helped in time—that is, if infections are treated and the dietary pattern becomes plentiful in protein, calories, and other essential nutrients—then the disease process reverses. They begin to grow again and may even show no signs of their previous condition, except perhaps shortness of stature. Unfortunately, by the time many of these children reach a hospital or care center, they already have severe infections. Despite the best care, they still die. Or, if they survive, they return home only to become ill again.

MARASMUS

Marasmus (referred to as *protein-calorie malnutrition,* especially when experienced by older children and adults) typically occurs as an infant slowly starves to death. It is caused by diets containing minimal amounts of calories, as well as too little protein and other nutrients. The word *marasmus* means "to waste away," in Greek. Victims have a "skin-and-bones" appearance, with little or no subcutaneous fat (review Fig. 6-16). Marasmus commonly develops in infants who either are not breastfed or have stopped breastfeeding in the early months. When people are poor and sanitation is lacking, bottle feeding often leads to marasmus. Often the weaning formula used is improperly prepared because of unsafe water and because the parents cannot afford sufficient infant formula for the child's needs. If parents dilute the formula to provide more feedings, they will be providing only more water for the infant.

Marasmus in infants commonly occurs in the large cities of poverty-stricken countries. In cities, bottle feeding is often necessary because the infant is cared for by others when the mother is working or away from home. An infant with marasmus requires large amounts of calories and protein, similar to the needs of a **preterm** infant, and, unless the child receives them, full recovery from the disease may never occur. The majority of brain growth occurs between conception and the child's first birthday, with the brain growing at its highest rate after birth. If human milk or formula does not support brain growth during the first months of life, the brain may not grow to its full adult size, leading to diminished intellectual function. Both kwashiorkor and marasmus plague infants and children; mortality rates in developing countries are often 10 to 20 times higher than in North America.

preterm An infant born before 37 weeks of gestation; also referred to as *premature.*

✔ CONCEPT CHECK 6.8

1. What are the characteristics of kwashiorkor and marasmus?
2. Why are bottle-fed infants at high risk for marasmus in poverty-stricken countries?

6.9 Nutrition and Your Health
Vegetarian and Plant-Based Dietary Patterns

© D. Hurst/Alamy

There are many documented health benefits of following a vegetarian diet. Studies show that death rates from some chronic diseases, such as certain forms of cardiovascular disease, hypertension, many forms of cancer, type 2 diabetes, and obesity, are lower for vegetarians than for nonvegetarians. Vegetarians often live longer, as shown in religious groups that practice vegetarianism. Other factors of healthful lifestyles, such as not smoking, abstaining from alcohol and drugs, and regular physical activity, are typical of vegetarians and probably partially account for the lower risks of chronic disease and longer lives seen in this population.

As you learned in Sections 2.2 and 2.3, the Dietary Guidelines for Americans and MyPlate emphasize a plant-based diet of whole-grain breads and cereals, fruits, and vegetables. In addition, the American Institute for Cancer Research promotes "The New American Plate," which includes plant-based foods covering two-thirds (or more) of the plate and meat, fish, poultry, or low-fat dairy covering only one-third (or less) of the plate. Although these recommendations allow the inclusion of animal products, they are definitely more "vegetarian-like" than typical North American diets.

Vegetarianism has evolved over the centuries from a necessity into an option. It is difficult to know exactly how many Americans follow a vegetarian or plant-based diet. A 2012 study from the Vegetarian Resource Group found 4% of U.S. adults (9 million people) to be vegetarian with only 2 million being strictly vegan (see Further Reading 11). Vegetarianism is popular among college students. According to a 2009–2010 survey, 12% of college students consider themselves vegetarian.

Vegetarian diets have evolved to include many soy-based meat alternatives. In addition, cookbooks that feature the use of a variety of fruits, vegetables, and seasonings are enhancing food selection for vegetarians of all degrees.

The growing popularity of vegetarian diets has prompted changes in the marketplace. Many restaurants offer vegetarian meals in response to the growing number of customers who want a vegetarian option when they eat out (see Further Reading 11). Campus dining services offer vegetarian options at every meal.

As nutrition science has grown, new information has enabled the design of nutritionally adequate vegetarian diets. It is important for vegetarians to take advantage of this information because a diet of only plant-based foods has the potential to promote various nutrient deficiencies and substantial growth retardation in infants and children. People who choose a vegetarian diet can meet their nutritional needs by following a few basic rules and knowledgeably planning their diets.

▲ Meatless Monday is a nonprofit initiative that began in the United States in 2003 to reduce dietary saturated fat. The Meatless Monday campaign recommends that we cut meat from our diet on Monday and thus encourages us to increase our consumption of fruits, vegetables, whole grains, and legumes. The Meatless Monday campaign (www.meatlessmonday.com) is now worldwide, active in 36 countries. Ideally, this eating pattern will flow into other days of the week and translate into healthier eating habits (see Further Reading 9). © Getty Images/Jonelle Weaver

Why Do People Become Vegetarians?

People choose vegetarianism for a variety of reasons including ethics, religion, economics, and health. Some believe that killing animals for food is unethical. Hindus and Trappist monks eat vegetarian meals as a practice of their religion. In North America, many Seventh Day Adventists base their practice of vegetarianism on biblical texts and believe it is a more healthful way to live.

Some advocates of vegetarianism base their food preference upon the inefficient use of animals as a source of protein. In the United States, nearly 70% of the grain crop is used for animal feed, and globally 35% of the grain harvest is used to produce animal protein. Although animals that humans eat sometimes eat grasses that humans cannot digest, many also eat grains that humans can eat. According to the United Nations Environment Programme, it takes approximately 3 kilograms of grain to produce 1 kilogram of animal protein in cereal-fed animals (see Further Reading 7). An advantage of grass-fed livestock that eat from a pasture is that they convert grass into protein more efficiently than those raised on grains.

People might also practice vegetarianism because it limits saturated fat and cholesterol intake, while encouraging a high intake of complex carbohydrates; vitamins A, E, and C; carotenoids; magnesium; and fiber.

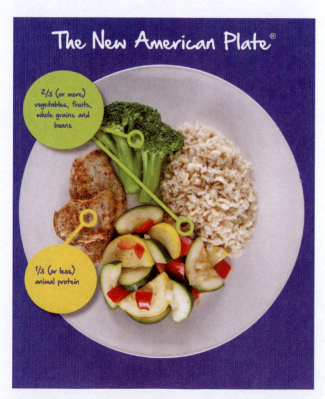

▲ "The New American Plate" published by the American Institute for Cancer Research was a forerunner of and embodies the same concepts as the MyPlate program.

Source: http://www.aicr.org/reduce-your-cancer-risk/recommendations-for-cancer-prevention/. Reprinted with permission from the American Institute for Cancer Research.

Good for Disease Prevention

Plant sources of proteins can positively impact heart health in several ways. First, the plant foods we eat contain no cholesterol nor *trans* fat and little saturated fat. As noted in Chapter 5, a vegan diet coupled with regular exercise and other lifestyle changes can lead to a reversal of atherosclerotic plaque in various arteries in the body. The major types of fat in plant foods are monounsaturated and polyunsaturated fats. Nuts in particular are high in monounsaturated fat, which helps to keep blood cholesterol low.

Beans and nuts contain soluble fiber, which binds to cholesterol in the small intestine and prevents it from being absorbed by the intestinal cells. Also, due to the activity of some phytochemicals, foods made from soybeans can lower production of cholesterol by the liver. The effect is modest (about a 2% to 6% drop). Since 1999, the Food and Drug Administration has allowed health claims for the cholesterol-lowering properties of soy foods, and the American Heart Association has recommended inclusion of some soy protein in the diets of people with high blood cholesterol. As noted in Chapter 2, to list a health claim for soy on the label, a food product must have at least 6.25 grams of soy protein and less than 3 grams of fat, 1 gram of saturated fat, and 20 milligrams of cholesterol per serving.

There are several other heart-protective compounds in plant foods. Some of the phytochemicals may help to prevent blood clots and relax the blood vessels. Nuts are an especially good source of nutrients implicated in heart health, including vitamin E, folate, magnesium, and copper. Frequent consumption of nuts (about 1 ounce of nuts five times per week) is associated with a decreased risk of cardiovascular disease. Recall from Chapter 2 that FDA allows a provisional health claim on food labels to link nuts with a reduced risk of developing cardiovascular disease.

The numerous phytochemicals in plant foods are also thought to aid in preventing cancers of the breast, prostate, and colon. Many of the proposed anticancer effects of foods containing plant protein are through antioxidant mechanisms (see Newsworthy Nutrition). Plants also may be particularly good sources of protein for people with diabetes or impaired glucose tolerance because the high fiber content of plant foods leads to a slower increase in blood glucose. Frequent nut consumption may even reduce the risk of developing gallstones, obesity, and type 2 diabetes.

▲ Plant proteins, like those in walnuts, can be incorporated into one's diet in numerous ways, such as adding them to banana nut muffins. © YAY Media AS/Alamy

Newsworthy Nutrition

Vegetarian Dietary Patterns Decrease Risk of Colorectal Cancers

Because colorectal cancers are a leading cause of cancer deaths, it is of great interest to determine if eating patterns can decrease their risk. The hypothesis of this study presented an association between vegetarian dietary patterns and the incidence of cancers of the colon and rectum. The study design was a dietary assessment, using a validated quantitative food frequency questionnaire, of 77,659 Seventh-Day Adventist men and women for 7 years who were categorized into four vegetarian dietary patterns (vegan, lactoovovegetarian, pescovegetarian [a vegetarian who also eats aquatic animal protein], and semivegetarian) and a nonvegetarian dietary pattern. State cancer registries were used to identify cases of colorectal cancer. The results included 380 cases of colon cancer and 110 cases of rectal cancer during the 7.3-year follow-up of participants. As a group, vegetarians were 22% less likely to get colorectal cancers (19% for colon cancer; 29% for rectal cancer) than meat-eaters. When the risk was broken down by diet type, pescovegetarians had a 43% lower risk; vegans, 16%; lactoovovegetarians, 18%; and semivegetarians, 8% lower risk than meat-eaters. All of these effects were similar for men and women and for black and nonblack participants. These results support the hypothesis that vegetarian dietary patterns are associated with an overall lower incidence of colorectal cancers. Pescovegetarians had a much lower risk compared with nonvegetarians, suggesting that compounds in fish such as omega-3 fatty acids may play a protective role in the prevention of colorectal cancers.

Source: Orlich MJ and others: Vegetarian dietary patterns and the risk of colorectal cancers. *Journal of American Medical Association Internal Medicine* 175:767, 2015.

INCREASING PLANT PROTEINS IN YOUR DIET

The following are some suggestions for including plant proteins in your diet.

- Try a veggie burger instead of a hamburger. These are usually made from beans and come in a variety of delicious flavors. They are available in the frozen foods section of the grocery store and many restaurants have added them to their menus.
- Sprinkle sunflower seeds or chopped almonds on top of your salad to add taste and texture.
- Mix chopped walnuts into the batter of your banana bread to boost your intake of monounsaturated fats.
- Eat soy nuts (oil-roasted soybeans) or edamame as a snack.
- Use peanut butter as your spread on bagels instead of butter or cream cheese.
- Make taco filling using a can of great northern beans heated with one-half packet of taco seasoning and chopped tomatoes.
- Use calcium-fortified soy milk, especially if you have lactose malabsorption or lactose intolerance.

FOOD PLANNING FOR VEGETARIANS

Of the estimated 5% of American adults who call themselves vegetarians, less than 2% are total vegetarians, or **vegans,** who eat only plant foods. **Fruitarians** primarily eat fruits, nuts, honey, and vegetable oils. This plan is not recommended because it can lead to nutrient deficiencies in people of all ages. **Lactovegetarians** are more liberal than vegans; they allow dairy products in their plant-based diet. **Lactoovovegetarians** modify the diet even further and eat dairy products and eggs, as well as plant foods. These inclusions make food planning easier because the dairy and eggs are rich in some nutrients that are missing or minimal in plants, such as vitamin B-12 and calcium. The more variety in the diet, the easier it is to meet nutritional needs.

OPTIMIZING A VEGAN PLAN

Planning a vegan dietary pattern requires knowledge and creativity to yield high-quality protein and other key nutrients without animal products. In Section 6.3, you learned about complementary proteins, whereby the essential amino acids deficient in one protein source are supplied by those of another consumed at the same meal or the next (see Fig. 6-8). Many legumes are deficient in the essential amino-acid methionine, whereas grains are limited in lysine. Eating a combination of legumes and grains, such as beans and rice, will supply the body with adequate amounts of all essential amino acids (see Fig. 6-8). As with any meal plan, variety is an especially important characteristic of a nutritious vegan dietary pattern. Table 6-3 exemplifies vegetarian food plans, which emphasize grains, legumes, nuts, and seeds to help meet protein needs.

Aside from amino acids, low intakes of certain micronutrients can be a problem for the vegan. At the forefront of nutritional concerns

▲ Keep in mind that amino acids in vegetables are best used when a combination of sources is consumed. © Mitch Hrdlicka/Getty Images

vegan A person who eats only plant foods.

fruitarian A person who primarily eats fruits, nuts, honey, and vegetable oils.

lactovegetarian A person who consumes plant products and dairy products.

lactoovovegetarian A person who consumes plant products, dairy products, and eggs.

TABLE 6-3 ■ **Food Plan for Vegetarians Based on MyPlate**

| Food Group | MyPlate Servings | | Key Nutrients Supplied‡ |
	Lactovegetarian*	Vegan†	
Grains	6–11	8–11	Protein, thiamin, niacin, folate, vitamin E, zinc, magnesium, iron, and fiber
Beans and other legumes	2–3	3	Protein, vitamin B-6, zinc, magnesium, and fiber
Nuts, seeds	2–3	3	Protein, vitamin E, and magnesium
Vegetables	3–5 (include 1 dark-green or leafy variety daily)	4–6 (include 1 dark-green or leafy variety daily)	Vitamin A, vitamin C, folate, vitamin K, potassium, and magnesium
Fruits	2–4	4	Vitamin A, vitamin C, and folate
Dairy	3	____	Protein, riboflavin, vitamin D, vitamin B-12, and calcium
Fortified soy milk	____	3	Protein, riboflavin, vitamin D, vitamin B-12, and calcium

*This plan contains about 75 grams of protein in 1650 kcal.

†This plan contains about 79 grams of protein in 1800 kcal.

‡One serving of vitamin- and mineral-enriched ready-to-eat breakfast cereal is recommended to meet possible nutrient gaps. Alternatively, a balanced multivitamin and mineral supplement can be used. Vegans also may benefit from the use of fortified soy milk to provide calcium, vitamin D, and vitamin B-12.

are riboflavin, vitamins D and B-12, iron, zinc, iodine, and calcium. Although use of a balanced multivitamin and mineral supplement can help, the following dietary advice should be implemented.

Riboflavin can be obtained from green leafy vegetables, whole grains, yeast, and legumes—components of most vegan plans. Alternate sources of vitamin D include fortified foods (e.g., margarine), some mushroom varieties, and regular sun exposure.

Vitamin B-12 only occurs naturally in animal foods. Plants can contain soil or microbial contaminants that provide trace amounts of vitamin B-12, but these are negligible sources of the vitamin. Because the liver can store vitamin B-12 for about 4 years, it may take a long time after removal of animal foods from the dietary pattern for a vitamin B-12 deficiency to surface. If dietary B-12 inadequacy persists, deficiency can lead to anemia, nerve damage, and mental dysfunction. These deficiency consequences have been noted in the infants of vegetarian mothers whose breast milk was low in vitamin B-12. Vegans can prevent a vitamin B-12 deficiency by finding a reliable source of this vitamin, such as fortified soybean milk, ready-to-eat breakfast cereals, and special yeast grown on media rich in vitamin B-12.

For iron, the vegan can consume whole grains and ready-to-eat breakfast cereals, dried fruits and nuts, and legumes. The iron in these foods is not absorbed as well as iron in animal foods but consuming these foods with a good source of vitamin C can enhance iron absorption. Cooking in iron pots and skillets can also add iron to food.

The vegan can find zinc in whole grains (especially ready-to-eat breakfast cereals), nuts, and legumes, but phytic acid and other substances in these foods limit zinc absorption. Breads are a good source of zinc because the leavening process (rising of the bread dough) reduces the influence of phytic acid. Iodized salt is a reliable source of iodine. It should be used instead of plain salt, both of which are found in U.S. supermarkets.

Of all nutrients, calcium and vitamin D are the most difficult to consume in sufficient quantities for vegans. Fortified foods including fortified soy milk, fortified orange juice, calcium-rich tofu (check the label), and certain ready-to-eat breakfast cereals and snacks are the vegan's best option for obtaining these nutrients. Green leafy vegetables and nuts also contain calcium, but the mineral is either not well absorbed or not very plentiful from these sources. Dietary supplements are another option. Special diet planning is always required because even a multivitamin and mineral supplement will not supply enough calcium to meet the needs for bone health.

Consuming adequate quantities of omega-3 fatty acids is yet another nutritional concern for vegetarians, especially vegans. Fish and fish oils, abundant sources of these heart-healthy fats, are omitted from many types of vegetarian plans. Alternative plant sources of omega-3 fatty acids include canola oil, soybean oil, seaweed, microalgae, flax seeds, chia seeds, and walnuts.

Special Concerns for Infants and Children

Infants and children, notoriously picky eaters in the first place, are at highest risk for nutrient deficiencies as a result of improperly planned vegetarian and vegan dietary patterns. With the use

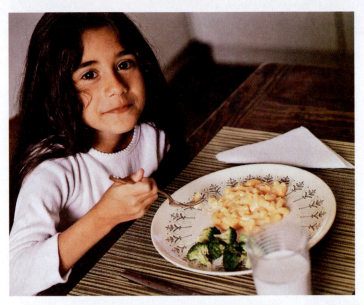

▲ Children can safely enjoy vegetarian and vegan diets as long as certain adjustments are made to meet their age-specific nutritional needs. © Brand X Pictures/Getty Images

of complementary proteins and good sources of the problem nutrients just discussed, the calorie, protein, vitamin, and mineral needs of vegetarian and vegan infants and children can be met (see Further Reading 1). The most common nutritional concerns for vegetarian and vegan infants and children are deficiencies of iron, vitamin B-12, vitamin D, and calcium.

Vegetarian and vegan plans tend to be high in bulky, high-fiber, low-calorie foods that cause a feeling of fullness. While this is a welcome advantage for most adults, children have small stomach capacity and relatively high nutrient needs compared to their size and thus may feel full before their calorie needs are met. For this reason, the fiber content of a child's dietary pattern may need to be decreased by replacing high-fiber sources with some refined grain products, fruit juices, and peeled fruit. Other concentrated sources of calories for vegetarian and vegan children include fortified soy milk, nuts, dried fruits, and avocados.

CASE STUDY   Planning a Vegetarian Dietary pattern

Jordan is a freshman in college. He lives in a campus residence hall and teaches martial arts in the afternoon. He eats two or three meals a day at the residence hall cafeteria and snacks between meals. Jordan and his roommate both decided to become vegetarians because they recently read an article on a fitness website describing the health benefits of a vegetarian dietary pattern. Yesterday Jordan's vegetarian plan consisted of a Danish pastry for breakfast and a tomato-rice dish (no meat) with pretzels and a diet soft drink for lunch. In the afternoon, after his martial arts class, he had a milkshake and two cookies. At dinnertime, he had a vegetarian sub sandwich consisting of lettuce, sprouts, tomatoes, cucumbers, and cheese, with two glasses of fruit punch. In the evening, he had a bowl of popcorn.

Answer the following questions and check your response at the end of this chapter.

▲ Has Jordan planned a healthy and nutritious vegetarian dietary pattern? © Purestock/SuperStock

1. What type of health benefits can Jordan expect from following a well-planned vegetarian dietary pattern?
2. What is missing from Jordan's current dietary plan in terms of foods that should be emphasized in a vegetarian dietary pattern?
3. Which nutrients are missing in this current dietary plan?
4. Are there any food components in the current diet plan that should be minimized or avoided?
5. How could he improve his new dietary pattern at each meal and snack to meet his nutritional needs and avoid undesirable food components?

Summary (Numbers refer to numbered sections in the chapter.)

6.1 Amino acids, the building blocks of proteins, contain a very usable form of nitrogen for humans. Of the 20 common types of amino acids found in food, nine must be consumed in food (essential) and the rest can be synthesized by the body (nonessential).

6.2 Individual amino acids are bonded together to form proteins. The sequential order of amino acids determines the protein's ultimate shape and function. This order is directed by DNA in the cell nucleus. Diseases such as sickle cell anemia can occur if the amino acids are incorrect on a polypeptide chain. When the three-dimensional shape of a protein is unfolded—denatured—by treatment with heat, acid or alkaline solutions, or other processes, the protein also loses its biological activity.

6.3 Almost all animal products are nutrient-dense sources of protein. The high quality of these proteins means that they can be easily converted into body proteins. Rich plant sources of protein, such as beans, are also available.

High-quality (complete) protein foods contain ample amounts of all nine essential amino acids. Lower quality (incomplete) protein foods lack sufficient amounts of one or more essential amino acids. This is typical of plant foods, especially cereal grains. Different types of plant foods eaten together often complement each other's amino-acid deficits, thereby providing high-quality protein in the diet.

6.4 Protein digestion begins in the stomach, where stomach acid and pepsin break down proteins into shorter polypeptide chains of amino acids. In the small intestine, these polypeptide chains eventually separate into amino acids in the absorptive cells. The free amino acids then travel via the portal vein that connects to the liver. Some then enter the bloodstream.

6.5 Important body components—such as muscles, connective tissue, transport proteins in the bloodstream, visual pigments, enzymes, some hormones, and immune cells—are made of proteins. These proteins are in a state of constant turnover. The carbon chains of proteins may be used to produce glucose (or fat) when necessary.

6.6 The protein RDA for adults is 0.8 gram per kilogram of healthy body weight. This corresponds to 56 grams of protein daily for a 70-kilogram (154-pound) person and 46 grams per day for a 57-kilogram (125-pound) person. The North American diet generally supplies plenty of protein with men consuming about 100 grams of protein daily, and women consuming closer to 65 grams. These protein intakes are also of sufficient quality to support body functions. To maintain a state of protein balance, people need to balance protein intake with losses. A positive protein balance is needed to supply the raw materials required to build new tissues during growth or recovery from an illness or injury. To achieve this, a person must eat more protein daily than he or she loses. Consuming less protein than needed leads to negative protein balance, such as when acute illness reduces the desire to eat.

6.7 Excessive protein intakes primarily stem from eating patterns rich in animal products. Excessive intake of red meat, especially processed forms, has been linked to colon cancer and deaths caused by cardiovascular disease and cancer. A high-protein intake may overburden the kidneys by forcing them to excrete the extra nitrogen as urea. Due to this potential for imbalances and toxicities, the best practice to ensure adequacy is to stick to whole foods as sources of amino acids rather than supplements.

6.8 Undernutrition can lead to protein-calorie malnutrition in the form of kwashiorkor or marasmus. Kwashiorkor results primarily from an inadequate protein intake in comparison with body needs, which often increase with concurrent disease and infection. Kwashiorkor often occurs when a child is weaned from human milk and fed mostly starchy gruels. Marasmus results from extreme starvation—a negligible intake of both protein and calories. Marasmus commonly occurs during famine, especially in infants.

6.9 Vegetarian and other plant-based dietary patterns provide many health benefits, including lower risks of such chronic diseases as cardiovascular disease, diabetes, and certain cancers. The benefits associated with the plant-based diets appear to stem from the lower content of saturated fat and cholesterol and the higher amount of fiber, vitamins, minerals, and phytochemicals.

Check Your Knowledge (Answers are available at the end of this question set.)

1. The "instructions" for making proteins are located in the
   a. cell membrane.
   b. cell nucleus.
   c. cytoplasm.
   d. lysosome.

2. A nutrient that could easily be deficient in the diet of a vegan would be
   a. vitamin C.
   b. folic acid.
   c. calcium.
   d. carbohydrate.

3. An example of protein complementation used in vegetarian dietary planning would be the combination of
   a. cereal and milk.
   b. bacon and eggs.
   c. rice and beans.
   d. macaroni and cheese.

4. If an essential amino acid is unavailable for protein synthesis,
   a. then the cell will make the amino acid.
   b. then protein synthesis will stop.
   c. then the cell will continue to attach amino acids to the protein.
   d. then the partially completed protein will be stored for later completion.

5. An individual who eats only plant food is referred to as a
   a. planetarium.
   b. vegan.
   c. lactovegetarian.
   d. lactoovovegetarian.

6. Which of the following groups accounts for the differences among amino acids?
   a. amine group
   b. side chain
   c. acid group
   d. keto group

7. Absorption of amino acids primarily takes place in the
   a. stomach.
   b. liver.
   c. small intestine.
   d. large intestine.

8. Jack is not an athlete and weighs 176 pounds (80 kilograms). His RDA for protein is _____ grams.
   a. 32
   b. 40
   c. 64
   d. 80

9. The basic building block of a protein is called a(n)
   a. fatty acid.
   b. monosaccharide.
   c. amino acid.
   d. gene.

10. Which of the following is true about protein intake of people in the United States?
   a. Most do not consume enough protein.
   b. Most consume the amount needed to balance losses.
   c. Athletes do not get enough protein without supplementation.
   d. Most consume more than is needed.

Answer Key: 1. b (LO 6.2), 2. c (LO 6.3), 3. c (LO 6.3), 4. b (LO 6.2), 5. b (LO 6.9), 6. b (LO 6.1), 7. c (LO 6.4), 8. c (LO 6.6), 9. c (LO 6.1), 10. d (LO 6.7)

Study Questions (Numbers refer to Learning Outcomes)

1. Discuss the relative importance of essential and nonessential amino acids in the diet. Why is it important for essential amino acids lost from the body to be replaced in the diet? (LO 6.1)

2. What is the role of cholecystokinin (CCK) in protein digestion? (LO 6.4)

3. What is a limiting amino acid? Explain why this concept is a concern in a vegetarian diet. How can a vegetarian compensate for limiting amino acids in specific foods? (LO 6.8)

4. Briefly describe the organization of proteins. How can this organization be altered or damaged? What might be a result of damaged protein organization? (LO 6.2)

5. Describe four functions of proteins. Provide an example of how the structure of a protein relates to its function. (LO 6.5)

6. How are DNA and protein synthesis related? (LO 6.2)

7. What would be one health benefit of reducing high-protein intake(s) to RDA amounts for some people? (LO 6.6)

8. Which eight foods are the major sources of proteins that cause food allergies? (LO 6.3)

9. Outline the major differences between kwashiorkor and marasmus. (LO 6.8)

10. What are the possible long-term effects of an inadequate intake of dietary protein among children between the ages of 6 months and 4 years? (LO 6.8)

What the Dietitian Chose

Consuming adequate protein is important for muscle repair and synthesis, but consuming excessive protein from any source provides no advantage. Excess protein is not stored in the body but may be metabolized as fuel or stored as fat, not muscle. In fact, some excess subcutaneous fat is probably the reason you have not seen your toned muscles yet.

Cutting back on calories or including more endurance exercise in your routine can help to reduce body weight and body fat as you tone your muscles. Animal protein, in particular, is often a source of excess total and saturated fat. Not only will this hinder efforts at weight loss, but it is detrimental to heart health.

Americans typically consume two to three times as much protein as they actually need. The average American intake of 100 grams per day for men or 65 grams per day for women easily meets even the highest protein recommendations for resistance exercise (1.7 grams of protein per kilogram). Also, omnivorous dietary patterns and appropriately planned vegan diets can supply ample amino acids to support muscle recovery and synthesis.

It is not a good idea to take individual amino-acid supplements. Your digestive tract is adapted to handle whole proteins: hydrochloric acid and enzymes break polypeptides into amino acids that can be absorbed by the cells of the small intestine. Taking large doses of one amino acid can impair the absorption and/or metabolism of other amino acids.

Whey protein, a by-product of cheese production from cow's milk, is considered to be a high-quality protein because it is easily digested and contains all of the essential amino acids. It is a source of the BCAAs valine, leucine, and isoleucine. BCAAs can be used for fuel by exercising muscles and are particularly important for synthesizing muscle tissue. The rationale is that whey protein supports muscle recovery and anabolism after exercise. Protein and amino-acid supplements are expensive and may be detrimental to health. It is safer and more economical to focus on a diet that provides 10% to 35% of calories from a variety of lean sources of protein.

▲ This 4-ounce grilled chicken breast is an excellent choice, providing 38 grams of high-quality yet inexpensive lean protein. © Ingram Publishing/SuperStock

CASE STUDY SOLUTION Planning a Vegetarian Dietary pattern

1. Studies show that the incidence of and the death rates from some chronic diseases, such as certain cardiovascular diseases, hypertension, many forms of cancer, type 2 diabetes, and obesity, are lower for vegetarians than for nonvegetarians.

2. Many components of a healthy vegetarian diet—whole grains, nuts, soy products, beans, two to four servings of fruits, and three to five servings of vegetables per day—are missing. With so few fruits and vegetables, Jordan's diet is also low in the many phytochemicals under study for numerous health benefits.

3. Protein appears to be low in the diet because Jordan has not replaced meat with a good plant source of protein. Vitamin B-12, iron, and zinc are also missing from the foods

he is choosing. His diet seems to be adequate in calcium and riboflavin because he is including dairy products (milkshake and cheese).

4. Some of Jordan's food choices are high in fat (Danish pastry, milkshake, and cookies) and sugar (fruit punch).

5. A healthy vegetarian diet includes whole grains, nuts, soy products, beans, two to four servings of fruits, and three to five servings of vegetables per day. It is apparent that he has not yet learned to implement the concept of complementary proteins, so the quality of protein in his diet is low. Meals that combine legumes or vegetables with grains or nuts (see Fig. 6-8) will provide the needed amounts of all amino acids.

Further Readings

1. ADA Reports: Position of the American Dietetic Association and Dietitians of Canada: Vegetarian diets. *Journal of the American Dietetic Association* 109:1266, 2009.

2. Burlingame B, Dernini S: Sustainable diets: The Mediterranean diet as an example. *Public Health Nutrition* 14:2285, 2011.

3. Cooper CC: Gluten free and healthy. *Today's Dietitian* 14(5):24, 2012.

4. Fessler TA: Malnutrition: A serious concern for hospitalized patients. *Today's Dietitian* 10(7):44, 2008.

5. Fleischer DM and others: Primary prevention of allergic disease through nutritional interventions. *Journal of Allergy and Clinical Immunology: In Practice* 1:29, 2013.

6. Micha R and others: Red and processed meat consumption and risk of incident coronary heart disease, stroke, and diabetes mellitus: A systemic review and meta-analysis. *Circulation* 121:2271, 2010.

7. Moomaw WT and others: The critical role of global food consumption patterns in achieving sustainable food systems and food for all. *A UNEP*

Discussion Paper, United Nations Environment Programme, Division of Technology, Industry and Economics, Paris, France, 2012. http://www.humanmedia.org/dcc/pdf/unep_food_report_2012.pdf. Accessed April 12, 2013.

8. Nierenberg D, Reynolds L: Farm animal populations continue to grow. *Vital Signs,* Worldwatch Institute, March 23, 2012. http://vitalsigns.worldwatch.org/vs-trend/farm-animal-populations-continue-grow. Accessed April 12, 2013.

9. Palmer S: Meatless Monday. *Today's Dietitian* 15(1):38, 2013.

10. Pan A and others: Red meat consumption and mortality: Results from two prospective cohort studies. *Archives of Internal Medicine* 172:555, 2012.

11. Stahler C: How often do Americans eat vegetarian meals? And how many adults in the U.S. are vegetarian? *Vegetarian Journal* 31:12, 2012.

12. Williams CD and others: Associations of red meat, fat, and protein intake with distal colorectal cancer risk. *Nutrition and Cancer* 62(6):701, 2010.

 To get the most out of your study of nutrition, go to McGraw-Hill's online resources: Connect www.mcgrawhillconnect.com, where you will find NutritionCalc Plus, LearnSmart, and many other dynamic tools.

Rate Your Plate

Protein and the Vegetarian

Alana weighs 110 pounds and is excited about all the health benefits that might accompany a vegetarian dietary pattern. However, she is concerned that she will not consume enough protein to meet her needs. She is also concerned about possible vitamin and mineral deficiencies. Use NutritionCalc Plus or a food composition table to calculate her protein intake and see if her concerns are valid.

	Protein (grams)
Breakfast Calcium-fortified orange juice, 1 cup Soy milk, 1 cup Fortified bran flakes, 1 cup Banana, medium	
Snack Calcium-enriched granola bar	
Lunch Garden burger, 4 ounces Whole-wheat bun Mustard, 1 tbsp Soy cheese, 1 ounce Apple, medium Green leaf lettuce, 1 ½ cups Peanuts, 1 ounce Sunflower seeds, 1/4 cup Tomato slices, 2 Mushrooms, 3 Vinaigrette salad dressing, 2 tbsp Iced tea	
Dinner Kidney beans, 1/2 cup Brown rice, 3/4 cup Fortified margarine, 2 tbsp Mixed vegetables, 1/4 cup Hot tea	
Dessert Strawberries, 1/2 cup Angel food cake, 1 small slice Soy milk, 1/2 cup	
	Total Protein (grams) _____

Alana's dietary plan contained 2150 kcal, with _____ grams (you fill in) of protein (Is this plenty for her?), 360 grams of carbohydrate, 57 grams of total dietary fat (only 9 grams of which came from saturated fat), and 50 grams of fiber. Her vitamin and mineral intake with respect to those of concern to vegetarians—vitamin B-12, vitamin D, calcium, iron, and zinc—met her needs.

© Ingram Publishing

Student Learning Outcomes

Chapter 7 is designed to allow you to:

7.1 Describe energy balance and the uses of energy by the body.

7.2 Compare methods to determine energy use by the body.

7.3 Discuss methods for assessing body composition and determining whether body weight and composition are healthy.

7.4 Explain factors associated with the development of obesity and outline the risks to health posed by being overweight or obese.

7.5 List and discuss characteristics of a sound weight-loss program.

7.6 Describe why reduced calorie intake is the main key to weight loss and maintenance.

7.7 Discuss why physical activity is a key component in weight loss and especially important for later weight maintenance.

Chapter 7
Energy Balance and Weight Control

7.8 Describe why and how behavior modification fits into a weight-loss program.

7.9 Outline the benefits and hazards of various weight-loss methods for severe obesity.

7.10 Discuss the causes and treatment of being underweight.

7.11 Evaluate popular weight-reduction diets and determine which are safe and successful.

In the last 25 years, there has been a dramatic increase in the percentage of individuals who are overweight or obese. Recall from Chapter 1 that the obesity epidemic remains a crisis, not only in the United States but also globally among affluent people and in developing countries where Westernized diets (high saturated fat, high sugar) are increasing in popularity and more sedentary lifestyles are adopted. Excess body fat increases the likelihood of many health problems, such as cardiovascular disease, cancer, hypertension, stroke, bone and joint disorders, and type 2 diabetes, especially if a person performs minimal physical activity.

Currently, most weight-reduction efforts fail before dieters reach a healthy weight range. Typical popular ("fad") diets are generally monotonous and highly restrictive. The more restrictive diets may even endanger some populations, such as children, teenagers, pregnant women, and individuals with various health conditions. A more logical "total dietary pattern" approach to weight loss is straightforward: (1) reduce calorie intake; (2) increase physical activity; and (3) change eating behaviors and patterns (see Further Reading 1).

A variety of groups, including government agencies, the food industry, health professionals, and community organizations, have begun to address the growing weight problem in North America. It is expected that without this national effort to promote effective new approaches to maintaining healthy weight, the current trends will continue (Fig. 7-1; see Further Readings 1, 3, and 20). This chapter will lead you to an understanding of the causes, consequences, and potential treatments of obesity.

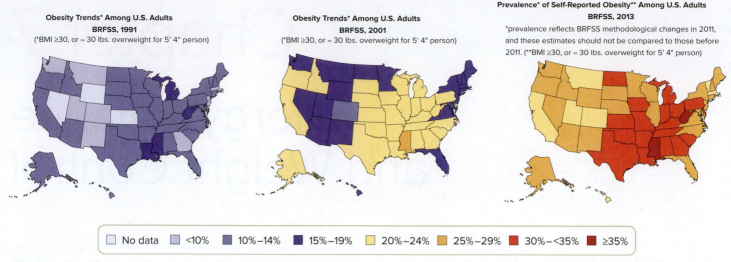

Obesity Trends* Among U.S. Adults
BRFSS, 1991
(*BMI ≥30, or ~ 30 lbs. overweight for 5' 4" person)

Obesity Trends* Among U.S. Adults
BRFSS, 2001
(*BMI ≥30, or ~ 30 lbs. overweight for 5' 4" person)

Prevalence* of Self-Reported Obesity** Among U.S. Adults
BRFSS, 2013
*prevalence reflects BRFSS methodological changes in 2011, and these estimates should not be compared to those before 2011. (**BMI ≥30, or ~ 30 lbs. overweight for 5' 4" person)

☐ No data ☐ <10% ☐ 10%–14% ☐ 15%–19% ☐ 20%–24% ☐ 25%–29% ☐ 30%–<35% ☐ ≥35%

FIGURE 7-1 ▲ Obesity trends among U.S. adults: 1991, 2001, 2013.
Source: CDC Behavioral Risk Factor Surveillance System (see Further Reading 3).

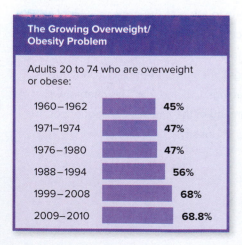

©Marty Bucella www.martybucella.com

"How many calories do you burn by downloading diet apps?"

▲ What components make up a successful weight-loss plan? What constitutes a "fad" diet? Why are overweight and obesity rates rising worldwide? What might be the future consequences of this trend? This chapter provides some answers. Reprinted with permission of Marty Bucella.

The Growing Overweight/Obesity Problem

Adults 20 to 74 who are overweight or obese:

Year	Percent
1960–1962	45%
1971–1974	47%
1976–1980	47%
1988–1994	56%
1999–2008	68%
2009–2010	68.8%

7.1 Energy Balance

We begin this chapter with both good and bad news. The good news is that if you stay at a healthy body weight, you increase your chances of living a long and healthy life. The bad news is that over 65% of all North American adults are overweight, significantly more than in the 1980s. Of those, about 50% (36% of the total population) are obese. There is a good chance that any of us could become part of those statistics if we do not pay attention to the prevention of significant weight gain in adulthood. Rapid weight gain (>10 pounds) signals that a reevaluation of lifestyle may be in order.

The prevalence and trends in obesity rates in the United States have been analyzed in several recent studies. One study estimated the prevalence of adult obesity and severe obesity through the year 2030 using statistical models of CDC obesity data. The study estimated a 33% increase in obesity prevalence and a 130% increase in severe obesity prevalence over the next two decades, with 51% of the population projected to be obese by 2030 if current trends continue. If obesity rates stop climbing and remain at current levels, the savings in medical expenditures over the next two decades would be over $549 billion (see Further Reading 5).

There is good news regarding our obesity trends as seen in two other studies. In the first, the prevalence of adult obesity in the United States was estimated from the 2009–2010 National Health and Nutrition Examination Survey (NHANES) and compared to adult obesity and body mass index (BMI) from earlier years of NHANES data. In 2011 to 2012, obesity rates were 33% among adult men and 36% among adult women, which was not a significant change since 2003 to 2008. These results suggest a slowing or leveling off of the obesity and BMI trends compared to increases observed between 1980 and 1999 (see Further Reading 7).

Because energy intake is a key determinant of weight, another study examined trends in energy intake using NHANES surveys from 1971–1975 to 2009–2010. They found that while energy intake increased from 1955 kcal per day during 1971–1975 to 2269 kcal per day during 2003–2004, it has declined more recently to 2195 kcal per day during 2009–2010. In fact, from 1999–2000 to 2009–2010, a downward trend in energy intake was observed (see Further Reading 7). These recent results suggest that the decrease in energy intakes over the past 10 years or more has had a minimal effect on slowing the obesity trend. There is no quick cure for overweight, despite what the advertisements claim. The most reliable and successful weight loss comes from hard work and commitment. A combination of decreased calorie intake, increased physical activity, and behavior modification is considered to be the most reliable treatment for the overweight condition. And without a doubt, the prevention of the overweight condition in the first place is the most successful approach.

POSITIVE AND NEGATIVE ENERGY BALANCE

A healthy weight can result from paying more attention to the important concept of **energy balance** (Fig. 7-2). Think of energy balance as an equation consisting of energy input and energy output:

> Energy input   Energy output
> (calories from food intake) = (metabolism; digestion, absorption, and transport
>   of nutrients; physical activity)

energy balance The state in which energy intake, in the form of food and beverages, matches the energy expended, primarily through basal metabolism and physical activity.

Intake	Output	Weight Change	Energy Balance
			Energy balance (equilibriuim) — Calories in / Calories out
3000 kcal	3000 kcal	No change	
			Positive energy balance — Calories in / Calories out
4000 kcal	2000 kcal	Increase	
			Negative energy balance — Calories in / Calories out
2000 kcal	3000 kcal	Decrease	

FIGURE 7-2 ▲ A model for energy balance: Intake versus output. This figure depicts energy balance in practical terms.

positive energy balance The state in which energy intake is greater than energy expended, generally resulting in weight gain.

negative energy balance The state in which energy intake is less than energy expended, resulting in weight loss.

bomb calorimeter An instrument used to determine the calorie content of a food.

Thermometer

Ignite food

Insulation around chamber

Oxygen-filled chamber for food

Air space

Water

FIGURE 7-3 ▲ Bomb calorimeters measure calorie content by igniting and burning a dried portion of food. The burning food raises the temperature of the water surrounding the chamber holding the food. The increase in water temperature indicates the number of calories in the food because 1 kcal equals the amount of heat needed to raise the temperature of 1 kilogram of water by 1 degree Celsius.

The balance of calories (measured in kilocalories) on the two sides of this equation can influence energy stores, especially the amount of triglyceride stored in adipose tissue. When energy input is greater than energy output, the result is **positive energy balance.** The excess calories consumed are stored, which results in weight gain. There are some situations in which positive energy balance is normal and healthy. During pregnancy, a surplus of calories supports the developing fetus. Infants and children require a positive energy balance for normal growth and development. In adults, however, even a small positive energy balance is usually in the form of fat storage rather than muscle and bone and, over time, can cause body weight to climb.

On the other hand, if energy input is less than energy output, there is a calorie deficit and **negative energy balance** results. A negative energy balance is necessary for successful weight loss. It is important to realize that when we lose weight, we lose some lean tissue in addition to adipose tissue.

The maintenance of energy balance substantially contributes to optimal health and well-being in adults by minimizing the risk of developing many common health problems associated with overweight and obesity. Adulthood is often a time of subtle weight gain over time, which eventually turns into obesity and a greater risk of disease if left unchecked. Aging does not directly cause weight gain; rather the problem stems from a pattern of excess energy intake coupled with limited physical activity and slower metabolism. Let us look in detail at the factors that affect the energy balance equation.

ENERGY INTAKE

Energy needs are met by dietary intake, represented by the number of calories consumed each day. Determining the appropriate amount and type of food to match our energy needs is a challenge for many of us. Our desire to consume food and the ability of our bodies to use it efficiently are survival mechanisms that have evolved with humans. However, because of current North American food supplies and accessibility, many of us are now too successful in obtaining excessive energy. The abundance of food and high-calorie beverages lead to overconsumption and excess stores of body fat. Given the cheap cost and wide availability of palatable food in vending machines, drive-through windows, social gatherings, and fast-food restaurants—combined with *supersized* portions—it is no wonder that the average adult is 8 pounds heavier than just 10 years ago. In response to this cultural trend of food being widely available, "defensive eating" (i.e., making careful and conscious food choices, especially in regard to portion size) on a continual basis is important for many of us.

The number of calories in a food is determined with an instrument called a **bomb calorimeter.** This calorie determination is shown in Figure 7-3. The bomb calorimeter measures the amount of calories (kilocalories) coming from carbohydrate, fat, protein, and alcohol. Recall that carbohydrates and proteins each yield about 4 kcal per gram, fats yield about 9 kcal per gram, and alcohol yields 7 kcal per gram. These energy figures have been adjusted for (1) our ability to digest the food; and (2) substances in food, such as fibrous plant parts, that burn in the bomb calorimeter but are not absorbed and do not provide calories to the human body. The figures are then rounded to whole numbers. However, today it is also possible and more common to determine the calorie content of a food by quantifying its carbohydrate, protein, and fat (and possibly alcohol) content from the food label. Then the calories per gram are used to calculate the total calories. (Recall that Section 1.4 showed how to do this calculation.)

ENERGY OUTPUT

So far, some factors concerning energy intake have been discussed. Now let us look at the other side of the equation: energy output.

The body uses energy for three general purposes: (1) basal metabolism; (2) physical activity; and (3) digestion, absorption, and processing of ingested nutrients. A fourth minor form of energy output, known as adaptive thermogenesis, refers to energy expended during fidgeting or shivering in response to cold (Fig. 7-4).

FIGURE 7-4 ▲ The components of energy intake and expenditure. This figure incorporates the major variables that influence energy balance. *Remember that alcohol is an additional source of energy.* The size of each component shows the relative contribution of that component to energy balance.

Basal Metabolism. **Basal metabolism** is expressed as basal metabolic rate (BMR) and represents the minimal amount of calories expended in a fasting state to keep a resting, awake body alive in a warm, quiet environment. For a sedentary person, basal metabolism accounts for about 60% to 75% of total energy use by the body. Some of the processes that utilize energy include the beating of the heart, respiration by the lungs, and the activity of other organs such as the liver, brain, and kidney. It does not include energy used for physical activity or digestion, absorption, and processing of recently consumed nutrients. If the person is not fasting or completely rested, the term **resting metabolism** is used and expressed as resting metabolic rate (RMR). An individual's RMR is typically higher than his or her BMR.

basal metabolism The minimal amount of calories the body uses to support itself in a fasting state when resting and awake in a warm, quiet environment. It amounts to roughly 1 kcal per kilogram per hour for men and 0.9 kcal per kilogram per hour for women; these values are often referred to as *basal metabolic rate (BMR)*.

resting metabolism The amount of calories the body uses when the person has not eaten in 4 hours and is resting (e.g., 15 to 30 minutes) and awake in a warm, quiet environment. It is usually slightly higher (10%) than basal metabolism due to the less strict criteria for the test; often referred to as *resting metabolic rate (RMR)*.

To see how basal metabolism contributes to energy needs, consider a 130-pound woman. First, knowing that there are 2.2 pounds (lb) for every kilogram (kg), convert her weight into metric units:

$$130 \text{ lb} \div 2.2 \text{ lb/kg} = 59 \text{ kg}$$

Then, using a rough estimate of BMR of 0.9 kcal per kilogram per hour for an average female (1 kcal per kilogram per hour is used for an average male), calculate her BMR:

$$59 \text{ kg} \times 0.9 \text{ kcal/kg} = 53 \text{ kcal/hr}$$

Finally, use this hourly BMR to find her BMR for an entire day:

$$53 \text{ kcal/hr} \times 24 \text{ hr} = 1272 \text{ kcal/day}$$

These calculations provide an estimate of basal metabolism, as it can vary as much as 25% to 30% among individuals. Factors that increase basal metabolism include:

- Greater **lean body mass**
- Larger body surface area per body volume (e.g., for a given weight, a tall person has greater body surface area compared to a short person)

lean body mass Body weight minus fat storage weight equals lean body mass. This includes organs such as the brain, muscles, and liver, as well as bone and blood and other body fluids.

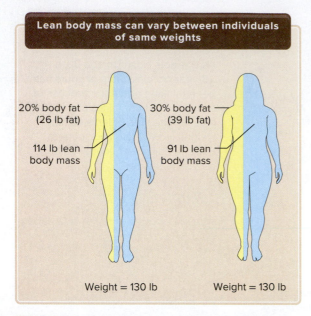

Lean body mass can vary between individuals of same weights

20% body fat
(26 lb fat)

114 lb lean
body mass

30% body fat
(39 lb fat)

91 lb lean
body mass

Weight = 130 lb   Weight = 130 lb

FIGURE 7-5 ▲ Lean body mass (LBM), the most important determinant of the basal metabolic rate, varies greatly between individuals. Persons of the same body weight can have different amounts of LBM and body fat and, therefore, have varying energy needs.

- Male gender (caused by greater lean body mass)
- Body temperature (fever or cold environmental conditions)
- Thyroid hormones (elevated or hyperthyroid condition)
- Stress (release of norepinephrine)
- Pregnancy
- Caffeine and tobacco use (Using the practice of smoking to control body weight is not recommended as too many health risks are increased.)

Of those factors, the amount of lean body mass a person has is the most important one. Persons with higher amounts of lean body mass have a higher BMR because lean tissue is more metabolically active than fat. The lean tissue, therefore, requires more energy to support its activity. Although overweight and obese persons have an increased amount of body fat, they also typically have a high amount of lean body mass and therefore a high BMR to go along with it (Fig. 7-5).

In contrast to factors that increase basal metabolism, a low calorie intake, such as an extreme diet regime, decreases basal metabolism by about 10% to 20% (about 150 to 300 kcal per day) as the body shifts into a conservation mode. This is a barrier to sustained weight loss during dieting that involves extremely low calorie diets. In addition, the effects of aging make weight maintenance a challenge. As lean body mass slowly and steadily decreases, basal metabolism declines 1% to 2% for each decade past the age of 30. However, because physical activity aids in maintenance of lean body mass, remaining active as one ages helps to preserve a higher basal metabolism and, in turn, aids in weight control.

Energy for Physical Activity. Physical activity increases energy expenditure above and beyond basal energy needs by as much as 15% to 35%. In choosing to be active or inactive, we determine much of our total calorie expenditure for a day. Calorie expenditure from physical activity varies widely among people. For example, climbing stairs rather than riding the elevator, walking rather than driving to class, and standing at a workstation rather than sitting all increase physical activity and, hence, energy use. The alarming incidence of and recent increase in obesity in North America are partially the result of our inactivity and sedentary lifestyles. Jobs demand less physical activity, and leisure time is often spent in front of a television or computer screen.

thermic effect of food (TEF) The increase in metabolism that occurs during the digestion, absorption, and metabolism of energy-yielding nutrients. This represents 5% to 10% of calories consumed.

Thermic Effect of Food In addition to basal metabolism and physical activity, the body uses energy to digest food, and absorb and further process the nutrients recently consumed. Energy used for these tasks is referred to as the **thermic effect of food (TEF).** TEF is similar to a sales tax; it is like being charged about 5% to 10% for the total amount of calories you eat to cover the cost of processing that food eaten. We may even recognize this increase in metabolism as a warming of the body during and right after a meal. Because of this "tax," you must eat between 5 and 10 kcal extra for every 100 kcal needed for basal metabolism and physical activity. If your daily calorie intake was 3000 kcal, for example, TEF would account for 150 to 300 kcal. As with other components of energy output, the total amount can vary somewhat among individuals.

Food composition influences TEF. For example, the TEF value for a protein-rich meal is 20% to 30% of the calories consumed and is higher than that of a carbohydrate-rich (5% to 10%) or fat-rich (0% to 3%) meal. Lean protein foods such as chicken breast, egg whites, and white fish have the highest TEF at almost 30%. This means that if you eat 100 kcal of chicken breast, almost 30 of those calories are burned off just to digest it. This is because it takes more energy to metabolize amino acids (from protein sources) into fat than to convert glucose (from carbohydrate sources) into glycogen or transfer absorbed fat into adipose stores. In addition, large meals result in higher TEF values than the same amount of food eaten over many hours. The TEF value for alcohol is approximately 20%.

While a person (130-pound woman) is resting, the percentage of total energy use and corresponding energy use by various organs are approximately as follows:

Brain	19%	242 kcal/day
Skeletal muscle	18%	229 kcal/day
Liver	27%	343 kcal/day
Kidney	10%	127 kcal/day
Heart	7%	89 kcal/day
Other	19%	242 kcal/day
Total	100%	1272 kcal/day

Adaptive Thermogenesis **Adaptive thermogenesis** represents the increase in nonvoluntary physical activity triggered by cold conditions or overeating. Some examples of nonvoluntary activities include shivering when cold, fidgeting, maintenance of muscle tone, and maintaining body posture when not lying down. Studies have shown that some people are able to resist weight gain from overfeeding by inducing thermogenesis, whereas, to a great extent, others are not.

The contribution of thermogenesis to overall calorie output is fairly small. The combination of basal metabolism and TEF accounts for 70% to 85% of energy used by a sedentary person. The remaining 15% to 30% is used mostly for physical activity, with a small amount used for thermogenesis.

Brown adipose tissue is a specialized form of adipose tissue that participates in thermogenesis. The brown appearance results from its greater number of mitochondria. Brown adipose tissue contributes to thermogenesis by releasing some of the energy from energy-yielding nutrients into the environment as heat instead of producing ATP. Hibernating animals use brown adipose tissue to generate heat to withstand a long winter. In infants, brown adipose tissue is metabolically active and contributes as much as 5% of body weight and regulates heat to protect internal organs. Adults have very little brown adipose tissue, and its role in adulthood remains unknown.

▲ A few foods, such as celery, have been hypothesized to use more calories for TEF than they contain, making them negative calorie foods. Despite its recurring popularity in fad diet plans, there is no scientific evidence supporting the idea that any food is calorically negative. Although these foods still yield some calories, they remain excellent choices to include in a weight-loss plan because they have such low energy density. © Ingram Publishing

adaptive thermogenesis This term encompasses the ability of humans to regulate body temperature within narrow limits (thermoregulation). Two visible examples of thermogenesis are fidgeting and shivering when cold.

brown adipose tissue A specialized form of adipose (fat) tissue that produces large amounts of heat by metabolizing energy-yielding nutrients without synthesizing much useful energy for the body. The unused energy is released as heat.

✓ CONCEPT CHECK 7.1

1. What are the main components of energy balance?
2. How is the energy content of food determined and expressed?
3. What are the four main purposes for which the body uses energy? Approximately how much does each component contribute to overall energy use by the body?

7.2 Determination of Energy Use by the Body

The amount of energy a body uses can be measured by both direct and indirect calorimetry or can be estimated based on height, weight, degree of physical activity, and age.

DIRECT AND INDIRECT CALORIMETRY

Direct calorimetry measures the amount of body heat released by a person. The person is put into an insulated metabolic chamber, often the size of a small bedroom, and body heat released raises the temperature of a layer of water surrounding the chamber. A calorie (kilocalorie), as you recall, is related to the amount of heat required to raise the temperature of water. By measuring the water temperature in the direct calorimeter before and after the body releases heat, the energy expended can be calculated. Direct calorimetry works because almost all the energy used by the body eventually leaves as heat. However, because of its expense and complexity, direct calorimetry is rarely used.

The most commonly used method of **indirect calorimetry** measures the respiratory gas exchange, which is the amount of oxygen a person consumes and the amount of carbon dioxide he or she expels (Fig. 7-6). A predictable relationship exists between the body's use of energy and oxygen. For example, when metabolizing a typical mixed diet of the energy-yielding nutrients (carbohydrate, fat, and protein), the human body uses 1 liter of oxygen to yield about 4.85 kcal of energy.

Instruments to measure oxygen consumption for indirect calorimetry are widely used. They can be mounted on carts (metabolic carts) and rolled up to a hospital bed or carried in

▲ The cultural trend of serving large quantities of high-calorie foods can easily lead to positive energy balance. Sharing your meal with another person is a good way to avoid overeating when served large portions. © Mitch Hrdlicka/Getty Images

direct calorimetry A method of determining a body's energy use by measuring heat released from the body. An insulated chamber is typically used.

indirect calorimetry A method to measure energy use by the body by measuring oxygen uptake and carbon dioxide output. Formulas are then used to convert this gas exchange value into energy use, estimating the proportion of energy nutrients that are being oxidized for energy in the fuel mix.

FIGURE 7-6 ▲ Indirect calorimetry measures oxygen intake and carbon dioxide output from respirations to determine energy expended during activities.
© Samuel Ashfield/SPL/Science Source

a backpack while a person engages in physical activity to measure how many calories are burned during these activities. There are even portable handheld instruments to estimate indirect calorimetry. Tables presenting energy costs of various forms of exercises rely on information gained from indirect calorimetry studies. You will also see an estimation of calories burned during a workout on most exercise equipment. The accuracy of these values is discussed in Section 7.7.

ESTIMATES OF ENERGY NEEDS

As covered in Section 2.6, the Food and Nutrition Board has published a number of formulas to estimate energy needs, referred to as Estimated Energy Requirements (EER). Those for adults are shown here. As you calculate your own EER, remember to do multiplication and division before addition and subtraction! (Specific information regarding energy needs for pregnant women, lactating women, and children is covered in Sections 18.4, 18.7 and Section 19.2.) The calories used for basal metabolism are already factored into these formulas.

The variables in the formulas correspond to the following:

$$EER = \text{Estimated Energy Requirement}$$
$$AGE = \text{age in years}$$
$$PA = \text{physical activity estimate (see following table)}$$
$$WT = \text{weight in kilograms (pounds divided by 2.2)}$$
$$HT = \text{height in meters (inches divided by 39.4)}$$

Estimated Energy Requirement Calculation for Men 19 Years and Older:

$$EER = 662 - (9.53 \times AGE) + PA \times (15.91 \times WT + 539.6 \times HT)$$

Estimated Energy Requirement Calculation for Women 19 Years and Older:

$$EER = 354 - (6.91 \times AGE) + PA \times (9.36 \times WT + 726 \times HT)$$

Physical Activity (PA) Estimates

Activity Level	PA (Men)	PA (Women)
Sedentary (e.g., no exercise)	1.00	1.00
Low activity (e.g., walks the equivalent of 2 miles per day at 3 to 4 mph)	1.11	1.12
Active (e.g., walks the equivalent of 7 miles per day at 3 to 4 mph)	1.25	1.27
Very active (e.g., walks the equivalent of 17 miles per day at 3 to 4 mph)	1.48	1.45

The following is a sample calculation for a man who is 25 years old, 5 feet 9 inches (1.75 meters), 154 pounds (70 kilograms), and has an active lifestyle. His EER is as follows:

$$EER = 662 - (9.53 \times 25) + 1.25 \times (15.91 \times 70 + 539.6 \times 1.75) = 2997 \text{ kcal}$$

The next equation is a sample calculation for a woman who is 25 years old, 5 feet 4 inches (1.62 meters), 120 pounds (54.5 kilograms), and has an active lifestyle. Her EER is as follows:

$$EER = 354 - (6.91 \times 25) + 1.27 \times (9.36 \times 54.5 + 726 \times 1.62) = 2323 \text{ kcal}$$

Track Your Energy Needs

Use the forms in Appendix C to track your energy expenditure and estimate your energy needs. List all of your activities for a 24-hour period. Record the number of minutes spent in each activity to total 1440 minutes (24 hours in a day). Record the energy cost, in calories, for each activity and multiply the energy cost by the minutes to obtain the energy expended for each activity. Total all the calorie values for your estimated energy expenditure for the day.

You have determined the man's EER to be about 3000 kcal and the woman's EER to be about 2300 kcal per day. Remember that this is only an estimate; many other factors, such as genetics and hormones, can affect actual energy needs.

The www.ChooseMyPlate.gov website provides an interactive tool to estimate your calorie needs called Daily Food Plan. Figure 7-7 shows the range of activity levels and calorie recommendations for age and gender groups.

✓ CONCEPT CHECK 7.2

1. What methods can be used to measure energy use by the body?
2. Estimated Energy Requirement (EER) can be calculated based on which five factors?

7.3 Assessing Healthy Body Weight

Numerous methods are used to establish what body weight should be, typically called *healthy weight*. Healthy weight is currently the preferred term to use when describing a weight associated with optimal health. Older terms, such as *ideal weight* and *desirable body weight*, are subjective and are no longer used in the literature. Several tables exist, generally based on weight-for-height criteria. These tables arose from studies of large population groups. When applied to a population, they provide good estimates of weight associated with health and longevity; however, they do not necessarily indicate the healthiest body weight for each individual. For example, *athletes with more lean muscle mass but low fat mass will often have higher body weights than sedentary individuals.*

Listening to the body's hunger cues, regularly eating a balanced and healthy dietary pattern, and remaining physically active are all positive behaviors that help one maintain an appropriate height/weight value over time. Healthy body weight is based upon both personal and individual factors. Body weight must be considered in terms of overall health, not a mathematical calculation. Under the guidance of a clinician, an individual should establish a "personal" healthy weight based on weight history, body fat distribution patterns, physical activity, dietary habits, family history of obesity, and current health status. Indications that your weight may be unhealthy include the following weight-related conditions:

- Hypertension
- Elevated non-HDL cholesterol
- Family history of obesity, cardiovascular disease, or certain cancers
- Pattern of upper-body (apple) fat distribution
- Elevated blood glucose

These criteria and current height/weight standards serve only as a rough guide. On a more practical note, other questions can be pertinent: What is the least one has weighed as an adult for at least one year? What weight has one been able to maintain during previous diets without feeling constantly hungry? A healthy lifestyle may make a more important contribution to a person's health status than the number on the scale. Being fit and overweight are not necessarily mutually exclusive, and neither is thin synonymous with healthy if the person is not also physically active.

BODY MASS INDEX

Currently, **body mass index (BMI)** is the most widely used weight-for-height standard because it is a noninvasive clinical measurement closely related to body fat content for most individuals (Fig. 7-8).

MyPlate Calorie Guidelines		
Children	**Sedentary** ⟶	**Active**
2–3 years	1000 ⟶	1400
Females	**Sedentary** ⟶	**Active**
4–8 years	1200 ⟶	1800
9–13	1400 ⟶	2200
14–18	1800 ⟶	2400
19–30	1800 ⟶	2400
31–50	1800 ⟶	2200
51+	1600 ⟶	2200
Males	**Sedentary** ⟶	**Active**
4–8 years	1200 ⟶	2000
9–13	1600 ⟶	2600
14–18	2000 ⟶	3200
19–30	2400 ⟶	3000
31–50	2200 ⟶	3000
51+	2000 ⟶	2800

FIGURE 7-7 ▲ MyPlate Calorie Guidelines for age and gender.

▲ Physical activity, such as walking, is an important component of our energy expenditure. © Ronnie Kaufman/Blend Images LLC

body mass index (BMI) Weight (in kilograms) divided by height (in meters) squared; a value of 25 and above indicates overweight and a value of 30 and above indicates obesity.

Women Men

BMI 20

BMI 25

BMI 30 +

FIGURE 7-8 ▲ Estimates of body shapes at different BMI values.

Body mass index is calculated as $\dfrac{\text{body weight (in kilograms)}}{\text{height}^2 \text{ (in meters)}}$

An alternate method for calculating BMI is $\dfrac{\text{weight (pounds)} \times 703}{\text{height}^2 \text{ (inches)}}$

BMI weight categories are shown in Table 7-1. A healthy weight for height is defined by a BMI between 18.5 and 24.9. Health risks from excess weight may begin when the BMI is 25 or more. These are general cutoff values for the presence of overweight and obesity, respectively. What is your BMI? How much would your weight need to change to yield a BMI of 25? or 30? Figure 7-9 lists the BMI for various heights and weights.

The concept of BMI is convenient to use because the values apply to both men and women (i.e., gender neutral). However, any weight-for-height standard remains a crude measure. Keep in mind that a BMI of 25 to 29.9 is a marker of *overweight* (compared to a standard population) and not necessarily a marker of excessive body fatness. Many men (especially athletes) have a BMI greater than 25 because of extra muscle mass. Also, very short adults (under 5 feet tall) may have a high BMI that may not necessarily reflect overweight or fatness. For this reason, BMI should be used only as a screening tool for overweight or obesity. Adult BMIs should not be applied to children, growing adolescents, frail older adults, pregnant and lactating women, and highly muscular individuals. Pregnant women and children have unique BMI standards (see Section 18.4 and Section 19.1).

Still, overfat and overweight conditions generally appear together. The focus is on BMI in clinical settings mainly because this is much easier and cheaper to measure than total body fat.

ESTIMATING BODY FAT CONTENT AND DIAGNOSING OBESITY

If calorie intake exceeds output over time, overweight (and often obesity) is a likely result. Often, obesity-related health problems eventually follow (Table 7-2) (see Further Reading 16). As mentioned, BMI values can be used as a convenient clinical tool to screen for overweight (BMI ≥ 25), obesity (BMI ≥ 30), and severe obesity (BMI ≥ 40) in individuals older than 20 years of age. Medical experts, however, recommend that an individual's diagnosis of obesity should not be based primarily on body weight but rather on the total amount of fat in the body, the location of body fat, and the presence or absence of weight-related medical conditions.

Body fat varies widely among individuals. Good to acceptable amounts of body fat are about 11% to 20% for men and 16% to 30% for women. Men with over 24% body fat and women with over 37% body fat are considered obese. The higher range of body fat percentage

◄ A high BMI may not reflect overweight or fatness. Extra muscle mass can result in a BMI >25. © McGraw-Hill Education

TABLE 7-1 ■ **Body mass index categories.**

Category	BMI
Underweight	< 18.5
Healthy weight	18.5–24.9
Overweight	25–29.9
Obese	30–39.9
Severely (morbidly) obese	≥ 40

BMI is a useful measure of weight-for-height standards and estimated body fat. It is a good gauge of risk for diseases associated with body fat.

TABLE 7-2 ■ Health Problems Associated with Excess Body Fat

Health Problem	Potentially Attributable To:
Surgical complications	Increased anesthesia needs; greater risk of wound infections (decrease in immune function)
Pulmonary disease and sleep disorders	Excess weight stressing the lungs and pharynx
Type 2 diabetes	Enlarged adipose (fat) cells poorly bind insulin and inadequately respond to insulin signals; reduced synthesis of factors that promote insulin action and increased synthesis of factors that counter insulin action
Hypertension	Increased miles of blood vessels found in the adipose tissue, increased blood volume, and increased resistance to blood flow related to hormones made by adipose cells
Cardiovascular disease (e.g., coronary heart disease and stroke)	Increased LDL cholesterol and triglycerides; reduced HDL cholesterol; increased synthesis of blood clotting and inflammatory factors by enlarged adipose cells; potential for altered heart rhythm
Bone and joint disorders (including gout)	Excess pressure placed on knees, ankles, and hip joints
Gallstones	Increased cholesterol content of bile
Skin disorders	Accumulation and trapping of moisture and microorganisms in tissue folds
Various cancers	Estrogen and other hormones contribute to tumor growth by adipose cells; increased hyperinsulinemia or insulin resistance; systemic inflammation associated with cancer risk; excess calorie intake may encourage tumor development (animal studies)
Shorter stature (in some forms of obesity)	Earlier onset of puberty
Pregnancy risks	More difficult delivery; increased birth defects and gestational diabetes; greater anesthesia needs
Reduced physical agility and increased risk of accidents and falls	Excess weight impairs physical movement and gait
Menstrual irregularities and infertility	Hormone imbalances; insulin resistance; increased oxidative stress
Vision problems	Higher rates of cataracts and other eye disorders
Premature death	Comorbidities and greater risk factors for numerous chronic diseases and complications
Infections	Reduced immune system activity
Liver damage and eventual failure	Excess fat accumulation in the liver (fatty liver)
Erectile dysfunction in men	Low-grade inflammation caused by reduced function of the cells lining the blood vessels and impaired blood circulation

The greater the degree of obesity, the more likely and the more serious these health problems generally become. They are much more likely to appear in people who show an upper-body fat distribution pattern and/or are greater than twice their healthy body weight.

for women is needed physiologically to maintain reproductive functions, including estrogen production.

To measure body fat content accurately using typical methods, both body weight and body volume of the person are used to calculate body density. Body weight is easy to measure on a conventional scale. Of the typical methods used to estimate body volume, **underwater weighing** remains the most accurate. This technique determines body volume using the difference between conventional body weight and body weight measured under water, along with the relative densities of fat tissue and lean tissue, using a mathematical formula. This procedure requires that an individual be totally submerged in a tank of water, with a trained technician directing the procedure (Fig. 7-10). **Air displacement** is another method of determining body volume. Body volume is quantified by measuring the space a person takes up inside a measurement chamber, such as the BodPod (Fig. 7-11).

underwater weighing Also known as hydrostatic weighing, this is a method of estimating total body fat by weighing the individual on a standard scale and then weighing him or her again submerged in water. The difference between the two weights is used to estimate total body volume.

air displacement A method for estimating body composition that makes use of the volume of space taken up by a body inside a small chamber. This tool is also known as air displacement plethysmography.

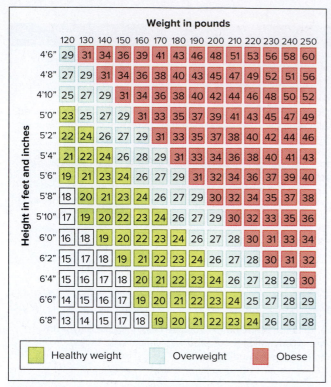

Weight in pounds

Height	120	130	140	150	160	170	180	190	200	210	220	230	240	250
4'6"	29	31	34	36	39	41	43	46	48	51	53	56	58	60
4'8"	27	29	31	34	36	38	40	43	45	47	49	52	51	56
4'10"	25	27	29	31	34	36	38	40	42	44	46	48	50	52
5'0"	23	25	27	29	31	33	35	37	39	41	43	45	47	49
5'2"	22	24	26	27	29	31	33	35	37	38	40	42	44	46
5'4"	21	22	24	26	28	29	31	33	34	36	38	40	41	43
5'6"	19	21	23	24	26	27	29	31	32	34	36	37	39	40
5'8"	18	20	21	23	24	26	27	29	30	32	34	35	37	38
5'10"	17	19	20	22	23	24	26	27	29	30	32	33	35	36
6'0"	16	18	19	20	22	23	24	26	27	28	30	31	33	34
6'2"	15	17	18	19	21	22	23	24	26	27	28	30	31	32
6'4"	15	16	17	18	20	21	22	23	24	26	27	28	29	30
6'6"	14	15	16	17	19	20	21	22	23	24	25	27	28	29
6'8"	13	14	15	17	18	19	20	21	22	23	24	26	26	28

Height in feet and inches

🟩 Healthy weight   ⬜ Overweight   🟥 Obese

Developed by the National Center for Health Statistics in collaboration with the National Center for Chronic Disease Prevention and Health Promotion

FIGURE 7-9 ▲ Convenient height/weight table based on BMI. A healthy weight for height generally falls within a BMI range of 18.5 to 24.9 kg/m² (shown in green).

bioelectrical impedance The method to estimate total body fat that uses a low-energy electrical current. The more fat storage a person has, the more impedance (resistance) to electrical flow will be exhibited.

dual energy X-ray absorptiometry (DEXA) A scientific tool used to measure bone mineral density.

The total annual cost attributable to obesity-related disease is about $200 billion in the United States. This is double what it was nearly a decade ago. At least half of this cost is supported by the taxpayers, who fund Medicare and Medicaid.

upper-body obesity The type of obesity in which fat is stored primarily in the abdominal area; defined as a waist circumference more than 40 inches (102 centimeters) in men and more than 35 inches (88 centimeters) in women; closely associated with a high risk for cardiovascular disease, hypertension, and type 2 diabetes. Also known as android obesity.

Once body volume is known, it can be used along with body weight in the following equation to calculate body density. Then using body density, body fat content finally can be determined.

$$\text{Body density} = \frac{\text{body weight}}{\text{body volume}}$$

$$\% \text{ body fat} = (495 \div \text{body density}) - 450$$

For example, assume that the individual in the underwater weighing tank in Figure 7-10 has a body density of 1.06 grams per cubic centimeter. We can use the second formula to calculate that she has 17% body fat ([495 ÷ 1.06] − 450 = 17).

Skinfold thickness measurements are also a common anthropometric method to estimate total body fat content, although there are some limits to its accuracy. Clinicians use calipers to measure the fat layer directly under the skin at multiple sites and then plug these values into a mathematical formula (Fig. 7-12).

The analysis of **bioelectrical impedance** is also used to estimate body fat content. The instrument sends a painless, low-energy electrical current through the body via wires and electrode patches to estimate body fat. This estimation is based on the assumption that adipose tissue resists electrical flow more than lean tissue because it has a lower electrolyte and water content than lean tissue. More adipose tissue has proportionately greater electrical resistance. Within a few seconds, bioelectrical impedance analyzers convert body electrical resistance into an approximate estimate of total body fat, as long as body hydration status is normal (Fig. 7-13). Body composition monitors, better known as body fat calculators, which use bioelectric impedance, are now available for home use. These machines are similar in shape and use to bathroom scales, but their main purpose is to measure body fat. An electrical current passes easily through conductive foot pads and/or handheld electrodes. These in-home devices will hopefully encourage individuals to be less concerned with what they weigh than whether their weight comes from fat or muscle.

A more advanced determination of body fat content can be made using **dual energy X-ray absorptiometry (DEXA).** DEXA is considered the most accurate way to determine body fat, but the equipment is expensive and not widely available. This X-ray system allows the clinician to separate body weight into separate components: fat, fat-free soft tissue, and bone mineral. Additional software can be used to determine body fat distribution. The usual whole-body scan requires about 10 to 25 minutes, and the dose of radiation is less than a chest X ray. An assessment of bone mineral density and the risk of osteoporosis can also be made using this method (Fig. 7-14).

There are a few other methods of assessing body composition, but those listed are the ones you are most likely to encounter in health clinics, fitness centers, and research articles referenced in this book. In the hands of a trained clinician, these assessments provide valuable information about body fat beyond simple measures of height and weight.

USING BODY FAT DISTRIBUTION TO FURTHER EVALUATE OBESITY

In addition to the amount of fat we store, the location of that body fat is an important predictor of health risks. Some people store fat in upper-body areas, whereas others store fat lower on the body. **Upper-body obesity,** characterized by a large abdomen or waist, is more often called *abdominal* or *central* obesity and is related to insulin resistance and fatty liver leading to diabetes, high blood lipids, and heart disease. Because men more

FIGURE 7-10 ◄ Underwater weighing. In this technique, the subject exhales as much air as possible and then holds his or her breath and bends at the waist to become totally submerged. Once submerged, the underwater weight is recorded. Using this value, body volume can be calculated. © David Madison/Getty Images

FIGURE 7-11 ► BodPod. This device determines body volume based on the volume of displaced air, measured as a person sits in a sealed chamber. © BOD POD® Body Composition Tracking System photo provided courtesy of COSMED USA, Inc.

Fat

Caliper

Triceps brachii muscle

Skin

Bone

FIGURE 7-12 ◄ Skinfold measurements. With proper technique and calibrated equipment, skinfold measurements taken at various sites around the body can be used to predict body fat content in about 10 minutes. Measurements are made at several locations, including the triceps (pictured here). © Tamara Lackey/fstop/Corbis

FIGURE 7-13 ▲ Bioelectrical impedance estimates total body fat in less than 5 minutes and is based on the principle that body fat resists the flow of electricity, since it is low in water and electrolytes. The degree of resistance to electrical flow is used to estimate body fatness. This handheld device sends an electrical current through the body and gives a percentage of body fat when it has completed its process.

FIGURE 7-14 ► Dual energy X-ray absorptiometry (DEXA). This method measures body fat by passing small doses of radiation through the body. The radiation reacts differently with fat, lean tissue, or bone, allowing these components to be quantified. The scanner arm moves from head to toe and in doing so can determine body fat and bone density. DEXA is currently considered the most accurate method for determining body fat (as long as the person can fit under the arm of the instrument). The radiation dose is minimal. © Science Photo Library/Alamy

Upper-body fat
distribution
(android: apple shape)

Lower-body fat
distribution
(gynoid: pear shape)

FIGURE 7-15 ▲ Body fat stored primarily in the upper body (android) brings higher risks of obesity-related diseases than lower-body (gynoid) obesity. Here, the woman's waist circumference of 32 inches and the man's waist circumference of 44 inches indicate that the man has upper-body fat distribution but the woman does not, based on the risk factors of 35 inches for women and 40 inches for men.

lower-body obesity The type of obesity in which fat storage is primarily located in the buttocks and thigh area. Also known as gynoid or gynecoid obesity.

▲ Waist circumference is an important measure of weight-related health risk.
© Science Photo Library/Alamy

typically develop upper-body obesity, it is also known as *android* obesity. While other adipose cells empty fat into general blood circulation, the fat released from abdominal adipose cells goes directly to the liver, by way of the portal vein. This influx of fat interferes with the liver's ability to use insulin and negatively affects lipoprotein metabolism by the liver. These abdominal adipose cells are not just storage depots; they are metabolically active and release many hormones and other peptides, called adipokines, involved in long-term energy regulation. When they fill with excess fat, the cells become dysfunctional and release altered secretions, resulting in inflammation, insulin resistance, and other adverse health conditions leading to chronic disease.

High blood testosterone levels encourage upper-body obesity, as does excessive alcohol intake, and smoking. This pattern of fat storage is commonly known as the apple shape (large abdomen and small buttocks and thighs). Upper-body obesity is assessed by measuring the circumference of the abdomen at the waist. A waist circumference more than 40 inches (102 centimeters) in men and more than 35 inches (88 centimeters) in women indicates risk for upper-body obesity (Fig. 7-15). If BMI is also 25 or more, health risks are significantly increased.

Estrogen and progesterone encourage **lower-body (gynoid) obesity**—the typical female pattern. The small abdomen and much larger buttocks and thighs give a pearlike appearance. Fat deposited in the lower body is not mobilized as easily as the other type and often resists being released. After menopause, blood estrogen levels fall, encouraging greater upper-body fat distribution and raising the risk of chronic disease dramatically for postmenopausal females.

✓ CONCEPT CHECK 7.3

1. How is body mass index determined?
2. What are the BMI, body fat percentage, and waist circumference values for men and women that are associated with increased risk of health problems related to being overweight?
3. What are five methods by which body fat content can be estimated?
4. Obesity leads to an increased risk of which diseases?

7.4 Why Some People Are Obese—Nature Versus Nurture

The energy imbalance that promotes obesity stems from cultural, economic, and social factors (see Further Reading 6). Many studies of obesity attribute the increasing trends to the growth of the global food system, including advancements in energy-dense food processing, marketing, and the widespread availability of more affordable energy-dense foods.

Both genetic (nature) and environmental (nurture) factors can increase the risk for obesity (Table 7-3). The location of fat storage is strongly influenced by genetics. For example, research studies have found that offspring born to obese mothers are at heightened risk of obesity later in life. Consider the possibility that obesity is nurture allowing nature to express itself. Some obese people begin life with a slower basal metabolism, maintain a sedentary lifestyle, and consume highly refined, calorie-dense diets. These people are nurtured into gaining weight, promoting their natural genetic predisposition toward obesity. Even with a genetic tendency toward obesity, individuals can attain a healthier body weight by engaging in positive lifestyle behaviors with increased physical activity and decreased calorie consumption.

TABLE 7-3 ■ What Encourages Excess Body Fat Stores and Obesity?

Factor	How Fat Storage Is Affected
Age	Excess body fat is more common in adults and middle-age individuals due to loss of lean body mass and reduction in physical activity.
Menopause	Hormonal changes result in increased abdominal fat deposition.
Gender	Females have more fat mass than males due to less lean body mass and reduced surface area.
Energy balance	Over a long period, dietary patterns consistent with positive energy balance promote storage of excess body fat.
Dietary consumption	Excess calorie intake from saturated fat, alcohol, and calorie-dense foods and beverages contribute to obesity.
Physical activity	Sedentary behavior leads to positive energy balance and promotes body fat storage.
Basal metabolism	A low BMR due to factors such as thyroid problems or energy restriction is linked to weight gain.
Thermic effect of food	Some obese individuals metabolize nutrients more efficiently, and thus expend fewer calories for digestion and absorption.
Increased hunger sensations	Some individuals appear to have blunted satiety, which may be linked to various brain signals involved in food reward pathways.
Ratio of fat to lean tissue	A high ratio of fat mass to lean body mass is correlated with weight gain.
Fat uptake by adipose tissue	Efficiency of fat storage is high in some obese individuals and may even increase with weight loss.
Social and behavioral factors	Obesity is associated with socioeconomic status; familial conditions; social networks; lifestyles; binge eating; availability of inexpensive, "supersized" high-fat food; patterns of leisure activities; increased screen time; smoking cessation; excessive alcohol intake; and meals eaten away from home.
Genetic predisposition	Genetic factors may affect energy expenditure, deposition of adipose tissue or lean tissue, and the relative proportion of fat and carbohydrate used by the body.
Ethnicity	In some groups, higher body weight may be more socially acceptable, which may promote overeating.
Certain medications	Increased hunger/appetite can be a side effect of many medications.
Childbearing	A pattern of weight gain during the childbearing years can occur to support fetus. Fat stored during pregnancy to support lactation may not be lost in women who do not breastfeed.
Region of residence	Regional environmental and lifestyle differences, such as high-fat diets and sedentary lifestyles, especially in the South and Midwest, lead to higher rates of obesity.

HOW DOES NATURE CONTRIBUTE TO OBESITY?

Studies in pairs of **identical twins** give us insight into the contribution of nature (genetics) relative to obesity. Even when identical twins are raised apart, they tend to show similar weight gain patterns, both in overall weight and body fat distribution. It appears that nurture (environment), which includes dietary patterns and lifestyle behaviors, varies slightly between twins raised apart. Nurture appears to have less to do with obesity than nature. A child with no obese parent has only a 10% chance of becoming obese. When a child has one obese parent (very common in our society), that risk advances up to 40%, and with two obese parents, it soars to 80%. Our genes play a role in our metabolic rate, fuel use, and differences in brain chemistry—all of which ultimately affect body weight.

We also inherit specific body types. Tall, thin people appear to have an inherently easier time maintaining healthy body weight. This is probably because basal metabolism increases as body surface increases; therefore, taller people use more calories than shorter people, even at rest.

Humans have inherited a so-called "thrifty" metabolism that enables us to store fat readily. In early human history, our genes adapted to an environment where food was sometimes scarce; thus, a metabolism that efficiently stored fat would have been a safeguard against starvation in times of famine. Now, with a constant overabundance of food, we require wise

identical twins Two offspring that develop from a single ovum and sperm and, consequently, have the same genetic makeup.

▲ Studies in identical twins give us insight into the genetic contribution to obesity. © Ingram Publishing/SuperStock

set-point Theory of weight status that refers to the close regulation of body weight. It is not known what cells control this set point or how it functions in weight regulation. There is evidence, however, that complex mechanisms exist that help regulate weight.

hypothalamus A region at the base of the brain that contains cells that play a role in the regulation of energy intake, respiration, body temperature, satiety, and other body functions.

leptin A hormone made by adipose tissue in proportion to total fat stores in the body that influences long-term regulation of fat mass. Leptin also influences reproductive functions, as well as other body processes, such as release of the hormone insulin.

food choices and regular physical activity to maintain energy balance. Depending on genetic traits we inherit from our parents, some of us are more prone to weight gain in the modern food environment than others.

Does the Body Have a Set Point for Weight? The **set-point** theory of weight maintenance proposes that humans have a genetically predetermined body weight or body fat content, which the body closely regulates. Several physiological changes that occur during calorie reduction and weight loss support this theory. For example, research suggests that the **hypothalamus** monitors the amount of body fat in humans and tries to keep that amount constant over time. The release and circulation of the hormone **leptin,** from adipose cells, promotes a satiety and a sense of fullness, thus reducing appetite. As adipose cells increase in size and number, overall production of leptin increases, which should suppress appetite. If adipose mass is reduced, leptin levels are reduced, so appetite should be increased. This system, however, is not foolproof. Research has shown that overweight persons have large amounts of leptin coming from the excess body fat, but their brains seem to be "leptin resistant" and are not getting the signal to stop eating.

Thyroid hormone levels change in relation to body fatness, too. When calorie intake is reduced, the blood concentration of thyroid hormones falls, which slows basal metabolism. Also, the calorie cost of weight-bearing activity decreases, so that an activity that burned 100 kcal before weight loss may only burn 80 kcal after weight loss. Furthermore, as weight loss occurs, the body becomes more efficient at storing fat by increasing the activity of the enzyme lipoprotein lipase, which permits fat entry into cells. All of these changes protect the body from losing weight.

If a person overeats, in the short term, basal metabolism tends to increase. This causes some resistance to weight gain. In the long run, however, resistance to weight gain is much less than resistance to weight loss. When a person gains weight and stays at a stable weight for some time, the body tends to establish energy balance at a new set point.

Opponents of the set-point theory argue that weight does not remain constant throughout adulthood: the average person gains weight slowly through old age. Also, if an individual is placed in a different social, emotional, or physical environment, weight can be altered and maintained at a markedly higher or lower point. These arguments suggest that humans, rather than having a set point determined by genetics or the number of adipose cells, settle into a particular stable weight based on their circumstances, often regarded as a "settling point."

The size-acceptance nondiet movement, "Health at Every Size," indirectly refers to a set point for weight by defining healthy weight as the natural weight the body adopts, given a healthy diet and meaningful levels of physical activity. Overall, the set point is weaker in preventing weight gain than in preventing weight loss. Even with a set point helping us, the odds are in favor of eventual weight gain unless we commit to a healthy lifestyle.

DOES NURTURE PLAY A ROLE?

Environmental factors, such as consuming an energy-dense diet and failing to meet physical activity guidelines, literally shape us. This seems likely when we consider that our gene pool has not significantly changed in the past 25 years, whereas according to the U.S. Centers for Disease Control and Prevention, the ranks of obese people have grown to epidemic proportions over the last 25 years.

Some would argue that body weight similarities between family members stem more from learned behaviors than genetic similarities. Even couples, who have no genetic link, may behave similarly toward food and eventually assume similar degrees of leanness or fatness. Adult obesity in women is often rooted in childhood obesity. In addition, relative inactivity and periods of stress or boredom, as well as excess weight gain during pregnancy, contribute to female obesity. (Section 18.7 notes that breastfeeding one's infant contributes to loss of some excess fat associated with pregnancy.) These patterns suggest both social and genetic interactions contribute to body weight. Male obesity, however, is not strongly linked to childhood obesity and, instead, tends to appear after age 30. This powerful and prevalent pattern suggests a primary role of nurture in obesity, with less genetic influence.

Is poverty associated with obesity? Ironically, in developed nations, the answer is *yes*. North Americans of lower socioeconomic status, especially minorities, are more likely to be obese than those of higher socioeconomic status. Several social and behavioral factors promote fat storage and support the link between socioeconomic status and obesity. These factors may include lower socioeconomic status, overweight friends and family, a cultural/ethnic group that prefers higher body weight, a lifestyle that discourages healthy meals and adequate exercise, easy availability of inexpensive high-calorie food, limited access to fresh fruits and vegetables, excessive screen time, lack of adequate sleep, emotional stress, meals frequently eaten away from home, and smoking cessation. Weight gain associated with cessation of smoking has been shown to be a result of increased calorie consumption, with 96% of the weight gain as fat.

▲ Body weight is influenced by many factors related to both nature and nurture. We resemble our parents because of the genes we have inherited, as well as the lifestyle habits, including diet, that we have learned from them.
© Jack Hollingsworth/Getty Images

✓ CONCEPT CHECK 7.4

1. Explain how body weight is influenced by nature (genetics).
2. What role does nurture (environment) play in determining body weight?

7.5 Treatment of Overweight and Obesity

Treatment of overweight and obesity should be long term and similar to that for any chronic disease. Treatments require sustainable lifestyle changes, rather than quick fixes promoted by many popular "fad" diets. We often view a "diet" as something one attempts temporarily, only to resume prior (typically poor) habits once satisfactory results have been achieved. This is a primary reason so many people regain lost weight. Instead, an emphasis on healthy, active living with acceptable dietary patterns and behaviors will promote weight loss and sustained weight maintenance. Maintenance of a healthy weight requires lifelong changes in habits, not short-term and rapid weight loss as seen in so-called crash diets.

LOSING BODY FAT

One pound of weight loss includes adipose tissue plus supporting lean tissues and fluids, and represents approximately 3300 kcal per pound (about 7.2 kcal per gram). Because there are approximately 3500 kcal in 1 pound of fat, the past 50 years of weight-loss advice has centered on the notion that a deficit of approximately 500 kcal per day is required to lose 1 pound of adipose tissue per week. This fairly simple "3500-kcal rule," however, may be an inaccurate predictor of weight change, resulting in unrealistic expectations. Over the years, energy balance research has shown that weight loss occurs more gradually than would be predicted by the 3500-kcal rule because of several factors, including the loss of muscle along with fat during weight loss. Experts have developed new weight-loss prediction formulas that estimate a much slower and realistic pattern of weight loss. Researchers emphasize that weight change is not linear. Rather, it occurs most rapidly during the first year after a change in energy balance and tapers off over the next 2 years. In addition, changes in energy intake and physical activity must be strictly maintained over time. Research has also shown that individuals have a tendency to overestimate their self-reported physical activity levels and underestimate their dietary intakes. Clearly, such inaccuracies in energy intake and output would result in much slower, if any, weight loss over time.

You can read more about weight-loss prediction formulas in Further Reading 8. A web-based "body weight simulator" can help predict expected weight loss over time. The Body Weight Planner, which can be found at **http://bwsimulator.niddk.nih.gov,** projects weight loss over time based on an individual's height, weight, age, current calorie intake, calorie reduction, and activity level. As always, guidelines emphasize that the daily calorie deficit can come from decreased calorie intake, increased physical activity, or ideally, a combination of both.

▲ Student life is often full of physical activity. This is not necessarily true for a person's later sedentary work life; hence, weight gain is highly possible. © Getty Images/SW Productions

As you read brochures, blogs, articles, or research reports about specific diets, look beyond the initial weight loss to see if the reported weight loss was maintained over time. If weight loss was not maintained, then the program was not successful.

The 2015–2020 Dietary Guidelines for Americans provide the following recommendations related to "Consume a healthy eating pattern that accounts for all foods and beverages within an appropriate calorie level."

- Choose a healthy eating pattern at an appropriate calorie level to help achieve and maintain a healthy body weight, support nutrient adequacy, and reduce the risk of chronic disease.
- To meet nutrient needs within calorie limits, choose a variety of nutrient-dense foods across and within all food groups in recommended amounts.
- Consume an eating pattern low in added sugars, saturated fats, and sodium.
- Choose nutrient-dense foods and beverages across and within all food groups in place of less healthy choices.
- Aim to achieve and maintain a healthy body weight. The relationship between diet and physical activity contributes to calorie balance and managing body weight.

WHAT TO LOOK FOR IN A SOUND WEIGHT-LOSS PLAN

Individuals can develop a weight-management plan by seeking advice from a health professional such as a registered dietitian nutritionist (RDN). Interactive tools such as www.ChooseMyPlate.gov can also aid in weight loss and maintenance. Overall, a sound weight-loss program (Fig. 7-16) should include these components:

A one-sided approach that focuses only on restricting calories is a difficult plan of action. Instead, adding physical activity and an appropriate behavioral component will contribute to success in weight loss and eventual weight maintenance (Fig. 7-17). The 2015–2020 Dietary Guidelines for Americans recommendations focus on healthier dietary patterns translating to reduced discretionary calorie intake and meeting physical activity recommendations.

RATE OF LOSS

- ☐ Encourages slow and steady weight loss, rather than rapid weight loss, to promote lasting weight management
- ☐ Sets goal of 1 pound of fat loss per week
- ☐ Includes a period of weight maintenance for a few months after 10% of body weight is lost
- ☐ Evaluates need for further dieting before more weight loss begins

FLEXIBILITY

- ☐ Supports participation in normal activities (e.g., parties, and restaurants)
- ☐ Adapts to individual habits and tastes

INTAKE

- ☐ Meets nutrient needs (except for energy needs)
- ☐ Includes common foods, with no foods being promoted as magical or special
- ☐ Recommends a fortified ready-to-eat breakfast cereal or balanced multivitamin/mineral supplement, especially when intake is less than 1600 kcal per day
- ☐ Uses MyPlate or a comparable food guide as a pattern for food choices

BEHAVIOR MODIFICATION

- ☐ Focuses on maintenance of healthy lifestyle (and weight) for a lifetime
- ☐ Promotes reasonable changes that can be maintained
- ☐ Encourages social support
- ☐ Includes plans for relapse, so that one does not quit after a setback
- ☐ Promotes changes that control problem eating behaviors
- ☐ Promotes self-monitoring pratices such as keeping food diaries and setting goals

OVERALL HEALTH

- ☐ Requires screening by a physician for people with existing health problems, those over 40 (men) to 50 (women) years of age who plan to increase physical activity substantially, and those who plan to lose weight rapidly
- ☐ Encourages regular physical activity, sufficient sleep, stress reduction, and other healthy changes in lifestyle
- ☐ Addresses underlying psychological weight issues, such as depression or marital stress

FIGURE 7-16 ▶ Characteristics of a sound weight-loss plan. Use this checklist to evaluate any weight-loss plan before putting it into practice.

Control calorie intake

Engage in positive behaviors

Perform regular physical activity

FIGURE 7-17 ◄ Weight-loss triad. The key to weight loss and maintenance can be thought of as a triad, which consists of three interrelated components: (1) controlling calorie intake, (2) performing regular physical activity, and (3) engaging in positive behaviors. Without one component of the triad, weight loss and later maintenance becomes highly unlikely.

(1): © Jon Feingersh/Blend Images/Corbis RF;
(2): © Jose Luis Pelaez Inc/Blend Images LLC;
(3): ©chrisgramly/Getty Images

For more information on weight control, obesity, and nutrition, visit the Weight-control Information Network (WIN) at http://win.niddk.nih.gov/index.htm. Complete guidelines for weight management are available at www.nhlbi.nih.gov/guidelines. Other websites include www.nutrition.gov and www.heart.org.

ASK THE RDN   Biggest Loser Eating Plan

Dear RDN: *I'm a fan of The Biggest Loser TV show and see they have a diet and exercise plan. After reading all about the perils of fad diets in this chapter, I want to be sure this program is safe. Can you help?*

Sure! *The Biggest Loser* program has a popular diet and exercise plan. The first *Biggest Loser* book, released in 2005, has been expanded to include a *30-Day Jump Start* edition, *6 Weeks to a Healthier You,* and *The Biggest Loser: The Weight Loss Program to Transform Your Body, Health and Life* (released in 2013). In addition, there is now an online 6-week express program, "Biggest Loser Club," which costs approximately $20 per month.

Overall, the Biggest Loser plan is based on sound nutrition and physical activity principles, but it does require some effort and discipline. This program is based on eating small, frequent meals of nutrient-dense and high-fiber foods. It follows the *Biggest Loser*'s 4-3-2-1 Pyramid: four servings of fruits and vegetables, three servings of lean protein, two servings of whole grains, and 200 kcal of "extras." This plan also recommends drinking six to eight glasses of water per day, limiting sodium and saturated fats, and avoiding caffeine.

Limitations: Although supplements are not recommended, some of the meal plans may fall below 1200 kcal per day and require a supplement. If you select the more interactive online version (Biggest Loser Club), there is a fee to participate.

Strengths: This plan focuses on both diet and physical activity, which are essential components for long-term weight management. All food groups are well represented and the foods may be purchased at any grocery store. Vegetarian, vegan, and gluten-free options are all possible within this plan. The online version includes additional support, recipes, videos, and tracking tools.

In sum, choosing dietary and physical activity patterns that closely align with evidence-based recommendations is always the goal! The combination of diet and exercise has been shown to improve success in long-term weight loss and maintenance.

Eat well, exercise, and prosper,

Colleen Spees, PhD, RDN, LD, FAND (author)

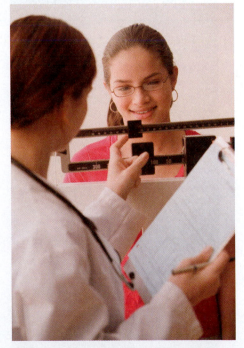

▲ Slow, steady weight loss is one of the characteristics of a sound weight-loss program.
© Jose Luis Pelaez Inc/Blend Images LLC

WEIGHT LOSS IN PERSPECTIVE

The following three principles point to the importance of preventing obesity. This concept has wide support because conquering obesity is so difficult. Public health strategies to address the current obesity problem must speak to all age groups. There is a particular need to focus on children and adolescents because patterns of excess weight and sedentary lifestyles developed during youth may form the basis for a lifetime of weight-related conditions and increased mortality. In the adult population, attention should be directed toward weight management and maintenance by encouraging healthy dietary patterns and increasing physical activity.

1. **Decrease calorie intake** by approximately 500 kcal per day to allow for slow and steady weight loss.
2. **Increase physical activity** to the equivalent of more than 150 minutes of moderate-intensity aerobic activity each week.
3. **Make positive behavior changes** to sustain lifestyle modifications promoting health.

✓ **CONCEPT CHECK 7.5**

1. What are the characteristics of an appropriate weight-loss program?
2. What are the Dietary Guidelines related to "Consume a healthy eating pattern that accounts for all foods and beverages within an appropriate calorie level"?

7.6 Control of Calorie Intake Is Essential for Weight Management

Per day, the average woman requires approximately 1800 to 2400 kcal and the average male requires 2200 to 3000 kcal. A goal of losing 1 pound or so of stored fat per week may require limiting calorie intake to 1200 kcal per day for women and 1500 kcal per day for men. Although the number of calories allowed could be higher for very active people, decreasing calorie intake is necessary in our increasingly sedentary society. Keep in mind that this calorie intake is restrictive, especially for those who have been eating in excess of their calorie requirements. In addition, any calorie reduction will promote the loss of lean mass along with fat tissue. With regard to consuming fewer calories, some experts suggest consuming less fat (especially saturated fat and *trans* fat); others suggest consuming less carbohydrate, especially refined (non-whole-grain) carbohydrates. Protein intakes in excess of what is typically needed by adults are also receiving attention. At this time, a primarily plant-based, high-fiber dietary pattern has been the most successful in long-term studies. A recent report (see Newsworthy Nutrition) confirms that the kinds of food we eat have a large effect on weight gain over the years. Finding what works for you is a process of trial and error. The notion that any type of diet promotes significantly greater calorie use by the body is unfounded (see Further Readings 17, 18, and 19).

Portion control is another challenge that influences our calorie intake and requires a change in our approach to eating. The concept of energy density can help dieters choose more nutrient-rich foods with fewer calories per gram. With this technique, we can fill our plates with larger portions of low-energy-density foods, which are low in calories but high in volume. These low-energy-density foods enable us to eat fewer calories without eating less volume and help us feel full and satisfied while we are losing weight. Fruits and vegetables are great examples of low-energy-density foods. The Volumetrics Diet (see Further Reading 7) is based on this energy-density approach to eating. Although no foods are off limits, dieters are encouraged to eat foods similar to the ones they are craving such as crunchy carrots and hummus instead of potato chips and dip.

One way to monitor calorie intake at the start of a weight-loss program is by reading labels. Label reading is important, because many foods are more energy dense than people understand (Fig. 7-18). Another method is to write down everything you eat and drink for 24

For interactive dietary and physical activity tools, see SuperTracker and Daily Food Plan at www.ChooseMyPlate.gov.

Newsworthy Nutrition

Plant-Based Dietary Pattern Promotes Healthy Body Weight

Over 146,000 participants from the Nurses' Health Study (NHS), Health Professionals Follow-Up Study (HPFS), and Nurses' Health Study II (NHS II) were assessed for the effect of diet quality over time on body weight. Healthy diet quality scores were correlated with greater intakes of fruits and vegetables, whole grains, and nuts. Subjects who had greater adherence to a plant-based dietary pattern, especially younger women or overweight individuals, gained significantly less weight over a 4-year period. The results of this study underscore the importance of healthy dietary patterns in promoting healthy body weight.

Source: Fung TT and others: Long-term change in diet quality is associated with body weight change in men and women. *Journal of Nutrition* 145:1850, 2015.

Nutrition Facts

7.5 servings per container

Serving size	2/3 cup (65g)

Amount per serving

Calories	134

	% Daily Value*
Total Fat 3g	5%
Saturated Fat 1.5g	9%
Trans Fat 0g	
Cholesterol 0mg	3%
Sodium 42mg	2%
Total Carbohydrate 23g	8%
Dietary Fiber 0g	0%
Total Sugars 18g	
Includes 12g Added Sugars	24%
Protein 4g	
Vitamin D 0.1mcg	1%
Calcium 80mg	8%
Iron 0mg	0%
Potassium 204mg	6%

Nutrition Facts

7.5 servings per container

Serving size	2/3 cup (106g)

Amount per serving

Calories	362

	% Daily Value*
Total Fat 23g	35%
Saturated Fat 15g	75%
Trans Fat 0g	
Cholesterol 160mg	53%
Sodium 114mg	5%
Total Carbohydrate 27g	9%
Dietary Fiber 0g	0%
Total Sugars 20g	
Includes 16g Added Sugars	32%
Protein 7g	
Vitamin D 0.2mcg	2%
Calcium 112mg	11%
Iron 0mg	0%
Potassium 175mg	5%

hours (Appendix C) and then calculate calorie intake by using your diet-analysis software. With knowledge of current calorie intake, future food choices can be adjusted as needed. People often underestimate portion sizes when recording food intake, so measuring cups and a food scale can help.

Table 7-4 shows how to start reducing calorie intake. As you should realize, it is best to consider healthy eating a lifestyle change, rather than a fad diet or rapid weight-loss plan. Also, liquids deserve attention because liquid calories do not stimulate satiety mechanisms to the same extent as solid foods. The corresponding advice from experts is to use beverages that have few or no calories and limit sugar-sweetened beverages.

FIGURE 7-18 ▲ Reading labels helps you choose foods with fewer calories. Which of these frozen desserts is the best choice, per ½-cup serving, for a person on a weight-loss diet? The % Daily Values are based on a 2000-kcal diet. Read more about these dessert choices in What the Dietitian Chose.

CONTROLLING HUNGER

A challenge to most weight-loss programs is to regulate hunger while eating less and exercising more. Separating true hunger from habit or emotional eating is the first step toward controlling the hunger that can sabotage a diet. Hormones and your nervous system tell you when you are hungry. The hormone ghrelin in your blood, along with an empty stomach, signals the brain that you are hungry. Likewise, nerves in the stomach signal the brain when you are full, but it can take up to 20 minutes for these satiety signals to reach the brain. The goal is to be hungry at mealtime but not so ravenous that you are tempted to binge. Eat slowly and stop eating when you are comfortably full. If hunger strikes between meals, determine if you are feeling true hunger; and if you are, then choose a small, high-fiber snack to hold you over until the next

TABLE 7-4 ■ **Saving Calories: Ideas for Getting Started**

Save This Much	By Choosing This	Instead of This
45 kcal	1 cup 1% milk	1 cup whole milk
50 kcal	12 oz light beer	12 oz regular beer
60 kcal	1 cup cornflakes cereal	1 cup sugar-coated flakes cereal
65 kcal	½ cup boiled potatoes	½ cup fried potatoes
135 kcal	1 cup plain popcorn	1 oz potato chips
140 kcal	3 oz lean beef	3 oz marbled beef
140 kcal	1 cup raw vegetables	½ cup potato salad
150 kcal	2 tbsp low-calorie salad dressing	2 tbsp regular salad dressing
150 kcal	1 English muffin	1 Danish pastry
150 kcal	6 oz wine cooler made with sparkling water	6 oz gin and tonic
150 kcal	12 oz sugar-free soft drink	12 oz regular soft drink
175 kcal	½ broiled chicken	½ batter-fried chicken
185 kcal	1 slice angel food cake	1 slice white cake with icing
210 kcal	3 oz lean roast beef	½ cup beef stroganoff
310 kcal	1 apple	1 slice apple pie

meal. Drinking a glass of water can also help decrease hunger pangs between meals. Including lean protein (nuts, low-fat dairy, soy protein, or lean meat, fish, or chicken) in meals and snacks will also keep hunger at bay. Eating high-volume foods that are rich in water and fiber will provide bulk with fewer calories, fill your stomach, and send satiety signals to the brain. Becoming more mindful of what you eat will go a long way to controlling hunger and overall calorie intake (read more about mindful eating in Section 7.8). When you slow down, you will not only enjoy each mouthful but also give your stomach time to signal your brain that you are full.

CONQUERING THE WEIGHT-LOSS PLATEAU

It is important for anyone on a weight-loss program to know that healthy weight loss is slow, sometimes erratic, and it is normal to reach a weight-loss plateau. After losing weight for weeks, suddenly the pounds cease to budge. Fortunately, there are some strategies to overcome these plateaus and start obtaining results again. There are several reasons why weight loss may stall. During the first part of a weight-loss program, individuals are typically losing fluid in addition to fat, causing a weight loss larger than the expected 1 to 2 pounds per week. Because a healthy weight-loss program is designed to cause fat loss rather than loss of muscle or fluid, your weight loss will begin to slow after the first week or so. Also the level of calorie deprivation needed to lose weight is hard to maintain, and you may begin to eat more calories. This "calorie creep" can contribute to the weight-loss plateau and eventually lead to weight gain. When this happens, it is important to go back to tracking your calories by logging what you eat and drink and weighing yourself frequently. Another possible reason for the weight-loss plateau is that your metabolism is adjusting to your lower calorie intake. In this case, it may be time to reduce your calories somewhat and drink plenty of water. Your metabolism may also be adapting to your physical activity routine. Varying the intensity of your workout routine, therefore, will help your muscles burn more calories and can help get you past the weight plateau. Strength training, along with the calorie-burning cardio exercises, is important to build muscle mass, which ultimately uses more calories for metabolism.

✓ **CONCEPT CHECK 7.6**

1. How are hormones involved in hunger control?
2. What are "calorie creep" and the weight-loss plateau, and how can they lead to weight gain?

Calorie Estimation on Exercise Machines

The control panel of your exercise machine will typically display your time, speed, distance covered, and calories burned. Time, speed, and distance are generally accurate values, but calories burned is a rough estimate based on the weight you enter before you start your workout. The calories burned are estimates that are not completely accurate because they do not consider factors other than weight, such as body fat percentage, fitness level, form, and running efficiency.

Treadmills and other cardio machines have been shown to overestimate calories burned by up to 20%. A heart rate monitor or fitness tracker is usually more accurate at estimating the number of calories you burn during a workout than are calorie estimators on cardio machines.

7.7 Regular Physical Activity Promotes Weight Loss and Maintenance of a Healthy Weight

Regular physical activity is important for everyone, especially those trying to lose weight or maintain a lower body weight. Calorie burning is enhanced both during and after physical activity. Therefore, activity greatly complements a reduction in calorie intake for weight loss. Many of us rarely do more than sit, stand, and sleep. More calories are used during physical activity than at rest. Expending only 100 to 500 extra kilocalories per day above and beyond normal daily activity, while controlling calorie intake, can lead to a steady and sustained weight loss. Furthermore, physical activity has many other benefits, including a boost for overall self-esteem and quality of life. A Key Recommendation from the 2015–2020 Dietary Guidelines is to meet physical activity guidelines and reduce time spent in sedentary behaviors. The Dietary Guidelines point to the 2008 Physical Activity Guidelines for Americans for specific recommendations. Weight management, as well as other health outcomes including diseases and risk factors for disease, were considered in developing the Physical Activity Guidelines. Although some adults will need a higher level of physical activity than others, it is recommended that adults perform a minimum of 150 minutes

TABLE 7-5 ■ Approximate Calorie Costs of Various Activities and Specific Calorie Costs Projected for a 150-Pound (68-Kilogram) Person

Activity	Kcal per kg per hour	Total kcal per hour	Activity	Kcal per kg per hour	Total kcal per hour
Aerobics—heavy	8.0	544	Ice skating (10 mph)	5.8	394
Aerobics—light	3.0	204	Jogging— medium	9.0	612
Basketball—vigorous	10.0	680	Jogging— slow	7.0	476
Calisthenics—light	4.0	272	Lying down	1.3	89
Cleaning	3.6	243	Jogging (10 mph)	13.2	897
Cooking	2.8	190			
Cycling (13 mph)	9.7	659	Swimming (0.25 mph)	4.4	299
Cycling (5.5 mph)	3.0	204	Tennis	6.1	414
Dressing/showering	1.6	106	Walking (3.75 mph)	4.4	299
Driving	1.7	117	Weight lifting—heavy	9.0	612
Eating (sitting)	1.4	93	Weight lifting—light	4.0	272
Golf (using power cart)	3.6	244	Writing (sitting)	1.7	118

The values in Table 7-5 refer to total energy expenditure, including that needed to perform the physical activity, plus that needed for basal metabolism, the thermic effect of food, and thermogenesis. You can find the calorie costs of additional activities using the Physical Activity Calorie Counter at http://www.acefitness.org/acefit/tools-and-calculators/.

of moderate-intensity aerobic activity each week to achieve and maintain a healthy body weight. Some individuals may need more than the equivalent of 300 minutes per week.

Adding any of the activities in Table 7-5 to one's lifestyle can increase calorie expenditure, promote health, and reduce body fat over time. Duration and regular performance, rather than intensity, are the keys to success with this approach to weight loss. One should search for activities that can be continued over time. In this regard, walking vigorously 3 miles per day can be as helpful as aerobic dancing or jogging if it is maintained. Moreover, activities of lighter intensity are less likely to lead to injuries. Some resistance (weight-training) exercises should also be added to increase and retain lean body mass and, in turn, fat use (see Section 14.2). As lean muscle mass increases, so will one's overall metabolic rate. Keep in mind that aerobic activity, including brisk walking, jogging, or cycling, burns more fat than resistance activity. An added benefit of including exercise in a weight-reduction program is maintenance of bone health. In sum, any type of exercise is better than no exercise at all.

Unfortunately, opportunities to expend calories in our daily lives are diminishing as technology systematically eliminates almost every reason to move our muscles. The easiest way to increase physical activity is to make it an enjoyable part of a daily routine. To start, one might pack a pair of athletic shoes and walk around the block before coming home after school or work every day. Other ideas are avoiding elevators in favor of stairs and parking the car farther away from the shopping mall.

Pedometers or wearable fitness trackers are inexpensive devices that monitor activity and steps. A recommended goal for activity is to take at least 10,000 steps per day; typically, we take half that many or less. A pedometer tracks steps and often distance. Fitness trackers (like FitBits and Jawbones) are wearable devices that often track steps, distance, sleep patterns, and calorie expenditures throughout the day. Fitness trackers calculate calories by measuring heart rate, sweat rate, or heat loss and production. Like pedometers, these devices can motivate users to do more activity.

▲ Physical activity complements any weight-loss or maintenance plan. © Zefa RF/Alamy

✓ CONCEPT CHECK 7.7

1. What should individuals remember about physical activity as part of their weight-loss plan?

7.8 Behavioral Strategies for Weight Management

Setting realistic goals should be the first step toward successful weight loss and management. Realistic weight-loss goals will keep you more focused and motivated, and help to guarantee success. A successful weight-loss program is all about transitioning to a healthier lifestyle. The most helpful goals will focus on changes to your behavior, such as exercising 150 minutes per week, drinking plenty of water, or eating five servings of vegetables a day, rather than reaching a certain weight. Making lifestyle changes means identifying the behaviors and barriers that led to weight gain in the first place. Controlling calorie intake means addressing those barriers and modifying *problem* behaviors. Only you can decide what behaviors may be preventing weight management and calorie control. What triggers you to start (or stop) eating? What factors influence your food choices?

The 2015 Dietary Guidelines identify ways to empower people to make healthy *shifts* in their dietary patterns to encourage weight management:

- Consume more fruits and vegetables.
- Make half of all grains consumed be whole grains.
- Consume more dairy products, in nutrient-dense forms.
- Increase variety in protein food choices and make more nutrient-dense choices.
- Shift from solid fats to oils.
- Replace high-calorie, high-sodium intakes with more nutrient-dense options:
  - Reduce added sugar consumption to less than 10% of calories per day.
  - Reduce saturated fat intake to less than 10% of calories per day
  - Reduce sodium intake to less than 2300 milligrams per day.
- Consume no-sugar-added beverages.
- Reduce portion sizes of nonnutrient-dense foods and beverages.
- Meet the Physical Activity Guidelines for America.

MINDFUL EATING

As we mentioned in the previous section on calorie control, becoming more mindful of your dietary patterns will help you maintain weight and caloric intake. The concept of eating mindfully has become increasingly popular since publication in 2006 of the best-selling book *Mindless Eating: Why We Eat More Than We Think*. Making the break from mindless eating focuses on making changes to avoid triggers that may tempt you to eat less healthy food or to eat too much, or both. In contrast, the principles of mindful eating include being aware of the entire eating experience from food preparation to consumption, including recognizing and respecting the physical hunger and satiety cues, and being wise in eating decisions. Today, there are many publications, websites, and programs associated with the art of eating mindfully. The "Mindful Eating Cycle" from the book *Eat What You Love, Love What You Eat* includes the following key questions that can help you discern if you are eating for reasons other than physical hunger (see Further Reading 9). The answers to these questions will be instrumental in changing problem eating behavior.

- Why do I eat?
- When do I want to eat?
- What do I eat?
- How do I eat?
- How much do I eat?
- Where does the energy go?

A key component of mindful eating is a nonjudgmental awareness of eating patterns that will hopefully lead to a healthier relationship between you and food.

OTHER BEHAVIORAL STRATEGIES

Chain-breaking, stimulus control, cognitive restructuring, contingency management, and self-monitoring are behavior modification strategies used by clinicians that help put problem behaviors in perspective and organize the intervention into manageable steps.

▲ Fruit is a great snack—high in nutrients and low in calories. © Dennis Gray/Cole Group/Getty Images

Chain-breaking separates behaviors that tend to occur together (e.g., overindulging on potato chips while watching television). Although these activities do not have to occur together, they often do. Individuals need to identify and break these chain reactions.

Stimulus control puts us in charge of temptations. Options include covering tempting food with foil, removing energy-dense snacks from the kitchen counter, and avoiding bringing home especially tempting items. Provide a positive stimulus by keeping healthier snacks available to satisfy hunger/appetite.

Cognitive restructuring changes our frame of mind. For example, after a hard day, avoid using alcohol or comfort foods as quick relief for stress. Instead, plan for healthful, relaxing activities for stress reduction. Find a positive outlet like taking a walk or catching up with a good friend.

Labeling some foods as "off limits" sets up an internal struggle to resist the urge to eat that food. This hopeless battle can make us feel deprived, and we eventually lose the fight. Managing food choices with the principle of moderation is best. If a favorite food becomes troublesome, place it off limits only temporarily, until it can be enjoyed in moderation.

Contingency management prepares one for situations that may trigger overeating (e.g., when snacks are served at a party) or hinder physical activity (e.g., rain).

Self-monitoring can reveal problem eating behaviors—such as unconscious overeating—that may lead to weight gain. Records of dietary and physical activity behaviors can encourage new habits that will counteract unwanted behaviors. Obesity experts note this is the key behavioral tool to use in any weight-loss program (see Further Reading 10). Several of these online tools and others are also available as apps for smartphones and other mobile devices (see Further Reading 4 for a review of smartphone apps for heart-healthy living).

Overall, it's important to address specific problems such as snacking, compulsive eating, and mealtime overeating. Behavior modification principles (Table 7-6) are critical components of weight reduction and maintenance. Without them, it is difficult to make lifelong lifestyle changes needed to achieve weight-control goals.

RELAPSE PREVENTION IS IMPORTANT

Preventing relapse is thought to be the hardest part of weight control—even harder than losing weight. Successful weight managers plan for lapses, do not overreact, and take charge immediately. Change responses such as "I ate that cookie; I'm a failure" to "I ate that cookie, but I did well to stop after only one!" When individuals lapse from their plan, newly learned food habits should steer them back on track. Without a strong behavioral program for **relapse prevention** in place, a lapse frequently turns into a relapse and a potential collapse. Once a pattern of poor food choices begins, individuals may feel failure and stray farther from the plan. As the relapse lengthens, the entire plan collapses and falls short of the weight-loss goal. Losing weight is difficult. Overall, maintenance of weight loss is fostered by the "3 *M*s": motivation, movement, and monitoring.

SOCIAL SUPPORT AIDS BEHAVIORAL CHANGE

Healthy social support is helpful in weight control. Helping others understand how they can be supportive can make weight management easier. Family and friends can provide praise and encouragement. Unfortunately, your social network can also sabotage your efforts, so be aware of whom you can rely on for support. A registered dietitian nutritionist (RDN) or other trained interventionist can keep you accountable and help you learn from difficult situations. Long-term contact with a professional can be helpful for later weight maintenance. Groups of individuals attempting to lose weight or maintain losses can also provide empathetic support.

SOCIETAL EFFORTS TO REDUCE OBESITY

The incidence of obesity in the United States is now considered an epidemic. An epidemic is a public health problem, and such problems call for collective action. In fact, improvement in the health of our nation requires an approach that includes many sectors. Partnerships, programs, and policies that support healthy eating and active living must be coordinated.

chain-breaking Breaking the link between two or more behaviors that encourage overeating, such as snacking while watching television.

stimulus control Altering the environment to minimize the stimuli for eating (e.g., removing foods from sight by storing them in kitchen cabinets).

cognitive restructuring Changing one's frame of mind regarding eating; for example, instead of using a difficult day as an excuse to overeat, a person would substitute other pleasures for rewards, such as a relaxing walk with a friend.

contingency management Forming a plan of action to respond to a situation in which overeating is likely, such as when snacks are within arm's reach at a party.

self-monitoring Tracking foods eaten and conditions affecting eating; actions are usually recorded in a diary, along with location, time, and state of mind. This is a tool to help people understand more about their eating habits.

relapse prevention A series of strategies used to help prevent and cope with weight-control lapses, such as recognizing high-risk situations and deciding beforehand on appropriate responses.

Food and Activity Tracking

Here are some websites where you can record your food and physical activity online for free:

- http://www.myfitnesspal.com/
- https://www.supertracker.usda.gov/
- www.fitday.com
- http://www.livestrong.com
- http://nutritiondata.self.com
- www.sparkpeople.com

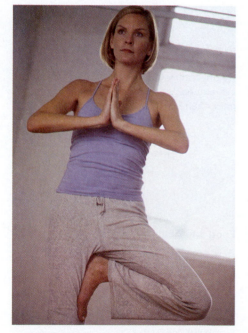

Successful weight losers and maintainers from the National Weight Control Registry:

- Eat a low-fat, high-carbohydrate diet (on average 25% of calorie intake as fat).
- Eat breakfast almost every day.
- Self-monitor by regularly weighing oneself and keeping a food journal.
- Exercise for about 1 hour per day.
- Eat at restaurants only once or twice per week.

Other recent studies support this approach, especially the last four characteristics.

▲ Individuals who successfully maintain their weight loss employ a variety of strategies, such as physical activity or meditation, to cope with the stresses and challenges of changing problem behaviors. © Royalty-Free/Corbis

TABLE 7-6 ■ Behavioral Tactics for Weight Loss

Shopping
1. Shop for food after eating so you are not hungry.
2. Shop from a list or use a shopping app.
3. Limit purchases of irresistible "problem" foods.
4. Shop for fresh foods around the perimeter of the store first.
5. Avoid highly processed, ready-to-eat foods.
6. Put off food shopping until absolutely necessary.

Planning
1. Plan meals in advance; keep healthy foods washed and prepared.
2. Substitute periods of physical activity for snacking.
3. Eat meals and snacks at scheduled times; don't skip meals.
4. Drink plenty of water throughout the day.

Activities
1. Store food out of sight to discourage impulsive eating.
2. Eat all food in a designated "dining" area; avoid buffet-type meals.
3. Keep serving dishes off the table, especially dishes of sauces and gravies.
4. Use smaller dishes and utensils.

Holidays and Parties
1. Drink fewer alcoholic beverages; alternate water with alcohol.
2. Eat a low-calorie snack before parties.
3. Plan eating behavior before parties.
4. Practice polite ways to decline food.
5. Don't get discouraged by an occasional setback.

Eating Behavior
1. Put the fork down between bites; chew thoroughly and slowly before taking the next bite.
2. Leave some food on the plate.
3. Pause in the middle of the meal and be mindful of the eating experience.
4. Do nothing else while eating (e.g., reading, watching television).

Rewards
1. Plan specific rewards for specific behavior (behavioral contracts); allow for small treat on exercise days.
2. Solicit help from family and friends; engage in exercise and healthy cooking together.
3. Use self-monitoring records (diet, physical activity, body weight) as basis for rewards. Many tracking apps are available.

Self-Monitoring
1. Note the time and place of eating.
2. List the type and amount of food and beverages consumed.
3. Record who is present and how you feel.
4. Use the dietary intake diary to identify problem areas.
5. Use online or mobile apps to track your progress, including your new nutrition and health goals and habits (see Further Reading 4).

Cognitive Restructuring
1. Avoid setting unreasonable goals; focus on small and manageable steps.
2. Focus on long-term progress, not occasional setbacks.
3. Avoid imperatives such as *always* and *never.*
4. Counter negative thoughts with positive restatements.

Portion Control
1. Make healthy substitutions, such as small fries instead of large fries or add cucumbers instead of croutons to salads.
2. Think small. Order the entrée and share it with another person. Order a cup of soup instead of a bowl or an appetizer in place of an entrée.
3. Use a take-home box. Ask your server to pack half the entrée in a take-home box before bringing it to the table.

As we said at the start of this chapter, many of us need to become "defensive eaters." Know when to refuse food after satiety registers and reduce portion sizes.

The 2015–2020 Dietary Guidelines Strategies for Action include:

1. Identifying and addressing successful approaches for change.
2. Improving knowledge of what constitutes healthy eating and physical activity patterns.
3. Enhancing access to adequate amounts of healthy, safe, and affordable food choices.
4. Promoting change in social and cultural norms and values to embrace, support, and maintain healthy eating and physical activity behaviors.

Public, private, and nonprofit organizations have begun to work together to address and reverse this public health crisis. For example, the U.S. Food and Drug Administration has brought together leaders from industry, government, academia, and the public health community to seek solutions to the obesity epidemic by making changes in foods eaten outside the home (restaurant and carry-out foods). These groups have collaborated and made recommendations to support the consumer's ability to manage calorie intake. Recommendations include "social marketing" programs that promote healthy eating and active living.

▲ Large portions of food, such as this steak, provide us with many opportunities to overeat. It takes much perseverance to eat sensibly. How do the portion sizes shown here compare to those recommended by MyPlate?
© Ernie Friedlander/Cole Group/Getty Images

✅ **CONCEPT CHECK 7.8**

1. What behavior modification steps are helpful in changing problem eating behaviors to increase weight-loss success?
2. How does mindful eating help control hunger?

7.9 Professional Help for Weight Loss

The first professional to see for advice about a weight-loss program is a primary care provider. This person is equipped to assess overall health and current weight status by examining health parameters such as blood pressure, blood lipids, and blood glucose that can be altered because of excess weight. Your clinician may then recommend a registered dietitian nutritionist (RDN) for a specific behavioral weight-loss plan and answers to nutrition-related questions. RDNs are uniquely qualified to help design a weight-loss plan because they understand both food composition and the psychological importance of food. Exercise physiologists can provide advice about programs to improve physical activity. The expense for such professional interventions is tax deductible in the United States in some cases (see a tax advisor) and often covered by health insurance plans if prescribed by a primary care provider or covered by a student wellness plan.

Many communities have a variety of weight-loss organizations. These include self-help groups, such as Weight Watchers, which offer social support and education. Other programs, such as Jenny Craig and Physicians' Weight Loss Center, are less desirable for the average person because they require expensive food purchases and don't encourage healthy food preparation. Often, the leaders are not credentialed dietitians or other trained professionals. These programs tend to be expensive because of their requirements for intense counseling or mandatory diet foods and supplements. These commercial diet products as well as diet programs that require product purchases promote weight cycling, sometimes called "yo-yo dieting," and ultimately result in rebound weight gain at a higher body fat level. In addition, the Federal Trade Commission has charged these and other commercial diet-program companies with misleading consumers through unsubstantiated weight-loss claims and deceptive testimonials.

MEDICATIONS FOR WEIGHT LOSS

Candidates for medications for obesity include those with a BMI ≥30 or BMI ≥27 with at least one obesity-associated comorbid condition (e.g., type 2 diabetes, cardiovascular disease, hypertension) and who are motivated to lose weight. For specific populations, medication, also known as pharmacotherapy, may be considered to supplement lifestyle interventions to help achieve targeted weight loss and health goals. Drug therapy alone has not been found to be successful for long-term weight maintenance. Success with medications

▲ All weight-loss programs should begin with a visit to your primary care provider. © Dynamic Graphics/JupiterImages RF

Fat Digestion Without Orlistat

Enzymes called lipases help digest fat.

Lipase enzyme

Triglyceride

Lipase enzyme

Free fatty acid

Monoglyceride

Free fatty acid

Monoglycerides and free fatty acids are ready to be absorbed.

Fat Digestion With Orlistat

Orlistat attaches to lipases and blocks them from digesting some of the fat.

Triglyceride

Orlistat

Lipase enzyme

Intact triglycerides are not absorbed.

FIGURE 7-19 ▲ Orlistat is a weight-loss drug that works in the digestive system to block digestion and subsequent absorption of about one-third of the fat in the food we eat. A low-dose form of this drug (alli) is now available without a prescription.

amphetamine A group of medications that induce stimulation of the central nervous system and have other effects in the body. Abuse is linked to physical and psychological dependence.

▲ alli (orlistat) is an over-the-counter weight-loss drug that blocks fat digestion and absorption. © McGraw-Hill Education/Jill Braaten, photographer

has been shown only in those who also modify their behavior, decrease calorie intake, and increase physical activity. For a drug to be considered effective in treating obesity, it must pass FDA guidelines and prove to be relatively safe.

Three main classes of medications have been used. An **amphetamine**-like medication (phentermine [Fastin® or Ionamin®]) prolongs the activity of epinephrine and norepinephrine in the brain. This therapy is effective for some people in the short run but has not yet been proven effective in the long run. The medication should not be used by pregnant or nursing women or those under 18 years of age.

The second class of medication approved by FDA for weight loss is orlistat (Xenical®). This medication reduces fat digestion by about 30% by inhibiting lipase enzyme action in the small intestine (Fig. 7-19). This cuts absorption of dietary fat by one-third for about 2 hours when taken along with a meal containing fat. This malabsorbed fat is deposited in the feces. Fat intake has to be controlled, however, because large amounts of fat in the feces cause numerous side effects, such as diarrhea, gas, bloating, and oily discharge. The malabsorbed fat also carries fat-soluble vitamins (vitamins A, D, E, K) into the feces, so the person taking orlistat must take a multivitamin and mineral supplement at bedtime. In this way, any micronutrients not absorbed during the day can be replaced. A low-dose form of orlistat (alli™) is now available over the counter without a prescription.

Approved weight-loss medications work in various ways to curb appetite. Lorcaserin hydrochloride (Belviq®) suppresses appetite by altering serotonin receptors found within the feeding center of the hypothalamus in the brain (see Further Reading 14). It works similarly to the banned drugs fenfluramine (Fen-Phen™) and sibutramine (Meridia®), which caused various heart problems (see Further Reading 11). However, because lorcaserin is more selective, none of the heart issues have been documented in clinical tests. Documented side effects of lorcaserin include bleeding/bruising, mental/mood changes, shaking/twitching, shortness of breath, irregular heartbeat, swelling, and fever. If you are taking medication to treat diabetes, lorcaserin can increase your risk for hypoglycemia.

Qsymia® is a combination of phentermine and the seizure/migraine drug topiramate. Topiramate is effective in causing weight loss because it enhances satiety, makes foods taste less appealing, and helps you burn more calories. Qsymia has serious side effects, however, including the potential to cause birth defects if taken during pregnancy.

The most recent drug approved for weight loss is Saxenda® (liraglutide). It slows gastric emptying and enhances the feeling of fullness. Another recently approved medication is Contrave®. Contrave combines bupropion (the active ingredient in the antidepressant Wellbutrin™) and naltrexone (an anti-addiction drug). The drug includes a warning about increased risk of suicidal thoughts or seizures. All of these new drugs continue to be tested and long-term effects are not known.

Sometimes, physicians may prescribe medications that are not approved for weight loss but have weight loss as a side effect. Such an application is termed "off-label." Over-the-counter medications and supplements are widely marketed as miracle cures for obesity, but in some cases, they do more harm than good. Today more than ever, let the buyer beware concerning any purported weight-loss aid not prescribed by a physician.

Overall, in skilled hands, prescription medications can aid weight loss in some instances. However, they do not replace the need for reducing calorie intake, modifying "problem" behaviors, and increasing physical activity, both during and after therapy. Often, any weight loss during drug treatment can be attributed mostly to the individual's hard work at balancing calorie intake with calorie output.

TREATMENT OF SEVERE OBESITY

Severe (morbid) obesity—having a BMI ≥40 or weighing at least 100 pounds over healthy body weight (or twice one's healthy body weight)—requires professional treatment. Because of the serious health implications of severe obesity, drastic measures may be necessary. Such treatments are recommended only when traditional diets and medications fail. Drastic weight-loss procedures are not without side effects, both physical and psychological, making careful monitoring by a primary care provider a necessity.

Very-Low-Calorie Diets If more traditional diets have failed, treating severe obesity with a **very-low-calorie diet (VLCD)** is possible, especially if the person has obesity-related diseases that are not well controlled (e.g., hypertension, type 2 diabetes). Some researchers believe that people with body weight greater than 30% above their healthy weight are appropriate candidates. The VLCD is dangerous because of its rapid weight loss and potential for severe health complications, including heart problems and gallstones. Often providing less than 800 kcal per day, all VLCD programs should be administered under strict medical supervision, as careful monitoring by a trained clinician is crucial throughout this very restrictive form of weight loss.

Optifast® and other VLCD meal replacements are commercial programs. In general, these diets allow a person to consume only 400 to 800 kcal per day, often in liquid form. (These diets were previously known as protein-sparing modified fasts.) Of this amount, approximately 30 to 120 grams (120 to 480 kcal) are carbohydrates. The rest are from high-quality protein in the amount of 70 to 100 grams per day (280 to 400 kcal). This low carbohydrate intake often causes ketosis, an acidic state caused by inadequate glucose for fuel, which may decrease hunger. The main reasons for weight loss, however, are the minimal energy consumption and restricted food choices. About 3 to 4 pounds can be lost per week, often due to water and lean body mass losses. Men tend to lose at a faster rate than women. When physical activity and resistance training augment this diet, a greater loss of adipose tissue occurs.

Weight regain remains a nagging problem, especially without a behavioral and physical activity component. If behavioral therapy and physical activity supplement a long-term support program, maintenance of the weight loss is more likely but still difficult. Any program under consideration should include a detailed maintenance plan. Today, antiobesity medications may also be included in this phase of the program.

Intermittent Fasting The dietary practice known as intermittent fasting, where one cycles days of so-called normal eating with a day or days of eating little to nothing, is gaining popularity. Despite evidence that intermittent fasting can promote weight loss in some individuals, most dietitians and clinicians remain skeptical of this approach for any length of time. Until more evidence is available, focus on the recommended evidence-based principles you've learned in this chapter.

Bariatric Surgery **Bariatrics** is the medical specialty focusing on the treatment of obesity. Bariatric surgery is only considered for people with severe obesity (BMI ≥40 or BMI ≥35 with obesity-related comorbid conditions) and includes surgery aimed at promoting weight loss. Two types of bariatric operations are now common and effective for eligible clients (see Further Reading 12). Both procedures can be performed using an open (8- to 10-inch) incision in the middle of the abdomen or a laparoscopic approach in which several smaller (½- to 2-inch) incisions are used that allow cameras and instruments to enter the abdomen. **Adjustable gastric banding** (also known as the lap-band® procedure) is a restrictive procedure in which the opening from the esophagus to the stomach is reduced by a hollow gastric band. This creates a small pouch and a narrow passage into the rest of the stomach and thus decreases the amount of food that can be eaten comfortably. The band can be inflated or deflated via an access port placed just under the skin. Studies have shown that adjustable gastric banding is more effective long term than a very-low-calorie diet (400 to 800 kcal) for people who are about 50 pounds overweight.

very-low-calorie diet (VLCD) Known also as *protein-sparing modified fast (PSMF)*, this diet allows a person less than 800 calories per day, often in liquid form. Of this, 120 to 480 calories are typically from carbohydrate, and the rest are mostly from high-quality protein.

bariatrics The medical specialty focusing on the treatment of obesity.

adjustable gastric banding A restrictive procedure in which the opening from the esophagus to the stomach is reduced by a hollow gastric band.

gastroplasty Gastric bypass surgery performed on the stomach to limit its volume to approximately 30 milliliters. Also referred to as stomach stapling.

sleeve gastrectomy Surgical reduction of stomach by about 75% (to about the size of a banana). Also known as the gastric sleeve.

Gastric bypass (also called **gastroplasty** or stomach stapling) is another bariatric surgical procedure used for treating severe or morbid obesity. The most common bariatric procedure is vertical sleeve gastrectomy (VSG) followed by the Roux-en-Y gastric bypass (RYGBP). RYGBP works by reducing the stomach capacity to about 30 milliliters (the volume of one egg or a shot glass) and bypassing a short segment of the upper small intestine. VGS surgically restricts the stomach to a long tubular shape with a reduced volume of 150 to 200 milliliters and alters both appetite hormones and gastric acid. The excluded stomach, representing about 85% of the original capacity, is removed. **Sleeve gastrectomy,** or gastric sleeve, reduces the size of the stomach by about 75% (to about the size of a banana) by removal of a large portion of the stomach following the major curve (Fig. 7-20). With both of these procedures, weight loss is promoted mainly because overeating of solid foods is now less likely due to rapid satiety and discomfort or vomiting after overeating.

Patient selection criteria for bariatric surgery include:

- BMI >40
- BMI >35 when accompanied by obesity-related comorbidities.
- Obesity present for a minimum of 5 years, with failure of nonsurgical weight loss.
- Absence of contraindications (medical).
- No history of alcoholism or major untreated psychiatric disorders.
- Well-informed, compliant, and motivated patient.

The risks of bariatric surgery are serious and include death and both early and late postoperative complications, such as bleeding, blood clots, hernias, electrolyte imbalances, and severe infections. Risk of death from these demanding and complex surgeries can be as high as 2%. These risks depend on many factors related to the surgeon and facility, the patient, and the procedure. The procedures that are simply restrictive (e.g., adjustable gastric banding and sleeve gastrectomy) do not cause malabsorption and rarely affect bowel function. However, for those procedures that induce malabsorption (e.g., Roux-en-Y gastric bypass),

Normal stomach — Esophagus, Stomach, Small intestine

Gastric bypass — Stomach pouch, Esophagus, Unused portion of stomach, Staple line, Small intestine

Gastric banding (e.g., LAP-BAND® procedure) — Esophagus, Small stomach pouch, Gastric band, Larger stomach portion, Port for injecting saline solution, Small intestine

Sleeve gastrectomy — Pylorus, Gastric "sleeve", Excised stomach

Vertical-banded gastroplasty — Esophagus, Staple line, Stomach pouch, Banded outlet, Unused portion of stomach, Small intestine

FIGURE 7-20 ◀ The normal stomach and the most common forms of gastroplasty for treating severe obesity. The gastric bypass is the most effective method. In banded gastroplasty, the band prevents expansion of the outlet for the stomach pouch.

nutrient deficiencies are of greater concern if the person is not adequately treated in the years following the surgery. Anemia and bone loss might then be the result.

Bariatric surgery is costly and may not be covered by medical insurance. The average cost for gastric bypass procedures is $18,000 to $35,000 and for adjustable gastric banding is $17,000 to $30,000. In addition, follow-up surgery is often needed after weight loss to correct stretched skin, previously filled with fat. Furthermore, the surgery necessitates major lifestyle changes, such as the need to plan frequent, small meals. Therefore, the dieter who has chosen this drastic approach to weight loss faces months of difficult adjustments.

Despite potential adverse effects, the benefits of bariatric surgery for those who are eligible usually outweigh the risks. In terms of long-term weight-loss success, bariatric surgeries have the best results of any intervention. Weight-loss statistics vary by surgical method, but on average, about 75% of people with severe obesity eventually lose and keep off 50% or more of excess body weight. In addition, many patients experience significant improvements in blood sugar, cholesterol, and blood pressure. By no means is bariatric surgery a quick and easy fix for obesity, but with a serious commitment to permanent lifestyle changes and long-term follow-up with a health professional, these procedures can positively impact both quality and quantity of life.

Lipectomy Spot reducing by using diet and physical activity is not possible. "Problem" local fat deposits can be reduced in size, however, using suction lipectomy. Lipectomy, or liposuction, involves surgical removal of fat. A pencil-thin tube is inserted into an incision in the skin, and the fat tissue, often in the buttocks and thigh area, are suctioned out through a tube and discarded. This procedure involves risks, such as infection, permanent depressions in the skin, nerve damage, and blood clots which can lead to kidney failure and sometimes death. The procedure is designed to help a person lose about 4 to 8 pounds per treatment. The costs vary greatly and are dependent upon site and clinician but may cost $1800 per site with total costs ranging from $2600 to $9000.

✔ CONCEPT CHECK 7.9

1. What are the surgical options for morbidly obese people who have failed to lose weight with other weight-loss strategies?
2. How restrictive is a very-low-caloric diet plan? Why is monitoring by a qualified health professional important?

7.10 Treatment of Underweight

Underweight is defined by a BMI less than 18.5 and can be caused by a variety of factors, such as cancer, infectious disease (e.g., tuberculosis), digestive tract disorders (e.g., chronic inflammatory bowel disease), and excessive dieting or physical activity. Genetic background may also lead to a higher RMR, a slight body frame, or both. Health problems associated with underweight include the loss of menstrual function, low bone mass, complications with pregnancy and surgery, and slow recovery after illness. Significant underweight is also associated with increased death rates, especially when combined with cigarette smoking. We frequently hear about the risks of obesity but seldom of underweight. In our culture, being underweight is much more socially acceptable than being overweight or obese.

Sometimes being underweight requires medical intervention. A clinician should be consulted first to rule out hormonal imbalances, depression, cancer, infectious disease, digestive tract disorders, excessive physical activity, and other hidden disease such as a serious eating disorder (see Chapter 15 for a detailed discussion of eating disorders).

The causes of underweight are not altogether different from the causes of obesity. Internal and external satiety-signal irregularities, the rate of metabolism, genetic factors, and psychological traits can all contribute to underweight.

underweight A body mass index below 18.5. The cutoff is less precise than for obesity because this condition has been less studied.

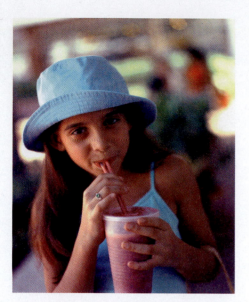

▲ Underweight people should increase their consumption of calorie-dense foods, such as smoothies, that are also loaded with nutrients. © Dynamic Graphics Group/Creatas/Alamy

In growing children, the high demand for calories to support physical activity and growth can cause underweight. During growth spurts, active children and adolescents may not take the time to consume enough calories to support their needs. Moreover, gaining weight can be a formidable task for an underweight person. An extra 500 kcal per day may be required to gain weight, even at a slow pace, in part because of the increased expenditure of energy in thermogenesis. In contrast to the weight loser, the weight gainer may need to increase portion sizes and include frequent snacks.

When underweight requires a specific intervention, one approach for treating adults is to gradually increase their consumption of calorie-dense foods, especially those high in vegetable fats. Nuts and granola can be good calorie sources with low saturated fat content. Dried fruits and bananas are good fruit choices. If eaten at the end of a meal, they don't cause early satiety. The same advice applies to salads and soups. Underweight people should replace such foods as diet soft drinks with good calorie sources, such as 100% fruit juices and nutrient-rich smoothies.

Encouraging a regular meal and snack schedule also aids in weight gain and maintenance. Sometimes underweight individuals have experienced stress at work or have been too busy to eat. Making regular meals a priority may not only help them attain an appropriate weight but also help with digestive disorders, such as constipation, sometimes associated with irregular eating times.

GAINING WEIGHT AS MUSCLE, NOT FAT

A combination of high-quality nutrition and strength training is needed to gain weight as muscle. Strength training slows muscle loss that comes with dieting and aging, increases the strength of your muscles and connective tissues, and increases bone density. When weight is lost, up to a quarter of the loss may come from muscle mass, which can slow basal metabolism. Strength training helps protect against lean body mass losses and rebuilds any muscle lost by dieting—or prevents it from being lost in the first place. The best bet when starting a strength-training program is to seek individualized counseling from a qualified sports dietitian or certified fitness trainer who can address personal goals and limitations and can help with alignment and execution of each exercise.

There are several things to consider when designing dietary patterns to accompany training. During a workout, it is normal for the body to break down some muscles due to the stress placed on them. Once you're finished strength training, you want to repair and build muscle again. It is very important to get proper nutrients into the body after a workout to promote recovery and muscle building. Immediately before and again after strength training, a serving of high-quality protein should be consumed to optimize performance and build lean muscle mass. It is also important to have some carbohydrate along with protein to increase the protein absorption, replete glycogen stores, and provide future fuel for workouts. Although a quick protein bar or shake is great when you're at the gym, it should not be the only source of protein. During meals, lean protein sources such as tuna, lean chicken, soy, and beans are the most appropriate. Those who work out but eat nothing but food high in saturated fat and calories will gain fat in addition to any muscle gains. To gain lean muscle mass, one needs a balanced diet rich in protein and carbohydrates, including plenty of fruits, vegetables, and whole grains. The number of calories you require each day varies greatly and will depend on your weight, activity level, age, and muscle mass. If you are working out 3 days a week, you can eat about 15 kcal per pound of body weight. If you work out 5 days a week, you can increase that calorie count to 20 kcal per pound.

✓ CONCEPT CHECK 7.10

1. How is underweight defined and what are some of its primary causes?
2. What are the components necessary to gain weight as muscle and not as fat?

7.11 Nutrition and Your Health

Popular Diets—Cause for Concern

© BananaStock/PunchStock

People on diets often fall within a healthy BMI of 18.5 to 25. Rather than worrying about weight loss, these individuals should focus on a healthy lifestyle that allows for weight maintenance. Incorporating necessary lifestyle changes, especially regular physical activity, and learning to accept one's individual body characteristics should be the overriding goals.

The dieting mania can be viewed as mostly a social problem, stemming from unrealistic weight expectations (especially for women) and lack of appreciation for the natural variety in body shape and size. Not every woman can or should look like a fashion model, nor can every man look like a Greek god, but all of us can strive for good health and, if physically possible, an active lifestyle.

The size-acceptance nondiet movement, "Health at Every Size," has attempted to shift the paradigm away from the use of "popular" weight-loss diets. Goals of the movement are all independent of body weight and include improvement of self-image, normalization of eating behavior, and increase in physical activity.

How to Recognize an Unreliable Diet

The criteria for evaluating weight-loss programs with regard to their safety and effectiveness were discussed in Section 7.5 (review Fig. 7-16). In contrast, unreliable fad diets typically share some common characteristics:

1. They promote rapid weight loss. This is the primary temptation that attracts the dieter. As mentioned, this initial weight loss primarily results from water loss and lean muscle mass depletion.
2. They often limit food selections and dictate specific rituals, such as eating only fruit for breakfast or cabbage soup every day.
3. They use testimonials from famous people and tie the diet to well-known cities, such as Beverly Hills or South Beach.
4. They bill themselves as cure-alls. These diets claim to work for everyone, whatever the type of obesity or the person's genetic or environmental makeup.
5. They often recommend expensive supplements or meals.
6. No attempts are made to change eating habits permanently. Dieters follow the diet until the desired weight is reached and then revert to old behaviors; they are told, for example, to eat rice for a month, lose weight, and then return to old habits.
7. They are generally critical of and skeptical about the scientific community. The lack of a quick fix from medical and dietetic professionals has led some of the public to seek advice from those who appear to have the answer.
8. They claim that there is no need to exercise.

Many overweight people try to help themselves by using the latest popular (also called "fad") diets. But, as you will see, most of these fad diets do not help, and some can actually harm those who follow them (Table 7-7). Research has shown that early dieting and unhealthful weight-control practices in adolescents can lead to an increased risk of weight gain, overweight, and eating disorders.

At the request of USDA, researchers were convened to evaluate weight-loss diets. They came to this conclusion: forget these fad diets when it comes to dieting. Most of the popular diets are nutritionally inadequate and include certain foods that people would not normally choose to consume in large amounts. The experts stated that eating less of one's favorite foods and becoming more physically active can be much more effective when trying to implement a weight-loss strategy. People need a plan they can live with in the long run so that a healthy weight becomes permanent. The goal should be weight management over a lifetime, not immediate weight loss. Every popular diet leads to some immediate weight loss simply because daily intake is monitored and monotonous food choices are typically part of the plan. Overall, a healthy dietary pattern coupled with regular physical activity is adequate for weight loss.

Probably the cruelest characteristic of these diets is that they essentially guarantee failure for the dieter. Fad diets are not designed for permanent weight loss. Habits are not changed, and the food selection is so limited that the person cannot follow the diet in the long run. Although dieters assume that they have lost fat, they have lost mainly muscle mass and body fluids. As soon as they begin eating normally again, much of the lost tissue is replaced as fat mass. In a matter of weeks or months, most of the lost weight is back. The dieter appears to have failed, when actually the *diet* has failed. The gain and loss cycle is called weight cycling

TABLE 7-7 ■ Summary of Popular Diet Approaches to Weight Control

Approach	Examples*	Characteristics	Dietitian's Review
Moderate calorie restriction	• *Dieting for Dummies* (2003) • Flat Belly Diet (2008) • Jenny Craig (1980s) • Slim-fast (1980s) • *Ultimate Volumetrics Diet* (2012) • Weight Watchers (1960s)	• Generally 1200 to 1800 kcal per day • Moderate fat intake • Reasonable balance of macronutrients • Encourage exercise • May use behavioral approach	These diets may be acceptable if a multivitamin and mineral supplement is used and permission of primary care provider is granted
Carbohydrate focused	• *Dr. Atkin's Diet Revolution* (1973, 2002) • *G.I. (Glycemic Index) Diet* (2003) • Nutrisystem (2003) • *South Beach Diet* (especially initial phases) (2003) • *Sugar Busters Diet* (1998, 2003) • *Zone Diet* (1995)	• Restricted carbohydrate diets generally advise consumption of fewer than 100 grams of carbohydrate per day • Some plans focus on carbohydrate choices (e.g., choosing low rather than high glycemic index foods).	Selecting high-fiber, whole-grain sources of carbohydrates is advisable. Severe carbohydrate restriction may lead to ketosis, reduced exercise capacity, excessive animal fat intake, constipation, headaches, bad breath, and muscle cramps. Severe carbohydrate restriction is not recommended.
Low fat	• *Eat More, Weigh Less* (1993, 2001) • *Fit or Fat* (1977, 2005) • *T-Factor Diet* (1989, 2001)	• Generally less than 20% of calories from fat • Limited (or elimination of) animal protein sources; also limited plant oils, nuts, and seeds	Some aspects of low-fat diet plans may be unacceptable. Negative outcomes may include flatulence, poor mineral absorption, and a sense of deprivation.
Novelty diets	• *Alkaline Cure* (2014) • *Beverly Hills Diet* (1981, 1996) • *Eat Right 4 Your Type* (1996) • Fast Metabolism Diet (2013) • Paleo Diet (2010)	• Promote certain nutrients, foods, or combinations of foods as having unique, magical, or previously undiscovered qualities	Novelty diets are usually not nutritionally balanced, thus malnutrition is possible. Failure to make long-term changes may lead to relapse, and unrealistic food choices lead to possible bingeing.

*Dates listed are original release date followed by most recent release date, if applicable.

or "yo-yo" dieting. This whole scenario can add more blame and guilt, challenging the self-worth of the dieter. It can also come with some health costs, such as increased upper-body fat deposition. If someone needs help losing weight, consult a nutrition expert, like a registered dietitian nutritionist. It is unfortunate that current trends suggest that people are spending more time and money on "quick fixes" than on such professional help.

The hCG diet is an example of an unsafe fad diet that fits these characteristics. Human chorionic gonadotropin (hCG) is a hormone found in the urine of pregnant women and has been associated with dieting because, theoretically, it is supposed to suppress hunger and trigger the body's use of fat for fuel. The fact is, clinical studies have shown hCG to be ineffective as a weight-loss aid. Not only has FDA not approved any hCG weight-loss products, but FDA and Federal Trade Commission have issued warning letters to companies marketing over-the-counter hCG products labeled as "homeopathic" for weight loss. Companies have been warned that they are violating federal law by selling drugs that have not been approved and by making unsupported claims for the products. It is true that individuals will lose weight on the hCG diets, but only because most hCG diets limit dieters to only 500 calories per day in addition to the hCG injections or serum drops under the tongue. These extremely low-calorie diets are virtually impossible to maintain and can lead to nutrient deficiencies and harmful side effects.

Types of Popular Diets

THE BOTTOM LINE

During the last decade, only a few independent clinical trials have compared types of diets (such as high protein or low carb). Most find very modest differences in sustained weight loss and no consistent winner. One consistent finding is that overall adherence to the lower calorie regimen over time, despite the specific composition of the diet, is a stronger predictor of weight loss.

HIGH-PROTEIN, LOW-CARBOHYDRATE APPROACHES

High-protein, low-carbohydrate diets are a popular approach to losing weight. These diets typically recommend at least 30% to 50% of their total calories from protein and drastically restrict carbohydrate. Low-carbohydrate intake leads to less glycogen synthesis and therefore less water in the body (about 3 grams of water are stored per gram of glycogen). As discussed in Chapter 4, a very-low-carbohydrate intake also forces the liver to produce needed glucose. The source of carbons for this glucose is mostly proteins from tissues such as muscle, resulting in loss of protein tissue, which is about 72% water. Essential ions such as potassium

▲ In time, the very-low-carbohydrate, high-protein diets typically leave a person fatigued and wanting more variety in meals, and so the diets are abandoned. Dropout rates are high on these diets. © Ernie Friedlander/Cole Group/Getty Images

are also lost in the urine. In the initial stages of a low-carbohydrate diet, losses of glycogen stores, lean tissue, and water cause rapid weight loss. When a normal diet is resumed, the protein tissue is rebuilt and the weight is regained.

In addition, restricting carbohydrate causes your body to burn fat instead of carbohydrate for fuel. In theory, this burning of excess fat stores makes a lot of sense for weight loss. Remember, however, that when we burn fat without carbohydrate, it causes the body to go into the metabolic state called ketosis. This disruption in the body's acid-base balance has the short-term benefit of making you feel less hungry, yet long-term ketosis can become dangerous when ketones build up. High levels of ketones lead to dehydration and alterations in the chemical balance of your blood.

For most dieters, a low-carb plan is such a major change from normal habits that it is very difficult to maintain. However, research indicates that low-carbohydrate diets may be an effective alternative to low-fat diets for some people (see Further Reading 2). In a recent 2-year study published in the *New England Journal of Medicine,* moderately obese adults on a low-carbohydrate diet lost and kept off about 12 pounds, compared to 10 pounds for those following the traditional Mediterranean diet and 7 pounds for those on a restricted-fat plan. This study suggested that the ability to stick with moderate calorie restriction over the long term is a better determinant of success than the exact macronutrient composition of the diet (see Further Reading 17). The most popular diet using a low-carbohydrate approach is Dr. Atkins' New Diet Revolution. More moderate approaches are found in the various Zone diets (40% of calorie intake as carbohydrate), Sugar Busters diet, and the South Beach diet (especially initial phases).

CARBOHYDRATE-FOCUSED DIETS

Several recent diets, including Sugar Busters, the Glucose Revolution, and Eat, Drink, and Weigh Less, do not restrict carbohydrates but rather emphasize the "good" carbohydrates in place of the "bad" or "harmful" ones. These diets recommend eating plenty of fruits, vegetables, whole grains, and cutting out simple sugars and processed or refined grains. The carbohydrate-focused diets rely largely on low glycemic index foods. In theory, these foods will cause a slow, steady rise and fall in blood sugar after a meal, which may help control hunger.

LOW-FAT APPROACHES

The very-low-fat diets contain approximately 5% to 10% of calories as fat and are often very high in carbohydrates. The most notable are the Pritikin Diet and the Dr. Dean Ornish "Eat More, Weigh Less" diet plans. If followed consistently, these approaches lead to weight loss and may be helpful for reducing heart disease risks; however, they are difficult to follow. People are quickly bored with this type of diet because they cannot eat many of their favorite foods. These dieters eat primarily plant-based foods (grains, fruits, and vegetables), which most people cannot do for very long. Eventually, the person wants some foods higher in fat or protein. Furthermore, such diets may have too much carbohydrate for some people who have a family history of diabetes.

NOVELTY DIETS

A variety of diets are built on gimmicks. Some novelty diets emphasize one food or food group and exclude almost all others. A rice diet was designed in the 1940s to lower blood pressure; now it has resurfaced as a weight-loss diet. The first phase consists of eating only rice and fruit. On the Beverly Hills Diet, you eat mostly fruit. The Paleo Diet is designed to mimic the diets of cavemen and includes meats, seafood, vegetables, fruits, and nuts.

The most questionable of the novelty diets propose that "food gets stuck in your body." Fit for Life, the Beverly Hills Diet, and Eat Great, Lose Weight are examples. The supposition is that food gets stuck in the intestine, putrefies, and creates toxins, which invade the blood and cause disease. In response, recommendations are to not consume meat with potatoes or to consume fruits only after noon. These recommendations are based on no scientific merit, make no physiological sense, and promote unnecessary weight cycling.

MEAL REPLACEMENTS

Meal replacements come in many forms, including beverages or formulas, frozen or shelf-stable entrees, and meal or snack bars. Most meal replacements are fortified with vitamins and minerals and are appropriate to replace one or two regular meals or snacks per day. Although they are not a "magic bullet" for weight loss, they have been shown to help some people lose weight. Advantages of these convenient products are that they provide portion- and calorie-controlled foods that can serve as a visual education on appropriate portion sizes. A disadvantage is that when dieters rely on foods selected and prepared by someone else, they do not learn behaviors necessary to select and prepare healthy foods on their own.

QUACKERY IS CHARACTERISTIC OF MANY POPULAR DIETS

Many popular diets fall under the category of quackery—people taking advantage of others. They usually involve a product or service that costs a considerable amount of money. Often, those offering the product or service don't realize that they are promoting quackery because they were victims themselves. For example, they tried the product and by pure coincidence, felt it worked for them, so they promote it to all their friends and relatives.

Numerous other gimmicks for weight loss have come and gone and are likely to resurface. If in the future an important aid for weight loss is discovered, you can feel confident that major journals, such as the *Journal of the Academy of Nutrition and Dietetics, Journal of the American Medical Association,* or *New England Journal of Medicine,* will report it. Quackwatch.com is an online resource for consumers to help identify quackery.Further Readings

CASE STUDY   Choosing a Weight-Loss Program

Joe has a hectic schedule. During the day, he works full time at a warehouse distribution center filling orders. At night, three times a week, he attends class at the local community college in pursuit of computer certification. On weekends, he likes to watch sports on television, spend time with family and friends, and study. Joe has little time to exercise or think about what he eats—that is, convenience rules. He stops for coffee and a pastry on his way to work, has a burger or pizza for lunch at a fast-food restaurant, and for dinner picks up fried chicken or fish at the drive-through on his way to class. Unfortunately, over the past few years, Joe's weight has been climbing. He is 5 feet, 10 inches tall and weighs 200 pounds. Lately, he has frequently been short of breath during his shift at work. Watching a game on television a few nights ago, he saw an infomercial for a weight-loss supplement that promises to increase his energy level and allow him to continue to eat large portions of tasty foods but not gain weight. A famous actor supports the claim that this product allows one to eat at will and not gain weight. This claim is tempting to Joe.

Answer the following questions, then check your responses at the end of the chapter.

1. Has Joe been experiencing positive or negative energy balance over the past few years? What is his current BMI?
2. What aspects of Joe's lifestyle (other than diet) are causing this effect on his energy balance?
3. What changes could Joe make to his diet and physical activity patterns that would promote weight loss or maintenance?
4. Why should Joe be skeptical of the claims he heard about the weight-loss product in the infomercial?
5. Referring back to the characteristics of unreliable diets, what advice can you offer Joe for evaluating weight-loss programs?

▲ What changes can Joe make in his daily routine and diet to prevent weight gain? © Ryan McVay/Getty Images

Summary (Numbers refer to numbered sections in the chapter.)

7.1 Energy balance considers energy intake and energy output. Negative energy balance occurs when energy output surpasses energy intake, resulting in weight loss. Positive energy balance occurs when calorie intake is greater than output, resulting in weight gain.

Basal metabolism, the thermic effect of food, physical activity, and adaptive thermogenesis account for total energy use by the body. Basal metabolism, which represents the minimum amount of calories required to keep the resting, awake body alive, is primarily affected by lean body mass, surface area, and thyroid hormone concentrations. Physical activity is energy use above that expended at rest. The thermic effect of food describes the increase in metabolism that facilitates digestion, absorption, and processing of the nutrients recently consumed. Adaptive thermogenesis includes nonvoluntary activities, such as shivering and fidgeting, that increase energy use and may counter extra calories from overeating. In a sedentary person, about 70% to 85% of energy use is accounted for by basal metabolism and the thermic effect of food.

7.2 Energy use by the body can be measured as heat given off by direct calorimetry or as oxygen used by indirect calorimetry. A person's Estimated Energy Requirement can be calculated based on the following factors: gender, height, weight, age, and amount of physical activity.

7.3 A body mass index (weight in kilograms ÷ height^2 in meters) of 18.5 to 24.9 is one measure of healthy weight. A healthy weight is best determined in conjunction with a thorough health evaluation by a clinician or dietitian. A body mass index of 25 to 29.9 represents overweight. Obesity is defined as a body mass index of 30 or move or a total body fat percentage over 25% (men) or 35% (women).

Fat distribution greatly determines health risks associated with obesity. Upper-body fat storage (android), as measured by a waist circumference greater than 40 inches (102 centimeters) for men or 35 inches (88 centimeters) for women, typically results in higher risks of hypertension, cardiovascular disease, and type 2 diabetes than lower-body fat storage (gynoid).

7.4 Both genetic (nature) and environmental (nurture) factors can increase the risk of obesity. The set-point theory proposes that we have a genetically predetermined body weight or body fat content, which the body strives to regulates.

7.5 A sound weight-loss program should meet the individual's nutritional needs by emphasizing a wide variety of low-calorie, high-fiber foods; adapts to one's habits; consists of readily obtainable foods; strives to change poor eating behaviors; stresses regular physical activity; and stipulates the supervision by a clinician if weight is to be lost rapidly, if the person is obese (body mass index over 40), or if the individual is over the age of 40 (men) or 50 (women) and plans to perform substantially greater physical activity than recommended.

7.6 New weight-loss formulas predict a much slower and realistic pattern of weight loss, with a calorie deficit of 10 kcal per day resulting in a 1-pound weight loss over 3 years. Weight change is not linear; it occurs most rapidly during the first year after a change in energy balance, but tapers off over the next 2 years if changes in energy intake and physical activity are strictly maintained over time.

7.7 Physical activity as part of a weight-loss program should be focused on duration rather than intensity. Ideally, about 60 minutes of moderate-intensity physical activity should be part of each day to prevent adult weight gain.

7.8 Behavior changes are a vital part of a weight-loss program because individuals may have many habits that discourage successful weight loss and maintenance. Specific behavior modification techniques, such as stimulus control and self-monitoring, can be used to help change problem behavior.

7.9 Medications to blunt appetite, such as phenteramine (Fastin) and lorcaserin (Belviq), can aid weight loss. Orlistat (Xenical) reduces fat absorption from a meal when taken with the meal. Weight-loss drugs are reserved for those who are obese or have weight-related problems, and they must be administered under close physician supervision.

The treatment of severe obesity may include very-low-calorie diets containing 400 to 800 kcal per day or bariatric surgery to reduce stomach volume to approximately 30 milliliters (1 ounce). Both of these measures should be reserved for people who have failed at more conservative approaches to weight loss. They also require close medical supervision.

7.10 Underweight can be caused by a variety of factors, such as excessive physical activity and genetics. Sometimes being underweight requires medical attention. A primary care provider should be consulted first to rule out underlying health issues. The underweight person may need to increase portion sizes, learn to incorporate calorie-dense foods frequently, and drink fluids between meals. In addition, encouraging a regular meal and snack schedule aids in both weight gain and weight maintenance.

7.11 Many overweight people try popular diets that most often are not helpful and may actually be harmful. Unreliable diets typically share some common characteristics, including promoting quick weight loss, limiting food selections, using personal testimonials as proof, and requiring no physical activity.

Check Your Knowledge (Answers are available at the end of this question set.)

1. An energy deficit of 100 kcal per day would result in a total weight loss of about 10 pounds over a _____ period.
   a. 1-week
   b. 4-week
   c. 1-year
   d. 3-year

2. Thermic effect of food represents the energy cost of
   a. chewing food.
   b. peristalsis.
   c. basal metabolism.
   d. digesting, absorbing, and packaging nutrients.

3. A well-designed weight-loss diet should
   a. increase physical activity.
   b. alter problem behaviors.
   c. reduce energy intake.
   d. do all of the above.

4. All of the following factors are associated with a higher basal metabolic rate *except*
   a. stress.
   b. low calorie intake.
   c. fever.
   d. pregnancy.

5. The intent of bariatric surgery is to
   a. reduce stomach volume.
   b. slow transit time.
   c. surgically remove adipose tissue.
   d. prevent snacking.

6. Basal metabolism
   a. represents about 30% of total energy expenditure.
   b. is energy used to maintain heartbeat, respiration, other basic functions, and physical activities.
   c. represents about 60% to 75% of total calories used by the body during a day.
   d. includes energy to digest food.

7. It is recommended that adults should do the equivalent of _____ minutes of moderate-intensity aerobic activity each week for weight loss and to achieve and maintain a healthy body weight.
   a. 60
   b. 90
   c. 150
   d. 300

8. Probably the most important contributing factor for obesity rates today in the United States is
   a. food advertising.
   b. snacking practices.
   c. inactivity.
   d. eating processed food.

9. The major goal for weight reduction in the treatment of obesity is the loss of
   a. weight.
   b. body fat.
   c. body water.
   d. body protein.

10. For most adults, the greatest portion of their energy expenditure is for
    a. physical activity.
    b. sleeping.
    c. basal metabolism.
    d. the thermic effect of food.

Answer Key: 1. d (LO 7.6), 2. d (LO 7.2), 3. d (LO 7.6), 4. b (LO 7.1), 5. a (LO 7.10), 6. c (LO 7.1), 7. c (LO 7.8), 8. c (LO 7.5), 9. b (LO 7.6), 10. c (LO 7.1)

Study Questions (Numbers refer to Learning Outcomes)

1. Explain how nurture and nature can contribute to the development of obesity. What are the two most convincing pieces of evidence that both genetic and environmental factors play significant roles in the development of obesity? **(LO 7.4)**

2. How does energy imbalance, including the role of physical activity, lead to weight gain and obesity? **(LO 7.1)**

3. Define how a healthy weight may be determined. **(LO 7.3)**

4. Describe a practical tool to define obesity in a clinical setting. **(LO 7.3)**

5. List three health issues that are related to obesity and the mechanism or reason that each condition occurs. **(LO 7.3)**

6. List three key characteristics of a sound weight-loss program? **(LO 7.5)**

7. Why is the claim for quick, effortless weight loss by any method always misleading? **(LO 7.5)**

8. Define the term *behavior modification*. Relate it to the terms *stimulus control, self-monitoring, chain-breaking, relapse prevention,* and *cognitive restructuring*. Give examples of each. **(LO 7.8)**

9. Why should obesity treatment be viewed as a lifelong commitment rather than a short diet or episode of weight loss? **(LO 7.5)**

10. What steps are important to remember when an underweight person wants to gain muscle but not fat? **(LO 7.10)**

What the Dietitian Chose

© Ingram Publishing/SuperStock

In this case, the dietitian starts with the Nutrition Facts panel (label) on the package when making a dessert choice. Research has shown that reading labels plays a role in decreasing obesity, especially in women, who were found to be more likely to read nutrition labels (see Further Reading 13). Regular varieties of ice cream contain at least 10% milk fat by weight and are therefore a source of saturated fat and cholesterol. The milk fat gives the product the smooth, creamy texture for which ice cream is famous. You can see that the regular ice cream has 180 kcal, 10 grams fat, 6 grams saturated fat, and 65 mg cholesterol. The sugar content is 19 grams; some of this comes from natural milk sugar (lactose), and some sugar is added for flavor.

Premium ice cream varieties, such as those you would find in an ice cream shop, may have up to 300 kcal, 18 grams fat, and 30 grams sugar per ½-cup serving! That's equivalent to 4 teaspoons of butter and 7 teaspoons of sugar. Such decadent treats can be enjoyed in moderation but are best reserved for special occasions.

Reduced-fat, low-fat, light, or fat-free varieties of ice cream have less than 10% milk fat. This can be accomplished by starting with lower-fat milk, using gelatin instead of eggs, using fat replacers, incorporating more air into the product (e.g., "churned"), or any combination thereof. "Reduced fat" means the product has at least 25% less fat than the original product. "Low fat" sets the standard at 3 grams of fat or less per ½-cup serving.

"Light" ice cream has at least 50% less fat than the original product. "Fat free" signifies 0.5 gram of fat or less per ½-cup serving. The brand shown here is "light": it contains lower fat and sugar than the regular ice cream. It has 110 kcal, 3 grams fat, 2 grams saturated fat, 10 milligrams cholesterol, and 14 grams sugar per serving. For weight-management purposes, this saves you 70 kcal, 7 grams of fat, and 5 grams of sugar per serving compared to regular ice cream. Reducing the fat content of ice cream might also reduce the creamy texture, but for most reduced-fat, low-fat, and light products, the change is barely noticeable.

© Comstock Images

Frozen yogurt is not always a lower-calorie option than ice cream. It does not have to comply with the same 10% milk fat standard as ice cream does, so there may be a wide range of fat and sugar contents. This brand of frozen yogurt has 180 kcal, 3 grams fat, 1 gram saturated fat, and 45 milligrams cholesterol. The product is marketed as "low fat"—and it does only contain 3 grams of fat per ½-cup serving—but there are still 22 grams of sugar. This is a great example of how low fat does not necessarily mean low calorie.

Serving size is the most important part of the Nutrition Facts panel when it comes to calorie control. No matter how low the calorie, fat, and sugar contents are, if you consume multiple servings of any product, you are likely to take in too many calories. Likewise, you can control your calorie intake by choosing a smaller portion of premium ice cream.

Nutrition Facts

Kroger Private Selection—Country Made Vanilla Ice Cream

Serving Size:			2/3 cup
Calories			**240**

Total Fat	13 g	**Total Carbs**	25 g
Saturated	8 g	Dietary Fiber	0 g
Trans	0 g	Total Sugars 25g	
Polyunsaturated	0 g	Includes 19g	
Monounsaturated	0 g	Added Sugars	38%
Cholesterol	87 mg	**Protein**	8 g
		Sodium	60 mg

Vitamin D 0.2mcg	2%	Iron 0.4mg	2%
Calcium 100mg	10%	Potassium 175mg	5%

The % Daily Value (DV) tells you how much a nutrient in a serving of food contributes to a daily diet. 2,000calories a day is used for general nutrition advice.

Nutrition Facts

Kroger Deluxe—Vanilla Bean Light Ice Cream

Serving Size:			2/3 cup
Calories			**145**

Total Fat	4 g	**Total Carbs**	23 g
Saturated	2.5 g	Dietary Fiber	0 g
Trans	0 g	Total Sugars 19g	
Polyunsaturated	0 g	Includes 12g	
Monounsaturated	0 g	Added Sugars	24%
Cholesterol	13 mg	**Protein**	4 g
		Sodium	67 mg

Vitamin D 0.1mcg	1%	Iron 0mg	0%
Calcium 100mg	10%	Potassium 211mg	5%

The % Daily Value (DV) tells you how much a nutrient in a serving of food contributes to a daily diet. 2,000calories a day is used for general nutrition advice.

Nutrition Facts

Haagen-Dazs—Yogurt Frozen Low Fat Vanilla

Serving Size:			2/3 cup
Calories			**240**

Total Fat	4 g	**Total Carbs**	40 g
Saturated	1.3 g	Dietary Fiber	0 g
Trans	0 g	Total Sugars 30g	
Polyunsaturated	0 g	Includes 23g	
Monounsaturated	0 g	Added Sugars	46%
Cholesterol	64 mg	**Protein**	12 g
		Sodium	60 mg

Vitamin D 0.2mcg	2%	Iron 0mg	0%
Calcium 200mg	20%	Potassium 180mg	5%

The % Daily Value (DV) tells you how much a nutrient in a serving of food contributes to a daily diet. 2,000calories a day is used for general nutrition advice.

CASE STUDY SOLUTION Choosing a Weight-Loss Program

1. Joe's weight has been climbing, so he has been experiencing positive energy balance.
2. When Joe is not working, his activity level is low. His time watching television and studying does not use much energy. Joe should try to find time for physical activity after work and on weekends.
3. Balancing calorie intake with energy expenditure is the main key to weight loss and weight maintenance. Changes that Joe could make to his diet include a decrease in high saturated-fat and high-calorie items in his take-out meals. He should include more fruits, vegetables, and whole grains in his meals. A whole-grain cereal with fruit would be a healthy and convenient substitute for his breakfast pastry.

   A grilled chicken sandwich on a whole-grain bun or a nutritious salad would be a healthy option for lunch. Grilled fish or chili with a sweet potato or salad would be healthier choices for dinner. Table 7-4 includes many ideas for food substitutions that will lower calories.
4. Joe will be wasting his money if he buys the product seen in the infomercial. Unfortunately, regulation of the supplement industry is woefully lacking. In the future, if there is a meaningful breakthrough in weight loss and weight control, health authorities such as the Surgeon General's Office or the National Institutes of Health will make North Americans aware of that fact.
5. The characteristics of a sound weight-loss plan are shown in Figure 7-16. These characteristics include a slow and steady rate of weight loss, flexibility relative to your habits and tastes, nutritional adequacy, behavior modification, physical activity, and maintenance of overall health.

Further Readings

1. Academy of Nutrition and Dietetics: Position of the Academy of Nutrition and Dietetics: Total diet approach to healthy eating. *Journal of the Academy of Nutrition and Dietetics* 113:307, 2013.

2. Bazzano LA and others: Effects of low-carbohydrate and low-fat diets: A randomized trial. *Annals of Internal Medicine* 161(5):309, 2014.

3. Centers for Disease Control and Prevention (CDC). Overweight and obesity. November 12, 2015. http://www.cdc.gov/obesity/data/ prevalence-maps.html. Accessed November 14, 2015.

4. Dyczkowski CT, Seher CL: Smartphone apps for heart-healthy living—clients can track diet and exercise habits at their fingertips. *Today's Dietitian* 14(8):18, 2012.

5. Finkelstein EA and others: Obesity and severe obesity forecasts through 2030. *American Journal of Preventive Medicine* 42(6):563, 2012.

6. Flegal KM and others: Prevalence of obesity and trends in the distribution of body mass index among U.S. adults, 1999–2010. *Journal of the American Medical Association* 307(5):491, 2012.

7. Ford ES, Dietz WH: Trends in energy intake among adults in the United States: Findings from NHANES. *American Journal of Clinical Nutrition* 97(4):848, 2013.

8. Hall KD and others: Energy balance and its components: Implications for body weight regulation. *American Journal of Clinical Nutrition* 95:989, 2012.

9. Harris C: Mindful eating—studies show this concept can help clients lose weight and better manage chronic disease. *Today's Dietitian* 15(3):42, 2013.

10. Hollis JF and others: Weight loss during the intensive intervention phase of the weight-loss maintenance trial. *American Journal of Preventive Medicine* 35:118, 2008.

11. James WPT and others: Effect of sibutramine on cardiovascular outcomes in overweight and obese subjects. *New England Journal of Medicine* 363(10):905, 2010.

12. Keidar A: Bariatric surgery for type 2 diabetes reversal: The risks. *Diabetes Care* 34:S361, 2011.

13. Loureiro ML and others: The effects of nutritional labels on obesity. *Agricultural Economics* 43:333, 2012.

14. Miller LE: Lorcaserin for weight loss: Insights into U.S. Food and Drug Administration approval. *Journal of the Academy of Nutrition and Dietetics* 113:25, 2013.

15. National Center for Chronic Disease Prevention and Health Promotion: *Obesity: Halting the epidemic by making health easier.* Centers for Disease Control and Prevention, Department of Health and Human Services, 2009.

16. See R and others: The association of differing measures of overweight and obesity with prevalent atherosclerosis: The Dallas Heart Study. *Journal of the American College of Cardiology* 50:752, 2007.

17. Shai I and others: Weight loss with a low-carbohydrate, Mediterranean, or low-fat diet. *New England Journal of Medicine* 359:229, 2008.

18. Slavin J and others: How fiber affects weight regulation. *Food Technology* 62:34, 2008.

19. Svetkey LP and others: Comparison of strategies for sustaining weight loss: The weight-loss maintenance randomized controlled trial. *Journal of the American Medical Association* 299:1139, 2008.

20. Trust for America's Health: F as in fat: How obesity threatens America's future 2012. Robert Wood Johnson Foundation. 2012. http://healthyamericans.org/report/100/. Accessed April 5, 2013.

 To get the most out of your study of nutrition, go to McGraw-Hill's online resources: Connect www.mcgrawhillconnect.com, where you will find NutritionCalc Plus, LearnSmart, and many other dynamic tools.

Rate Your Plate

A Close Look at Your Weight Status

Determine the following two indices of your body status: body mass index and waist circumference.

Body Mass Index (BMI)

Record your weight in pounds: _____ pounds

Divide your weight in pounds by 2.2 to determine your weight in kilograms: _____ kilograms

Record your height in inches: _____ inches

Divide your height in inches by 39.4 to determine your height in meters: _____ meters

Calculate your BMI using the following formula:

BMI = weight (kilograms)/height^2 (meters)

BMI = _____ kg/ _____ m^2 = _____

Waist Circumference

Use a tape measure to measure the circumference of your waist (just above the hip bone with your stomach relaxed; see http://www.cdc.gov/healthyweight/assessing/). Circumference of waist (umbilicus) = _____ inches

Interpretation

1. When BMI is greater than 25, health risks from obesity often begin. It is especially advisable to consider weight loss if your BMI exceeds 30. Does yours exceed 25 (or 30)?

   Yes _____ No _____

2. When a person has a BMI greater than 25 and a waist circumference of more than 40 inches (102 centimeters) in men or 35 inches (88 centimeters) in women, there is an increased risk of cardiovascular disease, hypertension, and type 2 diabetes. Does your waist circumference exceed the standard for your gender?

   Yes _____ No _____

3. Do you feel you need to pursue a program of weight loss?

   Yes _____ No _____

Application

From what you have learned in Chapter 7, list three specific actions you can take to move toward (or maintain) a healthy weight.

_____

_____

_____

Student Learning Outcomes

Chapter 8 is designed to allow you to:

8.1 Define the terms *micronutrient, vitamin, mineral,* and *functional foods,* and list characteristics of each.

8.2 Classify the vitamins according to whether they are fat soluble or water soluble.

8.3 Classify the minerals as major, trace, or ultratrace.

8.4 Discuss the digestion, absorption, and storage of micronutrients, particularly as these processes relate to risk of toxicity.

8.5 Explain how food-handling practices, conditions of the body, dietary components, and other factors influence the availability of micronutrients from food.

8.6 Summarize the basic functional roles of micronutrients, providing two examples of micronutrients that participate in each role.

8.7 Explain several health benefits of phytochemicals and identify main sources of phytochemicals.

8.8 Understand appropriate uses of dietary supplements.

Chapter 8
Overview of Micronutrients and Phytochemicals

"Let food be thy medicine and medicine be thy food."
—Hippocrates

Is food medicine? Consider the following examples:

- Fatigue, bleeding gums, bruising, and scaly skin—these are the symptoms of **scurvy,** which plagued seamen during long ocean voyages until 1753 when James Lind, a physician in the British navy, found that consumption of citrus fruits could prevent this disease.
- An epidemic of **rickets** occurred among children in post–Industrial-Revolution Britain during the late eighteenth century. They suffered from bone pain, frequent fractures, weakness, and deformities such as bowed legs. In 1922, cod-liver oil was determined to be an effective treatment for rickets.
- First noted in medical literature in the mid-sixteenth century, **chlorosis** was a disorder characterized by a green skin color, extreme weakness, and poor appetite. Chlorosis was mainly described among adolescent women, and some physicians of the era declared it to be a hysterical condition. In the early 1700s, British physician Thomas Sydenham prescribed that afflicted women drink "mineral water impregnated with the Iron Mine" that alleviated the symptoms.

How do citrus fruits, cod-liver oil, and mineral water prevent or cure such serious ailments? As nutrition science has evolved, the discovery of essential compounds in the foods and beverages we consume has overturned old misconceptions about the origins of some diseases. Citrus fruits (sure cures for scurvy) contain vitamin C. Cod-liver oil, a preventive treatment for rickets, is an excellent source of vitamin D. The mineral water prescribed by Sydenham supplied iron for his patients suffering from chlorosis, a form of iron-deficiency anemia.

Vitamins C and D and iron are just a few examples of **micronutrients**—nutrients that yield no energy and are required in small amounts (milligrams or micrograms). However slight its requirement, each micronutrient is essential for one or more functions in the body (Fig. 8-1). In this chapter, we will present an overview of the micronutrients. You will gain knowledge about the micronutrients and begin to see how vitamins and minerals work together to perform various physiological functions. Later, in Chapters 9 through 13, the functional roles of these micronutrients will be examined in greater detail.

scurvy The vitamin C deficiency disease characterized by weakness, fatigue, slow wound healing, opening of previously healed wounds, bone pain, fractures, sore and bleeding gums, diarrhea, and pinpoint hemorrhages on the skin.

rickets A disease characterized by poor mineralization of newly synthesized bones because of low calcium content. Arising in infants and children, this deficiency is caused by insufficient amounts of the vitamin D hormone in the body.

FIGURE 8-1 ▶ Micronutrients contribute to many functions in the body. © John Lund/ Getty Images

chlorosis In traditional medical terminology, a form of iron-deficiency anemia characterized by pale or greenish skin, weakness, fatigue, and shortness of breath. In modern medical literature, chlorosis is termed *hypochromic anemia*.

micronutrient A nutrient needed in milligram or microgram quantities in a diet.

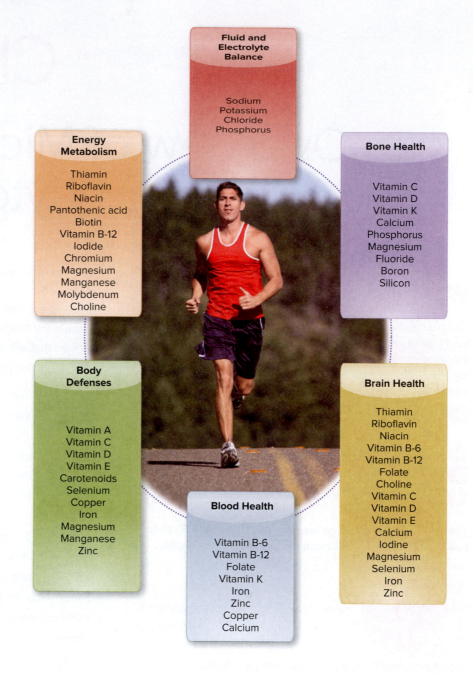

Fluid and Electrolyte Balance

Sodium
Potassium
Chloride
Phosphorus

Energy Metabolism

Thiamin
Riboflavin
Niacin
Pantothenic acid
Biotin
Vitamin B-12
Iodide
Chromium
Magnesium
Manganese
Molybdenum
Choline

Bone Health

Vitamin C
Vitamin D
Vitamin K
Calcium
Phosphorus
Magnesium
Fluoride
Boron
Silicon

Body Defenses

Vitamin A
Vitamin C
Vitamin D
Vitamin E
Carotenoids
Selenium
Copper
Iron
Magnesium
Manganese
Zinc

Blood Health

Vitamin B-6
Vitamin B-12
Folate
Vitamin K
Iron
Zinc
Copper
Calcium

Brain Health

Thiamin
Riboflavin
Niacin
Vitamin B-6
Vitamin B-12
Folate
Choline
Vitamin C
Vitamin D
Vitamin E
Calcium
Iodine
Magnesium
Selenium
Iron
Zinc

8.1 Vitamins: Vital Dietary Components

vitamin An essential organic (carbon-containing) compound needed in small amounts in the diet to help regulate and support chemical reactions and processes in the body.

fat-soluble vitamins Vitamins that dissolve in fat and such substances as ether and benzene but not readily in water. These vitamins are A, D, E, and K.

water-soluble vitamins Vitamins that dissolve in water. These vitamins are the B vitamins and vitamin C.

By definition, **vitamins** are essential organic (carbon-containing) substances needed in small amounts in the diet for normal function, growth, and maintenance of the body. In general, humans require a total of about 1 ounce (28 grams) of vitamins for every 150 pounds (70 kilograms) of food consumed. Vitamins can be divided into two broad classes based on solubility: vitamins A, D, E, and K are **fat-soluble vitamins** (Table 8-1), whereas the B vitamins and vitamin C are **water-soluble vitamins** (Table 8-2). The B vitamins include thiamin, riboflavin, niacin, pantothenic acid, biotin, vitamin B-6, folate, and vitamin B-12. Although choline is not classified as a vitamin, it is an essential nutrient so will be discussed in this chapter.

Vitamins are generally *essential* in human diets because they cannot be synthesized in the human body, and their synthesis may be reduced by environmental factors. This means we must obtain these nutrients in our diets. Notable exceptions are vitamin A, which we

TABLE 8-1 ■ Summary of the Fat-Soluble Vitamins

Vitamin	Major Functions	RDA or AI	Dietary Sources	Deficiency Symptoms	Toxicity Symptoms
Vitamin A (preformed and provitamin A)	• Required for normal vision • Gene expression • Growth, development, reproduction • Embryonic development • Immune function • Cancer prevention	*Men:* 900 micrograms RAE (3000 IU preformed vitamin A) *Women:* 700 micrograms RAE (2300 IU preformed vitamin A)	• Liver • Fortified dairy • Fish, fish oils • Darkly colored fruits and leafy vegetables • Fortified milk • Eggs	• Night blindness • Xerophthalmia • Inadequate growth • Dry skin • Inadequate immune function	• Birth defects • Bone pain and fractures • Liver toxicity • Nervous system disorders • Nausea and vomiting UL = 3000 micrograms (10,000 IU) of preformed vitamin A
Vitamin D (calciferol)	• Maintain serum calcium and phosphorus concentrations • Bone health • Gene expression and cell growth	15 micrograms (600 IU)	• Fish liver oils • Flesh of fatty fish • Egg yolk • Fortified dairy • Fortified cereals	• Rickets in children • Osteomalacia in adults • Delayed growth • Reduced immunity	• Hypercalcemia • Decreased renal function and hypercalciuria • Kidney failure • Cardiovascular system failure • Calcification of soft tissues UL = 100 micrograms (4000 IU)
Vitamin E	• Antioxidant • Prevents breakdown of vitamin A and unsaturated fatty acids	15 milligrams alpha-tocopherol (22 IU natural form, 33 IU synthetic form)	• Vegetable oils • Unprocessed cereal grains • Nuts • Fruits • Vegetables • Fortified cereals	• Hemolysis of red blood cells • Nerve damage • Anemia	• Hemorrhagic toxicity UL = 1000 milligrams (1100 IU synthetic form, 1500 IU natural form)
Vitamin K	• Coenzyme during the synthesis of proteins involved in blood clotting and bone metabolism	*Men:* 120 milligrams *Women:* 90 milligrams	• Green leafy vegetables • Liver • Plant oils and margarine	• Hemorrhage • Fractures	• Disruption of anticlotting medications No UL

Abbreviations: RDA= Recommended Dietary Allowance; AI = adequate intake; RAE = retinol activity equivalents; IU = international units; UL = Upper Intake Level

can synthesize from certain pigments in plants; vitamin D, which we can synthesize in the body if the skin is exposed to adequate sunlight; niacin, synthesized from the amino acid tryptophan; and vitamin K and biotin, synthesized to some extent by bacteria in the intestinal tract.

To be classified as a vitamin, a compound must meet the following criteria: (1) the body is unable to synthesize enough of the compound to maintain health; and (2) absence of the compound from the diet for a defined period produces deficiency symptoms that, if caught in time, are quickly alleviated when the essential compound is reintroduced. A compound does not qualify as a vitamin merely because the body cannot make it. Evidence must suggest that deficiency occurs and health may decline when the substance is not consumed.

As scientists began to identify various vitamins, related deficiency diseases, such as scurvy and rickets, were dramatically corrected. For the most part, as the vitamins were discovered, they were named alphabetically: A, B, C, D, E, and so on. Later, many substances

TABLE 8-2 ■ **Summary of the Water-Soluble Vitamins and Choline**

Vitamin	Major Functions	RDA or AI	Dietary Sources*	Deficiency Symptoms	Toxicity Symptoms
Thiamin	• Coenzyme in metabolism of carbohydrates and branched-chain amino acids	*Men:* 1.2 milligrams *Women:* 1.1 milligrams	• Enriched, fortified, or whole grains • Ready-to-eat cereals • Pork	• Beriberi resulting in nervous system dysfunction	• Unknown No UL
Riboflavin[†]	• Coenzyme in numerous redox reactions	*Men:* 1.3 milligrams *Women:* 1.1 milligrams	• Organ meats • Milk • Bread products and fortified cereals	• Inflammation of the mouth and tongue • Eye disorders	• Unknown No UL
Niacin	• Coenzyme in many biological reduction and oxidation reactions required for energy metabolism	*Men:* 16 milligrams (NE) *Women:* 14 milligrams (NE)	• Meat, fish, poultry • Enriched and whole grains • Fortified ready-to-eat cereals	Pellagra: • Diarrhea • Dermatitis • Dementia • Death	• Flushing and itchy skin • GI distress UL = 35 milligrams
Pantothenic acid	• Coenzyme in fatty acid metabolism	5 milligrams	• Organ meats • Poultry • Beef • Potatoes • Broccoli • Whole grains • Tomato products • Yeast • Egg yolk	No natural deficiency disease or symptoms	• Unknown No UL
Biotin	• Coenzyme in synthesis of fat, glycogen, and amino acids	30 micrograms	• Liver • Small amounts in fruits and meats	• Dermatitis • Tongue soreness • Anemia • Depression	• Unknown No UL
Vitamin B-6[†]	• Coenzyme for amino-acid metabolism • Neurotransmitter synthesis • Red blood cell synthesis	*Men (up to 50 years):* 1.7 milligrams *Women (up to 50 years):* 1.3 milligrams	• Fortified cereals • Organ meats • Fortified soy-based meat substitutes	• Anemia • Convulsions • Nausea • Dermatitis • Depression	• Sensory neuropathy UL = 100 milligrams
Folate (folic acid)[†]	• Coenzyme in nucleic- and amino-acid metabolism • Red blood cell synthesis	400 micrograms (DFE)	• Enriched cereal grains • Dark leafy vegetables • Enriched and whole grains • Fortified ready-to-eat cereals	• Megaloblastic anemia • Neural tube birth defects • Diarrhea • Depression • Fatigue	• Masks vitamin B-12 deficiency UL = 1000 micrograms synthetic folic acid (exclusive of food folate)
Vitamin B-12[†]	• Coenzyme in nucleic-acid metabolism • Red blood cell synthesis	2.4 micrograms Older adults and vegans may need fortified foods or supplements	• Fortified cereals • Meat • Fish • Poultry	• Megaloblastic anemia • Nerve damage • Fatigue	• Unknown No UL

TABLE 8-2 ■ *(continued)*

Vitamin	Major Functions	RDA or AI	Dietary Sources[*]	Deficiency Symptoms	Toxicity Symptoms
Vitamin C (Ascorbic acid)	• Connective tissue synthesis • Hormone and neurotransmitter synthesis • Antioxidant • Immune function • Improves nonheme iron absorption	*Men:* 90 milligrams *Women:* 75 milligrams Smokers should add 35 milligrams	• Citrus fruits • Potatoes • Brussels sprouts • Cauliflower • Broccoli • Spinach • Strawberries	• Scurvy • Poor wound healing • Pinpoint hemorrhages • Bleeding gums • Fatigue • Infections • Bruises	• GI disturbances • Kidney stones • Excess iron absorption UL = 2 grams
Choline[†]	• Neurotransmitter and phospholipid synthesis	*Men:* 550 milligrams *Women:* 425 milligrams	• Milk • Liver • Eggs • Peanuts	No natural deficiency	• Fishy body odor • Sweating • Hypotension • Hepatotoxicity UL = 3.5 grams per day, based on development of fishy body odor and reduced blood pressure

Abbreviations: RDA =Recommended Dietary Allowance; AI = adequate intake; RAE = retinol activity equivalents; IU = international units; UL = Upper Intake Level; NE = niacin equivalents; DFE = dietary folate equivalents; UL = Upper Intake Level

[*]Fortified ready-to-eat breakfast cereals are good sources for most of these vitamins and a common source of B vitamins for many of us.

[†]These nutrients also participate in homocysteine metabolism; meeting the RDA or AI may reduce the risk of developing cardiovascular disease.

originally classified as vitamins were found not to be essential for humans and were dropped from the list. Other vitamins, thought at first to be only one chemical, turned out to be essential chemicals, so the alphabetical names had to be broken down by letter and number (B-6, B-12, and so on).

In addition to correcting deficiency diseases, a few vitamins have also proved useful in treating several nondeficiency diseases. For example, **megadoses** of a form of niacin can be prescribed as part of blood cholesterol-lowering treatment for certain individuals. Still, any claimed benefits from use of vitamin supplements, especially intakes in excess of the Upper Level (if set), should be viewed critically because unproved supplement claims are quite common. Remember, whenever you take a supplement at high doses, you are taking it at a pharmacological dose—that of a drug. Expect side effects as you would from any drug.

Vitamins isolated from foods ("natural") or synthesized in the laboratory ("synthetic") are the same chemical compounds and work equally well in the body. Contrary to claims in the health-food literature, "natural" vitamins isolated from foods are, with very few exceptions, no more healthful or effective than those synthesized in a laboratory. Of note, the natural form of vitamin E is more potent than the synthetic form. In contrast, synthetic folic acid, the form of the vitamin added to ready-to-eat breakfast cereals and flour, is 1.7 times more potent than the natural vitamin form (see Further Reading 3).

megadose Large intake of a nutrient beyond estimates of needs or what would be found in a balanced diet; 2 to 10 times human needs is a starting point.

ABSORPTION AND STORAGE OF VITAMINS IN THE BODY

The fat-soluble vitamins (A, D, E, and K) are absorbed along with dietary fat. Special carriers in the bloodstream help distribute some of these vitamins. These vitamins travel together with dietary fats as part of chylomicrons through the bloodstream to reach body cells. Fat-soluble vitamins are stored mostly in the liver and fatty tissues.

▲ It's time for a healthy snack! Store fresh produce in the refrigerator to preserve vitamin content and reduce spoilage. © Jill Giardino/Getty Images

bioavailability The degree to which an ingested nutrient is absorbed and available to be utilized by the body.

tissue saturation The limited storage capacity of water-soluble vitamins in the tissues.

When fat absorption is efficient, about 40% to 90% of the fat-soluble vitamins are absorbed. Anything that interferes with normal digestion and absorption of fats, however, also interferes with fat-soluble vitamin absorption. For example, people with cystic fibrosis, a disease that often hampers fat absorption, may develop deficiencies of fat-soluble vitamins. Some medications, such as the weight-loss drug orlistat (alli®), discussed in Section 7.9, also interfere with fat absorption. Unabsorbed fat carries these vitamins to the large intestine, and they are excreted in the feces. People with such conditions are especially susceptible to vitamin K deficiency because body stores of vitamin K are lower than those of the other fat-soluble vitamins. Vitamin supplements, taken under a primary care provider's guidance, are part of the treatment for preventing a vitamin deficiency associated with fat malabsorption. Finally, people who use mineral oil as a laxative at mealtimes risk fat-soluble vitamin deficiencies. Fat-soluble vitamins dissolve in the mineral oil, but the intestine does not absorb mineral oil. Hence, the fat-soluble vitamins are eliminated with the mineral oil in the feces.

Water-soluble vitamins are handled much differently than fat-soluble vitamins. After being ingested, the B vitamins are first broken down from their active coenzyme forms into free vitamins in the stomach and small intestine. The vitamins are then absorbed, primarily in the small intestine. Typically, about 50% to 90% of the water-soluble vitamins in the diet are absorbed, which means they have relatively high **bioavailability.** Water-soluble vitamins are transported to the liver via the hepatic portal vein and are distributed to body tissues. Once inside the cells, the active coenzyme forms are resynthesized. Although some supplement manufacturers sell vitamins in their coenzyme forms, there is no benefit of consuming the coenzyme forms, as these are broken down during digestion and activated inside cells when needed.

Excretion of vitamins varies primarily on their solubility. Except for vitamin K, fat-soluble vitamins are not readily excreted from the body. Hence, toxicity can become an issue. Water-soluble vitamins are excreted based on **tissue saturation,** the degree to which the tissue vitamin stores are full. Tissue storage capacity is limited. As the tissues become saturated, the rate of excretion via the kidney increases sharply, preventing potential toxicity. Unlike other water-soluble vitamins, B-6 and B-12 are stored in the liver and not easily excreted in the urine.

In light of the limits of tissue saturation for many water-soluble vitamins, these vitamins should be consumed in the diet daily. However, an occasional lapse in the intake of even water-soluble vitamins causes no harm. Symptoms of a vitamin deficiency occur only when that vitamin is lacking in the diet and the body stores are essentially exhausted. For example, for an average person, the diet must be devoid of thiamin for 10 days or lacking in vitamin C for 20 to 40 days before developing the first symptoms of deficiencies of these vitamins.

VITAMIN TOXICITY

For most water-soluble vitamins, when you consume more than the Recommended Dietary Allowances (RDA) or Adequate Intake (AI), the kidneys efficiently filter the excess from the blood and excrete these compounds in urine. Notable exceptions are vitamins B-6 and B-12, which are stored in the liver. Although they are water soluble, these two B vitamins may accumulate to toxic levels.

In contrast to the water-soluble vitamins, fat-soluble vitamins are not readily excreted, so they can accumulate in the body and cause toxic effects. Although a toxic effect from an excessive intake of any vitamin is theoretically possible, toxicity of the fat-soluble vitamin A is the most frequently observed. Vitamin A causes toxicity at intakes as little as two times the RDA. Vitamin E and the water-soluble vitamins niacin, vitamin B-6, and vitamin C can also cause toxic effects but only when consumed in very large amounts (15 to 100 times above recommended). Overall, vitamins are unlikely to cause toxic effects unless taken in supplement (usually pill) form. It is rare to develop a toxicity from consuming food sources of vitamins.

Some people believe that consuming vitamins far in excess of their needs provides them with extra energy, protection from disease, and prolonged youth. They seem to think that if a little is good, then more must be better. A "one-a-day" type of multivitamin and mineral supplement usually contains less than two times the Daily Values of its components, so daily use of these products is unlikely to cause toxic effects in men and non-pregnant women. However, consuming multiple supplements, especially potent sources of vitamin A, can cause serious health issues. See Section 8.4 to learn more about appropriate uses of dietary supplements.

PRESERVATION OF VITAMINS IN FOODS

Good sources of vitamins can be found in all food groups, especially fruits and vegetables (Fig. 8-2). However, storage time and several environmental factors can affect vitamin content of foods. The riper the food, the more vitamins it will contain, but substantial amounts of vitamins can be lost from the time a fruit or vegetable is harvested until it is eaten. Therefore, it is best to eat fresh produce as soon as possible after harvest. The water-soluble vitamins, particularly thiamin, vitamin C, and folate, can be destroyed with improper storage and excessive cooking. Heat, UV light, exposure to oxygen, cooking submersed in water, and alkalinity are factors that can destroy vitamins.

There are several steps you can take to preserve nutrients when you are purchasing, storing, and preparing fruits and vegetables (Table 8-3). Frozen vegetables and fruits are often as nutrient rich as freshly harvested produce, because fruits and vegetables are typically frozen immediately after harvesting. As part of the flash-freezing process, vegetables are quickly blanched in boiling water. Blanching destroys the enzymes that would otherwise degrade the vitamins. If a food is not to be eaten within a few days, freezing is the best preservation method to retain nutrients.

MyPlate:

Sources of Vitamins and Choline

Grains	Vegetables	Fruits	Dairy	Protein
• Thiamin	• Vitamin A	• Vitamin A	• Vitamin D	• Thiamin
• Riboflavin	• Vitamin K	• Vitamin C	• Riboflavin	• Riboflavin
• Niacin	• Folate		• Vitamin B-12	• Niacin
• Folic acid	• Vitamin C		• Choline	• Biotin
				• Vitamin B-6
				• Vitamin B-12
				• Choline

FIGURE 8-2 ▲ Certain food groups on MyPlate are especially rich sources of various vitamins and choline. This is true for those listed. Each may be also found in other MyPlate groups but in lower amounts. In addition to those vitamins listed here, pantothenic acid is present in moderate amounts in many groups, and vitamin E is abundant in plant oils.

TABLE 8-3 ■ Tips for Preserving Vitamins in Produce

Preservation Methods	Why?
Keep fruits and vegetables cool until eaten.	Enzymes in fruits and vegetables begin to degrade vitamins once they are harvested. Chilling limits this process.
Refrigerate fruits and vegetables (except bananas, onions, potatoes, and tomatoes) in moisture-proof, airtight containers or in the vegetable drawer.	Nutrients keep best at temperatures near freezing, at high humidity, and away from air.
Trim, peel, and cut fruits and vegetables minimally—just enough to remove inedible parts.	Oxygen breaks down vitamins faster when more of the food surface is exposed. Whenever possible, cook fruits and vegetables in their skins.
Microwave, steam, or stir-fry vegetables.	More nutrients are retained when there is less contact with water.
Minimize cooking time.	Prolonged cooking (slow simmering) and reheating reduce vitamin content.
Avoid adding fats to vegetables during cooking if you plan to discard the liquid.	Fat-soluble vitamins will be lost in discarded fat. If you want to add fats, do so after vegetables are fully cooked and drained.
Do not add baking soda to vegetables to enhance the green color.	Alkalinity destroys vitamin D, thiamin, and other vitamins.
Store canned and frozen fruits and vegetables carefully.	To protect canned foods, store them in a cool, dry location. To protect frozen foods, store them at 0 °F (−32 °C) or colder. Eat within 12 months.

✓ **CONCEPT CHECK 8.1**

1. What is a megadose? Are there any negative consequences of consuming megadoses of vitamins? Are there any situations in which megadoses of vitamins are useful?

2. List at least three differences between fat-soluble and water-soluble vitamins.

3. List three ways to preserve vitamin content when storing, preparing, or cooking foods.

8.2 Minerals: Essential Elements for Health

mineral Element used in the body to promote chemical reactions and to form body structures.

Whereas vitamins are compounds consisting of many elements (e.g., carbon, oxygen, and hydrogen), **minerals** are individual chemical elements. They cannot be broken down further. The mineral content of foods is sometimes called "ash" because it is all that remains after the whole food has been destroyed by high temperatures or chemical degradation. In humans, minerals make up about 4% of adult body weight (Fig. 8-3). A mineral is essential if a dietary inadequacy results in a physiological or structural abnormality and its addition back into the diet reinstates normal health and function. Sixteen minerals are known to be essential in the diet.

Minerals are categorized based on the amount we need per day. Recall from Section 1.3 that if we require greater than 100 milligrams (1/50 of a teaspoon) of a mineral per day, it

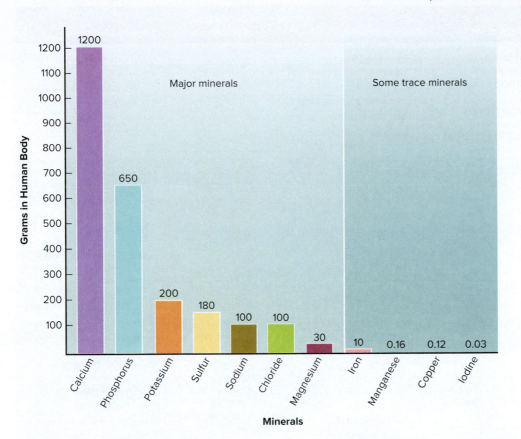

FIGURE 8-3 ◄ Approximate amounts of various minerals in the average human body. Other trace minerals of nutritional importance not listed here include chromium, fluoride, molybdenum, selenium, and zinc.

is considered a **major mineral** (Table 8-4). These include calcium, phosphorus, magnesium, sulfur, sodium, potassium, and chloride. **Trace minerals** are required at levels less than 100 milligrams per day (Table 8-5). Nine essential trace minerals (iron, zinc, copper, iodine, selenium, molybdenum, fluoride, manganese, and chromium) have been identified for humans.

Information about trace minerals is rapidly expanding. With the exceptions of iron and iodine, the importance of trace minerals to humans has been recognized only within the last 50 years or so. Although we need 100 milligrams or less of each trace mineral daily, they are as essential to good health as are major minerals.

In some cases, discovering the importance of a trace mineral reads like a detective story, and the evidence is still unfolding. In 1961, researchers linked dwarfism in Middle Eastern villagers to a zinc deficiency. Other scientists recognized that a rare form of heart disease in an isolated area of China was linked to a selenium deficiency. In North America, some trace mineral deficiencies were first observed in the late 1960s and early 1970s when the minerals were not added to synthetic formulas used for intravenous feeding.

It is difficult to precisely define our trace mineral needs because we need only minute amounts. Highly sophisticated technology is required to measure such small amounts in both food and body tissues.

There are several additional trace minerals (sometimes called **ultratrace minerals**) found in the human body, but many of them have no known requirements. These include arsenic, boron, nickel, silicon, and vanadium.

ABSORPTION AND STORAGE OF MINERALS IN THE BODY

Foods offer us a plentiful supply of many minerals, but the ability of our bodies to absorb and use them varies. The bioavailability of minerals depends on many factors, including many nonmineral components of foods. Age, gender, genetic variability, nutritional status, and diet will all affect mineral absorption and bioavailability. Numerous prescription drugs

major mineral Vital to health, a mineral that is required in the diet in amounts greater than 100 milligrams per day.

trace mineral Vital to health, a mineral that is required in the diet in amounts less than 100 milligrams per day.

ultratrace mineral A mineral present in the human diet in trace amounts but that has not been shown to be essential to human health.

Sulfur is unique among the major minerals because it has no known dietary requirement. Proteins supply all the sulfur we need. Sulfur is found in many important compounds in the body, such as some amino acids (e.g., methionine) and vitamins (e.g., biotin and thiamin). It helps to maintain acid-base balance in the body and is an important part of the liver's drug-detoxifying pathways.

TABLE 8-4 ■ Summary of the Major Minerals

Mineral	Major Functions	RDA or AI	Dietary Sources	Deficiency Symptoms	Toxicity Symptoms
Sodium	• Maintains fluid volume outside of cells and thus normal cell function	*Age 19–50 years:* 1500 milligrams *Age 51–70 years:* 1300 milligrams	• Processed foods to which sodium chloride (salt) has been added • Salted meats, nuts, cold cuts • Margarine, butter • Salt added to foods in cooking or at the table	• Muscle cramps	• Hypertension • Increased risk of cardiovascular disease and stroke UL = 2300 milligrams
Potassium	• Maintains fluid volume • Acts to blunt the rise of blood pressure in response to excess sodium intake • Decrease markers of bone turnover and recurrence of kidney stones	4700 milligrams	• Fruits • Vegetables • Dried peas • Dairy products • Meats • Nuts	• Irregular heartbeat • Loss of appetite • Muscle cramps	• None documented from food alone • Supplements or salt substitutes can result in hyperkalemia and possibly sudden death in susceptible individuals No UL
Chloride	• With sodium, maintains fluid volume outside of cells and thus normal cell function	2300 milligrams	• Foods to which sodium chloride (salt) has been added	• Convulsions in infants	• In concert with sodium, results in hypertension UL = 3600 milligrams
Calcium	• Blood clotting • Muscle contraction • Nerve transmission • Bone and tooth formation	*Age 9–18 years:* 1300 milligrams *Age >18 years:* 1000–1200 milligrams	• Dairy • Corn tortillas • Calcium-set tofu • Chinese cabbage • Kale • Broccoli • Fortified foods and beverages	• Increased risk of osteoporosis	• Kidney stones • Hypercalcemia • Hypercalciuria • Prostate cancer • Constipation • Soft tissue calcification UL = 2500 milligrams
Phosphorus	• Maintenance of pH • Storage and transfer of energy • Nucleotide synthesis	*Age 9–18 years:* 1250 milligrams *Age >18 years:* 700 milligrams	• Dairy products • Soft drinks • Peas • Meat • Nuts • Eggs • Some cereals and breads	• Possibility of poor bone maintenance	• Metastatic calcification • Skeletal porosity • Interference with calcium absorption UL = 4 grams
Magnesium	• Cofactor for enzyme systems and vitamin D activation • Reduces tooth decay	*Men:* 400–420 milligrams *Women:* 310–320 milligrams	• Green leafy vegetables • Beans and peas • Nuts • Meat • Peanut butter • Milk	• Weakness • Muscle pain • Irregular heartbeat • Seizures	• Osmotic diarrhea UL = 350 milligrams (nonfood sources only)
Sulfur	• Part of vitamins and amino acids • Aids in drug detoxification • Acid-base balance	None established	• Protein foods • Dried fruit • Soy flour • Fruit juices • Coconut milk • Red and white wine • Bread • Meats that are high in sulfur amino acids	• None observed	• Osmotic diarrhea where water supply has high levels No UL

Abbreviation: UL = Upper Intake Level; RDA= Recommended Dietary Allowance; AI = adequate intake

TABLE 8-5 ■ Summary of Key Trace Minerals

Mineral	Major Functions	RDA or AI	Dietary Sources	Deficiency Symptoms	Toxicity Symptoms
Iron	• Component of hemoglobin and numerous enzymes • Immune function • Cognitive development	*Men:* 8 milligrams *Premenopausal women:* 18 milligrams	Nonheme plant sources: • Fruits • Vegetables • Fortified bread and grain products Heme animal sources: • Meat and poultry	• Fatigue • Microcytic hypochromic anemia	• GI distress UL = 45 milligrams
Zinc	• Component of multiple enzymes and proteins • Regulation of gene expression • Protein metabolism • Wound healing and growth	*Men:* 11 milligrams *Women:* 8 milligrams	• Fortified cereals • Red meats • Seafood	• Skin rash • Diarrhea • Decreased appetite and sense of taste • Hair loss • Poor growth and development • Poor wound healing	• Reduced copper status UL = 40 milligrams
Selenium	• Defense against oxidative stress • Regulation of thyroid hormone action • Reduction and oxidation status of vitamin C and other molecules	55 micrograms	• Organ meats • Seafood • Plants (depending on soil selenium content)	• Muscle pain • Weakness • Form of heart disease	• Hair and nail brittleness and loss UL = 400 micrograms
Iodine	• Component of the thyroid hormones	150 micrograms	• Foods of marine origin • Processed foods • Iodized salt	• Goiter • Mental retardation • Congenital hypothyroidism: Poor growth in infancy when mother is iodine deficient during pregnancy	• Elevated thyroid stimulating hormone (TSH) concentration UL = 1.1 milligrams
Copper	• Component of enzymes in iron metabolism • Collagen synthesis	900 micrograms	• Organ meats • Seafood • Nuts and seeds • Wheat bran cereals, whole-grain products • Cocoa	• Anemia • Low white blood cell count • Poor growth	• GI distress • Liver damage UL = 8 to 10 milligrams
Fluoride	• Inhibits the initiation and progression of dental caries • Stimulates new bone formation	*Men:* 4 milligrams *Women:* 3 milligrams	• Fluoridated water • Fluoridated dental products • Tea • Marine fish	• Increased risk of dental caries	• Enamel and skeletal fluorosis UL = 10 milligrams
Chromium	• Helps to maintain normal blood glucose levels	*Men (up to 50 years):* 35 micrograms *Women (up to 50 years):* 25 micrograms	• Some cereals • Meats • Poultry • Fish • Beer	• High blood glucose after eating	• Chronic renal failure No UL
Manganese	• Involved in the formation of bone • Cofactor for enzymes involved in amino acid, cholesterol, and carbohydrate metabolism	*Men:* 2.3 milligrams *Women:* 1.8 milligrams	• Nuts • Legumes • Tea • Oats	None observed in humans	• Elevated blood concentration and neurotoxicity UL = 11 milligrams
Molybdenum	• Cofactor for enzymes involved in catabolism of sulfur amino acids, purines, and pyridines	45 micrograms	• Legumes • Grain products • Nuts	• None observed in healthy humans	• Reproductive effects observed in animal studies UL = 2 milligrams

Abbreviation: RDA = Recommended Dietary Allowance; AI = adequate intake; UL = Upper Intake Level

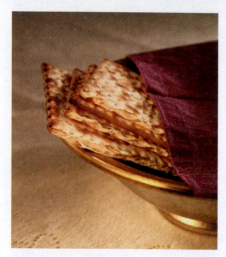

▲ The zinc deficiencies found among some Middle Eastern populations are attributed partly to their consumption of unleavened breads, such as matzo, resulting in low bio-availability of dietary zinc. If grains are leavened with yeast, as they are in bread making, enzymes produced by the yeast can break some of the bonds between phytic acid and minerals. This increases mineral absorption.
© Nancy R. Cohen/Getty Images

phytic acid (phytate) A constituent of plant fiber that chemically binds minerals and prevents their absorption. Phytic acid can depress calcium absorption from other foods present in the GI tract.

oxalic acid (oxalate) An organic acid found in spinach, rhubarb, beet greens, chard, and sweet potatoes. It can depress the absorption of certain minerals, such as calcium, but only in the food itself.

CRITICAL THINKING

Gwen follows a vegetarian diet. What factors in foods of plant origin may limit the bioavailability of minerals, such as calcium and zinc, in her diet?

---

also adversely affect mineral absorption. The mineral content listed in a food composition table is a starting point for estimating the contribution the food will make to our mineral needs.

Components of fiber, such as **phytic acid (phytate)** and **oxalic acid (oxalate),** can limit absorption of some minerals by binding to them. Spinach, for example, contains plenty of calcium, but only about 5% of it (compared to the average 25% bioavailability of calcium from foods) can be absorbed because of its high concentration of oxalic acid, which binds calcium. High-fiber diets—particularly those in excess of current daily recommendations of 25 grams (adult women) to 38 grams (adult men)—can decrease the absorption of iron, zinc, and possibly other minerals.

Many minerals, such as magnesium, calcium, iron, and copper, are of similar sizes and electrical charges ($^+2$ charge). Having similar sizes and the same electrical charge causes these minerals to compete with each other for absorption; therefore, an excess of one mineral may decrease the absorption and metabolism of other minerals. For example, a large intake of zinc decreases copper absorption. Therefore, people should avoid taking individual mineral supplements unless a dietary deficiency or medical condition specifically warrants it. Whole foods, however, pose little risk for these mineral interactions, giving us another reason to emphasize foods in meeting our nutrient needs.

Several beneficial vitamin-mineral interactions occur during nutrient absorption and metabolism. When consumed in conjunction with vitamin C, absorption of certain forms of iron, such as that in plant products, improves. The active form of the vitamin D hormone improves calcium absorption. Many vitamins also require specific minerals to act as components in their structure and as cofactors for their function. For example, without magnesium or manganese, the thiamin coenzyme cannot function efficiently.

The average North American diet derives minerals from both plant and animal sources. Overall, minerals from animal products are better absorbed than those from plants because binders, such as fiber, are not present to hinder absorption. However, the mineral content of plants greatly depends on mineral concentrations of the soil in which they are grown. Vegans should be aware of the potentially poor mineral content of some plant foods and choose some concentrated sources of minerals. Soil conditions have less of an influence on the mineral content of animal products because livestock usually consume a variety of plant products grown from soils of differing mineral contents.

Like vitamins, the majority of the minerals are absorbed in the small intestine. Minor amounts may be absorbed in the stomach, and some sodium and potassium are absorbed in the large intestine. After minerals are absorbed, some travel freely in the bloodstream, but many are carried by specific transport proteins to their sites of action or storage. Calcium is one example of a mineral that can travel as an ion in the blood or bound to a blood protein called albumin. Iron, on the other hand, has damaging effects in its unbound form, so it is transported bound to proteins, such as transferrin.

Minerals are stored in various tissues throughout the body. Some minerals must remain in the bloodstream to maintain fluid balance and aid body functions. Others, such as calcium, phosphorus, magnesium, and fluoride, are stored mainly in bones. Iron, copper, zinc, and many trace minerals are stored in the liver. Still others are stored in muscle tissue, organs, or glands.

MINERAL TOXICITIES

Excessive mineral intake, especially of trace minerals such as iron and copper, can have toxic results. For many trace minerals, the gap between just enough and too much is quite small. Taking minerals in supplement form poses the biggest threat for mineral toxicity, whereas food sources are unlikely culprits. Mineral supplements exceeding current standards for mineral needs—especially those that supply more than 100% of the Daily Values on supplement labels—should be taken only under a primary care provider's supervision. The Daily Values are, for the most part, higher than our current standards (e.g., Recommended Dietary Allowances [RDA]) for mineral needs. Without close monitoring, doses of minerals should not exceed established Upper Level values.

MyPlate:

Sources of Minerals

ChooseMyPlate.gov

FIGURE 8-4 ◄ Certain groups of MyPlate are especially rich sources of various minerals. This is true for the minerals listed. Each mineral may also be found in other groups but in lower amounts. Other trace minerals are also present in moderate amounts in many groups. With regard to the grains group, whole-grain varieties are the richest sources of most trace minerals listed.

Grains	Vegetables	Fruits	Dairy	Protein
• Sodium chloride • Calcium (fortified products) • Phosphorus • Magnesium • Iron • Zinc • Copper • Selenium • Chromium	• Potassium • Magnesium	• Potassium • Boron	• Calcium • Phosphorus • Zinc	• Sodium chloride (processed foods) • Potassium • Phosphorus • Magnesium • Selenium • Iron • Zinc • Copper

The potential for toxicity is not the only reason to carefully consider the use of mineral supplements. Harmful interactions with other nutrients are possible. Also, contamination of mineral supplements—with lead, for example—is a possibility. Use of brands approved by the United States Pharmacopeial Convention (USP) lessens this risk (see Section 8.5). Even with the best intentions, people can harm themselves using mineral supplements.

PRESERVATION OF MINERALS IN FOODS

Minerals are found in plant and animal foods (Fig. 8-4), but as you previously read, the bioavailability of minerals varies widely. Minerals are not typically lost from animal sources during processing, storage, or cooking; but for plant sources, significant amounts may be lost during food processing. When grains are refined, the final products have lost the majority of their vitamin E, many B vitamins, and many trace minerals. The more refined a plant food, as in the case of white flour, the lower its mineral content. During the enrichment of refined grain products, iron is the only mineral added, whereas the selenium, zinc, copper, and other minerals lost during refinement are not replaced. Following the recommendation of the 2015–2020 Dietary Guidelines for Americans to "make half your grains whole" will effectively preserve the mineral content of foods.

✓ CONCEPT CHECK 8.2

1. Define nutrient bioavailability.
2. Are ultratrace minerals essential in the human diet? List three examples of ultratrace minerals.
3. Should people take individual mineral supplements? Why or why not?
4. Where are minerals stored in the body?

CASE STUDY   Getting the Most Nutrition from Your Food

In the dietary supplements aisle of the grocery store, the choices are endless—and expensive. Julie, a college sophomore, just read the Academy of Nutrition and Dietetics' Position Paper on nutrient supplementation for her class. She learned that dietary supplements, such as a basic multivitamin and mineral supplement, can be a good backup plan to ensure adequate nutrition, but the jury is still out when it comes to demonstrating a long-term benefit of dietary supplements. About one-third of U.S. adults regularly take nutrient supplements, but interestingly, it is usually the people who already consume a healthy diet who take them. Getting more than the recommended amount of a nutrient does not confer additional health benefits. In fact, too much of some vitamins and minerals can lead to ill health and toxicities.

Julie decides she would rather focus on getting her nutrients from foods. How can she get the most vitamins and minerals out of the foods she eats? Answer the following questions and check your responses at the end of the chapter.

1. What factors can damage or reduce vitamins in food?
2. To maximize vitamin content, what should Julie keep in mind as she selects fresh produce for purchase?
3. How does food processing affect vitamin and mineral content? Does it make a difference if Julie chooses products with whole grains or refined grains?
4. When storing fruits and vegetables in her apartment, what steps can Julie take to minimize nutrient losses?
5. Which cooking methods are best for preserving vitamin content?

© Tanya Constantine/Blend Images LLC

8.3 The Functional Roles of Micronutrients

The next five chapters will explore the vitamins and minerals from a functional perspective. The micronutrients will be grouped and discussed as they apply to various roles and functions in the body. Keep in mind that each vitamin and mineral has multiple roles in metabolism. For example, calcium, best known for its role in bone formation, is also crucial for the transmission of nerve impulses through the body and plays a key role in blood clotting. Vitamin C contributes to cellular antioxidant function, bone health, and metabolism of proteins. At all levels—cellular, tissue, organ, and whole body—vitamins and minerals clearly play important and interrelated roles in maintaining healthy body functions.

ENZYMES, COENZYMES, AND COFACTORS

enzyme A compound that speeds up the rate of a chemical reaction but is not altered by the reaction. Almost all enzymes are proteins (some are made of genetic material).

Before moving ahead in your study of the functional roles of vitamins and minerals, it is important to understand how enzymes work. **Enzymes** are catalysts for biochemical reactions in living organisms. A catalyst is a compound that speeds the rate of a reaction but is not altered by the reaction. Think about starting a fire manually. This process can be quite cumbersome, unless you have lighter fluid. Enzymes are like lighter fluid for chemical reactions. In fact, most of the chemical reactions in the body would not occur (or would occur at very slow rates) in the absence of enzyme catalysts. As you will learn in Chapter 10, enzymes are crucial players in antioxidant reactions, which help neutralize free radicals in the body. In Chapter 12, you will see that enzymes are necessary for the normal breakdown of carbohydrates, lipids, and proteins to generate energy. They also catalyze synthetic reactions, such as the assembly of triglycerides for storage in adipose tissue. These are the roles of just a few of the enzymes in the human body; thousands of other enzymes have been identified and studied!

cofactor An inorganic compound (e.g., mineral) that combines with an inactive enzyme to form a catalytically active form.

Typically, enzymes are made of proteins, but many such proteins require the aid of another compound—a **cofactor**—for biological activity (Fig. 8-5). Frequently, the assisting compounds are one or more vitamins or minerals. A cofactor is a general term referring to any organic or inorganic substance that binds to an enzyme to aid enzyme activity. A **coenzyme** is one type of organic cofactor. In our discussions of vitamins and minerals, vitamins (organic molecules) are called coenzymes and minerals (inorganic molecules) are called cofactors.

Requirements for an enzyme and its cofactors are specific, with little or no enzymatic activity observed if another cofactor is substituted for the required one. The B vitamins function as coenzymes in many chemical reactions of energy metabolism. For example, thiamin is part of the coenzyme thiamin pyrophosphate, which catalyzes several reactions in carbohydrate and protein metabolism. Minerals are required as cofactors for activation of about 30% of all known enzymes. Selenium's role in the function of glutathione peroxidase, one of the body's antioxidant enzyme systems, is one example.

FLUID AND ELECTROLYTE BALANCE

Chapter 9 focuses on the roles of the micronutrients in fluid and electrolyte balance. Water balance requires sodium, potassium, chloride, and phosphorus. Levels of these minerals in the blood are tightly regulated by the body, and imbalances can have dire consequences. In addition to maintaining the delicate balance between intracellular and extracellular water, these minerals participate in nerve impulse transmission and acid-base balance, which are discussed briefly in Chapter 9.

BODY DEFENSES

Recall from Section 3.8 that the immune system is the body's defense against pathogens. Chapter 10 will enhance your understanding of the body's defense systems and how various vitamins, minerals, and phytochemicals protect tissues from pathogens, damaging oxidant chemicals, and tumors. Several micronutrients—especially vitamin A and zinc—are important for the proper growth and development of the tissues that make up the immune system. Other vitamins and minerals assist immune function by virtue of their antioxidant roles. These include vitamins E and C, carotenoids, and selenium.

BONE HEALTH

In Chapter 11, you will learn how micronutrients are vital to bone health. When we think of bone, we often imagine the hard, lifeless architecture of a skeleton hanging in the back of our high school science classroom. However, bone is a living and dynamic tissue that supports growth, houses nerves and blood vessels, produces blood cells, and helps regulate blood levels of certain minerals. Chapter 11 explores the roles of vitamins D and K, calcium, phosphorus, magnesium, and fluoride in bone health.

ENERGY METABOLISM

Chapter 12 delves into the roles of vitamins and minerals in energy metabolism. Although vitamins and minerals yield no energy to fuel body functions, they often participate as cofactors or coenzymes in energy-yielding reactions, as introduced previously. The B vitamins, iodine, chromium, manganese, and molybdenum are integrally involved in metabolism of the macronutrients.

BLOOD AND BRAIN HEALTH

Chapter 13 presents the roles of micronutrients in the maintenance of blood and brain health. Blood health encompasses clotting ability and the transport of oxygen, nutrients, and waste products. Vitamin K and calcium participate in blood clotting. The health of blood cells is influenced by iron, copper, folate, vitamin B-6, and vitamin B-12.

Eating for brain health encompasses supporting brain growth and development early in life as well as protecting the brain from damage (e.g., from oxidative stress) throughout

coenzyme An organic compound that combines with an inactive enzyme to form a catalytically active form. In this manner, coenzymes aid in enzyme function.

FIGURE 8-5 ▲ Coenzymes, such as those formed from B vitamins, aid in the function of various enzymes. Without the coenzyme, the enzyme cannot function properly, and deficiency symptoms associated with the missing vitamin eventually appear. Health-food stores sell the coenzyme forms of some vitamins. These expensive forms of vitamins are completely unnecessary. The body produces all the coenzymes it needs from vitamin precursors.

▲ Is it better to get nutrients from foods or dietary supplements? © Comstock Images

ASK THE RDN — Raw Food Diet Plan

Dear RDN: *My roommate follows a raw food diet and claims that cooking foods destroys key nutrients and makes foods toxic. Is this true?*

This highly restrictive diet includes consuming uncooked, unprocessed, mostly organic fruits, vegetables, and spouted grains. Some may consume unpasteurized dairy products and raw eggs, meat, and fish. Advocates of this diet believe that heat destroys key nutrients and enzymes that are necessary to fight disease. Although some phytochemicals and nutrients are more bioavailable in raw form, there are many plant-based foods (e.g., tomatoes) that actually become more digestible once exposed to heat. In addition, many uncooked and unpasteurized products are sources of foodborne pathogens. Food poisoning is of particular concern for pregnant women, young children, older adults, immunocompromised individuals, and those with chronic disease.

Limitations: This diet is extremely difficult to maintain, especially when dining out, because of its many restrictions. Complete exclusion of food groups (e.g., dairy and meat) may lead to nutrient deficiencies, so supplements (e.g., iron, calcium, and vitamin B-12) may be necessary. Also, the cost and limited availability of organic foods may be prohibitive.

Strengths: This plan is compatible with vegetarian, vegan, and gluten-free dietary patterns. Raw food adopters often lose or maintain weight given most of the foods allowed are low in calories and fat.

In sum, a plant-based dietary pattern is recommended for Americans; however, there is no evidence to support the nutritionally inadequate, extreme, and potentially harmful raw food practices.

Warm regards,

Colleen Spees, PhD, RDN, LD, FAND (author)

life. As you will learn in Chapter 13, the B vitamins support brain health because they are essential for energy and amino-acid metabolism. Antioxidant nutrients, including vitamins C and E, selenium, and some phytochemicals, may protect the brain from oxidative stress. In addition, adequate intake of the essential fatty acids supports optimal brain development and cognitive function.

MICRONUTRIENTS ARE MULTITASKERS

Micronutrients are vital to every aspect of human health. Although requirements for vitamins and minerals are small, depriving the body of any one of these important dietary components can be debilitating or even deadly. Although dietary supplements may be useful under some circumstances, foods are safe, effective, and enjoyable sources of vitamins and minerals for most healthy children and adults. As you study the next five chapters, prepare to be amazed by the intricate interplay of micronutrients and human health.

✓ CONCEPT CHECK 8.3

1. Which micronutrients help to regulate fluid balance in the body?
2. Which micronutrients are involved in antioxidant reactions and immune function in the body?
3. Provide three examples of nutrients that support bone health.
4. List the micronutrients that function as coenzymes in energy metabolism.
5. Which micronutrients are implicated in the health of blood cells?

8.4 Phytochemicals

In addition to the approximately 45 essential nutrients, there are thousands of other substances in food. For many years, a great deal of nutrition research concentrated on gaining knowledge about carbohydrates, lipids, proteins, vitamins, and minerals. Now, there is growing interest about the potential health benefits of other substances found in food (see Further Reading 1). Foods that are sources of the chemicals that provide health benefits beyond being essential dietary nutrients are termed **functional foods.** Oatmeal is an example of a functional food as it contains soluble fiber that can lower cholesterol levels. Other foods are modified to improve health benefits. For example, some orange juice is fortified with calcium for bone health. Functional foods can be placed into two categories: (1) **zoochemicals,** health-promoting compounds found in animal food; and (2) phytochemicals, health-promoting compounds found in plant foods (*phyto* means "plant" in Greek). Phytochemicals are responsible for the unique colors, flavors, and odors observed in plants. For plants, phytochemicals serve as an environmental protective mechanism to help plants survive the elements (UV exposure, insects, and other predators). Interestingly, these chemicals improve human health when diets high in plant foods are consumed. In addition to the carotenoids discussed in Section 10.5, some of the phytochemicals being studied include allicin, phytosterols, isothiocyanates, lignans, stanols, ellagic acid, flavonoids, saponins, glucosinolates, polyphenols, phytoestrogens, sulphides, lectins, and many more. Examples of foods that are rich sources of phytochemicals include fruits, vegetables, whole grains, legumes, beans, herbs, spices, nuts, and seeds.

Over 4000 phytochemicals have been identified in a single black raspberry, and over 600 carotenoids are found in plants. The full extent of these health benefits are just beginning to be elucidated. See Table 1-3 to review food sources of a variety of phytochemicals. Phytochemicals cannot be synthesized in the body, so we must obtain them from food; however, they are not considered essential nutrients because a deficiency disease is not observed when they are removed from the diet. Thus, even though you may see the word "phytonutrient" in some sources, "phytochemical" is the most accurate term.

functional foods Foods that have health benefits beyond basic nutrition.

zoochemicals Chemicals found in animal products that have health-protective actions.

PHYTOCHEMICAL FUNCTIONS

Although the study of the metabolic actions of phytochemicals is relatively new, numerous mechanistic protective health benefits of these plant-based foods and beverages have been noted, beyond those conferred by their vitamin and mineral contents:

- Stimulate the immune system
- Reduce inflammation
- Prevent DNA damage and aid in DNA repair
- Reduce oxidative damage to cells
- Regulate intracellular signaling of hormones and gene expression
- Activate insulin receptors
- Inhibit the initiation and proliferation of cancer, and stimulate spontaneous cell death
- Alter the absorption, production, and metabolism of cholesterol
- Mimic or inhibit hormones and enzymes
- Decrease the formation of blood clots

PHYTOCHEMICAL RECOMMENDATIONS

There are no specific dietary recommendations for the amount of phytochemicals that should be consumed, except that they should be consumed as food. At present, we know that phytochemicals have protective functions with minimal side effects when consumed naturally in a variety of foods. Therefore, it is wise to eat a wide variety of whole plant foods to obtain the optimum amount of macronutrients, vitamins, minerals, fiber, and phytochemicals. A combination of different plant foods will also increase the antioxidant capacity of the total diet, and there is no doubt that we need to consume a greater variety and quantity of antioxidant-rich foods. Tens of thousands of phytochemicals have been identified, and researchers believe that there are many more yet to discover. We can bet that building meals that resemble MyPlate, with at least five servings of fruits and vegetables per day, will provide a diet rich in phytochemicals.

In the United States, average consumption of fruits and vegetables falls far short of these recommendations. It is estimated that the average American diet has a total antioxidant capacity of about 3000 to 5000 oxygen radical absorbance capacity (ORAC) units (see Chapter 10). This should be closer to 12,000 units, which we could achieve by eating eight to nine servings of fruits and vegetables each day (see Further Reading 10). The message is also getting out that we should be choosing more fruits and vegetables that have rich colors, which are an indication of their phytochemical content.

Many phytochemicals are available as single and combined supplements on grocery, pharmacy, and health-food store shelves. The research, however, suggests that the bioactive phytochemicals are only beneficial when they are present in whole plant foods, not as isolated compounds or extracts in dietary supplements. Indeed, there is very little evidence to support the use of these supplements. In fact, when some of these plant chemicals, including antioxidants, are isolated in pill form, they can actually have the opposite effect. They become prooxidants, meaning they will promote oxidative stress rather than reduce it.

Phytochemicals are widely distributed in the food supply, yet because of the lack of an accurate, comprehensive database, estimating intake remains difficult. This affects researchers' ability to determine what level of phytochemical intake is optimal or what level of intake could potentially pose a health risk.

✓ CONCEPT CHECK 8.4

1. Give one example of a functional food.
2. Which food group has the richest supply of phytochemicals?
3. Diets rich in phytochemicals have been associated with a decreased risk of which diseases?

8.5 Nutrition and Your Health
Dietary Supplements—Who Needs Them?

© Nancy R. Cohen/Getty Images

The phrase *multivitamin and mineral supplement* (MVM) has been mentioned many times so far in your readings. Often, these and other supplements are marketed as cures for anything and everything. This cure-all approach is promoted by the supplement industry and countless health-food stores, pharmacies, and supermarkets.

According to the Dietary Supplement Health and Education Act (DSHEA) of 1994, a supplement in the United States is a product intended to supplement the diet that bears or contains one or more of the following ingredients:

- A vitamin
- A mineral
- An herb or other botanical
- An amino acid
- A dietary substance to supplement the diet, which could be an extract or a combination of the first four ingredients in this list

The definition is broad and covers a wide variety of nutritional substances. The use of dietary supplements is a common practice among North Americans and generates about $34 billion annually for the industry in the United States (Fig. 8-6). Supplements can be sold without proof that they are safe and effective. Unless FDA has evidence that a supplement is inherently dangerous or marketed with an illegal claim, it will not regulate such products closely (the vitamin folate is an exception). FDA has limited resources to police supplement manufacturers and has to act against these manufacturers one at a time. Thus, we cannot rely on the FDA to protect us from vitamin and mineral supplement overuse and misuse. We bear that responsibility ourselves, with the help of professional advice from a primary care provider or registered dietitian nutritionist.

Supplement manufacturers and distributors can make broad claims about their products under the "structure or function" provision of the law. The products, however, cannot claim to prevent, treat, or cure a disease. Because menopause and aging are not diseases per se, products alleging to treat symptoms of these conditions can be marketed without FDA approval. For example, a product that claims to treat hot flashes arising during menopause can be sold without any evidence to prove that the product actually works, but a product that claims to decrease the risk of cardiovascular disease by reducing blood cholesterol must have results from scientific studies that justify the claim.

Why do people take supplements? Frequently given reasons include to:

- Maintain overall health and wellness
- Fill nutrient gaps in the diet
- Reduce susceptibility to health problems (e.g., colds)
- Prevent disease (heart attacks, cancer, osteoporosis, etc.)
- Reduce stress
- Increase "energy"

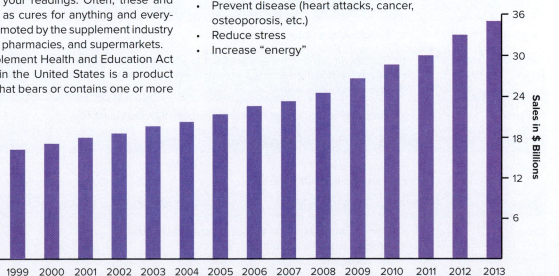

FIGURE 8-6 ▲ The dietary supplement industry is a growing multibillion-dollar business.

Should You Take a Supplement?

Multivitamin and mineral supplements (MVMs) are popularly regarded as a simple backup plan or an insurance policy, even for people who consciously try to consume a balanced diet. Users aim to prevent nutrient deficiencies or chronic diseases by filling any gaps between dietary intake and nutrient needs. However, evidence to support the widespread use of MVMs is mixed. While there is little risk of harm from consuming a balanced MVM that supplies no more than 100% of the Daily Value for the nutrients it contains, most studies indicate no discernible advantage. The National Institutes of Health (NIH), in its State-of-the-Science report, concluded that the present evidence is insufficient to recommend either for or against the use of MVMs to prevent chronic disease (see Further Readings 4, 5, 6, and 9).

Do specific vitamin or mineral supplements provide any benefit? The experts found that only a few studies of vitamin and mineral supplements demonstrate beneficial effects for the prevention of deficiencies or chronic diseases. For example, postmenopausal women may benefit from taking calcium and vitamin D supplements to increase bone mineral density and decrease fracture risk. Table 8-6 outlines the population groups who are most likely to benefit from taking dietary supplements.

While there may be moderate benefits of consuming dietary supplements, uninformed use of supplements can be risky. Indeed, most cases of nutrient toxicity are a result of supplement use. High doses of one nutrient can affect absorption or metabolism of other nutrients. For example, excessive zinc intake can inhibit copper absorption, and large amounts of folate can mask signs and symptoms of a vitamin B-12 deficiency (see Chapter 13). Also, some supplements can interfere with medications. For instance, high intakes of vitamin K or vitamin E alter the action of anticlotting medications, vitamin B-6 can offset the action of L-dopa (used in treating Parkinson's disease), and large doses of vitamin C might interfere with certain cancer therapy regimens.

For most Americans, finding ways to incorporate the recommended servings of fruits, vegetables, and whole grains into their dietary patterns is the safest and healthiest way to ensure nutrient adequacy (see Further Reading 1). Many of the health-promoting effects of foods cannot be found in a bottle. Recall the discussions of phytochemicals in Section 1.3 and the benefits of fiber in Section 4.2. Few or no phytochemicals and no fiber are present in most supplements. Multivitamin and mineral supplements also contain little calcium to keep the pill size small. Furthermore, the oxide forms of magnesium, zinc, and copper used in many supplements are not as well absorbed as forms found in foods. Overall, supplement use is not a replacement for sound dietary patterns.

TABLE 8-6 ■ Who Is Most Likely to Benefit from Dietary Supplements?

Type of Supplement	Who May Benefit
MVM	• People on restrictive diets (<1200 kcal per day), vegans, vegetarians • Older adults (over 50) • Those with unbalanced or inadequate diets (e.g., in cases of food insecurity, "picky" eaters) • Pregnant women or those of childbearing age • People with malabsorptive diseases • People who take medications that interfere with nutrient absorption or metabolism
Various B vitamins	• People who abuse alcohol
Folic acid	• Women of childbearing age (especially during pregnancy and breastfeeding)
Vitamin B-12	• Older adults • Strict vegans
Vitamin C	• People who smoke
Vitamin D	• People with limited milk intake (due to allergies or lactose intolerance) • People with limited exposure to sunlight or darker skin pigment (e.g., infants, many African-Americans, and some older adults)
Vitamin E	• People who follow diets low in fat (especially low in plant oils)
Vitamin K	• Newborns (given by injection shortly after birth)
Calcium	• Strict vegans • Older adults with bone loss
Fluoride	• Some older infants and children (as recommended by a dentist)
Iron	• Women with excessive bleeding during menstruation • Women who are pregnant • Strict vegans
Zinc	• Strict vegans

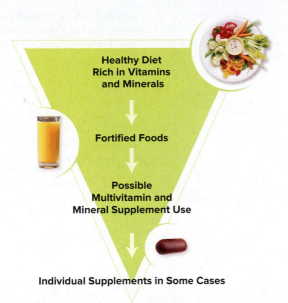

Healthy Diet Rich in Vitamins and Minerals

Fortified Foods

Possible Multivitamin and Mineral Supplement Use

Individual Supplements in Some Cases

FIGURE 8-7 ▲ Supplement savvy—an approach to the use of nutrient supplements. Emphasizing healthy dietary patterns rich in vitamins and minerals should always be the first option, while individual supplements should be the last. (salad): © C Squared Studios/Getty Images; (orange juice): © Ingram Publishing; (vitamin pill): © Getty Images

As illustrated in Figure 8-7, when it comes to improving nutrient intake, emphasize foods before considering dietary supplements. First, you should assess your current dietary habits. The Dietary Guidelines for Americans and MyPlate are two tools consumers can use to plan a healthy diet (see Chapter 2). If nutrient gaps still remain, identify food sources that can fill these gaps. For example, ready-to-eat breakfast cereals supply a variety of micronutrients, including vitamin E, folic acid, vitamin B-6, and highly absorbable forms of vitamin B-12. Other fortified foods, such as calcium-fortified orange juice, may also be useful. Be mindful of portion sizes of highly fortified foods, however, as multiple servings could lead to excessive intakes of some nutrients such as vitamin A, iron, and synthetic folic acid. Lastly, if supplement use is desired, educate yourself and discuss this choice with your primary care provider or registered dietitian nutritionist.

Which Supplement Should You Choose?

If you decide to take a multivitamin and mineral supplement, start by choosing a nationally recognized brand (from a supermarket

Top Five Dietary Supplements in 2014

1. Multivitamins
2. Vitamin D
3. Calcium
4. Vitamin C
5. Vitamin B / B Complex

Source: Council for Responsible Nutrition

Believing that supplements provide the nutrition her body needs, Janice regularly takes numerous supplements while paying relatively little attention to daily food choices. How would you explain to Janice that this practice may lead to health problems?

or pharmacy) that contains about 100% of the Daily Values for the nutrients present. A multivitamin and mineral supplement should generally be taken with or just after meals to maximize absorption. It is important to be sure that total intake from this supplement, any additional supplements, and highly fortified foods (such as ready-to-eat breakfast cereals) provides no more than the Upper Level for each vitamin and mineral. This is especially important with regard to preformed vitamin A intake. Always consult your primary care provider or registered dietitian nutritionist and read all labels carefully (Fig. 8-8). The Newsworthy Nutrition in this section highlights some of the dangers of supplement overuse.

Because research on a variety of nutrient supplements has revealed a lack of product quality, FDA now requires supplement makers to test the identity, purity, strength, and composition of all their products. As an extra protection, select supplements that bear the logo of the United States Pharmacopeial Convention (USP). The USP is an independent, nonprofit group of scientists that reviews products for strength, quality, purity, packaging, labeling, speed of dissolution, and shelf-stability. The USP designation on a supplement label indicates that the product has been evaluated and meets professionally accepted standards of supplement quality.

Another consideration in choosing a supplement is avoiding superfluous ingredients, such as para-aminobenzoic acid (PABA),

▲ Look for the USP symbol on your vitamin or mineral supplement.
© McGraw-Hill Education/Jill Braaten, photographer

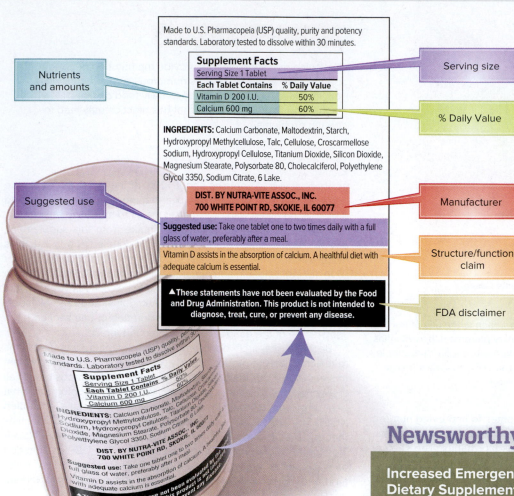

Made to U.S. Pharmacopeia (USP) quality, purity and potency standards. Laboratory tested to dissolve within 30 minutes.

Nutrients and amounts

Supplement Facts
Serving Size 1 Tablet

Each Tablet Contains	% Daily Value
Vitamin D 200 I.U.	50%
Calcium 600 mg	60%

Serving size

% Daily Value

INGREDIENTS: Calcium Carbonate, Maltodextrin, Starch, Hydroxypropyl Methylcellulose, Talc, Cellulose, Croscarmellose Sodium, Hydroxypropyl Cellulose, Titanium Dioxide, Silicon Dioxide, Magnesium Stearate, Polysorbate 80, Cholecalciferol, Polyethylene Glycol 3350, Sodium Citrate, 6 Lake.

**DIST. BY NUTRA-VITE ASSOC., INC.
700 WHITE POINT RD, SKOKIE, IL 60077**

Manufacturer

Suggested use

Suggested use: Take one tablet one to two times daily with a full glass of water, preferably after a meal.

Vitamin D assists in the absorption of calcium. A healthful diet with adequate calcium is essential.

Structure/function claim

▲These statements have not been evaluated by the Food and Drug Administration. This product is not intended to diagnose, treat, cure, or prevent any disease.

FDA disclaimer

FIGURE 8-8 ◄ Nutrient supplements display a nutrition label that is different from food labels. This Supplement Facts label must list the ingredient(s), amount(s) per serving, serving size, suggested use, and % Daily Value if one has been established. In addition, this label includes structure/function claims, which are not mandatory elements of the supplement label. When structure/function claims are made, however, the label also must include the FDA warning that these claims have not been evaluated by the agency.

hesperidin complex, inositol, bee pollen, and lecithins. These compounds are not needed in our diets. These potentially harmful components are especially common in expensive supplements sold in many health-food stores and online. In addition, use of l-tryptophan and high doses of beta-carotene or fish oils is discouraged.

A few websites to help you evaluate ongoing claims and the safety of supplements are:

- www.acsh.org
- www.quackwatch.com
- www.ncahf.org
- ods.od.nih.gov
- www.usp.org/dietary-supplements/overview

These sites are maintained by groups or individuals committed to providing reasoned and authoritative nutrition and health advice to consumers.

Newsworthy Nutrition

Increased Emergency Department Visits for Dietary Supplement Users

Intake of dietary supplements, including herbals, vitamins, and mineral supplements, continues to increase in the United States, yet few studies have investigated safety of these products. The aim of this study was to evaluate adverse events directly related to dietary supplement intake that resulted in emergency department visits. Surveillance data were collected from 63 nationally representative emergency departments from 2004 to 2013. Over 23,000 emergency department visits per year were attributed to adverse events related to dietary supplement intake, resulting in 2154 hospitalizations annually. Of emergency department visits, 28% related to supplement use involving young adults (ages 20 to 34). After excluding dietary supplement intake by unsupervised children, 66% of supplement-related emergency department visits involved herbal or complementary nutritional products and 32% involved micronutrients. Herbals and complementary nutritional products for weight loss and enhanced energy were prevalent. These products resulted in complaints of heart palpitations, chest pain, or tachycardia. In light of the fact that the dietary supplement industry is not well regulated, supplement users must be extremely cautious and stay well informed of the potential health risks.

Source: Geller A and others: Emergency department visits for adverse events related to dietary supplements. *New England Journal of Medicine* 15:373, 2015.

Summary (Numbers refer to numbered sections in the chapter.)

8.1 Vitamins are organic substances required in small amounts in the diet for growth, function, and body maintenance. These can be categorized as fat soluble (vitamins A, D, E, and K) or water soluble (B vitamins and vitamin C). Vitamins cannot be synthesized by the body in adequate amounts to support health, and the chronic absence of a vitamin from the diet leads to development of a deficiency disease or state. Fat-soluble vitamins require dietary fat for absorption and are carried by lipoproteins in the blood. Vitamin toxicity is most likely to occur from megadoses of fat-soluble vitamins because they are readily stored in the body. Intakes of water-soluble vitamins that exceed the storage ability of tissues are typically excreted in urine. Some vitamins are susceptible to destruction by light, heat, air, or alkalinity, or may be lost from foods in cooking water or fats.

8.2 Minerals are inorganic elements, some of which are required for human health. Major minerals are required in amounts of 100 milligrams or more per day. These include calcium, phosphorus, magnesium, sulfur, sodium, potassium, and chloride. Trace minerals are required in amounts less than 100 milligrams per day and include iron, zinc, copper, iodine, selenium, molybdenum, fluoride, manganese, and chromium. Other minerals that are present in small amounts in the diet but have no known requirements are called ultratrace minerals. Mineral bioavailability is affected by age, gender, heredity, nutritional status, and other components of the diet. Any toxicities are likely to result from dietary supplementation, not whole food sources. The process of refinement greatly reduces mineral content of grain products.

8.3 Vitamins and minerals serve multiple roles in the body but can be grouped by their common functions. The B vitamins, iodine, chromium, magnesium, manganese, molybdenum, and choline are involved in energy metabolism. Body defense mechanisms depend on vitamins A, C, D, and E; copper; iron; selenium; and zinc. Bone health relies on vitamins C, D, and K; calcium; phosphorus; magnesium; fluoride; boron; and silicon. Fluid and electrolyte balance is regulated by sodium, potassium, chloride, and phosphorus. The health of blood cells requires vitamins B-6, B-12, and K; folate; iron; copper; and zinc. Optimal brain health requires adequate intake of the B vitamins and antioxidant nutrients.

8.4 Functional foods, such as oatmeal, provide health benefits beyond basic nutrition. Functional foods often contain large amounts of plant-derived compounds known as phytochemicals. These nonessential compounds are what provides plants with their unique color, odor, and flavor. Human consumption is linked to numerous protective health benefits.

8.5 To meet nutrient needs and prevent chronic disease, foods should be emphasized, but dietary supplements can be useful in some circumstances. For example, women of childbearing age, older adults, vegans, and people with malabsorptive diseases are most likely to benefit from dietary supplements. Consumers should educate themselves about possible benefits and risks and discuss concerns with their primary care provider.

Check Your Knowledge (Answers are available at the end of this question set.)

1. An organic compound needed in small amounts by the body for normal growth, function, and maintenance is a
   a. vitamin.
   b. functional food.
   c. trace mineral.
   d. phytochemical.

2. An inorganic element used by the body in chemical reactions and to form body structures is a
   a. vitamin.
   b. mineral.
   c. coenzyme.
   d. phytochemical.

3. Which of the following is a water-soluble vitamin?
   a. vitamin A
   b. vitamin K
   c. thiamin
   d. choline

4. Which of the following is an essential trace mineral?
   a. selenium
   b. phosphorus
   c. calcium
   d. silicon

5. Fat-soluble vitamins are absorbed from the small intestine into
   a. plasma.
   b. serum.
   c. lymph.
   d. urine.

6. A megadose of which of the following micronutrients is most likely to lead to toxicity?
   a. vitamin A
   b. niacin
   c. vitamin K
   d. magnesium

7. Certain compounds in plant foods, such as phytic acid, can limit the bioavailability of
   a. vitamins.
   b. minerals.
   c. phytochemicals.
   d. choline.

8. Which of the following cooking methods is best for preservation of vitamins in foods?
   a. boiling
   b. deep-frying
   c. stir-frying
   d. pressure cooking

9. Vitamin A participates in
   a. immunity.
   b. fluid and electrolyte balance.
   c. bone health.
   d. all of the above.

10. Supplementation with certain vitamins or minerals is most likely to be useful for
    a. college students studying for finals.
    b. older adults with low stomach acid production.
    c. curing cancer.
    d. preventing AIDS.

Answer Key: 1. a (LO 8.1), 2. b (LO 8.1), 3. c (LO 8.1), 4. a (LO 8.3), 5. c (LO 8.4), 6. a (LO 8.4), 7. b (LO 8.5), 8. c (LO 8.5), 9. a (LO 8.6), 10. b (LO 8.7)

Study Questions (Numbers refer to Learning Outcomes)

1. Compare and contrast vitamins and minerals. **(LO 8.1)**

2. What are two defining characteristics of vitamins? **(LO 8.1)**

3. List two examples of fat-soluble vitamins and two examples of water-soluble vitamins. **(LO 8.2)**

4. Provide two examples of major minerals and two examples of trace minerals. **(LO 8.3)**

5. What are ultratrace minerals? **(LO 8.3)**

6. Explain why fat-soluble vitamins are more likely to cause toxicity than water-soluble vitamins. **(LO 8.4)**

7. List two components of plant foods that limit mineral bioavailability. **(LO 8.5)**

8. Contrast the micronutrient content of whole versus refined grains by listing three examples of differences in vitamin or mineral content. **(LO 8.5)**

9. Provide one example of a micronutrient that has more than one functional role in the body. List its multiple functional roles. **(LO 8.6)**

10. Diets rich in phytochemicals have been associated with which protective health benefits? **(LO 8.7)**

11. Are dietary supplements recommended for the general population? Why or why not? **(LO 8.8)**

What the Dietitian Chose

Which is healthiest: fresh, frozen, or canned produce? To answer this question, it helps to know a little bit about ripening and harvesting. While fruits and vegetables are still on the plant, their vitamin content (as well as flavor) increases as they ripen. The maximal nutrient content coincides with the peak of ripeness. Thus, your peach will have its highest vitamin and phytochemical content if it is harvested at peak ripeness. However, once harvested, this ripe fruit is easily damaged and spoils rather quickly: moisture is lost and the flesh deteriorates due to the actions of natural plant enzymes as well as microbes. To avoid damage and ensure optimal appearance on the grocery shelf, many growers harvest their produce a few days early. So the fruit at the grocery store may have been picked before it was fully ripe, meaning it did not achieve maximal nutrient content. This prematurely harvested fruit will become softer and sweeter sooner, but the nutrient content cannot increase after it has been harvested.

Besides that, consider that growers may ship their products thousands of miles before they get to your grocery store. Depending on the product, this may mean days or even weeks have passed from the time your peach was harvested until you purchase it at the store. Then, the fruit may sit on your counter or in your refrigerator for several more days. In this chapter, you learned that exposure to light, heat, and oxygen can destroy some vitamins. The longer a fresh fruit or vegetable is exposed to these elements, the greater the nutrient losses. Storing fresh produce under refrigeration slows down, but does not stop, nutrient losses.

Are all vitamins lost as fresh produce is shipped, stored, and displayed in the produce section? A few of the water-soluble vitamins are extremely susceptible to losses. These losses vary by product and storage conditions, but one study showed that fresh green peas can lose about half of their vitamin C within 1 week of storage and fresh spinach loses nearly all of its vitamin C within a similar time frame (see Further Reading 7). To a lesser extent, thiamin, riboflavin, and folate content also decrease during storage. Fat-soluble nutrients, such as vitamin E and carotenoids, are more stable.

For fresh produce, you will find the highest vitamin content in fruits and vegetables that: (1) have been recently harvested; (2) are in season; and (3) are at peak ripeness. Although you may not be

able to grow your own fruits and vegetables at home, finding a local farmer's market is an excellent way to obtain high-quality, fresh produce. Realize, however, that the out-of-season, out-of-state produce on grocery store displays may not be your best choice.

Are canned or frozen products healthy alternatives? Produce that is destined for canning or freezing will be harvested at the peak of ripeness and will be quickly transported to food-processing facilities after it is harvested. This allows less time for light, heat, and oxygen to destroy vitamins. The initial steps of freezing and canning also induce some nutrient losses.

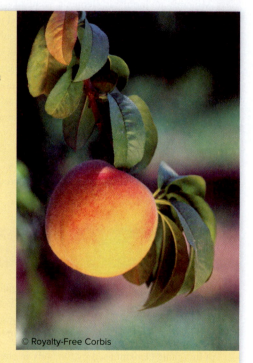
© Royalty-Free Corbis

The canning process exposes food to high temperatures to kill pathogens that might otherwise cause spoilage while the food is stored. This exposure to heat destroys an average of 60% of vitamin C, as well as some of the B vitamins. However, once the canned fruit is on the shelves, it is largely protected from light and oxygen. Depending on storage temperatures, nutrient content will be retained better than in fresh produce.

Some of the preservatives and other additives in canned fruits and vegetables give rise to additional nutritional concerns. Sodium is often added to canned vegetables for flavor and as a preservative. As you will learn in Chapter 9, many Americans exceed the Upper Level for this nutrient, placing themselves at risk for hypertension.

Draining and rinsing canned vegetables can remove about half of the added sodium, but it is likely that other minerals and water-soluble nutrients will be discarded as well. For canned fruit, on the other hand, added sugar is a concern. A 1/2 cup of sliced peaches packed in heavy syrup provides 100 kilocalories and 23 grams of sugar. In comparison, the same portion of fresh peaches provides about 30 kilocalories and 6 grams of natural fruit sugar. If you select canned fruit, be sure to choose products that are packed in light syrup or fruit juice. A 1/2 cup of sliced peaches in extra-light syrup provides a more reasonable 60 kilocalories and 13 grams of sugar.

Canning, then, leads to some initial nutrient losses, but over time, nutrients are fairly well preserved. Additions of sodium or sugar could negatively impact nutritional status. How does frozen produce compare?

Prior to being frozen, most vegetables (and a few fruits) are blanched. Blanching—the process of quickly heating foods in boiling water or steam, followed by rapid cooling with ice or cold water—is used to inactivate enzymes in fresh produce that would otherwise degrade the plant tissues. This process preserves the flavor, color, and texture of the food. This quick exposure to heat does destroy some vitamin C (about 50%) and other water-soluble vitamins, but losses from continued enzyme activity would be greater over time if the food were not blanched. Once frozen, some nutrients are still susceptible to oxidation, but vitamin content is preserved quite well over time. Despite the initial losses of some water-soluble nutrients during blanching, freezing is the best way to preserve nutrients. Plus, most frozen fruits and vegetables do not have added sodium or sugar, but always check food labels (review Section 7.6) to be sure!

If available, recently harvested, fully ripe, locally grown fruits or vegetables will deliver optimal taste, texture, and nutrient content. However, if produce is out of season and not local, then canned or frozen fruits or vegetables have similar nutrient content as the "fresh" produce at the grocery store. In addition, canned or frozen fruits and vegetables (without added ingredients) are often more economical and convenient choices. In this case locally grown produce was not available, so the dietitian chose frozen peaches based on their well-preserved vitamin content, low added sugars, overall convenience, and low cost.

CASE STUDY SOLUTION Getting the Most Nutrition from Your Food

1. Exposure to light, heat, oxygen, or alkalinity leads to destruction of some vitamins, particularly the water-soluble vitamins. In addition, some vitamins can be leached into cooking water or fat during food preparation.

2. Because light, heat, and oxygen can destroy some vitamins, prolonged storage of produce can reduce vitamin content. Imported (i.e., not in season) produce in the grocery store may have been harvested several days or even weeks before it reaches the shopping cart. If Julie focuses on buying fruits and vegetables that are in season for her area and have been grown locally, the total time from harvest to purchase is likely to be less. Finding fresh, local produce at a farmer's market also decreases the number of steps from the field to Julie's plate, so vitamin content will be higher.

3. Food processing dramatically decreases the nutrient content of grains. Discarding the bran and germ parts of the grain reduces vitamin E, the B vitamins, and minerals such as magnesium, iron, and zinc. The enrichment of grains adds back some B vitamins and iron, but refined grains are still lower than whole grains in many micronutrients. Choosing to make half your grains whole will help in meeting micronutrient needs without dietary supplements.

4. Decreasing exposure to light, heat, and air will limit destruction of vitamins. Most produce should be stored in closed containers in the refrigerator. Julie shouldn't peel or chop her fruits and vegetables until just before consuming them to limit exposure to air. Foods that will not be eaten within a few days should be frozen to maintain nutrient content.

5. Steaming, microwaving, and stir-frying are the best cooking methods for preserving vitamin content of foods. During food preparation, some vitamins may be destroyed by heat or leached into cooking water or fat, thus reducing nutrient availability. Boiling vegetables, for example, results in losses of B vitamins, especially folate. Higher temperatures and longer cooking times increase vitamin losses. Using quick cooking methods, such as microwaving, and avoiding overcooking vegetables can help to retain nutrients. Using a lid on the cooking pot can reduce cooking time, helping to preserve vitamin content. When vegetables are steamed, fewer water-soluble vitamins are lost in cooking water. Fat-soluble vitamins, such as vitamin A and carotenoids, can be lost in fat used for cooking, so use minimal fat during cooking or add any fats for flavoring after food is cooked.

Further Readings

1. ADA Reports: Position of the American Dietetic Association: Nutrient supplementation. *Journal of the American Dietetic Association* 109:2073, 2009.

2. Alexander DD and others: A systematic review of multivitamin-multimineral use and cardiovascular disease and cancer incidence and total mortality. *Journal of the American College of Nutrition* 32:5, 2013.

3. Fulgoni VL III and others: Foods, fortificants, and supplements: Where do Americans get their nutrients? *Journal of Nutrition* 141:1847, 2011.

4. Martini LA and others: Role of vitamins and minerals in prevention and management of type 2 diabetes mellitus. *Nutrition Reviews* 68:341, 2010.

5. NIH State-of-the-Science Conference Statement on Multivitamin/Mineral Supplements and Chronic Disease Prevention. *NIH Consensus State-of-the-Science Statements* 23(2):1, 2006.

6. Palmer S: Dietary antioxidants—Do foods and supplements with high antioxidant values guarantee better health? *Today's Dietitian* 15:4, 2013.

7. Rickman JC, Barrett DM, Bruhn CM: Nutritional comparison of fresh, frozen and canned fruits and vegetables. Part 1. Vitamins C and B and phenolic compounds. *Journal of the Science of Food and Agriculture* 87:930, 2007.

8. Rickman JC, Barrett DM, Bruhn CM: Nutritional comparison of fresh, frozen, and canned fruits and vegetables. Part II. Vitamin A and carotenoids, vitamin E, minerals, and fiber. *Journal of the Science of Food and Agriculture* 87:1185, 2007.

9. Sesso HD and others: Multivitamins in the prevention of cardiovascular disease in men: The Physician's Health Study II randomized controlled trial. *Journal of the American Medical Association* 308:1751, 2012.

10. Webb D: Phytochemicals' role in good health. *Today's Dietitian* 15:9, 2013.

 To get the most out of your study of nutrition, go to McGraw-Hill's online resources: Connect www.mcgrawhillconnect.com, where you will find NutritionCalc Plus, LearnSmart, and many other dynamic tools.

Rate Your Plate

© The McGraw-Hill Education/Andrew Resek, photographer

Throughout the chapters on vitamins and minerals, you will see breakfast cereals described as enriched, fortified, cold, or ready to eat. What do these terms mean? The cereal you pour out of a carton, add milk to, and enjoy is called ready-to-eat or cold cereal. Any addition of nutrients to a food product is called *fortification*. In the United States, FDA strictly defines *enrichment* as a special type of fortification of refined grain products. Per pound of flour, all refined grains must contain at least 2.9 milligrams of thiamin, 1.8 milligrams of riboflavin, 24 milligrams of niacin, 0.7 milligram of folic acid, and 20 milligrams of iron. Enrichment replaces some (but not all) of the nutrients lost during the milling of grains.

You can tell if a product is fortified by reading the Nutrition Facts panel. In the following table, **Cereal A** has been enriched to levels mandated by FDA. **Cereal B,** the enriched or fortified choice, contains 100% of the DV for select vitamins and minerals, especially the B vitamins and iron. Whereas all refined grain products are enriched with thiamin, riboflavin, niacin, folic acid, and iron, many food manufacturers choose to fortify their products with additional nutrients. In this text, when we refer to fortified breakfast cereals, we are referring to this latter group of food products.

Nutrient	Cereal A (1 ounce) % DV	Cereal B (1 ounce) % DV	Your Favorite Cereal % DV	Nutrient	Cereal A (1 ounce) % DV	Cereal B (1 ounce) % DV	Your Favorite Cereal % DV
Vitamin A	25	15		Niacin	25	100	
Vitamin C	25	100		Vitamin B-6	25	100	
Calcium	0	0		Folic acid	25	100	
Iron	50	100		Pantothenic acid	—*	100	
Vitamin D	10	10		Phosphorus	4	4	
Vitamin E	25	100		Magnesium	—*	4	
Thiamin	25	100		Zinc	—*	100	
Riboflavin	25	100					

*Information not provided on label.

Locate a Nutrition Facts panel for one of your favorite breakfast cereals. In the blank spaces in the table, record the % DV for each nutrient provided by one serving. If some data are missing, fill in the blanks with an asterisk. Based on your observations, answer the following questions.

1. Is your favorite cereal fortified? How can you tell?

   _____

   _____

2. Examine the calorie, fat, and sugar content listed on your Nutrition Facts panel. How does the cereal compare to the recommendations of the Dietary Guidelines for Americans and other health authorities to limit calories, fat, and added sugars?

   _____

   _____

3. Which special population groups can especially benefit from daily use of a fortified breakfast cereal?

   _____

   _____

4. What could you eat with your breakfast cereal to build a meal that meets MyPlate standards?

   _____

   _____

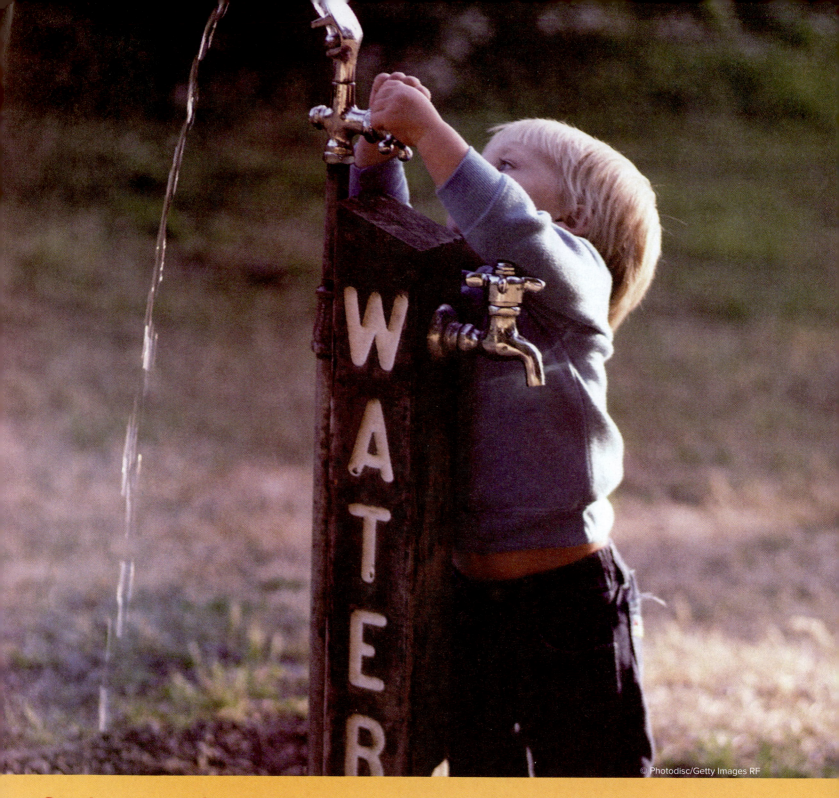

© Photodisc/Getty Images RF

Student Learning Outcomes

Chapter 9 is designed to allow you to:

9.1 List and explain the functions of water in the body.

9.2 Describe the control mechanisms that regulate water intake and output.

9.3 Identify recommended intakes and sources of water.

9.4 Describe the health consequences of dehydration.

9.5 List the four minerals that function as electrolytes.

Chapter 9
Fluid and Electrolyte Balance

What Would You Choose?

Water is the best choice for everyday hydration because it quenches thirst without calories. There are currently many "water" choices available. Do you need water that contains vitamins and minerals? What is the difference between spring water and mineral water? Is bottled water safer to drink than tap water? As you peruse the store shelves, which is the healthiest choice to take along to the student recreation center for your workout?

a Reusable bottle filled with tap water

b Aquafina® Pure Water

c San Pellegrino® Mineral Water

d Vitaminwater®

Think about your choice as you read Chapter 9, then see What the Dietitian Chose at the end of the chapter.

Despite ongoing changes in our nutrient intake, environmental conditions, and level of physical activity, the internal and external composition of the trillions of cells in the human body remains relatively constant. This balanced environment is vital for cells to function properly. In humans, three key factors are under tight intracellular and extracellular control: water, electrolyte distribution, and pH.

Water (H_2O) is the most abundant molecule in the human body, yet it cannot be stored in the body. Fluids must be consumed daily to replenish what is lost through respiration (lungs), perspiration (skin), and excretion (urine and feces). The body has several intricate mechanisms to ensure fluid conservation.

Maintenance of fluid balance relies on strict control of dissolved mineral levels inside and outside the cells. These dissolved minerals—sodium, chloride, potassium, and phosphorus—are called *electrolytes*. Not only do they regulate the distribution of water throughout the body, but they are also involved in maintenance of acid-base balance and in the conduction of nerve impulses. In this chapter, you will learn about the importance of water and how the electrolytes work together to regulate fluid balance, acid-base balance, and nerve function. Sodium, potassium, and chloride will be discussed in detail. The importance of phosphorus will be noted, but a detailed discussion of phosphorus appears in Chapter 11, as it relates to bone health.

9.6 Describe how electrolytes control fluid balance, acid-base balance, and nerve impulse transmission.

9.7 List dietary sources and daily requirements of the electrolyte minerals.

9.8 Describe factors that can contribute to the development of hypertension.

FIGURE 9-1 ▶ Although the percentages vary for men and women, the main constituent of the body is water.
© Digital Vision/Getty Images

Healthy Man (170 pounds)	Healthy Woman (130 pounds)
1 pound of glycogen (<1%)	1 pound of glycogen (<1%)
10 pounds of minerals (6%)	7 pounds of minerals (5%)
27 pounds of fat (16%)	17 pounds of protein (13%)
27 pounds of protein (16%)	32 pounds of fat (25%)
105 pounds of water (62%)	74 pounds of water (57%)

WHERE'S THE WATER?

The percentage of water varies tremendously among tissues. For example, muscle is 73% water, adipose tissue is 10% to 20% water, and bone contains approximately 20% water. As the fat content of the body increases, the percentage of lean muscle decreases, and subsequently the percentage of body water decreases. When body composition measurements are performed on extremely lean athletes, the percentage of body water will be around 70%.

9.1 Water: Essential to Human Life

Every cell, tissue, and organ contains some water. Overall, water comprises 50% to 70% of the human body (Fig. 9-1). Indeed, water is essential for life. Whereas humans can live for several weeks without food, we can survive for only a few days without water. The simple H_2O molecule has some amazing properties: it is a versatile solvent, a coolant, and a lubricant. As detailed in the next few sections, these properties make water uniquely suited to carry out a number of essential roles in the human body (Fig. 9-2).

WATER IS THE UNIVERSAL SOLVENT

solvent A liquid substance in which other substances dissolve.

Water is often called the "universal **solvent**" because so many different solutes can be dissolved in it. This property of water makes it first, an ideal transport vehicle for nutrients and wastes; and second, a medium for many chemical reactions of human metabolism.

Water Transports Nutrients and Wastes The majority of the nutrients we consume—carbohydrates, proteins, minerals, and many vitamins—are water soluble. As described in Chapter 5, lipids, although they are not soluble in water, can be surrounded by a layer of water-soluble protein so they can be dispersed throughout the water-based environment within and around cells and tissues. As the primary component of blood and lymph, water acts to transport nutrients to all the cells of the body.

The metabolism of nutrients generates some waste products, most of which can dissolve in water and exit the body as part of urine. For example, when proteins are broken down as fuel, the nitrogen portion of amino acids cannot be used for energy production. Recall from Chapter 6 that these nitrogenous waste products are converted into urea by the liver and excreted in urine. In addition, when we consume more than we need of some nutrients, such as sodium, the excess can be dissolved in water and excreted in urine. Typical urine output ranges from 1 to 2 liters per day, depending mostly on our intakes of fluid, protein, and sodium.

FIGURE 9-2 ▲ Water has many essential functions in the body.
© Ingram Publishing / Fotosearch

Water Is a Medium for Chemical Reactions Because so many compounds dissolve in water, it provides a medium in which chemical reactions take place in the body. Furthermore, water itself (H_2O) is an important participant in many chemical reactions. When carbohydrates, lipids, and proteins are metabolized as sources of energy, water is one of the by-products. In fact, this **metabolic water** (1 cup or more per day) contributes to the maintenance of fluid balance in the body.

metabolic water Water formed as a by-product of carbohydrate, lipid, and protein metabolism.

WATER CONTRIBUTES TO BODY TEMPERATURE REGULATION

Water temperature changes slowly because it has a great ability to hold heat. Water molecules are polar (charged), so they are attracted to each other. This attractive force is strong, and energy is required during heating to separate the water molecules. Because the human body is 50% to 70% water, it takes a lot of energy to change body temperature.

When overheated, the body secretes fluids in the form of perspiration, which evaporates through skin pores, releasing heat energy. So, as perspiration evaporates, heat energy is removed from the skin, cooling the body in the process (Fig. 9-3). In response to an increased body temperature, blood vessels in the skin become larger, allowing greater water loss through perspiration. Each quart (approximately 1 liter or 2 pounds) of perspiration that evaporates represents approximately 600 kilocalories of energy lost from the skin and surrounding tissues.

When carbohydrates, lipids, and proteins are used by cells in the body, energy is released in the form of heat. About 60% of this energy is turned into body heat; the other 40% is converted to forms of energy that cells can use (principally ATP). Almost all of that energy eventually leaves the body in the form of heat. Perspiration is the primary way to prevent this rise in body temperature. If this heat could not be dissipated, the body temperature would rise enough to prevent enzyme systems from functioning efficiently, ultimately leading to death.

Should you feed a fever? Fever is an increase in body temperature caused by an infection. When you have a fever, you do need more energy. For every increase of 1°F (0.5°C) in internal temperature above normal, your basal metabolic rate (BMR) increases by 7%. Although BMR is elevated for a person with a fever, physical activity will likely be lower than normal, which lowers overall energy needs. Thus, having a fever is not a reason to overeat.

WATER MOISTENS, LUBRICATES, AND CUSHIONS

The body secretes many fluids that are primarily water. Water-based secretions are produced by the digestive tract, respiratory tract, urogenital tract, eyes, and skin. Saliva acts as

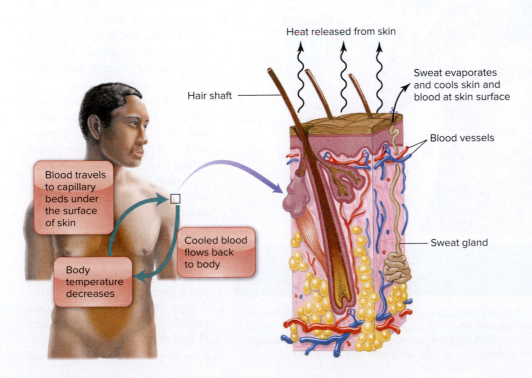

Heat released from skin

Hair shaft

Sweat evaporates and cools skin and blood at skin surface

Blood vessels

Blood travels to capillary beds under the surface of skin

Cooled blood flows back to body

Body temperature decreases

Sweat gland

FIGURE 9-3 ◄ Body temperature is reduced when heat is transported from the body through the bloodstream to the surface of the skin. As perspiration evaporates from the surface of the skin, heat is dissipated. This cools the blood, which circulates back to the body, reducing body temperature.

▲ Tears are one example of water's role as a lubricant. This fluid allows the eyeball to move smoothly in its socket and helps to flush away foreign particles. Lack of tear production is a symptom of dehydration. © Danil Chepko/123

a lubricant, allowing food to pass through the esophagus to the stomach. Mucus provides a protective fluid coating throughout the digestive tract. The lungs are coated with a layer of mucus that provides an important immunologic function. Water helps form the lubricant found in knees and other joints of the body. The spinal cord and brain are cushioned by cerebrospinal fluid. Water is also the basis of amniotic fluid, which functions as a shock absorber surrounding the growing fetus in the mother's womb. Without adequate availability of water, the ability of the body to produce these critical secretions will be limited.

✓ CONCEPT CHECK 9.1

1. Why is it significant that water is the "universal solvent"?
2. Describe how water regulates body temperature.
3. Provide two examples of water's role as a lubricant.

9.2 The Water Balancing Act

Despite its critical importance for human survival, water is not stored in the body. It is continually lost through respiration (lungs), perspiration (skin), and excretion (urine and feces). Through mechanisms that monitor blood pressure and the concentration of solutes in body fluids, the nervous, endocrine, digestive, and urinary systems work elegantly together to maintain fluid balance and support life.

WATER INTAKE

The Adequate Intake (AI) for *total* water is 2.7 liters (11 cups) for adult women and 3.7 liters (15 cups) for adult men. This amount is based primarily on average water intake from fluids and foods. For *fluid* alone, this corresponds to about 2.2 liters (9 cups) for women and about 3 liters (13 cups) for men.

Fluid intake—including water, juice, coffee, tea, soft drinks, milk, and even alcoholic beverages—makes the biggest contribution to our total water needs. For the woman in Figure 9-4, fluid intake adds up to about 9 cups. In addition, nearly all foods contain water. Many fruits and vegetables are more than 80% water, and many meats contain at least 50% water (Fig. 9-5). In Figure 9-4, water from foods supplies another 2 cups. As mentioned, the body produces 250 to 350 milliliters (1 to 1.5 cups) of water each day as a by-product of the chemical

Water Intake

Fluids:
2150 milliliters (~9 cups)

+

Water content in food:
500 milliliters (~2 cups)

+

Water produced from metabolism:
300 milliliters (~1.25 cups)

Water Output

Urine:
1950 milliliters (~8.25 cups)

+

Skin perspiration:
600 milliliters (~2.5 cups)

+

Lung respiration:
300 milliliters (~1.25 cups)

+

Feces:
100 milliliters (~0.4 cup)

Total Water Intake
2950 milliliters
(approximately ~12.25 cups)

Total Water Output
2950 milliliters
(approximately ~12.25 cups)

FIGURE 9-4 ▲ Estimate of water balance—intake versus output—in a woman. We primarily maintain body fluids at an optimum amount by adjusting water intake to output. As you can see for this woman, most water comes from the liquids we consume. Some comes from the moisture in foods, and the remainder is manufactured during metabolism. Water output includes that lost via urine, skin, lungs, and feces.

MyPlate:
Sources of water

Grains	Vegetables	Fruits	Dairy	Protein
• Bread • Pasta (cooked) • Rice (cooked)	• Potatoes • Lettuce • Tomatoes • Squash • Green beans • Vegetable juices	• Oranges • Apples • Bananas • Melons • Plums • Fruit juices	• Milk • Yogurt	• Beef • Poultry • Seafood • Beans

FIGURE 9-5 ▲ Sources of water from MyPlate. The fill of the background color (none, 1/3, 2/3, or completely covered) within each group on the plate indicates the average nutrient density for water in that group. Overall, the vegetables, fruits, dairy, and protein groups contain many foods that are nutrient-dense sources of water. Although not depicted on MyPlate, all beverages are nearly 100% water. Fats and oils, on the other hand, have almost no water. (milk) © D. Hurst/Alamy; (vegetables) © Ingram Publishing; (oranje juice) © Ingram Publishing

reactions used to metabolize energy. In Figure 9-4, metabolic water amounts to 1.25 cups; however, the amount of metabolic water produced can double in physically active people.

WATER OUTPUT

Usually, urinary excretion of water accounts for the greatest source of output. Average urinary water loss per day is approximately 1650 milliliters (7.5 cups), but may vary based on intake of fluids, protein, and sodium. Removal of waste products requires at least 500 milliliters (2 cups) of urine production per day. Urine output consistently below this level is often a sign of chronic dehydration due to low fluid intake.

Water is lost through the skin in the form of perspiration. On days of low physical activity, these losses amount to about 1 liter. Under hot, humid conditions or with strenuous physical activity, losses can be much greater. Some water is also lost from the lungs in the form of water vapor in exhaled air. Together with perspiration, the fluid lost through lung respiration is sometimes called "insensible" water loss because it is difficult to measure.

A relatively small amount of water is lost daily in the feces. When we consider the large amount of water used to lubricate the digestive tract, the loss of only 100 milliliters (0.5 cup) of water each day through the feces is remarkable. In addition to the variable amount of water ingested in the form of foods and fluids, about 8000 milliliters (35 cups) of water enters the digestive tract daily through secretions from the mouth, stomach, intestine, pancreas, and other organs. The small intestine absorbs most of this water, while the colon takes up a lesser but important amount. The kidneys also greatly conserve water. They can reabsorb as much as 97% of the water filtered each day. The volumes of water intake and output shown in Figure 9-4 are estimates. Altitude, ambient temperature, humidity, physical activity, and intake of caffeine and alcohol will influence water loss.

FLUID CONSERVATION

Blood pressure and the concentration of solutes in the blood are closely monitored by receptors in the kidneys, blood vessels, and brain. Once the body registers a shortage of available water, it increases fluid conservation (Fig. 9-6). Hormones that participate in this process are **antidiuretic hormone (ADH), angiotensin,** and **aldosterone.** The pituitary gland, located in the brain, senses the concentration of solutes in the blood. When blood concentration of solutes is high, the pituitary gland releases ADH. The kidneys respond to ADH by reducing urine production and output. ADH also causes blood vessel constriction, which acts to raise blood pressure. Meanwhile, the kidneys possess receptors that monitor blood pressure. Low blood pressure triggers the release of an enzyme that activates angiotensin and, eventually, aldosterone, two hormones that signal the kidneys to retain more sodium and, in turn, more water via osmosis. As sodium and water are retained, blood pressure increases back to normal.

DEHYDRATION

Despite mechanisms that work to conserve water, fluid continues to be lost via the feces, skin, and lungs. Those losses must be replaced. In addition, there is a limit to how concentrated urine can become. Eventually, if fluid is not consumed, the body becomes dehydrated and suffers ill effects.

By the time a person loses 1% to 2% of body weight in fluids, he or she will be thirsty (Fig. 9-7). Even this small water deficit can cause one to feel tired and dizzy and to experience headaches. At a 4% loss of body weight, muscles lose significant strength and endurance, and central nervous system function is negatively affected (e.g., memory and reaction time are compromised and one becomes impatient). By the time body weight is reduced by

antidiuretic hormone (ADH) A hormone that is secreted by the pituitary gland when blood concentration of solutes is high. It causes the kidneys to decrease water excretion, which increases blood volume.

angiotensin A hormone produced by the liver and activated by enzymes from the kidneys. It signals the adrenal glands to produce aldosterone also and directs the kidneys to conserve sodium (and therefore water). Both of these actions have the effect of increasing blood volume.

aldosterone A hormone produced by the adrenal glands when blood volume is low. It acts on the kidneys to conserve sodium (and therefore water) to increase blood volume.

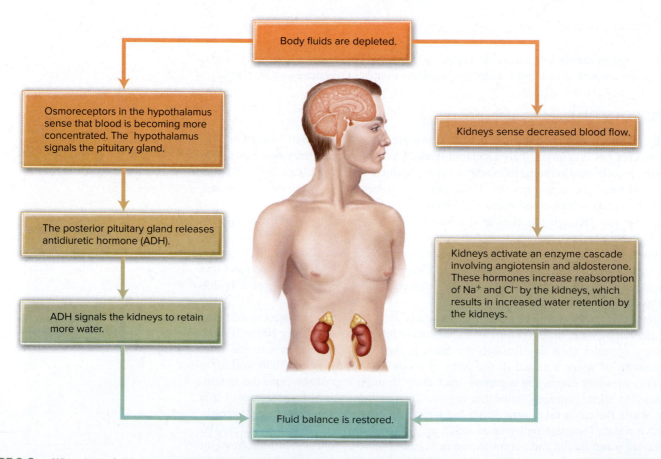

FIGURE 9-6 ▲ When body fluids are depleted, hormonal signals from the pituitary gland and the kidneys work together to increase fluid retention by the kidneys and thereby restore fluid balance.

Body weight lost (%)	
0	Thirst
2	Stronger thirst; vague discomfort and sense of oppression; loss of appetite; increasing hemoconcentration
4	Less movement; lagging pace; flushed skin; impatience; drowsiness; apathy; nausea; emotional instability
6	Tingling in arms, hands, and feet; stumbling; headache; heat exhaustion (faintness, dizziness, fatigue, nausea, elevated body temperature and elevated respiratory rate)
8	Labored breathing; dizziness; cyanosis (bluish color of skin caused by poor oxygen flow in body); indistinct speech; increasing weakness; mental confusion
10	Muscle cramps; inability to balance with eyes closed; general incapacity; delirium and wakefulness; swollen tongue; circulatory insufficiency; marked hemoconcentration and decreased blood volume; failing kidney function
> 10	Increasing risk of death, especially if associated with illness or extreme heat and exercise

FIGURE 9-7 ▶ The effects of dehydration can range from thirst to death, depending on the extent of water weight lost.

10%, heat tolerance is decreased and weakness results. Ultimately, **dehydration** will lead to kidney failure, coma, and death. Dehydration is a contributing factor to the development of heatstroke, a serious condition. Performing strenuous physical activity in hot, humid conditions can lead to dehydration and the inability to control body temperature. Heart rate is increased and the skin becomes dry. Unassisted, the individual will become unconscious and die. Adequate fluid intake and, if possible, avoidance of physical activity in hot, humid conditions are the best steps to prevent heat illness.

Another potential consequence of inadequate fluid intake is kidney stones. When urine production is lower than about 500 milliliters per day, the urine is concentrated, increasing the risk of kidney stone formation in susceptible people (generally men). Kidney stones form from minerals and other substances that have precipitated out of the urine and accumulate in the kidney.

The simplest way to determine if water intake is adequate is to observe urine color (Fig. 9-8). If hydration is adequate, urine should be clear or pale yellow (like lemonade); concentrated urine is dark yellow (like apple juice). Urine color can be influenced by consuming supplements (especially some B vitamins), medications, and food. Lots of carotenoid-containing items (e.g., carrot juice, pumpkin, winter squash) can tint the urine orange. Too many fava beans or too much rhubarb will turn it dark brown. A reddish or pinkish urine results from eating too many beets or blackberries. Asparagus not only makes the urine smell like asparagus, but can also turn it a bit green.

IS THIRST A GOOD INDICATOR OF HYDRATION STATUS?

If you do not drink enough water, your brain communicates the need to drink by signaling thirst. In most cases, drinking fluids in response to the thirst sensation will result in adequate hydration. However, the thirst mechanism can lag behind actual water loss during prolonged exercise and illness, as well as in older adults. Sick children, especially those with fever, vomiting, diarrhea, and increased perspiration, and older persons often need to be reminded to drink plenty of fluids because their thirst mechanism may be duller.

dehydration Inadequate intake of water to replace losses.

FIGURE 9-8 ▲ Monitoring the color of urine is a good gauge of hydration.

As you will learn in Chapter 14, athletes need to monitor fluid status. They should weigh themselves before and after training sessions to determine their rate of water loss and, thus, their water needs. However, the body can absorb only about 60% of the water consumed. So athletes should drink about 50% more than what they lose through sweat in a workout. Their goal is to consume 2 to 3 cups of fluid for every pound lost.

CAN A PERSON CONSUME TOO MUCH WATER?

water intoxication Potentially fatal condition that occurs with a high intake of water, which results in a severe dilution of the blood and other fluid compartments.

hyponatremia Dangerously low blood sodium level.

Even though the kidneys of a healthy person can process up to 15 liters of urine per day, it is possible to drink too much water. As water intake increases above what is needed, kidneys process the excess fluid and excrete dilute urine. If water intake far exceeds the kidneys' processing ability, overhydration and sodium dilution in the blood result. This condition is commonly known as **water intoxication,** or more accurately, **hyponatremia.** Endurance athletes exercising for prolonged times, drinking large volumes of water to replace sweat losses, are especially at risk. Using sport drinks (see Chapter 14) will help replace the sodium lost in sweat. Water intoxication can happen to healthy people when they drink a great deal of water in a very short period of time. Severe hyponatremia results along with extreme and rapid blood dilution, causing tissue swelling. The heartbeat becomes irregular, allowing fluid to enter the lungs; the brain and nerves swell, causing severe headaches, confusion, seizure, and coma. Unless water is restricted and a concentrated salt solution administered under close medical monitoring, the person will die.

WHAT IS THE DIFFERENCE BETWEEN HARD AND SOFT WATER?

hard water Water that contains high levels of calcium and magnesium.

soft water Water that contains a high level of sodium.

In North America, 89% of homes have hard water. **Hard water** contains relatively high levels of the minerals calcium and magnesium, whereas **soft water** is high in sodium. Naturally occurring soft water is found in the Pacific North and Northwest, New England, South Atlantic-Gulf, and Hawaii. When washing with hard water, it is difficult to work up lather, and a pronounced ring is left around the bathtub or sink. Soft water does a better job of cleaning clothes and feels much better when bathing.

Hard water can be converted into soft water through the use of a commercial water softener. As water travels through the water softener, calcium and magnesium exchange with sodium found in the water softener device. The water that exits the softener has a low calcium and magnesium content; however, the sodium content is high. The additional intake of sodium from soft water is undesirable for people restricting sodium intake due to **hypertension.** The additional intake of calcium and magnesium afforded by consuming hard water would be more beneficial than increasing sodium intake through the use of softened water.

Water that comes out of your refrigerator dispenser or through a filter on your faucet typically runs through a charcoal (carbon) filter. The carbon attracts compounds present in tap water to remove off flavors. Importantly, it does not remove fluoride, a mineral essential to help fight tooth decay.

hypertension A condition in which blood pressure remains persistently elevated. Obesity, inactivity, alcohol intake, excess salt intake, and genetics may each contribute to the problem.

IS BOTTLED WATER HEALTHIER THAN TAP WATER?

Bottled water is a popular alternative to tap water; in 2014, Americans consumed 34 gallons of bottled water per person. Many people choose bottled water because they believe it is less likely to be contaminated with pathogens or impurities than tap water. Much of the bottled water produced in the United States, however, is actually processed municipal tap water. There are some differences in water treatment methods: rather than using chlorine to disinfect water, most bottled water is treated with ozone, which does not impart a flavor to the water. Although the Environmental Protection Agency regulates and monitors public water supplies, and the Food and Drug Administration regulates bottled water, the standards for quality and contaminant levels are identical for both.

Beyond the level of contaminants, there are some definite differences between bottled and tap water. As you'll learn in Chapter 11, a small amount of fluoride is added to municipal water supplies to prevent dental caries. Very few bottled water manufacturers add the mineral fluoride to the water. People who drink primarily bottled water should include regular tap water throughout the day in order to receive the benefits of fluoride. Trips to the drinking fountain or making coffee or tea with tap water should suffice.

Another big difference between bottled water and tap water is the way it is delivered. Tap water travels through pipes into your home, but bottled water requires extra packaging and more costly methods of transport and storage. The large amount of plastic used to package the more than 11 billion gallons of bottled water consumed in America each year creates huge energy use, recycling, and solid waste disposal concerns.

Beyond its impact on the environment, the use of plastics may pose additional threats to human health. Drinking water from a freshly washed or newly opened bottle is fine. But plastic, like the food we eat, has a shelf life. Over time, the chemicals that make up plastic break down and can leach into the liquid inside the container. Temperature, age of the bottle, acidity of the contents, and type of plastic (recycling code) all make a difference. Age of the consumer makes a difference, too, as babies and young children are more susceptible to problems than adults. Here are some guidelines for the proper use of water bottles:

1. Stainless steel bottles are best for the long run if you are going to use your bottles over and over.
2. If you choose plastic, look for recycling codes 2 and 4 (see Further Reading 5). When these types of plastics break down, they are the least harmful. You can also use a bottle with recycling code 7 as long as it also has "BPA free" molded into its bottom next to the recycle code.
3. Avoid bottles with recycle codes 3 and 7 without "BPA free" embedded in the plastic. These hard plastics may contain bisphenyl A (BPA). Since the 1930s, this organic compound has been used to make clear bottles. When such a bottle is cleaned with harsh (laboratory) detergents or used to hold acidic or high-temperature liquids, BPA can leach into the bottle's contents. Exposure can occur through air and skin in addition to diet. BPA is considered an endocrine disrupter, which at low doses can mimic the body's own hormones. Thus, there is concern about chronic exposure for infants and young children. BPA has been banned for use in Canada and many European countries. In the United States, FDA has banned use of BPA in the manufacture of baby bottles and sippy cups. Many manufacturers of reusable water bottles are switching to "BPA free" plastics. If the bottom of your water bottle does not have this phrase molded near the recycling symbol, your bottle contains BPA. Be careful to avoid putting acidic (lemonade, juices, etc.) or hot beverages in your bottle (see Further Readings 7 and 12).
4. Choose a reusable bottle with a wide mouth so you can easily clean it.
5. When your plastic bottle becomes scratched or cracked, throw it away. Bacteria can grow inside.
6. Do not store your containers of water in a hot garage or in the back of your hot car. The heat quickly breaks down the plastic. If a bottle has been open and exposed to heat, do not drink the contents. Pitch the water and recycle the bottle. If it is your reusable bottle, wash and soak it in a sanitizer, such as 4 milliliters (¼ teaspoon) bleach in 1 liter (1 quart) of water.

Read more about bottled water at www.nrdc.org/water/drinking/qbw.asp. To find a list of brands of bottled water that contain fluoride, check out the website of the International Bottled Water Association at www.bottledwater.org/fluoride.

✔ CONCEPT CHECK 9.2

1. List the components of water intake and water output.
2. What is the AI for fluid intake for adult men? For adult women?
3. In your own words, describe the hormonal regulation of water balance (see Figure 9-6).
4. List two situations in which thirst is not a reliable indicator of fluid needs.
5. What is water intoxication?

9.3 Electrolytes Regulate Fluid Balance

intracellular fluid Fluid contained within a cell; it represents about two-thirds of body fluid.

ion A positively or negatively charged atom.

electrolyte A mineral that separates into positively or negatively charged ions in water. They are able to transmit an electrical current.

extracellular fluid Fluid found outside the cells; it represents about one-third of body fluid.

osmosis The passage of water through a membrane from a less concentrated compartment to a more concentrated compartment.

isotonic Having equal concentration of solutes.

hypertonic Having high concentration of solutes.

hypotonic Having low concentration of solutes.

Each cell of the body is surrounded by a membrane that allows water to pass freely through it. Water found inside the cell membrane is part of the **intracellular fluid.** Intracellular fluid accounts for 63% of fluid in the body. The remaining body fluid is found outside of cells in one of two extracellular spaces: (1) the fluid portion of blood (plasma) and lymph, accounting for 7% of body fluid; or (2) the fluid between cells (interstitial), making up 30% of body fluid (Fig. 9-9).

Although water can freely travel into and out of cells across the cell membrane, the body controls the amount of water in the intracellular and extracellular compartments mainly by controlling ion concentrations. **Ions** are minerals that dissolve in water and are either positively (+) or negatively (−) charged. These charged ions allow the transfer of electrical current, so they are called **electrolytes.** Four electrolytes predominate: sodium (Na^+) and chloride (Cl^-) are primarily found in the **extracellular fluid,** and potassium (K^+) and phosphate (PO_4^-) are the principal electrolytes in the intracellular fluid.

The term **osmosis** is used to describe the passage of water through a membrane from an area of lower electrolyte concentration to an area of higher electrolyte concentration. Where ions move, water follows passively. Under normal conditions, the concentration of electrolytes on either side of the cell membrane is controlled in such a way that the intracellular fluid and extracellular fluid are **isotonic.** Thus, water movement into and out of the cell is in equilibrium (Fig. 9-10). However, if the intracellular concentration of electrolytes is greater than the extracellular concentration—that is, **hypertonic**—water will flow freely into the cell. If too much water flows in, the cell can burst, similar to filling a balloon with too much air. The opposite can also occur. When the intracellular concentration of electrolytes is relatively low or **hypotonic** compared to the extracellular environment, water will exit the cell, leading to cell shrinkage.

The principle of osmosis is used by the digestive tract to absorb water from the colon. Water from beverages, foods, and intestinal tract secretions makes the contents of the intestinal tract high in water as it enters the colon from the small intestine. Cells that line the colon lumen (inside the colon) actively absorb sodium. Water follows sodium, causing a large amount of water to be absorbed from the colon. As a result, daily water loss from feces is low—approximately 100 milliliters (0.5 cup).

During illness, when large volumes of fluid are lost through vomiting and diarrhea, osmosis can lead to a life-threatening condition. Fluid losses from the gastrointestinal tract result in an increased concentration of electrolytes in the extracellular space. As intracellular water exits the cells in an attempt to dilute the extracellular fluid, cells shrink and lose their ability to function normally. In the heart, this imbalance can lead to a decreased ability of the heart to pump blood and, ultimately, to cardiac failure. Infants and older adults are particularly susceptible to the effects of severe dehydration.

FIGURE 9-9 ▲ Fluid compartments in the body. Total fluid volume is about 40 liters (about 169 cups).

3 Liters
Blood plasma

14 Liters
Fluid between cells
Lymph
Gastrointestinal fluid
Spinal column fluid
Fluid in eyes
Tears
Synovial fluid (in joints)

25 Liters
Fluid found inside every type of cell (e.g., blood, bone, muscle, adipose)

Fluid compartments

Extracellular fluid (37%)

Intracellular fluid (63%)

Total fluid (40 liters)

Liters

Isotonic Solution	Hypotonic Solution	Hypertonic Solution

● Water molecules
● Solute molecules

The concentration of solute molecules inside the cells is the same as the concentration outside the cells.

The concentration of solute molecules is greater inside than outside. In order to gain equilibrium, water flows in (as shown by the arrows), which causes the cell to swell.

The concentration of solute molecules is greater outside than inside. Because the environment outside the cell is more concentrated, water flows out, causing the cell to shrink.

A normal (isotonic) concentration results in a typically shaped red blood cell. Water moves into and out of the cell in equilibrium (black arrows), but there is no net water movement.

A dilute (hypotonic) solution with a low ion concentration results in swelling and subsequent rupture (puff of red in lower left part of cell) of a red blood cell placed into the solution.

A concentrated (hypertonic) solution, with a high ion concentration, causes shrinkage of the red blood cell as water moves out of the cell and into the concentrated solution.

FIGURE 9-10 ▲ Effects of various ion concentrations in a fluid on human cells. This shows the process of osmosis. Fluid is shifting into and out of the red blood cell in response to changing ion concentrations in the fluid surrounding the cells.

✓ CONCEPT CHECK 9.3

1. Define osmosis.
2. Of the four main electrolytes, which two are in highest concentration inside the cell? Which are in highest concentration outside the cell?
3. What happens to fluid in the cells when the concentration of sodium in the blood is higher than the concentration of sodium inside the cells?

9.4 Electrolytes Are Essential for Nerve Impulse Transmission

Sodium, potassium, chloride, and phosphate ions are found in different concentrations on either side of the cell membrane. These ions are charged, creating an electrochemical gradient across the cell membrane. This gradient is maintained across membranes by an energy-dependent pump that can transfer sodium from inside to outside the cell. When Na^+ is actively pumped out of the cell, K^+ enters the cell in an attempt to balance the loss of the positively charged sodium ions, but the rate at which Na^+ ions are pumped out of the cell exceeds the rate at which K^+ ions flow into the cell. As a result, the inside of the cell has a slight negative charge relative to the outside. When the cell is in a resting state, this slight polarization of the cell membrane is maintained by the action of ion pumps.

A nerve impulse starts in response to stimulation, such as a needle pricking the finger (Fig. 9-11), causing positively charged sodium ions to rush into the cell, making the cell less

FIGURE 9-11 ▶ Electrolytes control the conduction of a nerve impulse. (a) Under resting conditions, the intracellular fluid has slightly more electrolytes with a negative charge. (b) Nervous stimulation causes the influx of sodium into the interior of the cell. The intracellular charge changes from slightly negative to slightly positive (depolarization). This results in an electrical signal (action potential) transmitted along the surface of the membrane. (c) The pumping of positive ions from intracellular to extracellular space allows the membrane to return to the resting state. This process is called repolarization.

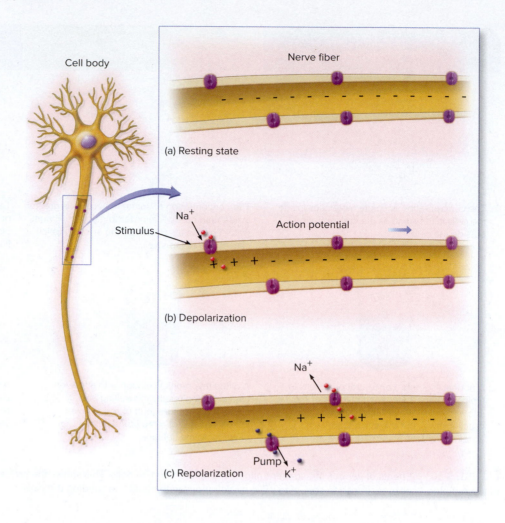

Cell body

Nerve fiber

(a) Resting state

Stimulus

Na^+

Action potential

(b) Depolarization

Na^+

Pump

K^+

(c) Repolarization

depolarization During nerve impulse transmission, the process in which the resting state of the nerve cell membrane (slightly negative inside the cell membrane) is temporarily disrupted.

action potential Change in the electrical charge of the nerve cell membrane resulting in an electrical signal that can be transmitted from one nerve cell to the next.

repolarization During nerve impulse transmission, the restoration of the resting state of the nerve cell membrane.

negatively charged. The change in electrical charge is known as **depolarization** of the nerve cell membrane. The depolarization of one area of the membrane will stimulate the influx of Na^+ into an adjacent area of the membrane. Thus, the electrical signal (**action potential**) is transmitted along the nerve cell and from one cell to the next (like dominoes falling). Immediately after the change in electrolyte balance, sodium is actively pumped out of the cell to reestablish the normal electrolyte balance. This restoration of the slightly negative charge inside the cell membrane is called **repolarization.**

✓ **CONCEPT CHECK 9.4**

1. What is an electrochemical gradient and how is it maintained?
2. Review Figure 9-11. In your own words, describe how an action potential is transmitted along a nerve cell.

9.5 Electrolytes Maintain Acid-Base Balance

pH A measure of relative acidity or alkalinity of a solution. The pH scale is 0 to 14. A pH of 7 is neutral; a pH below 7 is acidic; a pH above 7 is alkaline.

Electrolytes provide another critical function by maintaining fluid **pH** in a very narrow range. Even small deviations from the normal range of pH will negatively affect the rate at which chemical reactions take place within the body and the ability of hemoglobin to bind to oxygen. The pH of a fluid is determined by the concentration of hydrogen ions (H^+). The pH scale is logarithmic, which means that a change of 1 pH unit (e.g., 8 to 7) is equivalent

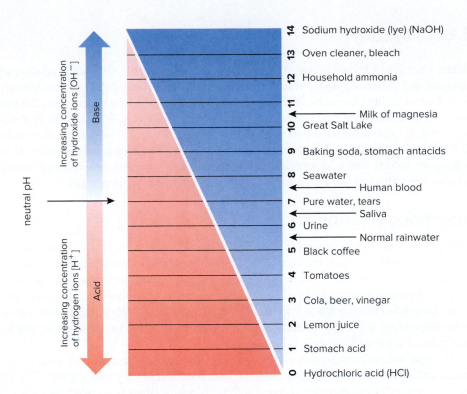

FIGURE 9-12 ◄ pH scale. The diagonal line indicates the proportionate number of hydrogen ions to hydroxide ions. Any pH value above 7 is basic, any pH value below 7 is acidic, and a pH equal to 7 is neutral.

to a 10-fold increase in the hydrogen ion concentration. The pH of blood, foods, and other common substances is shown in Figure 9-12.

Acids are continuously produced when carbohydrates, lipids, and proteins are used by the body to provide energy to the cells. These acids must be neutralized; otherwise, the pH of the body would become acidic. Under normal conditions, the body is easily able to maintain a pH of 7.4 in the extracellular fluids. A large production of acids results in acidosis, in which blood pH is 7.0 to 7.3. When that happens, people are often disoriented and fatigued. Acidosis can occur in poorly controlled diabetes, starvation, diarrhea, and conditions such as emphysema, in which there is excessive production of carbon dioxide for an extended time. Alkalosis (blood pH 7.5 or higher) occurs less often but is just as critical. Here, the body loses too much acid through diuretics, vomiting, or conditions in which you exhale too much carbon dioxide, such as pneumonia or altitude sickness. With alkalosis, you feel agitated and dizzy. Under these conditions, the control systems to maintain normal pH may be inadequate.

Regulation of pH is complex, involving **buffer** systems, the respiratory system, and kidney secretion of excess acid or base. Proteins have a critical function in the buffer system as they bind or release hydrogen ions to control pH. The respiratory system can increase or decrease the amount of carbon dioxide exhaled when breathing. Increased production and release of carbon dioxide can lower pH because CO_2 dissolves in blood or water, creating an acidic compound. Electrolytes, especially sodium, function in the kidney to control the release of acid and base in the urine to maintain pH balance. Phosphate is also an important buffering agent. Sodium and potassium salts of phosphoric acid are among the most widely used buffers in the scientific laboratory.

buffer Compounds that cause a solution to resist changes in acid–base conditions.

✓ CONCEPT CHECK 9.5

1. When we measure the pH of a solution, we are actually measuring the concentration of which ion?

2. List three conditions that could lead to acidosis.

3. How is sodium involved in maintenance of acid-base balance?

4. How is the respiratory system involved in maintenance of acid-base balance?

▲ How does this meal of a turkey club sandwich and French fries compare to MyPlate? How could you reduce the sodium content of this meal? © John A. Rizzo/Getty Images

9.6 Sodium

Sodium (Na) is best known as one of the elements in common table salt. Salt is nutritionally important and was once a highly valued chemical compound! Historically, salt was treasured because of its ability to preserve foods and it was used as a form of payment, thus the word *salary,* which comes from the Latin *salarium.* Salt is 40% sodium and 60% chloride by weight (the chemical symbol Na represents the Latin term *natrium).* One teaspoon of salt contains 2400 milligrams of sodium. What was once difficult to find, however, is now abundant in our food supply. Indeed, nearly all Americans exceed dietary requirements for sodium by so much that reducing sodium in our diets is the focus of major public health campaigns.

FUNCTIONS OF SODIUM

Nearly all the sodium we consume is absorbed by the digestive tract. When sodium chloride (NaCl) is dissolved in water, the chemical bond holding the two atoms together breaks and the charged ions Na^+ and Cl^- are released. These electrolytes, as well as others, attract water. The concentration of intracellular and extracellular water is controlled by the concentration of the electrolytes. Fluid balance is maintained by moving or actively pumping sodium ions where more water is needed. Sodium ions also function in nerve impulse conduction and absorption of some nutrients (e.g., glucose).

Although sodium consumption varies tremendously from day to day, even meal to meal (unless strictly controlled for health reasons), our blood levels vary only slightly. The kidneys function as a sodium filter. If blood sodium is low, sodium is secreted back into the blood as it flows through the kidney, resulting in a decreased urine output. Conversely, if our blood sodium levels are too high, the sodium is filtered out by the kidneys and excreted into the urine. When this excess sodium is removed, water follows, resulting in greater urine output. Without drinking extra water, dehydration can result. Fortunately, high-sodium (salty) foods make us thirsty and drive us to drink more fluids.

SODIUM DEFICIENCY

A low sodium intake, coupled with excessive perspiration and persistent vomiting or diarrhea, has the ability to deplete the body of sodium. This state can lead to muscle cramps, nausea, vomiting, dizziness, and later shock and coma. The likelihood of this occurring is low, because the kidney is efficient at conserving sodium under conditions of low-sodium status.

When excessive perspiration leads to weight loss that exceeds 2% to 3% of total body weight (or about 5 to 6 pounds), sodium losses should raise concern. Even then, adding salt to food or selecting some salty foods such as soup or crackers is sufficient to restore body sodium for most people. Athletes who perspire for hours during endurance activities need to consume sodium from electrolyte-replacement or sports drinks during exercise to avoid depletion of sodium and hyponatremia. Perspiration contains about two-thirds the sodium concentration found in blood or about 1 gram of sodium per liter.

GETTING ENOUGH SODIUM

About 77% of the sodium we consume is in the form of salt added during food manufacturing and food preparation at restaurants. Sodium added while cooking or at the table at home provides about 11% of our intake, and naturally occurring sodium in foods provides the remaining 12% (Fig. 9-13). Most unprocessed foods are relatively low in sodium; milk is one exception (about 120 milligrams per cup).

The more highly processed and restaurant food we consume, the higher our sodium intake. Conversely, the more unprocessed and home-cooked meals prepared, the more control a person has over sodium in the diet. Major contributors of sodium in the adult diet are white bread and rolls, hot dogs and lunch meat, cheese, soups, and foods with tomato

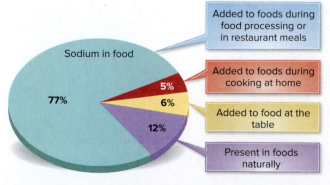

Sodium in food

77%

5% Added to foods during food processing or in restaurant meals

6% Added to foods during cooking at home

12% Added to food at the table

Present in foods naturally

FIGURE 9-13 ▲ Salt arrives in the American diet largely as a result of food processing.

sauce—partly because these foods are consumed so often. Other foods that can be major contributors to sodium intake include French fries, pretzels, potato chips, sauces, and gravies.

If we ate only unprocessed foods and added no salt, we would consume about 500 milligrams of sodium per day. The AI for sodium is 1500 milligrams for adults through age 50 but declines for older adults (see box). If we compare 500 milligrams of sodium from a diet of unprocessed foods with the typical 2300 to 4700 milligrams or more consumed by adults, it is clear that food processing, dining out, and salt added while cooking are the major contributors to sodium intake. When dietary sodium must be restricted, it is important to check the sodium content listed on food labels to monitor sodium intake.

Most people can adapt to wide variations in dietary sodium intakes; today's sodium intake is found in tomorrow's urine. However, approximately 10% to 15% of adults are *salt sensitive* or technically *sodium sensitive;* that is, sodium intake has a direct effect on their blood pressure. As their sodium intake increases, so does their blood pressure. Among these people, lower sodium diets (about 2000 milligrams daily) often decrease blood pressure. Groups that appear to be especially affected are African-Americans, Asian-Americans, and people who have diabetes and/or are overweight (see Section 9.9). Lifestyle factors such as being overweight and inactive are the major contributors to the development of hypertension.

Although current research suggests no association between sodium intake and risk of cardiovascular disease, heart failure, or death (see Newsworthy Nutrition), the medical community still recommends that adults reduce salt and sodium consumption to reduce the risk

Sodium
AI
9–50 years: 1500 milligrams
51–70 years: 1300 milligrams
>70 years: 1200 milligrams
DV: 2400 milligrams
UL: 2300 milligrams

ASK THE RDN   Pass the Salt?

Dear RDN: As a college student, do I need to be concerned about the amount of salt in my diet or are the limits just for older adults with high blood pressure?

Since the 1970s, Americans have been told to limit their salt, more specifically sodium, intakes to control blood pressure. For most Americans, this is a tough rule to follow because of our preference for salty foods. To complicate matters, the scientific community continues to debate this issue as the research presents conflicting evidence. Experts do agree that consuming too much salt may be harmful, especially for individuals with high blood pressure. Scientists disagree, however, on the definition of "too much" salt. The Dietary Guidelines define too much as >2300 milligrams of sodium per day, the amount in 1 teaspoon of salt. This guideline was confirmed in a recent review by the Institute of Medicine (Further Reading 6) that determined the evidence linking sodium intake and blood pressure to be compelling. The American Heart Association recommends 1500 milligrams per day for those over 50 and for all African-Americans (see Further Reading 3), but the Institute of Medicine found insufficient data to support such tight limits. Adding to the confusion, several new studies (see Further Reading 8) failed to conclusively link dietary sodium intake with health outcomes such as heart disease and stroke.

Remember that sodium is the culprit in salt but is an essential nutrient that affects every body system, including the cardiovascular system. Indeed, too little sodium may pose serious health risks. The typical American, however, consumes over 3500 milligrams of sodium per day!

Current evidence links excessive sodium intake with high blood pressure. Most Americans, including college-age students, should reduce sodium intakes to <2300 milligrams per day. To begin reducing overall sodium consumption, read food labels carefully and select foods low in sodium (140 milligrams or less per serving), consume more whole foods and fewer highly processed foods, cook at home, and ask for low-sodium options in restaurants. Deli meats and cheeses are very high in sodium. The sodium in breads, pizza, crackers, and snack foods add up quickly because we typically eat so much of them. Also, reducing sodium while at the same time eating foods rich in potassium, such as fruits and vegetables, might achieve greater health benefits than reducing sodium alone. In sum, choosing fewer highly processed foods and preparing most of your meals at home will result in a healthy, yet achievable, sodium intake.

With just a dash of salt,

Anne M. Smith, PhD, RDN, LD (author)

(a)

(b)

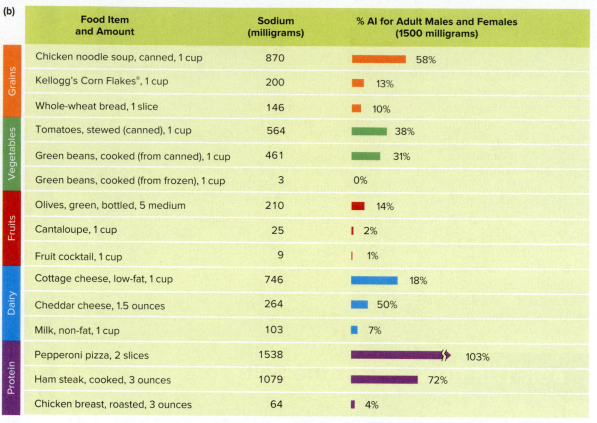

	Food Item and Amount	Sodium (milligrams)	% AI for Adult Males and Females (1500 milligrams)
Grains	Chicken noodle soup, canned, 1 cup	870	58%
	Kellogg's Corn Flakes®, 1 cup	200	13%
	Whole-wheat bread, 1 slice	146	10%
Vegetables	Tomatoes, stewed (canned), 1 cup	564	38%
	Green beans, cooked (from canned), 1 cup	461	31%
	Green beans, cooked (from frozen), 1 cup	3	0%
Fruits	Olives, green, bottled, 5 medium	210	14%
	Cantaloupe, 1 cup	25	2%
	Fruit cocktail, 1 cup	9	1%
Dairy	Cottage cheese, low-fat, 1 cup	746	18%
	Cheddar cheese, 1.5 ounces	264	50%
	Milk, non-fat, 1 cup	103	7%
Protein	Pepperoni pizza, 2 slices	1538	103%
	Ham steak, cooked, 3 ounces	1079	72%
	Chicken breast, roasted, 3 ounces	64	4%

FIGURE 9-14 ▲ Food sources of sodium. (a) The fill of the background color (none, 1/3, 2/3, or completely covered) within each food group on MyPlate indicates the average nutrient density for sodium for *natural, unprocessed foods* in that group. (b) The bar graph shows the sodium content of several natural and processed foods from each food group compared to the AI for adult males and females. Overall, the dairy group is the only food group that provides much sodium in its natural form. Food processing adds significant sodium to foods such as canned vegetables and cured meats.

Source: Nutrition data from USDA National Nutrient Database for Standard Reference, Release 26.

Is sea salt a healthier choice than common table salt? Sea salt is made by evaporating sea water. It is minimally processed, which gives it a coarser texture, and it may contain traces of magnesium, calcium, and potassium. In contrast, table salt is typically mined from the earth and processed into fine grains. Many consumers prefer the taste and texture of sea salt over table salt, but when it comes to heart health, there is no significant difference in sodium or chloride content. Furthermore, as you will learn in Chapter 13, most of the table salt sold in North America is fortified with iodine, an essential nutrient for thyroid function. Next time you purchase salt, compare the labels of several products to assess any nutritional differences for yourself.

of developing hypertension later in life (see Further Reading 2). It is also a good idea to have your blood pressure checked regularly. If you are diagnosed with hypertension, you should reduce sodium intake as you follow a comprehensive plan to treat this disease. Reducing sodium intake may also help maintain a healthy calcium status, as sodium intake greater than about 2000 milligrams per day may cause calcium to be lost in the urine along with the sodium excreted. The effect of this increased urinary calcium loss on bone health is controversial.

Adopting a reduced-salt diet is a significant lifestyle change for most people because many typical food choices will have to be limited (Fig. 9-14). At first, foods may taste bland, but eventually, you will perceive more flavor as the taste receptors in the tongue become more sensitive to the salt content of foods. It takes 6 to 8 weeks to retrain your taste buds to sense sodium at a lower level. Slowly reducing sodium intake by substituting lemon juice, herbs, and spices will allow you to become accustomed to a diet that contains minimal amounts of salt. Many cookbooks and online sources offer excellent recipes for flavorful dishes.

AVOIDING TOO MUCH SODIUM

The Upper Level (UL) for sodium for adults is 2300 milligrams (2.3 grams), approximately 1 teaspoon. Intakes exceeding this amount typically increase blood pressure. Current research also links excessive sodium consumption to overweight and obesity. As salt intake increases, fluid intake also increases; if calorie-laden beverages are chosen, weight gain may ensue (see Further Reading 4). About 95% of North American adults have sodium intakes that exceed that UL. It must be noted that the Daily Value (DV) of 2400 milligrams exceeds the UL for sodium. A healthier goal is to aim for the AI of 1500 milligrams (see Further Reading 11).

Newsworthy Nutrition

No Evidence for Extreme Sodium Restrictions for Older Adults

The relationship between dietary sodium and health outcomes in older adults remains unclear. The aim of this study was to examine the association between sodium intake and the incidence of cardiovascular disease (CVD), heart failure (HF), and death in older adults. Data was obtained from 2642 older adults, aged 71 to 80 years, participating in a 10-year study beginning in 1997–1998. A food frequency questionnaire was used to assess dietary sodium intake at baseline. Participants were categorized according to sodium intake: <1500 mg/d (291 participants [11.0%]), 1500 to 2300 mg/d (779 participants [29.5%]), and >2300 mg/d (1572 participants [59.5%]). During the 10-year study, 881 participants died, 572 developed CVD, and 398 developed HF. Sodium intake was not associated with 10-year mortality or risk of CVD or HF. Adjusting for caloric intake and body mass index did not affect the results. There were no consistent interactions with sex, race, or hypertensive status observed for any outcome. In conclusion, sodium intake in adults aged 71 to 80 was neither associated with 10-year mortality nor incidence of CVD or HF. The authors emphasize the need for additional rigorous studies before recommending any further restrictions of sodium intake beyond the current UL of 2300 mg/d for adults.

Source: Kalogeropoulos AP and others: Dietary sodium content, mortality, and risk for cardiovascular events in older adults: The Health, Aging, and Body Composition (Health ABC) Study. *Journal of the American Medical Association Intern Med.* 175(3):410-419, 2015.

✔ CONCEPT CHECK 9.6

1. List three high-sodium food sources in your dietary pattern.
2. Which organ regulates the amount of sodium in your blood?
3. Define *sodium sensitivity*.
4. List three specific changes you could make to your diet to decrease your sodium intake.

9.7 Potassium

FUNCTIONS OF POTASSIUM

Potassium (K) performs many of the same functions as sodium, such as water balance and nerve impulse transmission. (The chemical symbol K represents the Latin term *kalium*.) All membranes contain an energy-dependent pump that can transfer sodium from inside to outside the cell. When sodium (Na^+) is actively pumped out of the cell, potassium (K^+) enters the cell in an attempt to balance the loss of the positively charged sodium ions. That makes potassium the principal positively charged ion inside cells. Intracellular fluids contain 95% of the potassium in the body. Higher potassium intake is associated with *lower* rather than higher blood pressure values (see Newsworthy Nutrition in Section 9.9).

▲ Fruits and vegetables are rich sources of potassium. © C Squared Studios/Getty Images

POTASSIUM DEFICIENCY

Low blood potassium, also known as hypokalemia, is a life-threatening problem. Symptoms often include a loss of appetite, muscle cramps, confusion, and constipation. Eventually, the heart beats irregularly, decreasing its capacity to pump blood.

Hypokalemia can result from malnutrition and inadequate food intake, most commonly observed with chronic diarrhea or vomiting, or as a side effect of medications, including laxatives and some diuretics. Vulnerable populations include people with certain eating disorders (see Chapter 15) or alcohol use disorders (see Chapter 20). Other populations at increased risk for potassium deficiency include people on very-low-calorie diets and athletes who exercise for prolonged periods. In these situations, more potassium-rich foods should be consumed to compensate for potentially low body potassium. People who take potassium-wasting **diuretics** (water pills) for high blood pressure need to carefully monitor their dietary intake of this potassium. Increased intake of fruits and vegetables or potassium chloride supplements are typically prescribed by primary care providers.

diuretic A substance that increases the volume of urine.

GETTING ENOUGH POTASSIUM

Unprocessed foods, including fruits, vegetables, milk, whole grains, dried beans, and meats, are rich sources of potassium (Fig. 9-15). An easy guide is to remember that the more processed your food, the higher it is in sodium and the lower it is in potassium. Major contributors of potassium to the adult diet include milk, potatoes, beef, coffee, tomatoes, and orange juice.

Approximately 90% of the potassium we consume is absorbed, but dietary patterns are more likely to be lower in potassium than sodium because we add salt to our food, not

(a)

ChooseMyPlate.gov

(b)

	Food Item and Amount	Potassium (milligrams)	% AI for Adult Males and Females (4700 milligrams)
Grains	Raisin bran cereal, 1 cup	352	7%
	Quinoa, cooked, ½ cup	159	3%
	White bread, 1 slice	29	1%
Vegetables	Swiss chard, cooked, 1 cup	961	20%
	Potato, baked (with skin), 1 medium	926	20%
	Acorn squash, cooked, 1 cup	896	19%
Fruits	Orange juice, fresh, 1 cup	496	11%
	Cantaloupe, 1 cup	426	9%
	Banana, 1 medium	422	9%
Dairy	Yogurt, plain, non-fat, 1 cup	625	13%
	Milk, fat-free, 1 cup	382	8%
	Soymilk, 1 cup	296	6%
Protein	Kidney beans, cooked, ½ cup	358	8%
	Sirloin steak, grilled, 3 ounces	286	6%
	Pistachios, dry roasted, 1 ounce	285	6%

FIGURE 9-15 ▲ Food sources of potassium. (a) The fill of the background color (none, 1/3, 2/3, or completely covered) within each food group on MyPlate indicates the average nutrient density for potassium in that group. (b) The bar graph shows the potassium content of several foods in each food group compared to the AI for adult males and females. Overall, the richest sources of potassium are unprocessed foods of plant origin, such as fruits, vegetables, and beans.

Source: Nutrition data from USDA National Nutrient Database for Standard Reference, Release 26.

potassium. In fact, North Americans typically consume only 2000 to 3000 milligrams of potassium per day, much less than the AI (see box). Many of us need to increase potassium intake, preferably by increasing fruit and vegetable intake.

Potassium

AI: 4700 milligrams

DV: 3500 milligrams

UL: none

AVOIDING TOO MUCH POTASSIUM

If the kidneys function normally, typical food intakes will not lead to potassium toxicity. Thus, no Upper Level for potassium has been set. When the kidneys function poorly, potassium increases in the blood, inhibiting heart function and leading to a slowed heartbeat. If left untreated, the heart eventually stops beating, resulting in a cardiac arrest and death. Therefore, in cases of kidney failure or kidney disease, close monitoring of the levels of potassium in blood and in the diet becomes critical.

✓ CONCEPT CHECK 9.7

1. List two functions of potassium in the body.
2. How is potassium intake related to blood pressure?
3. List three specific changes you could make to your diet to increase your potassium intake.

9.8 Chloride

FUNCTIONS OF CHLORIDE

Chloride (Cl) is a negative ion found primarily in the extracellular fluid. Along with sodium and potassium, chloride helps to regulate fluid balance in the body. In fact, chloride itself may be partially responsible for increases in blood pressure that accompany high-salt diets.

Chloride ions are also a component of the acid produced in the stomach (hydrochloric acid) and are important for overall maintenance of acid-base balance in the body. This electrolyte is used during immune responses as white blood cells attack foreign cells. In addition, nervous system function relies on the presence of chloride.

CHLORIDE DEFICIENCY

Low levels of chloride in the blood can lead to a disturbance of the body's acid-base balance. A chloride deficiency is unlikely, however, because our dietary salt intake is so high. Frequent and lengthy bouts of vomiting, if coupled with a nutrient-poor diet, can contribute to a deficiency because stomach secretions contain a lot of chloride. Individuals with bulimia or severe cases of gastroenteritis are at risk for chloride deficiency. In addition, low chloride levels could occur as a side effect of some medications, such as diuretics or laxatives.

Like sodium, nearly all the chloride consumed is efficiently absorbed. The principal route of excretion is the kidneys, although some chloride is lost in perspiration.

GETTING ENOUGH CHLORIDE

When it comes to sources of chloride, it is important to make the distinction between the chloride ion, which is vital for body functions, and chlorine (Cl_2), which is a poisonous gas. Chlorine is used to disinfect municipal water supplies. A small amount of chlorine may remain in tap water, but the substance evaporates quickly. Municipal and well water supplies usually contain some chloride (leached from the earth) as well, but water does not represent a significant source of chloride in the diet.

A few fruits and vegetables, such as seaweed, celery, tomatoes, and olives, are naturally good sources of chloride. Most of our dietary chloride, however, comes from salt added to

▲ Chloride is likely part of the blood-pressure-raising property of sodium chloride (salt).

© Keith Brofsky/Getty Images

Chloride
AI: 2300 milligrams
DV: 3400 milligrams
UL: 3600 milligrams

foods. Knowing a food's salt content allows for a close prediction of its chloride content. Salt is 60% chloride by weight.

Like sodium, nearly all the chloride consumed is efficiently absorbed. The AI for chloride (see box) is based on the 40:60 ratio of sodium to chloride in salt (1500 milligrams of sodium to 2300 milligrams of chloride). If the average adult consumes about 9 grams of salt daily, that yields 5.4 grams (5400 milligrams) of chloride. The principal route of excretion is the kidneys, although some chloride is lost in perspiration.

AVOIDING TOO MUCH CHLORIDE

The average adult typically consumes an excess of this mineral. Because chloride has a role in raising blood pressure, it is important that aging adults consciously control salt intake to decrease risk of developing hypertension. Learning at a young age to select low-salt foods is the best way to start.

✓ CONCEPT CHECK 9.8

1. List two functions of chloride in the body.
2. How is chloride intake related to blood pressure?

9.9 Nutrition and Your Health

Minerals and Hypertension

© Picturenet/Blend Images LLC

In the United States, 78 million or an estimated one in five adults has hypertension. Over the age of 65, the number rises to one in every two adults. Only about half of cases are being treated. Blood pressure is expressed by two numbers. The higher number represents systolic blood pressure, the pressure in the arteries when the heart muscle is contracting and pumping blood into the arteries. Optimal systolic blood pressure is 120 mmHg or less. The second value is diastolic blood pressure, the artery pressure when the heart is relaxed. Optimal diastolic blood pressure is 80 mmHg or less. Elevations in both systolic and diastolic blood pressure are strong predictors of disease (Fig. 9-16).

Hypertension is defined as sustained systolic pressure exceeding 139 mmHg or diastolic blood pressure exceeding 89 mmHg. Most cases of hypertension (about 95%) have no clear-cut cause. Such cases are classified as **primary or essential hypertension.** Kidney disease, sleep-disordered breathing (sleep apnea), and other

primary hypertension Blood pressure of 140/90 mmHg or higher with no identified cause; also called *essential hypertension.*

secondary hypertension Blood pressure of 140/90 mmHg or higher as a result of disease (e.g., kidney dysfunction or sleep apnea) or drug use.

causes often lead to the other 5% of cases, classified as **secondary hypertension.** African-Americans and Asian-Americans are more likely than Caucasians to develop hypertension and to do so earlier in life.

Unless blood pressure is periodically measured, the development of hypertension is easily overlooked. Because it usually does not cause symptoms, it is described as a silent disorder.

Why Control Blood Pressure?

Blood pressure needs to be controlled mainly to prevent cardiovascular disease, kidney disease, strokes and related declines in brain function, poor blood circulation in the legs, problems with vision, and sudden death. These conditions are much more likely to be found in individuals with hypertension than in people with normal blood pressure. Smoking and elevated blood lipoproteins make these diseases even more likely. Individuals with hypertension need to be diagnosed and treated as soon as possible, as the condition generally progresses to a more serious stage over time and even resists therapy if it persists for years. The benefits of controlling blood pressure were confirmed by the results of a recent randomized study of patients at high risk for cardiovascular events (see Further Reading 10). Decreasing the systolic blood pressure of these patients to less than 120 mmHg, as compared with less than 140 mmHg, resulted in lower rates of fatal and nonfatal major cardiovascular events and death from any cause.

Contributors to Hypertension

Because we do not know the cause of 95% of the cases of hypertension, we can identify only risk factors that contribute to its development. A family history of hypertension is a risk factor, especially if both parents have (or had) the problem. In addition, blood

How High Is High?

If your systolic and diastolic pressures fall into different categories, your risk depends on the higher category

SYSTOLIC   DIASTOLIC

Hypertension (High)

140   90

Pre-hypertension

120   80

Normal

Numbers (in millimeters of mercury) apply to adults who aren't taking drugs to lower their blood pressure.

FIGURE 9-16 ▲ The cutoff for hypertension is 140/90 mmHg, but the risk of heart attacks and stroke precedes the rise in blood pressure.

pressure can increase as a person ages. Some increase is caused by atherosclerosis. As plaque builds up in the arteries, the arteries become less flexible and cannot expand. When vessels remain rigid, blood pressure remains high. Eventually, the plaque begins to make the problem worse by decreasing the blood supply to the kidneys, which decreases their ability to control blood volume and, in turn, blood pressure.

Overweight people have a much greater risk of having hypertension than lean people. Overall, obesity is considered the number one lifestyle factor related to hypertension. This is especially the case in minority populations. Additional blood vessels develop to support excess tissue in overweight and obese individuals, and these extra miles of associated blood vessels increase work by the heart and also blood pressure. Hypertension is also linked to obesity if elevated blood insulin levels result from insulin-resistant adipose cells. This increased insulin level augments sodium retention in the body and accelerates atherosclerosis. In such cases, a weight loss of as little as 10 to 15 pounds often can help treat hypertension.

Inactivity is considered the number two lifestyle factor related to hypertension. If an obese person can engage in regular physical activity (at least 5 days per week for 30 to 60 minutes) and lose weight, blood pressure often returns to normal.

Third, excess alcohol intake is responsible for about 10% of all cases of hypertension, especially in middle-age males and among African-Americans in general. When hypertension is caused by excessive alcohol intake, it is usually reversible. A sensible alcohol intake for people with hypertension is two or fewer drinks per day for men and one or no drinks per day for women and all older adults.

In some people, particularly African-Americans and older overweight persons, blood pressure is especially sensitive to sodium. In these people, excess salt leads to fluid retention by the kidney and a corresponding increase in blood volume, resulting in increased blood pressure. It is not clear whether sodium or chloride is more responsible for the effect. Because most of our sodium comes in the form of salt, if one reduces sodium intake, chloride intake naturally falls. For the most part, a recommendation to consume less sodium is equivalent to a call for less salt in the diet. Only some North Americans are susceptible to increases in blood pressure from salt intake, so it is only the number four lifestyle factor related to hypertension. It is unfortunate that salt intake receives the major portion of public attention with regard to hypertension. Efforts to prevent hypertension should also focus on obesity, inactivity, and excessive consumption of alcohol.

Other Minerals and Blood Pressure

Minerals such as calcium, potassium, and magnesium also deserve attention when it comes to prevention and treatment of hypertension (see Newsworthy Nutrition and Further Reading 9). Studies show that a dietary pattern rich in these minerals and low in salt can decrease blood pressure within days of beginning this type of diet, especially among African-Americans. The response is even similar to that seen with commonly used medications. The diet is called the Dietary Approaches to Stop Hypertension (DASH) diet (Table 9-1). The diet is rich in calcium, potassium, and magnesium and low in salt. Both magnesium and calcium are important for healthy blood pressure because they help blood vessels relax. It takes a standard MyPlate Daily Food Plan; adds one to two extra vegetables and fruits servings; and emphasizes consumption of nuts, seeds, or

TABLE 9-1 ■ What Is the DASH Diet?
The DASH diet is low in fat and sodium and rich in fruits, vegetables, and low-fat dairy products. Here is the breakdown:

Per Day	Per Week
6–8 servings of grains and grain products	4–5 servings of nuts, seeds, or legumes
4–5 servings of fruit	5 servings of sweets and added sugars
4–5 servings of vegetables	
2–3 servings of low-fat or fat-free dairy products	
2 or fewer servings of meats, poultry, and fish	
2–3 servings of fats/oils	

legumes (beans) 4 to 5 days of the week. In DASH studies, participants also consumed no more than 3 grams of sodium and no more than one to two alcoholic drinks per day. A DASH 2 diet trial tested three daily sodium intakes (3300 milligrams, 2400 milligrams, and 1500 milligrams). People showed a steady decline in blood pressure on the DASH diet as sodium intake declined. Overall, the

Newsworthy Nutrition

Slash Sodium, but Step Up Potassium to Control Blood Pressure

Studies have linked high sodium and low potassium intakes to increased blood pressure. There is limited research, however, on the association of sodium-to-potassium intake ratio with blood pressure and hypertension. The hypothesis of this study assumed the sodium-to-potassium ratio would be positively associated with blood pressure. Data on 10,563 participants in the 2005–2010 National Health and Nutrition Examination Survey (NHANES) were analyzed. Subjects were ≥20 years of age and were not taking antihypertensive medication or following a low-sodium diet. The average sodium intake (3569 mg/d), potassium intake (2745 mg/d), and sodium-to-potassium ratio (1.41) were all significantly associated with systolic blood pressure. For each 1000-mg/d increase in sodium intake, blood pressure increased by 1.04 mmHg, but for each 1000-mg/d increase in potassium intake, blood pressure decreased by 1.24 mmHg. Blood pressure also increased by 1.05 mmHg per 0.5-unit increase in sodium-to-potassium ratio. These results provide evidence that high sodium intakes combined with suboptimal potassium consumption are associated with hypertension.

Source: Zhang Z and others: Association between usual sodium and potassium intake and blood pressure and hypertension among U.S. adults: NHANES 2005–2010. *PLoS ONE* 8(10):e75289, 2013.

DASH diet is seen as a total dietary approach to treating hypertension, with the many healthful practices of the dietary pattern being responsible for the fall in blood pressure. It is also impressive that a panel of health experts has named the DASH diet the best overall eating plan, ranking it first for the sixth year in a row on the *U.S. News & World Report's* 2016 Best Diets list.

Other studies also show a reduction in stroke risk among people who consume a diet rich in fruits, vegetables, and vitamin C (recall that fruits and vegetables are rich in vitamin C). Overall, a diet low in salt and rich in low-fat and fat-free dairy products, fruits, vegetables, whole grains, and some nuts can substantially reduce hypertension and stroke risk in many people, especially those with hypertension (see Further Reading 1).

Medicine Cabinet

Diuretics are commonly prescribed to lower blood pressure. Diuretics cause the kidneys to excrete more urine but at the same time may increase urinary excretion of minerals and decrease blood levels of potassium, magnesium (see Chapter 11), and zinc (see Chapter 13). Those taking diuretics need to carefully monitor their dietary intake of these minerals, especially potassium, and increase intake of fruits and vegetables or potassium chloride supplements as prescribed by primary care providers.

Examples:

- Hydrochlorothiazide (Microzide®)
- Furosemide (Lasix®)

Beta-blockers decrease the heart's rate, as well as its workload and blood output.

Examples:

- Atenolol (Tenormin®)
- Metoprolol tartrate (Lopressor®)

ACE (angiotensin-converting enzyme) inhibitors cause the body to produce less **angiotensin,** which causes the blood vessels to relax and open up and thus lower blood pressure.

Examples:

- Benazepril hydrochloride (Lotensin®)
- Lisinopril (Prinivel®, Zestril®)

Source: American Heart Association. Prevention and treatment of high blood pressure, http://www.heart.org.

medicine cabinet pills - © Footage supplied by Goodshoot/Punchstock

angiotensin A hormone produced by the liver and activated by enzymes from the kidneys. It signals the adrenal glands to produce aldosterone also and directs the kidneys to conserve sodium (and therefore water). Both of these actions have the effect of increasing blood volume.

diuretic A substance that increases the volume of urine.

Medications to Treat Hypertension

There are a variety of high blood pressure medications otherwise known as antihypertensives. The different classes of these drugs are summarized in the Medicine Cabinet feature in this section. Diuretics, or "water pills," are one class that work to reduce blood volume (and therefore blood pressure) by increasing fluid output in the urine. Other medications act by slowing heart rate or by causing relaxation of the small muscles lining the blood vessels. A combination of two or more medications is commonly required to treat hypertension that does not respond to diet and lifestyle therapy.

Prevention of Hypertension

Many of the risk factors for hypertension and stroke are controllable, and appropriate lifestyle changes can reduce a person's risk (Fig. 9-17), depending on the severity of the hypertension. Experts also recommend that those with hypertension lower blood pressure through diet and lifestyle changes before resorting to blood pressure medications.

Advice	Details	Drop in Systolic Blood Pressure
Lose excess weight	For every 20 pounds you lose (if BMI > 25)	5 to 20 points
Adopt a DASH eating plan	Eat a lower-fat diet rich in vegetables, fruits, and low-fat dairy foods	8 to 14 points
Exercise daily	Get 30 minutes a day of aerobic activity (such as brisk walking)	4 to 9 points
Limit sodium	Eat no more than 2400 mg per day (1500 mg per day is better)	2 to 8 points
Limit alcohol	Have no more than 2 drinks per day for men, 1 drink per day for women (1 drink = 12 oz beer, 5 oz wine, or 1.5 oz 80-proof whiskey)	2 to 4 points

FIGURE 9-17 ▲ What works? If your blood pressure is high, here's how much lifestyle changes should lower it.

Source: *The Seventh Report of the Joint National Committee on Prevention, Detection, Evaluation, and Treatment of High Blood Pressure* (www.nhlbi.nih.gov/health-pro/guidelines/current/hypertension-jnc-7).

CASE STUDY Focus On The Positive

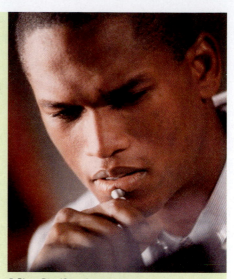

© PhotoDisc/Getty Images

Jerome enjoys listening to his nutrition professor's experiences with successes and failures in advising people on diet change. The instructor says that when people focus on doing something positive in their diet, they automatically start to do less of the negative—like substituting one behavior with another. While at the pharmacy the other day, Jerome stopped at the station to check his blood pressure. He did not like the results. He went to the student health center for a recheck, as advised by the American Heart Association. He was diagnosed as prehypertensive, with a blood pressure of 129/85. Jerome was sad but not shocked. He is African-American and has a family history of hypertension. He exercises four times per week, controls stress through playing piano, is close to his family, enjoys friends, and does not drink or smoke. Jerome lives in an apartment with three friends. His mom taught him to cook, which he does three nights per week. Jerome does not skip meals (eats breakfast) and packs a lunch to eat on campus. However, too often dinner is late and he grabs packaged snack foods to ward off hunger until he can fix dinner.

Jerome talks with his nutrition professor about his dilemma. She wants him to stay positive and asks him to focus on potassium. She tells him that if he focuses on including high-potassium foods, he will receive some added benefits.

Answer the following questions about Jerome's situation and check your responses at the end of the chapter.

1. Since Jerome is an African-American, why is it prudent for him to do something about his blood pressure right now?
2. In what other nutrients are potassium-rich foods high?
3. How might these foods be beneficial for Jerome in his desire to control his blood pressure?
4. What are some potassium-rich foods that Jerome could have readily available at home to help him ward off hunger until he is ready to eat his dinner? Can he pack any of these for a quick snack?

Summary (Numbers refer to numbered sections in the chapter.)

9.1 Water constitutes 50% to 70% of the human body. Its unique chemical properties enable it to dissolve substances as well as serve as a medium for chemical reactions, temperature regulation, and lubrication. Water also helps regulate the acid-base balance in the body.

9.2 Sources of water include beverages, foods, and metabolic water. Water is lost via urine, skin, lungs, and feces. Antidiuretic hormone, angiotensin, and aldosterone regulate fluid balance via the kidneys. For adults, daily water needs from the combination of food and drink are estimated at 11 cups (women) and 15 cups (men) per day. Both deficient water intake (dehydration) and excessive water intake (water intoxication) can lead to physical and mental impairment or death.

9.3 Intracellular fluid is fluid contained within cells, accounting for about two-thirds of total fluid. Extracellular fluid (e.g., plasma, lymph, gastrointestinal secretions, synovial fluid) makes up the remaining one-third of body fluid. Water moves freely across cell membranes by osmosis. The distribution of water in various body compartments is strictly regulated by the concentrations of electrolytes, including sodium, potassium, chloride, and phosphate. Intakes of sodium, potassium, and chloride are related to the development of hypertension.

9.4 Electrolytes are involved in transmission of nerve impulses. At rest, the inside of the nerve cell membrane has a slightly negative charge. Stimulation of the nerve cell leads to depolarization of the cell membrane: sodium ions flow into the cell, leading to a slightly positive charge within the cell membrane. Depolarization of one part of the nerve cell membrane triggers depolarization of an adjacent area, so an electrical signal can be transmitted along the cell. After nervous stimulation, sodium ions are pumped back into the cell and the membrane is repolarized.

9.5 The pH is a measure of the concentration of hydrogen ions in a solution. A pH of 7 is neutral, greater than 7 is basic, and less than 7 is acidic. The pH of the blood is maintained close to 7.4. Sodium and phosphate function in the pH regulation of body fluids.

9.6 Sodium, the major positive ion found outside cells, is vital in fluid balance and nerve impulse transmission. The North American diet provides abundant sodium through highly processed foods and table salt. About 10% to 15% of the adult population is sensitive to sodium intake. Overweight people and African-Americans are especially at risk for developing hypertension from consuming excessive sodium.

9.7 Potassium, the major positive ion found inside cells, has a similar function to sodium. Fruits, vegetables, and dairy are good sources.

9.8 Chloride is the major negative ion found outside cells. It is important in digestion as part of stomach acid and in immune and nerve functions. Table salt supplies most of the chloride in our diets.

9.9 Maintaining a healthy weight; limiting alcohol intake; exercising regularly; decreasing salt intake; and ensuring adequate potassium, magnesium, and calcium in the diet all can play a part in controlling high blood pressure.

Check Your Knowledge (Answers are available at the end of this question set.)

1. Which of the following is a function of water in the body?
   a. temperature regulation
   b. acid-base balance
   c. nerve impulse transmission
   d. all of the above

2. Minerals involved in fluid balance are
   a. calcium and magnesium.
   b. copper and iron.
   c. calcium and phosphorus.
   d. sodium and potassium.

3. The primary function of sodium is to maintain
   a. bone mineral content.
   b. hemoglobin concentration.
   c. immune function.
   d. fluid distribution.

4. Chloride is
   a. a component of hydrochloric acid.
   b. an intracellular fluid ion.
   c. a positively charged ion.
   d. converted to chlorine in the intestinal tract.

5. Hypertension is defined as a blood pressure of _____ or higher.
   a. 110/60
   b. 120/65
   c. 140/90
   d. 190/80

6. Fatigue, headaches, dizziness, and muscle weakness are signs of
   a. hypertension.
   b. dehydration.
   c. kidney stones.
   d. low blood potassium.

7. A hormone that causes the kidneys to conserve sodium is called
   a. glucagon.
   b. parathyroid hormone.
   c. antidiuretic hormone.
   d. aldosterone.

1. Total water needs are about _____ cups per day for women and about _____ cups per day for men.
   a. 8; 10
   b. 9; 13
   c. 11; 15
   d. 15; 18

9. The major intracellular positive ion is
   a. sodium.
   b. potassium.
   c. chloride.
   d. calcium.

10. Food sources of potassium include
    a. milk.
    b. kidney beans.
    c. orange juice.
    d. all of the above.

Answer Key: 1. a (LO 9.1), 2. d (LO 9.6), 3. d (LO 9.6), 4. a (LO 9.6), 5. c (LO 9.8), 6. b (LO 9.4), 7. d (LO 9.2), 8. c (LO 9.3), 9. b (LO 9.5), 10. d (LO 9.7)

Study Questions (Numbers refer to Learning Outcomes)

1. List five functions of water in the body. **(LO 9.1)**

2. Describe the effects of antidiuretic hormone (ADH) and aldosterone on body water. **(LO 9.2)**

3. Approximately how much water do you need each day to stay healthy? Identify at least two situations that increase the need for water. Then list three sources of water in the average person's diet. **(LO 9.3)**

4. List three consequences of mild (1% to 2% loss of body weight) dehydration. List three consequences of severe dehydration. **(LO 9.4)**

5. What are two similarities and differences between sodium and potassium? Between sodium and chloride? **(LO 9.5)**

6. What is the relationship between sodium and water balance, and how is that relationship monitored as well as maintained in the body? **(LO 9.6)**

7. How do sodium and potassium participate in nerve impulse transmission? **(LO 9.6)**

8. What metabolic processes affect the pH of body fluids? Why is it important for pH to be maintained within a narrow range? **(LO 9.6)**

9. Of the micronutrients discussed in this chapter, which are typically consumed in excess? Which of the micronutrients in this chapter are typically lacking in North American diets? **(LO 9.7)**

10. List three dietary strategies to lower blood pressure. **(LO 9.8)**

What the Dietitian Chose

Bottled water has become very popular. In 2014, each American consumed more than 34 gallons of bottled water, adding up to about 10.9 billion gallons for the nation. The public perception that bottled water is safer and healthier than tap water has stimulated the current bottle-toting habit. The truth is that bottled and tap water are both regulated: bottled water by FDA and tap water by the Environmental Protection Agency (EPA). FDA requirements for bottled water mimic those of the EPA for water quality, but in neither does the water have to be contaminant free.

"Pure" is an advertising term and means nothing about the quality of the water. Recent controversy over misleading advertising by major companies such as Pepsico® and Coca-Cola® that use public source water in their respective products, Aquafina® and Dasani®, has led to the printing of "Public Source Water" or "PSW" on labels.

Mineral water must contain consistent levels of natural elements from an underground source; no minerals may be added to the water. The precise mineral content varies by source, but common minerals found in water include calcium, magnesium, potassium, sodium, sulfur, iron, fluoride, zinc, and some ultratrace minerals. The minerals impart some taste to the water but are typically a minor contributor to overall mineral intake.

There is no legal definition for "vitamin water." Manufacturers of vitamin water (i.e., soft-drink companies) often use filtered or distilled water and add sweeteners (e.g., high-fructose corn syrup) and citric acid as flavoring agents, plus several vitamins (mostly vitamin C and an assortment of B vitamins). In 2010, a barrage of class action lawsuits were filed by a number of U.S. consumers against the Coca-Cola Bottling Company for false marketing of its popular vitaminwater® brand as a healthy drink containing nutrients and failing to adequately inform consumers of the amount of sugar in vitaminwater. These products are marketed as healthy because they contain added vitamins, but most of them also supply a surprising amount of sugar. Recall that the American Heart Association recommends that men and women get no more than 150 or 100 kcal per day, respectively, from added sugars. A 20-ounce bottle of vitaminwater has 33 grams of sugar, providing 132 kcal from added sugar. This is about half the sugar in a regular soft drink, but you can see how this can add up to excess. Furthermore, most North Americans consume adequate amounts of vitamin C and the B vitamins without the aid of these beverages. The class action lawsuits were settled in late 2014

© Comstock Images

ensuring that the misleading phrases on the vitaminwater labels and marketing will be removed and that the Coca-Cola products will state the amount of calories per vitaminwater bottle.

Consumers should also be aware of FDA definitions for other types of bottled water:

- Artesian water must come from a confined aquifer.
- Spring water must flow naturally to the surface.
- Purified water is produced through an approved process such as distillation or reverse osmosis.

Relying on bottled water is an expensive habit, personally and environmentally. If you use bottled water to meet your recommended fluid needs, you will spend close to $1500 per year compared with about 50 cents for the same volume of tap water. On a larger scale, it is estimated that close to 90% of water bottles end up in the trash, clogging our landfills or being shipped to other countries for recycling. It is well known that America has some of the cleanest, safest tap water in the world. While following the recommendations to drink more water, hydrate with tap or home-filtered water in a reusable container (see Further Reading 7).

CASE STUDY SOLUTION Focus On the Positive

1. African-Americans are at higher risk for hypertension than any other racial or ethnic group. Within this group, hypertension is more common, it occurs at an earlier age, and is more severe. Approximately 40% of African-Americans have hypertension. The longer it is left untreated, the more severe its complications become. These complications include stroke, heart attack, kidney disease, and congestive heart failure.

2. Fruits and vegetables that are high in potassium tend also to be high in vitamins A (especially beta-carotene) and C. The only exceptions are two white foods: bananas are high in potassium but low in vitamins A and C; potatoes are high in potassium and vitamin C but low in vitamin A. In addition, fruits and vegetables provide plenty of soluble fiber. Whole grains are higher in potassium than refined grains. With whole grains, there is more insoluble fiber. Beans (black, red, pinto) and peas (chickpeas, split peas, lentils) are high not only in potassium but also in proteins and soluble fiber. They are naturally low in fat. Low-fat dairy products provide plenty of potassium, calcium, and vitamin D.

3. Eating fruits, vegetables, whole grains, beans, and peas will provide plenty of fiber. Fiber helps with weight management by contributing to satiety. Additionally, soluble fiber helps to lower cholesterol. Beans provide Jerome with low-cost, low-fat sources of protein, so he can substitute them for meat at meals. When he includes high-potassium foods in his diet, he will naturally begin to increase his intake of fiber and vitamins A and C, while simultaneously lowering his intake of fat and sodium.

4. If Jerome has a time-bake feature on his oven at home, before he leaves for classes, he could set the oven to have a baked potato ready for him the minute he walks through the door. He could also learn to use a slow-cooker. By slow-cooking food while he is gone, Jerome would come home to a place filled with delicious aromas and healthy food. Carrots, peas, potatoes, chicken, canned tomatoes, celery, spices, and chickpeas can be combined the night before, refrigerated, poured into the slow-cooker in the morning, and set on low to cook in his absence. Jerome will come home to a meal that is high in potassium, vitamins A and C, soluble fiber, and protein, and low in fat and sodium. If he adds some crunchy whole-grain bread, he'll have a feast. For a heart-healthy snack, he could pack a mixture of dried fruit, nuts, and cereal, and buy a carton of low-fat milk.

Further Readings

1. Aburto NJ and others: Effect of lower sodium intake on health: Systematic review and meta-analyses. *British Medical Journal* 346:f1326, 2013.

2. Appel LJ and others: The importance of population-wide sodium reduction as a means to prevent cardiovascular disease and stroke: A call to action from the American Heart Association. *Circulation* 123:1138, 2011.

3. Cobb LK and others: Methodological issues in cohort studies that relate sodium intake to cardiovascular disease outcomes—A science advisory from the American Heart Association. *Circulation* 129:1173, 2014.

4. Grimes CA and others: Dietary salt intake, sugar-sweetened beverage consumption, and obesity risk. *Pediatrics* 131:14, 2013.

5. Howard BC: What do recycling symbols on plastics mean? *The Daily Green.* March 2008. http://www.thedailygreen.com/green-homes/latest/recycling-symbols-plastics-460321.

6. IOM (Institute of Medicine): *Sodium intake in populations assessment of evidence.* Washington, DC: National Academies Press, 2013.

7. Maid S: Should you drink tap or bottled water? *Scientific American.* October 21, 2015. http://www.scientificamerican.com/article/should-you-drink-tap-or-bottled-water/

8. O'Donnell M and others: Urinary sodium and potassium excretion, mortality, and cardiovascular events. *New England Journal of Medicine* 371:612, 2014.

9. Potassium and sodium out of balance: Too little potassium and too much sodium is bad for the heart and general health. *Harvard Health Letter* 19:4, 2009.

10. SPRINT Research Group: A randomized trial of intensive versus standard blood-pressure control. *New England Journal of Medicine.* Online. November 9, 2015. doi:10.1056/NEJMoa1511939

11. Thalheimer JC: Spotlight on sodium: How much is too much, and how little is too little? *Today's Dietitian* 16(11):26, 2014.

12. U.S. Food and Drug Administration. FDA continues to study BPA. *FDA Consumer Update.* March 2012. http://www.fda.gov/downloads/ForConsumers/ConsumerUpdates/UCM297971.pdf

 connect **To get the most out of your study of nutrition, go to McGraw-Hill's online resources: Connect www.mcgrawhillconnect.com, where you will find NutritionCalc Plus, LearnSmart, and many other dynamic tools.**

I. How High Is Your Sodium Intake?

Complete this questionnaire to evaluate your sodium habits with respect to typically rich sources.

How Often Do You . . .	Rarely	Occasionally	Often	Regularly (Daily)
1. Eat cured or processed meats, such as ham, bacon, sausage, frankfurters, and other luncheon meats?				
2. Choose canned or frozen vegetables with sauce?				
3. Use commercially prepared meals, main dishes, or canned or dehydrated soups?				
4. Eat cheese, especially processed cheese?				
5. Eat salted nuts, popcorn, pretzels, corn chips, or potato chips?				
6. Add salt to cooking water for vegetables, rice, or pasta?				
7. Add salt, seasoning mixes, salad dressings, or condiments—such as soy sauce, steak sauce, catsup, and mustard—to foods during preparation or at the table?				
8. Salt your food before tasting it?				
9. Ignore labels for sodium content when buying foods?				
10. When dining out, choose obviously salty sauces or foods?				

Source: Adapted from *USDA Home and Garden Bulletin* No. 232-6, April 1986.

The more checks you put in the "often" or "regularly" column, the higher your dietary sodium intake. However, not all the habits in the table contribute the same amount of sodium. For example, many natural cheeses such as cheddar are relatively moderate in sodium, whereas processed cheeses and cottage cheese are much higher. To moderate sodium intake, choose lower sodium foods from each food group more often and balance high-sodium food choices with low-sodium ones.

II. Rate Your Beverage Choices

Water is the key component in the beverage-consumption guidelines (Table 9-2). These recommendations give guidance on the health and nutritional benefits as well as the risks of various beverage categories. The basis of the Beverage Guidance System is that fluids should not provide a significant amount of the energy nutrients in a healthy diet. More specifically, the system recommends that beverages provide less than 10% of total calories consumed for a 2200-kcal diet.

TABLE 9-2 ■ The Beverage Guidance System

Level	Category *	Recommended Servings per Day
1	Water	50 fluid ounces (1.7 liters)
2	Tea or coffee, unsweetened	0 to 40 fluid ounces (0 to 1.4 liters)
3	Low-fat and skim milk and soy beverages	0 to 16 fluid ounces (0 to 0.5 liter)
4	Noncalorically sweetened beverages (diet drinks)	0 to 32 fluid ounces (0 to 1 liter)
5	Calorie beverages with some nutrients (100% fruit juices, alcoholic beverages, whole milk, sports drinks)	0 to 8 fluid ounces 100% fruit juices (0 to 0.25 liter); 0 to 1 alcoholic drink for women, 0 to 2 alcoholic drinks for men
6	Calorically sweetened beverages (regular soft drinks)	0 to 8 fluid ounces (0 to 0.25 liter)

*Categories established based on their possible health benefits or risks.

Source: Adapted from Popkin and others. A new proposed guidance system for beverage consumption in the United States. *American Journal of Clinical Nutrition* 83:529, 2006.

© Hoby Finn/Getty Images

1. Think of all the beverages you drank yesterday, from the time you woke up to the time you went to bed. Do your best to recall the types and amounts of your fluid intake in the space here.

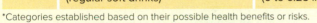

2. Next to each beverage choice you listed for question 1, indicate its category from the Beverage Guidance System.

3. Did you come close to the recommendation to consume 50 fluid ounces (1.5 liters) of fluid in the form of water yesterday?

4. How many fluid ounces of your beverages fit into categories 2, 3, 4, 5, or 6? Did you exceed the recommended servings per day for these categories?

5. What changes could you make in your beverage choices to follow the Beverage Guidance System more closely? How does following the Beverage Guidance System contribute to good health?

Student Learning Outcomes

Chapter 10 is designed to allow you to:

10.1 Summarize the functions of the immune system, including the roles of the skin, GI tract, white blood cells, and lymphoid tissue.

10.2 Understand *oxidation* and *reduction,* and describe how antioxidants function to neutralize free radicals.

10.3 Outline the functions of vitamin A and the carotenoids, list food sources of vitamin A, and describe signs and symptoms of vitamin A deficiency and toxicity.

10.4 Outline the functions of vitamin C, list its food sources, and describe signs and symptoms of vitamin C deficiency and toxicity.

10.5 Outline the functions of vitamin E, list its food sources, and describe signs and symptoms of vitamin E deficiency and toxicity.

Chapter 10
Nutrients Involved in Body Defenses

What Would You Choose?

With a class schedule that begins at 8 every morning, you are searching for a beverage that will jump-start your day as well as provide antioxidants that will boost your body's defense against stress. You know that coffee is the most common morning pick-me-up, but lately you have been hearing a lot about the health benefits of tea, especially green tea. Which of the following would you choose as the first drink of the day to make you alert while also decreasing your risk of oxidative stress and other health concerns?

a Tall 12-ounce cup of Starbucks® Pike Place Roast coffee

b 8-ounce cup of fresh-brewed green tea (from Lipton® Natural Green Tea bag)

c 8-ounce cup of fresh-brewed black tea (from Lipton 100% Natural Tea bag)

d 17-ounce bottle of Honest Tea® Honey Green Tea

Think about your choice as you read Chapter 10, then see What the Dietitian Chose at the end of the chapter.

From day to day, the human body is subject to harm from many sources. Bacteria and viruses would like to take up residence in the body. Free radical molecules—produced in the body or from the environment—batter our cell membranes and threaten our DNA. Cancerous cells invade our tissues and alter normal body functions.

In this chapter, you will learn about micronutrients that support the body's defense systems, including the immune system and the various antioxidant systems. The health of epithelial tissues, which form a barrier to the environment, requires adequate intake of vitamin A, several B vitamins, vitamin C, and zinc. White blood cells are needed to destroy any pathogens that make it beyond those barrier defenses. The formation and function of white blood cells are especially dependent upon vitamins A, C, D, and E, as well as the mineral zinc. Antioxidant defense systems rely on vitamins C and E, carotenoids and other phytochemicals, and a handful of minerals such as selenium and zinc.

Can antioxidants prevent disease? Can megadoses of vitamin C and zinc protect you from the common cold? Is it better to get antioxidants from food or supplements? Can you rationalize eating a lot of chocolate or blueberry pie if it contains phytochemicals? This chapter provides some answers.

10.6 Outline the functions of selenium, list its food sources, and describe signs and symptoms of selenium deficiency and toxicity.

10.7 Outline the functions of zinc, list food sources of zinc, and describe signs and symptoms of zinc deficiency and toxicity.

10.8 Describe the role of antioxidant phytochemicals.

10.9 Explain the benefits of probiotics for the development and maintenance of the immune system.

10.10 Describe the relationships between dietary patterns and cancer risk.

lymphoid tissue Specialized cells that participate in the immune response; includes the thymus, spleen, lymph nodes, and white blood cells.

lymph nodes Clusters of lymphoid tissue, situated along the lymph vessels, that trap and destroy pathogens.

lysozyme An enzyme produced by a variety of cells; it can destroy bacteria by rupturing their cell membranes.

gut-associated lymphoid tissues (GALT) Clusters of lymphoid cells located throughout the gastrointestinal tract that destroy pathogens.

macrophages Large white blood cells that arise from monocytes; one of several types of white blood cells that phagocytize pathogens and signal other white blood cells to mount an immune response.

10.1 Defending the Body Against Pathogens

THE IMMUNE SYSTEM

It can be difficult to visualize the immune system because it is really a collection of diverse tissues that work together to prevent infection, break down aged and dying cells, and remove abnormal cells (Fig. 10-1). **Lymphoid tissue** and white blood cells are specific to the immune system, but as you learned in Section 3.8, other body systems also support the immune system: the skin and GI tract provide physical and chemical barriers against invading pathogens. The lymphatic system, as well, is a major site of immune activity: the **lymph nodes** trap pathogens, and the lymph itself transports white blood cells through the body.

Skin The skin is a large component of the immune system, forming an almost continuous barrier surrounding the body. Invading microorganisms have difficulty penetrating the skin; however, if the skin is split by lesions, bacteria can easily pass through this barrier. Skin health is poor during deficiencies of nutrients such as essential fatty acids, vitamin A, niacin, and zinc. Vitamin A deficiency also decreases gland secretions in the skin that contain the enzyme **lysozyme,** which is capable of killing bacteria. Bacterial eye infections are common in developing countries, often as a result of a vitamin A deficiency.

Intestinal Cells The cells of the small and large intestines form another important barrier to invading microorganisms. The cells are packed closely together, producing a physical barrier to microorganisms. In addition, specialized **gut-associated lymphoid tissues (GALT)** are scattered throughout the intestinal tract. GALT assists the cells of the GI tract in keeping pathogens from entering the bloodstream.

Nutrient deficiencies can cause the intestinal cells to break down, weakening the mucosal membrane so that microorganisms can more easily enter the body and cause infections. Thus, two common results of undernutrition related to an impaired immune system are diarrhea and bacterial infections of the bloodstream. To protect the health of the intestinal tract, an adequate nutrient intake is necessary—especially of protein, vitamin A, vitamin B-6, vitamin B-12, vitamin C, folate, and zinc.

White Blood Cells Once a microorganism enters the bloodstream, white blood cells move in to attack it. There are several types of white blood cells that participate in this response and function in unique ways. Monocytes (which are precursors to **macrophages**), neutrophils, and eosinophils are part of a class of white blood cells called **phagocytes.** These cells circulate throughout the blood and lymph, ingesting and sometimes digesting microorganisms and foreign particles via lysosomes present in the cells (Fig. 10-2). This process of **phagocytosis** is one example of **cell-mediated immunity,** achieved when immune cells directly interact with and destroy pathogens. In **antibody-mediated immunity** (discussed in "Adaptive Immunity" later in this section), some types of lymphocytes produce **antibodies** in response to foreign proteins (**antigens**). These antibodies mark the invader for destruction by other immune cells.

Lymphoid Tissue The lymphoid tissues are specific to the immune system and include the thymus, bone marrow, spleen, lymph nodes, and other clusters of immune cells distributed throughout the body. The **thymus** is a gland that is located near the heart. Along with the cells of the bone marrow, the thymus is involved in the formation and maturation of white blood cells. The thymus is most active from infancy through adolescence, but its activity tapers off during adulthood.

The **spleen,** located near the stomach, contains many macrophages that remove foreign proteins and dead or damaged cells from the blood. The spleen is vital for the clearance of old red blood cells from circulation.

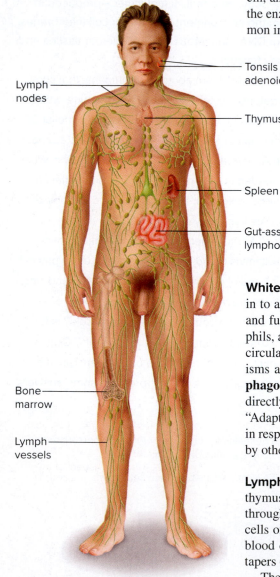

Lymph nodes

Bone marrow

Lymph vessels

Tonsils and adenoids

Thymus

Spleen

Gut-associated lymphoid tissue

FIGURE 10-1 ▲ Components of the immune system.

Lymph nodes appear along the vessels of the lymphatic system. Recall from Section 3.4 that the lymphatic system collects fluid that leaks from the blood vessels and returns it to the cardiovascular system through a vessel near the heart. As lymph flows through the lymphatic system, microorganisms and other foreign proteins will be trapped in the lymph nodes, where white blood cells can destroy them.

Lastly, there are clusters of lymphoid tissues located throughout the body, especially at sites where pathogens are likely to enter the body, such as the lungs and GI tract. As mentioned, patches of gut-associated lymphoid tissue (GALT), situated along the GI tract, are major sites of lymphocyte activity.

THE IMMUNE RESPONSE

Innate Immunity There are two different categories of immune responses: nonspecific (innate) immunity and specific (adaptive) immunity. Innate immunity refers to those physical and chemical defenses that keep any type of foreign substance out of the body. We are born with innate immunity and it is our first line of defense against infection. The physical and chemical barriers of the skin and the GI tract are part of innate immunity.

The **inflammatory response** is another nonspecific tactic used by the cells of the immune system to eradicate pathogens. When macrophages ingest a foreign protein or pathogen, they become activated. Activated macrophages and damaged tissues (in the case of injury) release chemical signals called **cytokines** that damage invading microorganisms and result in swelling, fever, and recruitment of many white blood cells to the site of invasion or trauma.

Typically, the inflammatory response is short lived, briefly boosting the activity of the immune system to quickly deal with pathogens. However, growing evidence links chronic, low levels of inflammation to many of the ailments that plague Americans. Typical American dietary patterns—high in refined carbohydrates, added sugars, solid fats, and overall calories—are thought to promote inflammation, thereby increasing risks for cardiovascular diseases, cancer, type 2 diabetes, and a long list of other infirmities. In contrast, dietary patterns that include plentiful fruits and vegetables, plant sources of protein, unsaturated fats from plant oils and fish, and whole grains are associated with lower inflammation and lower risks of chronic diseases (see Further Reading 17). This "anti-inflammatory" diet is consistent with the Dietary Guidelines for Americans and the advice of many health authorities, including the American Heart Association and American Institute for Cancer Research.

Adaptive Immunity Whereas innate immunity is nonspecific and offers immediate defense against pathogens, adaptive immunity is specific and must be developed over time as we are exposed to individual pathogens. Certain types of lymphocytes produce antibodies, which bind to antigens and thereby mark foreign proteins and microorganisms for destruction by other white blood cells. The primary adaptive response of the lymphocytes may take several days or weeks to eradicate a pathogen, but after an initial exposure to a particular antigen, the lymphocytes create a template (memory) that allows future recognition of the microorganism or foreign protein. Thus, upon subsequent exposure to the same antigen, the lymphocytes' response will be more vigorous and rapid.

NUTRIENTS THAT SUPPORT THE IMMUNE SYSTEM

Protein, B Vitamins, and Iron Help to Form New Cells Many of the cells that support the immune system—white blood cells, skin, and GI cells—are rapidly turned over. Their constant synthesis requires steady nutrient intake. In general, rapidly dividing cells need adequate protein, folate, vitamin B-6, vitamin B-12, and iron. Protein supplies the building blocks, and vitamin B-6 is involved in the metabolism of amino acids to make new cell proteins. As you will learn in Chapter 13, folate, vitamin B-12, and iron are necessary for the synthesis of new DNA.

Minerals Support Cell Structure and Help to Destroy Pathogens Zinc and copper (see Section 13.6) play structural roles and are critical for the synthesis of white blood cells.

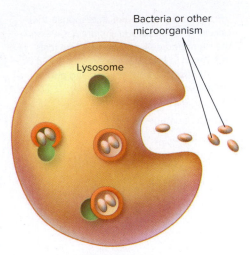

Phagocyte

FIGURE 10-2 ▲ One class of white blood cells, phagocytes, can ingest bacteria, fungi, viruses, and other foreign particles in the process of phagocytosis. An indentation is formed and the particle is engulfed by the cell. The foreign material is eventually digested by lysosomes in the cell.

phagocytes Immune cells (e.g., neutrophils and macrophages) that engulf substances.

phagocytosis A process in which a cell forms an indentation, and solid particles enter the indentation and are engulfed by the cell.

cell-mediated immunity A process in which certain white blood cells come in contact with the invading cells to destroy them.

antibody-mediated immunity A process in which one type of lymphocyte produces antibodies that bind to specific antigens, thus marking foreign proteins or pathogens for destruction by other white blood cells.

antibody Blood protein that binds foreign proteins found in the body.

antigen Any substance that induces a state of sensitivity and/or resistance to microorganisms or toxic substances after a lag period; a foreign substance that stimulates a specific aspect of the immune system.

thymus Lymphoid organ located near the heart that participates in maturation of white blood cells.

spleen Lymphoid organ located near the stomach that filters aged and dead cells and foreign proteins out of blood.

inflammatory response A response that occurs when tissues are injured, causing the damaged cells to release chemicals that result in blood vessels leaking fluid into the tissues, causing swelling and inflammation.

cytokines Chemical messengers that regulate immune responses.

Iron (see Section 13.5) and zinc are also required for the production of enzymes used by white blood cells to destroy pathogens.

Vitamins A and D Regulate Gene Expression By binding to receptors on DNA, the active forms of vitamins A and D can control immune system activity at the genetic level by switching various genes on or off. Vitamin D, covered in relation to bone health in Section 11.5, enhances the innate immune response by helping immune cells to proliferate and by promoting the expression of certain proteins involved in destroying pathogens. Conversely, adaptive immune responses are usually suppressed by vitamin D. Researchers link the ability of vitamin D to limit the action of certain white blood cells to a decreased risk for autoimmune diseases.

Antioxidant Nutrients Protect Immune Cells The white blood cells utilize oxidation to kill pathogens. For example, an iron-containing enzyme kills bacteria that have been engulfed by phagocytes. The antioxidant capabilities of vitamin C, vitamin E, and selenium help to protect the body's cells from being damaged by the oxidation reactions used to destroy pathogens. The roles of antioxidants are explored in further detail in Section 10.2.

The antioxidant nutrients appear to have other roles in immune function as well, such as increasing the proliferation of immune cells and regulating expression of proteins involved in the immune response. In this chapter, you will learn specifically about the roles of vitamins A, C, and E, zinc, and selenium in support of the immune system (see Further Reading 6). Table 10-1 summarizes the many nutrients involved in immune function.

TABLE 10-1 ■ Micronutrients That Support Immune Function

Nutrient	Primary Roles in Immunity
Vitamin A	• Maintains the health of epithelial cells • Contributes to function of mucus-secreting cells • Supports activity of white blood cells
Vitamin B-6	• Maintains the health of epithelial cells • Synthesis of white blood cells • Production of proteins involved in the immune response
Vitamin B-12	• Maintains the health of epithelial cells • White blood cell formation and activity
Vitamin C	• Antioxidant function protects immune cells from oxidative damage • Stimulates production and activity of white blood cells
Vitamin D	• Modulates gene expression in white blood cells • Possible role in prevention of autoimmune diseases
Vitamin E	• Antioxidant function protects immune cells from oxidative damage • May protect against age-related declines in immune function
Folate	• Maintains the health of epithelial cells • White blood cell formation and activity
Zinc	• Development and function of white blood cells • Supports ability of cells to use oxidation reactions to kill pathogens
Iron	• Development and function of white blood cells • Supports ability of cells to use oxidation reactions to kill pathogens
Copper	• Production of white blood cells, particularly phagocytes
Selenium	• Antioxidant function protects immune cells from oxidative damage • Involved in expression of cytokines that regulate the immune response

It is easy to see how nutrient deficiencies (undernutrition) can negatively impact immune function. Remarkably, research demonstrates that obesity (overnutrition) impairs immunity as well. Among obese people, diet and lifestyle choices contribute to chronic, low levels of inflammation throughout the body. Adipose tissue becomes infiltrated with white blood cells that secrete immune-stimulating chemicals that increase risk for insulin resistance, cardiovascular diseases, type 2 diabetes, cancer, and autoimmune diseases.

✓ **CONCEPT CHECK 10.1**

1. Describe two ways the GI tract assists the immune system.

2. What is the process by which cells can engulf particles, such as bacteria and fungi? What types of cells perform this function?

3. Differentiate between innate immunity and adaptive immunity.

4. What is the inflammatory response? What dietary patterns lead to chronic, low levels of inflammation?

10.2 Protecting the Body from Oxidative Damage

OXIDATION AND REDUCTION

To understand oxidation and reduction, let us first review the anatomy of an atom. The nucleus of an atom contains protons and neutrons. Electrons circle the nucleus and are found in pairs. The nucleus is positively (+) charged, and the electrons are negatively (−) charged. When the positive and negative charges are balanced, there is no overall charge to the atom. When the number of electrons does not equal the number of protons, the atom has a net positive or negative electrical charge and is called an ion.

Atoms join together (or bond) to form molecules. For example, hydrogen (H) and oxygen (O) bond to form a molecule of water (H_2O). Carbohydrates, lipids, and protein are examples of molecules. Approximately half of all enzymatic (chemical) reactions in the body involve the exchange of electrons between atoms and molecules. The gain of a negatively charged electron is called **reduction,** and the loss of an electron is termed **oxidation** (Fig. 10-3).

Oxidative stress occurs when there is an imbalance between the production of various reactive compounds and the ability of the organism's natural protective mechanisms to cope with these reactive compounds and prevent adverse effects (see Further Reading 10).

Normally, atoms are stable; they have an even number of electrons in the outermost shell from the nucleus. When an electron is lost from an atom during oxidation, the atom ends up with an unpaired electron in its outer shell. In most reactions, there is an immediate pairing of electrons from two atoms to form a stable molecule. However, sometimes a molecule or atom may be left with an unpaired electron in its outer shell.

The presence of the free electron results in a situation in which the number of positive charges contributed by the nucleus of the atom is no longer equal to the number of negative charges in the electrons surrounding the nucleus. These chemically unstable atoms are classified as **free radicals.** Free radicals are chemically reactive and sometimes aggressive. To reestablish a balance between positive and negative charges, the free radical steals an electron from an adjacent stable atom or molecule. Once this process starts, it leads to a chain reaction. With the loss of an electron, that nearby molecule now becomes an unstable free radical. In order to reestablish neutrality, it looks to acquire an electron from another adjacent molecule.

The production of free radicals is a normal consequence of cellular respiration and metabolism. To a degree, free radicals are purposefully produced to protect our health. For example, white blood cells produce highly reactive free radicals that assist in the destruction of bacteria, viruses, and fungi (see Section 10.1). The production of free radicals has also been shown to be an important component of the mechanism by which the body destroys altered cells, which could potentially progress to cancerous growth.

On the other hand, overproduction of free radicals can be harmful to healthy cells. The damage can happen within the cell membrane or inside the cell, disrupting cell function and growth. Remember, the cell membrane is a lipid bilayer. In the cell membrane, two layers of phospholipids are oriented so that their hydrophilic ("attracted to water") heads are exposed to the watery environment that makes up the cytoplasm of the cell and the extracellular fluid

reduction The process of gaining an electron during a chemical reaction.

oxidation The process of losing an electron during a chemical reaction.

oxidative stress Imbalance between the production of reactive compounds and the body's ability to protect against their adverse effects.

free radical An unstable atom with an unpaired electron in its outermost shell; also called *reactive oxygen species.*

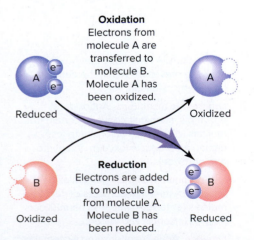

FIGURE 10-3 ▲ Electrons are transferred between molecules in oxidation-reduction reactions.

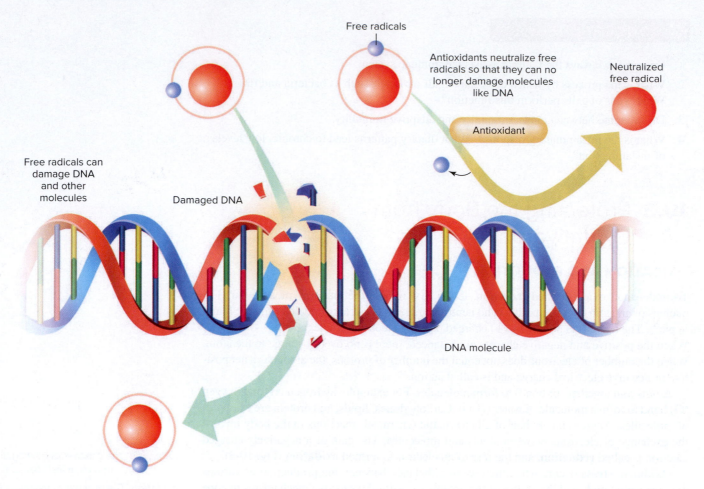

Free radicals

Antioxidants neutralize free radicals so that they can no longer damage molecules like DNA

Neutralized free radical

Antioxidant

Free radicals can damage DNA and other molecules

Damaged DNA

DNA molecule

FIGURE 10-4 ▲ Free radicals can damage specific structures, such as DNA, within cells. Antioxidants minimize the adverse effects of free radicals.

antioxidant A substance that has the ability to prevent or repair the damage caused by oxidation.

superoxide dismutase Antioxidant enzyme system that converts certain free radicals (superoxide anions) into less damaging products (oxygen and hydrogen peroxide).

glutathione peroxidase An antioxidant enzyme system that converts certain free radicals (peroxides) into less harmful compounds (alcohols and water).

catalase Antioxidant enzyme system that converts harmful reactive oxygen species (peroxides) into less harmful products (water and oxygen).

outside the cell. The tails, which are fatty acids, are hydrophobic (or lipophilic—"attracted to fat") and are aligned toward each other in the interior of the cell membrane. Many of the fatty acids within the cell membrane are polyunsaturated. Recall from Section 5.2 that the double bonds in polyunsaturated fatty acids are highly susceptible to oxidation. When free radicals interact with the electrons from those double bonds, the cell membrane loses its integrity and more reactive compounds are produced that further damage DNA, lipids, and proteins. The layer of phospholipids is "broken," and so is the cell's ability to regulate the flow of water and nutrients in and out of it. Eventually, with enough breakage, the cell will collapse.

When free radicals damage the DNA within cells, the genetic code can be altered. Oxidative damage of DNA is thought to contribute to the development of cancer (Fig. 10-4).

As you learned in Section 5.8, oxidation of low-density lipoproteins (LDLs) is thought to contribute to atherosclerosis. Oxidized LDLs are taken up by scavenger cells that are attached to the inner walls of blood vessels. Over time, the accumulation of fatty material leads to formation of plaque, which narrows the opening of the blood vessel and makes it less flexible (see Further Readings 1, 4, 5, and 24).

ANTIOXIDANT DEFENSES

The body has two principal defense mechanisms to limit or defend against the adverse effects of free radicals: antioxidant enzyme systems and **antioxidant** chemicals (Fig. 10-4). Antioxidant enzyme systems convert harmful free radicals into less damaging compounds at specific locations within cells. Examples of antioxidant enzymes include **superoxide dismutase, glutathione peroxidase,** and **catalase.** The activity of these antioxidant enzymes depends on the presence of mineral cofactors, such as selenium, manganese, zinc, iron, and copper.

Antioxidant chemicals are derived from food. They include vitamins (C and E), a vitamin precursor (beta-carotene), and some phytochemicals (see Chapter 8). These antioxidants principally function by donating an electron or hydrogen atom to reactive molecules to stabilize the molecule's structure (Fig. 10-5). The antioxidants then become temporarily unstable; but because of their own mechanisms to be reduced, either by enzymatic or nonenzymatic reactions, they are not reactive molecules that will induce cellular damage.

The antioxidant enzyme systems and dietary antioxidant chemicals work in concert to limit free radical formation, destroy free radicals, and assist in repairing oxidative damage induced by reactive molecules. Over time, however, these defense mechanisms can be overwhelmed by oxidative stress. An imbalance between production of free radicals and the cell's antioxidant defenses can lead to cell dysfunction and play a role in the development of cancer, cardiovascular disease, and many other age-related conditions (see box).

To limit the oxidative damage caused by free radicals, it is essential to optimize the supply of nutrients that support antioxidant function. Dietary recommendations, including those found in the Dietary Guidelines for Americans, MyPlate, and the Fruits & Veggies: More Matters® campaign, are based on the premise that increased consumption of fruits and vegetables will increase intake of the antioxidant vitamins, minerals, and phytochemicals that will help detoxify reactive molecules, including free radicals.

A dietary antioxidant, as defined in the Dietary Reference Intakes, is "a substance in foods that significantly decreases the adverse effects of reactive species such as reactive oxygen and nitrogen species on normal physiological function in humans" (see Further Reading 10). Antioxidants can work by delaying or inhibiting the initiation step of oxidation (primary antioxidants), by slowing the oxidation by removing the substrate, or by neutralizing free oxygen radicals (secondary antioxidants). Antioxidant vitamins, minerals, and phytochemicals may help to prevent or postpone diseases that are linked to oxidative stress. The nutrients that participate in the body's antioxidant defenses include vitamin C (ascorbic acid), vitamin E (**tocopherols**), and selenium (see Further Reading 16). These nutrients must be consumed in the diet as the body cannot synthesize them. Some phytochemicals may also act as antioxidants, including **carotenoids, isoflavones, flavonoids,** and **anthocyanins.** Several trace minerals—manganese, zinc, iron, and copper—are also involved in antioxidant activity by virtue of their roles as cofactors for antioxidant enzymes.

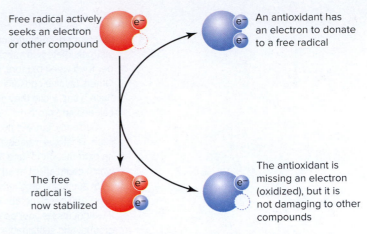

FIGURE 10-5 ▲ Antioxidants (in blue) stabilize free radicals (in red) by donating electrons to them. Free radicals are dangerous to cells because they seek to fill their outer shells by removing electrons from other substances such as DNA, proteins, and lipids.

tocopherols The chemical name for some forms of vitamin E. The alpha form is the most potent.

carotenoids Precursors of vitamin A found in plant foods.

isoflavones Phytochemicals produced in legumes, with soybeans being the most common source of isoflavones in food.

flavonoids Most common group of polyphenol phytochemicals; found in citrus fruits, berries, red onion, tea, red wine, and dark chocolate.

anthocyanins Flavonoid plant pigments that appear red, purple, or blue and are found in berries, grapes, and red cabbage.

ASK THE RDN   Detox Diets

Dear RDN: *I put on 10 pounds last year, and I can't seem to shed the extra weight. Can a detox diet help?*

There is little consensus about the definition of a detoxification diet, but in general, such plans are meant to assist the body's natural mechanisms to get rid of harmful toxins that arise from metabolism and from our environment (see Further Reading 22). When you look at the advocates of detox diets, it should raise a red flag that its praises are sung primarily by celebrities, tabloid magazines, and TV talk-show hosts who claim that detox diets cause weight loss, improve energy, and reduce risk of chronic diseases.

We are exposed to toxins every day. Some are produced by the body—such as the ammonia that arises from metabolism of amino acids. Many more are present in the foods we eat, the water we drink, and the air we breathe. Fortunately, the human body has several natural detoxification systems that convert harmful substances into water-soluble compounds that can be excreted via urine, sweat, bile, or feces.

Scientific evidence shows that the body's detoxification pathways are effective without any extra intervention. Popular culture detox diets have become a fad that features extreme,

The chemical damage produced by free radicals has been linked to numerous diseases, including:

- Age-related macular degeneration
- Alzheimer's disease
- Arthritis
- Atherosclerosis
- Cancer
- Cataracts
- Diabetes
- Emphysema
- Kidney disease
- Parkinson's disease

uninformed, and nutritionally inadequate dietary practices. One of the most harmful regimens instructs dieters to subsist on a liquid diet of lemon juice, maple syrup, water, and cayenne pepper for a week or more. Some plans rely on herbal laxatives to purge the colon of waste materials. Others involve consuming up to 8 cups per day of juice made from organic fruits and vegetables. Such plans, while they may boost certain nutrients and phytochemicals, are extremely low in calories and protein.

Currently, there is no clinical evidence to support the benefits of these detox diets. Side effects such as fatigue, headaches, or decreased mental acuity are signs of low blood sugar. Taken to an extreme, prolonged fasts and nutritionally inadequate diets can lead to chemical imbalances, which could affect heart function.

In summary, an overly restrictive diet is difficult to maintain and may end up decreasing lean mass and basal metabolic rate. Sustained weight loss requires a lifestyle change, not a quick fix! If weight loss is your goal, moderate calorie restriction combined with physical activity will support gradual and sustainable weight loss (see Chapter 7). B vitamins, antioxidant nutrients, phytochemicals (e.g., flavonoids), dietary fiber, and plenty of fluid are what the body requires to detoxify and flush harmful compounds from the body. The best prescription to support your body's detoxification pathways is to consume a diet rich in fruits, vegetables, and whole grains, and to emphasize plant sources of protein every day—not just for a few days a year.

Pure and simple,

Angela Collene, MS, RDN, LD (author)

✓ CONCEPT CHECK 10.2

1. What happens to electrons during the processes of reduction and oxidation?
2. What is a free radical? Why are free radicals thought to be harmful to cells?
3. How do antioxidant chemicals reduce cellular damage?

10.3 Vitamin A (Retinoids) and Carotenoids

Vitamin A was the first fat-soluble vitamin to be recognized as an important component of food essential for human health. Almost all (90%) of vitamin A is stored in the liver; the remaining 10% is in adipose tissue, kidneys, and the lungs. Either a deficiency or toxicity can cause severe problems, and there is a narrow range of optimal intakes between these two states.

Vitamin A is in a group of compounds known as **retinoids.** There are three active forms of vitamin A: **retinol, retinal,** and **retinoic acid.** These are often called preformed vitamin A. They exist only in animal products. When retinol is stored, it is esterified (joined to a fatty acid) and becomes **retinyl.** In supplements, you will often find vitamin A listed as retinyl acetate or retinyl palmitate.

Besides the retinoids, which come from animal sources, many foods of plant origin contain **carotenoids,** some of which can be converted into vitamin A in the body. Carotenoids are not essential nutrients; they are categorized as phytochemicals (review Chapter 8). More than 600 carotenoids have been identified, but just three can be converted to retinol in the body: alpha carotene, **beta-carotene,** and beta-cryptoxanthin. Because these carotenoids can be turned into vitamin A, they are termed **provitamin A.** Of these three, only beta-carotene serves as a significant source of vitamin A. Neither the absorption of carotenoids nor the conversion of the provitamin A carotenoids into vitamin A is an efficient process. Other carotenoids that may play a role in human health but are not vitamin A precursors include lycopene, zeaxanthin, and lutein.

retinoids Chemical forms of preformed vitamin A; one source is animal foods.

retinol Alcohol form of vitamin A.

retinal Aldehyde form of vitamin A.

retinoic acid Acid form of vitamin A.

retinyl Storage form of vitamin A.

carotenoids Precursors of vitamin A found in plant foods.

beta-carotene The orange-yellow pigment in carrots; beta-carotene is the only carotenoid that can be sufficiently absorbed and converted into retinol in the body.

provitamin A A substance that can be converted into vitamin A.

FUNCTIONS OF VITAMIN A AND CAROTENOIDS

Health of Epithelial Cells and Immune Function For many years, vitamin A has been dubbed the "anti-infection" vitamin. Vitamin A is covered in this chapter because it maintains the health of epithelial cells, which line internal and external surfaces of the lungs, intestines, stomach, vagina, urinary tract, and bladder, as well as those of the eyes and skin. Retinoic acid is required for immature epithelial cells to develop into mature, functional epithelial cells. Without vitamin A, mucus-forming cells such as those in the intestines and lungs deteriorate and lose function. For the eye, this can lead to blindness (see "Vision" in this section). Hyperkeratosis, also a result of vitamin A deficiency, is a condition in which skin cells produce too much keratin, blocking the hair follicles and causing "gooseflesh" or "toadskin" appearance. The excessive keratin in these skin cells causes the skin to be hard and dry.

The epithelial tissues just described serve as important barriers to infection. Vitamin A also supports the activity of certain immune system cells, specifically the T-lymphocytes, or T-cells. Together, these effects leave the vitamin A–deficient person at great risk for infections. Vitamin A–deficient animals and humans have an increased infection rate, but when they are supplemented with vitamin A, the immune response improves.

Vision The link between vitamin A and night vision has been known since ancient Egyptians used juice extracted from liver to cure **night blindness.** Vitamin A performs important functions in light-dark vision and, to a lesser extent, color vision. Light entering the back of the eye reaches a lining called the **retina.** The retina consists of rods, cones, and nerve cells. Rods detect black and white, and are responsible for night vision. Cones are responsible for color vision. Rods and cones require vitamin A for normal function. One form of vitamin A (retinal) allows certain cells in the eye to adjust to dim light (such as after seeing the headlights of an oncoming car; Fig. 10-6). Without sufficient dietary vitamin A, the cells in the eye cannot quickly readjust to dim light, causing night blindness.

If vitamin A deficiency progresses, the cells that line the cornea of the eye (the clear window of the eye) lose the ability to produce mucus. The eye then becomes dry. This disease is called **xerophthalmia,** which means dry eye. Eventually, dirt particles scratch the dry surface of the eye, leading to blindness. Xerophthalmia can progress to the stage where there is an accumulation of dead cells and secretions on the surface of the eye. This condition is called Bitot's spots (Fig. 10-7).

Vitamin A deficiency is the leading cause of blindness worldwide. North Americans are at low risk because typical American diets contain plentiful sources of preformed vitamin A, such as fortified milk and eggs. However, poor vitamin A intakes, low-fat intakes that do not allow for sufficient vitamin A absorption, and low stores of vitamin A lessen the ability of children to meet high needs during periods of rapid growth. Worldwide, about one-third of children suffer from vitamin A deficiency. Hundreds of thousands of children in developing nations, especially Southeast Asia and Africa, become blind each year because of vitamin A deficiency. Some of these children ultimately die from infections. Worldwide, attempts to reduce this problem have included promoting breastfeeding, giving large doses of vitamin A twice yearly, and fortifying sugar, margarine, and monosodium glutamate with vitamin A. These food vehicles are used because they are commonly consumed by the population of less-developed nations. This effort has proven effective in some countries.

Another effort is to treat maternal night blindness in these same areas of the world. Among pregnant women, night blindness is a marker of vitamin A deficiency that will likely lead to pregnancy-related deaths, malnutrition, anemia, and infant mortality. Screening and supplementing populations of pregnant women can be effective in treating and preventing this public health problem.

Some carotenoids are also important for vision. The macula (also known as the macula lutea, meaning "yellow spot") is in the central area of the retina and is responsible for the most detailed central vision. It contains the carotenoids lutein and zeaxanthin in high enough concentrations to impart a yellow color. Age-related macular degeneration (Fig. 10-8), the leading cause of blindness among older adults in North America, occurs because of changes in this macular area of the retina. In one study of older adults, the higher the total number of

night blindness Vitamin A deficiency disorder that results in loss of the ability to see under low-light conditions.

retina A light-sensitive lining in the back of the eye. It contains retinal.

xerophthalmia Hardening of the cornea and drying of the surface of the eye, which can result in blindness.

FIGURE 10-6 ▶ Vitamin A functions to maintain vision. Light enters the eye through the cornea and lens, and then hits the retina. The light reacts with vitamin A—containing rhodopsin, which is stored in the rod cells of the retina. Rod cells allow us to see black-and-white images. When light reacts with rhodopsin, retinal is cleaved from rhodopsin (bleaching), a process that stimulates an electrical impulse to the brain. A new molecule of vitamin A then combines with opsin to regenerate rhodopsin. The yellow background indicates the bleaching events that occur in the light; the gray background indicates the regenerative events that can occur in either light or dark conditions.

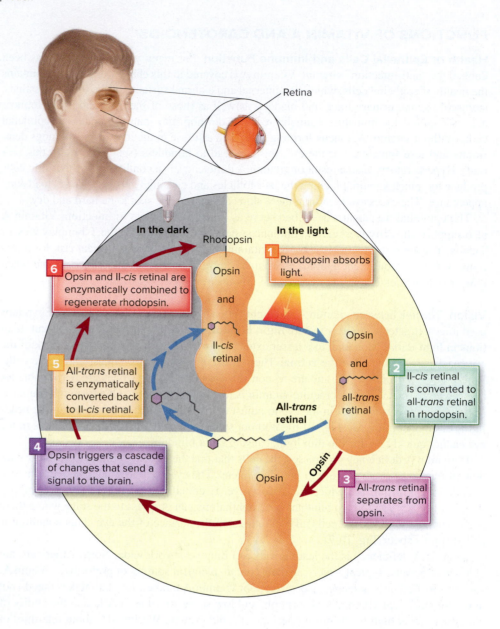

Retina

In the dark

In the light

Rhodopsin

1 Rhodopsin absorbs light.

6 Opsin and ll-*cis* retinal are enzymatically combined to regenerate rhodopsin.

Opsin

and

ll-*cis* retinal

Opsin

and

all-*trans* retinal

2 ll-*cis* retinal is converted to all-*trans* retinal in rhodopsin.

5 All-*trans* retinal is enzymatically converted back to ll-*cis* retinal.

All-*trans* retinal

4 Opsin triggers a cascade of changes that send a signal to the brain.

Opsin

Opsin

3 All-*trans* retinal separates from opsin.

FIGURE 10-7 ▲ Vitamin A deficiency eventually leads to blindness. Note the severe effects on this eye. This problem is commonly seen today in Southeast Asia. © Dr. Alfred Sommer

FIGURE 10-8 ▲ The blurry center of the image simulates the vision of a person with macular degeneration. National Eye Institute, National Institute of Health

carotenoids (beta-carotene, lutein, and zeaxanthin) consumed in the diet, the lower was the risk for age-related macular degeneration. The richest sources of lutein and zeaxanthin are green leafy vegetables (Table 10-2).

These carotenoids may also decrease the risk of cataracts in the eyes. Research studies point toward the actual fruit and vegetables with their high carotenoid content as contributing to reduced risk for eye disorders. Consuming just carotenoids as supplements for this purpose is not recommended. Multivitamin and mineral supplements formulated for older adults (e.g., Centrum Silver™) are being marketed as a source of lutein. Consumers must be aware that studies on carotenoids are generally conducted with food rather than supplements.

Growth, Development, and Reproduction Vitamin A participates in the processes of growth, development, and reproduction in several ways. At the genetic level, vitamin A binds to receptors on DNA to increase synthesis of a variety of proteins. Some of these proteins are required for growth. During early fetal growth, vitamin A functions in the differentiation and maturation of cells that will ultimately form tissues and organs. Vitamin A–deficient children experience stunted growth. For bones to grow and elongate, old bone must be remodeled (broken down) so that new bone can be formed. Vitamin A assists with the breakdown and formation of healthy bone tissue. Adequate intake of vitamin A is needed for reproduction; it aids in sperm production (associated with its epithelial role) and in a normal reproductive cycle for women.

Cardiovascular Disease Prevention   Carotenoids may play a role in preventing cardiovascular disease in individuals at high risk. This role may be linked to carotenoids' ability to inhibit the oxidation of low-density lipoproteins (LDLs). Until definitive studies are complete, many scientists recommend that we consume a total of at least five servings of a combination of fruits and vegetables per day as part of an overall effort to reduce the risk of cardiovascular disease. Other phytochemicals, including flavonoids, phenolic acids, and phytoestrogens, may have a more significant effect in cardiovascular disease prevention than carotenoids.

Cancer Prevention   Vitamin A and the carotenoids have potential benefits but also potential dangers where cancer prevention is concerned. Vitamin A plays a role in cellular differentiation and embryonic development. However, because of the potential for toxicity, unsupervised use of megadose vitamin A supplements to reduce cancer risk is not advised and can be potentially life threatening. For preformed vitamin A, dietary adequacy promotes optimal health, but toxicity can be dangerous.

Population studies show that regular consumption of foods rich in carotenoids decreases the risk of several types of cancer, including cancers of the lung, skin, oral cavity, and **prostate gland.** In particular, the dietary carotenoid lycopene (the red pigment found in tomatoes, watermelon, pink grapefruit, and guava) seems to protect against prostate cancer—one of the most common cancers among North American men. Some food companies have even marketed their tomato products as important sources of lycopene. Their role of carotenoids in cancer prevention is thought to be a by-product of their antioxidant activity.

While dietary carotenoid intake appears to be protective against cancer, supplementation with carotenoids has not proved to be beneficial. For example, recall from Section 1.5 that studies from the United States and Finland failed to show a reduction in lung cancer in male smokers and nonsmokers given supplements of the carotenoid beta-carotene for 5 or more years. In fact, beta-carotene use in male smokers increased the number of lung cancer cases compared with control groups. No comparable studies have been conducted with women. Although further research continues, most researchers are convinced that beta-carotene supplementation offers no protection against cancer. Overall, the best advice is to rely on food sources of both the retinoids and carotenoids to promote optimal health.

GETTING ENOUGH VITAMIN A

Preformed vitamin A (e.g., retinol, retinal, and retinoic acid) is found in liver, fish, fish oils, fortified milk, butter, yogurt, and eggs (Fig. 10-9). Margarine and spreads are also fortified with vitamin A.

About 65% of the vitamin A in the typical North American diet comes from preformed vitamin A sources, whereas provitamin A (carotenoids) dominates in the diet among poor people in other parts of the world. The provitamin A carotenoids are mainly found in dark-green and yellow-orange vegetables and some fruits. Carrots, spinach and other greens, winter squash, sweet potatoes, broccoli, mangoes, cantaloupe, peaches, and apricots are examples of such sources. Beta-carotene accounts for some of the orange color of carrots. In vegetables such as broccoli, this yellow-orange color is masked by dark-green chlorophyll

TABLE 10-2 ■ **Vegetables Rich in Lutein and Zeaxanthin**

Vegetables (serving size)	Lutein and Zeaxanthin (mg)
Kale (½ cup cooked)	11.9
Spinach (½ cup cooked)	10.2
Swiss chard (½ cup cooked)	9.6
Collard greens (½ cup cooked)	7.3
Spinach (1 cup raw)	3.7
Peas (½ cup cooked)	1.9
Broccoli (½ cup cooked)	1.2
Romaine lettuce (1 cup raw)	1.1
Brussels sprouts (½ cup cooked)	1.0
Zucchini (½ cup cooked)	1.0

▲ The carotenoid lycopene is the red pigment found in tomatoes, watermelon, guava, and pink grapefruit and seems to protect against prostate cancer. © FoodCollection

prostate gland   A solid, chestnut-shaped organ surrounding the first part of the urinary tract in the male. The prostate gland secretes substances into the semen.

▲ Provitamin A carotenoids from foods (not supplements) are the safest way to meet vitamin A needs. A serving of these carrots would be an excellent addition to the vegetable section of MyPlate. Cooking food sources of carotenoids actually makes them more bioavailable. © Ingram Publishing/SuperStock

(a)

(b)

Food Item and Amount	Vitamin A (micrograms RAE*)	% RDA for Adult Males (900 micrograms RAE)	% RDA for Adult Females (700 micrograms RAE)
Grains			
Cream of Wheat®, Cooked, ½ cup	280	31%	40%
Kellogg's® Raisin Bran® cereal, 1 cup	228	25%	33%
Corn muffin, 1 medium	59	7%	8%
Vegetables			
Sweet potato, baked, 1 large	1730	192%	247%
Spinach, cooked, 1 cup	943	105%	135%
Kale, cooked, 1 cup	885	98%	126%
Fruits			
Cantaloupe, 1 cup	300	33%	43%
Apricots, dried, ½ cup	117	13%	17%
Mango, 1 cup	90	10%	13%
Dairy			
Milk, fat-free, 1 cup	150	17%	21%
Soymilk (fortified), 1 cup	134	15%	19%
Cheese, cheddar, 1.5 ounces	113	13%	16%
Protein			
Beef liver, pan-fried, 3 ounces	6273	697%	896%
Tuna, bluefin, broiled, 3 ounces	643	71%	92%
Egg, hard-boiled, 1 large	74	8%	11%
Fats & Oils			
Butter, 1 teaspoon	34	4%	5%
Margarine, 1 teaspoon	0	0%	0%
Olive oil, 1 teaspoon	0	0%	0%

* Retinol activity equivalents.

FIGURE 10-9 ▲ Food sources of vitamin A and carotenoids. (a) The fill of the background color (none, 1/3, 2/3, or completely covered) within each food group on MyPlate indicates the average nutrient density for vitamin A and provitamin A carotenoids in that group. (b) The bar graph shows the vitamin A content of several foods from each food group compared to the RDA for adult males and females. Overall, the fruits and vegetables groups provide many rich sources of carotenoids, whereas fortified dairy products and certain choices in the protein group are good sources of preformed vitamin A. The grains group also contains some foods that are nutrient dense because they are fortified with vitamin A.

Source: *Nutrition data from USDA National Nutrient Database for Standard Reference, Release 26.*

Vitamin A

RDA
  Men: 900 micrograms RAE
  Women: 700 micrograms RAE
DV: 1000 micrograms (5000 IU)
UL: 3000 micrograms RAE

pigments. Still, green vegetables contain provitamin A. Green, leafy vegetables, such as spinach and kale, have high concentrations of lutein and zeaxanthin. Tomato juice and other tomato products, such as pizza or spaghetti sauce, contain significant amounts of lycopene. In contrast to many other nutrients, cooking food improves the bioavailability of carotenoids. In raw fruits and vegetables, carotenoids are bound to proteins. Cooking disrupts this protein bond and frees the carotenoid for better absorption.

The RDA for vitamin A (see box) is expressed in retinol activity equivalents (RAE). These RAE units take into account the activity of both preformed vitamin A and the carotenoids that are synthesized into vitamin A in humans. The total RAE value for a food is calculated by adding the concentration of preformed vitamin A to the amount of provitamin A carotenoids in the food that will be converted into vitamin A.

You may have noticed that the RDA for vitamin A is given in micrograms, whereas the vitamin A content on Supplement Facts labels is given in international units (IU) . Legally, supplement manufacturers still must provide amounts of vitamin A in IU, which is a measure of the biological activity of a nutrient rather than its absolute quantity (see the following conversion factors).

The diets of North American adults typically contain adequate vitamin A. Most adults in North America have liver reserves of vitamin A three to five times higher than needed to provide good health. Thus, the use of vitamin A supplements by most people is unnecessary. Populations in North America that may be at risk for vitamin A deficiency include those with low vegetable intakes (e.g., some children, older adults, and the urban poor); people with alcoholism or liver disease; or people with severe fat malabsorption.

AVOIDING TOO MUCH VITAMIN A

Intakes in excess of the UL for vitamin A are linked to birth defects and liver toxicity. Other possible side effects include an increased risk of hip fracture and poor pregnancy outcomes.

During the early months of pregnancy, a high intake of preformed vitamin A is especially dangerous because it may cause fetal malformations and spontaneous abortions. This is because vitamin A binds to DNA and influences cell development. Women of childbearing age should limit their overall intake of preformed vitamin A from food and dietary supplements to no more than about 100% of the Daily Value. Thus, it is important to limit consumption of rich food sources of preformed vitamin A, such as liver. In addition, medications that contain derivatives of vitamin A should be avoided during pregnancy (see Medicine Cabinet). These precautions apply to women who are pregnant and also those who may possibly become pregnant; vitamin A is stored in the body for long periods, so women who ingest large amounts during the months before pregnancy place their fetus at risk.

In contrast, ingesting large amounts of vitamin A-yielding carotenoids does not cause toxic effects. A high carotenoid concentration in the blood (called hypercarotenemia) can occur if someone routinely consumes large amounts of carrots or takes pills containing beta-carotene (more than 30 milligrams daily) or if infants eat a great deal of squash. The skin turns yellow-orange, particularly the palms of the hands and soles of the feet. It differs from jaundice, a sign of liver failure. In jaundice, the yellow discoloration extends to the sclera (whites) of the eye, whereas in hypercarotenemia it does not. Hypercarotenemia does not appear to cause harm and disappears when carotenoid intake decreases. Dietary carotenoids do not produce toxic effects because (1) their rate of conversion into vitamin A is relatively slow and regulated, and (2) the efficiency of carotenoid absorption from the small intestine decreases markedly as oral intake increases.

---

1 RAE =

- 1 microgram of retinol (or retinal or retinoic acid; all the same)
- 12 micrograms of beta-carotene from foods or supplements
- 24 micrograms of other carotenoids from food

Converting IU to RAE

- IU ÷ 3.3 if the supplement is preformed vitamin A (such as retinyl acetate)
- IU ÷ 6.6 if the supplement is carotenoids (usually beta-carotene)

▲ Inuits long knew and explorers soon learned to avoid eating the liver of polar bears. Just 4 ounces (120 grams) of polar bear liver will deliver a toxic dose of 1.36 million RAE of vitamin A. That's 136 times the RDA! © Digital Vision/Getty Images

▲ As little as four to five large carrots daily can produce hypercarotenemia. Taking a break from carrots, squash, and pumpkins will turn the skin back to normal. © Ingram Publishing/SuperStock

---

Medicine Cabinet

Two derivatives of vitamin A are used to treat moderate to severe acne. Tretinoin (Retin-A) is used topically (applied to the skin), and isotretinoin (Roaccutane) is taken orally. These drugs appear to work by altering genes expressed by the skin cells. However, taking vitamin A supplements or making a paste from supplements and applying it to your skin will have no effect on acne. In fact, high doses of vitamin A can induce toxic symptoms, including birth defects. Isotretinoin's label clearly advises against the use of the medication during pregnancy, and its use is strictly monitored by the Food and Drug Administration (FDA). In order for women to receive this medication, they must have two negative pregnancy tests; sign a patient information/consent form; agree to use two effective forms of birth control; register, along with their doctors and pharmacists, with iPLEDGE (https://www.ipledgeprogram.com); and agree to follow all instructions of the program.

Medicine Cabinate - pills: Footage supplied by Goodshoot/Punchstock

1. What are the consequences of vitamin A deficiency?
2. How are the carotenoids related to vitamin A?
3. What are the names of four carotenoids known to have antioxidant functions?
4. List two rich food sources of retinoids and two rich food sources of carotenoids.

10.4 Vitamin C (Ascorbic Acid)

FUNCTIONS OF VITAMIN C

Supporting Body Defenses Vitamin C (also known as ascorbic acid or ascorbate) functions as a powerful antioxidant because it can readily accept and donate electrons. Its antioxidant properties have been postulated to reduce the formation of cancer-causing nitrosamines in the stomach. Vitamin C also aids in the reactivation of vitamin E after vitamin E has donated an electron to a free radical. Population studies suggest that the antioxidant properties of vitamin C may be effective in the prevention of certain cancers (esophagus, mouth, and stomach) and cataracts. The extent to which vitamin C functions in the reduction of diseases is debatable based on the scientific studies to this point.

As part of its antioxidant role, vitamin C assists the immune system. Recall from Section 10.1 that certain white blood cells use oxidation reactions to destroy pathogens. Vitamin C protects the body's cells from the harmful oxidants that are generated as part of the immune response. Beyond this antioxidant activity, vitamin C appears to stimulate the proliferation and function of various types of white blood cells.

Nobel laureate Dr. Linus Pauling claimed that supplementation with large doses of vitamin C could combat the common cold. In the 1970s, he advocated consumption of at least 1000 milligrams of vitamin C daily. It is unclear if illnesses and infections actually increase vitamin C requirements beyond the RDA, but as a result of the popularity of Pauling's books and the respectability of his scientific credentials, millions of North Americans supplement their diets with vitamin C. A recent meta-analysis showed that routine vitamin C supplementation moderately reduces the severity and duration of the common cold, particularly among children. However, taking vitamin C supplements after the onset of a cold does not seem to offer any benefit (see Further Reading 8).

collagen Hard, insoluble and fibrous protein found in connective tissue, bone, teeth, tendons, and blood vessels.

Formation of Body Proteins Perhaps the best understood function of vitamin C is its role in the synthesis of **collagen.** This protein is highly concentrated in connective tissue, bone, teeth, tendons, and blood vessels. The important function of vitamin C in the formation of connective tissue is exemplified in the early symptoms of a deficiency: pinpoint hemorrhages under the skin (Fig. 10-10), bleeding gums, and joint pain. Vitamin C is very important for wound healing; it strengthens structural tissues by increasing the cross-connections between amino acids found in collagen. Without adequate vitamin C, wounds will not heal.

Vitamin C has a specific function in the synthesis of numerous other compounds in the body. It is required for the synthesis of carnitine, a compound that transports fatty acids into the mitochondria. In addition, it takes part in the formation of two neurotransmitters, serotonin and norepinephrine.

FIGURE 10-10 ▲ Pinpoint hemorrhages of the skin—an early symptom of scurvy. The spots on the skin are caused by slight bleeding. The person may experience poor wound healing. These are signs of defective collagen synthesis.
© Dr. P. Marazzi/Science Source

Enhancing Iron Absorption Vitamin C enhances iron absorption by keeping iron in its most absorbable form, especially as the mineral travels through the alkaline environment of the small intestine. Consuming 75 milligrams or more of vitamin C at a meal significantly increases absorption of the iron consumed at that meal. Increasing intake of vitamin C–rich foods is beneficial for those with poor iron status or for those who choose to limit iron-rich food sources. As you will learn in Chapter 13, iron-deficiency anemia is common in the United States and is the number one nutritional deficiency worldwide.

VITAMIN C DEFICIENCY

On long sea voyages before the mid-eighteenth century, half or more of sailing crews died owing to scurvy, the vitamin C deficiency disease. The symptoms of scurvy, which include bleeding gums, tooth loss, bruising, and scaly skin, illustrate the important function of vitamin C in the formation of connective tissue. Without vitamin C, the skin and blood vessels weaken and wounds will not heal. In 1740, the Englishman Dr. James Lind first showed that citrus fruits—two oranges and one lemon a day—could prevent the development of scurvy. Fifty years after Lind's discovery, daily rations for British sailors included limes (thus their nickname, limeys). Even after this discovery, scurvy continued to affect many people as thousands died during the American Civil War owing to inadequate intake of vitamin C.

▲ Citrus fruits are good sources of vitamin C.
© Purestock/SuperStock

GETTING ENOUGH VITAMIN C

Fresh, ripe fruits and vegetables are loaded with vitamin C. Besides the foods listed in Figure 10-11, other citrus fruits, papayas, broccoli, cauliflower, and many types of peppers pack a lot of vitamin C into a low-calorie package. Ready-to-eat breakfast cereals, potatoes, and fortified fruit drinks are also good sources of vitamin C. The five to nine servings of fruit and vegetables suggested by MyPlate's Daily Checklist can easily provide enough vitamin C to meet the RDA. The brighter the fruit or vegetable, the higher it tends to be in vitamin C. For example, while a green bell pepper has 96 milligrams of vitamin C, a red bell pepper provides 152 milligrams of vitamin C. Keep in mind, however, that vitamin C is rapidly lost in processing and cooking as it is unstable in the presence of heat, iron, copper, or oxygen and is water soluble. Boiling fruits and vegetables can destroy much of the vitamin C or cause it to leach out of the food. Extended time on grocery store shelves or on your countertop at home will also decrease vitamin C content. Thus, you should consume fresh fruits and vegetables as soon after harvest as possible.

> **Vitamin C**
> RDA
> Men: 90 milligrams
> Women: 75 milligrams
> DV: 60 milligrams
> UL: 2000 milligrams

The adult RDA of vitamin C is 75 milligrams for women and 90 milligrams for men per day. The Daily Value used

(a)

(b)

	Food Item and Amount	Vitamin C (milligrams)	% RDA for Adult Males (90 milligrams)	% RDA for Adult Females (75 milligrams)
Grains	Whole Grain Total® cereal, 1 cup	60	67%	80%
Grains	Tortellini with cheese filling, ½ cup	0	0%	0%
Grains	Brown rice, cooked, ½ cup	0	0%	0%
Vegetables	Red peppers, raw, 1 cup	190	211%	253%
Vegetables	Brussels sprouts, cooked, 1 cup	97	108%	129%
Vegetables	Spinach, raw, 2 cups	17	19%	23%
Fruits	Strawberries, 1 cup	89	99%	119%
Fruits	Orange, 1 medium	83	92%	111%
Fruits	Grapefruit juice, canned, 1 cup	72	80%	96%

FIGURE 10-11 ▲ Food sources of vitamin C. (a) The fill of the background color (none, 1/3, 2/3, or completely covered) within each food group on MyPlate indicates the average nutrient density for vitamin C in that group. (b) The bar graph shows the vitamin C content of several foods compared to the RDA for adult males and females. Overall, fruits and vegetables are the richest sources of vitamin C. Foods in the dairy and protein groups (not shown) are poor sources of vitamin C.

Source: *Nutrition data from USDA National Nutrient Database for Standard Reference, Release 26.*

▲ A daily serving of which three of these seven fruits will easily provide the recommended amount of vitamin C? © Ingram Publishing/SuperStock

on food and supplement labels is 60 milligrams. Tobacco users need to add an extra 35 milligrams per day to the RDA. The toxic by-products of cigarette smoke and the oxidizing agents found in tobacco products increase the need for the antioxidant action of vitamin C. Average daily consumption of vitamin C in the United States is in the range of 70 to 100 milligrams, and at this level of intake, absorption efficiency is about 80% to 90%.

AVOIDING TOO MUCH VITAMIN C

The Upper Level (UL) of vitamin C is 2000 milligrams. Note that when vitamin C is consumed in large doses, the amount in excess of daily needs mostly ends up in the feces or urine. The kidneys start rapidly excreting vitamin C when intakes exceed 100 milligrams per day. As the amount ingested increases, absorption efficiency decreases precipitously—to approximately 50% with intake of 1000 milligrams per day and to 20% with intakes of 6000 milligrams daily. Regular consumption of more than 2000 milligrams per day may cause stomach inflammation and diarrhea. Even 1000-milligram supplement pills can cause some nausea and GI distress. A recent study found that men who said they took a vitamin C supplement regularly were at higher risk of developing kidney stones; therefore, ingesting large amounts of vitamin C supplements is discouraged in people predisposed to kidney stones. Because vitamin C enhances the absorption of iron, vitamin C supplements are also not recommended for those who overabsorb iron or have excessive iron stores. High doses of vitamin C may interfere with medical tests for diabetes or blood in the feces. If you take vitamin C supplements at any dose, be sure to inform your doctor. Physicians may misdiagnose conditions if they do not realize the influence of large doses of vitamin on your medical test results.

✓ CONCEPT CHECK 10.4

1. How does the antioxidant role of vitamin C assist the immune system?
2. How do the signs of vitamin C deficiency relate to the many roles of the vitamin discussed in this chapter?
3. Why are fresh foods the best sources of vitamin C?

10.5 Vitamin E (Tocopherols)

In the 1920s, a fat-soluble compound was found to be essential for fertility in rats. This compound was named tocopherol from the Greek words *tokos,* meaning "birth," and *phero,* meaning "to bring forth." Later, this essential nutrient was named vitamin E, which is a family of four tocopherols and four tocotrienols called alpha, beta, gamma, and delta. They differ in that tocopherols have a saturated side chain, whereas the tocotrienols have an unsaturated side chain. Tocotrienols have not been as extensively studied as tocopherols, but current research explores their potential roles in prevention of cancer, diabetes, and cardiovascular diseases. Of these eight forms of vitamin E, alpha (α)-tocopherol is the most biologically active and the most potent.

FUNCTIONS OF VITAMIN E

Antioxidant The principal function of vitamin E in humans is as an antioxidant. Vitamin E is a fat-soluble vitamin found primarily in adipose tissue and in the lipid bilayers of cell membranes (Fig. 10-12). Many of the lipids within these membranes are polyunsaturated fatty acids (PUFA), which are particularly susceptible to oxidative attack by free radicals. The formation of free radicals may destabilize the cell membrane, which may ultimately alter the ability of the cell to function properly. Vitamin E can donate electrons or hydrogen to free radicals found in membranes, thereby making them more stable. The antioxidant function of vitamin E appears to be critical in cells continually exposed to high levels of oxygen, particularly red blood cells and the cells lining the lungs.

Increasing vitamin E intake has also been suggested as a way to prevent several chronic diseases that are linked to oxidative damage. For example, oxidized LDL cholesterol is a major component of the plaque that develops in arteries, which leads to atherosclerosis. Vitamin E is thought to attenuate the development of atherogenic plaque due to its ability to prevent or reduce the formation of oxidized LDL cholesterol (see Further Reading 5). Also, oxidative damage to proteins in the eye leads to the development of cataracts. Oxidized proteins cloud the lens of the eye and decrease visual acuity. Insufficient consumption of antioxidants from foods increases risk for these diseases.

Experts do not know whether supplementation with **megadoses** of vitamin E can confer any significant protection against diseases linked to oxidative damage. The consensus among the scientific community is that the established benefits of lifestyle choices have a far greater effect than any proposed benefits of antioxidant supplementation. The position of scientific research groups (e.g., American Heart Association, U.S. Preventive Services Task Force) is that it is premature to recommend vitamin E supplements to the general population, based on current knowledge and the failure of large clinical trials to show any consistent benefit. This conclusion is in agreement with the latest report on vitamin E by the Food and Nutrition Board of the National Academy of Sciences. In addition, the Food and Drug Administration has denied the request of the dietary supplement industry to make a health claim that vitamin E supplements reduce the risk of cardiovascular disease and cancer.

Other Roles of Vitamin E Although vitamin E has an essential function in fertility in many animal species, it does not appear to have this function in humans. It is, however, important for the formation of muscles and the central nervous system in early human development. Vitamin E has been shown to improve vitamin A absorption if the dietary intake of vitamin A is low. Vitamin E also functions in the metabolism of iron within cells, and it helps maintain nervous tissue and immune function.

VITAMIN E DEFICIENCY

Specific population groups are especially susceptible to developing marginal vitamin E status. Preterm infants tend to have low vitamin E stores because this vitamin is transferred from mother to baby during the late stages of pregnancy. Hence, the potential for oxidative damage, which could cause the cell membranes of red blood cells to break (hemolyze), is of particular concern for preterm infants. The rapid growth of preterm infants, coupled with the high oxygen needs of their immature lungs, greatly increases the stress on red blood cells. Special vitamin E–fortified formulas and supplements designed for preterm infants compensate for lack of vitamin E. Smokers are another group at high risk for vitamin E deficiency, as smoking readily destroys vitamin E in the lungs. One study showed that megadosing will not correct this vitamin E destruction by smokers. Others at risk of vitamin E deficiency include adults on very-low-fat diets (<15% total fat) or those with fat malabsorption.

GETTING ENOUGH VITAMIN E

Because vitamin E is only synthesized by plants, plant products (especially the oils) are the best sources. In the North American diet, nearly two-thirds of vitamin E is supplied by salad oils, margarines, spreads (low-fat margarine), and shortening (Fig. 10-13). Nuts and seeds

Phospholipid bilayer of cell membrane

Damaged phospholipids

Free radical

Phospholipids

Vitamin E

Neutralized free radical

Unsaturated fatty acids

FIGURE 10-12 ▲ Because it is fat soluble, vitamin E can insert itself into cell membranes, where it halts oxidative damage caused by free radicals.

megadose Large intake of a nutrient beyond estimates of needs or what would be found in a balanced diet; 2 to 10 times human needs is a starting point.

▲ The avocado in guacamole and the oil in the tortilla chip are good sources of vitamin E.
© BananaStock/PunchStock

(a)

(b)

Food Item and Amount	Vitamin E (milligrams)	Vitamin E (IU)	% RDA for Adult Males and Females (15 milligrams)
Grains			
Total® Raisin Bran cereal, 1 cup	13.5	20.1	90%
Whole-wheat bread, 1 slice	0.9	1.3	6%
Quinoa, cooked, ½ cup	0.6	0.9	4%
Vegetables			
Spinach, cooked, 1 cup	3.7	5.5	25%
Asparagus, cooked, 1 cup	2.7	4.0	18%
Sweet potato, baked, 1 cup	1.4	2.1	9%
Fruits			
Blackberries, 1 cup	1.7	2.5	11%
Mango, 1 cup	1.5	2.2	10%
Olives, 5 large	0.7	1.0	5%
Protein			
Sunflower seeds, dry roasted, 1 ounce	7.4	11.0	49%
Shrimp, cooked, 3 ounces	1.9	2.8	12%
Egg, hard-boiled, 1 large	0.5	0.8	3%
Fats & Oils			
Sunflower oil, 1 teaspoon	1.9	2.8	12%
Salad dressing, Italian, 2 tablespoons	0.6	1.0	4%
Butter, 1 teaspoon	0.1	0.2	1%

FIGURE 10-13 ▲ Food sources of vitamin E. (a) The fill of the background color (none, 1/3, 2/3, or completely covered) within each food group on MyPlate indicates the average nutrient density for vitamin E in that group.
(b) The bar graph shows the vitamin E content of several foods compared to the RDA for adult males and females. Overall, the richest sources of vitamin E are nuts, seeds, plant oils, and fortified breakfast cereals. The dairy group is not pictured in the bar graph because, except for plant-based dairy alternatives, foods in this group yield no vitamin E.
Source: *Nutrition data from USDA National Nutrient Database for Standard Reference, Release 26.*

are nutrient-dense sources of vitamin E. Breakfast cereals fortified with vitamin E are also good sources, but other than wheat germ, few other grain products provide much vitamin E. Milling of grains removes the germ, which is a source of PUFAs and vitamin E. By removing the germ, the resulting grain product has less chance of spoiling (i.e., rancidity of the PUFAs), but it loses most of its vitamin E.

Because plant oils contain mostly unsaturated fatty acids, the relatively high amount of vitamin E in plant oils naturally protects these unsaturated lipids from oxidation. Animal products (meat, dairy, eggs) and fish oils, on the other hand, contain very little vitamin E. Vitamin E is susceptible to destruction by oxygen, metals, light, and especially repeated use in deep-fat frying; thus, the vitamin E content of a food depends on how it is harvested, processed, stored, and cooked.

The RDA of vitamin E for adults is 15 milligrams per day of alpha-tocopherol, the most active, natural form of vitamin E (see box). This amount equals 22.4 milligrams of the less active, synthetic source. Typically, North American adults consume about two-thirds of the RDA for vitamin E from food sources. The Daily Value used on food and supplement labels is 30 milligrams.

Vitamin E

RDA: 15 milligrams
DV: 30 milligrams
UL: 1000 milligrams

As with vitamin A, the vitamin E content of dietary supplements is given in international units rather than simple metric measurements. International units reflect the different biological activity of natural vitamin E compared with synthetic preparations of vitamin E. Supplements may contain any of the variety of chemical forms of vitamin E, while only a fraction of these are biologically active. Therefore, a supplement containing synthetic vitamin E has lower biological activity (i.e., lower IU) than the same quantity of natural vitamin E. The more expensive natural vitamin E supplements contain only the biologically active form. See "Calculating Vitamin E Content of Dietary Supplements" for conversion factors used to calculate the vitamin E content of dietary supplements.

Calculating Vitamin E Content of Dietary Supplements

To find milligrams of *natural* vitamin E (d-alpha-tocopherol), multiply IU by 0.67. Conversely, to calculate IU from milligrams, multiply milligrams by 1.49.

Example: The RDA for vitamin E is 15 milligrams per day. This is equal to how many IU of natural vitamin E?

$$15 \text{ mg} \times 1.49 \text{ IU/mg} = 22.35 \text{ IU}$$

To find milligrams of *synthetic* vitamin E (dl-alpha-tocopherol), multiply IU by 0.45. Conversely, to calculate IU from milligrams, multiply milligrams by 2.22.

Example: If a vitamin E supplement contains 400 IU of dl-alpha-tocopherol, then how many milligrams of vitamin E does it contain?

$$400 \text{ IU} \times 0.45 \text{ mg/IU} = 180 \text{ mg}$$

AVOIDING TOO MUCH VITAMIN E

Unlike other fat-soluble vitamins, vitamin E is not stored in the liver. It is stored in adipose tissue throughout the body. The Upper Level for vitamin E is 1000 milligrams per day of supplemental alpha-tocopherol. Excessive intake of vitamin E can interfere with vitamin K's role in the clotting mechanism, leading to hemorrhage. The risk of insufficient blood clotting is especially high if vitamin E is taken in conjunction with anticoagulant medications (e.g., Coumadin® or heavy aspirin use). Always be cautious about using dietary supplements. In addition to the significant risk of drug interference and prolonged bleeding, vitamin E supplements can produce nausea, gastrointestinal distress, and diarrhea.

✓ CONCEPT CHECK 10.5

1. How does vitamin E work to prevent oxidative damage?
2. What are some rich food sources of vitamin E?
3. Why are preterm infants, smokers, and people with fat malabsorption particularly susceptible to oxidative damage to cell membranes?
4. What are the possible results of vitamin E toxicity?

10.6 Selenium

FUNCTIONS OF SELENIUM

Selenium (Se) is a trace mineral that exists in many readily absorbed chemical forms. Selenium's best-understood role is aiding the activity of one of the body's natural antioxidant enzymes, glutathione peroxidase. Glutathione peroxidase chemically converts potentially damaging peroxides (hydrogen peroxide, for example) into water. In functioning as part of our natural antioxidant enzyme system, selenium spares vitamin E and indirectly helps maintain cell-membrane integrity. Selenium is also a component of an enzyme essential for the activation of thyroid hormone (T3).

SELENIUM DEFICIENCY

Selenium content of foods is strongly dependent on the selenium content of the soil where plants are raised or animals graze. Worldwide, only one region—the Keshan province in China—has such low soil selenium levels that selenium deficiencies result. Such deficiencies were first reported by Chinese scientists in 1979. (Of note, communication and relations between the West and China were closed from 1949 until 1972. In the mid- and late 1970s, medical dialogue opened significantly.) Selenium deficiency symptoms in humans include muscle pain and wasting, and a certain form of heart damage. Also, due to its role in thyroid hormone metabolism, selenium deficiency may impair thyroid function, thereby limiting growth. In China's Keshan province, unless they receive supplements, children and adults develop characteristic muscle and heart disorders associated with inadequate selenium intake.

Low blood levels of selenium have been linked with an increased incidence of some forms of cancer, specifically prostate cancer (see Newsworthy Nutrition). Although selenium could prove to have a role in prevention of cancers in those with low or marginal selenium stores, it is premature to recommend selenium supplementation for this purpose. Animal studies in this area are conflicting. Current studies examine the interaction of selenium and vitamin E on **gene expression** in some cancers.

gene expression Use of DNA information on a gene to produce a protein. Thought to be a major determination of cell development.

Selenium
RDA: 55 micrograms
DV: 70 micrograms
UL: 400 micrograms

GETTING ENOUGH SELENIUM

Fish, meat (especially organ meats), shellfish, and eggs are good animal sources of selenium (Fig. 10-14). Brazil nuts, and grains and seeds grown in soils containing selenium are good plant sources. Major selenium contributors to the adult diet are animal and grain products.

(a)

(b)

	Food Item and Amount	Selenium (micrograms)	% RDA for Adult Males and Females (55 micrograms)
Grains	Egg noodles, cooked, ½ cup	19	35%
	Puffed wheat cereal, 1 cup	19	34%
	White rice, cooked, ½ cup	7	13%
Vegetables	Mushrooms, crimini, raw, 1 cup	19	35%
	Asparagus, cooked, 1 cup	11	20%
	Spinach, cooked, 1 cup	3	5%
Dairy	Swiss cheese, 1.5 ounces	8	14%
	Milk, fat-free, 1 cup	8	14%
	Soymilk, 1 cup	6	10%
Protein	Brazil nuts, 2 each	192	349%
	Tuna, grilled, 3 ounces	92	167%
	Oysters, steamed, 3 ounces	34	62%

FIGURE 10-14 ▲ Food sources of selenium. (a) The fill of the background color (none, 1/3, 2/3, or completely covered) within each food group on MyPlate indicates the average nutrient density for selenium in that group. (b) The bar graph shows the selenium content of several foods compared to the RDA for adult males and females. Overall, the richest sources of selenium are found in the protein foods and grains groups. Foods from the fruits group (not shown) provide very little selenium.

Source: *Nutrition data from USDA National Nutrient Database for Standard Reference, Release 26.*

Newsworthy Nutrition

Selenium and vitamin E supplements offer no benefit for cancer prevention

In the late 1990s and early 2000s, secondary results of two large trials of nutrient supplementation in cancer prevention hinted at possible roles for micronutrients in the prevention of prostate cancer. As a result, the 12-year Selenium and Vitamin E Cancer Prevention Trial (SELECT) was designed to further explore the roles of selenium and vitamin E for the prevention of prostate cancer. After just 7 years, the trial was stopped due to lack of evidence of any beneficial effect of the supplements on endpoints related to cancer. Follow-up of prostate cancer development in the men in this study showed a higher number of prostate cancer cases in the groups receiving vitamin E, selenium, or a combination of both, when compared to those receiving the placebo. The authors concluded that dietary supplementation with vitamin E significantly increased the risk of prostate cancer among healthy men. This trial demonstrated that neither selenium (200 micrograms per day of selenomethionine) nor vitamin E (400 IU per day of dl-alpha-tocopherol), either alone or in combination, reduced risk for prostate cancer. This is an example of why replication of research results is so important. The results of one study are not sufficient to inform clinical practice.

Source: Klein EA and others: Vitamin E and the risk of prostate cancer: The Selenium and Vitamin E Cancer Prevention Trial (SELECT). *Journal of the American Medical Association* 306:1549, 2011.

CASE STUDY   Choosing a Dietary Supplement

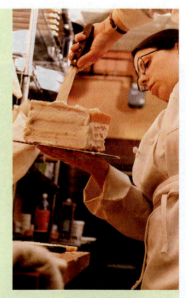

© Adam Crowley/Getty Images

Amy works the predawn shift as a baker at a popular bistro. Amy is also a full-time student, and the combination of taking a full course load at college and working early hours while her friends are sleeping has created a lot of stress for her. Amy's many commitments also make it important that she not become ill. Recently, one of her coworkers suggested that she take Nutramega antioxidant supplement to help prevent oxidative damage and illness. The product's label suggests that Nutramega helps prevent such problems, especially those associated with the changing of seasons. The label recommends taking two to three tablets daily for health maintenance and two to three tablets every 3 hours at the first sign of feeling ill. Amy looks at the Supplement Facts label on the bottle and finds that each tablet contains (as percent of the DV): 600% for vitamin E, 700% for vitamin C, and 10% for selenium. A month's supply costs about $50.

Answer the following questions and check your responses at the end of the chapter.

1. Are there any health risks associated with taking the "maintenance" dose of two to three tablets per day? How does this dose compare with the Tolerable Upper Intake Levels for the three nutrients?
2. How many tablets would be taken per day if Amy were feeling ill?
   a. For vitamin E, use the % Daily Value to calculate the milligrams that would be in this larger dose. How does this compare to the UL for vitamin E?
   b. Use the % Daily Value to calculate the milligrams of vitamin C in this larger dose. How does this compare to the UL for vitamin C?
   c. Use the % Daily Value to calculate the micrograms of selenium in this larger dose. How does this compare to the UL for selenium?
   d. Does the recommended dosage of any of these nutrients pose any health risks?
3. Does the cost of this supplement seem reasonable? How does it compare to the cost of a typical multivitamin/mineral supplement available at your local drug store?
4. Should Amy be concerned about meeting her nutrient needs? Does the type of stress she is under increase her nutrient needs?
5. After studying this chapter, what diet and supplement advice would you offer to Amy?

Supplement Facts

Serving Size 1 Tablet	
Each Tablet Contains	**% Daily Value**
Vitamin E	600%
Vitamin C	700%
Selenium	10%

▲ Be careful with Brazil nuts. This portion of 10 nuts contains 960 micrograms of selenium, which exceeds the Upper Limit for selenium of 400 micrograms per day. © Image Source/Getty

Some geographic regions identified with low-selenium soil in North America include the Northeast, Pacific, Southwest, and coastal plain of the Southeast in the United States; and the north central and eastern regions in Canada. We eat a variety of foods from many geographic areas, so it is unlikely that local areas with low soil selenium will mean inadequate selenium in our dietary patterns.

The RDA for selenium is 55 micrograms per day for adults. This intake maximizes the activity of selenium-dependent enzymes. Adults meet the RDA, consuming on average 105 micrograms each day.

AVOIDING TOO MUCH SELENIUM

High concentrations of selenium are rarely found in food, with the exception of Brazil nuts. Therefore, selenium toxicity has not been reported from eating food. Excessive selenium supplementation for an extended period has been shown to be toxic. The UL for selenium is 400 micrograms per day for adults. This is based on overt signs of selenium toxicity, such as hair loss, weakness, nausea, vomiting, and cirrhosis. Because Brazil nuts are such a concentrated source of selenium, it is recommended to avoid consuming them daily, thus preventing an inadvertent overload.

✓ CONCEPT CHECK 10.6

1. How does selenium play an antioxidant role?
2. What other functions does selenium play in the body?
3. What are the signs of a selenium deficiency?
4. What food groups are the best sources of selenium?
5. What are the signs of selenium toxicity?

10.7 Zinc

Zinc (Zn) deficiency was first recognized in the early 1960s in Egypt and Iran where it was linked to growth retardation and poor sexual development (Fig. 10-15). Even though the zinc content of their diets was fairly high, absorption of the mineral was limited by the phytic acid in unleavened bread. Parasite infestation and the practice of eating clay and other parts of soil also contributed to the severe zinc deficiency.

FUNCTIONS OF ZINC

Zinc appears in this chapter because it is vital for white blood cell formation and function. However, intakes in excess of the RDA do not provide any extra benefit for immune function. In fact, chronic excessive intakes can actually depress immune function.

Other roles of zinc in the body include:

- DNA synthesis and function
- Protein metabolism, wound healing, and growth
- Development of sexual organs and bones
- Storage, release, and function of insulin
- Cell membrane structure and function
- Component of superoxide dismutase (SOD), an enzyme that aids in the prevention of oxidative damage to cells (zinc, therefore, has an indirect antioxidant function)

In addition, zinc may slow the progression of macular degeneration of the eye and reduce the risk for developing certain forms of cancer.

FIGURE 10-15 ▲ Low intakes of zinc limit growth in people worldwide. On the right, an Egyptian farm boy, 16 years old and 49 inches tall, experienced limited growth and sexual development associated with zinc deficiency. Photo courtesy of Harold H. Sandstead, M.D.

ZINC DEFICIENCY

Symptoms of adult zinc deficiency include an acne-like rash, diarrhea, lack of appetite, delayed wound healing, impaired immunity, reduced sense of taste (metallic like) and smell, and hair loss. In children and adolescents with zinc deficiency, growth, sexual development, and learning ability may also be hampered.

GETTING ENOUGH ZINC

Protein-rich diets, especially those that include many animal sources of protein, are high in zinc. The average North American consumes 10 to 14 milligrams of zinc per day, about 80% of which is provided by meat, fish, poultry, fortified cereal, and dairy products (Fig. 10-16). There are no indications of moderate or severe zinc deficiencies in an otherwise healthy adult population. It is likely, however, that some North Americans—especially some poor children, vegans, and older people with alcoholism—have marginal zinc status (see Further Reading 14). These and other people who show deterioration in taste sensation, recurring infections, poor growth, or depressed wound healing should have their zinc status checked.

Overall, about 40% of dietary zinc is absorbed. Absorption efficiency depends on the body's need for zinc and the form of the mineral in foods. When zinc status is poor, absorption of the mineral increases. The zinc found in animal foods is better absorbed than that found in plants. Worldwide, however, most people rely on unfortified cereal grains (low in zinc) as their source of protein, calories, and zinc. As described, phytic acid in plant foods binds to zinc and limits its availability. Adding yeast to grains (leavening) breaks down phytic acid, increasing zinc bioavailability

Zinc
RDA:
Men: 11 milligrams
Women: 8 milligrams
DV: 15 milligrams
UL: 40 milligrams

(a)

ChooseMyPlate.gov

(b)

	Food Item and Amount	Zinc (milligrams)	% RDA for Adult Males (11 milligrams)	% RDA for Adult Females (8 milligrams)
Grains	White rice, enriched, ½ cup	1.1	10%	14%
Grains	Quinoa, cooked, ½ cup	1.0	9%	13%
Grains	Special K cereal, 1 cup	0.4	4%	5%
Vegetables	Asparagus, cooked, 1 cup	1.1	10%	14%
Vegetables	Zucchini, cooked, 1 cup	0.6	5%	7%
Vegetables	Spinach, raw, 2 cups	0.3	3%	4%
Dairy	Mozzarella cheese, part skim, 1.5 ounces	1.2	11%	15%
Dairy	Milk, fat-free, 1 cup	1.0	9%	13%
Dairy	Soymilk, 1 cup	0.6	6%	8%
Protein	Oysters, steamed, 3 ounces	66.8	607%	835%
Protein	Beef pot roast, 3 ounces	7.9	71%	98%
Protein	Peanuts, dry roasted, 1 ounce	0.9	9%	12%

FIGURE 10-16 ▲ Food sources of zinc. (a) The fill of the background color (none, 1/3, 2/3, or completely covered) within each food group on MyPlate indicates the average nutrient density for zinc in that group. (b) The bar graph shows the zinc content of several foods compared to the RDA for adult males and females. Overall, the richest sources of zinc are in the protein group. Foods in the fruits group (not shown) provide very little zinc.

Source: *Nutrition data from USDA National Nutrient Database for Standard Reference, Release 26.*

from leavened grain products. In populations that consume mainly unleavened bread, zinc deficiency can be a problem.

The form generally used in multivitamin and mineral supplements (zinc oxide) is not as well absorbed as zinc found naturally in foods, but still contributes to meeting zinc needs. High-dose calcium supplementation decreases zinc availability if taken too close to mealtime. Finally, zinc competes with copper and iron for absorption, and vice versa, when supplemental sources are consumed. Supplements with more than 100% of the Daily Value for individual minerals are not advised without medical supervision.

AVOIDING TOO MUCH ZINC

Excessive zinc intake over time can lead to problems by interfering with copper metabolism. The interference with copper metabolism is the basis for setting the UL. Zinc toxicity can occur from zinc supplements and overconsumption of zinc-fortified foods. A person using megadose supplementation should be under close medical supervision and take a supplement containing copper (2 milligrams per day). Zinc intakes over 100 milligrams result in diarrhea, cramps, nausea, vomiting, loss of appetite, and depressed immune system function, especially if intake exceeds 2000 milligrams per day. Intakes consistently over 2000 milligrams per day can lead to a depressed immune system and decreased high-density lipoproteins (HDLs).

> ### ✓ CONCEPT CHECK 10.7
>
> 1. List three good sources of zinc.
> 2. What are the consequences of zinc deficiency?

10.8 Antioxidant Phytochemicals

A number of phytochemicals are strong antioxidants. A diet rich in fruits and vegetables is an excellent source of antioxidant phytochemicals, including carotenoids, flavonoids, and phenolics. Beta-carotene has been shown to exert powerful antioxidant properties and lycopene, a red carotenoid found in tomatoes and pink grapefruit, appears to have even stronger antioxidant properties than beta-carotene. Other commonly eaten carotenoids that have antioxidant properties include alpha-carotene, beta-cryptoxanthin, lutein, and zeaxanthin. Polyphenols are the largest group of phytochemicals and consist mainly of flavonoids. Flavonoids function as antioxidants by inhibiting the oxidation of cholesterol, an initial step in the development of plaques in atherosclerosis. Rich sources of flavonoids include blueberries, chocolate, citrus fruit, and raspberries.

Because of their potential health-promoting effects, foods that are rich in antioxidants have been of great interest in the past few years. The antioxidant levels of 326 foods were analyzed and published by scientists at the USDA, most recently in 2010 (see Further Reading 25). The antioxidant activity of each food was measured as oxygen radical absorption capacity (ORAC), a standard assay that measures the inhibition of oxidation. The USDA has reported concern, however, that the ORAC values and the term *antioxidant* are being misused by food and dietary supplement manufacturers in an effort to promote their products. There are limitations of the ORAC method that are important to understand. For example, the ORAC assay measures the antioxidant capacity of foods in a test tube, not in humans, and therefore does not account for the ability of the antioxidants to be absorbed, get into tissues, and be metabolized. The fear is that marketing of so-called antioxidant-rich foods has confused consumers, especially those looking for a quick guide to foods with health benefits. It is certainly too simple to suggest that the reason fruits and vegetables are good for you is because they contain antioxidants and that those with the most antioxidants are

▲ Many fruits and vegetables, including red onion and garlic, contain phytochemicals with high antioxidant capacity. © James Gathany/CDC

"superfoods." It is important to remember that plant foods are good for us because of the combination of ingredients they contain, including vitamins, minerals, fiber, and the numerous phytochemicals. This is why the Dietary Guidelines for Americans encourage us to consume a variety of fruits, vegetables, and whole grains. A recent study of women age 18 to 44 years confirmed that meeting the recommendation to consume at least five fruits and vegetables daily (5-A-Day program) was associated with lower oxidative stress and improved antioxidant status (see Further Reading 20).

Despite its limitations, the ORAC value is a good way to estimate antioxidant capacity, especially when we keep in mind that antioxidant activity is just one of the benefits of phytochemicals. Much of the phytochemical research that began with ORAC values has now moved on to clinical studies in humans with or without chronic diseases. These studies are showing positive relationships between ORAC levels in foods and intake of dietary antioxidants and the effects on chronic diseases, including cancer and metabolic syndrome (see Further Reading 19). One recent study of 31,000 women in Sweden found that those with the lowest risk of stroke, whether they had a history of cardiovascular disease or not, had the diets with the highest total antioxidant capacity (see Newsworthy Nutrition in this section).

Table 10-3 lists the antioxidant activity of 48 common foods with the highest ORAC values, as well as the phytochemical categories present in each group. The fruit group offers the most options that have high antioxidant activity, with raspberries (black and red),

▲ The red, blue, and purple pigments in berries are anthocyanins that function as antioxidants and seem to protect us from disease.
© M. Lamotte/Cole Group/Getty Images RF

TABLE 10-3 ■ Antioxidant Activity of Common Foods

Food Group (Antioxidant Phytochemicals)	Serving Size	Total Antioxidant Capacity*
Fruits (Anthocyanins, Carotenoids, Flavonoids, Phenolic Acids)		
Raspberries, black	1 cup	23,641
Raisins, golden, seedless	1 cup (not packed)	15,153
Blueberries, wild, raw	1 cup	14,239
Plums, raw	1 cup	10,065
Cranberries, raw	1 cup	9090
Blackberries, raw	1 cup	8503
Apples, Red Delicious, raw, with skin	1 medium	7780
Strawberries, raw	1 cup	7141
Apples, Granny Smith, raw, with skin	1 medium	7094
Blueberries, raw	1 cup	6910
Pomegranate juice	1 cup	6676
Raspberries, raw	1 cup	6330
Juice, Concord grape	1 cup	6044
Cherries, sweet, raw	1 cup (no pits)	5770
Raisins, seedless	1 cup (not packed)	4939
Oranges, raw	1 cup (sections)	3785
Avocados, Hass, raw	1 cup cubed	2883
Grapes, red, raw	1 cup	2774
Mangos, raw	1 cup	2145

TABLE 10-3 ■ *(continued)*

Food Group (Antioxidant Phytochemicals)	Serving Size	Total Antioxidant Capacity*
Vegetables (Allyl Sulfides, Anthocyanins, Carotenoids, Flavonoids)		
Artichokes, hearts, boiled	1 cup	7909
Asparagus, raw	1 cup	3018
Spinach, frozen, chopped or leaf, unprepared	1 cup	2631
Beets, raw	1 cup	2415
Sweet potato, baked in skin	1 medium	2411
Cabbage, red, boiled	1 cup	2359
Onions, red, raw	1 cup	1749
Broccoli, boiled	1 cup	1684
Broccoli raab, raw	1 cup	1233
Ginger root, raw	1 tbsp	888
Garlic, raw	3 cloves	513
Nuts (Flavonoids, Phenolic Acids)		
Pecans	1 ounce/19 halves	5086
Walnuts, English	1 ounce/14 halves	3839
Hazelnuts or filberts	1 ounce/21 kernels	2734
Pistachio nuts, raw	1 ounce/49 kernels	2176
Almonds	1 ounce/23 kernels	1273
Chocolate (Flavonoids)		
Baking chocolate, unsweetened, squares	1 square (29 g)	14,484
Candies, chocolate, dark	1 ounce (28.35 g)	5901
Candies, semisweet, chocolate	1 ounce (28.35 g)	5118
Candies, milk chocolate	1 bar (44 g)	3308
Cocoa, dry powder, unsweetened	1 tbsp (5.4 g)	3005
Legumes (Isoflavones)		
Beans, black, mature seeds, boiled	1 cup (172 g)	3868
Beans, pinto, mature seeds, boiled	1 cup (171 g)	1546
Peanut butter, smooth style	2 tbsp (32 g)	1098
Peanuts, all types, raw	1 ounce (28.35 g)	898
Beverages (Flavonoids, Nonflavonoid Polyphenols)		
Wine, table, red, Cabernet Sauvignon	5 fluid ounces (147 g)	6649
Wine, table, red, Merlot	5 fluid ounces (147 g)	3925
Tea, green, brewed	1 cup	2970
Chocolate syrup	2 tbsp (39 g)	2469

*Total oxygen radical absorption capacity (ORAC).

raisins, blueberries, plums, cranberries, blackberries, apples, and strawberries ranked highest. Berries, including blueberries and strawberries, are colorful thanks to red, blue, and purple pigments called anthocyanins. These phytochemicals function as antioxidants and may protect the heart. A recent analysis of women in the Nurses' Health Study found that women who got the most anthocyanins from their food had a lower risk of heart attack compared to women who had the lowest intake of anthocyanins. In this study, 60% of the anthocyanins consumed came from blueberries and strawberries (see Further Reading 4). Anthocyanins are also found in blackberries, cherries, raspberries, red cabbage, red grapes, and black plums.

Apples are a fruit that offers tremendous potential because they are widely consumed and contain several phytochemicals that are strong antioxidants. Furthermore, epidemiological studies have found a relationship between the consumption of apples and a reduced risk of some cancers, cardiovascular disease, asthma, and diabetes. Although the type of phytochemicals varies greatly among varieties of apples, storage of apples has little to no effect on their phytochemical content. Artichokes, black beans, asparagus, spinach, beets, sweet potato, and red cabbage have the highest antioxidant activity among vegetables and legumes, and pecans, walnuts, hazelnuts, and pistachios ranked highest among nuts. Chocolate (dark and semisweet) and red wine, high in flavonoids and polyphenols, had some of the highest antioxidant activities of all the foods tested.

▲ Which would you choose, a brownie made with rich dark chocolate or a Granny Smith apple? Both foods contain phytochemicals with high antioxidant capacity. The apple will also supply vitamins and mineral and fiber, whereas the brownie will be significantly higher in calories from sugar and fat. © JGI/Jamie Grill/Getty Images

Newsworthy Nutrition

Antioxidant-rich foods reduce the risk of stroke

The hypothesis of this study of Swedish women was that consumption of antioxidant-rich foods will decrease the risk of stroke by inhibiting oxidative stress and inflammation. The antioxidant activity of foods was measured as total antioxidant capacity (TAC), which takes into account all antioxidants and the synergistic effects between them. The association between dietary TAC and stroke incidence was examined in 31,035 women aged 49 to 83 years who were free of cardiovascular disease (CVD) and in 5680 women with CVD history at the beginning of the study. Diet was assessed with a food frequency questionnaire, and the dietary TAC was calculated using oxygen radical absorbance capacity (ORAC) values. The results included 1322 stroke cases among CVD-free women and 1007 stroke cases among women with a CVD history. Women who were CVD free at baseline and had the highest dietary TAC had the lowest risk of total stroke. Among women with a CVD history, those with highest dietary TAC had a lower risk of hemorrhagic stroke but not total stroke. The major contributors to dietary TAC were fruit and vegetables, which contributed 50% of total TAC. Women with high dietary TAC consumed more fruits and vegetables and tea but less coffee. The authors conclude that dietary TAC is inversely associated with total stroke among CVD-free women and hemorrhagic stroke among women with CVD history, and therefore *supports* their hypothesis that consumption of antioxidant-rich foods may reduce the risk of stroke by inhibition of oxidative stress and inflammation.

Source: Rautiainen S and others: Total antioxidant capacity of diet and risk of stroke: A population-based prospective cohort of women. *Stroke* 43:335, 2012.

✓ CONCEPT CHECK 10.8

1. What categories of phytochemicals function as antioxidants?

2. Which food group has the richest supply of antioxidant phytochemicals?

3. What phytochemical group is responsible for the color of berries?

4. What is the ORAC assay, and what are the limitations to using its values to estimate antioxidant activity?

10.9 Probiotics and the Immune System

lactic acid bacteria Strains of bacteria that produce lactic acid from fermentation of dairy products; may confer health benefits when consumed as probiotics.

probiotic Live microorganisms that, when administered in adequate amounts, confer health benefits on the host.

prebiotic Selectively fermented ingredient that results in specific changes in the composition and/or activity of the gastrointestinal microbiota, thus conferring benefits upon the host.

synbiotic Combination of pro- and prebiotics taken to confer health benefits on the host.

microbiota Community of microorganisms living in a particular region; with regard to our discussion of probiotics, the community of microorganisms coexisting on and within the human body.

Microorganisms have been used for thousands of years to produce food and beverages, such as alcohol, bread, cheese, fermented soy, and yogurt. Over a century ago, Russian scientist Elie Metchnikoff noticed that Bulgarian peasants, who ate a lot of fermented dairy products (e.g., yogurt), lived long lives and rarely got sick. He began drinking "sour milk" daily as he researched the immune system. In 1907, he wrote about the digestive and immune benefits of consuming dairy foods fermented with **lactic acid bacteria.** He theorized that there are some bacteria in the human colon that lead to aging and illness, but by consuming these beneficial lactic acid bacteria, we could replace harmful bacteria and thereby avoid sickness. Although the term **probiotics**—used to describe these beneficial bacteria—was not defined until 1965, Metchnikoff is regarded as the "father of probiotics." His pivotal research on the mutually beneficial relationship between bacteria and their human hosts continues today.

Yogurt became popular in the United States in the 1960s, when it was promoted as a health food. The term *probiotic* literally means "for life." Consumption of probiotics and **prebiotics** has been linked to prevention and treatment of diarrhea, respiratory infections, vaginal and urinary tract infections, allergies, and many autoimmune diseases. Research on probiotics and prebiotics, which serve as food for probiotic microorganisms, has increased dramatically over the last decade, and the market for probiotic foods and supplements topped $2.25 billion in 2012.

PROBIOTICS, PREBIOTICS, AND SYNBIOTICS

Probiotics are live microorganisms that have positive effects on human health if they are consumed in sufficient quantities. These live microorganisms can be ingested as part of foods (e.g., yogurt and kefir), or they can be administered as supplements (e.g., pills, powders, or suppositories). Common probiotic bacteria used in foods and supplements include species of *Lactobacillus, Lactococcus,* and *Streptococcus* (commonly grouped together as lactic acid bacteria because they produce lactic acid when they are used to ferment dairy foods), as well as some species of the *Bifidobacterium* genus. Notice that the definition of probiotics is not limited to bacteria; although many probiotic microorganisms are bacteria, *Saccharomyces boulardii* is a strain of yeast that can also promote human health.

Prebiotics, on the other hand, are not living microorganisms. Prebiotics are ingredients (typically carbohydrates) that are not well digested by human enzymes but serve as fuel for beneficial bacteria in the gut. Fructooligosaccharides (FOS) are short chains of carbohydrates that can be broken down and used for energy by probiotic bacteria. Some other examples of prebiotics are galactooligosaccharides (GOS), trans-galactooligosaccharides (TOS), and lactulose. Human milk, as you will read in Chapter 18, contains prebiotics that selectively promote the growth of bifidobacteria in the digestive tracts of infants.

Synbiotics are food products or dietary supplements that contain both probiotics and prebiotics. The two components may work in the same or different parts of the GI tract, but they both work to improve human health.

THE GUT MICROBIOTA IS A DIVERSE COMMUNITY

At birth, humans have a sterile gut. As soon as they are exposed to the world outside the womb, however, a community of microorganisms moves into the GI tract and begins to multiply. The human GI tract gradually becomes colonized over the first year of life (Fig. 10-17). The makeup of the **microbiota** varies from person to person. In fact, of about 500 different strains of bacteria that have been identified in human colons, each person is home to a unique community of only about

The stomach is sparsely populated by about 1000 CFU per gram of contents. The low pH limits growth of most microorganisms.

As the pH of the small intestine increases through the duodenum, jejunum, and ileum, microorganisms begin to flourish. There are at least 1 million CFU per gram of contents inside the ileum.

The large intestine houses more than 100,000,000,000 CFU per gram of contents.

FIGURE 10-17 ▲ Bacteria in the gastrointestinal tract.

160 species. That unique community has been established by the age of 3. The exact composition of bacteria in your GI tract depends on a variety of factors: genetics, age, geographic environment, diet, and other lifestyle factors (see Further Reading 12). The way you came into the world (vaginal or caesarian birth) and the way you were fed as an infant (breast milk or formula) were choices that have directed the development of your gut microbiota throughout your lifetime. There are now studies indicating that the relative proportions of bacterial species in the gut are linked to obesity and risks for various diseases (see "Much More to Learn" later in this section).

Whatever the specific composition, bacterial cells in and on the human body outnumber human cells by 10 to 1! Some of these bacteria are beneficial. For example, when bifidobacteria and lactobacilli ferment undigested carbohydrates in the colon, they produce short-chain fatty acids that can serve as an energy source for the cells of the GI tract. Other bacteria can cause disease. For instance, some strains of *Escherichia coli* and *Clostridium difficile* can lead to diarrhea, dehydration, and, possibly, death. Some bacteria produce toxins that are linked to development of colon cancer. As Metchnikoff proposed over a century ago, if we shift the balance of the microbiota by consuming the beneficial bacteria (or prebiotics that promote their growth), we can crowd out the pathogenic bacteria.

The diversity of the microbiota has widespread effects on health. Data from the Human Genome Project indicate that humans have 20,000 to 25,000 genes that can code for proteins. Taking the human microbiota as a whole, the **microbiome** contains about 100 times as many genes as the human genome (see Further Reading 12). Many of these bacterial genes code for proteins that affect human health. Some affect the rate of cell turnover in the large intestine. Some enhance the absorption of minerals, such as calcium. Others may affect cholesterol synthesis. Many of the probiotic bacteria, including lactic acid bacteria and bifidobacteria, enhance immune function. The influence of the microbiome on immune function occurs at several levels.

▲ When we consume the lactic acid bacteria used to ferment dairy foods, these friendly bacteria can colonize the large intestine and enhance digestive and immune health.
© BananaStock/PunchStock

microbiome Entire collection of microorganisms, their genes, and their environment.

"BUGS" THAT BOOST IMMUNE FUNCTION

In laboratory animals that are born and raised in a sterile environment, the immune system is underdeveloped and more susceptible to autoimmune diseases and allergies. Based on this research, it is evident that a healthy gut microbiota is crucial for proper immune system development and maintenance.

Probiotics can influence the immune functions of the intestinal lining in several ways (see Further Reading 9). First, exposure of GALT to microorganisms promotes the maturation of the immune cells. GALT (review Section 10.1) makes up about 70% of all immune tissue in the body, and much of the GALT is situated in the large intestine, where the microbiota flourishes. Through early interactions with microorganisms in the gut, the cells of the immune system "learn" to recognize and differentiate between what is harmful and what is not. Production of certain antibodies by the mucosal cells is increased.

Second, probiotics help to reinforce the integrity of the GI tract, which provides a barrier against invasion by pathogens. The cells that line the intestines are knitted together by tight junctions, which are a network of tiny strands of protein that regulate the absorption of nutrients and block the entry of large molecules and pathogens. If the integrity of these tight junctions is compromised, the intestinal lining becomes more permeable, a condition commonly called a "leaky gut." A leaky gut allows large molecules, including microorganisms, to move from the lumen of the GI tract into body tissues. This can lead to infections or promote allergies and autoimmune diseases. Some strains of lactobacilli have been shown to influence the production of proteins that form tight junctions, thus decreasing the permeability of the gut. Some strains may promote the production of mucus proteins to further reinforce the gut barrier. Also, probiotic bacteria may enhance production of antioxidants and thereby protect those cells from oxidative damage.

In addition to promoting the integrity of the intestinal barrier, probiotics enhance immune function because they transiently alter the composition of the microbiota. As Metchnikoff suggested, consuming more of the healthy bacteria can crowd out the pathogenic strains. This occurs by several mechanisms. The metabolic activity of probiotic strains changes the acidity of the environment in the gut, which makes it less hospitable to the pathogenic strains. Increasing loads of probiotic bacteria will compete with pathogenic bacteria for binding sites and sources of food. Finally, some probiotic strains directly bind to pathogens or secrete substances that kill them.

Many of these actions of probiotics are mediated by cytokines (review Section 10.1). Probiotics generally enhance anti-inflammatory cytokines and decrease pro-inflammatory cytokines (see Further Reading 26). Given the detrimental effects of chronic inflammation you learned about in this chapter, the ability of probiotics to decrease the inflammatory response in the gut could have positive implications for the prevention of chronic diseases.

PREVENTING AND TREATING INFECTIOUS DISEASES

The most extensively studied benefit of probiotics is on the reduction of diarrhea. Diarrheal disease is a major cause of death in developing countries, especially among children. Even in developed nations, about 30% of the population is affected each year by at least one episode of diarrhea. By changing the microbiota, enhancing the integrity of the gut lining, and altering the inflammatory response, probiotics can be used to prevent or treat episodes of acute infectious diarrhea. The probiotic strains that have been tested in this regard include several strains of *Lactobacilli* and the yeast *Saccharomyces boulardii.* Use of these probiotics has been shown to reduce the risk of acute diarrhea by 57% among children and 26% among adults. As a treatment, probiotics can reduce the duration of acute infectious diarrhea (caused by rotavirus) by about 1 day (see Further Reading 3).

Probiotics have also proven useful for the prevention or treatment of antibiotic-associated diarrhea (see Further Reading 7). Chronic or repeated use of antibiotics (e.g., ciprofloxacin) greatly disturbs the microbiota; many strains of both harmful and beneficial bacteria are wiped out, while some hardy and opportunistic pathogens (e.g., *Clostridium difficile*) continue to flourish. *C.difficile* bacteria produce a toxin that causes severe inflammation in the colon, abdominal pain, and watery stools. Spores of *C. difficile* are hard to kill; this strain of bacteria is often transmitted in hospitals and has become increasingly resistant to antibiotic treatment. *C.difficile* infection causes diarrhea in about 336,000 people and kills about 14,000 people each year in the United States. Numerous trials support the use of probiotics for the prevention of antibiotic-associated diarrhea. Probiotics can be taken along with antibiotics to support the population of beneficial microorganisms.

There is evidence that probiotics may be useful for prevention or treatment of infections other than diarrhea, as well. Moderate improvements in rates of respiratory, vaginal, and urinary tract infections are seen with probiotic use (see Further Reading 21). Simply shortening the duration of the common cold by 1 or 2 days means that workers are absent less often (see Further Reading 18).

ALLERGIES AND AUTOIMMUNE DISEASES

Some researchers think that alterations in the microbiota contribute to the development of allergies and autoimmune diseases. Genetics alone cannot explain the increased rates of these disorders in recent years, leading researchers to suspect that environmental factors are at work. Blame may rest with changes in diet, infectious disease rates, use of antibiotics, or the makeup of the microbiota (see Further Reading 2).

Allergies and autoimmune disorders (e.g., type 1 diabetes and inflammatory bowel diseases) are various forms of immune system dysfunction. The gut microbiota is one of our immune system's first interactions with microorganisms. As you just learned, exposure to these microorganisms stimulates proper development of the immune system. If the diversity of the microbiota is limited or skewed toward a particular type of bacteria, then perhaps the immune system does not develop properly; in addition to attacking foreign proteins, antibodies attack the body's own cells.

This theory fits in with the **hygiene hypothesis.** According to the hygiene hypothesis, our tendency to sanitize every surface and treat every infection with antibiotics reduces exposure of the immune system to a diverse community of microorganisms. The understimulated

hygiene hypothesis Assumption that reduced exposure to microorganisms in the environment (e.g., as a result of overuse of antibacterial soaps and antibiotics) impairs proper development of the immune system, making a person more susceptible to allergies and autoimmune diseases.

immune system becomes sensitized to harmless proteins, such as food proteins, beneficial bacteria, or the body's own cells.

Indeed, there is mounting evidence that specific patterns in the microbiota are linked to allergies and autoimmune disorders. Specific patterns in the species and diversity of the microbiota have been observed, for example, among children with type 2 diabetes and people with certain bowel diseases (e.g., Crohn's disease and celiac disease). Is it possible that probiotics and prebiotics could be used to correct these imbalances in the microbiota and, thus, alleviate the burdens of allergies and autoimmune diseases?

One of the best-studied examples is the use of probiotics for the prevention of atopic dermatitis. This condition, most common in children, is characterized by red, scaly, and itchy skin rashes. Its exact cause is unknown, but it falls into the category of diseases of immune dysfunction and is highly associated with seasonal and food allergies. Although evidence does not support probiotics as a treatment of established atopic dermatitis, administration of probiotics to infants has been shown to be effective for prevention of atopic dermatitis (see Further Reading 3).

Emerging evidence indicates that use of probiotics may reduce seasonal allergies (see Further Reading 18). Among people with existing seasonal allergies, use of probiotics is associated with fewer allergy symptoms and reduced use of allergy medications. In addition, there is much interest in administering probiotics during pregnancy, infancy, or childhood to prevent allergies from developing.

Most people who develop type 1 diabetes have a specific genetic trait that predisposes them to the disease. Simply having the genetic trait does not guarantee development of type 1 diabetes; about 90% of whites in North America have this trait. However, when individuals with this genetic trait are exposed to an environmental trigger (e.g., a viral disease during childhood), they develop an autoimmune response that ends up destroying the beta cells of the pancreas. Some interesting research shows how probiotic bacteria may influence gut permeability and inflammatory responses in the intestines, thereby reducing some environmental triggers for development of type 1 diabetes (see Further Reading 2).

Similarly, inflammatory bowel diseases, such as Crohn's disease and ulcerative colitis, are thought to be caused by dysregulated immune responses that cause the immune system to attack the bacteria native to the GI tract. Some preliminary research indicates that probiotics can reduce symptoms in patients with ulcerative colitis, but further research is required to determine if probiotics are an effective way to prevent or treat inflammatory bowel diseases (see Further Reading 26). For now, it seems best to recommend probiotics as adjunct therapy for inflammatory bowel diseases; they may help to relieve symptoms of bloating and abdominal pain, but they are not considered a substitute for medical therapy.

CHOOSING A SAFE AND HIGH-QUALITY PRODUCT

The market for probiotics and prebiotics is expanding rapidly. New functional food products hit the shelves every week, and dietary supplements of single or combination probiotics abound (Table 10-4). Is it better to use a food or a supplement? There are benefits to each.

Probiotics Fermented dairy products, including yogurt, cheese, buttermilk, and kefir, are the most common examples of probiotic food products. Nondairy alternatives include fermented soy products (e.g., soy, miso, and tempeh), fermented vegetables (e.g., sauerkraut or kimchi), and juices or other foods with added live cultures. Probiotic-containing functional food products offer the advantage of providing nutrients in addition to beneficial microorganisms. Some research indicates that the food matrix may help to promote the survival of probiotic strains as they travel through the GI tract so that they make it to the colon intact.

TABLE 10-4 ■ **Probiotic Products**

Food Products	Probiotic Microorganisms
Activia® Greek yogurt	Bifidobacterium lactis
Good Belly® probiotic fruit drink	Lactobacillus plantarum
Lifeway® kefir	Lactobacillus lactis Lactobacillus rhamnosus Streptococcus diacetylactis Lactobacillus plantarum Lactobacillus casei Saccharomyces florentinus Leuconostoc cremoris Bifidobacterium longum Bifiobacterium breve Lactobacillus acidophilus Bifidobacterium lactis Lactobacillus reuteri
Attune® probiotic bar	Bifidobacterium lactis Lactobacillus acidophilus Lactobacillus casei
Supplements	
Culturelle®	Lactobacillus
Florastor®	Saccharomyces boulardii
Align®	Bifidobacterium infantis

▲ Whereas all yogurt is made by fermenting dairy products with bacteria, not all brands contain live and active cultures by the time they make it to store shelves. Check the label to see if your favorite brand contains live and active cultures. © McGraw-Hill Education/Christopher Kerrigan

Foods that contain probiotic microorganisms are functional foods; they supply benefits beyond the nutrients they contain.

It is important to note that not all fermented dairy products contain live strains of probiotics. To prolong shelf-life, some food manufacturers heat-treat yogurt after it has been cultured. Heat treatment will inactivate any live cultures. For this reason, yogurt-covered pretzels or similar baked snack foods do not contain live cultures. Look for brands of yogurt that are labeled with the voluntary statement "contains live and active cultures."

Freezing, on the other hand, does not destroy active cultures. As long as a frozen yogurt product was made from yogurt containing live cultures without further heat treatment, the microorganisms, although they may be dormant at freezing temperatures, will be active inside your body.

Supplements usually contain a higher dose of probiotic strains than food products. Dairy foods, which are the most common food sources of probiotics, are inaccessible for some people with lactose intolerance, food allergies, or taste aversions. Some may view supplements as a low-calorie way to obtain the health benefits of probiotics. Supplemental sources contain freeze-dried bacteria and usually come in the form of capsules or packets.

If you decide to try probiotic supplements, the International Scientific Association for Probiotics and Prebiotics offers a few recommendations to guide your selection (see Further Reading 11).

First, find out which strain or strains of microorganisms are in the product. The strain is important because not every strain has the same effects on human health. Some manufacturers of probiotic supplements or food products use a trademarked name, so you may have to dig deeper to find out which strain of bacteria is present. For example, Culturelle is the trademarked name of a product containing *Lactobacillus rhamnosus GG*.

Next, determine how much of the probiotic you should take. The dose of bacteria per recommended serving will be given as colony forming units (CFU). When clinical studies are conducted to determine the efficacy of a probiotic, they are tested at a specific dose. The effective dose—on the order of millions to billions of CFU per serving—depends on the strain. Dosing schedules vary from one serving per week to several times per day.

Recall that food labeling laws are strict about the information that can appear on a food or supplement label (Fig. 10-18). At this time, no statements have been approved by FDA for claims to cure, treat, or prevent disease. However, the label will include a statement about the intended use of the supplement, such as "promotes digestive health" or "supports immune function." Look for the words "clinically proven" on the product label, insert, or website to determine the strain and dose that have been shown to be effective to address your health concerns.

Prebiotics A good prebiotic should (1) make it to the colon without being degraded by our digestive enzymes or stomach acid, (2) be fermentable by microbes that live in the intestine, and (3) work selectively on a strain of beneficial bacteria. Natural sources of prebiotics include plants such as leeks, asparagus, chicory, Jerusalem artichoke, garlic, artichoke, onion, wheat, oats, bananas, and soybeans. However, you would need to eat a large quantity of these

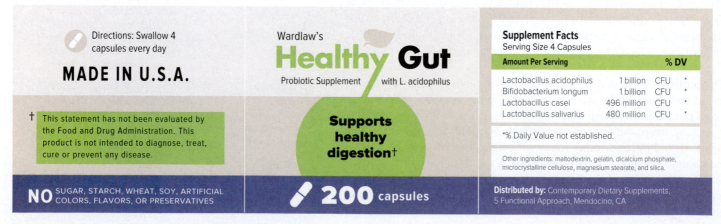

FIGURE 10-18 ▲ Probiotic supplement label.

foods to have an effect on the intestinal microbiota. Thus, most people get their prebiotics from supplements or functional foods with added prebiotics. A typical dose of prebiotics is about 5 to 10 grams per day, depending on the product.

SAFETY

Are probiotics and prebiotics safe? Recall from Chapter 2 that dietary supplements, although they fall under the jurisdiction of FDA, are not regulated as tightly as medications. This means that there is no real guarantee of safety or quality. The USP Verified mark, seen on some supplement labels, can provide consumers with some confidence about the identity, quality, purity, and strength of probiotic supplements.

Over many years and many trials, there have been very few reports of serious adverse effects of probiotic or prebiotic supplements. About three dozen cases of systemic infections have been documented. For this reason, caution should be taken in using these probiotics for premature infants and individuals with a compromised immune system. The most common side effects of probiotics are gas and abdominal bloating. Even these mild effects are only seen at very high doses, such as 20 grams per day or more. If there is any question about safety, just ask your health care provider. Never replace medications with supplements, and inform your health care provider about all medications and supplements you take.

MUCH MORE TO LEARN

Continued study of the microbial genome will help researchers to understand how microorganisms exert their influences on human health. The Human Microbiome Project in the United States and the Metagenomics of the Human Intestinal Tract program in Europe are two large-scale efforts to map the microbial genome and understand the interactions between human and microbial genes. Research efforts focus on the effects of the microbiome on development of type 1 diabetes and atopic diseases, such as eczema.

There is great interest in the potential for probiotics to reduce obesity and its comorbid conditions. Researchers have noticed distinct patterns of microbial populations when comparing the microbiota of lean and obese subjects. In animals, transplanting the microbiota of an obese mouse into a germ-free lean mouse is enough to induce obesity. There have been some human studies but not enough yet to make conclusive recommendations (see Further Reading 21).

We have learned much about the ways probiotics and prebiotics can affect the function of the immune system, yet there are many things left to uncover.

▲ Miso is a traditional Japanese seasoning made from fermented soybeans. It contains live cultures of a type of fungus. Besides its use to flavor foods such as the miso soup pictured here, it is also a source of vitamin B-12. Miso should be added to foods at the end of the cooking process or the live cultures will be destroyed. © L. Mouton/PhotoAlto

✓ CONCEPT CHECK 10.9

1. What is the difference between a probiotic and a prebiotic?
2. Other than yogurt, list two food sources of probiotic microorganisms.
3. Describe two ways probiotic microorganisms may work to support immune health.

Nutrition and Cancer

© Foodcollection

Cancer is the second leading cause of death for North American adults. It is estimated that more than 1620 people die each day of cancer in the United States, accounting for one in four deaths. Cancer-related medical expenses exceed $88 billion each year and are projected to reach $158 billion by 2020. The top four cancers, causing more than 50% of cancer deaths, are lung, colorectal, breast, and prostate.

Cancer is many complex diseases; each differs in the types of cells affected and, in some cases, in the factors contributing to cancer development and progression (Fig. 10-19). For example, the environmental and genetic factors leading to skin cancer often differ from those leading to breast cancer. Similarly, the treatments for the different types of cancer must also vary.

Cancer Progression

The initiation of cancer occurs when a DNA mutation occurs in a cell. Promotion and progression of cancer occurs when mutated cells multiply and proliferate uncontrollably. Without prompt and effective treatment, cancer continues to grow and spread. Most cancers take the form of tumors, although not all tumors are

cancers. A **tumor** is spontaneous new tissue growth that appears to serve no physiological purpose. It can be either **benign,** like a wart, or **malignant,** like most lung cancers. The terms *malignant tumor* and *malignant neoplasm* are synonymous with cancer.

Whereas benign (noncancerous) tumors are dangerous if their presence interferes with normal bodily functions, malignant (cancerous) tumors invade surrounding structures, including blood vessels, the lymph system, and nervous tissue. Cancer can spread, or **metastasize,** to distant sites via the blood and lymphatic circulation, thereby producing invasive tumors in almost any part of the body. Cancer metastasis is much more difficult to treat as each new cancer takes on distinct characteristics in response to its new environment. The fact that uncontrolled cancers spread explains why early detection and targeted treatment is critical. Cancers that are often diagnosed in the early stages, mainly due to widespread screening programs, are those in the colon, breast, and cervix.

Early Detection of Cancer

The CAUTION acronym listed here is a useful aid for remembering many early warning signs for cancer. Unexplained weight loss can be an additional symptom that should not be ignored.

- **C**hange in bowel or bladder habits
- **A** sore that does not heal
- **U**nusual bleeding or discharge
- **T**hickening or lump in the breast or elsewhere
- **I**ndigestion or difficulty in swallowing
- **O**bvious change in a wart or mole
- **N**agging cough or hoarseness

▲ Cruciferous vegetables such as cabbage and cauliflower are rich in anticancer phytochemicals. © C Squared Studios/Getty Images

tumor Mass of cells; may be cancerous (malignant) or noncancerous (benign).

benign Noncancerous; tumors that do not spread.

malignant Malicious; in reference to a tumor, the property of spreading locally and to distant sites.

metastasize The spreading of disease from one part of the body to another, even to parts of the body that are remote from the site of the original tumor. Cancer cells can spread via blood vessels, the lymphatic system, or direct growth of the tumor.

| Estimated % of Cancer Deaths for 2013 | | |
Male		Female
	Brain	2%
4%	Esophagus	
28%	Lung	26%
	Breast	14%
5%	Liver and bile duct	2%
6%	Pancreas	7%
7%	Leukemia and lymphomas	7%
9%	Colon and rectum	9%
4%	Urinary	
	Ovary	5%
10%	Prostate	
	Uterus and cervix	3%
27%	All others (e.g., oral and skin) (e.g., oral, skin, and bladder)	25%

FIGURE 10-19 ▲ Cancer is many diseases. Numerous types of cells and organs are its target. Over one-third of all cancers arise from smoking (primarily lung cancer).

Routine screenings are important for early detection of cancer. The American Cancer Society publishes current cancer screening guidelines based upon expert recommendations and research (see http://www.cancer.org/healthy/findcancerearly/cancerscreeningguidelines/american-cancer-society-guidelines-for-the-early-detection-of-cancer). Families with genetic predispositions to cancer should consult their primary care provider to discuss enhanced surveillance.

Factors That Influence the Development of Cancer

Genetics, environment, and lifestyle are potent forces that influence the risk for developing cancer. Of cancers, 5% to 10% are thought to be inherited and 90% to 95% are related to environmental factors. Genetic predispositions to cancer are most prevalent in colon, breast, and prostate cancers (35%, 27%, and 42% of all cases, respectively). Modifiable lifestyle and environmental exposures explain the huge variation in cancer rates from country to country. Excessive body fatness and dietary patterns account for over half of all environmentally related cancers.

Although we have little control over our genetic risk factors for cancer, we have tremendous influence over our lifestyle behaviors, especially with regard to smoking, alcohol intake, physical activity, UV exposure, and dietary patterns. Indeed, over one-third of all cancers in North America are due to tobacco use. About half of the cancers of the mouth, pharynx, and larynx are associated with heavy use of alcohol. The combined use of both alcohol and tobacco increases cancer risks even higher than either alone.

A Closer Look at the Influence of Diet on Cancer

Some food constituents may contribute to cancer development, whereas others have a protective effect (Table 10-5). Next, the association between body fat/calorie intake and cancer risk is presented, followed by a list of food constituents that may reduce the risk for cancer (see Further Reading 15).

Body Fatness Linked to Cancer Risk

An estimated one of every three cancer deaths in the United States is linked to excess body fat, poor nutrition, and inadequate physical activity. Of these, body weight appears to have the greatest impact on cancer risk. Excess body weight alone contributes to one of five cancer-related deaths. This includes cancer of the breast (post-menopausal), colon and rectum, esophagus, kidney, pancreas, gallbladder, liver, non-Hodgkin's lymphoma, multiple myeloma, cervix, ovary, **endometrium,** and aggressive prostate cancer.

There are several ways excess body fat can influence cancer risk. Adipose tissue secretes hormones, such as estrogen and insulin, that promote the development of cancer. Other proteins are secreted as well that regulate hormonal actions. Also, chronic and

endometrium The membrane that lines the inside of the uterus. It increases in thickness during the menstrual cycle until ovulation occurs. The surface layers are shed during menstruation if conception does not take place.

TABLE 10-5 ■ Food Constituents Associated with Cancer

Constituent	Dietary Sources	Action
Protective when consumed in recommended ranges*		
Vitamin A	Liver, fortified milk, fruits, vegetables	Encourages normal cell development
Vitamin D	Fortified milk, fatty fish	Increases production of a protein that suppresses cell growth
Vitamin E	Whole grains, vegetable oils, green leafy vegetables	Prevents formation of nitrosamines; antioxidant
Vitamin C	Fruits, vegetables	Can block conversion of nitrites and nitrates to potent carcinogens; antioxidant
Folate	Fruits, vegetables, whole grains	Encourages normal cell development; reduces the risk of colon cancer
Selenium	Meats, whole grains	Part of antioxidant system that inhibits tumor growth and kills cancer cells
Carotenoids, such as lycopene	Fruits, vegetables	Antioxidant-like properties; possibly influences cell metabolism
Flavonoids, indoles, phenols, and other phytochemicals	Vegetables, especially cabbage, cauliflower, broccoli, Brussels sprouts, garlic, onions, tea	May reduce cancer in the stomach and other organs
Calcium	Milk products, green vegetables	Slows cell division in the colon and binds bile acids and free fatty acids, thus reducing colon cancer risk
Omega-3 fatty acids	Cold-water fish, such as salmon and tuna	May inhibit tumor growth
Soy products	Tofu, soy milk, tempeh, soy nuts	Phytic acid possibly binds carcinogens in the intestinal tract; genistein component possibly reduces growth and metastasis of malignant cells
Conjugated linoleic acid	Milk products, meats	May inhibit tumor development and act as an antioxidant
Fiber-rich foods	Fruits, vegetables, whole-grain breads and cereals, beans, nuts	Colon and rectal cancer risk may be decreased by accelerating intestinal transit or binding carcinogens such that they are excreted
Possibly carcinogenic		
Excessive calorie intake	All macronutrients can contribute	Excess fat mass leading to obesity; increased synthesis of estrogen and other sex hormones, which may increase the risk for some cancer; resulting excess insulin output from creation of an insulin-resistant state is also implicated
Total fat	Meats, high-fat milk and milk products, animal fats, and vegetable oils	The strongest evidence is for excessive saturated and polyunsaturated fat intake; saturated fat is linked to an increased risk of prostate cancer
High glycemic load carbohydrates	Cookies, cakes, sugared soft drinks, candy	Insulin surges associated with these foods may increase tumor growth, such as in the colon
Alcohol	Beer, wine, liquor	Contributes to cancers of the throat, liver, bladder, breast, and colon (especially if the person does not consume enough folate)
Nitrites, nitrates	Cured meats, especially ham, bacon, and sausages	Under very high temperatures will bind to amino-acid derivatives to form nitrosamines, potent carcinogens
Multiring compounds: aflatoxin	Formed when mold is present on peanuts or grains	May alter DNA structure and inhibit its ability to properly respond to physiologic controls; aflatoxin in particular is linked to liver cancer
Benzo(a)pyrene and other heterocyclic amines	Charcoal-broiled foods, especially meats	Linked to stomach and colon cancer; to limit this risk, trim fat from meat before cooking, cut barbecuing time by partially cooking meat (such as in a microwave oven) prior to grilling, and don't consume blackened parts

*Many of the actions listed for these possibly protective agents are speculative and have been verified only by experimental animal studies. The best evidence supports obtaining these nutrients and other food constituents from foods. The U.S. Preventive Services Task Force supports this statement, noting there is no clear evidence that nutrient supplements provide the same benefits.

systemic inflammation and oxidative stress often typical among overweight and obese individuals contribute to carcinogenesis.

A strong link exists between cancer risk and excess calories in the diet. In animal experiments, restricting total calorie intake to about 70% of usual intake results in about a 40% reduction in tumor development, regardless of the macronutrient composition of the diet. Currently, calorie restriction appears to be the most effective technique for preventing cancer in laboratory animals. Unfortunately, it is difficult for humans to reduce dietary calories to 70% of usual intake. While the data obtained from animal studies are interesting, dietitians understand that severe calorie restrictions are not feasible and sustainable for most individuals. In addition, once cancer is present, calorie restriction may no longer be helpful.

Cancer-Fighting Foods

Many nutrients and plant compounds exhibit anticancer properties. These include antioxidants and phytochemicals (review Table 10-3). The antioxidant activity of vitamins C and E helps to prevent the formation of **nitrosamines** in the GI tract, thus reducing carcinogen exposure. Vitamin E also helps protect unsaturated fatty acids from damage by free radicals. Overall, carotenoids, vitamin E, vitamin C, and selenium from whole foods function as or contribute to antioxidant protection for the body. Some of these protective systems prevent DNA mutations by electron-seeking compounds, the main factor promoting cancer initiation.

Research shows that fruits and vegetables protect against a range of cancers. As well as containing key vitamins and minerals, which strengthen our immune system, they are good sources of biologically active phytochemicals. Foods containing fiber are also linked to a reduced risk of cancer. Fiber is thought to speed up "gut transit time," or the length of time it takes food to move through the digestive system. It has been suggested that an adequate intake of vitamin D may prevent the risk for some forms of cancer. Vitamin D can "turn on" (express) or "turn off" (silence) a host of genes that regulate cell growth and inflammation. The exact role of vitamin D relative to carcinogenesis continues to be an active area of research.

Although no single food or food component can fully protect you against cancer, evidence clearly shows that dietary patterns that are rich in a variety of plant foods—vegetables, fruits, whole grains, beans—help to reduce the risk for many cancers. MyPlate is aimed at cancer and disease prevention. It is likely that consumption of a wide variety of plant-based foods and adequate physical activity result in a "cocktail" effect that, together, are more potent and protective than either in isolation (see Further Reading 15).

Evidence-Based Recommendations for Cancer Prevention

Given the devastating toll of cancer treatment and lack of a definitive cure, efforts at prevention are of prime importance. Several health organizations have issued their own sets of diet and lifestyle guidelines for cancer prevention and survivorship. Here, we present the recommendations of the American Institute for Cancer Research, which are consistent with the recommendations of other cancer organizations.

nitrosamine A carcinogen formed from nitrates and breakdown products of amino acids; can lead to cancer.

AMERICAN INSTITUTE FOR CANCER RESEARCH RECOMMENDATIONS FOR CANCER PREVENTION

1. *Be as lean as possible without becoming underweight.* Maintaining a healthy body weight is one of the most important things you can do to reduce your risk of cancer. Aim to be at the lower end of the healthy BMI range.
2. *Be physically active for at least 30 minutes every day.* Physical activity in any form helps to lower cancer risk. Aim to build more activity, like brisk walking, into your daily routine. Limit sedentary habits such as excessive screen time.
3. *Avoid sugary drinks. Limit consumption of energy-dense foods.* Choosing healthy foods and drinks instead of those that are high in refined carbohydrates and often in added sugar and fat can help us avoid overweight and obesity and thereby reduce cancer risk.
4. *Eat more of a variety of vegetables, fruits, whole grains, and legumes.* For good health, base all of your meals on plant foods. When preparing a meal, aim to fill at least two-thirds of your plate with vegetables, fruits, whole grains, and beans.
5. *Limit consumption of red meats and avoid processed meats.* Red meat refers to beef, pork, and lamb—foods such as hamburgers, steaks, pork chops, and roast lamb. The term *processed meat* refers to meats preserved by smoking, curing, or salting or by the addition of preservatives. Examples include ham, bacon, pastrami, salami, hot dogs, and sausages. To reduce risk, limit intake to no more than 18 ounces per week.
6. *If consumed at all, limit alcoholic drinks to two (men) or one (women) per day.* For cancer prevention, it is best to avoid alcohol completely, but alcohol does afford some protection against cardiovascular disease.
7. *Limit consumption of salty foods and foods processed with salt.* Consuming too much salt can be harmful to our health, increasing the risk of stomach cancer as well as hypertension.
8. *Don't use supplements to protect against cancer.* To reduce your risk of cancer, choose a balanced dietary pattern rich in a variety of whole foods rather than supplements.
9. *It is best for mothers to breastfeed exclusively for up to 6 months and then add other liquids and foods.* Breastfeeding reduces the risk of breast and other reproductive cancers for the mother and lowers the risk of future obesity in the infant.
10. *After treatment, cancer survivors should follow the recommendations for cancer prevention.* Anyone diagnosed with cancer should receive specialized nutritional advice from a registered dietitian nutritionist or clinician. Once active treatment is complete, aim to adhere to the cancer-prevention recommendations.

And always remember . . . Do not smoke or chew tobacco.

Nutrition Concerns During Active Cancer Treatment

Diet and lifestyle changes can exert a powerful influence on the risk for developing cancer, but it is important to note that they are no substitute for preventive screening and appropriate medical care. Once cancer has developed, diet and lifestyle changes will not be adequate to prevent cancer growth or metastasis. Nutrition concerns during active cancer treatment (chemotherapy, radiation, surgery) vary depending on the site and stage of the cancer, but the overall goals of nutrition therapy are to minimize weight fluctuations and prevent nutrient deficiencies.

Weight loss, particularly loss of muscle mass, is a major concern during cancer treatment because malnutrition can interrupt treatment regimens and impede recovery. Common effects of cancer and/or cancer treatments include fatigue, mouth sores, dry mouth, taste abnormalities, nausea, and diarrhea—all of which can lead to inadequate food intake.

During active treatment, the most appropriate food choices are those that the cancer patient craves and can tolerate. Although food choices vary widely based on each patient's individual symptoms, cool, nonacidic liquids and soft, mildly flavored foods are generally well accepted. Small, frequent meals and foods with high nutrient and calorie density should be emphasized to meet calorie and protein needs. Often, liquid nutritional supplements

are needed. Because many cancer patients are immunocompromised as a result of their treatment, safe food handling practices are extremely important (see Chapter 17).

To learn more about cancer, review these sources of credible cancer information on the Internet:

American Cancer Society
www.cancer.org
National Cancer Institute
www.cancer.gov
American Institute for Cancer Research
www.aicr.org
Abramson Cancer Center's Oncolink
www.oncolink.org
Harvard School of Public Health's Disease Risk Index
www.diseaseriskindex.harvard.edu

Summary (Numbers refer to numbered sections in the chapter.)

10.1 The immune system is comprised of white blood cells, the thymus, the spleen, and lymphoid tissue, and is supported by a healthy GI tract, skin, and lymphatic system. There are two main types of immune responses: innate immunity and adaptive immunity. Innate immunity refers to nonspecific physical and chemical barriers that are present from birth. Adaptive immunity depends on the specific targeting of antigens by antibodies produced by white blood cells.

10.2 Many chemical reactions involve the transfer of electrons between molecules. A molecule is oxidized when it loses an electron; a molecule is reduced when it gains an electron. Production of free radicals (molecules with unpaired electrons) is a normal consequence of metabolism, but an overabundance of free radicals can cause damage to cells, especially cell membranes and DNA. This damage can lead to many diseases, including cancer and atherosclerosis. Antioxidant enzyme systems detoxify free radicals, often with the aid of mineral cofactors such as selenium and zinc. Antioxidant chemicals such as vitamins C and E can donate electrons to free radicals without becoming reactive themselves, a process that halts cellular damage.

10.3 Vitamin A, sometimes called the "anti-infection vitamin," maintains the health of epithelial tissues and is responsible for the function of mucus-secreting cells. It is also vitally important for normal vision. Vitamin A is found in meats, fortified dairy products, fish, eggs, and a variety of red, orange, or leafy green vegetables.

Carotenoids are phytochemicals that can be converted to vitamin A in the body. Three forms of carotenoids can yield vitamin A in humans: beta-carotene, alpha-carotene, and betacryptoxanthin. Although carotenoids are not essential nutrients, some have health-promoting qualities for humans. In addition to their contribution to vitamin A

intake, carotenoids are powerful antioxidants. Carotenoids are plentiful in dark green and orange vegetables.

10.4 Vitamin C is a potent antioxidant and also takes part in the synthesis of collagen, carnitine, and neurotransmitters, and can modestly enhance iron absorption. A vitamin C deficiency results in scurvy, evidenced by pinpoint hemorrhages in the skin, bleeding gums, and joint pain. Smoking increases the possibility of vitamin C deficiency. Fresh fruits and vegetables, especially citrus fruits, are good sources.

10.5 Vitamin E functions primarily as an antioxidant and is found in plant oils. By donating electrons to electron-seeking free-radical (oxidizing) compounds, it neutralizes them. This effect shields cell membranes and red blood cells from breakdown.

10.6 Selenium is a cofactor in the glutathione peroxidase system, which detoxifies free radicals. It acts along with vitamin E to provide antioxidant protection. Muscle pain, wasting, and a form of heart damage may result from a selenium deficiency. Meats, eggs, fish, and shellfish are good animal sources of selenium. Good plant sources include grains and seeds.

10.7 Zinc is a cofactor for more than 200 enzymes. It participates in DNA synthesis, protein metabolism, immune function, normal growth and development, insulin function, cell membrane structure and function, and antioxidant reactions. Food sources of zinc include beef, fortified grain products, and many other protein-rich foods.

10.8 In addition to carotenoids, other phytochemicals have health benefits related to their effects in antioxidant activity, DNA expression, cholesterol metabolism, and the inflammatory process, among others. Notable health-promoting phytochemicals include lycopene (in tomatoes, watermelon, and pink grapefruit) and flavonoids (in blueberries, raspberries, citrus fruit, and chocolate).

10.9 The microbiota makes an important contribution to the development and maintenance of the immune system. Probiotics are live microorganisms, such as strains of lactobacilli and bifidobacteria, that promote the health of the colon as well as other aspects of human health. Prebiotics are substances that are indigestible by humans, but which serve as fuel for probiotic microorganisms in the body.

10.10 Given the toll of cancer treatment and lack of a definitive cure, efforts at prevention are key. A variety of dietary changes will reduce your risk for cancer. Start by making sure that your dietary pattern is rich in fruits and vegetables, whole grains, beans, some fish, and low-fat or fat-free dairy products. In addition, remain physically active; avoid obesity; consume alcohol in moderation (if at all); and limit intake of red meat and salt-cured, smoked, and nitrate-cured foods.

Check Your Knowledge (Answers are available at the end of this question set.)

1. Megadoses of _____ are likely to enhance immune function.
   a. vitamin A
   b. vitamin C
   c. zinc
   d. none of the above

2. Some carotenoids are considered provitamins because they can be converted to
   a. vitamin K.
   b. vitamin E.
   c. vitamin D.
   d. vitamin A.

3. A deficiency of zinc could lead to
   a. stunted growth.
   b. increased risk of infections.
   c. increased risk of cancer.
   d. all of the above.

4. Vitamin C is necessary for the production of
   a. stomach acid.
   b. collagen.
   c. hormones.
   d. clotting factors.

5. Damage caused by free radicals is thought to contribute to
   a. atherosclerosis.
   b. Alzheimer's disease.
   c. diabetes.
   d. all of the above.

6. Good food sources of vitamin E include
   a. meats.
   b. white bread.
   c. nuts.
   d. all of the above.

7. Blueberries and chocolate are rich sources of the phytochemical group called
   a. flavonoids.
   b. carotenoids.
   c. allyl sulfides.
   d. isoflavones.

8. Which of the following meals is most compatible with AICR guidelines for cancer prevention?
   a. Flame-broiled chicken breast, baked potato, and mixed vegetables
   b. Poached salmon, steamed broccoli, and whole-grain bread
   c. Baked ham, sweet potato casserole, and spinach salad
   d. Cheese pizza and breadsticks with marinara sauce

9. Selenium is an antioxidant micronutrient because it
   a. donates electrons to free radicals.
   b. accepts electrons from free radicals.
   c. aids glutathione peroxidase activity.
   d. enhances the absorption of vitamin E.

10. Probiotic microorganisms may assist with the prevention or treatment of
    a. diarrhea.
    b. type 1 diabetes.
    c. obesity.
    d. all of the above.

Answer Key: 1. d (LO 10.1), 2. d (LO 10.3), 3. d (LO 10.7), 4. b (LO 10.4), 5. d (LO 10.2), 6. c (LO 10.5), 7. a (LO 10.8), 8. b (LO 10.10), 9. c (LO 10.6), 10. d (LO 10.9)

Study Questions (Numbers refer to Learning Outcomes)

1. List two ways the digestive system assists the immune system. **(LO 10.1)**

2. Describe the process by which an antioxidant can prevent a free radical from damaging cells. **(LO 10.2)**

3. How would you determine which fruits and vegetables displayed in the produce section of your supermarket are likely to provide plenty of carotenoids? **(LO 10.3)**

4. Describe three functions of vitamin C. **(LO 10.4)**

5. What is the role of vitamin E in the prevention of cardiovascular disease? Should people at risk for cardiovascular disease take vitamin E supplements? **(LO 10.5)**

6. Are selenium supplements recommended for prevention of cancer? Why or why not? **(LO 10.6)**

7. Describe at least two ways zinc supports body defense systems. **(LO 10.7)**

8. Plan a meal, using MyPlate as a guide, that includes at least three sources of antioxidant phytochemicals. **(LO 10.8)**

9. Describe at least two ways the gut microbiota may benefit immune function. **(LO 10.9)**

10. What is the relationship between consumption of foods that are rich sources of antioxidants and a decreased risk for cancer? **(LO 10.10)**

What The Dietitian Chose

©Ingram Publishing/SuperStock

Coffee and tea products are both effective at relieving mental and physical fatigue, and increasing mental alertness. Coffee is one of the most commonly consumed beverages in the world and has grown in popularity over recent years. The United States is the world's largest coffee consumer with about 83% of adults drinking coffee, and 63% of adults drinking it every day (data from the National Coffee Association). Coffee is made from roasted beans from the *Coffea arabica* bush, and its effects are largely due to its caffeine content. Caffeine works by stimulating the central nervous system, heart, and muscles. Of our choices, a 12-ounce cup of Starbucks coffee would provide about 260 milligrams of caffeine, significantly more caffeine than any of the tea choices. In addition, coffee contains hundreds of other chemicals, many of which have potential activities in the body. Some of these coffee compounds, including the phenolic acids, are known to have potent antioxidant properties. Although information about the availability of these antioxidant compounds from coffee is limited, coffee consumption has been shown to have several beneficial health effects.

Recent studies have shown an association between drinking coffee and a lower risk of stroke, basal cell carcinoma, and incidence of depression. In all of these studies, the protective effects of coffee peaked at 3 to 4 cups per day. Studies have also found an association between coffee consumption and reduced risk of Parkinson's and Alzheimer's diseases, dementia, type 2 diabetes, and liver cancer (see Further Reading 13). Decreases in markers of oxidative stress and inflammation have also been shown in coffee drinkers. Research has suggested that caffeine may be the key protective compound in coffee, because in studies, consumption of decaffeinated coffee was not associated with health benefits. Based on this information, a cup of coffee in the morning may give you more than just a quick energy boost.

A few warnings must also be included when we recommend coffee. First, you can become dependent on coffee for energy, resulting in headaches and anxiety when you try to go without it. The caffeine in coffee can also interfere with restful sleep and exacerbate acid reflux symptoms. Caffeine also has a mild diuretic effect, but caffeinated beverages do still contribute to hydration. Finally, remember that creating lattes and mochas by adding cream, chocolate, or other sweeteners to your coffee adds a significant number of calories and fat to your beverage.

If coffee has been shown to have so many health benefits and a good dose of caffeine, you are probably thinking that tea must be even better. For sure, all types of tea have been touted as healthy beverages. Black, green, white, and oolong tea all come from the *Camellia sinensis* tea plant, but differ in the ways their leaves are processed. Whereas green tea leaves are just withered and steamed, oolong and black tea leaves are crushed and then oolong is partially fermented and black tea leaves are fully fermented. Teas have been studied in humans, animals, and laboratory experiments, and shown to have many health benefits. The evidence suggests that regular tea drinkers who drink 2 or more cups per day have lower total and LDL cholesterol, less heart disease and stroke, and recover from heart attacks faster. Studies have also shown that drinking tea may also help lower the risk of breast or ovarian cancer recurrence. Memory also appears to benefit from tea drinking, with those drinking tea (green or black) at least five times per week having a slower rate of cognitive decline among adults 65 years or older. Green tea contains 2% to 4% caffeine, as well as polyphenols.

If you are looking for a greater shot of caffeine in your morning drink, coffee wins out over all of the tea products. An 8-ounce cup of brewed green tea delivers only 35 milligrams of caffeine. At double the volume, you get double the caffeine (70 milligrams) in the 17-ounce Honest Tea iced green tea product. Brewed black tea provides a bit more caffeine at 55 milligrams per 8-ounce cup but still significantly less than coffee. As with coffee, the caffeine in tea affects thinking and alertness, increases urine output, and stimulates the nervous system, heart, and muscles by increasing the release of neurotransmitters in the brain.

Tea is unique in that it is a rich source of the antioxidant group called **flavonoids.** Flavonoids are part of a broader category of chemicals called polyphenols and are found in many foods, including tea, cocoa, fruits, and vegetables. All of the teas from the *Camellia* plant contain polyphenol antioxidants at levels about 8 to 10 times greater than the amount of polyphenols found in fruits and vegetables. The flavonoids are just one of the families of tea polyphenols, and the catechins are an even smaller group of disease-fighting tea flavonoids. The catechins and antioxidants are thought to be the keys to the health benefits of tea. Epigallocatechin gallate (EGCG) is the catechin found in the greatest concentration in tea and the one most studied for its health benefits. (To avoid confusion, most tea companies simply use the term *antioxidants* on their package labels when describing this group of polyphenols in their tea products.)

With the beneficial evidence mounting for tea, despite its lower caffeine content, is green tea a better choice than black tea? Many of the studies on tea drinkers have not distinguished between green or black tea consumption. In addition, analysis shows that green and black tea have almost identical amounts of polyphenols/flavonoids. Lipton tea bags claim to have 175 milligrams of flavonoids per 8-ounce cup of black tea compared to 150 milligrams for their green tea. Researchers at Purdue University have found that an 8-ounce cup of fresh-brewed green tea contains about 320 milligrams of polyphenols, including about 190 milligrams of EGCG. To get the most health benefits from tea, most studies suggest steeping the tea bag or tea leaves for at least 3 minutes, and drinking 3 or more cups per day to keep your blood levels of polyphenols high. It takes time for the polyphenols to dissolve in water, so the longer you steep the tea, the more

flavonoids Most common group of polyphenol phytochemicals; found in citrus fruits, berries, red onion, tea, red wine, and dark chocolate.

flavonoids will be in your tea. Tea is a healthy substitute for soft drinks, which do not offer the antioxidants. If choosing a bottled tea, choose one made from brewed tea, not tea extracts or concentrate. Steer away from ready-to-drink or instant products because they will have only a fraction of the phytochemicals in brewed tea. Many bottled green teas are not 100% tea and are sweetened with sugar, high-fructose corn syrup, or honey. The Honest Tea choice in our list provides 70 calories per 17-ounce bottle due to the addition of honey. Lemon is a safe addition to tea because it adds the antioxidant vitamin C, which also protects the polyphenols from being oxidized and degraded. For further discussion of the merits of tea and of some additional bottled green tea products, see Further Reading 23.

© Foodcollection

While all of the choices given have merits as an early-morning beverage, the dietitian chose brewed black tea. The black tea will provide a moderate amount of caffeine to increase alertness without the drawback of producing a strong dependency. The black tea also has a healthy dose of flavonoids that appear to have antioxidant effects that will help fight disease-causing oxidative stress.

CASE STUDY SOLUTION   Choosing a Dietary Supplement

1. The maintenance dose of two to three tablets per day does not pose risk per se, because this dose of Nutramega does not exceed the Tolerable Upper Intake levels for vitamins E and C, zinc, or selenium.

2. a. **Vitamin E**
   600% (6 times) of the Daily Value of 13.5 milligrams (30 IU) equals 81 milligrams per tablet (Daily Value: 30 IU × 0.45 mg/IU = 13.5 mg). Sixteen tablets would yield 1296 milligrams of vitamin E. **This would be 1.3 times the Upper Level of 1000 milligrams (1296/1000 = 1.3).**

   b. **Vitamin C**
   700% (7 times) of the Daily Value of 60 milligrams equals 420 milligrams per tablet. Sixteen tablets would yield 6720 milligrams. The Upper Level is 2000 milligrams. **This would then yield 3.4 times the Upper Level (6720/2000 = 3.4).**

   c. **Selenium**
   10% of the Daily Value of 70 micrograms equals 7 micrograms per tablet. Sixteen tablets would yield 112 micrograms. **This is less than the Upper Level of 400 micrograms.**

   d. The suggested use of Nutramega "at the first sign of feeling ill" poses some health risks for Amy. Taking two to three tablets every 3 hours would mean taking at least sixteen tablets per day. This dosage would provide an intake of vitamins E and C in excess of the Upper Levels for these nutrients. The UL has been set for these nutrients because of the potential detrimental effects of chronically high doses, especially in supplement form.

3. Nutramega is expensive compared to the cost of the typical multivitamin and mineral supplement (a 1-month supply of the latter would cost about $3/month compared to about $50 for Nutramega).

4. Overall, Amy is smart to be concerned about meeting her nutrient needs, but the stress she is under does not increase nutrient needs.

5. A healthy diet as suggested by MyPlate should be Amy's primary focus. Taking a balanced multivitamin and mineral supplement is also a reasonable practice.

Further Readings

1. Basu A and others: Berries: Emerging impact on cardiovascular health. *Nutrition Reviews* 68:168, 2010.

2. Boerner BP, Sarvetnick NE: Type 1 diabetes: Role of intestinal microbiome in humans and mice. *Annals of the New York Academy of Sciences* 1243:103, 2011.

3. Cabana M: American Gastroenterological Association Institute's GI Lifelong Education and Resource Network: Probiotics and Prebiotics Webinar Series: Practical Guidelines on Probiotics and Prebiotics Use. http://www.gastro.org/probiotics-and-prebiotics-webinars

4. Cassidy A and others: High anthocyanin intake is associated with a reduced risk of myocardial infarction in young and middle-aged women. *Circulation* 127(2):188, 2013.

5. Cordero Z and others: Vitamin E and risk of cardiovascular diseases: A review of epidemiologic and clinical trial studies. *Critical Reviews in Food Science and Nutrition* 50:420, 2010.

6. Drake VJ: Micronutrient Information Center of the Linus Pauling Institute at Oregon State University: Nutrition and immunity. September 2, 2010. http://lpi.oregonstate.edu/infocenter/immunity.html

7. Goldenberg JZ and others: Probiotics for the prevention of Clostridium difficile-associated diarrhea in adults and children (review). *Cochrane Database of Systematic Reviews* 5, 2013.

8. Hemila H, Chalker E: Vitamin C for preventing and treating the common cold. *Cochrane Database of Systematic Reviews,* 2013.

9. Howarth GS, Wang H: Role of endogenous microbiota, probiotics and their biological products in human health. *Nutrients* 5:58, 2013.

10. Institute of Medicine of the National Academies. *Dietary Reference Intakes for vitamin C, vitamin E, selenium, and carotenoids.* Washington, DC: National Academy Press, 2000.

11. International Scientific Association for Probiotics and Prebiotics: Prebiotic/Probiotic Science. http://www.isapp.net/pp_intro.asp

12. Kelly D, Mulder IE: Microbiome and immunological factors. *Nutrition Reviews* 70:S18, 2012.

13. Kempf K and others: Effects of coffee consumption on subclinical inflammation and other risk factors for type 2 diabetes: A clinical trial. *American Journal of Clinical Nutrition* 91:950, 2010.

14. King JC: Zinc: An essential but elusive nutrient. *American Journal of Clinical Nutrition* 94:679S, 2011.

15. Kushi LH and others: American Cancer Society guidelines on nutrition and physical activity for cancer prevention: Reducing the risk of cancer with healthy food choices and physical activity. *CA: A Cancer Journal for Clinicians* 62:30, 2012.

16. National Institutes of Health, Office of Dietary Supplements: Dietary supplement fact sheet: Vitamin E. October 11, 2011. http://ods.od.nih.gov/factsheets/vitaminE.asp; Vitamin C. June 24, 2011. http://ods.od.nih.gov/factsheets/vitaminc.asp; Selenium. October, 12, 2012. http://ods.od.nih.gov/factsheets/Selenium.asp

17. Palmer S: Inflammation—can't stand the heat? Then get in the kitchen. *Today's Dietitian* 13(2):36, 2011.

18. Palmer S: Probiotics' potential—Research suggests beneficial bacteria may support immune health. *Today's Dietitian* 13(1):20, 2011.

19. Prior RL, Wu X: Diet antioxidant capacity: Relationships to oxidative stress and health. *American Journal of Biomedical Sciences* 5(2):126, 2013.

20. Rink SM and others: Self-report of fruit and vegetable intake that meets the 5 a day recommendation is associated with reduced levels of oxidative stress biomarkers and increased levels of antioxidant defense in premenopausal women. *Journal of the Academy of Nutrition and Dietetics* 113:776–85, 2013.

21. Rowland I and others: Current level of consensus on probiotic science: Report of an expert meeting—London, November 23, 2009. *Gut Microbes* 1:436, 2010.

22. Schaeffer J: Diet and detoxification. *Today's Dietitian* 16:34, 2014.

23. Schardt D: Tea time: What's all the fuss about green tea? *Nutrition Action Healthletter,* p. 9, May 2011.

24. Sesso HD and others: Vitamins E and C in the prevention of cardiovascular disease in men. The Physicians' Health Study II Randomized Controlled Trial. *Journal of American Medical Association* 300:2123, 2008.

25. U.S. Department of Agriculture, Agricultural Research Service. *Oxygen radical absorbance capacity (ORAC) of selected foods, release 2.* Nutrient Data Laboratory, 2010. http://www.ars.usda.gov/nutrientdata/orac

26. Veerappan GR, Betteridge J: Probiotics for the treatment of inflammatory bowel disease. *Current Gastroenterology Reports* 14:324, 2012.

Rate Your Plate

I. Spotting Fraudulent Claims on the Internet

Search for vitamins and vitaminlike substances sold over the Internet. Then write a report concerning any fraudulent or misleading claims made on behalf of these products. Are the websites selling vitamins, or are they a cover for selling something else? Compare the price of the vitamins from these sites with the price you would pay at the local supermarket or drugstore. Do any of these sites display any disclaimers or warnings about the products?

II. A Closer Look at Supplement Use

With the popularity of vitamin and mineral supplements, it is important to understand how to evaluate a supplement. Study the label of a supplement you use or one readily available from a friend or the supermarket. Then answer the following questions.

1. What is the recommended dosage of this supplement?

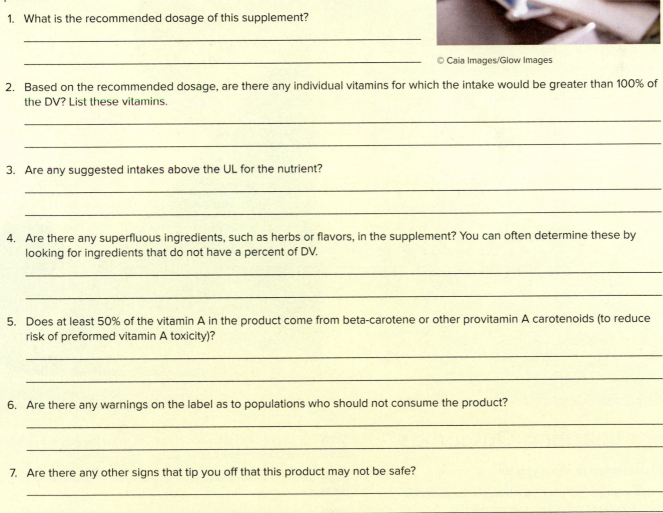

© Caia Images/Glow Images

2. Based on the recommended dosage, are there any individual vitamins for which the intake would be greater than 100% of the DV? List these vitamins.

3. Are any suggested intakes above the UL for the nutrient?

4. Are there any superfluous ingredients, such as herbs or flavors, in the supplement? You can often determine these by looking for ingredients that do not have a percent of DV.

5. Does at least 50% of the vitamin A in the product come from beta-carotene or other provitamin A carotenoids (to reduce risk of preformed vitamin A toxicity)?

6. Are there any warnings on the label as to populations who should not consume the product?

7. Are there any other signs that tip you off that this product may not be safe?

© Imagestate Media (John Foxx)/Imagestate

Student Learning Outcomes

Chapter 11 is designed to allow you to:

11.1 Describe the process of bone synthesis and degradation and classify bone as either cortical or trabecular.

11.2 List hormonal, lifestyle, and nutritional factors that influence bone health.

11.3 List sources and functions of calcium, including its role in bone growth, maintenance, and repair.

11.4 Describe the functions, recommendations, and sources of phosphorus.

11.5 Explain the functions and sources of vitamin D, including its synthesis by the action of ultraviolet radiation and the signs and symptoms of vitamin D deficiency.

Chapter 11
Nutrients Involved in Bone Health

The skeletal system can be thought of as the bricks and mortar that provide structural support for the body. An unexpected feature of this structure, however, is that bone is a vibrant, living tissue that flexes and undergoes constant breakdown and synthesis, serving as a reservoir for mineral metabolism. It is estimated that in the middle-aged adult, 9% of bone is removed and replaced by new bone every year. In addition to being the architectural framework, bone contains nerves and cartilage, and is the source of red and white blood cells and platelets. Numerous minerals and vitamins are essential to synthesize and maintain bone. This chapter will explore how these nutrients function together to achieve optimal bone health.

Maintenance of healthy bone is critical for an active, productive life. The human body contains 206 bones, infiltrated by blood vessels that supply nutrients and hormones to the cells found in bone. The interactions among genes, hormones, body weight, physical activity, nutrition, and other lifestyle factors ultimately determine bone health.

Are supplements as good as food sources when it comes to getting proper nutrition for bone health? What if I am allergic to milk—can I still get enough bone-building nutrients? How can I find out if I am at risk for osteoporosis? Chapter 11 provides some answers.

11.6 List magnesium functions and sources.

11.7 Describe the role of fluoride in tooth development and bone health as well as primary sources of fluoride.

11.8 List other nutrients involved in bone health, including their primary function in bone and common food sources.

11.9 Describe the process of osteoporosis development and prevention.

11.10 Describe current methods used to assess bone health.

11.11 Identify sources of dairy-free milk substitutes.

Trabecular bone
(spongy,
open lattice,
contains marrow)

Marrow cavity
(found in flat
and long bones)

Cortical bone
(dense/compact)

Periosteum

Blood vessel and
nerve fibers (supply
nutrients and oxygen
to bones)

FIGURE 11-1 ▲ There are two types of bone: cortical and trabecular. Cortical bone forms the shafts of bones and the outer mineral covering. Trabecular bone supports the outer shell of cortical bone in various bones of the body.

periosteum A specialized connective tissue covering all bones and having bone-forming potential.

cortical bone The compact or dense bone found on the outer surfaces of bone.

trabecular bone The less dense, more open structure bone found in the inner layer of bones.

bone marrow The spongy tissue in flat bones and trabecular bone that contains stem cells.

hemopoietic Stem cells in the bone marrow that are capable of developing into blood cells.

stromal Stem cells that can produce bone, cartilage, and fat.

osteoblast Bone cells that initiate the synthesis of new bone.

11.1 Bone Physiology

BONE STRUCTURE

Bone has three major components, each with a specific function (Fig. 11-1):

1. **Periosteum:** This thick, fibrous vascular membrane covers most of the (cortical) bone surface. Muscles, tendons, and ligaments connect to it. The periosteum does not cover the ends of long bones, because you need cartilage there for joint movement.

2. **Cortical** and **trabecular bone:** Cortical bone is sometimes called dense or compact bone. It comprises 80% of adult bone mass. The outer portion of nearly all bones is composed of dense, strong, cortical bone. The principal function of cortical bone is to provide strength and stability. Microscopic openings in cortical bone allow blood vessels and nerves to pass through, providing nutrients and hormones to bone cells.

   Trabecular bone provides even more strength and structural stability. Because it is spongy and less rigid, it acts more like a shock absorber. It has an open structure, which lightens the weight of bones. The latticelike matrix of trabecular bone has small cavities that can be filled with marrow or connective tissue. Trabecular bone is predominant in the ends of long bones, vertebrae, rib cage, and flat bones of the pelvis. About 20% of adult bone mass is trabecular.

3. **Bone marrow:** Marrow is a spongy tissue that contains stem cells. These stem cells are one of two types: **hemopoietic,** meaning they are capable of developing into blood cells (see Chapter 13), or **stromal,** cells that can produce bone, cartilage, and fat. In infancy, all marrow is red in color due to the high number of blood-producing cells. With age, more and more marrow becomes yellow, reflecting a higher number of fat cells. By adulthood, only 50% of marrow is red. Bone marrow is primarily located in flat bones (hip, breast, rib, shoulder blade, and vertebrae), in the shafts of long bones, and in pockets of trabecular bone. It is in the head of the femur (ball joint at hip) and humerus (forearm at elbow).

Are teeth bone? Teeth have the same properties as bone plus a hard protective outer covering called enamel, not infiltrated by vessels or nerves.

BONE GROWTH AND REMODELING

The growth, maintenance, and repair of bone involve a complex relationship between the synthesis of new bone by the bone-building cells, **osteoblasts,** and the breakdown of bone by **osteoclasts.** The degradation and resynthesis of bone is termed **bone remodeling** (Fig. 11-2). When you remodel a room, you tear down first and then you rebuild or you add on. The same principle applies to bone. Osteoclasts produced from stem cell bone marrow break down or degrade small amounts of bone. This process is called **resorption.** In doing so, minerals embedded in bone matrix, including calcium, phosphorus, and magnesium, are freed and released into the blood. The resynthesis of new bone is then accomplished by the activity of osteoblasts from bone marrow. These osteoblasts embed within the dissolved "resorption bay" (see Fig. 11-2) provided by the osteoclasts. The osteoblasts take up free calcium and phosphorus and, along with collagen, form a complex mixture called **hydroxyapatite.** This mixture adds strength and structure to the bone. Some osteoblasts become embedded within the bone matrix and become **osteocytes.** Figure 11-2 shows the relationship of these three cells in the bone. Synthesis of bone, for repair or growth, is a function of the osteoblast.

Bone growth occurs in length and width during the first two decades of life. The rate of bone formation exceeds the rate of bone breakdown during infancy, childhood, and young adulthood. The majority of bone growth occurs before adulthood, although in both males and females, peak bone mass is usually achieved a few years before age 30. Genetics as well as nutrient intake, drugs, hormones, physical activity, and lifestyle choices will influence the age at which peak bone mass is achieved. People with a larger frame size and body weight will have a greater bone mass due to the additional stress on the bone associated with the extra weight.

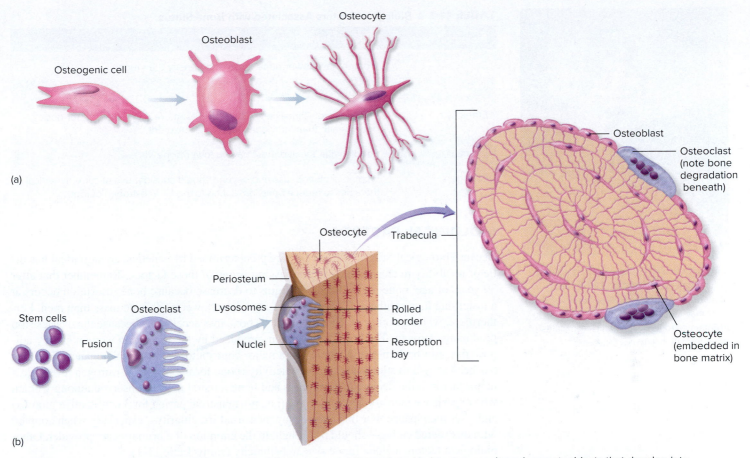

FIGURE 11-2 ▲ Bone remodeling. (a) Osteogenic cells (new bone cells produced in bone marrow) produce osteoblasts that develop into osteocytes. (b) Stem cells (from bone marrow) fuse together and form osteoclasts. These cells dissolve bone via the lysosomes and acids they contain. The osteoclasts degrade the bone (resorption) so that osteoblasts can embed and add more minerals and connective tissue (resynthesis).

The optimal situation throughout adulthood would be to maintain peak bone mass through an equal amount of bone resorption and resynthesis. However, after 30 years of age, bone resorption occurs at a faster rate than synthesis, resulting in a loss of bone mass and a decrease in bone mineral density. **Bone mineral density** is the concentration of minerals found in the bone and is used as an indicator of bone health. Bone is composed of approximately 65% minerals and 35% connective tissue. Minerals provide the strength and rigidity, whereas the connective tissue provides flexibility.

✓ CONCEPT CHECK 11.1

1. What are the roles of periosteum, cortical bone, trabecular bone, and bone marrow?
2. What types of cells are responsible for bone building and bone breakdown?

11.2 Factors That Influence Bone Health

Both biological and lifestyle factors influence the growth, maintenance, and overall health of bone. To optimize bone health, the goal is to maximize **bone mineral density** leading to the strongest bone. Trabecular bone is more responsive to factors that influence bone remodeling. This causes the breakdown and resynthesis of trabecular bone to occur at a faster rate when compared to cortical bone.

osteoclast Bone cells that break down bone and subsequently release bone minerals into the blood.

bone remodeling The chemical process by which bone is broken down and replaced by new bone.

resorption The process of losing substance. Bone resorption is part of the initial process for remodeling and growth.

hydroxyapatite Crystalline compound containing calcium, phosphorus, and sometimes fluoride, also known as bone mineral.

osteocyte Osteoblast embedded into the bone matrix.

bone mineral density Total mineral content of bone at a specific bone site divided by the width of the bone at that site, generally expressed as grams per cubic centimeter.

bone mineral density Total mineral content of bone at a specific bone site divided by the width of the bone at that site, generally expressed as grams per cubic centimeter.

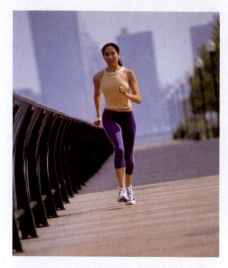

▲ Weight-bearing exercise such as walking or running is associated with increased bone density. Female athletes, however, must maintain an adequate energy intake to maintain estrogen levels, which stimulates bone formation. © Royalty-Free/Corbis

TABLE 11-1 ■ Biological Factors Associated with Bone Status

Biological Factors	Effect on Bone Status
Sex	Women have lower bone mass and density than men.
Age	Bone loss occurs after age 30.
Ethnicity	Individuals of Caucasian or Asian heritage are at greater risk for poor bone health than individuals of African descent.
Frame size	People with "small bones" have a lower bone mass.
Estrogen	Women at menopause and beyond should consider use of current medical therapies to reduce bone loss linked to the fall in estrogen output.

BIOLOGICAL FACTORS

Because biological factors (Table 11-1) are predetermined by genetics, an individual has little or no ability to change these factors. Aging is one of these factors. Remember that after 30 years of age, bone mineral density begins to decrease because bone resorption occurs at a faster rate than synthesis. Women, on average, have lower peak bone mass than men. Furthermore, when a woman reaches menopause, bone loss accelerates because the ovaries stop producing estrogen. The hormone estrogen, produced by the ovaries in women and by adipose tissue in both men and women, is a major contributor to bone maintenance. Estrogen has been shown to stimulate osteoblast activity (bone formation). Low estrogen levels are a major factor in the decline of bone mass and bone mineral density observed among women who experience menstrual irregularities (i.e., no menstrual period for 3 consecutive months) and after menopause. For this reason, any menstrual irregularity—especially when coupled with disordered eating—should be brought to the attention of a primary care provider. Other biological factors include frame size and ethnicity (study Table 11-1).

LIFESTYLE FACTORS

In contrast to the biological factors already described, we have the ability to influence bone health through various lifestyle choices (Table 11-2). Following a balanced dietary pattern that meets needs for calcium, vitamin D, protein, and other bone-building nutrients will provide the materials to synthesize and repair bone. Maintaining a healthy weight and active lifestyle are also important factors in bone health. The increased muscle mass that stems from weight-bearing physical activity, in particular, is associated with greater bone mineral density. Muscle keeps tension on bone, and the hormonal changes that occur with the stress associated with exercise cause bones to retain and possibly gain density (Fig. 11-3). Upper-body strength training is especially encouraged, as this area can be easily overlooked. Older adults especially need to stay physically active—including some weight-bearing and resistance activities.

At any age, smoking and excessive alcohol intake decrease bone mass. Smoking lowers the estrogen concentration in the blood in women, increasing bone loss. Smoking one pack of cigarettes per day throughout your adult life could result in a 5% to 10% acceleration of bone loss. Alcohol is toxic to bone cells for both men and women, and alcoholism is probably a major undiagnosed and unrecognized cause of low bone mineral density. Excessive intakes of phosphorus, caffeine, and sodium also adversely affect bone health but only if calcium intake is low or marginal.

At one point a high protein intake was assumed to have a negative influence on bone mass, because of its potential to generate acid in the bloodstream. The impact of protein intake and acid load on bone

Skeletal muscle pulls against the bone, causing it to rebuild and become more dense.

Biceps brachii muscle

FIGURE 11-3 ▲ The stress of muscles pulling on bone during exercise increases bone mineral density.

TABLE 11-2 ■ **Modifiable Lifestyle Factors Associated with Bone Status**

Lifestyle Factors	Call to Action
Adequate dietary pattern containing an appropriate amount of nutrients	• Follow MyPlate with special emphasis on adequate amounts of fruits, vegetables, and low-fat and fat-free dairy products. • Consider use of fortified foods (or supplements) to make up for specific nutrient shortfalls, such as vitamin D and calcium.
Healthy body weight	• Maintain a healthy body weight (BMI of 18.5–24.9) to support bone health.
Normal menses	• During childbearing years, seek medical advice if menses cease (such as in cases of anorexia nervosa or extreme athletic training).
Weight-bearing physical activity	• Perform weight-bearing activity as this contributes to bone maintenance, whereas bed rest and a sedentary lifestyle lead to bone loss. • Strength training, especially upper body, is helpful to bone maintenance.
Smoking	• Smoking lowers estrogen synthesis in women. Cessation is advised. Passive exposure is a risk.
Medications	• Some medications (e.g., thyroid hormone, cortisol, diuretics) stimulate urinary calcium excretion. • Some medications (e.g., alcohol, diuretics, cancer medications) stimulate urinary excretion of magnesium.
Excessive intake of protein, phosphorus, sodium, caffeine, wheat bran, or alcohol	• Moderate intake of these dietary constituents is recommended. Problems primarily arise when excessive intakes of these nutrients are combined with inadequate calcium consumption. • Excessive soft drink consumption is especially discouraged.
Inadequate UV-B exposure	• If sunlight exposure is limited (<10–15 minutes per day without sunscreen), focus on food or supplements to meet current RDA for vitamin D.

health has been debated, however, and recent studies suggest a bone-building influence of high protein intakes. Studies examining other aspects of acid-base status and bone health have also been inconsistent (see Further Reading 12).

✓ CONCEPT CHECK 11.2

1. What are the biological factors that influence bone mineral density?
2. What are the lifestyle factors that influence bone mineral density?

11.3 Calcium

FUNCTIONS OF CALCIUM

Bone Growth, Maintenance, and Repair Calcium (Ca) represents 40% of all the minerals present in the body and equals about 2.5 pounds (1200 grams) in the average person. All cells require calcium to function; however, more than 99% of the calcium in the body is used for growth, development, and maintenance of bones. Calcium is the main component of hydroxyapatite, the crystalline compound responsible for the structure and hardness of bone.

Muscle and Nerve Function Less than 1% of calcium is found in blood, but this circulating calcium is critical to supply the needs of cells other than bone cells. Forming and maintaining bone are calcium's major roles in the body, but it is critical for other processes as well. Muscle contraction is activated by calcium release and the flow of calcium along the surface of the muscle cell. In nerve transmission, calcium assists in the release of neurotransmitters and permits the flow of ions in and out of nerve cells.

▲ Ninety-nine percent of calcium in the body is in bones.
© Royalty-Free/Corbis

cellular differentiation The process of a less-specialized cell becoming a more specialized type. Think of stem cells in the bone marrow becoming red and white blood cells.

tetany A body condition marked by sharp contraction of muscles and failure to relax afterward; usually caused by abnormal calcium metabolism.

Many factors enhance calcium absorption, including:

- High need (e.g., during growth, pregnancy, lactation)
- Increased blood levels of **parathyroid hormone (PTH)** and vitamin D
- The presence of lactose in the diet
- Decreased flow rate (motility) of digestive contents through the intestine
- Acidic environment of the stomach

Many factors inhibit calcium absorption, including:

- Large amounts of **phytic acid (phytates)** and fiber from grains (if fiber intake exceeds 30 grams per day)
- **Oxalic acid (oxalates)** found in certain foods of plant origin (affects calcium absorption from its food source, but not calcium from other foods)
- Great excess of phosphorus, magnesium, sodium, and zinc in the diet (if calcium intake is very low)
- Tannins (polyphenols) in tea and some legumes (e.g., soy)
- A vitamin D deficiency
- Diarrhea
- Old age
- Some medications (anticonvulsants, cortisone, antacids)

parathyroid hormone (PTH) A hormone made by the parathyroid glands that increases synthesis of the vitamin D hormone and aids calcium release from bone and calcium conservation by the kidneys, among other functions.

phytic acid (phytate) A constituent of plant fiber that chemically binds minerals and prevents their absorption. Phytic acid can depress calcium absorption from other foods present in the GI tract.

oxalic acid (oxalate) An organic acid found in spinach, rhubarb, beet greens, chard, and sweet potatoes. It can depress the absorption of certain minerals, such as calcium, but only in the food itself.

Additional Functions and Health Benefits Calcium helps regulate cellular metabolism by influencing the activities of various enzymes and hormonal responses. Calcium also functions in the maintenance of cell membrane integrity, normal blood pressure, regulation of glucose concentration, and **cellular differentiation.** Calcium is essential for formation of a blood clot (see Section 13.2). It is the tight regulation of the concentration of calcium in the blood that keeps these processes going, even if a person fails to consume enough dietary calcium from day to day. There is some evidence that calcium has a role in preventing breast and colon cancer. Overall, the benefits of a diet providing adequate calcium extend far beyond bone health.

CALCIUM DEFICIENCY

The body tightly regulates blood calcium concentration within a narrow range, regardless of dietary intake. If dietary calcium intake is inadequate and blood calcium concentration begins to decrease, three hormonally controlled actions are stimulated to reestablish normal levels of calcium in the blood: (1) bones release calcium, (2) intestines absorb more calcium, and (3) the kidneys retain more calcium in the blood. Because of this tight hormonal regulation, poor dietary intake of calcium is not likely to result in low blood calcium. Rather, kidney diseases, hormonal abnormality, or medications are the likely culprits. If blood calcium falls below a critical point, muscles cannot relax after contraction and nerve function is disrupted. The result is a condition called **tetany** in which muscles become stiff or twitch involuntary.

You can see that the skeleton does more than simply provide the framework of the body; it also functions as a bank from which calcium can be added or withdrawn. Only about 1% of the calcium in bone is available at any time for this purpose. Over time, however, bone loss due to inadequate calcium intake and/or absorption may occur, though slowly. Clinical symptoms of the calcium loss from bones show after many years. By not meeting calcium needs, some people, especially women, are most likely setting the stage for osteoporosis and future bone fractures. Osteoporosis will be discussed in Section 11.9 of this chapter.

GETTING ENOUGH CALCIUM

Bone growth, development, and maintenance require an adequate calcium intake. Calcium requires an acidic environment in the gastrointestinal tract to be absorbed efficiently. Absorption occurs primarily in the upper part of the small intestine. This area tends to remain somewhat acidic because it receives the acidic stomach contents. After the first section of the small intestine, secretions from the pancreas enter the small intestine and the pH becomes neutral to slightly basic, causing calcium absorption to decrease. Efficient calcium absorption in the upper small intestine also depends on the presence of the active form of vitamin D. Adults absorb about 30% of the calcium in the foods eaten, but during times when the body needs extra calcium, such as in infancy and pregnancy, absorption increases to as high as 60%. Aging negatively influences the absorption efficiency of calcium. Due to decreased synthesis, absorption, and activation of vitamin D, as well as decreased acid secretion in the stomach, people over age 40 have a harder time meeting their needs for calcium.

The Recommended Dietary Allowance for calcium is 1000 milligrams per day for adults up through 50 years of age. For women older than age 50, and for both men and women over age 70, the RDA increases to 1200 milligrams per day. The RDA is based on the amount of calcium needed each day to offset calcium losses in urine, feces, and other routes. The RDA for young people ages 9 to 18 (1300 milligrams per day) includes an additional amount to allow for increases in bone mass during growth and development.

The calcium intakes of many Americans fall short of meeting the RDA. During late childhood and adolescence—a critical time for accretion of bone mass—sugar- and caffeine-laden beverages are frequently chosen instead of milk or dairy alternatives. This calcium deficit increases the risk for osteoporosis later in life. Into adulthood, average daily calcium intakes are approximately 800 milligrams for women and 1000 milligrams for men. Approximately half of adult women in the United States consume less than 60% of the recommended intake of calcium (Fig. 11-4). Some of this is due to their perception that dairy products are high in calories (although many reduced-fat dairy products are available). A growing number of Americans are choosing plant-based dietary patterns, including a vegan dietary pattern, which eliminates dairy products. Other adults simply lose their taste for milk as they age. In addition, lactose intolerance becomes more prevalent as people age.

Calcium is found in both plant and animal foods. Overall, dairy products provide about 75% of the calcium in North American dietary patterns. In fact, fat-free milk is the most nutrient-dense (milligrams per kcal) source of this bone-building nutrient. Calcium tends to have high **bioavailability** from dairy products because they contain vitamin D and lactose, which enhance calcium absorption. An exception is cottage cheese; most calcium is bound and unavailable for absorption. Bread, rolls, crackers, and foods made with milk products are secondary contributors. Other calcium sources are leafy greens (such as kale), almonds, some legumes, sardines, and canned salmon (Fig. 11-5).

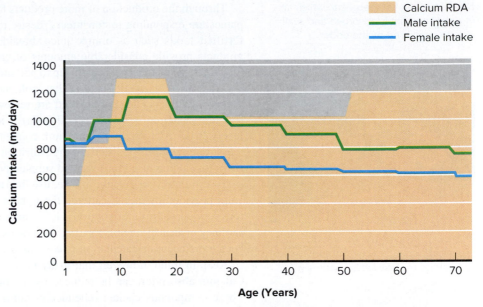

FIGURE 11-4 ▲ The gap between recommended dietary intake of calcium and daily consumption of calcium in males and females in the United States. Female calcium intake is low throughout the life span, whereas males' intakes drop below recommendations around age 50.

(a)

(b)

Food Item and Amount	Calcium (milligrams)	% RDA for Adult Males and Females (1000 milligrams)
Grains		
Total Raisin Bran cereal, 1 cup	1000	100%
English muffin, whole-wheat, 1 each	175	18%
Pancake, 4"	83	8%
Vegetables		
Spinach, cooked, 1 cup	245	25%
Butternut squash, cooked, 1 cup	84	8%
Broccoli, cooked, 1 cup	62	6%
Fruits		
Orange juice (fortified), 1 cup	349	35%
Figs, dried, ½ cup	121	12%
Raisins, ½ cup	36	4%
Dairy		
Yogurt, plain, non-fat, 1 cup	488	49%
Milk, fat-free, 1 cup	299	30%
Soymilk, (fortified), 1 cup	299	30%
Protein		
Tofu (with calcium sulfate), 3 ounces	574	57%
Salmon, canned with bones, 3 ounces	203	20%
Almonds, dry roasted, 1 ounce	76	8%

FIGURE 11-5 ▲ Food sources of calcium. (a) The fill of the background color (none, 1/3, 2/3, or completely covered) within each food group on MyPlate indicates the average nutrient density for calcium in that group. (b) The bar graph shows the calcium content of several foods in each food group compared to the RDA for adult males and females. Overall, the richest sources of calcium are dairy foods (and dairy alternatives), legumes, green leafy vegetables, and fortified foods.

Source: *Nutrition data from USDA National Nutrient Database for Standard Reference, Release 26.*

bioavailability The degree to which an ingested nutrient is absorbed and available to be utilized by the body.

▲ Calcium is found in plant sources such as green leafy vegetables but is in much higher concentration in dairy foods. © Mitch Hrdlicka/ Getty Images

Through the production of more products fortified with calcium, food and beverage companies are responding to consumers' desire to increase consumption of calcium. Calcium-fortified foods such as orange juice, breakfast cereals, breakfast bars, waffles, and soy products provide considerable amounts of calcium. In fact, an 8-ounce glass of calcium-fortified orange juice can provide up to 350 milligrams of calcium, whereas 8 ounces of milk has 300. Many dairy alternatives that look, feel, and taste like typical dairy foods are available in the grocery store today and are reviewed in Section 11.11 in this chapter. Another source of calcium is soybean curd (tofu) if it is made with calcium carbonate (check the label). It is easy to assess the calcium content of foods because it is among those nutrients that are required to be listed on the Nutrition Facts panel on food labels. The Daily Value (DV) for calcium used for food and supplement labels is 1000 milligrams.

To estimate your calcium intake, use the rule of 300s. Count 300 milligrams for the calcium provided by foods scattered throughout the diet. Add another 300 milligrams to that for every cup of milk or yogurt or 1.5 ounces of cheese. If you eat a lot of tofu, almonds, or sardines or drink calcium-fortified beverages, use Figure 11-5 or diet-analysis software to get a more accurate calculation of calcium intake.

Keep in mind, however, that many factors can influence the bioavailability of calcium. Calcium absorption can be reduced by the presence of oxalates, tannins, and phytic acid. These compounds chelate (chemically bind) calcium in the digestive tract. Oxalates are found in sweet potatoes, collard greens, spinach, and rhubarb. It is estimated that a person would have to consume over eight servings (8 cups) of spinach to absorb the same amount of calcium present in one serving (1 cup) of milk. Oxalates bind only the calcium in the food they are in; oxalate-containing foods do not affect the calcium availability from other foods. This does not hold true for phytates or tannins. Tea and some legumes are rich sources of tannins. Phytates are found in whole grains, raw beans, and nuts. Diets high in dietary fiber reduce mineral absorption. With this in mind, vegans should take extra care to include good sources of calcium in their dietary patterns.

Determining the Amount of Calcium in Food

Convert the percent Daily Value of calcium on food labels to milligrams by adding a "0" to the percentage. For example, if a food label states a serving supplies 30% of the DV for calcium, convert this to milligrams by adding a 0, so 30% is the same as 300 milligrams.

ASK THE RDN   **Coffee, Colas, and Bone Health**

Dear RDN: *I look forward to the caffeine boost I get from a cup of coffee in the morning and late afternoon, and I enjoy a diet cola with lunch. Could the caffeine in these drinks be damaging my bones and leading to osteoporosis?*

Coffee and colas are major sources of caffeine. An 8-ounce cup of coffee usually contains at least 95 milligrams of caffeine, and a 12-ounce cola typically has about 30 milligrams. High intakes of caffeine are known to decrease intestinal calcium absorption and simultaneously increase the amount of calcium excreted in the urine, suggesting that excessive use of caffeine can eventually contribute to bone loss. Research has confirmed that consuming 330 milligrams or more of caffeine daily (the amount found in about four cups of coffee) increases the risk of brittle or broken bones. The evidence shows both coffee and colas having effects on bone density that could contribute to osteoporosis. It is interesting that these associations appear only in women and are not linked to the consumption of black tea, which also contains caffeine. In fact, older women who drink tea have been shown to have greater bone density than women who do not drink tea at all. This effect may be related to unique compounds found in tea that may enhance bone health.

In addition to caffeine, regular and diet colas also contain phosphoric acid that can affect bones. Phosphorus is widespread in our food supply, both naturally and as an additive. The abundance of phosphorus in our food raises some concern that we may actually be getting too much of a good thing. Getting more phosphorus is generally considered safe in people with healthy kidney function who consume adequate calcium. However, high phosphorus intakes are a concern when they are combined with a low calcium intake, which creates an imbalance in the calcium-to-phosphorus ratio that can contribute to bone loss. This situation is more common when you regularly substitute soft drinks for milk.

The bottom line is that you can enjoy coffee and cola as long as you get enough calcium to meet your body's needs and make up for any caffeine-induced calcium losses. Be sure and include calcium-rich foods in your dietary pattern and consult your primary care provider or dietitian to discuss calcium supplementation if your intake falls short of the recommendations. Most importantly, make sure that your coffee and colas are not replacing milk and calcium-fortified juice consumption that promotes bone health. Practice moderation with your caffeine consumption to prevent caffeine from interfering with calcium absorption and excretion. Less than two cans of cola per day is advised and keep your coffee habit to no more than three (8-ounce) cups a day. Adding fat-free milk to your coffee can help offset any losses.

Start your day with café au lait,

Anne M. Smith, PhD, RDN, LD

▲ Chickpeas (garbanzo beans) are a good plant source of calcium at 80 milligrams per cup. A cup of hummus made from chickpeas provides 93.5 milligrams of calcium.
© L. Mouton/PhotoAlto

AVOIDING TOO MUCH CALCIUM

The Upper Level (UL) for calcium intake is 2500 milligrams per day for young adults, based on the observation that greater intakes increase the risk for some forms of kidney stones. Excessive calcium intakes by some people can also cause high blood and urinary calcium concentrations, irritability, headache, kidney failure, soft tissue calcification, and decreased absorption of other minerals, as noted previously.

Calcium Supplementation There has been much debate over the effectiveness of calcium and vitamin D supplementation for maintaining bone health. Although achieving the RDAs for calcium and vitamin D through dietary modifications has been found to improve bone mineral density and reduce rate of fractures, use of supplements to meet RDAs may actually impair skeletal health and worsen cardiovascular health. Recent studies have ignited controversy over these potential health risks of consuming large amounts of these nutrients, especially for older adults. One of these studies found that a dietary intake of calcium near the current recommendations was not related to higher bone mineral density of the hip or lumbar spine compared with lower intakes of calcium in elderly men and women in the United States. In addition, calcium intake beyond the RDA for elderly women and men, usually achieved by calcium supplements, did not provide any benefit for hip or lumbar spine bone mineral density in older adults (see Further Reading 2). Furthermore, the results of other studies, including the large Women's Health Initiative trial, have shown a small but statistically significant increase in the rate of heart attacks among older adults taking calcium supplements with or without vitamin D (see Further Reading 3). Although the observed relationships between calcium supplements and heart attack risk are small, the regular use of calcium supplements by so many older adults could translate into a large public health problem.

On the positive side, a recent report from the Women's Health Initiative study indicates that long-term use of a daily calcium and vitamin D supplement that is close to the RDA results in a substantial reduction in the risk of hip fracture among postmenopausal women. These authors also reported that the level of calcium and vitamin D supplementation did not result in an increase in other chronic diseases, including heart disease. The more positive effects of supplementation appear to happen when the level of total calcium and vitamin D intake is kept very close to the RDA (see Newsworthy Nutrition). Therefore, taking 1000 milligrams of calcium carbonate or calcium citrate daily as a supplement in divided doses (about 500 milligrams per tablet) is probably safe in many instances.

So which is better: calcium from food or supplements? The National Osteoporosis Foundation continues to encourage all individuals to consume the recommended amounts of calcium and vitamin D to protect bone health. Experts agree that we should strive to meet our calcium and vitamin D needs from foods first and that more research is needed to better comprehend the benefits and risks associated with calcium and vitamin D supplementation. Modification of eating habits to include foods that are good sources of calcium is a better

Newsworthy Nutrition

Calcium supplements decrease risk of hip fracture in women

The Women's Health Initiative (WHI) clinical trial randomly assigned 36,282 post-menopausal women in the United States to a placebo or 1000-milligram supplement of calcium carbonate plus 400 IU of vitamin D daily for 7 years. The hypothesis of this study was that calcium plus vitamin D supplementation would reduce hip fracture. This study also examined the health benefits and risks of calcium and vitamin D supplementation on total fractures, cardiovascular disease, cancer, and total mortality. Women in both groups were also allowed to take personal calcium and vitamin D supplements during the study, which was accounted for during the analysis of the data. Regarding bone health, the women who took the assigned calcium and vitamin D supplement but took no personal calcium supplements had a 75% lower risk of hip fracture than women who got the placebo and took no personal calcium supplements. The results also showed that women assigned to take calcium and vitamin D had no higher risk of heart disease, heart attacks, stroke, colorectal cancer, or total mortality. The supplement group did have a 17% increase risk of kidney stones. The authors concluded that long-term use of calcium and vitamin D appears to confer a substantial reduction in the risk of hip fracture among postmenopausal women. Because the risk reduction was significant only in women not taking any additional calcium supplements, it is recommended that women strive to consume the RDA for calcium (1200 milligrams per day) and vitamin D (600 IU per day up to age 70 and 800 IU per day over 70) from food and supplements combined.

Source: Prentice RL and others: Health risks and benefits from calcium and vitamin D supplementation: Women's Health Initiative clinical trial and cohort study. *Osteoporosis International* 24(2):567, 2013.

Vitamin D and Calcium Supplementation to Prevent Fractures Task Force Conclusions:

(1) There is not enough evidence to determine whether vitamin D and calcium supplements can prevent fractures in men and women who have not yet gone through menopause.

(2) There is not enough evidence to determine whether vitamin D and calcium supplements with greater than 400 IU of vitamin D and greater than 1000 mg of calcium can prevent fractures in noninstitutionalized postmenopausal women.

(3) There is enough evidence to recommend against daily supplementation with 400 IU or less of vitamin D and 1000 milligrams or less of calcium for the primary prevention of fractures in noninstitutionalized postmenopausal women because lower doses of vitamin D and calcium supplements do not prevent fractures in older women and may increase the risk of kidney stones. The full Task Force statement can be viewed at www.uspreventiveservicestaskforce.org/Page/Document/UpdateSummaryFinal/vitamin-d-and-calcium-to-prevent-fractures-preventive-medication.

plan of action and appears to be the safest means to prevent osteoporosis without jeopardizing heart health. In addition to this important mineral, foods that contain calcium also supply other vitamins, minerals, phytochemicals, and fats needed to support health. Problems associated with excessive consumption of calcium, such as constipation, are not likely when foods are the primary sources of calcium.

In an effort to provide guidance for the public, the U.S. Preventive Services Task Force recently reviewed current research studies on the use of vitamin D and calcium supplements to prevent fractures and issued recommendations in its *Vitamin D and Calcium Supplementation to Prevent Fractures* report in February 2013. The recommendations apply to adult men and women who live at home. They do not apply to those living in assisted living or skilled nursing facilities or who have been diagnosed with osteoporosis or vitamin D deficiency. The Task Force conclusions are listed in the adjacent box and are based on what they learned about the potential benefits and harms of using these supplements.

Keeping in mind the recommendations just discussed, increasing calcium intake through the use of a calcium supplement is beneficial if you have a milk allergy, do not like milk, are ovovegetarian, vegan, lactose intolerant, or cannot incorporate enough calcium-containing foods into your diet (see Further Reading 10). Always look for a supplement with added vitamin D, as it enhances calcium uptake. This additional vitamin D typically does not add to the cost of the supplement. Table 11-3 compares the two most common forms of calcium supplements. Calcium carbonate should be taken with meals because it requires an acid environment in the stomach to dissolve and maximize calcium absorption. Calcium citrate is indicated for people who cannot remember to take calcium carbonate with meals and for those who have low-acid stomach conditions, such as people who take acid-reducing medications for ulcers or reflux, or have had surgery for obesity reduction.

Calcium supplements have side effects, including gas, bloating, or constipation. Distributing small-dose supplements throughout the day, taking it with meals, or even changing the brand of supplement may alleviate some problems. Intake of calcium from supplements and/or food above 500 milligrams at any one time significantly reduces the percent absorbed.

TABLE 11-3 ■ Calcium Supplement Comparisons

	Calcium carbonate	Calcium citrate
Calcium content	40%	21%
Forms	Tablets, chewable tablets, soft chews	Pills (can be quite large) Liquid (sometimes easier to tolerate)
Cost	Least expensive, most common form	Most expensive
Bioavailability and meal timing	Needs acid environment in stomach, so take with acid food or take with meals	Best absorbed; does not need acid environment to be absorbed

With calcium supplements, interactions with other minerals are a concern. There is evidence that calcium supplements may decrease zinc, iron, and other mineral absorption. An effect of calcium supplementation on iron absorption is possible; however, this appears to be small over the long term. To be safe, people using a calcium supplement on a regular basis should notify their physician of the practice. Calcium supplements can also interfere with the body's ability to absorb certain antibiotics. If your doctor prescribes antibiotics, especially tetracycline, be sure to talk with your pharmacist about timing of your supplement, medication, and meals.

Tablet or liquid calcium supplements with the United States Pharmacopeia (USP) symbol are considered the safest. FDA has cautioned the public on the use of calcium supplements from dolomite, bone meal, coral, or oyster shell because of the potential for unhealthy levels of environmental contaminants, especially lead.

☑ **CONCEPT CHECK 11.3**

1. What percent of calcium in the body is found in bone and teeth?
2. Beyond its role in bone health, what are some other critical functions of calcium?
3. What role does vitamin D play in calcium metabolism?
4. What factors reduce calcium absorption?

11.4 Phosphorus

FUNCTIONS OF PHOSPHORUS

Phosphorus (P) is the second most abundant mineral in the body. Approximately 85% of phosphorus is found as a component of hydroxyapatite crystals that provide the functional component of bone and teeth. The remaining 15% of phosphorus is in the soft tissues, blood, and extracellular fluid (see Chapter 9). Phosphorus is part of DNA and RNA, the genetic material present in every cell. Therefore, phosphorus is critical for cellular replication and growth because DNA and RNA are responsible for mitosis and protein synthesis. Phosphorus is also a primary component of adenosine triphosphate (ATP), the energy molecule that fuels body functions. Phosphorus is essential for the activation and deactivation of certain enzymes and many of the B vitamins are functional only when a phosphate group is attached.

A major class of lipids contains phosphorus: phospholipids are the principal structural component of cell membranes, making up approximately 60% of membranes. These phospholipid membranes regulate the transport of nutrients and waste products into and out of cells. Phosphorus also serves as a buffer to maintain blood pH. Lastly, phosphorus (in the form of the phosphate ion) is the principal negatively charged ion in intracellular fluid and thus is essential for maintenance of fluid balance.

PHOSPHORUS DEFICIENCY

As a general rule, deficiencies of phosphorus are unlikely in healthy adults because it is so widespread in food and efficiently absorbed. If intakes of phosphorus are inadequate, the kidney compensates by increasing the reabsorption of phosphorus to prevent blood phosphorus levels from decreasing. Dietary phosphorus deficiency usually occurs only in cases of near-total starvation, including anorexia nervosa. Some health conditions such as diabetes and alcoholism, as well as medications such as antacids and diuretics, can cause phosphorus levels in the body to fall. Marginal phosphorus status can be found in preterm infants, vegans, older people on nutrient-poor diets, and people with long-term bouts of diarrhea, as occurs in Crohn's disease and celiac disease. A small percentage of older women undergoing osteoporosis treatment have been shown to be at high risk for phosphorus deficiency because phosphorus intake is low and phosphorus absorption is inhibited by calcium supplements. Symptoms of phosphorus deficiency include loss of appetite, anemia, muscle weakness, bone pain, fragile bones, increased susceptibility to infection, numbness and tingling of the extremities, difficulty walking, and irregular breathing (see Further Reading 8).

GETTING ENOUGH PHOSPHORUS

In contrast to calcium, phosphorus is naturally abundant in many foods. Milk, cheese, meat, and bread provide most of the phosphorus in the adult diet. Nuts, fish, breakfast cereals, bran, and eggs are also good sources (Fig. 11-6). About 20% to 30% of dietary phosphorus comes from food additives, especially in baked goods, cheeses, processed meats, and many soft drinks (about 75 milligrams per 12 ounces). As a food additive, phosphorus is considered a GRAS (generally recognized as safe) substance, and its function is to increase water binding and taste. Phosphoric acid, which gives a tangy, sour taste, will also significantly lower the pH of a food or beverage (pH of a soft drink is less than 3). Absorption of phosphorus is generally high, ranging from 55% to 80%. Phosphorus absorption from grains,

▲ Trail mix is rich in phosphorus. © imagebroker/Alamy

ChooseMyPlate.gov

(a)

(b)

	Food Item and Amount	Phosphorus (milligrams)	% RDA for Adult Males and Females (700 milligrams)
Grains	Trail mix (with chocolate, nuts, seeds), ½ cup	283	40%
Grains	Raisin bran cereal, 1 cup	205	29%
Grains	Oatmeal, prepared with water, ½ cup	90	13%
Vegetables	Potato, baked (with skin), 1 medium	121	17%
Vegetables	Asparagus, cooked, 1 cup	97	14%
Vegetables	Mushrooms, white, raw, 1 cup	60	9%
Dairy	Yogurt, plain, non-fat, 1 cup	385	55%
Dairy	Milk, fat-free, 1 cup	247	35%
Dairy	Soymilk, 1 cup	104	15%
Protein	Salmon, baked, 3 ounces	218	31%
Protein	Great northern beans, cooked, ½ cup	146	21%
Protein	Almonds, dry roasted, 1 ounce	134	19%

FIGURE 11-6 ▲ Food sources of phosphorus. (a) The fill of the background color (none, 1/3, 2/3, or completely covered) within each food group on MyPlate indicates the average nutrient density for phosphorus in that group. (b) The bar graph shows the phosphorus content of several foods in each food group compared to the RDA for adult males and females. Overall, the richest sources of phosphorus are dairy products and protein foods. Foods from the fruits group (not shown) are poor sources of phosphorus.

Source: *Nutrition data from USDA National Nutrient Database for Standard Reference, Release 26.*

however, is reduced because of the high phytic acid content. Vitamin D enhances phosphorus absorption.

The RDA for phosphorus is 700 milligrams for adult men and women (see box). The recommendation is higher (1250 milligrams per day) for young people ages 9 to 18 to support growth and development. Average daily adult consumption is about 1000 to 1600 milligrams.

Phosphorus
RDA: 700 milligrams
DV: 1000 milligrams
UL: 4000 milligrams

AVOIDING TOO MUCH PHOSPHORUS

The UL for phosphorus intake is 3 to 4 grams per day. Intakes greater than this can result in mineralization of soft tissues. Phosphorus levels in the blood are regulated primarily by the kidneys, and these organs are particularly sensitive to phosphorus toxicity. High intakes can lead to serious problems in people with certain kidney diseases. In addition, a high phosphorus intake coupled with a low calcium intake can cause a chronic imbalance in the calcium-to-phosphorus ratio in the dietary pattern and contribute to bone loss. This situation most likely arises when the RDA for calcium is not met, as can occur in adolescents and adults who regularly substitute soft drinks for milk or otherwise underconsume calcium.

✓ CONCEPT CHECK 11.4

1. What effect does vitamin D have on phosphorus absorption?
2. What are the key functions of phosphorus beyond bone health?
3. Is a deficiency of phosphorus likely? Why or why not?
4. What are the primary food sources of phosphorus?
5. What are the risks of excess intake of phosphorus?

7-dehydrocholesterol Precursor of vitamin D found in the skin.

vitamin D$_3$ (cholecalciferol) Previtamin form found naturally in some animal sources, including fish and egg yolks.

25-hydroxyvitamin D$_3$ (calcidiol or calcifediol) Form found in blood. Sometimes shortened to 25(OH)D$_3$.

1,25-dihydroxyvitamin D$_3$ (calcitriol) Biologically active form of vitamin D.

11.5 Vitamin D (Calciferol or Calcitriol)

Vitamin D is a fat-soluble vitamin with two unique qualities. First, vitamin D is the only nutrient that is also a hormone. A hormone is a compound manufactured by one organ of the body that then enters the bloodstream and has a physiological effect on another organ or tissue. The cells that participate in the synthesis of vitamin D are different from the cells that respond to vitamin D, namely bone and intestinal cells; therefore, vitamin D is considered a hormone.

Second, vitamin D is the only nutrient that can be produced in the skin upon exposure to ultraviolet light. The human production of vitamin D begins when the ultraviolet B (UVB) rays of the sun convert a cholesterol precursor of vitamin D (**7-dehydrocholesterol**) found in the skin into an inactive form of **vitamin D$_3$ (cholecalciferol)**. As illustrated in Figure 11-7, this compound must be activated to **25-hydroxyvitamin D$_3$ (calcidiol or calcifediol)** in the liver and to **1,25-dihydroxyvitamin D$_3$ (calcitriol)** in the kidney before it can function as the vitamin D hormone.

Our ability to absorb UVB rays and make vitamin D in the skin is affected by many factors. Dark skin pigmentation, geographic latitude, time of day, season of the year, weather conditions, and amount of body surface covered with clothing or sunscreen affect the skin's exposure to UVB rays and therefore influence vitamin D synthesis. Something as simple as complete cloud cover or severe pollution can reduce UVB rays by 50%. In addition, UVB rays will not penetrate glass. Aging reduces our ability to synthesize vitamin D—as much as 70% by age 70! Exposure of hands, face, and arms for about 15 minutes daily will support adequate vitamin D synthesis for most healthy children and adults. However, older adults and individuals

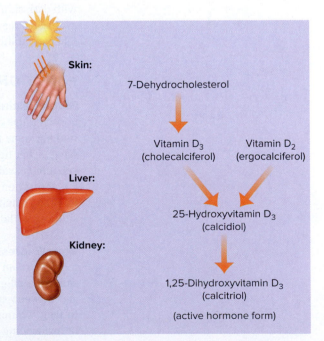

FIGURE 11-7 ▲ A precursor to vitamin D is synthesized when skin is exposed to sunlight. Previtamin D must be further modified by the liver and kidney for maximal activity.

TABLE 11-4 ■ **Factors That Impair Vitamin D Status**

Factor	Description
Inadequate sun exposure • Northern latitudes • Excess clothing (e.g., robes/veils) • Air pollution (i.e., smog) • Sunscreen with SPF > 8 • Excessive time spent indoors (e.g., due to health, work, or environmental conditions)	Limited exposure to UVB reduces the skin's ability to synthesize vitamin D.
Age	Vitamin D synthesis by the skin decreases. Vitamin D activation by the kidneys decreases.
Dark skin pigmentation	Melanin reduces the skin's ability to produce vitamin D, particularly for older adults and especially among women.
Inadequate dietary intake	Dietary intake of vitamin D is unable to compensate for inadequate skin synthesis of vitamin D.
Exclusive breastfeeding or low consumption of infant formula	Infants typically have limited sun exposure. Breast milk is a poor source of vitamin D. Infant formula contains vitamin D, but young infants may not consume adequate quantities to meet needs.
Fat malabsorption • Liver disease • Cystic fibrosis • Weight-loss medications	Poor absorption of dietary fat limits absorption of vitamin D from the small intestine.
Obesity	Release of vitamin D stored in subcutaneous fat is inefficient.
Liver diseases	Vitamin D activation by the liver decreases.
Kidney diseases	Vitamin D activation by the kidneys decreases.

with dark skin pigmentation require about three to five times this amount of sun exposure to synthesize an equivalent amount of vitamin D. Table 11-4 summarizes the various factors that can inhibit vitamin D synthesis, absorption, and activation.

FUNCTIONS OF VITAMIN D

Blood Calcium Regulation The main function of vitamin D (calcitriol) is to maintain the normal range of calcium and phosphorus in the blood. Together with the hormones parathyroid hormone (PTH) and calcitonin, vitamin D closely maintains blood calcium in a narrow range. This tight regulation of blood calcium level ensures that an appropriate amount of calcium is available to all cells. Vitamin D regulates calcium in three ways: (1) it influences the absorption of calcium and phosphorus from the small intestine; (2) in combination with PTH and calcitonin, it regulates calcium excretion via the kidney; and (3) it affects the deposition or withdrawal of minerals from the bones (Fig. 11-8).

Gene Expression and Cell Growth It is now accepted that the biological effects of vitamin D extend far beyond its role in bone health. Vitamin D is involved in gene expression and cell growth; it binds to and subsequently affects cells of the immune system, brain and nervous system, parathyroid gland, pancreas, skin, muscles, and reproductive organs. In fact, vitamin D is considered one of the most potent regulators of cell growth, capable of influencing normal development of some cells (e.g., skin, colon, prostate, and breast), in turn reducing cancer risk in these sites (see Further Reading 16). Besides its role in influencing cancer risk, evidence suggests that vitamin D has a role in the prevention of several chronic diseases, such as cardiovascular disease, diabetes, and hypertension.

(a) Increased production of calcium-absorbing proteins in the small intestine subsequently increases the amount of calcium absorbed from the intestinal tract.

(b) (with PTH) Decreased calcium excretion in the urine

(c) (with PTH) Increased osteoclast activity causes release of calcium from bones into blood

Active vitamin D hormone

FIGURE 11-8 ◄ Vitamin D regulates blood calcium. When blood levels of calcium begin to drop from the normal range, PTH stimulates the synthesis of the most active form of vitamin D (calcitriol) by the kidney. Calcitriol acts at three different sites to increase blood calcium: (a) small intestine, (b) kidney, and (c) bone. When blood calcium levels increase above the normal range, PTH release is inhibited and calcitonin is released, which has the opposite effects of PTH.

VITAMIN D DEFICIENCY

When vitamin D levels are adequate, about 30% to 40% of dietary calcium is absorbed by the small intestine. If blood levels of vitamin D are low, the small intestine is able to absorb only about 10% to 15% of calcium from the diet, which is not enough to maintain the calcium requirements for bone health and other functions. Without adequate levels of vitamin D in the blood, calcium absorption from the small intestine decreases. Subsequently, calcium and phosphorus deposition during bone synthesis is reduced, resulting in weak bones that do not develop properly. Vitamin D deficiency can be traced to poor dietary intake, poor absorption (e.g., fat malabsorption in children with cystic fibrosis), altered metabolism (e.g., liver or kidney disease), or inadequate sun exposure. Studies have shown that vitamin D deficiency can be a problem in individuals with dark skin and the elderly. Vitamin D deficiency is a concern among young infants who are not receiving (1) vitamin D supplementation, (2) sufficient exposure to sunlight, or (3) fortified food (e.g., cereal and dairy products).

Vitamin D deficiency can occur at any time, but when it occurs during infancy and early childhood, the resulting disease is known as rickets. The skeletal abnormalities of rickets include bowed legs, thick wrists and ankles, curvature of the spine, a pigeon chest (chest protrudes above the sternum), skull malformations, and pelvic deformities (Fig. 11-9). Studies show that vitamin D deficiency is prevalent among children and adolescents in the United States. It was estimated that 9% of children (7.6 million) in the United States were vitamin D deficient in 2009 (see Further Reading 5). For the prevention of rickets, infants should be provided supplemental vitamin D (under a physician's guidance). Keep in mind, however, that supplements need to be used carefully to avoid vitamin D toxicity in the infant.

Osteomalacia, which means soft bone, is an adult disease comparable to rickets. It can result from inadequate calcium intake, inefficient calcium absorption in the intestine, or poor conservation of calcium by the kidneys. It occurs most commonly in people with kidney, stomach, gallbladder, or intestinal disease (especially when most of the intestine has been removed) and in people with cirrhosis of the liver. These diseases affect both vitamin D activation and calcium absorption, leading to a decrease in bone mineral density. Bones become porous and weak and break easily. Research shows that treatment with 10 to 20 micrograms (400 to 800 IU) per day of vitamin D, in conjunction with adequate dietary calcium, can reduce fracture risk in older adults. Thus, vitamin D is just as important as calcium when it comes to bone health.

Individuals who are most at risk of a vitamin D deficiency are older than the age of 60, live in northern latitudes, have dark skin, are rarely outdoors or always wear sunscreen while outdoors, have chronic kidney disease, take medications that interfere with vitamin D absorption, have a condition that prevents fat absorption, or have had part of their stomach or intestine removed. A combination of sun exposure, dietary vitamin D intake, and vitamin D supplementation can prevent this problem.

osteomalacia Adult form of rickets. The bones have low mineral density and subsequently are at risk for fracture.

FIGURE 11-9 ▲ Vitamin D deficiency causes rickets, in which the bones and teeth do not develop normally. © Jeffrey I. Rotman/Corbis

▲ Solar radiation (UVB rays) on the skin is the most reliable way to maintain vitamin D status and provides about 80% to 100% of the vitamin D humans use. In the absence of adequate sun exposure, the body must rely on dietary sources of vitamin D to meet needs. To get the vitamin D value of 10 minutes of exposure to sunlight, you would have to eat 30 servings of fortified cereal or 30 cups of fortified orange juice. © Royalty-Free/Corbis

vitamin D-2 (ergocalciferol) Form found in nonanimal sources, such as in some mushrooms.

Vitamin D

RDA: 15 micrograms (600 IU)
DV: 10 micrograms (400 IU)
UL: 100 micrograms (4000 IU)

GETTING ENOUGH VITAMIN D

There are two forms of vitamin D: vitamin D-2 and vitamin D-3. **Vitamin D-2 (ergocalciferol)** is a synthetic product derived from the irradiation of plant sterols (ergosterol) and is used in some supplements. Vitamin D-3 (cholecalciferol)—the form synthesized in the human body—is more commonly used in supplements and fortified foods. Both forms of vitamin D must be modified by chemical reactions that occur in the kidney and liver (see Fig. 11-7) before they can be active in the body.

Sunlight is the best source of vitamin D. Unlike with supplements, you can never receive a toxic dose. With just 10 minutes of exposure of the arms and legs to sunlight, it is estimated that we synthesize roughly 3000 IU of vitamin D. To some extent, the vitamin D synthesized on sunny days can be stored "for a rainy day" in the liver and adipose cells. However, most people now limit sun exposure to decrease their risk of skin cancer. Unless you live in a year-round sunny climate and find yourself outside most days between 10 A.M. and 3 P.M., you are not meeting your vitamin D needs from sun exposure alone. Therefore, people residing in northern climates and with limited sun exposure in general should find alternative (dietary) sources, especially in the winter months (Fig. 11-10). Overall, anyone who does not receive enough direct exposure to sunshine to synthesize an adequate amount of vitamin D must have a dietary source of the vitamin.

The RDA for vitamin D (see box) is based on a daily intake that is sufficient to maintain bone health and normal calcium metabolism, assuming minimal sun exposure. The Dietary Guidelines for Americans recommend that all children over age 9 and adults should choose more foods that provide vitamin D, which is a nutrient of concern in American diets (see Further Reading 1).

Dietary sources of vitamin D are limited, with few foods being naturally high in vitamin D (Fig. 11-11). Fatty fish are considered the richest natural sources of vitamin D. Wild-caught salmon tops the list with around 600 to 1000 IU of vitamin D in a 3.5-ounce serving. Farmed salmon contains less: between 100 and 250 IU per 3.5-ounce serving. Canned salmon has even more vitamin D because it contains soft, edible bones. Tuna is a bit farther down the list with 6 ounces of canned light tuna providing about 300 IU. Eggs are another natural source with 1 large egg yolk delivering 41 IU. Although butter, liver, and a few brands of margarine contain some vitamin D, large servings must be eaten to obtain an appreciable amount of the vitamin; therefore, these foods are not considered significant sources.

Fortified foods are also an effective way to add vitamin D to your dietary pattern. Use of vitamin D–fortified milk, which began in the 1930s, effectively wiped out rickets in the United States. Because vitamin D is a fat-soluble vitamin, there is slightly more in a cup of whole milk (124 IU) compared to 1% (120 IU) or nonfat (115 IU) milk (this information will help you with the What Would You Choose feature in this chapter). Consumption of at least 2 cups of vitamin D–fortified milk a day is advisable for people at risk for vitamin D deficiency. Ready-to-eat breakfast cereals are also fortified with vitamin D and other vitamins

FIGURE 11-10 ▶ Seasonal variations to sunlight intensity. If you live north of 42 degrees N latitude, the angle of the winter sun is such that the sun's rays must pass through more of the atmosphere than at other times of the year. As a result, skin forms less pro-hormone vitamin D in the winter. The 42nd parallel crosses North America at the northern border of California on the West Coast and Boston on the East Coast. In the far North (e.g., Alaska), this effect can last up to 6 months. Living below the 34th parallel (i.e., south of Los Angeles to Columbia, South Carolina), UVB exposure is adequate year round.

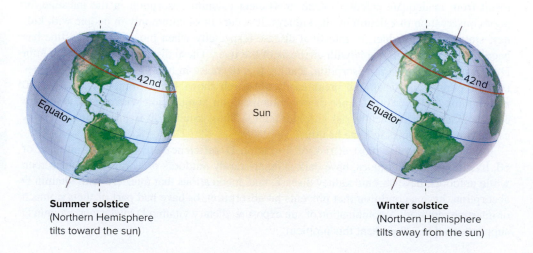

Summer solstice
(Northern Hemisphere tilts toward the sun)

Winter solstice
(Northern Hemisphere tilts away from the sun)

(a)

(b)

Food Item and Amount	Vitamin D (micrograms)	% RDA for Adult Males and Females (15 micrograms)
Grains Total® Raisin Bran cereal, 1 cup	2.5	17%
Cheerios® cereal, 1 cup	1.0	7%
White bread, 1 slice	0.0	0%
Fruits Orange juice (fortified), 1 cup	2.5	17%
Blackberries, 1 cup	0.0	0%
Kiwi, 1 cup	0.0	0%
Dairy Milk, whole, 1 cup	3.2	21%
Milk, fat-free, 1 cup	2.9	19%
Almond milk, sweetened, 1 cup	2.4	16%
Protein Salmon, baked, 3 ounces	11.0	73%
Egg, hard-boiled, 1 large	1.1	7%
Cod, baked, 3 ounces	1.0	7%
Fats & Oils Margarine (fortified), 1 teaspoon	0.5	3%
Butter, 1 teaspoon	0.1	1%
Olive oil, 1 teaspoon	0.0	0.0

FIGURE 11-11 ▲ Food sources of vitamin D. (a) The fill of the background color (none, 1/3, 2/3, or completely covered) within each food group on MyPlate indicates the average nutrient density for vitamin D in that group. (b) The bar graph shows the vitamin D content of several foods in each food group compared to the RDA for adult males and females. Overall, the richest sources of vitamin D are fish, fortified dairy products, and fortified breakfast cereals. Foods from the vegetables group (not shown) are not a source of vitamin D, except for a select variety of mushrooms.
Source: *Nutrition data from USDA National Nutrient Database for Standard Reference, Release 26.*

and minerals. A few provide about 100 IU per 1-cup serving, but most offer closer to 40 IU per serving. You will almost double your intake of vitamin D if you add milk on top of your fortified cereal. Some brands of orange juice are now available fortified with vitamin D (about 140 IU of vitamin D per 1-cup serving). You can count on foods fortified with vitamin D containing not much more than 100 IU per serving because U.S. government regulations cap the added amount at that level.

It takes some planning to meet daily vitamin D requirements from food sources. If you work indoors, live in a northern location, have a family history of skin cancer, and are not eating wild salmon every day, you are going to need a supplement. In supplements and fortified foods, vitamin D is available as vitamin D-2 and vitamin D-3; current research shows that vitamin D-3 is most effective at raising blood levels of vitamin D and reducing fracture risk.

During times of growth (i.e., from infancy through adolescence), consuming adequate vitamin D supports optimal bone mineralization. The American Academy of Pediatrics recommends that all infants, children, and adolescents should consume a minimum of 400 IU of vitamin D daily. Until such intake can be obtained from foods, vitamin D supplementation is endorsed (under a primary care provider's guidance). This recommendation includes all infants (exclusively breastfed, partially breastfed, or formula fed). As you will learn in Chapter 18, breast milk is a poor source of vitamin D, and exclusively breastfed infants with limited sun exposure are at risk for developing rickets. Even though infant formula contains vitamin D (60 IU per 100 kcal), the total intake of formula among young infants may not provide adequate vitamin D to meet needs. Evidence from clinical trials and

▲ The newest addition to foods naturally high in vitamin D is mushrooms. Mushrooms are the only vegetable to contain ergosterol, the precursor of vitamin D. Similar to humans, mushrooms also have the ability to make vitamin D when exposed to ultraviolet light. Although mushrooms are typically grown in the dark and do not contain the vitamin, some brands are now grown in ultraviolet light to stimulate vitamin D production. A vitamin D–rich Portobello mushroom that provides 400 IU of vitamin D per 3-ounce serving (about 1 cup of diced mushrooms) is already available in stores. © Foodcollection

▲ Milk is usually fortified with vitamin D as well as vitamin A. Note that the DV for vitamin D is lower than the RDA for adults. © Royalty-Free/ Corbis

historical precedence support this dosage of vitamin D for infants and children (see Further Reading 4). Keep in mind, however, that supplements need to be used carefully to avoid vitamin D toxicity in the infant.

For adults over the age of 70, the RDA increases to 20 micrograms per day because of the reduced ability to absorb vitamin D from the intestine and decreased ability to synthesize it in the skin. A number of experts suggest older adults, especially those over age 70 who have limited sun exposure or dark skin, receive about 1000 IU (25 micrograms) from a combination of vitamin D–fortified foods and a multivitamin and mineral supplement, with an individual supplement of vitamin D added if needed (see Further Reading 10).

Other population groups that have difficulty meeting vitamin D needs include vegans and people with milk allergies or lactose intolerance. Vitamin D supplements or vitamin D-fortified soy milk or fruit juices are options for people who do not consume dairy products.

AVOIDING TOO MUCH VITAMIN D

Too much vitamin D taken regularly can create serious health consequences in infants and children. Due to the role of vitamin D in calcium absorption, excretion, and release of calcium from bone, supplementation with high doses of vitamin D can cause calcium levels in the blood to increase above the normal range. The UL (see box in this section) is based on the risk of overabsorption of calcium and eventual calcium deposits in the kidneys and other organs. Calcium deposits in organs can cause metabolic disturbances and cell death. Toxicity symptoms also include weakness, loss of appetite, diarrhea, vomiting, mental confusion, and increased urine output. Please note that vitamin D toxicity does not result from excessive exposure to the sun because the body regulates the amount made in the skin (i.e., as exposure to sunlight increases, the efficiency of vitamin D synthesis decreases).

✔ **CONCEPT CHECK 11.5**

1. Why is vitamin D sometimes not considered an "essential" nutrient?
2. What is the association between vitamin D and sun exposure?
3. How is vitamin D activated in the body?
4. How does vitamin D work to maintain blood calcium levels?
5. What are some rich food sources of vitamin D?
6. Can vitamin D be toxic?

11.6 Magnesium

FUNCTIONS OF MAGNESIUM

Magnesium (Mg) is important for nerve and heart function, and aids in many enzyme reactions. Magnesium is similar to calcium and phosphorus in that most of the magnesium in the body is found in bones. Bone contains 60% of the body's magnesium. Magnesium in bones provides rigidity and it functions as a storage site that can be drawn upon by other tissues when dietary intake is inadequate to meet the body's needs. Magnesium functions to relax muscles after contraction. It promotes resistance to tooth decay by stabilizing calcium in tooth enamel. Over 300 enzymes use magnesium, and many energy-yielding compounds in cells require magnesium to function properly (e.g., ATP). Magnesium plays a critical role in the synthesis of DNA and protein. Another notable function of magnesium as it relates to bone health is that magnesium is required for the synthesis of vitamin D in the liver.

Other possible benefits of magnesium in relation to cardiovascular disease include decreasing blood pressure by dilating arteries and preventing heart abnormalities. People with cardiovascular disease should closely monitor magnesium intake, especially because they are often on medications such as diuretics that reduce magnesium status. A diet rich in food sources of magnesium and calcium is associated with lower risk of type 2 diabetes in some populations.

MAGNESIUM DEFICIENCY

In humans, a magnesium deficiency causes an irregular heartbeat, sometimes accompanied by weakness, muscle pain, disorientation, and seizures. In terms of bone health, low magnesium disrupts the hormonal regulation of blood calcium by parathyroid hormone and affects the activity of vitamin D. You might expect that magnesium deficiency would result in diminished bone mass, but to date, this has only been observed in animals. There is some evidence, however, that magnesium supplementation may improve bone density in postmenopausal women.

Magnesium deficiency develops very slowly. Not only is the mineral present in foods of both plant and animal origin, but the kidneys also are very efficient at retaining magnesium. Thus, it is uncommon for healthy people to suffer a clinically relevant magnesium deficiency due to dietary inadequacy alone. Poor magnesium status is most commonly found among people with abnormal kidney function, whether as a result of kidney disease or as a side effect of certain diuretics. Alcohol use disorders also can increase the risk of deficiency because dietary intake may be poor and because alcohol increases magnesium excretion in the urine. The disorientation and weakness associated with alcohol use disorders closely resembles the behavior of people with low blood magnesium. In addition, people with malabsorptive diseases (e.g., Crohn's disease), heavy perspiration, or prolonged bouts of diarrhea or vomiting are susceptible to low blood levels of magnesium.

GETTING ENOUGH MAGNESIUM

Magnesium is found in the plant pigment chlorophyll, so rich sources for magnesium are plant products, such as squash, whole grains (such as wheat bran), beans, nuts, seeds, and broccoli (Fig. 11-12). Animal products (e.g., milk and meats) and chocolate supply some magnesium, although not as much as foods of plant origin. Two other sources of magnesium are hard tap water, which contains a high mineral content, and coffee (espresso, not brewed).

The adult RDA for magnesium (see box) is based on the amount needed to offset daily losses. Adult men consume on average 320 milligrams daily, whereas women consume closer to 220 milligrams daily, suggesting that many of us should improve our intakes of magnesium-rich foods, such as whole-grain breads and cereals. The refined grain products that dominate the diets of many North Americans are poor sources of this mineral because refining reduces the magnesium content by as much as 80%. This low value also reflects poor intake of green and other brightly colored vegetables. If dietary intake of magnesium is inadequate, a balanced multivitamin and mineral supplement containing approximately 100 milligrams of magnesium can help close the gap between intake and needs. Nutrient-nutrient interactions can reduce magnesium absorption. Diets very high in phosphorus or fiber (phytate) limit intestinal absorption, as do diets too low in protein.

Magnesium
RDA:
Adult men: 400 milligrams
Adult women: 310 milligrams
DV: 400 milligrams
UL: 350 milligrams (nonfood sources only)

AVOIDING TOO MUCH MAGNESIUM

The UL for magnesium intake is 350 milligrams per day, based on the risk of developing diarrhea. This guideline refers only to *nonfood* sources such as antacids, laxatives, or supplements (see Further Reading 10). Food sources are not known to cause toxicity. Magnesium toxicity especially occurs in people who have kidney failure or who overuse over-the-counter medications that contain magnesium, such as certain antacids and laxatives (e.g., milk of magnesia). Older people are at particular risk, as kidney function may be compromised.

(a)

(b)

Food Item and Amount	Magnesium (milligrams)	% RDA for Adult Males (400 milligrams)	% RDA for Adult Females (310 milligrams)
Grains			
Raisin bran cereal, 1 cup	72	18%	23%
Whole-wheat bread, 1 slice	24	6%	8%
White bread, 1 slice	7	2%	2%
Vegetables			
Spinach, cooked, 1 cup	157	39%	51%
Okra, cooked, 1 cup	58	15%	19%
Sweet potato, baked, 1 cup	54	14%	17%
Fruits			
Banana, 1 medium	32	8%	10%
Blackberries, 1 cup	29	7%	9%
Pineapple, 1 cup	20	5%	6%
Dairy			
Yogurt, plain, non-fat, 1 cup	47	12%	15%
Soymilk, 1 cup	36	9%	12%
Milk, fat-free, 1 cup	27	7%	9%
Protein			
Peanut butter, 2 tablespoons	49	12%	16%
Navy beans, cooked, ½ cup	48	12%	15%
Chicken breast, roasted, 3 ounces	25	6%	8%

FIGURE 11-12 ▲ Food sources of magnesium. (a) The fill of the background color (none, 1/3, 2/3, or completely covered) within each food group on MyPlate indicates the average nutrient density for magnesium in that group. (b) The bar graph shows the magnesium content of several foods in each food group compared to the RDA for adult males and females. Overall, the richest sources of magnesium are vegetables and whole grains.

Source: *Nutrition data from USDA National Nutrient Database for Standard Reference, Release 26.*

✓ **CONCEPT CHECK 11.6**

1. What are the key functions of magnesium other than bone health?
2. What are the primary food sources of magnesium?
3. Who is at greatest risk of developing a magnesium deficiency?
4. When is magnesium toxicity most likely to occur?

11.7 Fluoride

The fluoride ion (F^-) is the form of this trace mineral essential for human health. Nearly all (about 95%) of the fluoride in the body is found in the teeth and skeleton. Dentists in the early 1900s noticed a lower rate of dental caries (cavities) in the southwestern United States. These areas contained high amounts of fluoride in the water. The amounts of fluoride were sometimes so high that small spots developed on the teeth (mottling). Even though mottled teeth were discolored, they contained few dental caries. Experiments in the early 1940s showed that fluoride in the water decreased the incidence of dental caries by 20% to 80% in children. Fluoridation of public water supplies in many parts of the United States has since been instituted (see Further Reading 13).

FUNCTIONS OF FLUORIDE

Fluoride functions in the following ways to prevent dental caries: (1) incorporates into tooth structure, causing it to be stronger and more resistant to acid degradation from bacteria found in plaque; (2) stimulates remineralization of enamel and inhibits tooth demineralization; and (3) has antibacterial effect on acid-producing microorganisms found in plaque.

GETTING ENOUGH FLUORIDE

The list of foods that are good sources of fluoride is rather short: marine fish, clams, lobster, crab, shrimp, tea, seaweed. Most of our fluoride actually comes from oral hygiene products and the water supply. Numerous products are available to apply fluoride to teeth topically. These include gels applied at a dentist's office, toothpaste, and mouth rinses for everyday use. Fluoride is also available in supplement form, although use should be directed by a dentist or pediatrician. The most economical method of distributing fluoride is to add the mineral to the community's drinking water.

In a few areas of the world, the fluoride content of groundwater is naturally high, but most groundwater supplies contain low levels of fluoride. In the 1950s, after researchers established a connection between fluoride and rates of dental caries, communities in the United States began adding fluoride to the municipal water supply to achieve a fluoride level of 0.7 to 1.2 milligrams per liter. (The lower levels are for communities in hotter climates, where total water consumption is higher.) About two-thirds of North Americans currently consume fluoridated water; these policies are made by individual municipalities. Because most people now have ample access to oral hygiene products with fluoride, in 2011, the U.S. Department of Health and Human Services and the Environmental Protection Agency issued new recommendations to lower the level of water fluoridation to just 0.7 milligram per liter.

The AI for fluoride for adults is 3.1 to 3.8 milligrams per day. This range of intake provides the benefits of resistance to dental caries without causing ill effects. As described, typical fluoridated water contains about 1 milligram per liter, which works out to about 0.25 milligram per cup. In communities without fluoridated water (e.g., those that rely on private well water), use of fluoride-containing oral hygiene products or dietary supplements is of heightened importance for combating dental decay. Note that fluoride is generally not added to bottled water. Frequent use of bottled water or a household reverse osmosis water purification system significantly restricts fluoride intake. A refrigerator or Brita® filter does not remove fluoride. When water fluoridation and fluoridated topical products are used in combination, the reductions in dental caries are additive.

▲ *Healthy People 2020* objectives for the nation set a target goal of 79.6% of the population using piped water to have that water optimally fluoridated. As of 2010, the benefits of community water fluoridation reached nearly 74% of the U.S. population served by community water systems. © Photodisc/Getty Images

fluorosis Discoloration of tooth enamel sometimes accompanied with pitting due to consuming a large amount of fluoride for an excessive period.

AVOIDING TOO MUCH FLUORIDE

The UL for fluoride is set at 1.3 to 2.2 milligrams per day for young children and 10 milligrams per day for children over 9 years of age and adults, based on skeletal and tooth damage seen with higher doses. Children may swallow large amounts of fluoride toothpaste as part of daily tooth care and develop **fluorosis.** During tooth development (first decade of life), fluorosis permanently damages teeth. Fluorosis leads to stained and pitted teeth (Fig. 11-13). Not swallowing toothpaste and limiting the amount used to "pea" size are the best ways to prevent this problem. In addition, children under 6 years should have tooth brushing supervised by an adult and should never use fluoride mouthwash. In adults, fluorosis is associated with hip fractures, weak/stiff joints, and chronic stomach inflammation.

There have been opponents to the fluoridation of public water supplies. Some people argue that water fluoridation standards were set at a time when much of the population did not have adequate access to fluoride-containing oral hygiene products, and that addition of fluoride to the water supply is no longer necessary. Other critics claim that chronic exposure to fluoridated water

FIGURE 11-13 ▲ Example of mottling (brown spots) in a tooth caused by overexposure to fluoride. Fluoride has been shown to increase protein synthesis in the osteoblast and subsequently have an effect on the production of new bone. © Paul Casamassimo, DDS, MS

Fluoride

AI: 3.1 to 3.8 milligrams

UL:

Young children: 1.3 to 2.2 milligrams

>9 years: 10 milligrams

is linked to a variety of health ailments affecting the skeletal, nervous, or endocrine systems. At this time, there is little scientific evidence to support claims that water fluoridation at current levels has adverse health effects other that dental fluorosis, but this is definitely an area for continued study. The updated recommendations for the level of water fluoridation aim to take advantage of the oral health benefits of fluoride while limiting unwanted health effects, including fluorosis (see Further Reading 11).

✓ CONCEPT CHECK 11.7

1. When is fluoride incorporated into teeth?
2. How does fluoride help reduce the development of dental caries?
3. What are our primary sources of fluoride?
4. What are the risks of excessive fluoride intake?

11.8 Other Nutrients Involved in Bone Health

In addition to those already discussed, there are several other vitamins and minerals that contribute to bone health (Table 11-5). For some, including vitamin K and boron, research clearly links dietary intake or blood nutrient levels to bone health outcomes. Others are still topics of current investigation (see Further Reading 14).

Both vitamins C and K are required for production of the organic phase of bone, which is comprised of collagen (90%) and other smaller matrix proteins, including **osteocalcin.** Other micronutrients that participate in the synthesis of collagen are iron, zinc, copper, and silicon. Vitamin C is essential for the formation of collagen, a hard, insoluble, fibrous protein found in connective tissue, bone, teeth, tendons, and blood vessels. Vitamin C deficiency in infants and children can impair bone growth. Aside from its role in collagen synthesis, vitamin C has been proposed to promote bone health through its antioxidant activity. High levels of oxidative stress contribute to bone resorption. Therefore, nutrients such as vitamin C and the carotenoids may preserve bone mineral density by limiting oxidative stress. Observational and experimental data regarding the antioxidant roles of vitamin C and carotenoids in bone health show mixed results and may depend on other factors, such as gender, smoking, and intake of other bone-building nutrients. Vitamin C and the carotenoids were discussed in relation to their antioxidant roles in Chapter 10.

Vitamin K activates proteins that are present in bone, muscle, and kidneys, thereby imparting calcium-binding potential to these organs. Vitamin K chemically modifies the protein osteocalcin, which is required for calcium to be added to and removed from bone. Osteocalcin is one of the most abundant small matrix proteins found in bones and the only matrix protein synthesized exclusively there. In one large study, men and women with the highest vitamin K intakes had a 65% lower risk of hip fractures compared to those with the lowest vitamin K intakes. Another study showed a relationship between high blood levels of vitamin K and reduced risk of vertebral fracture. Vitamin K will be discussed in more depth regarding its role in blood health in Chapter 13.

Two ultratrace minerals—boron and silicon—have been implicated in bone health. Recall that ultratrace minerals have no known dietary requirements, but they are present in the body in small amounts and participate in some body functions. Boron contributes to bone structure and strength due to its influences on osteoblast and osteoclast activity, transport of calcium across membranes, and vitamin D synthesis. Elderly women fed a low-boron diet had low blood levels of calcium and magnesium. Some studies indicate boron also participates in brain and immune functions, and other studies have examined a relationship between boron intake and cancer risk. There is no AI or RDA set, but an estimated daily requirement is 1 milligram per day. The UL for boron is 20 milligrams per day.

osteocalcin Small protein in the organic matrix of bone.

▲ This meal of almond chicken, broccoli, and brown rice provides several nutrients that are good for bone health. How does it compare to the MyPlate recommendations? © D. Fischer and P. Lyons/Cole Group/Getty Images

TABLE 11-5 ■ **Micronutrients That Function in Bone Health**

Nutrient	Primary Function in Bone	Common Food Sources
Calcium	Provides rigidity to bone; 99% of calcium in the human body is found in bones and teeth	Milk, yogurt, fortified orange juice, sardines, canned salmon, fortified foods and beverages
Phosphorus	Critical component of hydroxyapatite crystals in bone	Yogurt, almonds, milk, cheese, salmon, meats, eggs, soft drinks
Vitamin D	Regulates calcium and phosphorus levels for bone integrity and maintenance	Fish, milk, fortified cereals; best source is sunlight
Magnesium	Promotes resistance to tooth decay by holding calcium in tooth enamel; stored in bone like calcium; cofactor in vitamin D activation	Dark-green leafy vegetables, peanut butter, beans and peas, bananas, almonds
Fluoride	Strengthens bones and teeth; stimulates osteoblasts	Seafood, seaweed, tea; community water supplies have added fluoride; may not be present in bottled drinking water
Vitamin C	Participates in collagen synthesis; may protect bone from oxidative damage	Citrus fruits, strawberries, broccoli, leafy green vegetables
Vitamin K	Imparts calcium-binding ability to bone proteins	Green vegetables, liver, some plant oils, some calcium supplements
Zinc	Cofactor for enzymes in bone remodeling; contributes to collagen synthesis	Seafood, meats, green vegetables, whole grains
Copper	Contributes to collagen synthesis	Liver, cocoa, beans, nuts, whole grains, dried fruits
Iron	Cofactor in vitamin D activation; contributes to collagen synthesis	Meats, seafood, broccoli, peas, bran, enriched bread
Manganese	Cofactor for bone-remodeling enzymes	Nuts, oats, beans, tea
Potassium	Maintains alkaline blood pH, which prevents withdrawal of bone minerals for use as buffers	Spinach, squash, bananas, orange juice, milk, meat, legumes, whole grains
Boron	Influences osteoblast and osteoclast activity; participates in calcium transport; involved in synthesis of vitamin D	Fruits, vegetables, nuts, whole grains
Silicon	Contributes to collagen synthesis	Beer, bananas, string beans

Silicon, as already noted, participates in collagen synthesis. No UL for silicon has been established. Toxicity of silicon has been observed in people taking large amounts of silicon-containing antacids over a long period. The consequences are an increased incidence of kidney stones and decreased levels of some antioxidant enzymes. A serious respiratory condition called silicosis occurs with the inhalation of silicon dust.

Iron is required by an enzyme that converts vitamin D to its active form in the body. Manganese and zinc are examples of minerals that are required as cofactors for enzymes of bone remodeling. Iron, zinc, copper, and manganese will be explored further in Chapters 12 and 13. As you can see, dietary recommendations for bone health should extend beyond dairy products. Indeed, a diet rich in fruits and vegetables contains ample vitamin C, vitamin K, and several key trace minerals. Overall, following a dietary pattern that matches MyPlate will promote optimal bone health.

✔ **CONCEPT CHECK 11.8**

1. What is the role of vitamin K in bone health?
2. How does boron contribute to bone structure?

11.9 Osteoporosis

osteoporosis The presence of a stress-induced fracture or a T-score of −2.5 or lower. The bones are porous and fragile due to low mineral density.

Healthy People 2020 identified the prevention of the bone disease **osteoporosis** as one of its major focus areas. In 2014, the National Osteoporosis Foundation (NOF) reported that 54 million U.S. adults age 50 and older, more than one-half of the total U.S. adult population, is affected by osteoporosis and low bone mass (see Further Reading 17). Of those affected, 10.2 million currently have osteoporosis and another 43.4 have low bone mass. Of those with osteoporosis, it is estimated that 7.7 million are non-Hispanic White, 0.5 million are non-Hispanic Black, and 0.6 million are Mexican American. The numbers of adults over 50 with osteoporosis or low bone mass is increasing and expected to reach 64.4 million by 2020 and 71.2 million by 2030.

Osteoporosis continues to lead to approximately 2 million bone fractures per year in the United States, including nearly 300,000 broken hips. The health care costs associated with these fractures are projected to reach more than $25 billion by the year 2025, with the most rapid increases among minority populations (Fig. 11-14). The personal cost of a hip fracture surpasses any financial cost. Hip fractures are regarded as devastating. They result in loss of mobility and the need for long-term care. Women experience 80% of hip fractures, and the average age for hip fracture is 80 years (see Further Reading 6). Only 40% of people with hip fractures regain their earlier level of independence. More specifically, it is estimated that a year after fracturing a hip, 90% of those who needed no assistance climbing stairs before the fracture will not be able to climb five stairs; 66% will need help to get on or off a toilet; 50% will not be able to raise themselves from a chair; 31% will need assistance to get out of bed; and 20% will not be able to put on a pair of pants by themselves.

Hip fracture is associated with significant mortality. It is estimated that 20% to 30% of the 300,000 Americans 65 or older who fracture a hip each year will die within 12 months. Results from the national Fracture Intervention Trial showed a six times greater risk of mortality associated with a hip fracture among postmenopausal women with low bone mass. Other types of fractures or even fear of fracture due to osteoporosis can affect quality of life. Vertebral fractures, especially if there are several of them, cause significant pain, reduced lung function, loss of height, and a curved spine. Movement can be restricted and gait altered, increasing the risk and fear of falls and/or more fractures.

Women tend to lose 1% to 3% of their bone mass each year after menopause. Men also lose bone mass as they age, but the loss is more gradual. When the bone-demineralizing activities of osteoclasts exceed the bone-building activities of osteoblasts, bone mass

▲ Osteoporosis leads to millions of bone fractures each year, including debilitating fractures of the hip and spine. These fractures frequently result in the need for assistance with activities of daily living, as we see with this woman who needs a walker to help her navigate. © Realistic Reflections

FIGURE 11-14 ▶ Projected economic burden of osteoporosis by race/ethnicity, 2005–2025.

Source: Burge and others: Incidence and mortality of hip fractures in the United States. *Journal of Bone and Mineral Research* 22:465, 2007. Photo: ©Don Farrall/Getty Images.

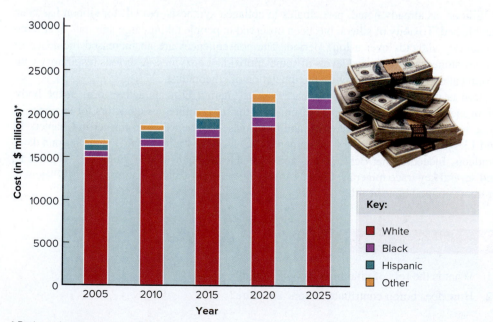

Key:
- ■ White
- ■ Black
- ■ Hispanic
- ■ Other

* Projected costs are not adjusted for inflation.

declines. This is a normal part of aging and does not always lead to unhealthy bones. However, if bone mass is low when this process begins, even moderate bone demineralization can lead to a condition called **osteopenia.** As more bone is lost, the entire matrix of the bone tissue also begins to break down. When this occurs, osteoporosis is likely to result. About 25% of women older than age 50 develop or have osteoporosis. Among people older than age 80, osteoporosis becomes the rule, not the exception. To young adults, it may sound benign to have osteoporosis. To older adults, the diagnosis presents the reality of life permanently changed.

TYPE 1 AND TYPE 2 OSTEOPOROSIS

There are two types of osteoporosis. **Type 1 osteoporosis,** also called postmenopausal osteoporosis, typically occurs in women between 50 and 60 years of age. This type of osteoporosis is directly linked to decreased estrogen concentrations that occur at menopause. Type 1 osteoporosis most dramatically affects trabecular bone, as this type of bone undergoes faster remodeling than cortical bone (Fig. 11-15).

A woman can lose 20% to 30% of trabecular bone and 5% to 10% of cortical bone between ages 50 and 60, unless intervention occurs (Fig. 11-16).

Trabecular bone has a much higher density of osteoblast and osteoclast cells than cortical bone. The osteoblast cells require estrogen for maximal activity. After menopause, osteoblast activity decreases; however, osteoclast activity remains high. The result is greater bone resorption than resynthesis. Minerals are released but not reincorporated into bone, so the locations where the osteoclasts left reserves or pockets for osteoblasts to rebuild the collagen mineral matrix will now become holes. The bones at greatest risk for osteoporotic fractures are the trabecular-rich bones of the

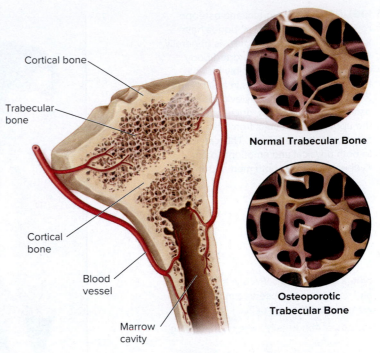

Normal Trabecular Bone

Osteoporotic Trabecular Bone

Cortical bone

Trabecular bone

Cortical bone

Blood vessel

Marrow cavity

FIGURE 11-15 ▲ Cortical and trabecular bone. Cortical bone forms the shafts of bones and their outer mineral covering. Trabecular bone supports the outer shell of cortical bone in various bones of the body. Note how the osteoporotic bone has much less trabecular bone. This leads to a more fragile bone and is not reversible to any major extent with current therapies.

osteopenia A bone disease defined by low mineral density.

type 1 osteoporosis Porous trabecular bone characterized by rapid bone demineralization following menopause.

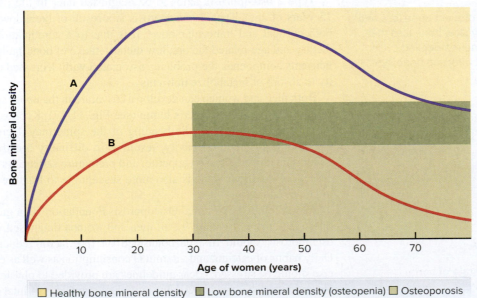

• **Woman A** had developed a high peak bone mass by age 30. Her bone loss was slow and steady between ages 30 and 50 and sped up somewhat after age 50 because of the effects of menopause. At age 75, the woman had a healthy bone mineral density value and did not show evidence of osteoporosis.

• **Woman B** with low peak bone mass experienced the same rate of bone loss as Woman A. By age 50, she already had low bone mineral density and by age 70, kyphosis and spinal fractures had occurred.

☐ Healthy bone mineral density ☐ Low bone mineral density (osteopenia) ☐ Osteoporosis

FIGURE 11-16 ▲ The relationship between peak bone mass and the ultimate risk of developing osteoporosis and related bone fractures.

Source: Based on data from R. Burge: Incidence and economic burden of osteoporosis related fractures in the United States, 2005–2025, Journal of Bone and Mineral Research, 22, 2007, 465.

FIGURE 11-17 ▶ Normal and osteoporotic woman. Osteoporotic bones have less substance, so osteoporosis generally leads to loss of height, distorted body shape, fractures, and possibly loss of teeth. Monitoring changes in adult height is one way to detect early evidence of osteoporosis. Kyphosis, or curvature of the upper spine, results from demineralization of the vertebrae. This can lead to both physical and emotional pain. Kyphosis occurs in both men and women.

type 2 osteoporosis Porous trabecular and cortical bone observed in men and women after the age of 70.

kyphosis Abnormally increased bending of the spine.

bisphosphonates Drugs that bind minerals and prevent osteoclast breakdown of bone. Examples are alendronate (Fosamax) and risedronate (Actonel).

Young woman

Elderly woman

Wedged upper vertebrae

Crushed lower vertebrae

Medicine Cabinet

Types of Osteoporosis Medications

Antiresorptive medications are used to prevent bone loss and decrease the risk of bone fractures. They slow bone loss that occurs during the breakdown phase of the remodeling cycle. These medicines slow bone loss without affecting bone synthesis so that bone density can increase.

- Bisphosphonates
- Alendronate (Fosamax® and Fosamax Plus D®)
- Ibandronate (Boniva®)
- Risedronate (Actonel®, Actonel® with Calcium, and Atelvia™)
- Zoledronic acid (Reclast®)
- Calcitonin (Fortical® and Miacalcin®)
- Denosumab (Prolia®)
- Estrogen therapy
- Estrogen agonists/antagonists (Evista®)

Anabolic drugs are used to increase the rate of bone formation and decrease the risk of fractures.

- Teriparatide (Forteo®) is currently the only osteoporosis medicine approved by FDA that rebuilds bone.

Circle of pills: © Footage supplied by Goodshoot/Punchstock.

pelvis (7% of fractures), vertebrae of the spine (27%) (Fig. 11-17), and portions of long bones such as the wrist (19%). People with either form of osteoporosis can lose significant height and experience severe pain, especially in the vertebrae. A woman may lose an inch or more in height as the bone is demineralized (see Fig. 11-17).

Type 2 osteoporosis tends to be diagnosed later in life (70 to 75 years of age). Type 2 osteoporosis is a result of breakdown of both cortical and trabecular bone. It is due to a combination of dietary and age-related factors; low dietary intake of bone-building nutrients compounds the problems associated with decreased ability to absorb or metabolize nutrients.

Both men and women can develop a curvature in the upper spine called **kyphosis** or dowager's hump (see Fig. 11-17). Kyphosis is a major concern because the bending of the spine may decrease the volume of the chest cavity, resulting in difficulty breathing, abdominal pain, decreased appetite, and premature satiety. As discussed, osteoporotic bone is also more susceptible to fracture following a fall.

According to the National Osteoporosis Foundation 2014 guidelines (see Further Reading 9), all men and women diagnosed with osteoporosis should first be counseled on risk factor reduction. Daily habits of calcium and vitamin D consumption as well as exercise should be stressed. Clear guidelines are provided to physicians for patients to be considered for pharmacological (drug) intervention. These drugs are indicated for postmenopausal women and men over 50 who meet specific standards for level of risk of future fracture as well as medical history (see Further Reading 7). Current medication options for men and women are **bisphosphonates** and

CASE STUDY   Worried About Grandma

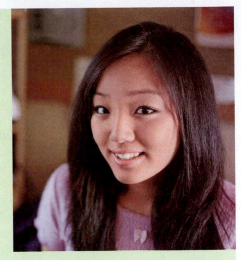

© Dennis Wise/Getty Images

Grace, a 23-year-old woman of Korean descent, is in her final year of nursing school in Boston. She also works 20 hours per week at a local pharmacy. Grace is worried about a phone call she just received from her mom. While out on her walk yesterday, Grandmother Kyon caught her toe on an uneven section of the sidewalk, fell, and broke her hip. The doctor diagnosed Grandmother Kyon with osteoporosis, and the family is worried about the long recovery ahead. As a nursing student, Grace knows how devastating a hip fracture can be. She also knows that osteoporosis can run in families. Grace resolves to do whatever she can to learn about osteoporosis and strengthen her bones now.

She starts by searching the Internet for a website that can help her determine if she is at high risk for osteoporosis. The New York State Department of Health Osteoporosis Education Prevention Program, http://www.health.ny.gov/publications/2047, offers a list of risk factors for osteoporosis. For herself, Grace sees a few risk factors that she cannot change, but there are a few that are glaringly obvious. She uses this website to "bone up" on ways to promote her bone health while she is still young.

Grace discovers she is probably pretty low in vitamin D intake. She also does not have much free time for exercise. She cooks traditional Korean dishes for half of her meals but eats fast food or sandwiches for the rest. Daily, she takes a multivitamin/mineral pill plus one calcium carbonate pill. She generally takes them when she brushes her teeth at night before bed. On weekends, she gets out with friends or her boyfriend and has a glass or two of wine. Grace does not smoke.

Answer the following questions about Grace's situation and check your responses at the end of the chapter.

1. Go to the URL that Grace visited and click on the link for Risk Factors for Osteoporosis. What risk factors do you see for Grace? What additional questions would you ask Grace to assess her risk for osteoporosis?
2. Grace went to the section "Keeping Your Bones and Teeth Strong for Life" to determine key actions she can take to strengthen her bones now. Which ones does she already do? Which lifestyle actions could Grace integrate into her daily life right now?
3. What are the environmental conditions that inhibit Grace from adequately synthesizing vitamin D? How can she overcome some of them?
4. What are some calcium and vitamin D sources in traditional Korean dishes?
5. Give Grace some tips to increase her calcium and vitamin D intake at fast-food restaurants without significantly increasing costs or calories.
6. Would you recommend any changes to her supplement regimen?

parathyroid hormone. Women may also use calcium and hormone replacement therapy (see Medicine Cabinet for a list of osteoporosis medications).

The incidence of osteoporosis increases as a person ages. Its significance as a personal and public health problem is intensifying as the U.S. population ages. It appears, however, that a large percentage of the cases of osteoporosis can be prevented. The key to prevention is to build dense bones during the first 30 years of life and then limit the amount of bone loss in adulthood. People with higher peak bone mass have more calcium to lose before bones become weak and fracture easily. A higher peak bone mass is also the reason males experience osteoporosis less often than females do; they have more bone mass to lose.

✓ CONCEPT CHECK 11.9

1. What type of injuries are most likely to happen as a result of osteoporosis?
2. What are the two types of osteoporosis and how do they differ?
3. What type of bone is most affected by osteoporosis?
4. Why is the achievement of peak bone mass as a young adult so important in preventing osteoporosis?
5. What are some current treatments for osteoporosis?

11.10 Bone Health Assessment

Until the 1990s, there were no convenient clinical measurement devices health care professionals could use to assess bone health. A routine X-ray could detect osteoporosis, but not until 30% or more of bone mass was already lost. A hairline fracture of the vertebrae also was used to diagnose osteoporosis. Both of these tools diagnosed the presence of osteoporosis, but did not predict risk. Today, we have tools that can quantitate bone mass and bone density, and, subsequently, the likelihood of a person's developing bone disease.

The most accurate test for assessing bone density is the central **dual energy X-ray absorptiometry (DEXA)** measurement of the hip and spine. The central DEXA procedure is simple, painless, safe, noninvasive, and generally takes less than 15 minutes. The ability of the bone to block the path of a low-level X ray is used as a measure of bone mineral density. A very low dose of radiation is used for the DEXA—about one-tenth of the exposure from a chest X ray. The hip and spine are measured because these sites are commonly affected by osteoporosis and are likely to result in more serious injuries.

From the DEXA measurement of bone density, a T-score is generated, which compares the observed bone density to that of a person at peak bone mass (e.g., age 30). The T-score is interpreted as shown in Figure 11-18.

dual energy X-ray absorptiometry (DEXA) A scientific tool used to measure bone mineral density.

THE T-SCORE SCALE

A bone mineral density test compares your bone density to that of a "young, normal" adult with peak bone density. Results are given as a T-score, which indicates how much your reading deviates from that desirable density. The World Health Organization defines T-scores on the scale below.

Normal bone density (> – 1.0):
Low risk of osteoporosis and/or fractures

Low bone density or osteopenia (–1.0 to –2.5):
Moderate risk of poor bone health

Osteoporosis (< – 2.5):
High risk of poor bone health

FIGURE 11-18 ▲ The classification for diagnosing osteoporosis is used by the World Health Organization. A T-score of −1.0 or higher is normal; a T-score from −1.0 to −2.5 indicates low bone mass and is known as osteopenia; and a T-score less than −2.5 indicates osteoporosis. Severe osteoporosis is diagnosed with a T-score of −2.5 or lower and a personal history of fragility fracture.

The National Osteoporosis Foundation 2014 recommendations call for DEXA testing for the following groups of people:

- All women age 65 and older and men age 70 and older
- Younger postmenopausal women and men (ages 50 to 69) who have risk factors
- Women going through perimenopause (transitioning into menopause) who have low body weight, have prior low-trauma fracture, or take high-risk medications, such as steroids
- Adults with fracture after age 50
- Adults with a health condition for which they take steroids for a prolonged period (e.g., rheumatoid arthritis, Crohn's disease, asthma)
- Anyone being considered for medication for osteoporosis or receiving therapy for osteoporosis

When DEXA measurements of the hip and spine are not feasible due to portability, expense, or morbid obesity, several peripheral measurements of bone density can be used as screening methods at various sites on the body. Peripheral DEXA uses the same technology as central DEXA but scans only the ankle or wrist. Peripheral quantitative computed tomography (pQCT) generates a three-dimensional scan of the radius in the arm or the tibia in the lower leg. It measures bone mineral density and can provide information on cortical and trabecular bone density, area, and thickness, as well as some measurements of bone strength. The quantitative ultrasound (QUS) technique uses sound waves to measure the density of bone in the heel, shin, and kneecap. These peripheral tests are sometimes used at health fairs, medical offices, and research settings. Although they cannot be used to diagnose osteoporosis, they can inform the health care provider if additional testing (i.e., central DEXA) is warranted.

Whether or not you have had your bone mineral density tested, you can also use the online Fracture Risk Assessment Tool (FRAX) to estimate your risk of fracture. You can calculate your FRAX score at http://www.shef.ac.uk/FRAX. The National Osteoporosis Foundation Guide recommends that doctors consider prescribing medication if your risk of a hip fracture is at least 3% over the next 10 years. The incidence of osteoporosis is far less in many other countries than in the United States. In reviewing Tables 11-1 and 11-2, you can see that the contributions for the greater incidence in the United States are mainly related to diet and other lifestyle behaviors. That means that osteoporosis can largely be prevented.

To summarize, the synthesis, maintenance, and repair of bone requires several vitamins, minerals, and hormones. The key nutrients include vitamin D and the minerals calcium, phosphorus, magnesium, and fluoride. Other nutrients that support bone health include vitamins C and K, boron, and silicon. In addition, adequate protein must be consumed, especially in the elderly, to reduce bone loss.

✓ CONCEPT CHECK 11.10

1. What is the most accurate test for bone density and how is it done?
2. According to the National Osteoporosis Foundation, who should have their bone density checked?
3. What are some less expensive tests of bone density or fracture risk that can be done?

Bone Health Without Dairy

▲ It is not just dairy! If you are lactose intolerant or just do not like dairy, you can still find calcium in foods. Soy and rice milks as well as some types of orange juice are fortified with calcium. © Stockbyte/Getty Images

© Food Passionates/Corbis

Why Go Dairy Free?

There are many reasons why you may choose to avoid dairy products. These include following a vegan diet or just trying to avoid the antibiotics and hormones that may be used in the dairy industry. You may have heard that a dairy-free diet will help lessen your digestive problems or increase weight loss. Or you may have no choice but to avoid dairy products because you have an allergy to milk protein or intolerance to lactose. Whatever the reasons for avoiding milk and other dairy products, you must understand the nutritional implications, especially related to bone health. The typical American diet relies on dairy products to provide several essential nutrients, including protein, calcium, potassium, and vitamin D. If you do not eat dairy products, it is critical that you know how to make healthy food substitutions to get the nutrients you need (see Further Reading 15).

Protein Quantity and quality must be considered when finding a substitute for the protein found in dairy foods. Dairy protein is a complete protein, meaning it provides all of the essential amino acids necessary for protein synthesis in the body. Quinoa and soy foods (e.g., soy milk, tofu, or edamame) are excellent plant protein choices because they also contain all of the essential amino acids. Rice products are used, too, but rice protein is not a complete protein source.

Calcium Leafy greens and broccoli are nondairy sources of calcium. Chia seeds, flaxseeds, and sesame seeds, as well as quinoa, also are rich sources. It is preferable to consume most of your nutrients in whole foods because they will be more easily absorbed by your body. The concentration of calcium in nondairy foods is significantly less than found in dairy products, making it difficult to get the calcium and other dairy nutrients just from whole foods. For example, you would have to eat 8 cups of cooked spinach or 3 cups of cooked Swiss chard to get the amount of calcium (300 milligrams) in 1 cup of milk. Foods fortified with calcium, such as soy milk and some types of orange juice, are usually necessary to fill in the gaps and bring calcium intake up to the RDA.

Vitamin D Exposure to sunlight for 10 minutes per day will ensure most of us are getting a full day's supply of vitamin D. Because this is not always possible, fortified breakfast cereals and orange juice are good nondairy sources of vitamin D.

Potassium Sweet potatoes, beet greens, and tomatoes are good plant sources of potassium.

Vitamin B-12 Because vitamin B-12 is found almost exclusively in meat and dairy foods, fortified foods will be a likely option when avoiding dairy. Foods fortified with vitamin B-12 include breakfast cereals, soy milk, and meat substitutes.

Dairy-Free Food Options

There are many dairy alternatives available in the grocery store today. These are products that look, feel, and taste like typical dairy foods but are not made from the milk of animals. They include dairy-free milks, sour creams, cheese, and ice cream. Not all of these substitutes, however, have the same nutritional profiles as the original milk-based product. It is very important, therefore, to know what nutrients you are looking for and then to read labels carefully to compare products. The following are examples of the dairy alternatives you can find in stores or online.

Milks Milk alternatives are now widely available and growing in popularity. In 2013, the *Bloomberg Businessweek* reported that sales of nondairy milk beverages made from rice, almonds, and coconut were nearly $1.4 billion, and expected to reach $1.7 billion by 2016. Growth in the market has been led by almond and coconut milk products. At the same time, interest in soymilk has waned. Most of the milk alternatives are healthy and delicious but not exact nutritional replicas of cow's milk (Table 11-6). Although fortified with calcium and vitamin D, most contain little if any protein because the protein remains in the pulp fraction that is strained out and discarded during the production of the plant-based milk. Several of the milk substitutes have unique health benefits. For example, almond milk is rich in vitamin E, magnesium, and potassium, and soy milk is a good source of protein.

Soy milk was one of the first and is now the most widely available dairy-free milk substitute in grocery stores. In the European Union, this product is commonly called "soy drink" because the term *milk* has been restricted to mammary secretions since 1987. Soy milk is made by soaking and grinding dry soybeans with water to make an emulsion of oil, water, and protein. Soy milk contains the highest quantity of protein of all the dairy alternatives with 6 to 10 grams per cup and also the best quality in that it contains all of the essential amino acids. It also has about the same proportion of protein (3.5%), fat (2%), and carbohydrate (3%) as cow's milk. It contains omega-3 fatty acids, fiber, magnesium, and manganese; and most brands are fortified with calcium (450 milligrams per cup), riboflavin, and vitamins A, D, and B-12. There are many brands of soy milk, including unsweetened and sweetened varieties, available at grocery and health food stores. Soy milk is a popular product for vegans because it is plant based, and for people with lactose intolerance because it is lactose free. Soy milk can be coagulated to produce tofu just as dairy milk can be made into cheese.

Rice milk has become another popular dairy alternative. It is made from boiled rice, brown rice syrup, and brown rice starch. It is naturally sweeter than cow's milk because the rice carbohydrates are broken down enzymatically in sugars during production. Additional sweeteners and flavors, such as vanilla, chocolate, or almond, may also be added to some varieties. Compared to cow's milk, rice milk is much higher in carbohydrates (24 grams per cup) and has

significantly less protein (1 gram per cup) and calcium, and no lactose. Most brands are fortified to contain about 300 milligrams of calcium per cup (30% DV) as well as iron, riboflavin, and vitamins A, D, and B-12. Rice milk is probably the most hypoallergenic of all the dairy alternatives and therefore is a good choice for people who are allergic to cow's milk or soy, in addition to those who are lactose intolerant. It is also a popular dairy substitute for vegans.

▲ Almonds are a natural source of calcium: 1 ounce contains 80 milligrams.
© Ingram Publishing/SuperStock

Almond milk is made from ground almonds and water, and has become a popular dairy alternative. On the positive side, a cup of almond milk contains about 200 milligrams of calcium (20% of Daily Value), 100 IU of vitamin D (25% of Daily Value), and 10 milligrams of vitamin E (50% of Daily Value). Almond milk is much lower in calories, however, than cow's milk. There are sweetened (60 calories per cup) and unsweetened varieties (40 calories per cup). Almond milk also contains very little protein (1 gram per cup), carbohydrate (2 grams per cup), and fiber (1 gram per cup), and has a fat content similar to that of rice milk (3 grams per cup). Because almond milk is low in fat and calories, and contains some essential vitamins and minerals, it can be used as a milk substitute by those who would like to lose weight. Many find the taste of almond milk more acceptable compared to other dairy substitutes.

Coconut milk is the liquid that is made from grated coconut meat. It has a high oil content and therefore is much higher in calories, fat, and saturated fat than other milks and milk substitutes. A 1-cup serving of canned coconut milk contains 552 calories and 57 grams of fat, of which 51 grams are saturated fat. Although it contains very little calcium, vitamin D, and other nutrients involved in bone health, coconut milk does contain about 22% of the Daily Value for iron. There are also coconut milk beverages available that compare closely to soy, rice, and almond milks. These beverages are a mixture of coconut cream and water, and per cup have only 4.5 grams of fat, 0 grams of protein, 70 calories, and 100 milligrams of calcium (10% DV).

Potato, oat, hemp, flax, and cashew milks are some more recent dairy-free alternatives. Potato milk, made simply from potatoes and water, is high in carbohydrates and low in protein. It is usually fortified with calcium and vitamins.

Oat milk, like rice milk, is considered a "grain milk," or nondairy beverage. It is made from oat groats mixed with water and potentially other grains and beans. It is low in calories (130 calories per cup) and fat but high in fiber and iron. It typically does not contain

TABLE 11-6 ■ How Nondairy Milk Beverages Compare to the Nutrient Content of Cow's Milk

Nutrients per 1-Cup Serving	Whole Milk	Soy Milk	Rice Milk	Almond Milk	Coconut Milk	Coconut Milk Beverage	Flax Milk	Cashew Milk
Calories	149	90	120	40–60	552	70	50	60
Total Fat (grams)	7.7	3.5	2.5	3	57	4.5	2.5	2.5
Protein (grams)	8	6	1	1	5	0	0	<1
Calcium (% Daily Value)	28	45	30	20	4	10	30	45

▲ Coconut milk is loaded with calories because of its high fat content, and contains very little calcium and vitamin D. © FoodCollection

calcium and is low in vitamin D (10% DV), so it would not be a good choice for maintaining bone health.

Hemp milk or hemp seed milk is made from hulled hemp seeds that are soaked and ground in water. The beverage is creamy and has a nutty flavor. A 1-cup serving contains about 160 calories, 24 grams of carbohydrate, 5 grams of fat, 3 grams of protein, and is fortified with calcium (50% DV) and vitamin D (30% DV).

Flax milk is cold-pressed flax oil mixed with filtered water. One cup unsweetened has 50 calories and provides 1200 milligrams of omega-3s but contains no protein. Flaxmilks are typically forti-fied with vitamin A (10%), vitamin D (25%), vitamin B-12 (25%), and calcium (30%).

Cashew milk is the most recent addition to the plant-based bev-erages industry. Although it has only 60 calories per cup and no saturated fat or cholesterol, it is creamier than skim milk and has nearly twice the calcium of cow's milk.

Cheeses Finding a dairy-free cheese that has the same taste, texture, and cooking qualities of regular cheeses is a challenge. Soy cheeses are the easiest to find, but nut-based cheeses made from cashews and macadamia nuts are also available in health food stores, some grocery stores, and online. Soy cream cheeses are available in grocery stores and are popular dairy substitutes because their taste and texture are similar to those of regular cream cheese. Likewise, soy-based sour creams are the most prevalent dairy-free sour creams. Recipes are available for cashew-based sour cream at http://www.savvyvegetarian.com/vegetarian-recipes/cashew-sour-cream-recipe.php.

Ice Cream, Yogurt, Smoothies, and Whipped Cream Soy-based ice creams are widely available in stores, and rice-based ice creams are also popular because of their sweetness. There are also almond and coconut ice creams available, and most sorbets and fruit-based sherbets are dairy free. As with most of the dairy-free products, soy-based yogurts are the most readily available in stores and are the only yogurt alternatives that will provide protein. Coconut- and nut-based yogurts can also be found in grocery stores and health food stores, and more consumers are looking for nondairy probiotic sources. Dairy-free smoothies are available at most grocery and health food stores. Rice milk is recommended for homemade smoothies because of its sweetness, whereas coconut and almond milk can provide their distinctive flavors. Soy-, rice-, and nut-based whipped toppings are also available but may contain high-fructose corn syrup and partially hydrogenated oils. Less processed whipping cream can also be made at home from coconut milk, almonds, or cashews.

Dairy-Free Shopping Guide: Things to Consider

- Replacing dairy milk with a plant-milk alternative can be part of a plant-based eating plan.
- Look for the unsweetened varieties available in most product lines.
- Choose plant-based milks that are fortified with vitamin D and calcium.
- Remember that most plant-based milks have negligible pro-tein. Only soy milk is similar to dairy milk in terms of protein. Be aware that almond milk that is extremely low in protein is becoming popular in coffee shops as a dairy-free creamer.
- Look for a dairy alternative with a short ingredient list (e.g., nuts, water, salt, and spices). Some dairy-free milks are full of additives, including stabilizers and thickening agents such as sugar, gums, inulin, and carrageenan.

Summary (Numbers refer to numbered sections in the chapter.)

11.1 The outermost layer of bone is the periosteum, a specialized type of connective tissue that covers most bone surfaces. Cortical and trabecular bone work together to provide strength, stability, and flexibil-ity. Cortical bone is dense and compact, providing strength and stability in the shafts of long bones. Trabecular bone is spongy and open, allow-ing for some flexibility and shock absorption. Bone marrow is the spongy tissue inside bones that contains stem cells, which can become blood, fat, cartilage, or bone cells. Teeth are bones covered with a pro-tective layer of enamel.

Bone remodeling is the continuous process of bone degradation and resynthesis of bone. Osteoclasts break down bone tissue by a process called resorption, which releases bone minerals into the blood. Osteo-blasts synthesize new bone tissue from collagen and hydroxyapatite.

Bone synthesis exceeds bone resorption until about age 30, after which bone mineral density is gradually lost throughout the rest of life.

11.2 Biological (i.e., nonmodifiable) factors that influence bone health include sex, age, ethnicity, and frame size. Lifestyle (i.e., modifiable) factors associated with bone status include several dietary components, body weight, normal menses, weight-bearing physical activity, smoking, certain medications, and exposure to UVB sunlight.

11.3 Calcium forms a part of bone structure and plays a role in blood clotting, muscle contractions, nerve transmission, and cell metab-olism. Calcium absorption is enhanced by stomach acid and the active vitamin D hormone. Dairy products are important calcium sources. Women are particularly at risk for not meeting calcium needs.

11.4 Phosphorus aids enzyme function and forms part of key metabolic compounds, cell membranes, and bone. It is efficiently absorbed, and deficiencies are rare, although there is some concern about possible poor intake by some older women. Good sources are dairy products, bakery products, and meats.

11.5 Vitamin D is both a hormone and a vitamin. Human skin synthesizes it using sunshine and a cholesterol-like substance. If we do not spend enough time in the sun, such foods as fish and fortified milk can supply the vitamin. The active hormone form of vitamin D helps regulate blood calcium in part by increasing calcium absorption from the intestine. Infants and children who do not get enough vitamin D may develop rickets, and adults with inadequate amounts in the body develop osteomalacia. Older people and infants often need a supplemental source. Toxicity may lead to calcification of soft tissue, weakness, and gastrointestinal disturbances.

11.6 Magnesium contributes to bone mineralization and vitamin D synthesis. It is also important for nerve and heart function and as an activator for many enzymes. Whole-grain breads and cereals (bran portion), vegetables, nuts, seeds, milk, and meats are good food sources.

11.7 Fluoride as part of regular intake of food sources and fluoridated water, as well as dental applications, makes teeth resistant to dental caries.

11.8 Trace minerals that participate in maintenance of bone health include boron, which affects calcium transport and vitamin D synthesis, and silicon, which influences connective tissue. In addition, vitamin C and protein are also required for proper synthesis of connective tissue in bone.

11.9 Osteoporosis is diagnosed when the T-score (a comparison of individual bone mineral density to age- and gender-specific averages) is 22.5 or lower or by the presence of a stress-induced fracture. Osteopenia is low bone mineral density that does not meet the diagnostic criteria of osteoporosis. Aside from bone fractures, osteoporosis causes kyphosis, pain, loss of mobility and independence, decreased lung capacity, fear of falling, and mortality. Women suffer greater loss of bone mineral density because they typically achieve lower peak bone mass during young adulthood and they lose more trabecular bone due to the hormonal effects of menopause. Type 1 osteoporosis is loss of trabecular bone that follows menopause. Type 2 osteoporosis is loss of cortical and trabecular bone that occurs in both men and women over age 60. Lifestyle factors (e.g., adequate dietary calcium, phosphorous, and vitamin D; exposure to UVB sunlight; and weight-bearing physical activity) are encouraged for prevention of osteoporosis. When lifestyle factors are not enough, medications (e.g., antiresorptive drugs and hormone therapies) may be used to prevent bone loss, but they are not without side effects.

11.10 The gold standard of bone health assessment is central dual energy X-ray absorptiometry (DEXA). Other methods of bone health assessment include peripheral DEXA, peripheral quantitative computed tomography, and quantitative ultrasound.

11.11 If avoiding milk and other dairy products, you must understand the nutritional implications for bone health. For protein, quinoa and soy foods are excellent choices because they contain all of the essential amino acids. There is significantly less calcium in nondairy foods than in dairy products. Exposure to sunlight for 10 minutes per day ensures a full day's supply of vitamin D. There are many dairy-free milks now available in grocery stores. Most of these milks are healthy and delicious but do not contain the exact nutrients found in cow's milk. Soy milk is the most widely available and has the highest quantity of protein of the dairy alternatives and about 45% of the DV of calcium.

Check Your Knowledge (Answers are available at the end of this question set.)

1. Vitamin D is called the sunshine vitamin because
   a. it is available in orange juice.
   b. exposure to sunlight converts a precursor to vitamin D.
   c. it can be destroyed by exposure to sunlight.
   d. it enhances the tanning process.

2. The most accurate measurement of bone mineral density is
   a. central DEXA.
   b. FRAX.
   c. peripheral QCT.
   d. QUS.

3. Which of the following is a lifestyle factor that increases bone mineral density?
   a. Smoking
   b. Physical activity
   c. Large frame size
   d. Use of SPF 50 sunscreen

4. At the end of long bones, inside the spinal vertebrae, and inside the flat bones of the pelvis, is a spongy type of bone known as _____ bone.
   a. osteoclastic
   b. osteoblastic
   c. trabecular
   d. compact

5. Individuals in which of the following groups are most likely to develop osteoporosis?
   a. Premenopausal women athletes
   b. Women taking estrogen replacement therapy
   c. Slender, inactive women who smoke
   d. Women who eat a lot of high-fat dairy products

6. Vitamin D enhances absorption of
   a. calcium.
   b. phosphorus.
   c. both calcium and phosphorus.
   d. neither calcium nor phosphorus.

7. Fatty fish is a source of
   a. vitamin C.
   b. vitamin D.
   c. vitamin K.
   d. magnesium.

8. All of the following sources of drinking water are poor sources of fluoride, except
   a. commercial bottled water.
   b. city household reverse-osmosis water purification system.
   c. city household refrigerator water filter system.
   d. well water from most regions in the United States.

9. Synthesis of the collagen matrix of bone requires all of the following, except
   a. silicon.   c. vitamin C.
   b. boron.   d. protein.

10. The dairy-free milk that has gained the most popularity and market share in the last few years is
    a. almond milk.   c. rice milk.
    b. oat milk.   d. soy milk.

Study Questions (Numbers refer to Learning Outcomes)

1. What are the differences between cortical and trabecular bone? (**LO 11.1**)

2. What are osteoclasts and osteoblasts? Describe the process of bone remodeling. (**LO 11.1**)

3. Describe the functions of two hormones that affect bone metabolism. (**LO 11.2**)

4. What is peak bone mass? At what age is peak bone mass achieved? List three lifestyle factors that affect peak bone mass. (**LO 11.2**)

5. Other than its role in bone structure, what are three functions of phosphorus? List three food sources of this mineral. (**LO 11.4**)

6. List three roles of magnesium in the body. Identify two chronic diseases that may be affected by magnesium status. (**LO 11.6**)

7. Describe the functions of fluoride in the body. List three sources of fluoride. (**LO 11.7**)

8. Describe two methods that can be used to assess bone density. What demographic groups should have bone density measured? (**LO 11.10**)

9. List three sources of dietary calcium. Identify two factors that negatively influence the absorption of calcium. Identify two factors that positively influence the absorption of calcium. (**LO 11.3**)

10. List and describe two vitamin D–deficiency diseases. Which groups of people likely need to supplement their diets with vitamin D, and on what do you base your answer? (**LO 11.5**)

What the Dietitian Chose

Vitamin D is important for regulation of calcium balance in the body: it increases absorption of calcium from the small intestine and helps to regulate the deposition of calcium into bones. For this reason, milk is fortified with vitamin D. For young adults, the RDA for vitamin D is now 15 micrograms per day.

Many people associate vitamin D with whole milk—and whole milk is a rich source of this nutrient. However, if you compare the Nutrient Facts panels from the various types of milk (Fig. 11-19), you will see that all commercial brands of milk contain about 250 milligrams of calcium and are fortified with 2.5 micrograms of vitamin D (25% Daily Value). Note that the Daily Value for vitamin D listed on food labels is still 10 micrograms (400 IU).

Is calcium-fortified orange juice a good source of vitamin D? Because vitamin D is so integral to calcium absorption, many calcium-fortified fruit juices, such as orange juice, also contain vitamin D (see Fig. 11-19). The level of fortification of orange juice with calcium and vitamin D varies by brand, but the calcium and vitamin D contents per serving are typically similar to those of milk.

Now that you have completed Chapter 11, you know that vitamin D is fat soluble. Does this mean you need the fat in whole milk to absorb the vitamin D? Researchers at Boston University compared the bioavailability of vitamin D from whole milk and skim milk and found no differences. Vitamin D bioavailability from calcium and vitamin D–fortified orange juice was also high. In addition, in the context of a meal, there are sure to be other sources of fat (e.g., egg yolk, vegetable oil) to aid fat-soluble vitamin absorption.

To sum up, milks with various fat contents and orange juice fortified with calcium and vitamin D are all rich sources of vitamin D and can help protect against bone loss. For the highest nutrient density, choose skim milk or fortified orange juice.

Skim Milk

Nutrition Facts

Serving size	1 cup (240ml)

Amount per serving

Calories	90

	% Daily Value*
Total Fat 0g	0%
Saturated Fat 0g	0%
Trans Fat 0g	0%
Cholesterol <5mg	1%
Sodium 125mg	5%
Potassium 410mg	12%
Total Carbohydrate 13g	
Dietary Fiber 0g	
Total Sugars 13g	
Includes 0g Added Sugars	0%
Protein 8g	17%
Vitamin D 100mcg	25%
Calcium 300mg	30%
Iron 0mg	0%
Potassium 382mg	11%
Vitamin A 150mcg	10%
Vitamin C 2.4mg	4%

The % Daily Value (DV) tells you how much a nutrient in a serving of food contributes to a daily diet. 2,000 calories a day is used for general nutrition advice.

2% Milk

Nutrition Facts

Serving size	1 cup (240ml)

Amount per serving

Calories	120

	% Daily Value*
Total Fat 5g	8%
Saturated Fat 3g	15%
Trans Fat 0g	0%
Cholesterol 20mg	7%
Sodium 125mg	5%
Potassium 400mg	11%
Total Carbohydrate 12g	4%
Dietary Fiber 0g	
Total Sugars 12g	
Includes 0g Added Sugars	0%
Protein 8g	16%
Vitamin D 100mcg	25%
Calcium 300mg	30%
Iron 0mg	0%
Potassium 366mg	11%
Vitamin A 150mcg	10%
Vitamin C 2.4mg	4%

The % Daily Value (DV) tells you how much a nutrient in a serving of food contributes to a daily diet. 2,000 calories a day is used for general nutrition advice.

Whole Milk

Nutrition Facts

Serving size	1 cup (240ml)

Amount per serving

Calories	150

	% Daily Value*
Total Fat 8g	12%
Saturated Fat 5g	25%
Trans Fat 0g	0%
Total Sugars 12g	
Includes 0g Added Sugars	0%
Protein 8g	16%
Vitamin D 100mcg	25%
Calcium 300mg	30%
Iron 0mg	0%
Potassium 366mg	10%
Vitamin A 90mcg	6%
Vitamin C 2,4mg	4%

The % Daily Value (DV) tells you how much a nutrient in a serving of food contributes to a daily diet. 2,000 calories a day is used for general nutrition advice.

Calcium-Fortified
100% Orange Juice

Nutrition Facts

8 servings per container

Serving size	8 fl oz (240ml)

Amount per serving

Calories	110

	% Daily Value*
Total Fat 0g	0%
Sodium 15mg	1%
Potassium 450mg	13%
Total Carbohydrate 27g	9%
Total Sugars 24g	
Includes 0g Added Sugars	0%
Protein 2g Not a significant source of protein	
Vitamin D 100mcg	25%
Calcium 350mg	35%
Iron 0mg	0%
Potassium 496mg	14%
Thiamin 0.15mg	10%
Vitamin B6 0.1mg	4%
Magnesium 24mg	6%

The % Daily Value (DV) tells you how much a nutrient in a serving of food contributes to a daily diet. 2,000 calories a day is used for general nutrition advice.

FIGURE 11-19 ▲ Milks of varying fat contents all contain the same amount of vitamin D. Many brands of orange juice are also fortified with calcium and vitamin D to match the nutrition found in milk.

CASE STUDY SOLUTION — Worried About Grandma

1. Grace's known risk factors:
   a. Race: Asian
   b. Relative with osteoporosis
   c. Little exercise
   What we don't know:
   a. Body weight: Is she under 127 pounds?
   b. What is her menstrual status? Has she had times of amenorrhea or irregular periods?
   c. Has she had any chronic illnesses, or does she take any medications that may affect her bone mineralization or absorption of calcium?
   d. What are the details about her calcium intake?
2. What Grace does right:
   a. Limits alcohol intake
   b. Does not smoke
   c. Has access to health care professionals (e.g., pharmacy, nursing instructors, and nursing training experience) for advice
   d. Is aware of the issue of calcium and vitamin D; already takes a calcium supplement
   Lifestyle changes Grace could make right now:
   a. Exercise. Grace needs to get moving! Because her time is limited, she can accomplish this objective through work. If she takes the bus to work, she could get off a few stops early and walk the remaining blocks. She could talk with her boss/supervisor to schedule her to stock shelves twice a week, allowing her to "lift weights" at work.
3. As a nursing student and employee in a pharmacy, Grace is inside most of the day; she cannot rely on sunlight to synthesize vitamin D. Boston is 42°21′ north of the equator, a location considered to have inadequate sunlight from November through March for vitamin D synthesis. Because Grace is Korean, her skin will take longer to synthesize vitamin D than if she were fair skinned. To overcome these limitations, Grace must work hard to expose her arms and face to sunlight (between the hours of 11 A.M. and 2 P.M. would be optimal) for 20 minutes, three to five times per week during the sunny months. She must also work to consciously consume foods with vitamin D or take a vitamin D supplement of 400 IU per day.
4. Traditional Korean fare includes plenty of rice, beans, vegetables, and fish. Dairy products are not popular in traditional Korean diets. Tofu, if prepared with calcium, can be a rich source of calcium. Other legumes provide some calcium—about 80 milligrams per 1/2 cup. Fish with edible bones are a good source of calcium. For example, 8 ounces of canned sardines provide 325 milligrams of calcium.
5. Instead of soft drinks, which have little nutritional value, Grace could choose low-fat milk or chocolate milk as her beverage. Some fast food restaurants offer yogurt as a side dish instead of fries. A baked potato topped with cheese and sour cream offers a bit more calcium than the typical serving of fries. If available, soup made with beans can provide some calcium.
6. Grace currently takes a balanced multivitamin and mineral supplement plus one calcium carbonate supplement each day. Food sources of calcium would be preferable, but if supplements are needed, Grace should make some changes to her routine to optimize absorption of bone-building nutrients. She currently takes the calcium carbonate when brushing her teeth at bedtime. Calcium carbonate should be taken with meals to enhance absorption. Alternatively, she could choose a supplement of calcium citrate, which can be taken without regard to food. In addition, choosing a calcium supplement with vitamin D will enhance absorption of calcium.

Further Readings

1. Adams JS, Hewison M: Update in vitamin D. *Journal of Clinical Endocrinology and Metabolism* 95:471, 2010.
2. Anderson JJ and others: Calcium intakes and femoral and lumbar bone density of elderly U.S. men and women: National Health and Nutrition Examination Survey 2005–2006 analysis. *Journal of Clinical Endocrinology and Metabolism* 97:4531, 2012.
3. a. Bolland MJ and others: Effect of calcium supplements on risk of myocardial infarction and cardiovascular events: Meta-analysis. *British Medical Journal* 341:c3691, 2010.
   b. Bolland MJ and others: Calcium supplements with or without vitamin D and risk of cardiovascular events: Reanalysis of the Women's Health Initiative limited access dataset and meta-analysis. *British Medical Journal* 342:d2040, 2011.
4. Casey CF and others: Vitamin D supplementation in infants, children, and adolescents. *American Family Physician* 81(6):745, 2010.
5. Keller M: Vitamin D deficiency in children. *Today's Dietitian* 14(12):26, 2012.
6. LeBlanc KE and others: Hip fracture: Diagnosis, treatment, and secondary prevention. *American Family Physician* 89:945, 2014.
7. Lewiecki EM: Current and emerging pharmacological therapies for the management of postmenopausal osteoporosis. *Journal of Women's Health* 19(10):1615, 2009.
8. Linus Pauling Institute Micronutrient Information Center. *Phosphorus.* June 2014. http://lpi.oregonstate.edu/mic/minerals/phosphorus. Accessed December 2015.
9. National Osteoporosis Foundation: *2014 Clinician's guide to prevention and treatment of osteoporosis.* Washington, DC: National Osteoporosis Foundation. www.nof.org. Accessed December 2015.
10. Office of Dietary Supplements, National Institutes of Health: Dietary supplement fact sheet: *Calcium fact sheet.* November 21, 2013. http://ods.od.nih.gov/factsheets/calcium; *Vitamin D fact sheet.* November 10, 2014. http://ods.od.nih.gov/factsheets/vitamind; and *Magnesium fact sheet.* November 4, 2013. http://ods.od.nih.gov/factsheets/magnesium. Accessed December 2015.
11. Palmer CA, Gilbert JA: Position of the Academy of Nutrition and Dietetics: The impact of fluoride on health. *Journal of the Academy of Nutrition and Dietetics* 112:1443, 2012.
12. Remer T and others: Dietary protein's and dietary acid load's influence on bone health. *Critical Reviews in Food Science and Nutrition* 54(9):1140, 2014. doi:10.1080/104008398.2011.627519
13. Rugg-Gunn AJ, Do L: Effectiveness of water fluoridation in caries prevention. *Community Dentistry and Oral Epidemiology* 240(Suppl. 2): 55, 2012.
14. Tucker KL: Osteoporosis prevention and nutrition. *Current Osteoporosis Reports* 7:111, 2009.
15. Schaeffer J: What's new in the dairy-free aisle. *Today's Dietitian* 17(2): 30, 2015.
16. Webb D: Vitamin D and cancer—Evidence suggests this vital nutrient may cut risk. *Today's Dietitian* 14(10):58, 2012.
17. Wright NC and others: The recent prevalence of osteoporosis and low bone mass in the United States based on bone mineral density at the femoral neck or lumbar spine. *Journal of Bone Mineral Research* 29:2520, 2014. doi:10.1002/jbmr.2269

Rate Your Plate

Working for Denser Bones

Osteoporosis and related low bone mass affect many adults in North America, especially older women. One-third of all women experience fractures because of this disease, amounting to about 2 million bone fractures per year.

Osteoporosis is a disease you can do something about. Some risk factors cannot be changed, but others, such as poor calcium intake, can. Is this true for you? To find out, complete this tool for estimating your current calcium intake. For all the following foods, write the number of servings you eat in a day. Total the number of servings in each category and then multiply the total number of servings by the amount of calcium for each category. Finally, add the total amount for each category to estimate your calcium intake for that day.

Does your intake meet your RDA set for calcium?

Food	Serving Size	Number of Servings	Calcium (mg)	Total Calcium (mg)
Plain low-fat yogurt	1 cup	_____		
Fat-free dry milk powder	½ cup	_____		
	Total servings	_____	× 400	= _____ mg
Canned sardines (with bones)	3 ounces	_____		
Fruit-flavored yogurt	1 cup	_____		
Milk: fat free, reduced fat, whole, chocolate, buttermilk	1 cup	_____		
Calcium-fortified soy, rice, or almond milk (e.g., Silk®)	1 cup	_____		
	¼ cup	_____		
Parmesan cheese (grated)	1 ounce	_____		
Swiss cheese	Total servings	_____	× 300	= _____ mg
Cheese (all other hard cheese)	1 ounce	_____		
Pancakes	3	_____		
	Total servings	_____	× 200	= _____ mg
Canned pink salmon	3 ounces	_____		
Tofu (processed with calcium)	4 ounces	_____		
	Total servings	_____	× 150	= _____ mg
Collards or turnip greens, cooked	½ cup	_____		
Ice cream or ice milk	½ cup	_____		
Almonds	1 ounce	_____		
	Total servings	_____	× 75	= _____ mg
Chard, cooked	½ cup	_____		
Cottage cheese	½ cup	_____		
Corn tortilla	1 medium	_____		
Orange	1 medium	_____		
	Total servings	_____	× 50	= _____ mg
Kidney, lima, or navy beans, cooked	½ cup	_____		
Broccoli	½ cup	_____		
Carrot, raw	1 medium	_____		
Dates or raisins	¼ cup	_____		
Egg	1 large	_____		
Whole-wheat bread	1 slice	_____		
Peanut butter	2 tablespoons	_____		
	Total servings	_____	× 25	= _____ mg
Calcium-fortified orange juice	6 ounces	_____		
Calcium-fortified snack bars	1 each	_____		
Calcium-fortified breakfast bars	½ bar	_____		
	Total servings	_____	× 200	= _____ mg
Calcium-fortified chocolate candies	1 each	_____	× 500	
Calcium supplements*	1 each	_____	Total calcium	= _____ mg
	Total servings	_____	intake	= _____ mg

Other calcium sources to consider include many breakfast cereals (100–250 mg per cup) and some vitamin/mineral supplements (200–500 mg or more per tablet).

*Amount varies, so check the label for the amount in a specific product and then adjust the calculation as needed.

Source: Adapted from *Topics in Clinical Nutrition*, "Putting Calcium into Perspective for Your Clients," G. Wardlaw and N. Weese, 11:1, © 1995 Aspen Publishers, Inc.

© BananaStock/Punchstock

Student Learning Outcomes

Chapter 12 is designed to allow you to:

12.1 Describe how vitamins and minerals function as coenzymes that are needed for metabolism reactions to occur.

12.2 Explain the functions of thiamin in carbohydrate metabolism and list its sources, recommendations, and deficiency symptoms.

12.3 Describe the functions of riboflavin in energy metabolism and the dietary sources of riboflavin that will prevent deficiency symptoms.

12.4 Describe the functions of niacin in energy metabolism and list its sources, recommendations, and deficiency symptoms.

12.5 Explain the functions of pantothenic acid in energy metabolism and list its sources and recommendations.

Chapter 12

Micronutrient Function in Energy Metabolism

What Would You Choose?

Since being accepted into the business program, your courses are getting tougher and you are staying up late doing homework. You also need work experience, so you are putting in 20 hours a week at the bookstore. With work, classes, homework, and hanging out with friends, you are only getting about 4 to 5 hours of sleep a night and barely have time to eat. You are feeling exhausted and looking for a good, quick energy source. Which of the following would you choose to get energized?

a Nature Made® B-Complex w/Vitamin C Dietary Supplement

b Centrum® Adults Under 50 Multivitamin and Mineral Supplement

c 2-ounce 5-Hour Energy® shot

d Several small meals throughout the day and 7 to 9 hours of sleep each night

Think about your choice as you read Chapter 12, then see What the Dietitian Chose at the end of the chapter.

How does the body convert the energy found in food into a form that the cells can use? Cells obtain energy from the chemical bonds found in the macronutrients (carbohydrates, lipids, and protein). You learned previously that during the process of digestion, these macronutrients are broken down chemically into smaller substances (monosaccharides, fatty acids, monoglycerides, glycerol, and amino acids). These smaller substances can be absorbed into the body via the small intestine. The circulatory system then transports these nutrients to the trillions of cells in the body. The cells use chemical reactions to further break down these substances into carbon dioxide and water. In the process, large amounts of energy are converted into a form (ATP) that the cells can use to perform work. The chemical processes used by cells to extract energy from these nutrients are termed *metabolism*. A major function of the micronutrients (vitamins and minerals) is to assist enzymes in the chemical reactions in energy metabolism. These micronutrients are called coenzymes (vitamins) (as you will see in Fig. 12-1) or cofactors (minerals) because they activate the enzymes and thus allow them to become functional.

12.6 Describe the functions of vitamin B-6 in amino-acid metabolism, and understand how to get enough vitamin B-6 in your dietary pattern and avoid too much from dietary supplements.

12.7 Describe the functions of biotin in chemical reactions and list its sources, recommendations, and deficiency symptoms.

12.8 Explain the functions of iodine in thyroid metabolism and list its sources, recommendations, and deficiency symptoms.

12.9 Describe the functions of chromium in glucose metabolism and its sources, recommendations, and deficiency symptoms.

12.10 Describe the functions of manganese and molybdenum, and understand how to get enough from dietary sources.

12.11 Understand the functions and sources of choline and why it is not considered an essential vitamin.

12.1 The Roles of B Vitamins in Energy Metabolism

coenzyme An organic compound that combines with an inactive enzyme to form a catalytically active form. In this manner, coenzymes aid in enzyme function.

cofactor An inorganic compound (e.g., mineral) that combines with an inactive enzyme to form a catalytically active form.

bioavailability The degree to which an ingested nutrient is absorbed and available to be utilized by the body.

The B vitamins and some minerals play key roles in metabolism as **coenzymes** or **cofactors,** respectively (recall Fig. 8-5). Several B vitamins are dependent on each other because they participate in the same metabolic pathways that convert macronutrients into usable energy (Fig. 12-1). Early symptoms of B vitamin deficiencies typically occur in the brain and nervous system, skin, and gastrointestinal (GI) tract because cells in these tissues are metabolically active. Cells in the skin and GI tract are also constantly being replaced.

After being ingested, the B vitamins are first broken down from their coenzyme forms into free vitamins in the stomach and small intestine. The vitamins are then absorbed, primarily in the small intestine. High **bioavailability** is a characteristic of the B vitamins, which means that, typically, about 50% to 90% of the B vitamins in the diet are absorbed. Once inside cells, the B vitamins are made into their coenzyme forms. Health-food stores sell the coenzyme forms of some vitamins, but these more expensive forms of vitamins are unnecessary. The body makes all the coenzymes it needs from vitamin precursors.

B VITAMIN INTAKES OF NORTH AMERICANS

The nutritional health of most North Americans with regard to the B vitamins is adequate. Typical diets contain plentiful and varied natural sources of these vitamins. In addition, many common foods, such as ready-to-eat breakfast cereals, are fortified with one or more of the B vitamins. In some developing countries, however, deficiencies of the B vitamins are more common and the resulting deficiency diseases pose significant health problems. (We will discuss these worldwide nutritional deficiencies in more detail in Chapter 16.)

FIGURE 12-1 ▲ B vitamins are essential components of many coenzymes involved in energy metabolism. (a) The B vitamins and their coenzymes (shown as their commonly used abbreviation). TPP, thiamin pyrophosphate; FAD, flavin adenine dinucleotide; FMN, flavin mononucleotide; NAD, nicotinamide adenine dinucleotide; NADP, nicotinamide adenine dinucleotide phosphate; PLP, pyridoxal phosphate; CoA, coenzyme A. (b) The coenzymes are shown associated with the metabolic pathways for which they are essential.

Because B vitamins are water soluble, very little is stored and excess ends up in the urine or stool. About 10% to 25% of these vitamins are lost from food during food processing and preparation because they dissolve in water. Light cooking methods, such as stir-frying, steaming, and microwaving, best preserve vitamin content (review Table 8-3).

Despite good B vitamin status of North Americans, marginal deficiencies of these vitamins may occur in some cases, especially among older adults who eat little food and in other people with poor dietary patterns. In the short run, such a marginal deficiency in most people likely leads only to fatigue or other unspecified physical effects. Although the long-term effects of such marginal deficiencies are yet unknown, increased risks of cardiovascular disease, cancer, and cataracts of the eye are suspected. With rare exceptions, healthy adults do not develop the more serious B vitamin-deficiency diseases from dietary inadequacy alone. The main exceptions are people with alcoholism. The combination of extremely unbalanced diets and alcohol-induced alterations of vitamin absorption and metabolism creates significant risks for serious nutrient deficiencies among people with alcoholism.

▲ Rapid cooking of vegetables in minimal fluids helps to preserve vitamin content. Steaming is one effective method. © C Squared Studios/Getty Images

B VITAMINS IN GRAINS

The production of refined grains, such as white flour from wheat, leads to the loss of B vitamins as well as other vitamins and minerals. When grains are milled to make refined products, seeds are crushed and the germ, bran, and husk layers are discarded, leaving just the starch-containing endosperm in the refined grains (recall Fig. 4-5). This starch is used to make white flour, bread, and cereal products. Unfortunately, many nutrients are lost in the discarded germ, bran, and husk materials. To counteract these losses, in the United States, bread and cereal products made from milled grains are enriched with four B vitamins (thiamin, riboflavin, niacin, and folic acid) and with the mineral iron.

Food enrichment was initiated by federal legislation in the 1930s to help combat nutrient deficiencies such as pellagra (niacin deficiency) and iron-deficiency **anemia.** Federal regulations included folate to the list of nutrients required to be added to refined grain products in 1998. Not all nutrients lost in milling are added back through enrichment such that products made with refined flour remain lower in vitamins E and B-6, potassium, magnesium, fiber, and other nutrients than products made with whole grains. This lower nutrient density is why nutrition experts and the Dietary Guidelines advocate daily consumption of whole-grain products, such as whole-wheat bread and brown rice, rather than refined grain products (Fig. 12-2).

The following sections focus on the B vitamins and trace minerals involved in energy metabolism.

anemia A decreased oxygen-carrying capacity of the blood. This can be caused by many factors, such as iron deficiency or blood loss.

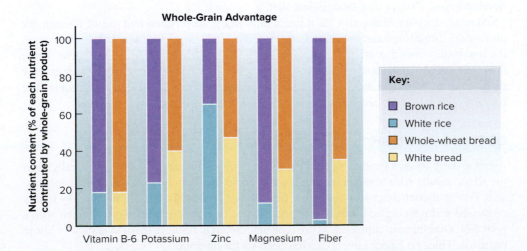

Whole-Grain Advantage

FIGURE 12-2 ◄ Comparison of the relative nutrient contents of refined versus whole grains. Nutrients are expressed as a percentage of the nutrient contribution of the whole-grain product.

Key:
- ■ Brown rice
- ■ White rice
- ■ Whole-wheat bread
- ■ White bread

Vitamin B-6   Potassium   Zinc   Magnesium   Fiber

✔ **CONCEPT CHECK 12.1**

1. What are the coenzymes associated with each of the B vitamins involved in energy metabolism?
2. What body organs or tissues are most likely to show symptoms if there is a deficiency of B vitamins?
3. Why are B vitamins lost when foods are cooked in water?
4. What group of people is at high risk of B vitamin deficiency?
5. What happens during the refining of grains that causes a decrease in nutrient density?
6. What is added during the "enrichment" of grain products, and why is it important?

12.2 Thiamin (Vitamin B-1)

FUNCTIONS OF THIAMIN

Thiamin was the first water-soluble vitamin to be discovered. One of its primary functions is to help release energy from carbohydrate. Its coenzyme form, thiamin pyrophosphate (TPP), participates in reactions in which carbon dioxide (CO_2) is released during the breakdown of carbohydrates and certain amino acids (see Fig. 12-1). These reactions are particularly important in the body's ATP-producing energy pathways. Thiamin also functions in chemical reactions that make RNA, DNA, and neurotransmitters.

THIAMIN DEFICIENCY

beriberi The thiamin-deficiency disorder characterized by muscle weakness, loss of appetite, nerve degeneration, and sometimes edema.

The thiamin-deficiency disease is called **beriberi,** a word that means "I can't, I can't" in the Sri Lanka language of Sinhalese. This disease was described long before thiamin was discovered to be a vitamin in 1910. The symptoms include weakness, loss of appetite, irritability, nervous tingling throughout the body, poor arm and leg coordination, and deep muscle pain in the calves. A person with beriberi often develops an enlarged heart and sometimes severe edema.

Beriberi is seen in areas where rice is a staple and polished (white) rice is consumed rather than brown (whole-grain) rice. In most parts of the world, even poor countries, white rice is preferred and is made by removing the bran and germ layer from brown rice. White rice is a poor source of thiamin, except for the enriched variety sold in the United States.

Beriberi results when glucose, the primary fuel for brain and nerve cells, cannot be metabolized to release energy because of the lack of thiamin. Because the thiamin coenzyme participates in glucose metabolism, problems with functions that depend on glucose such as brain and nerve action are the first signs of a thiamin deficiency. Symptoms can develop in just 10 days on a thiamin-free diet.

Alcohol abuse increases risk for thiamin deficiency. Absorption and use of thiamin are profoundly diminished and excretion is increased by consumption of alcohol. Furthermore, the low-quality diet that often accompanies severe alcoholism makes matters worse. There is limited storage in the body; therefore, an alcoholic binge lasting 1 to 2 weeks may quickly deplete already diminished amounts of the vitamin and result in deficiency symptoms. The beriberi associated with alcoholism is also called Wernicke-Korsakoff syndrome.

GETTING ENOUGH THIAMIN

Average daily intakes for men exceed the DV by 50% or more, and women generally meet the RDA. Adults with low incomes and older people may barely meet their needs for thiamin. Potential contributors to thiamin deficiency are dietary patterns dominated by highly processed and unenriched foods, sugar, and fat; and heavy alcohol intake combined with a poor diet. Oral thiamin supplements are typically nontoxic because thiamin is rapidly lost in the urine. Thus, no Upper Level (UL) has been set for thiamin.

▲ Pork is an excellent source of thiamin.
© D. Fischer and P. Lyons/Cole Group/Getty Images

(a)

ChooseMyPlate.gov

(b)

Food Item and Amount	Thiamin (milligrams)	% RDA for Adult Males (1.2 milligrams)	% RDA for Adult Females (1.1 milligrams)
Grains			
Cheerios® cereal, 1 cup	0.4	31%	34%
Wheat germ, 2 tablespoons	0.3	25%	27%
Flour tortilla, 8"	0.2	17%	18%
Vegetables			
Green peas, cooked, 1 cup	0.4	35%	38%
Acorn squash, cooked, 1 cup	0.3	29%	31%
Corn, cooked, 1 cup	0.1	12%	13%
Fruits			
Orange juice, fresh, 1 cup	0.2	17%	18%
Raisins, ½ cup	0.1	6%	7%
Watermelon, 1 cup	0.1	4%	5%
Dairy			
Yogurt, plain, non-fat, 1 cup	0.1	10%	11%
Milk, fat-free, 1 cup	0.1	9%	10%
Soymilk, 1 cup	0.1	6%	6%
Protein			
Ham, canned, 3 ounces	0.8	68%	74%
Kidney beans, cooked, ½ cup	0.1	12%	13%
Chicken breast, roasted, 3 ounces	0.1	5%	5%

FIGURE 12-3 ▲ Food sources of thiamin. (a) The fill of the background color (none, 1/3, 2/3, or completely covered) within each group on MyPlate indicates the average nutrient density for thiamin in that group. (b) The bar graph shows thiamin content of several foods in each group compared to the RDA for adult males and females. Overall, the richest sources of thiamin are meats (especially pork), whole grains, and fortified breakfast cereals.

Source: *Nutrition data from USDA National Database for Standard Reference, Release 26.*

Major sources of thiamin include pork products, whole grains (wheat germ), ready-to-eat breakfast cereals, enriched grains and flour, green beans, milk, orange juice, organ meats, peanuts, dried beans, and seeds (Fig. 12-3). When considering the sections of MyPlate, the protein and grain groups contain the most foods that are nutrient-dense sources of thiamin (see Fig. 12-3).

> **Thiamin**
> RDA
>   Men: 1.2 milligrams
>   Women: 1.1 milligrams
> DV: 1.5 milligrams
> UL: none

✓ CONCEPT CHECK 12.2

1. How is thiamin involved in energy metabolism?
2. What body organs or tissues are most likely to show symptoms if there is a deficiency of thiamin?
3. What group of people is at high risk of thiamin deficiency?
4. What are some excellent sources of thiamin?

12.3 Riboflavin (Vitamin B-2)

FUNCTIONS OF RIBOFLAVIN

Riboflavin derives its name from its yellow color (*flavus* means "yellow" in Latin). The coenzyme forms of riboflavin, flavin dinucleotide (FAD) and flavin mononucleotide (FMN), participate in many energy-yielding metabolic pathways, such as the breakdown of

FIGURE 12-4 ▲ Angular cheilitis, also called cheilosis or angular stomatitis, causes painful cracks at the corners of the mouth. © Dr. P. Marazzi/Science Photo Library/Science Source

fatty acids (see Fig. 12-1). Some metabolism of vitamins and minerals also requires riboflavin. Indirectly, riboflavin also has an antioxidant role in the body through its support of the enzyme glutathione peroxidase.

RIBOFLAVIN DEFICIENCY

Symptoms associated with riboflavin deficiency (ariboflavinosis) include inflammation of the mouth and tongue, dermatitis, cracking of tissue around the corners of the mouth (called cheilosis), various eye disorders, sensitivity to the sun, and confusion. Glossitis is a painful soreness or inflammation of the tongue that can signal a deficiency of riboflavin, niacin, vitamin B-6, folate, or vitamin B-12 (Fig. 12-4). Angular cheilitis, also called cheilosis or angular stomatitis, is inflammation of the corners of the mouth that may cause painful cracking. Both glossitis and angular cheilitis can be caused by other medical conditions; thus, further evaluation is required before diagnosing a nutrient deficiency. Such symptoms develop after approximately 2 months on a riboflavin-poor diet. Riboflavin deficiency typically would occur jointly with deficiencies of niacin, thiamin, and vitamin B-6 because these nutrients often occur in the same foods.

GETTING ENOUGH RIBOFLAVIN

On average, daily intakes of riboflavin are slightly above the RDA. As with thiamin, people with alcoholism risk riboflavin deficiency because they eat nutrient-poor diets. No specific symptoms indicate that riboflavin taken in megadoses is toxic, so no UL has been set. Riboflavin supplementation, including the riboflavin found in multivitamin supplements or in a heavily fortified breakfast cereal, can cause the urine to become bright yellow.

The grains, dairy, and protein groups of MyPlate contain the most nutrient-dense sources of riboflavin (Fig. 12-5). Major sources of riboflavin are ready-to-eat breakfast cereals, milk and milk products, enriched grains, meat, and eggs (see Fig. 12-5). Vegetables such

(a)

(b)

Food Item and Amount	Riboflavin (milligrams)	% RDA for Adult Males (1.3 milligrams)	% RDA for Adult Females (1.1 milligrams)
Grains			
Kellogg's All Bran® cereal, 1 cup	0.8	62%	73%
Egg noodles, cooked, ½ cup	0.1	8%	9%
Bread, white, 1 slice	0.1	8%	9%
Vegetables			
Mushrooms, raw, 5 medium	0.4	31%	36%
Spinach, cooked, 1 cup	0.4	31%	36%
Asparagus, cooked, 1 cup	0.3	23%	27%
Dairy			
Yogurt, plain, non-fat, 1 cup	0.5	38%	45%
Milk, fat-free, 1 cup	0.4	31%	36%
Cheese, feta, 1.5 ounces	0.4	31%	36%
Protein			
Beef liver, pan-fried, 3 ounces	2.8	215%	255%
Egg, hard-boiled, 1 large	0.3	23%	27%
Black beans, cooked, ½ cup	0.1	4%	5%

FIGURE 12-5 ▲ Food sources of riboflavin. (a) The fill of the background color (none, 1/3, 2/3, or completely covered) within each group on MyPlate indicates the average nutrient density for riboflavin in that group. (b) The bar graph shows riboflavin content of several foods in each group compared to the RDA for adult males and females. Overall, the richest sources of riboflavin are meats (especially liver), dairy products, and fortified breakfast cereals. Fruits (not shown) are not particularly good sources of riboflavin.

Source: *Nutrition data from USDA National Database for Standard Reference, Release 26.*

CASE STUDY Deficiency from a Vegan and Gluten-Free Diet?

Andrew has been a vegan for about 1 year; therefore, he does not consume any animal products, including meat, fish, poultry, eggs, or dairy. Earlier this year, Andrew began experiencing gastrointestinal problems such as bloating, cramping, and occasional diarrhea. He read that these symptoms may be caused by the gluten in his diet, so he is now also avoiding gluten altogether by eliminating bread, cereals, pasta, and all other products made from enriched or whole wheat. Within a week of eliminating gluten, Andrew's gastrointestinal tract is feeling better, but his mouth and tongue have become very sore and inflamed. He also has developed sores and cracks at the corners of his mouth.

Answer the following questions and check your responses at the end of the chapter.

1. What nutrients, including B vitamins, may be low or deficient in Andrew's vegan diet?
2. Why might the gluten in his diet be causing Andrew's gastrointestinal distress?
3. What nutrients may have been eliminated as a result of a gluten-free diet? (Refer back to discussion of the gluten-free diet in Section 3.12..)
4. What nutrient deficiency is most likely causing his problems around the mouth?
5. What food sources can be added to Andrew's vegan, gluten-free diet to alleviate his possible nutrient deficiencies?
6. Would a daily nutrient supplement be a possible remedy to avoid deficiencies?

---

as asparagus, broccoli, and various greens (e.g., spinach) are also good sources. Riboflavin is a relatively stable water-soluble vitamin; however, it is destroyed by light. Milk is sold in paper or opaque plastic containers rather than clear glass to protect the riboflavin. In the United States, many meet the riboflavin recommendation by consuming three servings of dairy products each day.

✓ CONCEPT CHECK 12.3

1. How is riboflavin involved in energy metabolism?
2. What body organs or tissues are most likely to show symptoms if there is a deficiency of riboflavin?
3. What types of foods are the best sources of riboflavin?

12.4 Niacin (Vitamin B-3)

FUNCTIONS OF NIACIN

Niacin functions in the body as one of two related compounds: nicotinic acid and nicotinamide. The coenzyme forms of niacin function in many cellular metabolic pathways. When you are generating energy (ATP) by burning carbohydrate and fat, a niacin coenzyme, nicotinamide dinucleotide (NAD) or nicotinamide dinucleotide phosphate (NADP), is used. Anabolic pathways in the cell—those that make new compounds—also often use a niacin coenzyme. This is especially true for fatty-acid synthesis (see Fig. 12-1).

Nicotinic acid has been promoted as a natural method to lower blood lipids including LDL cholesterol; however, due to potential adverse side effects, its use is discouraged without supervision by a primary care provider.

NIACIN DEFICIENCY

Because niacin coenzymes function in over 200 enzymatic reactions, niacin deficiency causes widespread problems in the body. Early symptoms include poor appetite, weight loss, and weakness. The distinct group of niacin-deficiency symptoms is known as **pellagra,** which

Riboflavin

RDA

   Men: 1.3 milligrams

   Women: 1.1 milligrams

DV: 1.7 milligrams

UL: none

pellagra Niacin-deficiency disease characterized by dementia, diarrhea, and dermatitis, and possibly leading to death.

▲ Corn is treated in an alkaline solution to release protein-bound niacin so it can be available in corn products such as tortillas, taco shells, tortilla chips, and corn flour. © Scott Bauer/USDA

dementia A general loss or decrease in mental function.

Niacin

RDA

   Men: 16 milligrams

   Women: 14 milligrams

DV: 20 milligrams

UL: 35 milligrams (nicotinic acid form)

(a)

means "rough or painful skin." The symptoms of the disease are **dementia,** diarrhea, and dermatitis (especially on areas of skin exposed to the sun). Left untreated, death often results.

Pellagra is the only dietary deficiency disease ever to reach epidemic proportions in the United States. It became a major problem in the southeastern United States in the late 1800s and persisted until the 1930s, when standards of living and diets improved. Pellagra was particularly prevalent in populations that consumed corn as a major part of their diet. Niacin in corn is bound by a protein that inhibits its absorption, making it less bioavailable. Soaking corn in an alkaline solution, such as lime water (water with calcium hydroxide), releases bound niacin and renders it more bioavailable. Hispanic people in North America traditionally soak corn in lime water before making tortillas. The treatment is one reason this Hispanic population never experienced much pellagra. Today, pellagra is rare in Western societies and is typically only seen associated with chronic alcoholism in conjunction with poverty and malnutrition and in those with rare disorders of tryptophan metabolism (e.g., Hartnup disease).

GETTING ENOUGH NIACIN

Besides the preformed niacin found in foods, we can synthesize niacin from the amino acid tryptophan. In this manner, we synthesize about 50% of the niacin required each day. This reaction requires two other vitamins (riboflavin and vitamin B-6) to function as coenzymes in this chemical conversion. The adult RDA of niacin is expressed as niacin equivalents (NE) to account for niacin received intact from the diet, as well as that synthesized from tryptophan: 60 milligrams of tryptophan in a diet yield about 1 milligram of niacin. The DV used on food and supplement labels is 20 milligrams.

Intakes of niacin by adults are about double the RDA, not including the contribution from tryptophan. Tables of food composition values also ignore tryptophan contribution. The best food sources of niacin are found in the protein group on MyPlate (Fig. 12-6). Major sources of niacin are tuna, poultry, peanuts, fish, ready-to-eat cereals, beef, and asparagus

(b)

	Food Item and Amount	Niacin (milligrams)	% RDA for Adult Males (16 milligrams)	% RDA for Adult Females (14 milligrams)
Grains	Total® Raisin Bran cereal, 1 cup	20	125%	143%
	Tortilla, flour, 8″	1.8	11%	13%
	Bread, whole wheat, 1 slice	1.4	9%	10%
Vegetables	Raw mushrooms, 5	4.7	29%	34%
	Potato, 1	2.1	13%	15%
	Asparagus, cooked, 1 cup	2.0	13%	14%
Fruits	Orange juice, fresh, 1 cup	1.0	6%	7%
	Banana, 1 medium	0.8	5%	6%
	Blueberries, 1 cup	0.6	4%	4%
Protein	Tuna, yellow fin, grilled, 3 ounces	18.8	118%	134%
	Chicken breast, roasted, 3 ounces	11.8	74%	84%
	Peanut butter, 2 tablespoons	4.2	26%	30%

FIGURE 12-6 ▲ Food sources of niacin. (a) The fill of the background color (none, 1/3, 2/3, or completely covered) within each group on MyPlate indicates the average nutrient density for niacin in that group. (b) The bar graph shows niacin content of several foods compared to the RDA for adult males and females. Overall, the richest sources of niacin are foods in the protein group and fortified breakfast cereals. Foods in the dairy group (not shown) contain very little niacin, but the tryptophan in dairy foods can be converted into niacin.

Source: *Nutrition data from USDA National Database for Standard Reference, Release 26.*

(see Fig. 12-6). Coffee and tea also contribute some niacin to the diet. Niacin is heat stable; little is lost in cooking.

AVOIDING TOO MUCH NIACIN

The UL for niacin pertains only to the nicotinic-acid form. Side effects include headache, itching, and increased blood flow to the skin because of blood vessel dilation or flushing in various parts of the body. These symptoms are especially seen when intakes are above 100 milligrams per day. In the long run, GI tract and liver damage are possible, so any use of megadoses, including large doses recommended for treatment for cardiovascular disease, requires close medical monitoring.

▲ Chicken is a good source of niacin. The tryptophan in chicken can also be metabolized to niacin. © Getty Images/iStock Exclusive RF

> ✔ **CONCEPT CHECK 12.4**
>
> 1. How is niacin involved in energy metabolism?
> 2. What are the three distinct signs of a niacin deficiency?
> 3. What are some excellent sources of niacin?
> 4. What is the relationship between tryptophan and niacin?

12.5 Pantothenic Acid (Vitamin B-5)

FUNCTIONS OF PANTOTHENIC ACID

Pantothenic acid is required for the synthesis of coenzyme A (CoA), a coenzyme in chemical reactions that allow the release of energy from carbohydrates, lipids, and protein. It also activates fatty acids so they can yield energy (see Fig. 12-1) and is used in the initial steps of fatty-acid synthesis. Pantothenic acid is so widespread in foods that a nutritional deficiency among healthy people who eat varied diets is unlikely. *Pantothen* means "from every side" in Greek.

PANTOTHENIC ACID DEFICIENCY

A deficiency of pantothenic acid might occur in alcoholism along with a nutrient-deficient diet. However, the symptoms would probably be hidden among deficiencies of thiamin, riboflavin, vitamin B-6, and folate, so the pantothenic acid deficiency might be unrecognizable.

GETTING ENOUGH PANTOTHENIC ACID

The Adequate Intake (AI) set for pantothenic acid is 5 milligrams per day for adults. Average consumption is well in excess of this amount. The DV on food and supplement labels is 10 milligrams. Rich sources of pantothenic acid are sunflower seeds, mushrooms, peanuts, and eggs (Fig. 12-7). Other rich sources are meat, milk, and many vegetables. No toxicity is known for pantothenic acid, so no UL has been set.

> **Pantothenic Acid**
> AI: 5 milligrams
> DV: 10 milligrams
> UL: None

> ✔ **CONCEPT CHECK 12.5**
>
> 1. What is the role of pantothenic acid in energy metabolism?
> 2. What are some rich sources of pantothenic acid?

	Food Item and Amount	Pantothenic Acid (milligrams)	% AI for Adult Males and Females (5 milligrams)
Grains	Whole Grain Total® cereal, 1 cup	10.0	200%
	Brown rice, cooked, ½ cup	0.4	8%
	White bread, 1 slice	0.1	2%
Vegetables	Mushrooms, raw, 5 medium	1.3	26%
	Acorn squash, cooked, 1 cup	1.0	20%
	Broccoli, cooked, 1 cup	1.0	20%
Fruits	Orange juice, fresh, 1 cup	0.5	10%
	Blueberries, 1 cup	0.2	4%
	Apple, Fuji, 1 medium	0.1	2%
Dairy	Yogurt, plain, non-fat, 1 cup	1.6	32%
	Milk, fat-free, 1 cup	0.9	18%
	Soymilk, 1 cup	0.3	6%
Protein	Power bar, 1 each	10.8	216%
	Beef liver, pan-fried, 3 ounces	5.6	112%
	Sunflower seeds, dry roasted, ¼ cup	2.6	52%

FIGURE 12-7 ▲ Food sources of pantothenic acid. (a) The fill of the background color (none, 1/3, 2/3, or completely covered) within each group on MyPlate indicates the average nutrient density for pantothenic acid in that group. (b) The bar graph shows the pantothenic acid content of several foods compared to the AI for adults. Overall, fortified foods and foods rich in protein are the best sources of pantothenic acid.

Source: *Nutrition data from USDA National Database for Standard Reference, Release 26.*

12.6 Vitamin B-6 (Pyridoxine)

FUNCTIONS OF VITAMIN B-6

This vitamin is known by its number, rather than its general name. Vitamin B-6 is a family of three structurally similar compounds. All can be converted into the active vitamin B-6 coenzyme pyridoxal phosphate (PLP). The coenzymes of vitamin B-6 are needed for the activity of numerous enzymes involved in carbohydrate, protein, and lipid metabolism. One of the primary functions is as a coenzyme in over 100 chemical reactions that involve the metabolism of amino acids and protein (see Fig. 12-1). The B-6 coenzyme, PLP, participates in reactions that allow the synthesis of nonessential (dispensable) amino acids by helping to split the nitrogen group ($-NH_2$) from an amino acid and making it available to another amino acid.

Vitamin B-6 also plays a role in **homocysteine** metabolism. Among the other important functions of vitamin B-6 are synthesis of neurotransmitters such as serotonin and gamma aminobutyric acid (GABA); conversion of tryptophan to niacin; breakdown of stored glycogen to glucose; and synthesis of white blood cells and the heme portion of **hemoglobin.**

VITAMIN B-6 DEFICIENCY

Because of the role of vitamin B-6 in hemoglobin synthesis, a deficiency in vitamin B-6 would affect multiple body systems, including the cardiovascular, immune, and nervous systems, as well as overall energy metabolism. Vitamin B-6 deficiency also results in widespread symptoms, including depression, vomiting, skin disorders, irritation of the nerves, anemia, and impaired immune response.

homocysteine An amino acid that arises from the metabolism of methionine. Vitamin B-6, folate, vitamin B-12, and choline are required for its metabolism. Elevated levels are associated with an increased risk of cardiovascular disease.

hemoglobin The iron-containing part of the red blood cell that carries oxygen to the cells and carbon dioxide away from the cells. The heme iron portion is also responsible for the red color of blood.

People with alcoholism are susceptible to a vitamin B-6 deficiency. A metabolite formed in alcohol metabolism can displace the coenzyme form of vitamin B-6, increasing its tendency to be destroyed. In addition, alcohol decreases the absorption of vitamin B-6 and decreases the synthesis of its coenzyme form. Cirrhosis and hepatitis (both can accompany alcoholism) also destroy healthy liver tissue. Thus, a cirrhotic liver cannot adequately metabolize vitamin B-6 or synthesize its coenzyme form.

GETTING ENOUGH VITAMIN B-6

With their ample consumption of animal products, North Americans have an average daily consumption of vitamin B-6 that is greater than the RDA. There is some research to indicate that athletes may need slightly more vitamin B-6 than sedentary adults. The athlete's body processes large quantities of glycogen and protein, and the metabolism of these compounds requires vitamin B-6. However, unless athletes restrict their food intake, they are likely to consume plenty of this B vitamin.

Major sources of vitamin B-6 are animal products and fortified ready-to-eat breakfast cereals (Fig. 12-8). Other sources are vegetables and fruits such as potatoes, spinach, bananas, and cantaloupes. Overall, the protein group of MyPlate offers most of the food sources of vitamin B-6 and animal sources and fortified grain products are the most reliable because the vitamin B-6 they contain is more absorbable than that in plant foods. Vitamin B-6 is rather unstable; heating and freezing can easily destroy it.

AVOIDING TOO MUCH VITAMIN B-6

The UL for vitamin B-6 is 100 milligrams per day, based on the risk of developing nerve damage. Studies have shown that intakes of 2 to 6 grams of vitamin B-6 per day for 2 or more months can lead to irreversible nerve damage. Symptoms of vitamin B-6 toxicity include walking difficulties and hand and foot tingling and numbness. Some nerve damage

▲ Bananas are a plant source of vitamin B-6.
© Royalty-Free/Corbis

Vitamin B-6

RDA
 Men: 1.7 milligrams
 Women: 1.3 milligrams
DV: 2 milligrams
UL: 100 milligrams

ChooseMyPlate.gov

(a)

(b)

	Food Item and Amount	Vitamin B-6 (milligrams)	% RDA for Adult Males and Females (1.3 milligrams)
Grains	Special K® cereal, 1 cup	2.0	154%
Grains	Kellogg's® Eggo® waffles, homestyle, 2 each	0.4	31%
Grains	Brown rice, cooked, ½ cup	0.1	8%
Vegetables	Potato, baked with skin, 1 medium	0.5	38%
Vegetables	Spinach, cooked, 1 cup	0.4	31%
Vegetables	Butternut squash, cooked, 1 cup	0.3	23%
Fruits	Banana, 1 medium	0.4	31%
Fruits	Raisins, ½ cup	0.1	8%
Fruits	Watermelon, 1 cup	0.1	8%
Protein	Beef liver, pan-fried, 3 ounces	0.8	62%
Protein	Turkey breast, roasted, 3 ounces	0.7	54%
Protein	Sunflower seeds, dry roasted, 1 ounce	0.2	15%

FIGURE 12-8 ▲ Food sources of vitamin B-6. (a) The fill of the background color (none, 1/3, 2/3, or completely covered) within each group on MyPlate indicates the average nutrient density for vitamin B-6 in that group. (b) The bar graph shows the vitamin B-6 content of several foods compared to the RDA for adults. Overall, the richest and most bioavailable sources of vitamin B-6 are animal sources of protein and fortified breakfast cereals. However, dairy foods (not shown) are not a particularly good source of vitamin B-6.

Source: *Nutrition data from USDA National Database for Standard Reference, Release 26.* Photo: ©Ivary Inc./Alamy.

in individual sensory neurons is probably reversible, but damage to the ganglia (where many nerve fibers converge) appears to be permanent. With 500-milligram tablets of vitamin B-6 available in health-food stores, taking a toxic dose is possible (see Further Reading 6).

> ✓ **CONCEPT CHECK 12.6**
>
> 1. What is the role of vitamin B-6 in energy metabolism and other body functions?
> 2. What are the primary sources of vitamin B-6?
> 3. Are vitamin B-6 supplements safe?

12.7 Biotin (Vitamin B-7)

FUNCTIONS OF BIOTIN

In its coenzyme form, biotin aids in dozens of chemical reactions. Biotin assists in the addition of carbon dioxide to other compounds, a reaction critical in synthesizing glucose and fatty acids, as well as breaking down certain amino acids.

BIOTIN DEFICIENCY

Symptoms of biotin deficiency include a scaly inflammation of the skin, changes in the tongue and lips, decreased appetite, nausea, vomiting, a form of anemia, depression, muscle pain and weakness, and poor growth.

GETTING ENOUGH BIOTIN

Our food supply is thought to provide 40 to 60 micrograms per person per day, more than the AI. The DV for biotin was set years before the vitamin had an AI level set and is based on outdated recommendations. The DV is used on food and supplement labels and is 10 times the estimate of needs. However, biotin is relatively nontoxic. Large doses (up to 1 milligram per day) have been given over an extended period without harmful side effects to children who exhibit defects in biotin metabolism. Thus, no UL for biotin has been set.

Protein sources, such as egg yolks, peanuts, and cheese, are good sources of biotin (Fig. 12-9). The biotin content of food is typically not measured and therefore is often not available in food composition tables or nutrient databases. Because intestinal bacteria synthesize some biotin that you can absorb, a biotin deficiency is unlikely. Scientists are not sure how much of the bacteria-synthesized biotin in our intestines is absorbed, so we still need to consume some in our diet. If bacterial synthesis in the intestines is not sufficient, as in people who are missing a large part of the colon or who take antibiotics for many months, special attention must be paid to meeting biotin needs.

Biotin's bioavailability varies significantly among foods based on the food's biotin-protein complex. In raw egg whites, biotin is bound to avidin, which inhibits absorption of the vitamin. Consuming many raw egg whites can eventually lead to biotin-deficiency disease. Cooking, however, denatures the protein avidin in eggs so it cannot bind biotin. In addition to food safety concerns (see Chapter 17), this is one of the important reasons to avoid consuming raw eggs.

Biotin
AI: 30 micrograms
DV: 300 micrograms
UL: None

> ✓ **CONCEPT CHECK 12.7**
>
> 1. What is the role of biotin in energy metabolism?
> 2. What are the signs and symptoms of biotin deficiency?
> 3. What are the best sources of biotin?
> 4. Why does consumption of raw eggs lead to biotin deficiency?

(a)

(b)

	Food Item and Amount	Biotin (micrograms)	% AI for Adult Males and Females (30 micrograms)
Vegetables	Sweet potato, baked, 1 cup	2.9	■ 10%
Vegetables	Mushrooms, canned, ½ cup	1.7	■ 6%
Vegetables	Carrots, cooked, 1 cup	0.9	▌ 3%
Fruits	Strawberries, 1 cup	2.3	■ 8%
Fruits	Orange juice, from concentrate, 1 cup	1.0	▌ 3%
Fruits	Raisins, ½ cup	0.3	▏ 1%
Dairy	Cheese, American, 2 ounces	1.7	■ 6%
Dairy	Cheese, cheddar, 1.5 ounces	0.6	▎ 2%
Dairy	Milk, non-fat, 1 cup	0.3	▏ 1%
Protein	Beef liver, pan-fried, 3 ounces	35.0	████████◇▶ 106%
Protein	Egg, hard-boiled, 1 large	10.0	█████ 33%
Protein	Peanuts, dry roasted, 1 ounce	4.9	██ 16%

FIGURE 12-9 ▲ Food sources of biotin compared to the Adequate Intake for adults. (a) The fill of the background color (none, 1/3, 2/3, or completely covered) within each group on MyPlate indicates the average nutrient density for biotin in that group. (b) The bar graph shows the biotin content of several foods compared to the AI for adults. Overall, foods rich in protein are the best sources of biotin. Grains (even fortified varieties) contain very little biotin, so they are not shown in the bar graph.

Source: *Nutrition data from Staggs CG and others: Determination of the biotin content of select foods using accurate and sensitive HPLC avidin binding.* Journal of Food Composition and Analysis *17:767, 2004.*

12.8 Iodine

FUNCTIONS OF IODINE

The thyroid gland actively accumulates and traps iodine from the bloodstream to support thyroid hormone synthesis. Thyroid hormones are synthesized using iodine and the amino acid tyrosine. Because these hormones help regulate metabolic rate and promote growth and development throughout the body, iodine (I) adequacy is important for overall energy metabolism.

IODINE DEFICIENCY

During World War I, a link was discovered between a deficiency of iodine and an enlarged thyroid gland, a condition called **goiter.** Men drafted into the military from areas such as the Great Lakes Region of the United States had a much higher rate of goiter than did men from other areas of the country. The soils in these areas have low iodine contents. In the 1920s, a researcher in Ohio found that low doses of iodine given to children over a 4-year period could prevent goiter. That finding led to the addition of iodine to salt beginning in the 1920s, the first time a nutrient was purposely added to food to prevent a disease.

Today, many nations, such as Canada, require iodine fortification of salt. In the United States, salt can be purchased either iodized or plain. Check for this on the label when you purchase salt. Some areas of Europe, such as northern Italy, have very low soil levels of iodine but have yet to adopt an iodine-fortification program. People in these areas, especially women, still suffer from goiter, as do people in areas of Latin America, the Indian subcontinent, Southeast Asia, and Africa. About 2 billion people worldwide are at risk of iodine deficiency, and approximately 800 million of these people have suffered the widespread effects of such a deficiency. Eradication of iodine deficiency is a goal of many health-related organizations worldwide.

goiter An enlargement of the thyroid gland; this is often caused by insufficient iodine in the diet.

▲ This woman has an enlargement of the thyroid gland (also known as goiter) caused by insufficient iodine in the diet. © Scott Camazine/ Science Source

congenital hypothyroidism A birth defect that impairs thyroid hormone synthesis. If untreated, this can lead to mental retardation and stunting of growth.

Iodine
RDA: 150 micrograms
DV: 150 micrograms
UL: 1.1 milligrams

If a person's iodine intake is insufficient, the thyroid gland enlarges as it attempts to take up more iodine from the bloodstream. This eventually leads to goiter. Simple goiter is a painless condition but, if uncorrected, can lead to pressure on the trachea (windpipe), which may cause difficulty in breathing. Although iodine can prevent goiter formation, it does not significantly shrink a goiter once it has formed. Surgical removal may be required in severe cases.

If a woman has an iodine-deficient diet during the early months of her pregnancy, the fetus suffers iodine deficiency because the mother's body uses up the available iodine. The infant may be born with stunted growth and developmental delays that collectively are known as **congenital hypothyroidism** (formerly called cretinism). Cretinism appeared in North America before iodine fortification of table salt began. Today, congenital hypothyroidism still appears in Europe, Africa, Latin America, and Asia. Recent studies have shown a link between mild iodine deficiency during pregnancy and decreased IQ (see Further Readings 2 and 4) in offspring in the United Kingdom and Australia. Marginal iodine status has been detected recently in women of childbearing years in the United States (see Newsworthy Nutrition).

GETTING ENOUGH IODINE

The RDA for iodine (see box) was set to support thyroid gland function. This is the same as the DV used on food and supplement labels. A half teaspoon of iodine-fortified salt (about 2 grams) supplies that amount. Most North American adults consume an estimated 190 to 300 micrograms of iodine daily, which is more than the RDA, not including that from use of iodized salt at the table. This extra amount of iodine adds up, because dairies use it as a sterilizing agent, bakeries use it as a dough conditioner, food producers use it as part of food colorants, and it is added to salt. There is concern, however, that vegans may not consume enough unless iodized salt is used. Iodized salt, dairy products, and grain products contain various forms of iodine (Fig. 12-10). Sea salt and kosher salt, however, are not typically iodized.

Newsworthy Nutrition

Marginal Iodine Status in Women Planning Pregnancies

Recent data has demonstrated a low urinary iodine concentration (UIC) and a high prevalence of subclinical hypothyroidism in women planning to become pregnant. Subclinical hypothyroidism during pregnancy has been associated with multiple adverse outcomes including spontaneous abortion, gestational hypertension, gestational diabetes, decreased IQ in the offspring, and preterm delivery. The purpose of this study was to assess the UIC and thyroid function levels of 141 women in Washington, D.C., who presented for prenatal screening and who were planning to become pregnant in the near future. This cohort of women exhibited a median UIC level of 100.5 micrograms/liter, the lowest value reported for women of childbearing age to date in the United States. A median UIC for a pregnant population below 150 micrograms/liter indicates inadequate iodine intake. In addition, 11% of the women had thyroid function test results consistent with subclinical hypothyroidism. Although 47% of the women reported taking prenatal vitamins, iodine is lacking in about half of the prenatal vitamins currently marketed in the United States. The authors conclude that this study demonstrates marginally inadequate iodine intake in women seeking preconception counseling and a high rate of prepregnancy subclinical hypothyroidism. This study provides evidence to support the inclusion of iodine in all prenatal vitamin and mineral supplements in the United States and that prenatal supplements should begin prior to conception.

Source: Stagnaro-Green A and others: Marginal iodine status and high rate of subclinical hypothyroidism in Washington DC women planning conception. *Thyroid* 25(10):1151, 2015.

(a)

ChooseMyPlate.gov

(b)

Food Item and Amount	Iodide (micrograms)	% RDA for Adult Males and Females (150 micrograms)
Iodized salt, ½ tsp	195	130%
White bread, 1 slice	29	19%
Corn muffin, 1 small	21	14%
Whole wheat bread, 1 slice	8	5%
Yogurt, plain, non-fat, 1 cup	106	71%
Milk, fat-free, 1 cup	103	69%
Cheese, cheddar, 1.5 ounces	22	15%
Pepperoni pizza, 1 slice	51	34%
Eggs, hard-boiled, 1 large	32	21%
Tuna, grilled, 3 ounces	13	9%

FIGURE 12-10 ▲ Food sources of iodine. (a) The fill of the background color (none, 1/3, 2/3, or completely covered) within each group on the MyPlate indicates the average nutrient density for iodine in that group. (b) The bar graph shows the iodine content of several foods compared to the RDA for adults. Overall, the richest sources of iodine are iodized salt (added to foods in any group), seafood and seaweed, and dairy products. Fruits and vegetables (not shown) are poor sources of iodine.

Source: *Nutrition data from USDA National Database for Standard Reference, Release 26.*

AVOIDING TOO MUCH IODINE

The UL for iodine is 1.1 milligrams per day. When high amounts of iodine are consumed, thyroid hormone synthesis is inhibited, as in a deficiency. This can appear in people who eat a lot of seaweed, because some seaweeds contain as much as 1% iodine by weight. Total iodine intake then can add up to 60 to 130 times the RDA.

CONCEPT CHECK 12.8

1. What is the role of iodine in thyroid metabolism?
2. What are the effects of iodine deficiency?
3. What is goiter?
4. Is salt always a good source of iodine?

12.9 Chromium

FUNCTIONS OF CHROMIUM

Chromium (Cr) enhances the function of insulin, so it is required for glucose uptake into cells. The mineral is involved in the metabolism of lipids and proteins as well, although the exact mechanisms are not known. Chromium supplements have been promoted for building muscle mass and for weight loss, but there is not much evidence to support these claims.

CHROMIUM DEFICIENCY

A chromium deficiency is characterized by impaired blood glucose control and elevated blood cholesterol and triglycerides. Low or marginal chromium intakes may contribute to an increased risk for developing type 2 diabetes, but opinions are mixed on the true degree

▲ Mushrooms are a good source of chromium.
© Comstock/PunchStock

Chromium

AI:

   Men: 35 micrograms

   Women: 25 micrograms

DV: 120 micrograms

UL: none

of this effect. Chromium deficiency appears in people maintained on intravenous nutrition solutions not supplemented with chromium and in children with malnutrition. Marginal deficiencies may go undetected because sensitive measures of chromium status are not available.

GETTING ENOUGH CHROMIUM

Specific data regarding the chromium content of various foods are scant, and most food-composition tables do not include values for this trace mineral. Because of two major limitations, we cannot accurately determine the amount of chromium in food: (1) the content is significantly affected by agricultural and manufacturing processes; and (2) when foods are analyzed, they may be "contaminated" by the chromium in the laboratory instruments themselves. Meat and whole-grain products, eggs, mushrooms, nuts, beer, and spices are relatively good sources of chromium. Brewer's yeast is also a good source.

Chromium absorption is quite low: only 0.4% to 2.5% of the amount consumed. Absorption is enhanced by vitamin C and niacin. Any unabsorbed chromium is excreted in the feces. Once absorbed, it is stored in the liver, spleen, soft tissue, and bone, and excreted via urine. Certain conditions can enhance urinary excretion of chromium: diets high in simple sugars (more than 35% of total calories), significant infection, acute prolonged exercise, pregnancy and lactation, and major physical trauma. If chromium intakes are already low, these states potentially can lead to deficiency.

The Adequate Intake (AI) for chromium is based on the amount present in a balanced dietary pattern (see box). Average adult intakes in North America are estimated at about 30 micrograms per day but could be somewhat higher.

No UL for chromium has been set because toxicity for that present in foods has not been observed. Chromium toxicity, however, has been reported in people exposed to industrial waste and in painters who use art supplies with high chromium content. Liver damage and lung cancer can result. Use of any supplement should normally not exceed the DV unless supervised by a physician because of the risk of toxicity.

✔ **CONCEPT CHECK 12.9**

1. How is chromium involved in carbohydrate metabolism?
2. Why is it hard to know the chromium content of foods?
3. Which foods are considered the best sources of chromium?

12.10 Other Trace Minerals Involved in Energy Metabolism

MANGANESE

The mineral manganese (Mn) is easily confused with magnesium (Mg). Not only are their names similar, but they also often substitute for each other in metabolic processes. As a participant in energy metabolism, manganese is required as a cofactor for synthesis of glucose and metabolism of some amino acids. Manganese is also needed by some enzymes, such as those used in free-radical metabolism (via superoxide dismutase). Manganese is also important in bone formation.

Manganese deficiency does not develop in humans unless the mineral is purposely removed from the diet. Animals on manganese-deficient diets suffer alterations in brain function, bone formation, and reproduction. If human diets were low in manganese, these symptoms would probably appear as well. As it happens, our need for manganese is low, and our diets tend to be adequate in this trace mineral.

The AI for manganese is 1.8 to 2.3 milligrams to offset daily losses (see box). Average intakes fall within this range. The DV used on food and supplement labels is 2 milligrams. Good food sources of manganese are nuts, rice, oats, and other whole grains, beans, and leafy vegetables.

Manganese

AI:

   Men: 2.3 milligrams

   Women: 1.8 milligrams

DV: 2 milligrams

UL: 11 milligrams

Manganese is toxic at high doses. Supplements are not recommended, as large doses can decrease absorption of other minerals. People with low iron stores must avoid manganese supplements or risk worsening anemia. The UL is 11 milligrams per day. This value is based on the development of nerve damage. Miners who have inhaled dust fumes high in manganese experience symptoms that mimic Parkinson's disease, including cognitive and muscular dysfunction.

MOLYBDENUM

Several human enzymes use molybdenum (Mo), including some involved in metabolism of amino acids that contain sulfur. No molybdenum deficiency has been reported in people who consume food orally. Deficiency symptoms have appeared in people maintained on intravenous nutrition devoid of this trace mineral. Symptoms include increased heart and respiratory rates, night blindness, mental confusion, edema, and weakness.

Good food sources of molybdenum include milk and dairy products, beans, whole grains, and nuts. The RDA for molybdenum is 45 micrograms to offset daily losses. The DV used on food and supplement labels is 75 micrograms. Our daily intakes average 76 micrograms (for women) and 109 micrograms (for men). The Upper Level for molybdenum is 2 milligrams per day. When consumed in high doses, molybdenum causes toxicity in laboratory animals, resulting in weight loss and decreased growth. Toxicity risk in humans is quite low.

▲ Nuts are rich in manganese. © Comstock/ PunchStock

Molybdenum
RDA: 45 micrograms
DV: 75 micrograms
UL: 2 milligrams

ASK THE RDN   Boosting your Metabolism

Dear RDN: I am concerned that my "slow metabolism" may be making it difficult to maintain a healthy weight. Are there things I can do that will increase my metabolism and help prevent my weight from creeping up?

Metabolism is an important component of weight control. Recall from Section 7.1 that your basal metabolic rate (BMR) or "metabolism" determines how quickly your body burns energy to maintain basic functions such as heartbeat and breathing. You may have inherited a "slow" metabolism, and after age 40, BMR steadily declines. This is a major contributor to age-related weight gain. Gaining fat mass while losing lean mass will slow metabolism even more.

Good news! You can speed up your metabolism, which will help manage your weight. Incorporating the following tips into your lifestyle will help boost your metabolism, burn more calories, and reduce extra body fat.

1. After a good nights *sleep*, simply *eating breakfast* is one of the most effective ways to improve your metabolism. While we sleep, BMR slows down to conserve energy. Depriving yourself of sleep, however, can lead to an overall slower metabolic rate because of negative effects on insulin and stress levels, appetite, and your body's ability to metabolize sugar. Eating a healthy breakfast in the morning jump-starts your metabolism, breaking it out of its fasting metabolic state. It is estimated that eating breakfast can increase resting metabolism by 10%. Because of this metabolic boost, it is not wise to skip breakfast to spare calories. Research shows that breakfast eaters are more likely to have a healthy BMI (under 25). A breakfast that combines complex carbohydrates, protein, and a little fat will get your metabolism going and will keep you satisfied until lunch (see Further Reading 8).

2. Believe it or not, *eating more often* and snacking can actually help you lose weight. As you go though your day, eating a small meal or snack every 3 to 4 hours will help you to burn more calories. In contrast, eating large meals with several hours between causes your metabolism to slow down. Skipping meals, following very-low-calorie diets, and fasting are not good strategies to boost your metabolism. These actions often decrease overall calorie intake but at the expense of a slower metabolism. Although very-low-calorie diets (<1,200 kcal a day for women or <1,800 for men) may help you lose weight at first, they will eventually fail because they are difficult to maintain and burn muscle, not fat.

high-intensity interval training (HIIT) Short, intense aerobic workout that alternates short periods of intense anaerobic exercise with less-intense recovery periods to provide improved athletic capacity and condition, improved glucose metabolism, and improved fat burning.

3. ***Eating more protein-rich foods*** will boost metabolism at mealtime, because more calories are burned digesting protein compared to fat or carbohydrates. Protein-rich foods, including lean meats, tofu, nuts, beans, eggs, and low-fat dairy products, will also provide building blocks for the growth and maintenance of muscle.

4. Muscle is more metabolically active than fat; every pound of muscle requires about 6 kcal a day just to sustain it, compared to only 2 kcal per pound of fat. Therefore, ***building muscle*** can cause a long-term increase in your resting metabolism. Resting metabolic rate (the calories your body burns even when you are at rest) is much higher in people with more muscle mass. Strength-training not only leads to muscle growth, but also raises your energy expenditure for the whole day. ***Aerobic exercise*** will increase your metabolism, not only during a workout, but also for a few hours afterward. Including **high-intensity interval training (HIIT)** will result in a greater, more sustained rise in resting metabolic rate compared to low- or moderate-intensity workouts.

5. As you are eating more protein and getting more exercise, remember to ***stay hydrated.*** Even mild dehydration will slow your metabolism. Research has shown that individuals who drink more water (eight or more glasses a day) burn more calories than those who drink less. Drinking a glass of water or other unsweetened beverage before every meal and snack will help you stay hydrated. Drinking caffeine-containing beverages such as coffee, tea, or energy drinks may cause a short-term rise in your metabolic rate. However, we do not recommend so-called "energy drinks" as part of your metabolism-boosting program (see What the Dietitian Chose at the end of this chapter for more on energy drinks). The high levels of caffeine and various other ingredients may cause more harm than good.

In a nutshell, to speed up your slow metabolism, start your day with breakfast, eat smaller meals more often, drink plenty of water, and exercise to stimulate and build muscle.

Kicking it up a notch,

Anne M. Smith, PhD, RDN, LD (author)

Table 12-1 lists snack ideas that are good sources of the energy nutrients along with the B vitamins and trace mineral cofactors needed for energy metabolism. Table 12-2 summarizes much of what we know about the B vitamins and trace minerals involved in energy metabolism.

TABLE 12-1 ■ Energy-Sustaining Snack Ideas

½ cup blueberries and 1 ounce walnuts
½ ounce almonds and ½ ounce dried apricots
½ cup apple slices dipped in 2 tablespoons almond butter or peanut butter
1 ounce multigrain tortilla chips with 1/4 cup tomato salsa
5 whole grain crackers with ¼ cup hummus
3 cups air-popped popcorn tossed with 1 teaspoon olive oil
Half of a sandwich made with whole-grain bread
6 ounces soy or dairy yogurt topped with 2 tablespoons natural granola
Smoothie made with frozen fruit, flaxseeds, and milk (soy, cow, rice, or hemp)

Source: Adapted from Aronson D: Eating for energy. *Today's Dietitian* 1(4):20, 2009 (see Further Reading 1).

✓ **CONCEPT CHECK 12.10**

1. What are the primary functions of manganese and molybdenum in metabolism of nutrients?
2. What are the good food sources of manganese and molybdenum?
3. Why is a deficiency of manganese or molybdenum possible when patients are fed intravenously?

TABLE 12-2 ■ **Summary of the Vitamins and Minerals Involved in Energy Metabolism**

Vitamin	Major Functions	Adult RDA or AI	Dietary Sources*	Deficiency Symptoms	Toxicity Symptoms
Thiamin	• Coenzyme of carbohydrate metabolism • Nervous system function	1.1–1.2 milligrams	• Sunflower seeds • Pork • Whole and enriched grains • Dried beans • Peas	*Beriberi* • Nervous tingling • Poor coordination • Edema • Heart changes • Weakness	None
Riboflavin	• Coenzyme of carbohydrate metabolism	1.1–1.3 milligrams	• Milk • Mushrooms • Spinach • Liver • Enriched grains	• Inflammation of the mouth and tongue • Cracks at the corners of the mouth • Eye disorders	None
Niacin	• Coenzyme of energy metabolism • Coenzyme of fat synthesis • Coenzyme of fat breakdown	14–16 milligrams (niacin equivalents)	• Mushrooms • Bran • Tuna • Salmon • Chicken • Beef • Liver • Peanuts • Enriched grains	*Pellagra* • Diarrhea • Dermatitis • Dementia • Death	Upper Level is 35 milligrams from supplements, based on flushing of skin
Pantothenic acid	• Coenzyme of energy metabolism • Coenzyme of fat synthesis • Coenzyme of fat breakdown	5 milligrams	• Mushrooms • Liver • Broccoli • Eggs *Most foods have some*	• No natural deficiency disease or symptoms	None
Biotin	• Coenzyme of glucose synthesis • Coenzyme of fatty-acid synthesis • Coenzyme of protein breakdown	30 micrograms	• Peanut butter • Lamb liver • Eggs • Milk • Whole grains	• Inflammation of the skin and mouth • Nausea/vomiting • Anemia • Depression • Muscle pain/weakness	None
Vitamin B-6	• Coenzyme of energy metabolism • Coenzyme of protein synthesis • Synthesis of heme	1.3–1.7 milligrams	• Salmon • Potato • Banana • Avocado • Chicken	• Irritability • Insomnia • Muscle weakness • Anemia	Upper Level is 100 milligrams, based on risk of developing nerve damage
Iodide	• Component of thyroid hormones	150 micrograms	• Iodized salt • White bread • Saltwater fish • Dairy products	• Goiter • Mental retardation • Congenital hypothyroidism: poor growth in infancy when mother is iodide deficient during pregnancy	Upper Level is 1.1 milligrams, based on inhibition of thyroid gland function
Chromium	• Aids insulin function	25–35 micrograms	• Meats • Whole grains • Brewer's yeast	• Impaired glucose tolerance • Elevated blood lipids	None from foods; environmental exposure leads to liver damage and lung cancer
Manganese	• Cofactor for glucose synthesis • Cofactor for amino-acid metabolism • Cofactor for anti-oxidant systems	1.8–2.3 milligrams	• Nuts • Whole grains • Beans • Leafy vegetables	None observed in humans	Upper Level is 11 milligrams based on development of nervous system disorders
Molybdenum	• Cofactor for amino-acid metabolism	45 micrograms	• Beans • Grains • Nuts	None observed in healthy humans	Upper Level is 2 milligrams based on poor laboratory growth in animals

*Fortified ready-to-eat breakfast cereals are good and readily available sources of vitamins and minerals for many of us.

12.11 Nutrition and Your Health
Choline: The Newest Vitamin?

▲ Choline is important for proper development of the fetal brain. Milk and other dairy products supply some choline. © Punchstock/BananaStock

Our knowledge of micronutrients continues to evolve. Although certain components of foods have been linked to prevention of diseases since ancient times, the first vitamin was not isolated until 1913—a mere century ago. Over the next 25 years, all the vitamins we know to be essential in the human diet—from A to E—were identified. For choline, a water-soluble compound that is important for many aspects of human health, the story is still unfolding.

In 1998, the Institute of Medicine recognized choline as an essential nutrient. When the Dietary Reference Intakes were released in 2000, only limited research on the dietary requirements for choline existed. One study of male volunteers showed decreased choline stores and liver damage when they were fed choline-deficient intravenous nutrition solutions. Based on this human study, plus laboratory animal studies, choline has been deemed essential, but it is not yet classified as a vitamin.

FUNCTIONS OF CHOLINE

Despite its lack of vitamin status, choline is needed by all cells and plays several important roles in the body.

Cell Membrane Structure Choline is a precursor for several phospholipids. Phosphatidylcholine (also known as lecithin) accounts

for about half of the phospholipids in cell membranes. Recall from Chapter 5 that phospholipids contribute to the flexibility of cell membranes and allow for the presence of both water- and fat-soluble compounds in cell membranes. With its role in cell membrane structure, choline is important for the health of every cell and particularly for the health of brain tissue, where it is present in high levels.

Single-Carbon Metabolism Choline is a precursor for betaine, a compound that participates in many chemical reactions that involve the transfer of single-carbon groups in metabolism. Important examples of metabolic pathways that involve the transfer of single-carbon groups include the synthesis of neurotransmitters, modifications of DNA during embryonic development, and the metabolism of homocysteine. As you learned in Section 12.6, high levels of homocysteine in the blood are related to increased risk of heart disease. Betaine and the B vitamin folate both donate single-carbon groups to convert homocysteine to another compound, thus reducing levels of homocysteine in the blood. The role of choline in single-carbon metabolism has broad implications, from embryonic development through old age.

Current research points to a role of adequate choline for the prevention of birth defects. Choline's purported role in prevention of birth defects is similar to that of folate. Both folate and choline are involved in formation of DNA during embryonic development. As you will read in Chapter 18, problems with DNA formation lead to birth defects. Indeed, animal studies show that maternal choline supplementation during critical stages of embryonic development can improve learning and memory in the offspring. In humans, as well, studies show that babies born to women with low choline intakes have four times higher rates of birth defects as babies born to women with high choline intakes.

Nerve Function and Brain Development Choline is part of acetylcholine, a neurotransmitter associated with attention, learning, memory, muscle control, and many other functions. Sphingomyelin, a choline-containing phospholipid, is part of the myelin sheath that insulates nerve cells. As already mentioned, brain tissue is particularly high in choline. During pregnancy, the concentration of choline in amniotic fluid is high, supplying choline to the developing brain of the fetus. Animal studies demonstrate that choline deficiencies during pregnancy lead to poor brain development, learning ability, and memory. The AI for choline is increased during pregnancy and breastfeeding to assist in proper brain development. Choline also may be useful for preventing or treating neurological disorders such as Alzheimer's disease.

Lipid Transport As part of phospholipids, choline is a component of lipoproteins, which carry lipids through the blood. Choline deficiencies in animals and humans lead to decreased production of lipid transport proteins, such as very-low-density lipoproteins (VLDLs). For certain, achieving adequate choline intake helps to avoid development of fatty liver. The inability of the liver to export fat to the rest of the body leads to the buildup of fat in the liver. A small amount of fat in the liver is normal, but excess fat leads to scarring of the liver tissue and eventual dysfunction. Fatty liver is a common cause of cirrhosis.

The roles of choline in lipid transport and homocysteine metabolism have implicated the nutrient in prevention of cardiovascular disease. However, research has also raised some concerns about possible negative effects of choline, namely an association between dietary choline intake and increased cardiovascular disease risk. Recent findings have shown that metabolism of dietary phosphatidylcholine, from foods such as eggs, by the intestinal microbiota produces an atherosclerosis-promoting compound that has been associated with an increased risk of major adverse cardiovascular events (see Further Reading 9).

GETTING ENOUGH CHOLINE

Choline is widely distributed in foods (Fig. 12-11). Soybeans, egg yolks, beef, cauliflower, almonds, and peanuts are good sources. In addition to natural food sources, lecithin is often added to food products as an emulsifier during processing, so many other foods are sources of choline.

Choline can exist in foods as free choline or as part of other compounds, such as phospholipids. Pancreatic enzymes break down some of the phospholipid forms prior to absorption. Free choline is water soluble and can be absorbed from the small intestine into portal circulation for transport to the liver. Choline that is part of phospholipids, on the other hand, is fat soluble and gets absorbed into the lymphatic system.

To some extent, choline also can be synthesized in the body by a process that involves other nutrients, such as folate and the amino acid methionine. If the body must synthesize choline to meet its needs, functional deficiencies of folate could result.

Eggs (with yolks) are by far the most nutrient-dense source of choline. One whole egg supplies about one-fourth of the daily choline needs in a 70-kcal package. However, dietary advice to limit saturated fat and cholesterol discourages frequent intake of egg yolks. Choline researchers suggest that an average of

▲ Dairy products, soy, almonds, and peanuts are natural sources of choline.
© C Squared Studios/Getty Images

one egg per day would assist in achieving the AI for choline while still supplying less than the 300-milligram-per-day limit for cholesterol.

An AI for choline has been set for adults (see box), but it is unknown whether a dietary supply is essential for infants or children. As noted, some choline can be synthesized in the body, but

Choline

AI
    Men: 550 milligrams
    Women: 425 milligrams
DV: not established
UL: 3.5 grams

(a)

(b)

Food Item and Amount	Choline (milligrams)	% AI for Adult Males (550 milligrams)		% AI for Adult Females (425 milligrams)	
Vegetables					
Swiss chard, cooked, 1 cup	50		9%		12%
Cauliflower, cooked , 1 cup	49		9%		12%
Mushrooms, shiitake, 4 each	30		5%		7%
Dairy					
Milk, fat-free, 1 cup	38		7%		9%
Yogurt, plain, non-fat, 1 cup	37		7%		9%
Cottage cheese, low-fat, ½ cup	18		3%		4%
Protein					
Beef liver, pan-fried , 3 ounces	339		62%		78%
Egg, hard-boiled, 1 large	147		27%		35%
Cod, baked, 3 ounces	71		13%		17%

FIGURE 12-11 ▲ Food sources of choline. (a) The fill of the background color (none, 1/3, 2/3, or completely covered) within each group on MyPlate indicates the average nutrient density for choline in that group. (b) The bar graph shows the choline content of several foods compared to the AI for adults. Overall, foods that are rich sources of protein are good sources of choline. Grains and fruits are not included in the bar graph because, in general, these are poor sources of choline.

Source: *Nutrition data from USDA National Database for Standard Reference, Release 26.*

current research indicates that synthesis by the body is not sufficient to meet the body's needs for choline. Nutrition surveys indicate that fewer than 10% of Americans meet the AI for choline. In addition, the AIs do not reflect wide genetic variation in individual choline requirements. Research suggests that at least half the population has genetic variations that increase dietary requirements for nutrients that serve in single-carbon metabolism, including choline and folate. Thus, even meeting the AI may not provide enough choline to support the body's needs for some people (see Further Reading 10). There are many proposed health benefits for adequate choline intake (see Further Reading 11).

The AI for choline increases during pregnancy (to 450 milligrams per day) and breastfeeding (to 550 milligrams per day) to support brain development of the fetus or infant. All prenatal vitamins do not contain choline; therefore, consumption of rich dietary sources of choline, such as eggs, is important for pregnant and breastfeeding women.

AVOIDING TOO MUCH CHOLINE

The UL for adults is set at 3.5 grams per day. Routinely exceeding the UL will result in a fishy body odor and low blood pressure.

Summary (Numbers refer to numbered sections in the chapter.)

12.1 The B vitamins yield no energy directly, but they contribute to energy-yielding chemical reactions in the body by virtue of their coenzyme functions. B vitamins are highly bioavailable. North American diets are typically adequate in B vitamins except in cases of poverty, metabolic disorders, or alcoholism. Whole grains are more nutrient-dense sources of B vitamins (as well as other nutrients) than refined grains. Several B vitamins function as coenzymes in energy metabolism. In addition, iodine, chromium, manganese, and molybdenum participate in various aspects of metabolism of carbohydrates, lipids, and protein.

12.2 Thiamin's coenzyme form is involved in metabolism of carbohydrates and proteins as well as synthesis of RNA, DNA, and neurotransmitters. Rich food sources of thiamin include pork, enriched or fortified grain products, and milk. Beriberi, the thiamin-deficiency disease, leads to muscle weakness and nerve damage. Thiamin toxicity is unknown, and no UL has been set.

12.3 The coenzymes of riboflavin participate in catabolism of fatty acids, metabolism of other vitamins and minerals, and the antioxidant activity of glutathione peroxidase. Dairy products, enriched and fortified grain products, meat, and eggs are rich food sources of riboflavin. Symptoms of ariboflavinosis include glossitis and angular cheilitis. There is no evidence of toxicity with high doses of riboflavin; no UL has been set.

12.4 Niacin's coenzymes function in the generation of ATP and in many anabolic pathways, especially fatty-acid synthesis. Rich food sources include seafood, poultry, meats, peanuts, and enriched or fortified grains. Pellagra, the disease of niacin deficiency, results in dermatitis, diarrhea, dementia, and eventual death. Megadoses of niacin have been used to lower blood lipids; but they cause side effects, such as flushing of the skin.

12.5 Pantothenic acid functions as a coenzyme in reactions that yield energy from carbohydrates, lipids, and protein, as well as

fatty-acid synthesis. It is widely distributed among foods, with sunflower seeds, mushrooms, peanuts, and eggs among the richest sources. A deficiency of pantothenic acid is unlikely, but symptoms would be similar to those seen with deficiencies of other B vitamins. There is no known toxicity and no UL for pantothenic acid.

12.6 Vitamin B-6 coenzymes activate many enzymes of carbohydrate, lipid, and especially protein metabolism. They also help synthesize neurotransmitters and participate in homocysteine metabolism. Rich food sources include animal products and enriched or fortified grain products, as well as some fruits and vegetables. A deficiency of vitamin B-6 leads to headaches, depression, gastrointestinal symptoms, skin disorders, nerve problems, anemia, and impaired immunity. Vitamin B-6 toxicity can result in nerve damage.

12.7 Biotin's coenzyme form aids in reactions that synthesize glucose and fatty acids and in the metabolism of amino acids. Egg yolks, peanuts, and cheese provide dietary biotin, but this vitamin is also synthesized by bacteria in the intestines. Consuming raw egg whites may lead to a biotin deficiency, because avidin in egg whites binds biotin and reduces its bioavailability. Biotin deficiency can lead to inflammation of the skin and mouth, gastrointestinal symptoms, muscle pain and weakness, poor growth, and anemia. No UL has been set for biotin as no toxicity has ever been observed.

12.8 Iodine is required for the formation and function of thyroid hormone. A dietary deficiency of iodine can lead to enlargement of the thyroid gland (goiter) or, for the offspring of deficient mothers, impaired physical and mental development (congenital hypothyroidism). Toxicity of iodine, like deficiency, also inhibits thyroid hormone synthesis. Iodized salt, some seafood, dairy products, and grain products are dietary sources of iodine.

12.9 Chromium participates in carbohydrate metabolism by aiding insulin function. Meat, whole-grain products, and Brewer's yeast are good sources of chromium, but data on chromium content of foods are limited. A chromium deficiency leads to impaired glucose tolerance and elevated blood lipids. There is no UL for chromium as toxicity has only been reported from exposure to environmental contamination.

12.10 Manganese is a cofactor for glucose synthesis and amino-acid metabolism. It also contributes to bone formation and antioxidant functions. Food sources include nuts, whole grains, beans, and leafy vegetables. Manganese deficiency is unknown in humans but would likely impair brain function, bone formation, and reproduction. Nerve damage may occur with manganese toxicity.

Molybdenum is a cofactor for enzymes that function in amino-acid metabolism. Food sources include dairy products, beans, whole grains,

and nuts. A deficiency, which has only been observed in people on total parenteral nutrition devoid of molybdenum, leads to problems with heart rate and respiration, mental confusion, and weakness. Risk for molybdenum toxicity in humans is low.

12.11 Choline is an essential nutrient, but has not yet been classified as a vitamin. As a component of phospholipids, it contributes to cell membrane structure, the myelin sheath that surrounds nerves, and functions in lipid transport. Like folate, choline plays a role in single-carbon metabolism, which has implications for prevention of birth defects, cancer, and heart disease. Egg yolks, meats, dairy products, soybeans, and nuts are good food sources of choline.

Check Your Knowledge (Answers are available at the end of this question set.)

1. A mineral that is required for activation or function of an enzyme is called
   a. a collagen.
   b. an organophosphate.
   c. a coenzyme.
   d. a cofactor.

2. B vitamins, including thiamin, riboflavin, and niacin, are called the "energy" vitamins because they
   a. can be broken down to provide energy.
   b. are part of coenzymes needed for release of energy from carbohydrates, fats, and proteins.
   c. are ingredients in energy drinks such as Powerade®.
   d. are needed in large amounts by competitive athletes.

3. Which of the B vitamins is sensitive to and can be degraded by light?
   a. Riboflavin
   b. Thiamin
   c. Niacin
   d. Pantothenic acid

4. Niacin can be synthesized in the body from the amino acid
   a. tyrosine.
   b. phenylalanine.
   c. tryptophan.
   d. glutamine.

5. A deficiency of iodine causes an enlargement of the thyroid called
   a. pellagra.
   b. goiter.
   c. beriberi.
   d. anemia.

6. Vitamin B-6 is an important coenzyme in the metabolism of
   a. fatty acids.
   b. bile acids.
   c. amino acids.
   d. pantothenic acid.

7. Avidin, a component of raw egg whites, may decrease the absorption of
   a. biotin.
   b. iron.
   c. thiamin.
   d. riboflavin.

8. Pantothenic acid functions as part of
   a. coenzyme A.
   b. PLP.
   c. NADP.
   d. coenzyme Q.

9. Choline is an important component of
   a. cholesterol.
   b. a phospholipid.
   c. an antioxidant.
   d. proteins.

10. Noodles, spaghetti, and bread are all made from wheat flour. This flour is enriched with all of the following nutrients except
    a. vitamin B-6.
    b. thiamin.
    c. niacin.
    d. iron.
    e. riboflavin.

Answer Key: 1. d (LO 12.1), 2. b (LO 12.1), 3. a (LO 12.3), 4. c (LO 12.4), 5. b (LO 12.8), 6. c (LO 12.6), 7. a (LO 12.7), 8. a (LO 12.5), 9. b (LO 12.11), 10. a (LO 12.1)

Study Questions (Numbers refer to Learning Outcomes)

1. Milling (refining) grains removes which vitamins and minerals? Which of these are replaced during processing? (**LO 12.1**)

2. What are the best food sources for thiamin? (**LO 12.2**)

3. What are the signs of a riboflavin deficiency? (**LO 12.3**)

4. Describe the three signs of the niacin deficiency pellagra. (**LO 12.4**)

5. How is pantothenic acid involved in energy metabolism? (**LO 12.5**)

6. Describe how the RDA, DV, and UL for vitamin B-6 should be used in everyday life. How do the RDA and DV for vitamin B-6 differ? (**LO 12.6**)

7. Why does the consumption of raw eggs lead to a biotin deficiency? (**LO 12.7**)

8. What is the relationship between iodine, the thyroid gland, and energy metabolism? (**LO 12.8**)

9. Explain the function of chromium in carbohydrate metabolism. (**LO 12.9**)

10. Why is choline not considered a vitamin? (**LO 12.11**)

What the Dietitian Chose

Everyone wants more energy, including college students. This may be one of the reasons energy supplements are the fastest-growing category of the supplement industry. The B-complex vitamins fall in this category and are typically marketed as being energy boosters. We know, however, that B vitamins do not give us energy directly. Rather, a supplement labeled as a B complex will contain the B vitamins that act as coenzymes in energy metabolism. The Supplement Facts label from the Nature Made® B-Complex w/Vitamin C Dietary Supplement indicates that one caplet contains thiamin, riboflavin, niacin, and vitamin B-6 in concentrations 2.5 to 10 times the Daily Value. The information provided for this Nature Made supplement states that "a combination of essential B *vitamins help produce cellular energy from the food you eat.*" Although this is an accurate statement about the role of the B vitamins in the conversion of carbohydrates, fat, and protein into energy, it also means that taking this supplement *alone* will not give you energy.

Nature Made B-Complex w/Vitamin C Dietary Supplement

Supplement Facts

Serving Size 1 Caplet

Amount Per Caplet	% Daily Value
Vitamin C 300 mg	500%
Thiamin 15 mg	1,000%
Riboflavin 10.2 mg	600%
Niacin 50 mg	250%
Vitamin B6 5 mg	250%
Pantothenic Acid 10 mg	100%

To produce energy, you must eat an adequate amount of calories. Even though this B-complex supplement has a big dose of B vitamins, they will not give you an energy boost unless you are deficient in them and are eating your recommended number of calories. Unless there is a specific medical need, it is not necessary to supplement with more than 100% of the Daily Value for any nutrient. If you have adequate B vitamin levels and take a supplement, you won't gain extra energy and your body will excrete the excess vitamin in your urine. In this case, you are wasting your money on something that is being flushed down the toilet.

If you feel that a supplement would be a good backup plan for days when your dietary intake is less than adequate, a balanced multivitamin-mineral supplement providing no more than 100% of the DV for nutrients is a prudent idea. Keep in mind, however, that for the majority of the healthy population, studies show that there is no overall benefit from taking multivitamin-mineral supplements (see Further Reading 5). Multivitamin and mineral supplements are also advertised as energy providers. Centrum® Adults provides the B vitamins involved in energy metabolism as well as all of the other essential vitamins and minerals. The Centrum product contains B vitamins and iron, claims that these nutrients "help support daily energy needs," and states the "B vitamins that can be found in Centrum Adults multivitamins play an important role in converting proteins, fats, and carbohydrates into energy." The Centrum product

Supplement Facts

Serving Size 1.93 fl. oz.

Amount Per Serving	% Daily Value
Niacin (as Niacinamide) 30mg	150%
Vitamin B6 (as Pyridoxine Hydrochloride) 40mg	2,000%
Folic Acid 400mcg	100%
Vitamin B12 (as Cyanocobalamin) 500mcg	8333%
Sodium 18mg	<1%
Energy Blend 1870mg	‡
Taurine, Glucuronic acid (as or from glucuronolactone), Malic Acid, N-Acetyl L-Tyrosine, L-Phenylalanine, Caffeine, Citicoline	

‡ Daily value not established.

© McGraw-Hill Education/Mark Dierker

contains just 100% of the Daily Value for B vitamins but would be beneficial only if you were deficient in these vitamins and had an adequate intake of calories.

Energy shots have become very popular with tired college students. A recent survey of U.S. adults found that almost one in four adults consumes sports and energy drinks at least once per week (see Further Reading 7). Annual sales of 5-Hour Energy® shots reached $1 billion in just 8 years, giving the product 90% of the energy shot market. In addition to three B vitamins, the 5-Hour Energy shot contains caffeine (220 milligrams) and the amino acid taurine. The 5-Hour Energy shot is artificially sweetened and has only 4 calories in the 2-ounce shot. Experts agree that caffeine provides most of the kick from an energy shot. Therefore, you should be cautious if using energy shots and also drinking coffee or other caffeinated drinks. Excess caffeine can cause nervousness, insomnia, nausea, vomiting, rapid heartbeat, and higher blood pressure.

Unfortunately, energy shot makers are not required to disclose their products' caffeine content on the Supplement Facts label. Most energy shots also have other ingredients, such as the taurine, tyrosine, and phenylalanine in 5-Hour. These ingredients raise concern because there is currently not enough research on how they react together. As we said for the B vitamin supplement and the multivitamin and mineral supplement, the B vitamins in the energy shot are not going to boost energy unless you're deficient in B vitamins.

The 5-Hour Energy shot may catch your eye, especially because it has the B vitamins niacin (150% DV), B-6 (2000%), and B-12 (8333%). Energy shots promise a quick, convenient boost of energy and have fewer calories than the full-size energy drinks.

So, even though this small shot has as much caffeine as a 12-ounce cup of coffee and 20 times the Daily Value of vitamin B-6, it still does not have the necessary source of sustained energy—that is, calories. Another problem with taking supplements that contain vitamins in unbalanced quantities is that vitamins often work closely together and levels of one vitamin affect how another vitamin works. This is especially true for the B vitamins, which are highly dependent on each other. For example, the 5-Hour Energy shot has only three B vitamins and very uneven levels of these, which will prevent them from working together.

As you have learned in the early chapters of this book, the nutrients that provide calories give you energy. Calories in the form of glucose are what our body cells prefer to use for energy. We know that glucose comes most directly from carbohydrate-containing foods, including grains, beans, vegetables, fruits, and dairy. Our body's cells break down glucose into ATP. Although the B vitamins play essential roles in the biochemical reactions that generate ATP from glucose, *they don't contain energy.*

A deficiency of B vitamins can affect your energy levels, but so can other things. Lack of sleep and inadequate calories are the first factors to consider. So, instead of reaching for one of the supplements, try to figure out what else may be causing the tiredness. If you are chronically tired, your body is telling you to make a change in your dietary pattern, exercise, stress level, or amount of sleep. To boost energy levels naturally:

- Eat several small meals throughout the day rather than three large ones.

- Avoid large amounts of sugar and fat.
- Don't skip meals, especially breakfast.
- Take a quick exercise break, such as a short walk.
- Exercise regularly.
- Reduce stress.
- Get 7 to 9 hours sleep each night.

Read more about boosting your metabolism in Ask the RDN in this chapter.

For the most part, typical American dietary patterns provide ample B vitamins. Fortified breakfast cereals are especially rich sources of B vitamins and many other micronutrients, and other grains, including breads, pasta, and rice, are enriched with thiamin, niacin, riboflavin, and folic acid, as well as iron. A dietary pattern that adheres to the Dietary Guidelines for Americans and MyPlate will provide enough B vitamins to meet daily needs. All of the B vitamins—thiamin, riboflavin, niacin, pantothenic acid, B-6, biotin, B-12, and folic acid—are frequently found in the same foods, including animal and plant sources. Good animal sources are fish, poultry, meat, eggs, and dairy products. Leafy green vegetables, lentils, beans, peas, and whole grains are rich plant sources of B vitamins. If you include these sources of calories in your diet, you will also be getting enough B vitamins.

CASE STUDY SOLUTION Deficiency from a Vegan and Gluten-Free Diet?

©Image Source/Getty Images

1. We know that Andrew's vegan dietary pattern contains no animal products. As a result, protein quantity and quality may be inadequate. Eliminating meat also removes a rich source of iron and several vitamins, including the B vitamins thiamin (especially in ham and pork), riboflavin, niacin, B-6, and B-12. The vegan's lack of dairy products excludes the richest source of calcium and a significant source of riboflavin. Without animal products in his dietary pattern, Andrew is dependent on beans, nuts, seeds, grains, fruits, and vegetables as his sources of the missing protein, vitamins, and minerals.

2. Andrew may be suffering from celiac disease, which is sensitivity to the gluten protein in wheat, barley, rye, and oats. Celiac disease results in problems involving multiple body systems, including an inflammation that damages the lining of the small intestine. This intestinal damage leads to malabsorption of nutrients from food and such symptoms as pain, bloating, diarrhea, or constipation. Andrew should be evaluated by his primary care physician and a gastroenterologist to determine if he has celiac disease and should be avoiding gluten.

3. Gluten-free diets must be designed carefully to be nutritious and healthy. Eliminating whole grains that contain gluten also eliminates a good source of fiber and several vitamins and minerals (see Further Reading 3). Gluten-free diets can be deficient in thiamin,

riboflavin, niacin, folate, and iron.

4. Andrew's sore, inflamed mouth and tongue, and sores and cracks at the corners of his mouth, are typical signs of a riboflavin deficiency. Because riboflavin is not found in many foods, more than one-third of Americans are assumed to get less than the recommended level of riboflavin. Riboflavin depletion or deficiency may have developed in Andrew as a result of his possible celiac disease, because damage to the small intestine can cause malabsorption of nutrients, including riboflavin. Riboflavin can also be lost through diarrhea in celiac disease sufferers. In addition, Andrew is a vegan and has been avoiding dairy products, a significant source of riboflavin, for at least 1 year.

5. If Andrew is diagnosed with celiac disease and continues to eliminate wheat and other gluten-containing grains from his diet, he needs to replace these grains with a nutrient-rich, gluten-free grain such as quinoa or

buckwheat. Because he seems to have developed a riboflavin deficiency, he should also balance the diet with lots of fruits and vegetables. Lean meat and low-fat dairy products would normally be recommended for a gluten-free diet but would not be included if Andrew continues to be a vegan. Some plant sources that are rich in riboflavin include mushrooms (especially portabella), soybeans such as edamame, almonds and almond butter, broccoli, and spinach. Other gluten-free "enriched" grains, such as rice, are also potential sources of riboflavin.

Andrew should shop for breads, cereals, and other baked products that are "enriched" with B vitamins such as riboflavin. Fortified ready-to-eat breakfast cereals are also a reliable source of vitamins and minerals. Gluten-free rice and corn Chex™ cereals are examples of fortified and affordable gluten-free offerings that are easy to find in the grocery store cereal aisle, whereas other specialty gluten-free products are harder to find and are expensive. Andrew also needs to cook foods that contain riboflavin, including enriched rice, broccoli, and spinach, in a way that minimizes the loss of the B vitamins. Because they are water soluble, riboflavin and the other B vitamins can be lost in the cooking water when we cook rice or pasta. To help retain the riboflavin

in these foods, Andrew should not rinse the rice or pasta after he has cooked it. When he cooks vegetables, he should use only a small amount of water and keep the lid on the pan so that riboflavin and other B vitamins are not lost in the steam. Riboflavin is also easily destroyed by exposure to light.

6. The RDA for riboflavin (1.3 milligrams per day for men and 1.1 milligrams per day for women) has been set to prevent deficiency in most individuals. This RDA can be easily met by eating a varied diet, which typically supplies 1.5 to 2 milligrams of riboflavin a day. Andrew, however, has many dietary restrictions because he is following a vegan dietary pattern and avoiding foods containing gluten. To ensure an adequate daily intake of riboflavin and other micronutrients, Andrew should consider a dietary supplement that contains riboflavin. The Linus Pauling Institute recommends taking a multivitamin-multimineral supplement that contains 100% of the Daily Values (DV) and will ensure an intake of at least 1.7 milligrams of riboflavin per day. Andrew can find riboflavin in both multivitamin and mineral supplements as well as B-complex vitamin supplements. He can read more about riboflavin at the Linus Pauling Institute website: http://lpi.oregonstate.edu/infocenter/vitamins/riboflavin/.

Further Readings

1. Aronson D: Eating for energy. *Today's Dietitian* 1(4):20, 2009.

2. Bath SC and others: Effect of inadequate iodine status in UK pregnant women on cognitive outcomes in their children: results from the Avon Longitudinal Study of Parents and Children (ALSPAC). *Lancet* 382:331, 2013.

3. Cooper CC: Gluten free and healthy—Dietitians can help reverse nutrition deficiencies common in celiac disease patients. *Today's Dietitian* 14(5):24, 2012.

4. Hynes KL and others: Mild iodine deficiency during pregnancy is associated with reduced educational outcomes in the offspring: 9-year follow-up of the Gestational Iodine Cohort. *Journal of Clinical Endocrinology Metabolism* 98:1954, 2013.

5. Kamangar F, Emadi A: Vitamin and mineral supplements: Do we really need them? *International Journal of Preventive Medicine* 3:221, 2012.

6. Office of Dietary Supplements, National Institutes of Health: Dietary supplement fact sheet: Vitamin B-6 fact sheet. September 15, 2011. http://ods.od.nih.gov/factsheets/vitaminb6. Accessed December 31, 2015.

7. Park S and others: Characteristics associated with consumption of sports and energy drinks among U.S. adults: National Health Interview Survey, 2010. *Journal of the Academy of Nutrition and Dietetics* 113:112, 2013.

8. Schaeffer J: Rise and dine!—A breakdown of breakfast's benefits with experts' best meal suggestions. *Today's Dietitian* 13(9):44, 2011.

9. Tang WH and others: Intestinal microbial metabolism of phosphatidylcholine and cardiovascular risk. *New England Journal of Medicine* 368(17):1575, 2013.

10. Webb D: Choline—rethinking the dietary requirement. *Today's Dietitian* 13:38, 2011.

11. Zeisel SH, da Costa K: Choline: An essential nutrient for public health. *Nutrition Reviews* 67:615, 2009.

 To get the most out of your study of nutrition, go to McGraw-Hill's online resources: Connect www.mcgrawhillconnect.com, where you will find NutritionCalc Plus, LearnSmart, and many other dynamic tools.

Rate Your Plate

Evaluating Claims for Vitamins and Vitamin-Like Substances in Energy Bars and Drinks

Using your favorite Internet search engine, search terms such as *energy boost, stress, mental acuity,* and *disease prevention,* along with *vitamin supplement, energy bar,* or *energy drink.* Answer the following questions regarding the products you find and the claims made on the products.

1. Identify claims for these products that you consider fraudulent or misleading.

2. What is the cost of these supplements?

3. Which of the energy vitamins do these products contain?

4. How do the amounts of vitamins they contain compare with the DRIs?

5. What compounds are included that are not considered essential nutrients?

6. What disclaimers or warnings are made about the products?

7. How likely is the supplement to improve a person's energy level and overall health?

© FoodCollection

Student Learning Outcomes

Chapter 13 is designed to allow you to:

13.1 Describe the composition of blood.

13.2 Describe the role of vitamin K in blood clotting and the signs and symptoms of deficiency and toxicity, understand its dietary requirements, and identify its food sources.

13.3 Summarize the functions of folate in cell metabolism, understand the dietary requirements needed to prevent megaloblastic anemia, and identify food sources of folate.

13.4 Understand the process of vitamin B-12 absorption and its role in folate metabolism, identify the dietary requirements for vitamin B-12 needed to avoid deficiency, and identify its food sources.

Chapter 13
Nutrients That Support Blood and Brain Health

What Would You Choose?

Since the World Health Organization recently categorized processed meat as carcinogenic and red meat as a probable carcinogen, you have been limiting your meat consumption to no more than once or twice a month. At the same time you are preparing for a hiking trip at high altitude and have heard that altitude sickness is a possibility if you have iron-deficiency anemia. What would you choose as a substitute for red meat to ensure adequate iron nutrition while cutting back on red meat consumption?

a 3 ounces of clams, mussels, or oysters

b 3 ounces of cooked turkey

c 1 cup of raw spinach

d 1 cup of Wheaties®

Think about your choice as you read Chapter 13, then see What the Dietitian Chose at the end of the chapter.

13.5 Describe the functions of iron in the maintenance of blood health and list its sources, dietary requirements, and deficiency and toxicity problems.

13.6 Describe the functions of copper and its potential for toxicity and list its sources, dietary requirements, and conditions that can lead to a deficiency.

13.7 Summarize the role of nutrition in the development and function of the brain and nervous system and understand how dietary patterns and other lifestyle choices may influence your risk of developing migraines, depression, and neurodegenerative diseases.

By now you have learned about almost all of the nutrients: where they come from and what they do in the body. Some of the nutrients supply chemical energy. Others provide building blocks to synthesize body structures. Still others regulate the many chemical reactions that keep us alive. How do these nutrients get from the digestive tract to the cells all throughout the body?

The answer is *blood*—an amazing transport medium for nutrients, oxygen, wastes, hormones, and cells. In this chapter, you will learn about micronutrients that support blood and brain health. The red and white blood cells are constantly being replaced, so the demands for nutrients that help to synthesize new cells—particularly folate and vitamin B-12—are high. When the health of red blood cells is compromised, poor physical and mental performance results. Healthy red blood cells that can efficiently carry oxygen require iron, vitamin B-6, and copper. When white blood cells are insufficient or dysfunctional, resistance to infections is compromised. We learned in Section 10.1 that the formation and function of white blood cells are especially dependent upon vitamins A, C, D, and E, as well as the mineral zinc.

To wrap up our study of the micronutrients, we will examine the influence of dietary patterns on brain health. Good nutritional status is essential for proper brain development and function. The brain requires a steady supply of micronutrients; deficiencies adversely affect the development and function of the brain.

13.1 Blood Cell Synthesis

erythrocyte Mature red blood cell. These have no nucleus and a life span of about 120 days; they contain hemoglobin, which transports oxygen and carbon dioxide.

hemoglobin The iron-containing part of the red blood cell that carries oxygen to the cells and carbon dioxide away from the cells. The heme iron portion is also responsible for the red color of blood.

The human body has a number of elaborate systems to keep its roughly 100 trillion cells alive and properly functioning. One of these marvels is the circulatory system. Blood is the conduit by which nutrients and oxygen are disseminated throughout the body. Stem cells within the bone marrow give rise to the red blood cells, white blood cells, and platelets that circulate in the blood (Fig. 13-1). Adequate levels of protein, several B vitamins, iron, copper, and zinc are particularly important for the formation of these blood components.

Red blood cells (**erythrocytes**) are the most prevalent type of blood cell (Fig. 13-2). Red blood cells contain a protein called **hemoglobin** that transports oxygen from the lungs to all the cells of the body. Iron, which is part of hemoglobin's structure, allows hemoglobin to

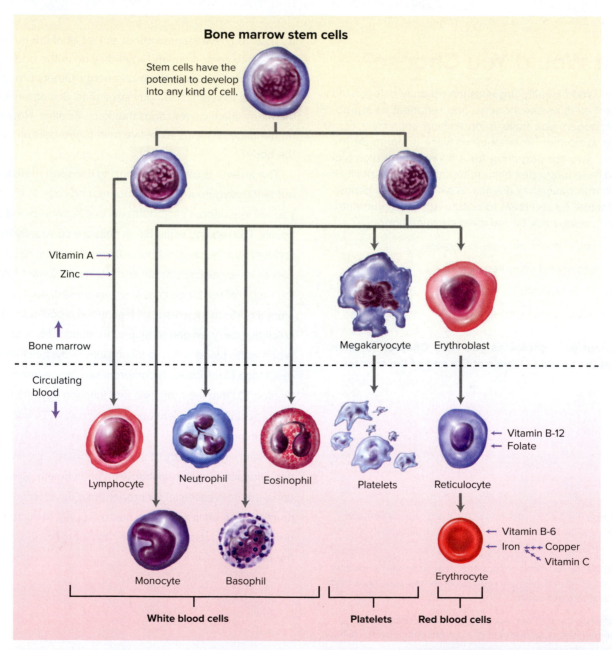

FIGURE 13-1 ▲ Blood cells are formed from stem cells in the bone marrow. Folate and vitamin B-12 are important for DNA synthesis and division of all cells. Red blood cells rely on vitamin B-6 and iron to form hemoglobin. Formation of white blood cells requires zinc.

bind to oxygen. In addition to iron, formation of hemoglobin also requires copper, vitamin C, and vitamin B-6.

What we commonly call white blood cells (**leukocytes**) are actually five types of cells, each with its own function: **neutrophils, lymphocytes, monocytes, eosinophils,** and **basophils.** White blood cells circulate through the blood and lymph, where they are key players in the body's immune defense systems. The lymphocytes are directly responsible for producing antibodies and destroying antigens. Adequate levels of protein, vitamin A, and zinc are especially important for the development of the white blood cells. Recall the discussion of the immune system system in Section 10.1.

Platelets (**thrombocytes**) are actually not cells; they do not have nuclei, so they are more accurately defined as cell fragments. When activated, platelets clump together at the site of an injury to form a plug, thus slowing the rate of bleeding until a permanent clot can form. If your platelet count is low, your clotting time is prolonged. In addition to forming clots, platelets also produce growth factors and chemicals that modulate inflammation. The cascade of events that leads to formation of a blood clot involves vitamin K and calcium (see Section 13.2).

The fourth component of blood, **plasma,** is the extracellular portion devoid of cells. It is the largest portion of blood, accounting for approximately 55% of total blood volume. Often, when you have blood tests done, it is your plasma levels that are measured. Plasma contains proteins, carbohydrates, lipids, micronutrients, hormones, enzymes, and electrolytes.

ERYTHROCYTES

Vitamins and minerals are key players in **erythropoiesis,** or the formation of red blood cells. The primary function of red blood cells is to carry oxygen from your lungs to all the tissues of your body. A secondary function is to carry the waste product, carbon dioxide, from tissues to your lungs. Unlike most cells, a red blood cell has no nucleus (Fig. 13-3). During maturation, the nucleus is lost to make room for hemoglobin. The iron in hemoglobin binds and carries four molecules of oxygen. Red blood cells have a flattened, concave surface to increase surface area. This allows more oxygen to diffuse through the membrane to bind to the iron. Red cells are also flexible, which allows them to squeeze through the tiny capillaries of the circulatory system.

serum Protein-rich portion of blood that separates out when blood coagulates.

leukocyte White blood cell; cell of the immune system.

neutrophil A common white blood cell that fights infections; levels rise during bacterial or fungal infections.

lymphocyte The white blood cell responsible for the immune response; regulates antibody production.

monocyte The white blood cell that ingests foreign cells; also called a phagocyte.

— Plasma

— White blood cells and platelets

— Red blood cells

FIGURE 13-2 ▲ When placed in a centrifuge, whole blood separates into its four components: red blood cells, white blood cells, platelets, and plasma. Blood tests often measure the levels of nutrients or their metabolites in the plasma or **serum,** that is, plasma from which clotting factors have been removed.

Heme group

Beta (β) chains

Alpha (α) chains

Iron (Fe++)

Oxygen (O₂)

FIGURE 13-3 ▲ The red color of blood comes from the iron-containing pigment protein called hemoglobin in red blood cells. Each molecule of hemoglobin contains four heme groups. The iron in heme is responsible for its ability to bind to oxygen. © Getty Images/iStock Exclusive

eosinophil This white blood cell is a type of phagocyte that increases in number during allergic reactions.

basophil The white blood cell that controls inflammation; level increases with poisoning.

thrombocyte (platelet) A protoplasmic disc smaller than a red blood cell; promotes coagulation.

plasma The fluid, extracellular portion of blood.

erythropoiesis Formation of red blood cells.

anemia A decreased oxygen-carrying capacity of the blood. This can be caused by many factors, such as iron deficiency or blood loss.

macrocytic (megaloblastic) Large cell size.

microcytic Small cell size.

hypochromic Pale in color (in reference to red blood cells), as could occur with inadequate hemoglobin content.

(a) Macrocytic
(or megaloblastic) anemia

(b) Microcytic, hypochromic anemia

FIGURE 13-4 ▲ (a) Macrocytic (or megaloblastic) anemia is characterized by large, immature red blood cells. Macrocytic anemia may indicate a deficiency of folate or vitamin B-12. (b) Microcytic, hypochromic anemia is characterized by small, pale-red blood cells. The pale color indicates a lack of hemoglobin. Microcytic, hypochromic anemia occurs with deficiencies of iron or vitamin B-6. a: © SPL/Science Source; b: © Omikron/Science Source

Anemia is a condition characterized by an inadequate number of healthy red blood cells. The following signs and symptoms of anemia can be traced to inadequate oxygen delivery to cells:

- Fatigue
- Rapid heart rate
- Shortness of breath
- Difficulty concentrating
- Pale skin
- Cold extremities

There are three main reasons anemia may occur: (1) blood loss; (2) destruction of blood cells (hemolysis); or (3) a decrease in production of red blood cells or of the hemoglobin in the cells. Micronutrient deficiencies could contribute to any of these. In Section 13.2, you will learn how a vitamin K deficiency can result in hemorrhage. A deficiency of vitamin E, an antioxidant nutrient you learned about in Section 10.5, leaves red blood cells susceptible to oxidative damage. The red blood cell membranes become fragile and break, losing their ability to transport oxygen. It is most likely, however, that nutrient deficiencies could impair erythropoiesis. Deficiencies of either folate or vitamin B-12 affect DNA synthesis, thereby impeding the maturation of red blood cells. Deficiencies of vitamin B-6 or iron could affect the synthesis of hemoglobin, which reduces the ability of red blood cells to transport oxygen. In addition, low levels of copper could affect iron metabolism and therefore limit hemoglobin synthesis.

Anemia is typically detected by symptoms resulting from a reduction in the *number* of healthy red blood cells. Further examining the *size* and *color* of the red blood cells can help an observer to determine the specific cause of the anemia. Healthy red blood cells are described as normocytic (normal size) and normochromic (normal color). Large red blood cells (**macrocytic or megaloblastic**) are signs of folate or vitamin B-12 deficiencies. Red blood cells that are small (**microcytic**) and pale in color (**hypochromic**) are indicative of iron or vitamin B-6 deficiencies (Fig. 13-4). In the following sections, you will learn more about the roles of folate, vitamin B-12, iron, and copper in erythropoiesis. (Vitamin B-6 was already covered in Section 12.6.) The roles of micronutrients in erythropoiesis and blood health are summarized in Table 13-1.

TABLE 13-1 ■ Micronutrients That Support Blood Health

Nutrient	Primary Roles in Blood Health
Vitamin B-6	• Synthesis of heme
Folate	• DNA synthesis; allows proper cell division
Vitamin B-12	• DNA synthesis; allows proper cell division
Vitamin C	• Enhances absorption of nonheme iron
Vitamin K	• Activates clotting factors
Iron	• DNA synthesis • Imparts iron-binding capacity to heme
Copper	• Transports iron

✓ **CONCEPT CHECK 13.1**

1. List the four components of blood and briefly describe their roles.

2. Where are blood cells formed?

3. In whole blood, which type of blood cell is most abundant?

4. List three possible causes of anemia.

5. Explain why macrocytic (megaloblastic) anemia occurs. Which nutrient deficiencies could be responsible for macrocytic anemia?

13.2 Hemostasis and Vitamin K

HEMOSTASIS

Damage to tissues leads to bleeding and blood loss. If blood loss is significant, the delivery of oxygen and nutrients to the cells will be impaired. Therefore, the body has several efficient mechanisms to quickly stop bleeding. Collectively, the following processes that stop blood loss are called **hemostasis:**

1. **Vasoconstriction:** narrowing of the blood vessels, which limits blood flow to the damaged tissue.
2. Formation of a **platelet** plug: platelets stick to the damaged tissue and to each other, creating a temporary seal that stops bleeding.
3. **Coagulation** (blood clotting): process by which blood changes from a liquid to a solid. The end result is reinforcement of the platelet plug with the protein, fibrin.

Coagulation of blood is a multistep process that involves the activation of a series of clotting factors that are always present in the plasma. Usually, platelets do not adhere to the inner lining of blood vessels and clotting factors remain in their inactive forms. This is important because inappropriate formation of blood clots could choke off the blood supply to living tissues. However, when activated by chemical signals released from damaged tissue, a cascade of reactions takes place in which one activated protein activates the next protein to its functional form, leading finally to the conversion of fibrinogen to fibrin (Fig. 13-5).

hemostasis The process of stopping blood loss.

vasoconstriction The narrowing of blood vessels. As part of hemostasis, this temporarily reduces the flow of blood to the site of injury while a clot is being formed.

platelet A protoplasmic disc smaller than a red blood cell that promotes coagulation; also called *thrombocyte.*

coagulation Formation of a blood clot.

What happens to a clot after the damaged tissue has healed? Enzymes break down the clot, releasing some proteins into the bloodstream. Eventually, these protein waste products are picked up by the liver and kidney, and their amino acids can be used to make other proteins.

FIGURE 13-5 ◄ Vitamin K works to activate clotting factors, which are then able to bind to calcium. The calcium binding to clotting factors is necessary for clot formation.

© Science Photo Library RF/Getty Images

Trigger:
Damage to Tissues
or
Blood Contacts Foreign Surface

Inactive Clotting Factors

Vitamin K

Calcium

Active Clotting Factors

Prothrombin activator

Prothrombin → Thrombin

Fibrinogen (soluble protein in blood) → Fibrin (insoluble protein in blood) →

Clot formed using threads of fibrin protein that trap blood cells, platelets, and fluid

hemorrhage An escape of blood from blood vessels.

Individual strands of fibrin join together to form a mesh that reinforces the platelet plug. At various points in the coagulation cascade, vitamin K and calcium are required as cofactors.

Hemorrhage is essentially the opposite of hemostasis. In hemorrhage, blood loss cannot be controlled and the blood supply to body tissues becomes depleted. Hemorrhage could result from insufficient vitamin K. Excessive vitamin E could also lead to hemorrhage because, at high doses, vitamin E interferes with the functions of vitamin K (see Section 10.5). In addition, excessive intakes of omega-3 fatty acids could cause hemorrhage because these fatty acids lead to the production of chemical messengers that inhibit blood clotting (see Section 5.6).

FORMS AND FUNCTIONS OF VITAMIN K

A family of compounds known collectively as vitamin K is found in plants, plant oils, fish oils, and animal products. Vitamin K is also synthesized by bacteria in the human colon, which normally fulfills approximately 10% of human requirements. Vitamin K has three forms: (1) phylloquinone, the most abundant form of vitamin K, is synthesized by green plants; (2) menaquinone is synthesized by gut bacteria; and (3) menadione is the synthetic form found in supplements. Interestingly, the synthetic menadione form of vitamin K is twice as biologically available as the other two!

Vitamin K serves as a cofactor in chemical reactions that add carbon dioxide (CO_2) molecules to various proteins, thus enabling these proteins to bind calcium. This is the biochemical basis for vitamin K's role in the life-and-death process of blood clotting. In the clotting cascade (see Fig. 13-5), vitamin K imparts calcium-binding ability to seven different proteins, eventually leading to the conversion of soluble fibrinogen into insoluble fibrin (i.e., the clot). The "K" stands for *koagulation* in the language spoken by the Danish researchers who first noted the relationship between vitamin K and blood clotting.

Besides its role in blood clotting, vitamin K is also important for bone health. The calcium-binding protein in the bone, osteocalcin, depends upon vitamin K for its function in bone mineralization (see Section 11.8).

VITAMIN K DEFICIENCY

At birth, a newborn has a relatively sterile gut—an intestinal tract with an insufficient amount of bacteria. Thus, the newborn cannot produce enough vitamin K to allow for effective blood clotting if the infant is injured or needs surgery. Therefore, vitamin K is routinely administered by injection shortly after birth. It is becoming more common, however, for parents to refuse vitamin K supplementation for their infants which, in some cases, has led to hemorrhagic complications, such as intracranial bleeding, due to vitamin K deficiency (see Further Reading 18). In adults, deficiencies of vitamin K have occurred when a person takes antibiotics for an extended time (this destroys the bacteria that normally produce some of the vitamin K that can be absorbed and used by humans) and when fat absorption is limited.

Medicine Cabinet

People who are prone to develop blood clots may take anticoagulants or "blood thinners." One example is Plavix® (clopidogrel), which works by inhibiting the activity of platelets. Another commonly prescribed anticoagulant is Coumadin® (warfarin). This medication inhibits vitamin K–dependent coagulation factors. When taking Coumadin or similar drugs, it is important to keep dietary intake of vitamin K consistent from day to day (see Further Reading 15).

medicine cabinet pills - © Footage supplied by Goodshoot/Punchstock

GETTING ENOUGH VITAMIN K

Major food sources of the phylloquinone form of vitamin K are green leafy vegetables, broccoli, asparagus, and peas (Fig. 13-6). The menaquinone form of vitamin K is found in some meats, eggs, and dairy products, and is the form synthesized by bacteria. Compared to that of plant sources, the nutrient density of vitamin K in foods of animal origin is rather low. Vitamin K is resistant to cooking losses.

As with other fat-soluble vitamins, absorption of vitamin K requires dietary fat and adequate liver and pancreatic secretions. Unlike other fat-soluble vitamins, though, not much vitamin K is stored in the body and excesses can be excreted via urine. Thus, a deficiency could develop rather quickly if dietary intake of this nutrient is poor, which can be a problem among older adults whose

(a)

(b)

Food Item and Amount	Vitamin K (micrograms)	% AI for Adult Males (120 micrograms)	% AI for Adult Females (90 micrograms)
Vegetables Spinach, cooked, 1 cup	889	741%	987%
Broccoli, cooked, 1 cup	220	183%	244%
Brussels sprouts, cooked, 1 cup	219	183%	243%
Fruits Rhubarb, cooked, 1 cup	51	42%	56%
Blueberries, 1 cup	29	24%	32%
Pomegranates, 1 cup arils	29	24%	32%
Dairy Cheese, cheddar, 1.5 ounces	6*	5%	7%
Soymilk, 1 cup	4	3%	4%
Milk 2%, 1 cup	1*	1%	1%
Protein Tofu, firm, cooked, 1 cup	6*	5%	7%
Egg, hard-boiled, 1 large	4*	3%	4%
Beef liver, pan-fried, 3 ounces	3	3%	4%
Fats & Oils Soybean oil, 1 teaspoon	8	7%	9%
Margarine, 1 teaspoon	4	4%	5%
Butter, 1 teaspoon	0	0%	0%

* Value includes phylloquinone and menaquinone.

FIGURE 13-6 ▲ Food sources of vitamin K. (a) The fill of the background color (none, 1/3, 2/3, or completely covered) within each food group on MyPlate indicates the average nutrient density for vitamin K in that group. (b) The bar graph shows the vitamin K content of several foods compared to the AI for adult males and females. Overall, the richest sources of vitamin K are green leafy vegetables. The grains group is not shown in the bar graph because grains provide very little vitamin K.

Source: *Nutrition data from USDA National Nutrient Database for Standard Reference, Release 26; and Elder SJ and others: Vitamin K contents of meat, dairy, and fast food in the U.S. diet.* Journal of Agricultural and Food Chemistry *54:463, 2006.*

diets lack vegetables. However, because vitamin K is fairly widespread in foods and some can be synthesized by bacteria in the colon, deficiencies of this vitamin rarely occur. No reports of toxicity have been published.

> **Vitamin K**
> Adequate Intake
>   Men: 120 micrograms
>   Women: 90 micrograms
> Daily Value: 80 micrograms
> Upper Level: None

✓ **CONCEPT CHECK 13.2**

1. List and describe the three steps of hemostasis.

2. What is the role of vitamin K in hemostasis?

3. Why is it important for people who take Coumadin to monitor their dietary intake of vitamin K?

ASK THE RDN   Mediterranean Diet

Dear RDN: *My father recently sent me the book* Eat Right for Your Type (4 Blood Types, 4 Diets): The Individualized Diet Solution to Staying Healthy, Living Longer & Achieving Your Ideal Weight *by Dr. Peter D'Adamo. This program sounds too good to be true. Should I be following a specific diet and exercise plan based upon my blood type?*

You are wise to question the "too good to be true" claims made by this book. Author D'Adamo, a doctor of naturopathy**,** proposes a direct connection between our blood type—O, A, B, and AB—and health problems we may have. In his book, D'Adamo suggests, "the secret to healthy, vigorous, and disease-free living might be as simple as knowing your blood type."

The basic premise of this diet is that the ABO blood groups are linked to the dietary habits of our ancestors and therefore determine what we should and should not eat today. According to the blood-type diet theory:

- Type O is considered the oldest blood type, so the optimal diet is the high-protein diet typical of hunter-gatherers—that is, heavy on lean meat, poultry, fish, and vegetables, and light on grains, beans, and dairy.
- Type A is believed to have evolved with the growth of agrarian societies. A vegetarian, meat-free diet is recommended, emphasizing organic fruits and vegetables, beans and legumes, and whole grains.
- Type B is believed to originate in nomadic tribes, therefore dairy products are beneficial, but corn, wheat, buckwheat, lentils, tomatoes, peanuts, and sesame seeds should be avoided.
- Type AB is considered more modern. A diet intermediate to those proposed for group A and group B is recommended, focusing on tofu, seafood, dairy, and green vegetables.

Although this book was a *New York Times* bestseller, scientists have concluded that no evidence exists to support the alleged health benefits of blood-type diets. Confusion may stem from the fact that people with certain blood types may have a higher or lower risk of some diseases (e.g., type Os have a lower risk of heart disease). There is no research, however, showing that this has anything to do with diet (see Further Reading 4).

Only one study has investigated the effects of these diets, and its results did not support the blood-type diet hypothesis. Although certain versions of The Blood Type Diet® were associated with improvements in heart health markers, the favorable effects were noted in everyone following the diet, not just those with a certain blood type (see Further Reading 20).

It is not surprising that persons have experienced positive results on The Blood Type Diet. All the versions of the diet promote calorie control and avoidance of highly processed foods. Positive results, however, cannot be attributed to the individual's blood type. Success on these diets, as with any eating pattern, typically stem from moderate calorie restriction and the ability to maintain the dietary pattern over time.

It is also important to note that diets based only on blood type may be risky for individuals with conditions such as diabetes, heart disease, or high blood pressure. Following the restrictions may conflict with the treatment plan for any of these chronic conditions. Dietary patterns recommended for these conditions—and for the general population—do not focus on specific foods and do not recommend cutting out any major food groups. Consult a RDN for more information.

So, in summary, it *is* too good to be true that we can design an individualized eating pattern based on something as simple as our blood type. Kudos to you for suspecting that there are many factors to consider when planning a dietary pattern that will help you stay healthy, live longer, and achieve a healthier body weight.

Not so simply,

Anne M. Smith, PhD, RDN, LD (author)

13.3 Folate (Vitamin B-9)

folate term to describe a variety of forms of this B vitamin found in foods and in the body.

The term **folate** is used to describe a variety of forms of this B vitamin found in foods and in the body. Folic acid is the synthetic form added to fortified foods and present in supplements.

FUNCTIONS OF FOLATE

A key role of the folate coenzyme is to supply or accept single carbon compounds. In this role, folate coenzymes help form DNA and metabolize amino acids and their derivatives, such as homocysteine. Folate works along with vitamin B-6 (see Section 12.6) and vitamin B-12 (see Section 13.4) to metabolize homocysteine. Folate also functions in the formation of neurotransmitters in the brain. Meeting folate needs can improve the depressed state in some cases of mental illness.

Research is also underway on the link between folate and cancer protection. Because folate aids in DNA synthesis, adequate folate status is important to maintain DNA integrity, including the control of certain cancer-promoting genes. Meeting the RDA for folate may be one way to reduce cancer risk.

FOLATE DEFICIENCY

One of the major results of a folate deficiency occurs in the early phases of red blood cell synthesis. With inadequate folate, immature red blood cells cannot divide because they cannot form new DNA. The cells grow progressively larger because they are still synthesizing protein and other cell parts to make new cells. When the time comes for the cells to divide, however, the amount of DNA is insufficient to form two nuclei. The cells thus remain in a large immature form, have a large nucleus, and are known as **megaloblasts.**

With the bone marrow of a folate-deficient person producing mostly immature megaloblast cells, few mature red blood cells arrive in the bloodstream. When fewer mature red blood cells are present, the blood's capacity to carry oxygen decreases, causing a condition known as **megaloblastic anemia** (also called macrocytic or large-cell anemia) (Fig. 13-7).

Medicine Cabinet

Methotrexate is a cancer drug that closely resembles a form of folate but cannot act in its place. Taken in high doses, methotrexate hampers folate metabolism. As a consequence, DNA synthesis is retarded and cell division decreases. Cancer cells are among the most rapidly dividing cells in the body, so they are among those first affected. However, other rapidly dividing cells, such as intestinal cells and skin cells, are also affected. Not surprisingly, typical side effects of methotrexate therapy—diarrhea, vomiting, and hair loss—are also symptoms of folate deficiency. Today, when patients are given methotrexate, they need to consume a folate-rich diet or take folic acid supplements in order to reduce the toxic side effects of the drug. High supplemental doses of folate have little or no influence on methotrexate's effectiveness as a cancer therapy.

medicine cabinet pills - © Footage supplied by Goodshoot/Punchstock

methotrexate A drug used to treat cancer, because it interferes with the growth of cells that reproduce quickly.

megaloblast A large, immature red blood cell that results from the inability of the cell to divide normally (*megalo* = large; *blast* = primitive or immature).

megaloblastic (macrocytic) anemia Anemia characterized by the presence of abnormally large red blood cells.

Red blood cell precursor (stem cell)

Folate or vitamin B-12 deficient

Folate and vitamin B-12 adequate

Cells are unable to divide

Cells divide normally

Megaloblastic blood cells seen here in the bone marrow are arrested at an immature stage of development. They still have their nuclei and are slightly larger than normal red blood cells.

Normal blood cells in the bloodstream. The size, shape, and color of the red blood cells show that they are normal. Mature red blood cells have lost their nuclei.

FIGURE 13-7 ◄ Megaloblastic (macrocytic) anemia occurs when red blood cells are unable to divide, leaving large, immature red blood cells. Either a folate or vitamin B-12 deficiency may cause this condition. Measurements of blood concentrations of both vitamins are taken to help determine the cause of the anemia. © Footage supplied by Goodshoot/Punchstock

Clinicians focus on red blood cells as an indicator of folate status because they are easy to collect and examine. Folate deficiency, however, disrupts cell division throughout the entire body. Other symptoms of folate deficiency are inflammation of the tongue, diarrhea, poor growth, mental confusion, depression, and problems in nerve function. One result of folate deficiency is elevated blood homocysteine levels which have been associated with cardiovascular risk and are considered an independent risk factor for atherosclerosis. Research is ongoing to examine the impact of folate (and other B vitamins) on cardiovascular disease risk.

Maternal folate deficiency (along with a genetic abnormality related to folate metabolism) has been linked to the development of **neural tube defects** in the fetus. These defects include **spina bifida** (spinal cord or spinal fluid bulge through the back) and **anencephaly** (absence of a brain). Low maternal plasma folate and vitamin B-12 levels result in high plasma homocysteine levels and are risk factors for neural tube defects. Adequate folate status is crucial for all women of childbearing age, pregnant or not, because the neural tube closes within the first 28 days of pregnancy, a time when many women are not even aware that they are pregnant. Research suggests that the risk for neural tube defects can be decreased by supplementation of mothers-to-be with folate (see Further Reading 17). Refer to Section 18.8 for more information on nutrition and birth defects.

Older people may be at risk for folate deficiency due to a combination of inadequate folate intake and decreased absorption. Perhaps these people fail to consume sufficient amounts of fruits and vegetables because of poverty or physical problems, such as poor dental health. In addition, folate deficiencies often occur with alcoholism, due mostly to poor intake and absorption. Symptoms of a folate-related anemia can alert a physician to the possibility of alcoholism.

GETTING ENOUGH FOLATE

Folate's name is derived from the Latin word *folium,* which means "foliage or leaves." Quite predictably, the richest sources of folate are green leafy vegetables. In addition, other vegetables, orange juice, dried beans, and organ meats are excellent sources of folate (Fig. 13-8). Fortified ready-to-eat breakfast cereals, bread, and milk are important sources of folic acid for many adults.

Folate is susceptible to destruction by heat and oxygen. The vitamin C present in some food sources of folate, such as orange juice, helps to reduce folate destruction, but food processing and preparation destroy 50% to 90% of the folate in food. This underscores the importance of regularly eating fresh fruits and raw or lightly cooked vegetables.

Pregnant women need extra folate (a total of 600 micrograms DFE) to accommodate the increased rates of cell division and DNA synthesis in their bodies and in the developing fetus. A healthy diet can supply this much. Still, prenatal care often includes a specially formulated multivitamin and mineral supplement enriched with folic acid to meet the higher RDA during pregnancy.

Prior to 1998, average daily folate intakes in the United States were approximately 320 micrograms for men and 220 micrograms for women. In 1998, the FDA mandated the fortification of grain products with folate with the aim of reducing birth defects of the spine. With this program, average intakes have increased by about 200 micrograms per day. Factors other than folate deficiency (e.g., genetics and environment) play a role in the development of neural tube defects, but studies have shown fortification of grain products with folic acid has decreased rates of neural tube defects in infants by an estimated 15% to 30% in the United States and up to 50% in other countries with higher background rates of neural tube defects (see Further Reading 10).

The folic acid enrichment of grains has also been accompanied by a noticeable decline in cardiovascular risk, especially risk for stroke, due to a drop in blood homocysteine levels among U.S. adults. Supplements of folic acid, B-12, and B-6 have been promoted to help lower homocysteine and decrease cardiac and stroke risk. This is only likely to be effective for individuals who start out with elevated homocysteine levels. Taking pharmacological

neural tube defect A defect in the formation of the neural tube occurring during early fetal development. This type of defect results in various nervous system disorders, such as spina bifida. Folate deficiency in the pregnant woman increases the risk that the fetus will develop this disorder.

spina bifida Birth defect resulting from improper closure of the neural tube during embryonic development. The spinal cord or fluid may bulge outside the spinal column.

anencephaly Birth defect characterized by the absence of some or all of the brain and skull.

Folate

RDA: 400 micrograms

DV: 400 micrograms

UL: 1000 micrograms (synthetic only)

▲ An objective of Healthy People 2020 is to increase by 10% the proportion of women of childbearing potential who take supplements containing folic acid prior to pregnancy.

© Banana Stock/Punchstock

(a)

(b)

	Food Item and Amount	Folate (micrograms DFE)	% RDA for Adult Males and Females (400 micrograms DFE)
Grains	Cheerios® cereal, 1 cup	336	84%
	Wheat germ, 2 tablespoons	150	38%
	Flour tortilla, 8″	98	25%
Vegetables	Asparagus, cooked, 1 cup	268	67%
	Spinach, cooked, 1 cup	263	66%
	Broccoli, cooked, 1 cup	168	42%
Fruits	Orange juice, fresh, 1 cup	74	19%
	Cantaloupe, 1 cup	37	9%
	Strawberries, raw, 1 cup	36	9%
Dairy	Yogurt, plain, 1 cup	29	7%
	Cottage cheese, low-fat, 1 cup	23	6%
	Soymilk, 1 cup	22	6%
Protein	Beef liver, pan-fried, 3 ounces	211	53%
	Lentils, cooked, ½ cup	179	45%
	Sunflower seeds, dry roasted, ¼ cup	76	19%

FIGURE 13-8 ▲ Food sources of folate. (a) The fill of the background color (none, 1/3, 2/3, or completely covered) within each group on MyPlate indicates the average nutrient density for folate in that group. (b) The bar graph shows folate content of several foods in each food group compared to the RDA for adult males and females. Overall, the richest sources of folate are green leafy vegetables and fortified grains.

Source: *Nutrition data from USDA National Nutrient Database for Standard Reference, Release 26.*

doses of folate is not likely to benefit people who have blood homocysteine levels in the normal range.

AVOIDING TOO MUCH FOLATE

The UL for folate (see box) only refers to synthetic folic acid, because folate, the natural form in food, has limited absorption. Some research indicates that too much folic acid could promote tumor development. Thus, even though folic acid fortification has been a public health success story for prevention of neural tube defects, there are concerns about the appropriate dose for the entire population (see Further Reading 10). In addition, large doses of folic acid can hide the signs of vitamin B-12 deficiency and therefore complicate its diagnosis. Specifically, regular consumption of large amounts of folate can prevent the appearance of an early warning sign of vitamin B-12 deficiency—the enlarged red blood cell size. For this reason, FDA limits the amount of folic acid in supplements (for nonpregnant adults) to 400 micrograms.

Folate recommendations for all but women of childbearing age are based on dietary folate equivalents (DFE). Synthetic folic acid, found in supplements and fortified foods, is more bioavailable than the folate that naturally occurs in food. The DFE unit takes into account these differences in bioavailability.

Dietary Folate Equivalents

1 DFE = 1 microgram folate from food

= 0.6 microgram folic acid from food

= 0.5 microgram folic acid from a supplement on an empty stomach

✓ CONCEPT CHECK 13.3

1. Explain what happens to red blood cells in macrocytic (megaloblastic) anemia.

2. Why do folate needs increase from 400 micrograms to 600 micrograms per day for pregnant women?

13.4 Vitamin B-12 (Cobalamin or Cyanocobalamin)

Vitamin B-12 is a unique vitamin. Its structure is the largest of all the vitamins and it is the only vitamin that contains a mineral as part of its structure. Unlike most water-soluble vitamins, B-12 can be stored to a significant extent in the liver, so it takes many months on a diet devoid of vitamin B-12 for a deficiency to occur. Vitamin B-12 is only found in foods of animal origin. Finally, the means by which the body absorbs vitamin B-12 is complex; a problem at any of its several absorption steps could impair absorption and lead to deficiency. To illustrate the multistep process by which vitamin B-12 is absorbed, we will trace the path of a meal containing vitamin B-12 through the digestive tract (Fig. 13-9).

In food, much of the vitamin B-12 is bound to protein and therefore cannot be absorbed. When food enters the mouth, **R-proteins** are secreted by the salivary glands. The bolus of food, including the R-proteins, travels down the esophagus to the stomach. Acid and enzymes present in the stomach release vitamin B-12 from food proteins, and the free vitamin B-12 then binds to R-protein. While food is in the stomach, the stomach cells release a protein-like compound called the **intrinsic factor.** When the **chyme** reaches the duodenum, pancreatic enzymes release vitamin B-12 from R-proteins. The free vitamin B-12 then combines with intrinsic factor. The vitamin B-12–intrinsic factor complex travels the length of the small intestine to the ileum, where vitamin B-12 is finally absorbed.

R-proteins Proteins produced by the salivary glands that bind to free vitamin B-12 in the stomach and protect it from stomach acid.

intrinsic factor A proteinlike compound produced by the stomach that enhances vitamin B-12 absorption.

chyme A mixture of stomach secretions and partially digested food.

FIGURE 13-9 ▶ The absorption of vitamin B-12 requires several compounds produced in the mouth, stomach, and small intestine. Defects arising in the stomach or small intestine can interfere with absorption and result in vitamin B-12 deficiency.

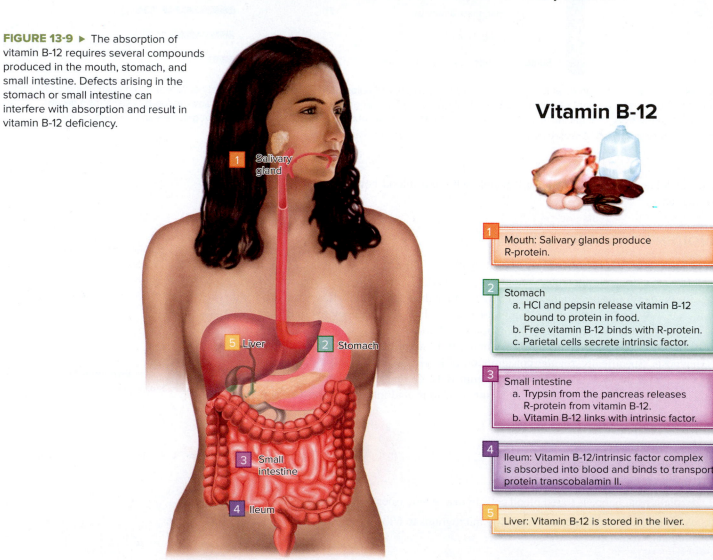

Vitamin B-12

1. Salivary gland
5. Liver   2. Stomach
3. Small intestine
4. Ileum

1 Mouth: Salivary glands produce R-protein.

2 Stomach
   a. HCl and pepsin release vitamin B-12 bound to protein in food.
   b. Free vitamin B-12 binds with R-protein.
   c. Parietal cells secrete intrinsic factor.

3 Small intestine
   a. Trypsin from the pancreas releases R-protein from vitamin B-12.
   b. Vitamin B-12 links with intrinsic factor.

4 Ileum: Vitamin B-12/intrinsic factor complex is absorbed into blood and binds to transport protein transcobalamin II.

5 Liver: Vitamin B-12 is stored in the liver.

If any of these steps fails or are altered, absorption can drop to 1% to 2%. In these cases, the person usually takes monthly injections of vitamin B-12, uses nasal gels of the vitamin to bypass the need for absorption, or takes megadoses of a supplemental form (300 times the RDA). In this latter case, the vitamin B-12 absorption defect is overcome by providing enough of the vitamin via simple diffusion across the intestinal tract.

About 95% of cases of vitamin B-12 deficiencies in healthy people result from defective absorption rather than from inadequate intakes. This is especially true for older people. As we age, stomach acid production declines and our stomachs have a decreased ability to synthesize the intrinsic factor needed for adequate vitamin B-12 absorption.

FUNCTIONS OF VITAMIN B-12

Vitamin B-12 participates in a variety of cellular processes. The most important function is participating in folate metabolism. B-12 is required to convert folate coenzymes to the active forms needed for metabolic reactions, such as DNA synthesis. Without vitamin B-12, reactions that require certain active forms of folate do not take place in the cell. Thus, a deficiency of vitamin B-12 can result in symptoms of a folate deficiency, including elevated homocysteine levels and macrocytic anemia.

Another vital function of vitamin B-12 is maintaining the myelin sheath that insulates neurons. Initial neurological symptoms of a vitamin B-12 deficiency include dysfunctional muscle control and impaired reflexes. Eventual destruction of the myelin sheath causes paralysis. If left untreated, vitamin B-12 deficiency eventually leads to death, mainly due to the destruction of nerves.

VITAMIN B-12 DEFICIENCY

The fatal consequences of vitamin B-12 deficiency can be observed in a disease known as **pernicious anemia.** The word *pernicious* means "leading to death." Indeed, before the discovery that consuming large doses of raw liver—a rich source of vitamin B-12—could be used to treat this particular disease, many people did die from it. Pernicious anemia is characterized by macrocytic anemia (with all the usual signs of anemia), sore mouth, depression, back pain, apathy, and severe nerve degeneration. Nerve damage can lead to tingling in the extremities, weakness, paralysis, and eventually death from heart failure. People with pernicious anemia usually do not lack vitamin B-12 in their dietary pattern. Instead, they suffer from an autoimmune disease that destroys the stomach cells that produce gastric acid and intrinsic factor. The resulting malabsorption of vitamin B-12 is responsible for all the symptoms of the disease.

Pernicious anemia affects about 2% of older adults. Other causes of vitamin B-12 malabsorption include age-related atrophy of the acid-producing cells of the stomach, inflammatory bowel disease, bariatric surgery, and bacterial overgrowth in the small intestine. (When acid production is low, bacteria normally present in the large intestine may colonize the small intestine and compete with our intestinal cells for vitamin B-12 absorption.) Because we are able to store some vitamin B-12, symptoms of nerve destruction do not develop until after about 3 years from the onset of the disease. Unfortunately, substantial nerve destruction often occurs before clinical signs of deficiency, such as anemia, are detected. The nerve destruction is irreversible.

Inadequate intake of vitamin B-12 is rarely responsible for deficiency, but it can occur. Infants breastfed by vegetarian mothers are at risk for vitamin B-12 deficiency. This may be accompanied by anemia and long-term nervous system problems, such as diminished brain growth, degeneration of the spinal cord, and poor intellectual development. The problems may have their origins during pregnancy, when the mother is deficient in vitamin B-12. Vegan diets supply little vitamin B-12 unless they include vitamin B-12–fortified food (e.g., soymilk) or supplements, so achieving an adequate vitamin B-12 intake is a key diet-planning goal for vegans.

GETTING ENOUGH VITAMIN B-12

Vitamin B-12 compounds are originally synthesized by bacteria, fungi, and other lower organisms, then become incorporated into animal tissues when animals consume them.

▲ With age, absorption of vitamin B-12 from food becomes less efficient, usually due to decreases in stomach-acid production.
© Dynamic Graphics/JupiterImages

pernicious anemia The anemia that results from a lack of vitamin B-12 absorption; it is pernicious because of associated nerve degeneration that can result in eventual paralysis and death.

▲ Salmon, rainbow trout and other types of seafood are excellent sources of vitamin B-12.
© Michael Lamotte/Cole Group/Getty Images

(a)

(b)

	Food Item and Amount	Vitamin B-12 (micrograms)	% RDA for Adult Males and Females (2.4 micrograms)
Grains	Cheerios® cereal, 1 cup	1.9	79%
	Egg noodles, cooked, ½ cup	0	0%
	Quinoa, cooked, ½ cup	0	0%
Dairy	Soymilk (fortified), 1 cup	2.1	86%
	Yogurt, plain, non-fat, 1 cup	1.5	63%
	Milk, fat-free, 1 cup	1.2	50%
Protein	Claims, baked, 3 ounces	84.1	3504%
	Beef liver, pan-fried, 3 ounces	67.3	2804%
	Kidney beans, cooked, ½ cup	0	0%

FIGURE 13-10 ▲ Food sources of vitamin B-12 compared to the RDA for adults. (a) The fill of the background color (none, 1/3, 2/3, or completely covered) within each group on MyPlate indicates the average nutrient density for vitamin B-12 in that group. (b) The bar graph shows the vitamin B-12 content of several foods in each food group compared to the RDA for adult males and females. Overall, foods of animal origin and fortified grains are the richest sources of vitamin B-12. Except for fortified grains, foods of plant origin (not shown) do not contain vitamin B-12.

Source: *Nutrition data from USDA National Nutrient Database for Standard Reference, Release 26.*

Vitamin B-12

RDA: 2.4 micrograms

DV: 6 micrograms

UL: None

Organ meats (especially liver, kidneys, and heart) are especially rich sources of vitamin B-12. Other major sources of vitamin B-12 include meat, seafood, ready-to-eat breakfast cereals, milk, and eggs (Fig. 13-10). Adults over age 50 are encouraged to seek a synthetic vitamin B-12 source to increase absolute absorption, which can be limited due to both reduced intrinsic factor and stomach-acid output (see Medicine Cabinet box). Synthetic vitamin B-12 is not food bound, so stomach acid is not required to release it from food. It will be more readily absorbed than the form found in food (see Further Reading 16). Ready-to-eat breakfast cereals and dietary supplements are two possible synthetic sources.

On average, adults consume two times the RDA or more (see box). This high intake provides the average meat-eating person with 2 to 3 years' storage of vitamin B-12 in the liver. A person would have to consume a diet essentially free of vitamin B-12 for approximately 20 years before exhibiting nerve destruction caused by a dietary deficiency. Still, vegans, who eat no animal products, should find a reliable source of vitamin B-12, such as fortified soy or rice milk, ready-to-eat breakfast cereals, and a form of yeast grown on media rich in vitamin B-12. Use of a multivitamin and mineral supplement containing vitamin B-12 is another option. Pernicious anemia most frequently develops after a few years of the loss of vitamin B-12 absorption capacity. The quicker appearance is because of the reduced ability to reabsorb vitamin B-12 excreted into the GI tract during digestion, coupled with reduced absorption of dietary sources. Vitamin B-12 supplements are essentially nontoxic, so no UL has been set.

Medicine Cabinet

Some medications may limit vitamin B-12 absorption. Antacids or other medications used to inhibit acid secretions will increase the pH within the stomach, thereby limiting release of vitamin B-12 from protein. People who have ulcers or reflux may take these drugs. Metformin, a popular medication for controlling diabetes, may reduce vitamin B-12 absorption. With any of these medications, you should check with your health care provider to see if supplemental vitamin B-12 is recommended.

medicine cabinet pills - © Footage supplied by Goodshoot/Punchstock

✓ CONCEPT CHECK 13.4

1. How does a vitamin B-12 deficiency lead to macrocytic anemia?

2. What role does vitamin B-12 play in the health of the brain and nervous system?

3. Identify two population groups that are at risk for vitamin B-12 deficiency. Explain why these people are at risk.

4. List some of the richest food sources of vitamin B-12.

13.5 Iron

Iron (Fe) is the trace mineral present in the largest amount in the body (see Fig. 8-3). Although the importance of dietary iron has been recognized for many years, iron deficiency is the most common nutrient deficiency worldwide. About 30% of the world's population is anemic; half of these cases are caused by iron deficiency. Iron is the only nutrient for which premenopausal women have a greater RDA than adult men.

FUNCTIONS OF IRON

Iron is part of the hemoglobin in red blood cells (Fig. 13-3) and **myoglobin** in muscle cells. Hemoglobin molecules in red blood cells transport oxygen (O_2) from the lungs to cells and then transport carbon dioxide (CO_2) from cells to the lungs for excretion. In addition, iron is used as part of many enzymes, some proteins, and compounds that cells use in energy production. Iron also is needed for brain and immune function, drug detoxification in the liver, and synthesis of collagen for bone health.

myoglobin Iron-containing protein that binds oxygen in muscle tissue.

IRON DEFICIENCY

If neither the diet nor body stores of iron can supply the iron needed for hemoglobin synthesis, the concentration of hemoglobin in red blood cells decreases. Medical professionals use both the percentage of blood that consists of red blood cells (**hematocrit**) and the hemoglobin concentration to assess iron status. Other measures indicative of poor iron status include the concentration of iron (serum iron) and iron-containing proteins in blood (**ferritin,** or **transferrin**).

When hematocrit and hemoglobin fall, an iron deficiency is suspected. In severe deficiency, hemoglobin and hematocrit fall so low that the amount of oxygen carried in the bloodstream is decreased. This condition is called iron-deficiency anemia.

Iron deficiency can be categorized into three stages:

- **Stage 1:** Iron stores become depleted, but no physiological impairment is observed.
- **Stage 2:** The amount of iron in transferrin is depleted; some physiological impairment occurs. Heme production is decreased, and activities of enzymes that require iron as a cofactor are limited.
- **Stage 3:** Red blood cells are small (microcytic), pale (hypochromic), and reduced in number; oxygen-carrying capacity of red blood cells declines.

Clinical symptoms of iron-deficiency anemia are associated with the lack of oxygen getting to the tissues. One experiences pale skin, fatigue upon exertion, poor temperature regulation (always cold, especially toes and fingers), loss of appetite, and apathy. Poor iron stores may decrease learning ability, attention span, work performance, and immune status even before a person is anemic. Children with chronic anemia have abnormal cognitive development (see Further Reading 21).

It is important to note that many more North Americans have an iron deficiency without anemia (stages 1 or 2) than have iron-deficiency anemia (stage 3). Their blood hemoglobin values are still normal, but they have little to no stores to draw from in times of growth or illness, and basic functioning may be marginally impaired. That could mean anything from too little energy to perform everyday tasks efficiently to difficulties staying mentally alert. In the United States, minority populations are more likely than whites to have iron-deficiency anemia. Compared to non-Hispanic white women, iron-deficiency anemia is at least two times more common among Hispanic and black women (see Further Reading 13).

There are many conditions that lead to an anemic state; iron-deficiency anemia is the most prevalent nutrient deficiency worldwide. Probably about 10% of North Americans in high risk categories have iron-deficiency anemia. This appears most often in infancy, the preschool years, and at puberty for both males and females. Growth—with accompanying expansion of blood volume and muscle mass—increases iron needs, making it difficult to

hematocrit The percentage of blood made up of red blood cells.

ferritin A protein that stores iron and releases it in a controlled manner. Acts as a buffer against iron deficiency and iron overload.

transferrin Iron-binding protein; controls the level of free iron in blood.

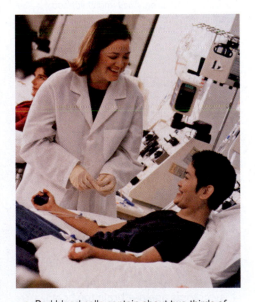

▲ Red blood cells contain about two-thirds of the body's total iron supply. Each time people donate blood, they sacrifice about 10% of their total blood volume, which removes about 7% of the body's iron supply. Over the next few weeks, the red blood cells will be replaced, so healthy people can usually donate blood two to four times a year without harmful consequences. As a precaution, blood banks first screen potential donors' blood for the presence of anemia (see Chapter 13 Case Study).
© Keith Brofsky/Getty Images

▲ During both pregnancy and childhood, demands for iron are high. Young children and women of reproductive age are at risk for iron-deficiency anemia. © Royalty Free/Corbis

heme iron Iron provided from animal tissues in the form of hemoglobin and myoglobin. Approximately 40% of the iron in meat is heme iron; it is readily absorbed.

myoglobin Iron-containing protein that binds oxygen in muscle tissue.

consume enough iron. Women are vulnerable to anemia during childbearing years due to menstrual blood losses. Anemia is also found in pregnant women because blood volume expands during pregnancy and extra iron is needed to synthesize red blood cells for the mother and the fetus. Iron-deficiency anemia in adult men is usually caused by blood loss from ulcers, colon cancer, or hemorrhoids. Athletes can have increased iron requirements due to increased blood loss in feces and urine, and chronic lysis of red blood cells in the feet due to the trauma of running.

To cure iron-deficiency anemia, a primary care provider should find the cause so that the anemia does not reoccur. A person will most likely need to take iron supplements (see Further Readings 12 and 16). Changes in eating patterns may prevent iron-deficiency anemia, but supplemental iron is the only reliable cure once it has developed. Supplements must be taken for 3 to 6 months or perhaps longer. Hemoglobin levels respond quickly to dietary changes and supplementation, but terminating supplements too soon means that iron stores (blood, bone marrow, etc.) will not be replenished. Remember, it takes longer than 1 month to become anemic, so it will take longer than 1 month to cure it.

ABSORPTION AND DISTRIBUTION OF IRON

Overall, iron absorption depends on three factors: (1) the person's iron status; (2) its form in food; and (3) other dietary components found in food. Controlling iron levels in the body is important because, when it comes to iron, there is a narrow gap between just enough and too much. As you've learned, too little iron can impair oxygen transport. To prevent deficiency, the human body highly conserves iron. Except for bleeding associated with menstruation, injury, or childbirth, body loss of iron is minimal. Approximately 90% is recovered and reused every day. On the other hand, too much iron in the body is also extremely damaging. It can accumulate in organs and promote oxidative damage. To avoid toxicity, iron absorption from the small intestine is tightly regulated.

The most important factor influencing iron absorption is body need. Iron needs are increased during pregnancy and growth. At high altitudes, the lower oxygen concentration of the air causes an increase in the hemoglobin concentration of blood and thus an increase in iron needs (see What Would You Choose?).

The principal mechanism to regulate iron content in the body is tight control of absorption. High doses of iron can still be toxic, but absorption is carefully regulated under most conditions. When iron stores are inadequate or needs are high due to growth or pregnancy, the main protein that carries iron, transferrin, more readily binds iron, shifting it from intestinal cells into the bloodstream. Absorption efficiency in times of need can be as high as 50%. On the other hand, if iron stores are adequate and the iron-binding protein in the blood is fully saturated with iron, absorption from the intestinal cells is minimal—as low as 2%. The iron remains in the intestinal cells, and it will be excreted in the feces when those intestinal cells slough off, which occurs every 5 to 6 days. In general, healthy people with adequate iron stores absorb between 5% and 15% of dietary iron, which is quite low compared to other nutrients.

The other major influence on iron absorption is the form of iron in food. **Heme iron,** derived from hemoglobin and **myoglobin,** comprises 40% of the iron in meat, fish, and poultry (MFP). Absorption of heme iron ranges from about 15% to 35%. Almost nothing affects its absorption. The absorption of **nonheme iron,** on the other hand, ranges from 2% to 8% because it is subject to many conditions that can either enhance or inhibit its absorption. Table 13-2 summarizes dietary factors that affect the bioavailability of nonheme iron and lists suggestions for enhancing its absorption. Nonheme iron makes up 60% of iron in MFP and 100% of the iron found in dairy, eggs, fruit, vegetables, grains, fortified foods, and supplements. Because most of our dietary iron is nonheme iron, our overall dietary iron absorption is 5% to 15%.

Acidity also affects iron absorption: an acidic environment solubilizes iron and keeps it in a form that can be readily absorbed. Therefore, any medication or health condition that lowers acid production of the stomach can decrease iron absorption. For example, acid-reducing medications that people take to control heartburn or ulcers can impair iron absorption.

TABLE 13-2 ■ Factors that Influence Nonheme Iron Absorption

Nonheme Enhancers	Nonheme Inhibitors
• Vitamin C • Add marinara sauce to your spaghetti noodles. • Drink orange juice with cereal. • MFP (meat, fish, poultry) protein • Add some tuna to your snack of crackers.	• Tannins (found in tea) • Can lower absorption by up to 60%, so drink tea between meals; does not apply to herbal "tea," which contains no tea leaves • Oxalates (spinach, rhubarb, chard) • Phytates (whole grains, bran, soybeans) • Megadoses of zinc, calcium, or copper

nonheme iron Iron provided from plant sources and animal tissues other than in the forms of hemoglobin and myoglobin. Nonheme iron is less efficiently absorbed than heme iron; absorption is closely dependent on body needs.

The iron added to foods and in most dietary supplements is nonheme iron.

Also, as people age, gastric acid secretion may decline. This puts older adults at risk for iron-deficiency anemia.

Other micronutrients also affect iron absorption and availability. Megadoses of zinc or calcium compete with iron for absorption in the small intestine. In contrast, adequate copper is important for iron metabolism and vitamin C is a powerful enhancer of iron absorption. Doses of 75 milligrams of vitamin C can increase nonheme absorption by 4%—a lot for nonheme. If you want to get the most iron out of your dietary supplement, take it with a glass of orange juice or other vitamin C–rich sources.

GETTING ENOUGH IRON

Animal sources contain approximately 40% heme iron, the most bioavailable form. The major iron sources in the adult diet are ready-to-eat breakfast cereals, beans, and animal products (Fig. 13-11). Iron is added to flour during the enrichment process. Other iron sources are peas and legumes, but the absorption of nonheme iron found in these products is relatively low. Milk and eggs are poor sources of iron. A common cause of iron-deficiency anemia in children is high consumption of milk coupled with insufficient meat intake. Vegans are particularly susceptible to iron-deficiency anemia because of their lack of dietary heme iron.

The adult RDA is based on a 10% absorption rate to cover average losses of about 0.8 milligram per day. For women of reproductive age, average menstrual losses are about 1 gram of additional iron per day. Thus, iron is the only nutrient for which premenopausal women have higher requirements than men. Most women do not consume the recommended 18 milligrams of iron daily. The average daily amount consumed by women is closer to 13 milligrams, while in men, it is about 18 milligrams per day. Women of reproductive age can close this gap between average daily intakes and needs by seeking out iron-fortified foods, such as ready-to-eat breakfast cereals that contain at least 50% of the DV. Use of a balanced multivitamin and mineral supplement containing up to 100% of the DV for iron is another option. Consuming more than 100% of the DV for iron from dietary supplements or fortified foods is not advised unless recommended by a primary care provider.

AVOIDING TOO MUCH IRON

The UL for iron is 45 milligrams per day. Higher amounts can lead to gastric distress. Although iron overload is not as common as iron deficiency, the consequences can be dire. Even a large single dose of 60 milligrams of iron can be life threatening to a 1-year-old. Children are frequently victims of iron poisoning (acute toxicity) because supplements, which look a lot like candy, may be easily accessible on kitchen tables and from cabinets. The FDA requires that all iron supplements carry a warning about toxicity. Furthermore, those with 30 milligrams of iron or more per tablet must be individually wrapped.

Iron toxicity accompanies the genetic disease, hereditary **hemochromatosis.** The disease is associated with a substantial increase in iron absorption from both food and supplements. The harshest effects are seen in iron-storing organs such as the liver and heart.

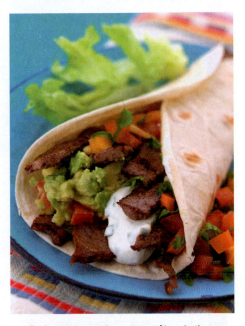

▲ Red meat is a major source of iron in the North American diet. Heme iron, which makes up about 40% of the iron in foods of animal origin, is better absorbed than nonheme iron.
© Ingram Publishing/SuperStock

Iron
RDA
  Men: 8 milligrams
  Women: 18 milligrams (8 milligrams after menopause)
DV: 18 milligrams
UL: 45 milligrams

hemochromatosis A disorder of iron metabolism characterized by increased iron absorption and deposition in the liver and heart. This eventually poisons the cells in those organs.

(a)

(b)

	Food Item and Amount	Iron (milligrams)	% RDA for Adult Males (8 milligrams)	% RDA for Adult Females (18 milligrams)
Grains	Frosted mini wheats, 24 biscuits	17.6	220%	98%
	Flour tortilla, 8"	1.0	13%	6%
	Whole-wheat bread, 1 slice	0.8	10%	4%
Vegetables	Spinach, cooked, 1 cup	6.4	80%	36%
	Parsley, raw, 1 cup	3.7	47%	21%
	Potato, baked (with skin), 1 medium	1.9	23%	10%
Fruits	Prune juice, 1 cup	3.0	38%	17%
	Raisins, ½ cup	1.6	19%	9%
	Orange, navel, 1 medium	0.2	2%	1%
Dairy	Soymilk, 1 cup	1.0	13%	6%
	Feta cheese, 1.5 ounces	0.3	4%	2%
	Milk, fat-free, 1 cup	0.1	1%	0%
Protein	Oysters, steamed, 3 ounces*	7.8	98%	44%
	Kidney beans, cooked, ½ cup	2.0	25%	11%
	Sirloin steak, grilled, 3 ounces*	1.5	18%	8%

*Contains heme iron

FIGURE 13-11 ▲ Food sources of iron. (a) The fill of the background color (none, 1/3, 2/3, or completely covered) within each group on MyPlate indicates the average nutrient density for iron in that group. (b) The bar graph shows the iron content of several foods in each food group compared to the RDA for adult males and females. Overall, the richest sources of iron are meats, legumes, and fortified grain products.

Source: *Nutrition data from USDA National Nutrient Database for Standard Reference, Release 26.*

Some iron is deposited in the pancreas and muscles. Blood levels remain high, too, which increases the likelihood of infections and may promote the development of cardiovascular disease.

Development of hereditary hemochromatosis requires that a person carry two defective copies of a particular gene. People with one defective gene and one normal gene (i.e., carriers) may also absorb too much dietary iron, but not to the same extent as those with two defective genes. About 5% to 10% of North Americans of Northern European descent are carriers of the genes leading to hemochromatosis. Approximately 1 in 250 North Americans have inherited both copies of the defective genes leading to hemochromatosis. These numbers are high, considering that many primary care providers regard it as a rare disease and therefore do not routinely test for it.

Anyone who has a blood relative (including uncles, aunts, and cousins) who has hemochromatosis or is a carrier should be screened for iron overload. At your next visit to a primary care provider, ask for a transferrin saturation test to assess iron stores. A ferritin test may also be added to assess your stores. Hemochromatosis can go undetected until a person reaches age 50 to 60, so some experts recommend screening for anyone over the age of 20.

If the disease goes untreated, iron accumulates and serious health problems may result: darkening of skin, arthritis, heart disease, diabetes, liver disease, and cancer (colon). Even with iron overload, the person may have anemia due to damage to the bone marrow or liver. Treatment of hemochromatosis is relatively easy, but it must be monitored consistently. Routine **phlebotomy** to remove excess iron is essential. One must be very careful about the diet. Few sources of heme iron should be eaten, and supplements with iron or vitamin C should be avoided. Highly fortified breakfast cereals must also be avoided.

phlebotomy Therapeutic blood removal, as a blood donation, for the purpose of ridding the body of excess iron.

✓ CONCEPT CHECK 13.5

1. What are heme and nonheme iron?
2. What can you do to enhance your absorption of nonheme iron?
3. What are some conditions that can lead to iron-deficiency anemia?

13.6 Copper

Copper (Cu) and iron are similar in terms of food sources, absorption, and functions. Copper is a component of blood. In the body, it is found in highest concentration in the liver, brain, heart, kidneys, and muscles. **Ceruloplasmin** is the name of the protein that carries most of the body's copper in the blood.

ceruloplasmin Copper-containing protein in the blood; functions in the transport of iron.

FUNCTIONS OF COPPER

Copper has been mentioned in several chapters already because it is a cofactor for many enzymes. In Section 10.2, you learned about the micronutrients involved in the body's antioxidant defenses. Copper serves as a cofactor for superoxide dismutase, an enzyme that defends the body against free-radical damage. In Section 11.8, we noted copper's role in the function of enzymes that create cross-links in connective tissue proteins, such as the collagen in bone. Copper also has a role as a cofactor in the last stage of energy metabolism, which converts the energy stored in carbohydrates, fats, and proteins into ATP.

Copper is important for blood health because of its role in making iron available for the formation of red blood cells. Copper is part of three different enzymes that assist in the transport of iron out of intestinal cells, through the blood, and to the bone marrow, where iron is incorporated into hemoglobin. Copper is also a cofactor for enzymes involved in blood clotting, immune system function (see Section 10.1), and blood lipoprotein metabolism. In addition, copper is needed for brain health through its role in enzymes involved in nerve myelination and neurotransmitter synthesis.

A genetic disease called **Menkes syndrome** decreases the amount of copper available to the brain and nervous system. Babies born with Menkes syndrome suffer from nervous system disorders, weak muscle tone, and delays in physical and cognitive development related to the lack of copper-containing enzymes that help to form nervous tissue and synthesize neurotransmitters. They usually do not live past the age of 3 years.

COPPER DEFICIENCY

Considering the many roles of copper, it is not surprising that copper deficiency affects so many different body systems. Symptoms of copper deficiency include a form of anemia, weakened immunity, bone loss, poor growth, and some forms of cardiovascular disease.

The groups most likely to develop copper deficiencies are preterm infants recovering from semistarvation on a milk-dominated diet (a poor source of copper) and people recovering from intestinal surgery. A copper deficiency can also result from the overuse of zinc supplementation, because zinc and copper compete with each other for absorption.

Menkes syndrome An inherited X-linked recessive pattern disorder that affects copper levels in the body.

	Food Item and Amount	Copper (micrograms)	% RDA for Adult Males and Females (900 micrograms)
Grains	Whole Grain Total cereal, 1 cup	140	▮ 16%
	Whole-wheat bread, 1 slice	73	▪ 8%
	White rice, cooked, ½ cup	35	▪ 4%
Vegetables	Spinach, cooked, 1 cup	313	▬ 35%
	Potato, baked (with skin) medium	185	▬ 21%
	Butternut squash, cooked, 1 cup	133	▪ 15%
Fruits	Blackberries, fresh, 1 cup	238	▬ 26%
	Red seedless grapes, 1 cup	192	▬ 21%
	Orange juice, fresh, 1 cup	109	▪ 12%
Dairy	Soymilk, 1 cup	401	▬ 45%
	Cottage cheese, 1 cup	68	▪ 8%
	Milk, fat-free, 1 cup	32	▪ 4%
Protein	Beef liver, pan-fried, 3 ounces	11816	▬▬▬▶ 1313%
	Walnuts, 1 ounce	386	▬ 43%
	Kidney beans, cooked, ½ cup	191	▬ 21%

FIGURE 13-12 ▲ Food sources of copper. (a) The fill of the background color (none, 1/13, 2/3, or completely covered) within each food group on MyPlate indicates the average nutrient density for copper in that group. (b) The bar graph shows the copper content of several foods in each food group compared to the RDA for adult males and females. Overall the richest sources of copper are found in the protein foods and grain groups.

Source: *Nutrition data from USDA National Nutrient Database for Standard Reference, Release 26.*

▲ Dark chocolate is a rich source of copper. These candies containing 53% cacao solids provide 1400 micrograms of copper, which is 72% of the Daily Value. © McGraw-Hill Education/ Mark Dierker

Copper

RDA: 900 micrograms

DV: 2 milligrams

UL: 10 milligrams

GETTING ENOUGH COPPER

Rich sources of copper include liver, legumes, seeds, whole-grain breads and cereals, and cocoa (Fig. 13-12). Milk and dairy products, fruits, and vegetables are generally poor sources of copper. Also, the form of copper typically found in multivitamin and mineral supplements (copper oxide) is not readily absorbed. It is best to rely on food sources to meet copper needs.

Copper absorption is highly variable, with higher intakes associated with lower absorption efficiency. Absorption takes place in the stomach and upper small intestine. Excess copper is not stored to a great extent, so when intake exceeds needs, the liver incorporates it into bile, which is excreted as part of the feces. Phytates, fiber, and excessive zinc and iron supplements may all interfere with copper absorption.

The copper status of adults appears to be good: the average daily adult intake is about 1 milligram for women and 1.6 milligrams for men. However, sensitive laboratory tests to determine copper status are lacking.

AVOIDING TOO MUCH COPPER

A single dose of copper greater than 10 milligrams can cause toxicity. Consequences of copper toxicity include GI distress, vomiting blood, tarry feces, and damage to the liver and kidneys. Toxicity cannot occur with food, only supplements or excessive exposure to copper salts used in agriculture.

© Stockbyte/PunchStock

CASE STUDY Anemia

Anita is a 60-year-old woman who prides herself on taking charge of her health. She exercises daily, whether it is walking her dog, playing golf, or participating in a tai chi class at the senior center. She follows the Dietary Guidelines for Americans, choosing a variety of whole grains; eating at least five servings per day of fruits and vegetables; and keeping her saturated fat, *trans fat,* and sodium intakes to a minimum. She eats lean sources of protein, choosing poultry, fish, or vegetable sources of protein instead of red meat. She maintains a healthy body weight, has never had high blood pressure or high blood sugar, and does not take medications or supplements. Last week, she went to a blood drive at her church with the intent of donating blood, but she was turned away because her hematocrit (a measure of the percentage of red blood cells in the blood) was slightly below the requirements for donation. Anita was surprised because she has never had a problem donating blood before. The nurse told Anita that her low hematocrit level was indicative of anemia, which has many possible causes. As Anita thought about it, she realized that she had been feeling more tired than usual.

Answer the following questions and check your responses at the end of the chapter.

1. Iron deficiency is the most common form of anemia. What role does iron play in the health of red blood cells? From the description, is it possible that Anita has low iron stores? What dietary changes could Anita make to improve her iron status?
2. Folate deficiency may lead to anemia. What role does folate play in the health of red blood cells? From the description, is it likely that Anita is deficient in folate?
3. Low vitamin B-12 may result in anemia. What role does vitamin B-12 play in the health of red blood cells? Suggest an explanation for why Anita may have low vitamin B-12 status even with adequate dietary intake of vitamin B-12. What dietary changes could Anita make to improve her vitamin B-12 status?
4. What should Anita do now that she knows she is anemic? Will changes to her food choices suffice to resolve the problem?

Wilson's disease is a genetic disease in which the liver cannot synthesize ceruloplasmin. In turn, copper accumulates in tissues, such as lungs and liver. People with Wilson's disease suffer damage to the liver and nervous system. A primary treatment for Wilson's disease is a vegan diet, as fruits and vegetables are low in copper. Researchers are currently interested in how excess copper in the blood may influence the development of Alzheimer's and Parkinson's diseases.

Wilson's disease A genetic disorder that results in accumulation of copper in the tissues; characterized by damage to the liver, nervous system, and other organs.

✓ CONCEPT CHECK 13.6

1. List three functions of copper.

13.7 Nutrition and Your Health

Brain Health: Food for Thought

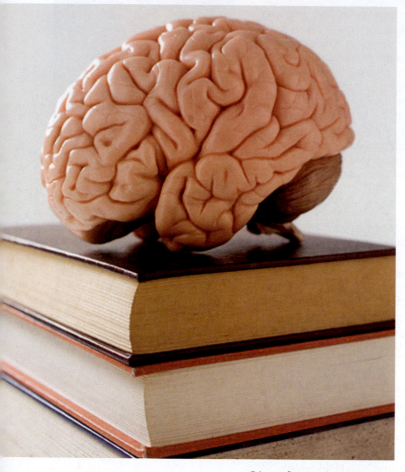

The human brain is a metabolically active organ that requires a continual supply of energy—preferably glucose—to meet its energy demands. Even though the average adult brain weighs only 3 pounds (about 2% of body weight), 20% of the body's blood is funneled to the brain to supply enough oxygen, glucose, and other nutrients necessary to support proper cognitive function. Indeed, your abilities to speak and understand others, focus on tasks, learn new information, and make decisions, as well as your overall mood, may be significantly impacted by your dietary choices.

So, what does it take to keep your brain's 100 billion neurons alive and functioning optimally? First, let's understand the roles of key nutrients—essential fatty acids, the B vitamins, choline, antioxidant nutrients, and some minerals—in brain function. Then, we'll examine how dietary patterns and other lifestyle choices may influence your risk of developing migraines, depression, and neurodegenerative diseases.

NUTRIENTS THAT FUNCTION IN BRAIN HEALTH

Formation of Brain Tissue Other than adipose tissue, nervous tissue is the fattiest tissue in the body—the brain is 60% fat by dry weight. Omega-3 and omega-6 fatty acids (including the two essential fatty acids, alpha-linolenic acid and linoleic acid) are used to form phospholipids, which are key players in the formation and maintenance of healthy cell membranes in the brain and nerve cells. Deficiencies of omega-3 or omega-6 fatty acids in the prenatal period or during infancy are detrimental to optimal brain health. Choline (see Section 12.11) is vital for the synthesis of two phospholipids, phosphatidylcholine and sphingomyelin, that are highly concentrated in nervous tissue.

Iodine is a vital nutrient during brain growth and development. As you read in Section 12.8, iodine is involved in the synthesis of thyroid hormones, which regulate growth, development, and metabolism. In utero and shortly after birth, iodine participates in the myelination of nerves. The consequences of a maternal iodine deficiency range from mild cognitive deficits to severe mental retardation and infant death.

Iron is another trace mineral that is vital during brain formation. Iron participates in the pathways that yield energy to fuel the brain, the myelination of nerve tissue, and the formation of neurotransmitters. A deficiency of iron during brain growth and development may result in impaired learning ability and behavioral problems.

Fueling the Brain The preferred source of fuel for the brain and nervous tissue is glucose, but the brain does not have any way to store appreciable amounts of this carbohydrate. Most of the time, the brain relies on the glucose that is circulating in the blood from your last meal. During times of fasting (e.g., overnight, very low carbohydrate diets), glucose can be derived from the breakdown of liver glycogen or the conversion of amino acids to glucose in the liver and kidneys. When the body is in a state of starvation, the brain is able to utilize ketone bodies (by-products of fatty-acid metabolism) as a source of fuel. However, ketones are acidic, so high levels of ketones can cause acidosis, which has negative and potential harmful implications for every body system.

As you learned in Chapter 12, the metabolism of glucose for fuel requires many micronutrient cofactors. Thus, deficiencies of thiamin, riboflavin, niacin, pantothenic acid, biotin, iron, magnesium, manganese, and vitamin B-12 can adversely affect brain function.

Nervous System: Communication Superhighway Communication between the brain and other body tissues occurs via nerve cells (also known as neurons), using a combination of electrical and chemical signals. Recall from Section 9.4 how sodium and potassium are involved in nerve impulse transmission. Shifts in the concentrations of these electrolyte nutrients across the nerve cell membrane allow for the transmission of an electrical signal along the length of the nerve cell. The speed at which electrical signals move depends on the **myelin** sheath that surrounds the nerve cell. Thiamin, folate, vitamin B-6, vitamin B-12, and iron are involved in the formation and function of the myelin sheath.

When an electrical signal reaches the end of a nerve cell, the message must be converted into a chemical signal. **Neurotransmitters** are chemical messengers that are released from nerve cells to

myelin A lipid and protein combination (lipoprotein) that covers nerve fibers.

neurotransmitter A compound made by a nerve cell that allows for communication between it and other cells.

▲ The brain and nervous system make up a communication superhighway. Sodium and potassium are essential for the proper transmission of electrical signals along the length of the nerve cell.
© MedicalRF.com

transmit a signal to a target cell, such as another nerve cell, an organ, or a gland. Acetylcholine, dopamine, norepinephrine, and serotonin are some examples of neurotransmitters. Amino acids are the building blocks of neurotransmitters. The synthesis and function of these chemical messengers also depends on several B vitamins, including thiamin, riboflavin, niacin, vitamin B-6, folate, and vitamin B-12.

Protecting Nervous Tissue As described, the brain is a metabolically active organ. Energy metabolism naturally generates some damaging free radicals. Recall from Section 10.2 that free radicals can cause oxidative damage to cell membranes and DNA. With its high concentration of polyunsaturated fatty acids, brain tissue is highly susceptible to the damaging effects of free radicals. Fortunately, the body's antioxidant systems are able to limit this type of cellular damage. An adequate supply of the antioxidant nutrients vitamin C, vitamin E, selenium, and zinc, as well as the phytochemical beta-carotene, help to protect the brain from oxidative damage.

Another metabolite that has been linked to declines in brain health is homocysteine. As you will recall from Section 13.3, high levels of homocysteine have been identified as a risk factor for poor health outcomes, including heart disease, cancer, stroke, and Alzheimer's disease. Metabolic pathways to convert homocysteine into less harmful amino acids require adequate levels of folate and vitamins B-6 and B-12. Choline may also participate in these metabolic processes.

Evidence clearly shows that in addition to specific dietary choices, the accumulation of excess body fat starting in childhood negatively impacts cognitive function (see Further Reading 9). Insulin resistance appears to be a mediating factor in the relationship between excess body fat and brain health. As you learned in Chapter 7, body weight management requires calorie control and physical activity. Independent of body weight, physical activity also improves brain development, cognition, attention, and memory (see Further Reading 14).

PROMOTING BRAIN HEALTH THROUGHOUT THE LIFE CYCLE

The brain is the body's command center. From brain development in utero until old age, food and lifestyle choices affect brain health. Now that you recognize the importance of nutrients for the growth, development, and function of the nervous system, let us examine how dietary patterns can affect brain health at various stages of the life cycle.

Gestation and Infancy Gestation and early infancy are critical periods for brain growth and development. Nutrient deficiencies

at this stage of the life cycle can profoundly affect neurological health throughout life. At this early phase, it is the biological mother's responsibility to ensure that the developing fetus has optimal nutrients for brain growth and development. Poor maternal intakes of folate, vitamin B-12, omega-3 fatty acids, and iron have all been related to reduced cognitive function in offspring (see Further Reading 5). As you will see in Chapter 18 , the RDAs for pregnant women for these nutrients increase to as much as 150% of the requirements for nonpregnant women. A

▲ Adequate maternal nutrition during gestation is necessary to ensure optimal brain growth and development.
© McGraw-Hill Education

dietary pattern that includes lean meats, legumes, fatty fish, and fortified breakfast cereals will support proper fetal brain growth and development. While good food sources of these nutrients are important, a pregnant woman is likely to require a dietary supplement, especially to meet her needs for iron and folic acid.

After birth, breastfeeding is the preferred method to nourish an infant (see Section 18.7). For brain health, the presence of long-chain polyunsaturated fatty acids (e.g., EPA and DHA) in human milk promotes optimal cognitive development. For a breastfed infant, the adequacy of the mother's diet will influence the nutrient content of the human milk and impact infant health. However, if breastfeeding is not possible or preferred, iron-fortified infant formula is a safe and healthy alternative. Infant formulas are designed to mimic the nutritional composition of human milk, which is the ideal food for infants.

Childhood and Adolescence Throughout childhood and adolescence, iron status is correlated with learning ability and behavior. Children who are deficient in iron experience decreased attention, poor memory, and may display disruptive behavior. In addition, good iron status can help to prevent lead poisoning, which is extremely detrimental to the nervous system. As you will learn in Section 19.4, young children are at heightened risk for iron deficiency. Overall intake of iron-rich foods can be poor because of low appetite, limited chewing ability, and food selectivity (i.e., picky eating). Caregivers should be sure to offer age-appropriate sources of iron, such as bite-size pieces of lean meat, legumes, and fortified cereals. In addition, ensure that excessive intakes of other foods (even nutrient-rich foods, like milk) do not crowd out rich food sources of iron. As children reach puberty, both boys and girls enter a growth spurt, which increases the demand for iron to build lean tissue and expand blood volume. Adolescent girls also require additional iron to compensate for monthly blood loss after menarche.

Adulthood

Eating Patterns and Migraine Headaches A migraine is a severe, intense, and recurring throbbing pain affecting one or both sides of the head in 38 million adults and children in the United States. Migraines interfere with quality of life in 90% of sufferers. Depression,

▲ The most commonly cited dietary triggers for migraine headaches are chocolate, cheese, citrus, alcohol, and coffee. © Ian Hooton/Science Source

anxiety, and sleep disturbances are common for those with chronic migraines. Other potentially debilitating neurological symptoms may include visual disturbances; nausea and vomiting; dizziness; sensitivity to sound, light, touch, and smell; and tingling or numbness in the extremities or face.

Both biologic and lifestyle factors contribute to migraines: family history, age, gender, hormonal changes, and lifestyle behaviors (Further Reading 1). Obese individuals are at increased risk of migraines, possibly related to higher levels of inflammation.

In susceptible individuals, potential dietary triggers for migraine headaches appear to be associated with foods that precipitate changes in blood flow and neurotransmitter release in the brain. Tyramine is a substance found naturally in foods such as aged cheese; aged, canned, cured, or processed meats; beans such as fava, garbanzo, pinto, and broad; pickles; and canned soups. Nitrates from processed meats and monosodium glutamate (MSG) from soy sauce, Asian dishes, and packaged foods have also been implicated as potential migraine triggers. Other food-related triggers include chocolate, nuts, olives, black tea, bananas, onions, raisins, apple skins, canned soups, red wine, and sulfites. Caffeine withdrawal, dehydration, meal skipping, supplements, and medications can also be overlooked culprits. Although there is some evidence that a low-fat, vegan dietary pattern reduces migraine frequency and severity (see Further Reading 3), a dietary pattern that complies with the Dietary Guidelines—that is, high in fruits, vegetables, whole grains, and legumes, but low in sodium, solid fats, alcohol, and added sugars—has also been linked to fewer complaints of migraine headaches (see Further Reading 6).

Nutrition and Depression Major depressive disorders affect nearly 1 in 10 adults in the United States. Clinical depression is more than just a "case of the blues." It is characterized by feelings of sadness, hopelessness, or despair that last for more than 2 weeks and interfere with daily living. Some symptoms of depression include loss of interest in activities that were once enjoyable (e.g., work, hobbies), changes in sleep habits (sleeping either too much or too little), and changes in appetite, which can lead to either weight loss or weight gain.

The causes of depression are varied. Stress, grief, illness, substance abuse, and some medications may certainly lead to depression, but biological changes in the brain are also implicated. For example, people who experience depression may have altered synthesis or activity of hormones (e.g., cortisol) or neurotransmitters (e.g., serotonin).

Does nutrition play a role in the biological basis for depression? The B vitamins, folic acid, vitamin B-6, and vitamin B-12 are involved in the synthesis and activity of neurotransmitters and have been studied most extensively in relation to depression. Research

also suggests that vitamin D and zinc may be particularly important in the prevention or treatment of depressive disorders.

Evidence supports a role of omega-3 fatty acids in the prevention or treatment of depression. The importance of omega-3 fatty acids to brain health is threefold. First, long-chain polyunsaturated fatty acids, particularly DHA, are incorporated into cell membranes throughout the brain. The fatty-acid composition of phospholipids affects the fluidity of cell membranes, which influences how well substances and signals are transported across the cell membrane. Membrane fluidity may affect how well chemical signals are transmitted by neurotransmitters from nerve cells to target cells. Second, omega-3 fatty acids improve vascular health by reducing the risk of blood clots and atherosclerosis. These changes ensure an adequate blood supply to the brain. Third, omega-3 fatty acids are involved in biochemical pathways that decrease inflammation and are associated with a reduction in depression (see Further Reading 7).

When it comes to overall dietary patterns, several studies have shown that following a plant-based diet—one naturally rich in folate and vitamin B-6—may reduce depression and anxiety. Emphasizing healthy sources of fat, such as walnuts, canola oil, flaxseed, oil, and fatty fish, will boost levels of omega-3 fatty acids in the body. In some cases, supplementation with omega-3 fatty acids may be appropriate. Conversely, dietary patterns that are high in added sugars may be a risk factor for depression. Rapid rises and falls in blood sugar may deprive the brain of glucose and negatively affect mood. Carbohydrates also influence the production of serotonin, a neurotransmitter that is associated with pleasure.

Preventing Neurodegenerative Diseases Neurodegenerative disease is a term that encompasses a variety of conditions characterized by gradual, progressive deterioration of neurons. Alterations of these cells result in abnormal functioning, plaque formation, and eventual cell death. The most common neurodegenerative diseases in the United States include Alzheimer's disease, **Parkinson's disease, Creutzfeldt-Jakob disease,** and **multiple sclerosis.** In the past, research focused on genetics and aging as the primary risk factors for diseases of the brain. Now, researchers are turning their focus to lifestyle choices, with energy balance and optimal body fatness viewed very important for optimizing brain health. Research actually links both undernutrition and overnutrition to reduced cognitive function, via mechanisms that involve changes in hormone levels in the body (see Further Reading 5).

Parkinson's disease Disease that belongs to a group of conditions called motor system disorders, which are the result of the loss of dopamine-producing brain cells. The four primary symptoms of PD are tremor, or trembling in hands, arms, legs, jaw, and face; rigidity, or stiffness of the limbs and trunk; bradykinesia, or slowness of movement; and postural instability, or impaired balance and coordination.

Creutzfeldt-Jakob disease A rare, degenerative, invariably fatal brain disorder. Symptoms include problems with muscular coordination, personality changes including progressive and severe mental impairment, impaired vision that may lead to blindness, and involuntary muscle jerks.

multiple sclerosis An unpredictable disease of the central nervous system that can range from relatively benign to somewhat disabling to devastating, as communication between the brain and other parts of the body is disrupted.

Obese adults are three times more likely to suffer impaired cognitive function and dementia.

The most common neurodegenerative disease is Alzheimer's disease, diagnosed in about 5.1 million adults in the United States. It is an irreversible, progressive deterioration of the brain that causes victims to steadily lose the ability to remember, reason, and comprehend, often taking a terrible toll on the mental and eventual physical health of older people. Scientists have proposed various causes, including alterations in cell development or protein production in the brain, strokes, altered blood lipoprotein composition, poor blood glucose regulation (e.g., diabetes), high blood pressure, viral infections, and high free radical levels. The 10 warning signs of Alzheimer's disease are listed here.

Early efforts at prevention of Alzheimer's disease should receive the most attention, because the process of cognitive decline begins 10 to 20 years before warning signs appear. Preventive measures for Alzheimer's disease focus on eating a diet rich in fruits and vegetables, maintaining brain activity through lifelong learning, and taking ibuprofen. Fruits and vegetables provide antioxidant nutrients, such as vitamin C, vitamin E, and selenium, that help to protect the body from the damaging effects of free radicals. In addition, various phytochemicals with antioxidant and anti-inflammatory properties, including polyphenols and carotenoids (e.g., lutein and zeaxanthin), have been shown to protect the brain throughout life (see Further Reading 8). Good food sources of lutein and zeaxanthin include green leafy vegetables, yellow-orange fruits and vegetables, and egg yolks. Polyphenols are found in foods such as berries, coffee, green or black tea, and chocolate.

Adequate intakes of folate, vitamin B-6, vitamin B-12, and choline are important to decrease blood homocysteine, which is a risk factor for neurodegenerative and cardiovascular disease (see Newsworthy Nutrition below). Dietary fats, too, may play a role in keeping Alzheimer's disease at bay. Individuals with diets rich in omega-3 fatty acids and low in saturated and *trans* fatty acids have a reduced risk of Alzheimer's disease (see Further Reading 5). The role of nutrition in preventing or minimizing the risk of this disease continues to be studied.

▲ The MIND Diet includes three servings of whole grains, a salad plus one other vegetable, and a glass of wine each day. © Ingram Publishing

The MIND Diet is a dietary intervention that shows promising results for protecting the brain against cognitive decline. MIND stands for Mediterranean-DASH Intervention for Neurodegenerative Delay, a hybrid of the nutrient-rich Mediterranean eating pattern (see Section 2.3) with the low-calorie, low-sodium DASH Diet (see Section 9.9). The MIND diet's 10 "brain-healthy" foods include green leafy vegetables, other vegetables, nuts, berries, beans, whole grains, fish, poultry, olive oil, and wine. The five foods to limit include red meats, butter and stick margarine, cheese, pastries and sweets, and fried or fast food. Each day, followers of the MIND Diet should consume a minimum of three servings of

Ten Warning Signs of Alzheimer's Disease

1. Recent memory loss that affects job performance
2. Difficulty performing familiar tasks
3. Problems with language
4. Faulty or decreased judgment
5. Problems with abstract thinking
6. Tendency to misplace things
7. Changes in mood or behavior
8. Changes in personality
9. Loss of initiative
10. Withdrawal from work or social activities

▲ Patients with advanced dementia may be easily distracted during meals, forget to eat, be unable to prepare food safely, and have trouble feeding themselves or swallowing. Caregivers and health care providers need to monitor the patient's weight to ensure maintenance of a healthy weight and nutritional state. © Ingram Publishing

Newsworthy Nutrition

Folic acid and Vitamin B-12 may prevent cognitive decline

Folic acid and vitamin B-12 may be effective in the prevention of cognitive impairment and dementia based on their ability to lower homocysteine concentrations and reduce vascular risk factors. This randomized controlled trial was designed to assess the effects of folic acid and vitamin B-12 on depression. Nine hundred and nine older adults in Australia (aged 60 to 74 years) received either a placebo or a dietary supplement containing 400 micrograms folic acid and 100 micrograms vitamin B-12 for 24 months. A secondary analysis revealed that subjects who received folic acid and vitamin B-12 performed better on tests of short- and long-term recall, which was also related to smaller increases in plasma homocysteine levels over time. Supplementation with these B vitamins may help older adults maintain cognitive functioning as they age.

Source: Walker JG and others: Oral folic acid and vitamin B-12 supplementation to prevent cognitive decline in community-dwelling older adults with depressive symptoms—the Beyond Ageing Project: A randomized controlled trial. *American Journal of Clinical Nutrition* 95:194, 2012.

whole grains, a salad plus one other vegetable, and one glass of wine. Nuts, beans, poultry, and berries are recommended regularly, but butter, cheese, and fast food are strictly limited (Further Reading 11). Adults that adhered to the MIND Diet had 54% lower rates of Alzheimer's disease. Even more surprising, those that followed the MIND pattern, even periodically, also reduced their risk of the disease by 35%. In 2016, the MIND Diet was ranked second in *U.S. News & World Report's* Best Diets Rankings, just behind the DASH Diet.

IN SUMMARY: FOOD FOR THOUGHT

When it comes to studies of individual nutrients and brain health, the results are not that impressive. Recognize, however, that we seldom eat just one nutrient. It is most relevant to examine how overall dietary patterns influence health. Time and time again, we see that dietary patterns rich in fruits, vegetables, legumes, nuts, whole grains, and fish are beneficial for brain health.

Now that you have studied the micronutrients and phytochemicals, you can understand that folate, vitamin B-6, and vitamin B-12 work together to keep homocysteine levels in check. You can describe how vitamins E and C from fruits and vegetables work as antioxidants to prevent damage and decrease inflammation. You understand the importance of polyunsaturated fatty acids in fish oils for brain function. Although a few studies have documented that micronutrient supplementation improves mood and psychological well-being, the overall evidence to support use of dietary supplements for brain health remains equivocal. Dietary supplements may seem like a quick fix to fill nutrient gaps to promote optimal brain health, but when we focus on isolated nutrients, we miss out on the synergistic effects of the full complement of brain-healthy nutrients and phytochemicals in whole foods (see Further Reading 2).

Summary (Numbers refer to numbered sections in the chapter.)

13.1 Blood consists of red cells (erythrocytes), white cells (leukocytes), platelets (thrombocytes), and plasma. The cellular components are formed in the bone marrow. Erythropoiesis is the formation of red blood cells, which requires vitamin B-6, folate, vitamin B-12, iron, and copper. A deficiency of any of these nutrients could lead to anemia.

13.2 Hemostasis describes the mechanisms that prevent blood loss, such as vasoconstriction, formation of a platelet plug, and blood coagulation. Vitamin K is essential for blood clotting and imparts calcium-binding ability to various proteins, including those in bone.

13.3 Folate plays an important role in DNA synthesis and homocysteine metabolism. Food sources are leafy vegetables, organ meats, and orange juice. Deficiencies of folate during pregnancy can lead to neural tube defects.

13.4 Vitamin B-12 is needed to metabolize folate and homocysteine, and to maintain the insulation surrounding nerves. Absorption of vitamin B-12 is a complex process that requires a salivary protein, adequate stomach-acid production, and an intrinsic factor produced by the stomach. A deficiency, which results in anemia and nerve degeneration, most likely results from poor absorption of vitamin B-12 rather than poor dietary intake. Pernicious anemia is one condition that can impair vitamin B-12 absorption. Vitamin B-12 is found in foods of animal origin, fortified foods, and supplements.

13.5 Iron is part of hemoglobin, which functions to transport oxygen and carbon dioxide in the blood. Also, iron participates as a cofactor for many enzymes. It is important for brain and immune function, detoxification of drugs, and bone health. Heme iron, found in meat, poultry, and seafood, is more efficiently absorbed than nonheme iron, which makes up some of the iron provided by animal sources and all of the iron provided by plant sources (e.g., whole grains, fortified grain products, and legumes). Hereditary hemochromatosis is a genetic condition that increases iron absorption, leading to accumulation of dangerously high levels of iron in the blood and organs.

13.6 Copper participates as a cofactor for enzymes with a broad range of functions: formation of red blood cells, release of iron from storage, antioxidant reactions, and synthesis of collagen in bone. It also participates in immune function, blood clotting, and blood lipid metabolism. Food sources of copper include beef liver, legumes, seeds, whole grains, and cocoa. Menkes syndrome and Wilson's disease are two genetic diseases that affect copper status.

13.7 Good nutritional status is essential for proper brain development and function. The brain requires a steady supply of glucose; micronutrient deficiencies adversely affect brain development and function. The key nutrients involved in brain function are the essential fatty acids, B vitamins, choline, antioxidant nutrients, and some minerals.

Check Your Knowledge (Answers are available at the end of this question set.)

1. A white blood cell is also known as
   a. an erythrocyte.
   b. a thrombocyte.
   c. a leukocyte.
   d. a cytokine.

2. An erythrocyte
   a. is a red blood cell.
   b. requires iron.
   c. transports carbon dioxide.
   d. is all of these.

3. The primary function of vitamin K is its role in
   a. carrying oxygen in hemoglobin.
   b. DNA synthesis.
   c. blood coagulation.
   d. antibody synthesis.

4. Strict vegetarians (vegans) are most at risk for deficiency of which of the following micronutrients?
   a. Vitamin K
   b. Vitamin B-12
   c. Folate
   d. Vitamin A

5. Dietary heme iron is derived from
   a. elemental iron in food.
   b. animal flesh.
   c. breakfast cereal.
   d. vegetables.

6. Which of the following micronutrients participates in DNA synthesis?
   a. Folate
   b. Vitamin B-12
   c. Iron
   d. All of these

7. Macrocytic anemia is likely the result of a deficiency of
   a. copper.
   b. zinc.
   c. vitamin B-6.
   d. vitamin B-12.

8. Choline is important for brain growth and development through its role in the synthesis of
   a. phospholipids.
   b. cholesterol.
   c. omega-3 fatty acids.
   d. amino acids.

9. The preferred energy source for the brain's metabolic activity is
   a. fatty acids.
   b. glucose.
   c. amino acids.
   d. fructose.

10. The MIND Diet is a hybrid of the Mediterranean Diet and the
    a. Blood-Type Diet.
    b. Paleo Diet.
    c. DASH Diet.
    d. Diabetes Diet.

Answer Key: 1. c (LO 13.1), 2. d (LO 13.1), 3. c (LO 13.2), 4. b (LO 13.4), 5. b (LO 13.5), 6. d (LO 13.1), 7. d (LO 13.4), 8. a (LO 13.4), 9. b (LO 13.7), 10. c (LO 13.7)

Study Questions (Numbers refer to Learning Outcomes)

1. Describe the four main components of blood. Where do blood cells come from? Which micronutrients affect blood cell formation? **(LO 13.1)**

2. How is vitamin K involved in hemostasis? What is the most life-threatening result of a vitamin K deficiency? **(LO 13.2)**

3. List three micronutrients that are required for erythropoiesis. Design a meal that would provide at least one source of each of these three nutrients. **(LO 13.2)**

4. Why does FDA limit the amount of folate that may be included in supplements and fortified foods? **(LO 13.3)**

5. Explain the difference between heme and nonheme iron. Name one food source of each. How does the body's need for iron influence the absorption of heme and nonheme iron? **(LO 13.5)**

6. List three symptoms of anemia. Explain the physiological basis for the symptoms of anemia. **(LO 13.1)**

7. Identify three micronutrient deficiencies that could be responsible for anemia. Describe the appearance of the red blood cells for each of these types of anemia. **(LO 13.1)**

8. Describe copper's role in blood health. **(LO 13.6)**

9. Describe at least two ways that nutrients are important for brain development and function. **(LO 13.7)**

10. Explain the components of the MIND Diet and the effect it has been shown to have on cognitive function. **(LO 13.7)**

What the Dietitian Chose

Many of us have been assessing our meat consumption since red meat was classified as "probably carcinogenic" to humans by a panel of experts convened by the World Health Organization. In 2015, this group reported that eating processed meat (e.g., hot dogs, ham, bacon) raises the risk of colon cancer and consuming other red meats "probably" raises the risk as well. This was based on limited evidence showing positive associations between eating red meat and developing colorectal cancer as well as links with pancreatic cancer and prostate cancer with the risk increasing with the amount of meat consumed.

Although the WHO panel did not offer specific guidelines on red meat consumption, its conclusions support recommendations made in 2002 by WHO and other scientific groups such as the U.S. Dietary Guidelines Advisory Committee, which also recommended in its 2015 Scientific Report that most people should reduce consumption of red and processed meats. Despite this recommendation and the scientific evidence, the actual 2015–2020 Dietary Guidelines for Americans do not include a similar recommendation to limit red meat consumption. Rather, the recommendation for the meats, poultry, and eggs subgroup at the 2000–calorie level is 26 ounce-equivalents per week (see Further Reading 19).

The Dietary Guidelines Report does admit there is evidence that eating patterns that include a lower intake of meats are associated with reduced risk of several conditions including cardiovascular disease, obesity, type 2 diabetes, and some types of cancer. With that said, it would be prudent to limit your red and processed meat consumption to no more than twice a month. Remember that the WHO Panel and the Dietary Guidelines define red meat as all beef, pork, lamb, veal, goat, and non-bird game (e.g., venison, bison, elk). Processed meats include those that have been transformed through salting, curing, fermentation, smoking, or other processes to enhance flavor or improve preservation.

How will this reduced meat intake affect your iron status? Optimal nutrition, in general, and iron status, specifically, will be very important for a success-ful hiking trip at high altitude. Without sufficient iron, your body cannot produce enough hemoglobin, making it impos-sible for the red blood cells to carry enough oxygen to the body's tissues. As a result, you may feel weak, tired, and irri-table at sea level, let alone at high altitude.

▲ To support optimal physical per-formance at high altitude, your body must manufacture additional red blood cells to transport oxygen to body tissues. © REB Images/Getty Images

There are several things to keep in mind when preparing to hike at high altitude and to prevent "altitude sickness." Climbing and hiking at high altitude can cause problems because the body must adjust to functioning with the lower oxygen level in the air. The best way to prevent altitude sick-ness is by acclimatization. This is a process that allows your

▲ Shellfish, such as the mussels and clams in this paella contain more iron per serving than red meat. © Image Source

body time to adapt to the change in oxygen concentration at a higher altitude. An important change that occurs in your body during this adaptation is the production of more red blood cells to carry more oxygen to be released from the blood to the body tissues.

To support the synthesis of hemoglobin for new red blood cells, you will need adequate stores of iron. Be sure to incorporate iron-rich foods into your eating pattern. Remember that there are two forms of dietary iron: heme and nonheme. Because heme iron is derived from hemoglobin, it is found in animal foods that originally contained hemoglobin, such as red meats, fish, and poultry. Heme iron, found in animal sources, is better absorbed than nonheme iron, found in plant sources.

If you choose to limit red meat in your dietary pattern, you will need an alternative source of iron in your diet. Beef is definitely a good source of heme iron, with 2.1 milligrams or more per 3-ounce serving. Some other foods that also have 2.1 milligrams or more per 3-ounce serving are sardines (canned in oil) and cooked turkey **(choice b)**. Chicken and fish also contain heme iron but at a much lower concen-tration (0.7 milligram or more per 3-ounce serving). There is another source of heme iron that is even greater than meat with 3.5 milligrams per 3-ounce serving—clams, mollusks, mussels, or oysters **(choice a)**.

If shellfish is not something you choose to consume several times a week, then you can look to add some nonheme iron from plant foods. Nonheme iron is also the form added to iron-enriched and iron-fortified foods. Although our bodies are less efficient at absorb-ing nonheme iron, most dietary iron is nonheme iron.

Very good sources of nonheme iron, with 3.5 milligrams or more per serving, are:

- Breakfast cereals enriched with iron, such as 1 cup of Wheaties® **(choice d)**
- 1/2 cup tofu
- 1 ounce pumpkin or sesame seeds

Good sources of nonheme iron, with 2.1 milligrams or more per serving, include:

- ½ cup canned lima beans, red kidney beans, chickpeas, or split peas

- 1 cup dried apricots
- 1 medium baked potato
- 1 medium stalk of broccoli
- 1 cup cooked enriched egg noodles
- ¼ cup wheat germ

Sources of nonheme iron, with 0.7 milligram or more, include:

- 1 ounce peanuts, pecans, walnuts, pistachios, roasted almonds, roasted cashews, or sunflower seeds
- ½ cup dried seedless raisins, peaches, or prunes
- 1 cup raw spinach (*choice c*)
- 1 medium green pepper
- 1 cup pasta
- 1 slice of bread, pumpernickel bagel, or bran muffin
- 1 cup rice

So the dietitian recommends you follow an eating pattern that would include 8 milligrams of iron per day for males, or

18 milligrams for females, by adding in a combination of rich sources of iron (see listing). To enhance absorption of iron from the foods you eat, include a good source of vitamin C, such as orange juice, broccoli, or strawberries; eat sources of nonheme iron with a food from the fish or poultry group; and avoid drinking coffee or tea or consuming calcium-rich foods or drinks with meals containing iron-rich foods.

Finally, it is important to find out where you are in terms of iron status so you can make the necessary adjustments. Make an appointment with your health care provider to have your iron status checked. If you are iron deficient or having trouble getting enough iron from food sources, you may need an iron supplement. If this is the case, speak to your clinician or RDN, and follow the instructions about the proper dosage of iron supplementation carefully. Fortunately, iron toxicity from food sources is rare, but overdoses are possible with supplements. Very little iron is excreted from the body, so too much iron can accumulate in body tissues and organs.

CASE STUDY SOLUTION   Anemia

1. Iron is part of hemoglobin, the protein in red blood cells that transports oxygen from the lungs to the body's cells and returns carbon dioxide to the lungs for excretion. At age 60, Anita is postmenopausal, so monthly losses of blood are not depleting her iron stores. Good sources of iron include ready-to-eat breakfast cereals, enriched grains, beans, and meats. Anita's food choices probably do supply adequate iron, but she could increase her absorption of iron by consuming iron-containing foods with a source of vitamin C, such as orange juice.

2. Vitamin B-6 is involved in the synthesis of hemoglobin, and a lack of vitamin B-6 may lead to microcytic, hypochromic anemia. Vitamin B-6 is widely available in the typical North American diet, found in ready-to-eat breakfast cereals, animal products, dairy products, fruits, and vegetables. Given Anita's nutrient-dense food choices, it is not likely that vitamin B-6 deficiency is the reason for her anemia.

3. Folate is involved in the maturation of red blood cells, and a deficiency leads to macrocytic (megaloblastic) anemia. Immature red blood cells are less efficient at carrying oxygen. Food sources of folate include green leafy vegetables, organ meats, and beans. Given Anita's healthy food choices, it is not likely that folate deficiency is the reason for her anemia.

4. Vitamin B-12 is involved in the metabolism of folate, so a lack of vitamin B-12 may lead to macrocytic anemia (described in answer 3). Vitamin B-12 is naturally found in foods of animal origin, including meats and dairy products, and is added to ready-to-eat breakfast cereals. With aging, many adults produce insufficient stomach acid and intrinsic factor, required for vitamin B-12 digestion and absorption. Thus, even though Anita's diet may appear adequate in vitamin B-12, her absorption of the vitamin may be low. Consuming a synthetic source of vitamin B-12, which does not require intrinsic factor for absorption, may improve her vitamin B-12 status. Fortified breakfast cereals or multivitamin supplements are typical sources of synthetic B-12.

5. Anita should talk with her health care provider to determine the cause and severity of her anemia. If Anita does have iron-deficiency anemia, the cause needs to be diagnosed. For a postmenopausal woman, a possible cause could be bleeding in the GI tract, which could be serious if left untreated. Dietary changes, such as consuming vitamin C to enhance iron absorption, can improve the health of her red blood cells and prevent future deficiencies, but in many cases, supplementation is necessary. A synthetic source of vitamin B-12 will overcome any absorption problems if vitamin B-12 deficiency is the cause of her anemia.

Further Readings

1. Appold K: Migraine headaches—here's how to identify food triggers and reduce debilitating symptoms. *Today's Dietitian* 14:14, 2012.

2. Barberger-Gateau P: Nutrition and brain aging: How can we move ahead? *European Journal of Clinical Nutrition* 68:1245, 2014.

3. Bunner AE and others: Nutrition intervention for migraine: A randomized crossover trial. *The Journal of Headache and Pain* 15:69, 2014.

4. Cusack L and others: Blood type diets lack supporting evidence: A systematic review. *American Journal of Clinical Nutrition* 98:99, 2013.

5. Dauncey MJ: Nutrition, the brain and cognitive decline: Insights from epigenetics. *European Journal of Clinical Nutrition* 68:1179, 2014.

6. Evans EW and others: Dietary intake patterns and diet quality in a nationally representative sample of women with and without severe headache or migraine. *Headache* 55:550, 2015.

7. Harrar S: Omega-3 fatty acids and mood disorders. *Today's Dietitian* 14:22, 2012.

8. Johnson EJ: Role of lutein and zeaxanthin in visual and cognitive function throughout the lifespan. *Nutrition Reviews* 72:605, 2014.

9. Khan NA and others: IV. The cognitive implications of obesity and nutrition in childhood. *Monographs of the Society for Research in Child Development* 79:51, 2014.

10. Krider KS and others: Folic acid food fortification—its history, effect, concerns and future directions. *Nutrients* 3:370, 2011.

11. Marcason W: What are the components to the MIND diet? *Journal of the Academy of Nutrition and Dietetics* 115:1744, 2015.

12. McDonagh M and others: Routine iron supplementation and screening for iron deficiency anemia in pregnant women: A systematic review to update the U.S. Preventive Services Task Force recommendation. Evidence Synthesis no. 123. AHRQ Publication no. 13-05188-EF-1. Rockville, MD: Agency for Healthcare Research and Quality; 2015.

13. Mei Z and others: Assessment of iron status in US pregnant women from the National Health and Nutrition Examination Survey (NHANES), 1999–2006. *American Journal of Clinical Nutrition* 93:1312, 2011.

14. Meeusin R: Exercise, nutrition and the brain. *Sports Medicine* 44:S47, 2014.

15. National Institutes of Health Clinical Center's Drug-Nutrient Interaction Task Force: Important information to know when you are taking: Coumadin and vitamin K. September 5, 2012. http://www.cc.nih.gov/ccc/patient_education/drug_nutrient/coumadin1.pdf

16. Office of Dietary Supplements, National Institutes of Health: Dietary supplement fact sheet: Iron. November 24, 2015. http://ods.od.nih.gov/factsheets/iron; Vitamin B-12 fact sheet. June 24, 2011.

17. Peker E and others: The levels of vitamın B12, folate and homocysteine in mothers and their babies with neural tube defects. *Journal Maternal and Fetal Neonatal Medicine* 23:1, 2015.

18. Schulte R and others: Rise in late onset vitamin K deficiency bleeding in young infants because of omission or refusal of prophylaxis at birth. *Pediatric Neurology* 50(6):564, 2014.

19. U.S. Department of Health and Human Services and U.S. Department of Agriculture. 2015–2020 Dietary Guidelines for Americans. 8th ed. December 2015. http://health.gov/dietaryguidelines/2015/guidelines/.

20. Wang J and others: ABO genotype, 'Blood-Type' diet and cardiometabolic risk factors. *PLoS One* 9(1):e84749, 2014. doi:10.1371/journal.pone.0084749

21. Yadav D, Chandra J: Iron deficiency: Beyond anemia. *Indian Journal of Pediatrics* 78:65, 2011.

 To get the most out of your study of nutrition, go to McGraw-Hill's online resources: Connect www.mcgrawhillconnect.com, where you will find NutritionCalc Plus, LearnSmart, and many other dynamic tools.

Rate Your Plate

Boosting Your Micronutrient Intake

For each of the following meal options, choose the one that would supply the most of the given micronutrient.

1. Which meal supplies the most iron?

A	B
• Roast beef sandwich on whole-grain bread with lettuce, tomato, and mustard	• Roast beef sandwich on whole-grain bread with lettuce, tomato, and mustard
• Grapes	• Grapes
• Skim milk	• Orange juice

2. Which meal supplies the most vitamin K?

A	B
• Pasta with shrimp, tomatoes, and spinach	• Pasta with shrimp, tomatoes, and feta cheese
• Italian bread with olive oil	• Italian bread with butter
• White wine	• White wine

3. Which meal supplies the most copper?

A	B
• Cheerios	• Blueberry bagel with cream cheese
• Banana	• Banana
• Orange juice	• Orange juice

4. Which meal supplies the most vitamin B-12?

A	B
• Cheeseburger	• Veggie burger
• Baked potato with sour cream	• Baked potato with sour cream
• Diet cola	• Iced tea

Answer Key:
1. B: The vitamin C in orange juice enhances absorption of the iron in the roast beef and enriched bread.
2. A: Spinach is a source of vitamin K, whereas cheese is not.
3. A: Fortified breakfast cereals are a good source of many trace minerals; although breads are enriched with some vitamins and minerals lost during the refining process, copper is not one of those.
4. A: Animal products are sources of vitamin B-12.

© Purestock/SuperStock

Student Learning Outcomes

Chapter 14 is designed to allow you to:

14.1 List five positive health-related outcomes of a physically active lifestyle.

14.2 Enumerate three key elements of a sound fitness regimen.

14.3 Describe the use of carbohydrates, fat, and protein to meet energy needs during different activities.

14.4 Differentiate between anaerobic and aerobic uses of glucose and identify advantages and disadvantages of each.

14.5 Explain how muscles and related organs adapt to an increase in physical activity.

14.6 Outline how to estimate an athlete's calorie needs and discuss the general principles for meeting overall nutrient requirements in the training diet.

14.7 Examine problems associated with weight loss by dehydration and outline the importance of fluids during exercise.

Nutrition: Fitness and Sports

14.8 Understand how athletes can optimize performance by consuming foods and fluids before, during, and after exercise.

14.9 List several ergogenic aids and describe their effects, if any, on an athlete's performance.

Are you a sedentary individual looking to start a personal exercise program? Do you participate in recreational sports, such as intramural volleyball? Or are you a competitive athlete who would like to take your performance to the next level? One thing is certain: at every level of fitness, sensible nutrition and physical activity complement each other in the pursuit of wellness.

Some athletes may fall into the trap of thinking that participation in sports alleviates the need to pay close attention to eating habits. Sports nutritionists and athletic trainers frequently remind their clients that "you can't out-train a poor diet." Indeed, as you will learn in this chapter, adequate intakes of overall calories and specific nutrients can have a big impact on physical performance.

On the other hand, good eating habits cannot substitute for physical training and genetic endowment. Most athletes are on the lookout for any advantage, whether real or perceived, that might enhance performance and give them the winning edge. For this reason, athletes are likely targets for nutrition marketing and misinformation. As you try to sort fact from fiction, be sure of this: no dietary practice or supplement can increase speed or promote gains in muscle mass without proper physical training.

Overall, making informed choices about foods, beverages, and dietary supplements can optimize many aspects of physical performance, from preventing fatigue to gaining muscle to recovering from workouts. In this chapter, you will discover how physical fitness benefits the entire body and how nutrition relates to physical performance. This information is important for the everyday, recreational athlete who exercises to manage weight or just to have fun. It is crucial, however, for elite athletes for whom a fraction of a second can make the difference between first and second place.

Healthy People 2020 objectives focus on reducing the proportion of adults who engage in no leisure time physical activity and increasing the proportion of adults who meet the 2008 Physical Activity Guidelines for aerobic and muscle-strengthening physical activity.

physical activity Any movement of skeletal muscles that requires energy.

exercise Physical activities that are planned, repetitive, and intended to improve physical fitness.

physical fitness The ability to perform moderate to vigorous activity without undue fatigue.

FIGURE 14-1 ▶ The benefits of regular, moderate physical activity and exercise.
© Rubberball Productions

14.1 An Introduction to Physical Fitness

Ravi and Chandra used to chat over a cup of coffee after their 8:00 A.M. nutrition class, but now they meet at the court for a game of racquetball. Terry listens to recorded political science lectures as he jogs around the track. Claudia takes the stairs instead of the elevator to her dorm room on the fourth floor. Marlie reviews her biology notes while she works out on the elliptical machine. What do these students have in common? They each have found inventive ways to incorporate physical activity into their crazy-busy college schedules.

Without a doubt, the benefits of **physical activity** outweigh the risks for most Americans. The potential benefits of regular physical activity include enhanced heart function, less injury, better sleep habits, and improvement in body composition. Physical activity also can reduce stress and positively affect blood pressure, blood cholesterol, blood glucose regulation, and immune function. In addition, physical activity aids in weight control, both by raising resting energy expenditure for a short time after exercise and by increasing overall energy expenditure. In fact, as physical fitness improves, so does your ability to mobilize fat as a source of energy. See Figure 14-1 and Further Reading 5 for a closer look at these and other benefits of a physically active lifestyle.

It is important to note that physical activity and exercise are not synonymous. Physical activity refers to any movement of skeletal muscles that requires energy. It includes exercise, sports, as well as all the simple, unplanned activities of daily living, such as raking the yard, walking up and down the stairs, and carrying bags of groceries into the house. **Exercise** specifically refers to those physical activities that are planned, repetitive, and intended to improve **physical fitness.** Examples of exercise include walking, biking, swimming, participating in team sports, and running.

Strengthens bones and joints

Reduces blood pressure

Improves blood glucose regulation

Increases cardiovascular function and improves blood lipid profile

Reduces stress and improves self-image

Aids in weight loss/weight control

Increases flexibility and balance

Increases muscle mass and strength

Improves immune function

Improves GI tract peristalsis

Reduces risk of colon cancer, prostate cancer, and likely breast cancer

Improves sleep (if activity is done in the morning or afternoon)

Improves cognitive function

Prevents or reduces mild depression or anxiety

The 2008 Physical Activity Guidelines for Americans recommend that all adults should avoid inactivity. Some physical activity is better than none, and adults who participate in any amount of physical activity gain some health benefits. The Physical Activity Guidelines set specific time goals for adults (review Section 2.2):

- For substantial health benefits, adults should do at least 150 minutes per week of **moderate-intensity,** or 75 minutes per week of **vigorous-intensity aerobic physical activity,** or an equivalent combination of moderate- and vigorous-intensity aerobic activity. Activity should be performed in episodes of at least 10 minutes, and preferably, it should be spread throughout the week.
- For additional and more extensive health benefits, adults should increase their physical activity to 300 minutes per week of moderate-intensity, or 150 minutes per week of vigorous-intensity aerobic physical activity, or an equivalent combination of moderate- and vigorous-intensity activity. Additional health benefits are gained by engaging in physical activity beyond this amount.
- Adults should also include **muscle-strengthening activities** that involve all major muscle groups on 2 or more days a week.

These recommendations are consistent with guidance from the American College of Sports Medicine (ACSM; see Further Reading 5).

Complying with the Physical Activity Guidelines is the first step toward managing weight, reducing risks for chronic diseases, and improving physical fitness. Losing excess weight and maintaining weight loss will require more than 150 minutes of physical activity per week.

Unfortunately, as noted in Chapter 7, many North American adults lead sedentary lives. A recent report from the Department of Health and Human Services revealed that only one in five American adults achieves the level of physical activity set forth by the Physical Activity Guidelines. When New Year's Day rolls around each year, many of us resolve to make exercise a priority in our lives, but statistics show that about half of all adults quit an exercise program within 3 months of initiation.

moderate-intensity aerobic physical activity Aerobic activity that increases a person's heart rate and breathing to some extent (4–6 on RPE scale). Examples include brisk walking, dancing, swimming, or bicycling on level terrain.

vigorous-intensity aerobic physical activity Aerobic activity that greatly increases a person's heart rate and breathing (7–8 on RPE scale). Examples include jogging, singles tennis, swimming continuous laps, or bicycling uphill.

muscle-strengthening activity Physical activity that increases skeletal muscle strength, power, endurance, and mass. Examples include lifting weights, using weight machines, and calisthenics (e.g., push-ups).

✓ CONCEPT CHECK 14.1

1. Differentiate between physical activity and exercise.
2. How much physical activity is recommended by the Physical Activity Guidelines for Americans to reduce risks for chronic diseases?
3. List the five benefits of regular physical activity that are most important to you.

14.2 Achieving and Maintaining Physical Fitness

Much of the nutrition advice that appears later in this chapter focuses on enhancing the performance of highly competitive athletes; however, only a few students would describe themselves as this type of athlete. Furthermore, in a health profession, most of your clients will be at a beginner or intermediate level of fitness. Certainly, proper nutrition supports physical performance at all levels. Perhaps more importantly, nutrition and physical activity complement each other when it comes to improving health outcomes. This section outlines how to get started with a plan to achieve physical fitness.

ASSESS YOUR CURRENT LEVEL OF FITNESS

Start by assessing your current level of fitness. In some cases, it is beneficial to seek medical advice before getting started. Men aged 40 years or older and women aged 50 years or older, anyone who has been inactive for many years, or those who have an existing health problem should discuss their fitness goals with their primary care provider before increasing activity. Health problems that require medical evaluation before beginning an exercise program include obesity, cardiovascular disease (or family history of it), hypertension, diabetes (or family history), chest pains or shortness of breath after mild exertion, and arthritis. Even if you do not have preexisting medical problems, enlisting the aid of a fitness professional (e.g., a qualified personal trainer) can help you to determine a safe starting point and establish realistic goals.

SET A GOAL

For any behavior change, goal setting will enhance your success. Taking into account your current level of fitness, choose a goal that is challenging yet attainable. For someone who has never exercised regularly, running a mile without stopping might be a worthwhile goal. An elite runner might strive to run that mile in under 4 minutes. Whatever goal you set, write it down and post it where you and everyone else can see it! Based on your long-term goal, also incorporate several smaller, short-term goals into your plan. Measurable, attainable, and realistic goals provide focus and motivation for any endeavor.

PLAN YOUR PROGRAM

What activities should you include in your fitness program? Although your goal may focus on just one aspect of fitness, such as being able to bench-press your body weight, a balanced fitness program will include three key types of activities: aerobic exercise, strength training, and flexibility.

Many fitness experts use the FITT principle to design a fitness program. FITT stands for *frequency, intensity, time,* and *type* of exercise. Frequency is the number of days per week you engage in a particular exercise. Intensity is how hard you work when you exercise—that is, how much you increase your heart rate or how much resistance you use when you lift weights. Type (also called *mode*) is your choice of activity, such as walking or running. Table 14-1 summarizes ACSM's guidance for planning a general fitness program (see Further Reading 5).

Aerobic Exercise Enhances Heart and Lung Function As you learned in Section 3.2, *aerobic* means "with oxygen." Aerobic exercises use large muscle groups in a rhythmic fashion and aim to increase your heart rate. The ability to perform aerobic exercise depends on the fitness of your heart and lungs—the organ systems that provide oxygen to the cells of the body.

TABLE 14-1 ■ **Elements of a Well-Rounded Fitness Program**

	Aerobic Fitness	Muscular Fitness	Flexibility
Frequency	5 days per week	2 to 3 days per week	2 to 3 days per week
Intensity	55% to 85% of MHR[a] or RPE[b] of 4 or higher (see Fig. 14-3)	40% to 80% of 1 RM[c] (lower to build endurance and higher to build strength)	To the point of tension
Time	20 to 60 minutes per day	1 to 3 sets of 8 to 12 repetitions of 8 to 10 different exercises	2 to 4 repetitions of 8 to 10 different exercises, held for 15 to 30 seconds each
Type (examples)	Brisk walking, running, cycling, swimming, basketball, tennis, and soccer	Bench press, squat, biceps curl, and abdominal crunch	Hamstring stretch, shoulder reach, and side bend

[a]Maximal heart rate

[b]Rating of perceived exertion

[c]1-repetition maximum

Aerobic activities usually form the backbone of a fitness program. Indeed, many of the benefits of fitness mentioned in Section 14.1 are direct effects of aerobic training. The ACSM recommends including at least 30 minutes per day of moderate-intensity aerobic activities on 5 days per week. Alternatively, less time spent in aerobic exercises of vigorous intensity can yield similar results. Walking, running, dancing, and biking are examples of aerobic activities.

There are a few ways to determine the intensity of aerobic exercise. A popular and simple method is to use a percentage of your age-predicted maximum heart rate (MHR) (Fig. 14-2). To find your MHR, subtract your age from 220. For a 20-year-old person, MHR equals 200 beats per minute ($220 - 20 = 200$).

At the initiation of an aerobic exercise program, aim for about 50% to 65% of MHR. Thus, (200×0.5) and (200×0.65) yield a target training zone of 100 to 130 beats per minute. As you progress and become more physically fit, you can work up to a higher heart rate. For an intermediate fitness enthusiast, 60% to 75% of MHR is recommended. For more experienced exercisers, 70% to 85% MHR is suitable.

Remember that heart rate is just an estimate of workout intensity. Medications, such as those for hypertension and other health conditions, may impact heart rate. If you have health concerns, a primary care provider can help to personalize your target zone.

Another way of determining the intensity of exercise is the Rating of Perceived Exertion (RPE) scale. One version includes a range of 0 to 10, with each number corresponding to a subjective feeling of exertion. For example, the number 0 is "nothing at all" (e.g., sitting at a table), and the number 10 is considered close to maximal effort or "very, very strong" (e.g., all-out sprint; Fig. 14-3).

When using the 10-point RPE scale, the goal is to aim for a rating of 4, which corresponds to the beginning of "somewhat strong." This is the point at which you begin to see significant fitness results. You should be working hard but still be able to talk to an exercise partner (sometimes called the "talk test").

Muscular Fitness Encompasses Strength, Endurance, and Power Muscles can be trained in several ways. *Muscular strength* is the maximal force a muscle can exert against a load at one time (one-repetition maximum or 1 RM). For example, a strength-trained

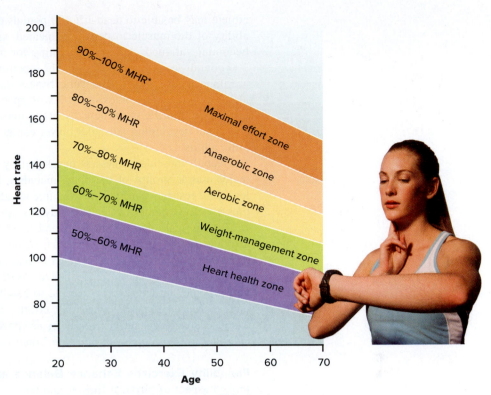

*MHR (maximum heart rate) = 220 - Age in years

FIGURE 14-2 ▲ Heart rate training chart. This chart shows the number of heart beats per minute that corresponds to various exercise intensities.
© Tetra Images/SuperStock

Measuring heart rate (pulse) is easy: Stop and count your pulse for 10 seconds and then multiply that number by 6 to determine beats per minute. Some exercise equipment and high-tech devices contain heart rate monitors.

RPE Scale*

Nothing at all | Very weak | Weak | Moderate | Somewhat strong | Strong | Very strong | Very, very strong

0 1 2 3 4 5 6 7 8 9 10

*Rating of perceived exertion (RPE) beyond 10 is considered maximal.

FIGURE 14-3 ◄ Rating of Perceived Exertion scale. When exercising, a rating of 4 or above is advocated for building/maintaining aerobic fitness.

athlete may be able to dead-lift 400 pounds one time. *Muscular endurance* refers to the ability of the muscle to perform repeated, submaximal contractions over time without becoming fatigued. An athlete training for muscular endurance may bench-press 80 to 100 pounds for several sets of 8 to 12 repetitions. Both muscular strength and endurance are important aspects of muscular fitness that relate to health for athletes of all levels. *Muscular power* combines strength with speed for explosive movements such as jumping or throwing. Power is a crucial aspect of muscular fitness for many athletes. Studies also show that developing muscular power can help to improve function and balance among older adults.

Overall, muscular fitness is developed by performing resistance exercises for all the major muscle groups of the body, including arms and shoulders, back, abdominals, and legs. This resistance may come from free weights (e.g., barbells), weight machines (e.g., leg press), or the weight of your own body (e.g., push-ups).

The Physical Activity Guidelines and ACSM recommend including muscle-strengthening activities in your fitness program on 2 to 3 nonconsecutive days per week (Fig. 14-4). (Taking a day or more to rest between bouts of resistance exercise is important to allow time for muscles to recover and increase in size.) Performing regular resistance exercises will help you become stronger and better able to handle the activities of daily living. It promotes increases in lean mass, which assist efforts at weight management. Compared to aerobic exercise alone, resistance exercise can also provide further reductions in risks for cardiovascular diseases, osteoporosis, and type 2 diabetes.

Flexibility Exercises Enhance Balance and Stability Flexibility is an often overlooked aspect of physical fitness, and tends to decline with age. Flexibility refers to the ability to move a joint through its full range of motion. Poor flexibility is often linked to chronic pain, especially in the lower back. Contrary to popular belief, research studies do not clearly support a role of flexibility exercises in preventing injury or muscle soreness from aerobic or strength-training activities. However, gains in flexibility can improve balance and stability, thereby reducing risks of falls and injuries, especially among older adults.

ACSM recommends performing flexibility exercises at least 2 to 3 days per week (see Fig. 14-4). It is best to perform stretches when the muscles have already been warmed up—after a few minutes of light-intensity aerobic activity. Examples of flexibility exercises include hamstring stretch, side bends, and shoulder reach. Some forms of exercise, such as Pilates or tai chi, combine stretching with strength moves.

Warm-Up and Cool-Down Be sure to plan for adequate warm-up and cool-down periods as part of your exercise routine. Begin by warming up with 5 to 10 minutes of low-intensity exercises, such as walking, slow jogging, or any slow version of the anticipated activity. This warms up your muscles so that muscle filaments slide over one another more easily, which increases range of motion and decreases the risk of injury. It is also thought to lower cardiovascular risks, particularly among people who are not accustomed to regular exercise. During cool-down, slow down for 5 to 10 minutes of low-intensity activity followed by 5 to 10 minutes of stretching. The same exercises performed during warm-up are appropriate. Although the cooldown does not actually prevent muscle soreness, it does reduce the dizziness or light-headedness that can occur with an abrupt end to a vigorous workout.

Josie's Fitness Plan

Monday
Spinning class (45 min)
Stretching routine (20 min)

Tuesday
Walking (30 min)
Weight machines (30 min)

Wednesday
Spinning class (45 min)
Stretching routine (20 min)

Thursday
Walking (30 min)
Weight machines (30 min)

Friday
Yoga (30 min)

Saturday
Trail hiking (60 min)

Sunday
Rest

FIGURE 14-4 ▲ Sample fitness plan. Josie's fitness plan incorporates aerobic, strength, and flexibility exercises. © John Lund/Sam Diephuis/Blend Images LLC

Get Started For sedentary people who are otherwise healthy, gradual **progression** toward a goal of regular physical activity is recommended. During the first phase of a fitness program to promote health, you should begin to incorporate short periods of physical activity into your daily routine. This includes walking, taking the stairs instead of the elevator, house cleaning, gardening, and other activities that cause you to "huff and puff" a bit. A sensible goal is a total of 30 minutes of this moderate type of physical activity on most (and preferably all) days of the week. If necessary, this can be broken up into increments lasting at least 10 minutes. If there is not much time for activity, you can get similar benefits from performing shorter sessions of increased intensity, such as running instead of walking or biking on hilly instead of flat terrain.

Once you can perform physical activity for 30 minutes per day, turn your attention to more specific goals, such as increasing muscle mass and strength, to reap even more benefits.

> **progression** Incremental increase in frequency, intensity, and time spent in each type of physical activity over several weeks or months.

✓ CONCEPT CHECK 14.2

1. Why is goal setting important for the success of an exercise program?
2. What is the FITT principle? Demonstrate how you would use the FITT principle to make a plan for aerobic fitness.
3. Differentiate between muscular strength, muscular endurance, and muscular power.
4. List two evidence-supported benefits of flexibility exercises.
5. Provide three tips for a person who needs help with long-term maintenance of a fitness program.

> **Stick with It!**
>
> Even after all the effort of assessing baseline fitness, setting goals, and designing a program, it turns out that maintaining an exercise program is the hardest part! To stick with an exercise program, experts recommend the following:
>
> - Start slowly.
> - Vary your activities; make it fun.
> - Include friends and family members.
> - Monitor progress and compare it to your goals.
> - Set aside a specific time each day for exercise; build it into your routine, but make it convenient.
> - Reward yourself for being successful in keeping up with your goals.
> - Don't worry about occasional setbacks; focus on the long-term benefits to your health.

14.3 Energy Sources for Exercising Muscles

Like other cells, muscle cells cannot directly use the energy released from breaking down glucose or triglycerides. Muscle cells need a specific form of energy for contraction. Body cells must first convert food energy (i.e., calories) to **adenosine triphosphate (ATP).**

The chemical bonds between phosphates in ATP and related molecules are high-energy bonds. Using the energy obtained from food, cells make ATP from its breakdown product **adenosine diphosphate (ADP)** and a phosphate group (abbreviated P_i). Conversely, to release energy from ATP, cells partially break the compound down into ADP and P_i. The released energy is used for many cell functions (Fig. 14-5).

> **adenosine triphosphate (ATP)** The main energy currency for cells. ATP energy is used to promote ion pumping, enzyme activity, and muscular contraction.
>
> **adenosine diphosphate (ADP)** A breakdown product of ATP. ADP is synthesized into ATP using energy from foodstuffs and a phosphate group (abbreviated P_i).

ANAEROBIC METABOLISM SUPPLIES ENERGY FOR SHORT BURSTS OF INTENSE ACTIVITY

Stored ATP Essentially, ATP is the immediate source of energy for body functions (Table 14-2). The primary goal in the use of any fuel, whether carbohydrate, fat, or protein, is to make ATP. A resting muscle cell contains only a small amount of ATP that can be used immediately. This amount of ATP could keep the muscle working maximally for only about 2 to 4 seconds if no resupply of ATP were possible. Fortunately, the cells have various mechanisms to resupply ATP. Overall, cells must constantly and repeatedly use and then reform ATP, using a variety of energy sources.

Phosphocreatine As soon as ATP stored in muscle cells begins to be used, another high-energy compound,

FIGURE 14-5 ▲ Food energy is stored in the chemical bonds between the phosphate groups in ATP. When a phosphate group is cleaved from ATP, energy to perform work is released. The product of the breakdown of ATP is adenosine diphosphate (ADP).

anaerobic Not requiring oxygen.
aerobic Requiring oxygen.

▲ Bursts of muscle activity, such as the 100-meter freestyle, use a variety of energy sources, including ATP, PCr, and glucose.
© Erik Isakson/Blend Images LLC

FIGURE 14-6 ▲ ATP yield from aerobic versus anaerobic glucose use. Encircled numbers indicate the number of carbons in each molecule.

TABLE 14-2 ■ **Energy Sources Used by Resting and Working Muscle Cells**

Energy Source*	When in Use	Activity
ATP	At all times	All types
Phosphocreatine (PCr)	All exercise initially; short bursts of exercise thereafter	Shotput, high jump, bench press
Carbohydrate (**anaerobic**)	High-intensity exercise, especially lasting 30 seconds to 2 minutes	200-yard (about 200-meter) sprint
Carbohydrate (**aerobic**)	Exercise lasting 2 minutes to several hours; the higher the intensity (e.g., running a 6-minute mile), the greater the use	Basketball, swimming, jogging, power walking, soccer, tennis
Fat (aerobic)	Exercise lasting more than a few minutes; greater amounts are used at lower exercise intensities	Long-distance running, long-distance cycling; much of the fuel used in a 30-minute brisk walk is fat
Protein (aerobic)	Low amount during all exercise; slightly more in endurance exercise, especially when carbohydrate fuel is depleted	Long-distance running

*At any given time, more than one source is used. The relative amount of use differs during various activities.

phosphocreatine (PCr), is used to resupply ATP. An enzyme in the muscle cell is activated to split PCr into phosphate and **creatine.** This releases energy that can be used to reform ATP from its breakdown products. If no other source of energy for ATP resupply were available, PCr could probably maintain maximal muscle contractions for about 10 seconds.

The main advantage of PCr is that it can be activated instantly and can replenish ATP at rates fast enough to meet the energy demands of the fastest and most powerful actions, including jumping, lifting, throwing, and sprinting. The disadvantage of PCr is that not much of it is made and stored in the muscles. Strength-training athletes sometimes use creatine supplements in an effort to increase PCr in muscles (see Section 14.6).

Anaerobic Glucose Breakdown Carbohydrates are an important fuel for muscles. The most useful form of carbohydrate fuel is the simple sugar glucose, available to all cells from the bloodstream. As you will recall from Section 4.2, glucose is stored as glycogen in the liver and muscle cells. Blood glucose is maintained by the breakdown of liver glycogen. Breakdown of glycogen stored in a specific muscle also helps meet the carbohydrate demand of that muscle, but the actual amount of glycogen stored in muscle is limited (about 350 grams for all the muscles in the body, which would yield about 1400 kcal).

When oxygen supply in the muscle is limited (anaerobic conditions), glucose is broken down into a three-carbon compound called **pyruvic acid.** The pyruvic acid accumulates in the muscle and is then converted to **lactic acid.** Only about 5% of the total amount of ATP that could be formed from complete breakdown of glucose is released through this anaerobic process (Fig. 14-6).

The advantage of anaerobic glucose breakdown is, it is the fastest way to resupply ATP, other than PCr breakdown. It therefore provides most of the energy needed for events that require a quick burst of energy, ranging from about 30 seconds to 2 minutes. Examples of activities that primarily rely on anaerobic glucose breakdown include sprinting 400 meters or swimming 100 meters.

The two major disadvantages of the anaerobic process are (1) the high rate of ATP production cannot be sustained for long periods; and (2) the rapid accumulation of lactic acid increases the acidity of the muscle. Normally, the pH of the muscle is about 7.1. Intense exercise that relies on anaerobic glucose breakdown can decrease the pH of muscle tissue to about 6.5. Acidity inhibits the activities of key enzymes in the muscle cells, slowing anaerobic ATP production and causing short-term fatigue. In addition, the acidity leads to a net potassium loss from muscle cells, which also contributes to fatigue. During exercise, you need to choose a sustainable pace according to the goals of the activity.

Before long, muscle cells release the accumulating lactic acid into the bloodstream. The liver (and the kidneys, to some extent) takes up the lactic acid and resynthesizes it into glucose. Glucose can then reenter the bloodstream, where it is available for cell uptake and breakdown. Individuals vary in their ability to clear lactic acid from the muscles and recycle it. Physical training may improve the ability of the body to remove and recycle lactic acid. Section 14.6 describes an ergogenic aid to neutralize lactic acid (also see Further Reading 3).

AEROBIC METABOLISM FUELS PROLONGED, LOWER-INTENSITY ACTIVITY

Carbohydrates If plenty of oxygen is available in the muscle (aerobic conditions), such as when the exercise is of low to moderate intensity, the bulk of the three-carbon pyruvic acid is shuttled to the mitochondria of the cell, where it is fully metabolized into carbon dioxide (CO_2) and water (H_2O) (Fig. 14-7). This aerobic breakdown of glucose yields

phosphocreatine (PCr) A high-energy compound that can be used to reform ATP. It is used primarily during bursts of activity, such as lifting and jumping.

creatine An organic (i.e., carbon-containing) molecule in muscle cells that serves as part of a high-energy compound (termed creatine phosphate or phosphocreatine) capable of synthesizing ATP from ADP.

pyruvic acid A three-carbon compound formed during glucose metabolism; also called *pyruvate*.

lactic acid A three-carbon acid formed during anaerobic cell metabolism; a partial breakdown product of glucose; also called *lactate*.

FIGURE 14-7 ◄ Simplified view of ATP formation from carbohydrate, fat, and protein. Along with phosphocreatine (PCr), all three macronutrients may be used for ATP synthesis, but glucose and fatty acids are primary sources. Glucose may be broken down anaerobically or may undergo complete aerobic metabolism. The products of fatty-acid breakdown are channeled into aerobic metabolism. Although limited, products of amino-acid breakdown are channeled into the aerobic pathway as well. Recall also from Chapter 12 that many vitamins and minerals participate in these metabolic pathways.

16-carbon
fatty acid

↓→ about 108 ATP
for cell use

↓

$CO_2 + H_2O$

▲ ATP yield from aerobic fatty-acid utilization.

▲ Fatty acids can come from all over the body, not necessarily from fat stored near the active muscles. *This is why spot reducing does not work.* Exercise can tone the muscles near adipose tissue but does not preferentially use those stores. © Comstock Images/Jupiterimages

approximately 95% of the ATP made from complete glucose metabolism (glucose → → $CO_2 + H_2O$).

Aerobic glucose breakdown supplies more ATP than the anaerobic process, but it releases the energy more slowly. This slower rate of aerobic energy supply can be sustained for hours. One reason is, the products are carbon dioxide and water, not lactic acid. Aerobic glucose breakdown makes a major energy contribution to activities that last anywhere from 2 minutes to several hours. Examples of such activities include jogging or distance swimming (review Table 14-2).

Endurance athletes sometimes reach a point in an event at which extreme physical and mental fatigue sets in; it feels impossible to stand up, let alone continue competing. Long-distance runners call this phenomenon "hitting the wall," and cyclists refer to it as "bonking." This occurs because muscle glycogen has been depleted and blood glucose has begun to decline during exercise, leading to deterioration of both physical and mental function. As you will learn in Section 14.5, maximizing glycogen storage before exercise, supplying carbohydrates during activity, and replenishing glycogen stores between events can help athletes avoid the game-stopping effects of glycogen depletion.

Fat When fat stores in body tissues begin to be broken down for energy, each triglyceride first yields three fatty acids and a glycerol molecule. The majority of the stored energy is found in the fatty acids. During physical activity, fatty acids are released from various adipose tissue depots into the bloodstream and travel to the muscles, where they are taken into each cell and broken down aerobically to carbon dioxide and water. Some of the fat stored in muscles (intramuscular triglycerides) also is used, especially as activity increases from a low to a moderate pace (see Further Reading 12).

Fat is an advantageous fuel for muscles: we generally have plenty of it stored, and it is a concentrated source of energy. For a given weight of fuel, fat supplies more than twice as much energy as carbohydrate does. However, the ability of muscles to use fat for fuel depends on the intensity of exercise. During intense, brief exercise, muscles may not be able to use much fat. The reason for this is that some of the steps involved in fat breakdown cannot occur fast enough to meet the ATP demands of short-duration, high-intensity exercise. However, fat becomes a progressively more important energy source as duration increases, especially when exercise remains at a low or moderate (aerobic) rate for more than 20 minutes (Fig. 14-8).

FIGURE 14-8 ▲ Generalized relationship between fuel use and exercise intensity. At rest or during light activity, nearly equal amounts of carbohydrate and fat are used to generate ATP. As activity intensifies (e.g., sprinting), anaerobic processes supply quick fuel, so the relative proportion of carbohydrates used for fuel increases. Except during endurance exercise, very little protein is used for fuel.

For lengthy activities at a moderate pace (e.g., hiking) or even sitting at a desk for 8 hours a day, fat supplies about 70% to 90% of the energy required. Carbohydrate use is much less. As intensity increases, carbohydrate use goes up and fat use decreases. During a 5-mile run at a moderate pace, muscles use about a 50:50 ratio of fat to carbohydrate. In comparison, for a sprint, the contribution of fat to resupply ATP is minimal. To summarize, remember that the only fast-paced (anaerobic) fuel we eat is carbohydrate; slow and steady (aerobic) activity uses fat in addition to carbohydrate.

Protein Although amino acids derived from protein can be used to fuel muscles, their contribution is relatively small, compared with that of carbohydrate and fat. Most protein is reserved for building and repairing body tissues and for synthesizing important enzymes, hormones, and transporters. As a rough guide, only about 5% of the body's ATP comes from the metabolism of amino acids.

During endurance exercise, proteins can contribute importantly to energy needs, perhaps as much as 10%, especially as glycogen stores in the muscle are exhausted. Most of the energy supplied from protein comes from metabolism of the branched-chain amino acids: leucine, isoleucine, and valine. A normal diet provides ample branched-chain amino acids to supply this amount of fuel; protein or amino-acid supplements are not typically needed.

CAN PHYSICAL TRAINING AFFECT FUEL USE?

As people start exercising regularly (e.g., a minimum of 150 minutes per week of moderate-intensity aerobic activity), they experience a "training effect." Initially, these individuals might be able to exercise for 20 minutes before tiring. Months later, exercise can be extended to an hour before they become fatigued. The training effect results from changes in the ability of exercising cells to use food fuel to generate ATP.

Almost immediately after a person begins a fitness program, both aerobic and strength training improve the insulin sensitivity of cells. In other words, more glucose can be transported from the bloodstream into the cells, where it can be broken down either anaerobically or aerobically. Improved blood glucose management is an added benefit for preventing or treating metabolic syndrome or type 2 diabetes.

Endurance aerobic activities also increase the ability of muscles to store glycogen. This highly branched polymer of glucose can be broken down into individual glucose units when the energy needs of the cell are high or when blood glucose levels start to drop. Increasing glycogen storage will help to delay fatigue during prolonged exercise.

Training induces elevations in muscle triglyceride content. This enhances the ability of muscles to use triglycerides to meet energy needs, particularly during low- or moderate-intensity endurance exercise. As you just learned, fat is a concentrated source of calories; complete oxidation of a long-chain fatty acid yields about three times as much ATP as metabolism of glucose. Many endurance athletes attempt to train their muscles to more readily use fat for fuel and thereby conserve muscle glycogen. In Section 14.5, you will learn more about this technique, known as **fat adaptation.**

Protein use becomes more efficient with training, too. Endurance training increases the ability of muscle cells to use branched-chain amino acids for fuel during prolonged activity. However, the ability to use carbohydrates and fats for fuel is also increased; as long as the diet is adequate in carbohydrates and fat, most protein is spared for muscle synthesis and repair.

In addition, training increases the number of mitochondria within muscle cells. Recall from Section 3.2 that mitochondria are the powerhouses of the cells; this is where glucose and fat are broken down aerobically to generate ATP. With more mitochondria, muscle cells can use carbohydrates and fat more efficiently.

Overall, the cardiovascular and respiratory systems become more efficient at providing oxygen to the cells of the body. Plasma volume increases shortly after a training program is started, and red blood cell volume eventually increases as well. The heart pumps more blood with each contraction. Training also increases the number of capillaries in muscles, which increases oxygen supply to the muscles. Meanwhile, lung capacity increases, so more

▲ The calories needed to perform come from carbohydrate, fat, and protein. The relative mix depends on the pace. © Realistic Reflections

CRITICAL THINKING

Marty started going to the gym about 8 weeks ago. At first, he noticed that he began "huffing and puffing" about 7 minutes into his aerobic workout. Now, however, he can work out for about 25 minutes without tiring. What is a possible explanation for this ability to work out longer?

fat adaptation Manipulating the diet and physical training regimen so that muscles become more efficient at metabolizing fat as fuel during aerobic activity.

oxygen is available. The increased supply of oxygen translates into more efficient aerobic metabolism of carbohydrates and fats. Thus, lactic-acid production from anaerobic glucose metabolism decreases. Lactic acid contributes to short-term muscle fatigue, so the less lactic acid produced, the longer the exercise can be sustained.

Through all these adaptations, physical training improves the ability of cells to convert food energy into fuel for exercise.

✓ CONCEPT CHECK 14.3

1. Describe one process used to resupply ATP during a short, intense burst of activity, such as a 100-meter sprint.

2. How does the ATP yield of anaerobic breakdown of glucose compare to that of aerobic breakdown of glucose?

3. Why is fat a useful source of energy during exercise? Name three types of activity during which fat supplies 50% or more of fuel.

4. Is protein a useful source of energy during exercise? Why or why not?

14.4 Tailoring Nutrient Recommendations for Athletes

Athletic training and genetic makeup are two important determinants of athletic performance. A good diet won't substitute for either factor, but diet can help to enhance and maximize an athlete's potential. On the other hand, a poor diet can seriously reduce performance (see Further Reading 19).

CALORIES

The daily calorie needs of athletes are highly individualized; genetics, hormones, age, sex, body size and composition, and training volume influence energy expenditure. A small, female gymnast may need only 1800 kcal daily to sustain her training regimen without losing body weight, whereas a large, muscular football player may need 4000 kcal per day. Because athletes are such a heterogeneous group, there is no perfect equation to estimate their daily calorie needs. Even for nonathletes, the Estimated Energy Requirement (EER) equation (see Section 7.2) provides only a rough approximation. However, you can use the EER equation as a starting point and individualize recommendations based on trial and error.

An estimate of the calories required to sustain moderate activity is 5 to 8 kcal per minute. The calories required for sports training or competition, then, must be added to those used to carry on normal activities. For example, consider a 135-pound young woman who requires 2200 kcal per day to fuel her normal activities. If she starts teaching two 45-minute Zumba classes each day, she will need about 500 extra kcal (a total of 2700 kcal per day) to maintain her current body weight. If an athlete experiences daily fatigue, the first consideration should be whether he or she is consuming enough food. Up to six meals per day may be needed, including one before each workout.

How can we know if an athlete is getting enough calories? Estimating daily intake from a food diary kept by the athlete is one way. Another option is to estimate the athlete's body fat percentage via skinfold measurements, bioelectrical impedance, or underwater weighing (review Section 7.3). Body fat should be the typical amount found for athletes in the specific sport practiced. This corresponds to 5% to 18% for most male athletes and 17% to 28% for most female athletes. The next step is to monitor body weight changes on a daily or weekly basis. If body weight starts to fall, calories should be increased; if weight rises and it is because of increases in body fat, the athlete should eat less.

Review Table 7-5 for the energy costs of typical forms of physical activity.

▲ Intense athletic training may require thousands of additional calories. This increased food intake should easily provide ample protein and other nutrients to support activity.
© Bernie McGroarty

If assessments of body composition show that an athlete has too much body fat, the athlete should lower food intake by about 200 to 500 kcal per day, while maintaining a regular exercise program, until the desirable fat percentage is achieved. On the other hand, if an athlete needs to gain weight, increasing food intake by 500 to 700 kcal per day will eventually lead to the needed weight gain. A mix of carbohydrate, fat, and protein is advised. Continuing to exercise will ensure that weight gain is mostly in the form of lean tissue rather than stored fat.

Historically, athletes who competed in sports with weight classes (e.g., wrestlers, boxers, judoists, and oarsmen) would try to lose weight before a competition. Being certified to compete in a lower weight class could help an athlete gain a mechanical advantage over an opponent of smaller stature. Many of the methods used to cut weight are unhealthy and dangerous. For example, an athlete could lose up to 22 pounds (10 kilograms) of body weight as water in 1 day by sitting in a sauna, exercising in a plastic sweatsuit, or taking diuretic drugs, which speed water loss via the kidneys. As you learned in Section 9.2, losing as little as 2% of body weight by dehydration can adversely affect physical and mental performance, especially in hot weather. A pattern of repeated weight loss or gain of more than 5% of body weight by dehydration carries risk of kidney malfunction and heat-related illness. Death is also a possibility.

To discourage such unhealthy practices and prevent future deaths, the National Collegiate Athletic Association and many states have authorized physicians or athletic trainers to set safe weight and body fat content minimums (e.g., 7% or more of total body weight for male athletes and 12% or more for females) in weight-class sports. Under current guidelines, athletes are assigned to weight classes at the beginning of the season and are not allowed to "cut weight" to gain a competitive advantage. In addition, urine specific gravity is measured prior to events to check for hydration status. This practice deters athletes from dehydrating themselves before weigh-in. Weight gain in the days after a competition (reflecting regain of body water) can now be no greater than 2 pounds. If athletes, such as wrestlers, wish to compete in a lower-bodyweight class and have enough extra fat stores, they should begin a gradual, sustained reduction in calorie intake months before the competitive season starts (see Further Reading 13).

CARBOHYDRATES

Anyone who exercises vigorously, especially for more than 1 hour per day on a regular basis, needs to consume a diet that includes moderate to high amounts of carbohydrate. Numerous servings of varied grains, starchy vegetables, and fruits provide enough carbohydrate to maintain adequate liver and muscle glycogen stores.

Depletion of carbohydrate ranks just behind depletion of fluid and electrolytes as a major cause of fatigue. Optimal carbohydrate intake depends on the size of the athlete and the type of physical activity. For light or skill-based sports, 3 to 5 grams of carbohydrate per kilogram of body weight will suffice. For exercise of moderate intensity, consume 5 to 7 grams of carbohydrate per kilogram. Athletes who train for several hours per day may need up to 12 grams of carbohydrates per kilogram of body weight, which may be 600 grams per day (or more). Attention to carbohydrate intake is especially important when performing multiple training bouts in one day (e.g., two-a-day swim practices) or heavy training on successive days (e.g., cross-country running).

Table 14-3 gives sample menus, based on MyPlate's Daily Food Plan recommendations, for diets providing food energy ranging from 1500 to 5000 kcal per day. In addition, the *Choose Your Foods* system designed for people with diabetes (see Appendix B) is a useful tool for planning all types of diets, including high-carbohydrate diets for athletes. As noted, athletes should obtain at least 60% of their total energy needs from carbohydrate (rather than the 50% typical of most North American diets), especially if exercise duration is expected to exceed 2 hours and total caloric intake is about 3000 kcal per day or less. Diets providing 4000 to 5000 kcal per day can be as low as 50% carbohydrate, as these will still provide sufficient carbohydrate (e.g., 500 to 600 grams or so per day).

▲ High-carbohydrate foods should form the basis of the diet for athletes.
© Royalty-Free/Corbis

TABLE 14-3 ■ Sample Daily Menus Based on MyPlate's Daily Food Plan*

1500 kcal	2000 kcal	3000 kcal	4000 kcal	5000 kcal
Breakfast Fat-free milk, 1 cup Cheerios®, 1/2 cup Bagel, 1/2 Cherry jam, 2 tsp Margarine, 1 tsp	**Breakfast** Fat-free milk, 1 cup Cheerios, 1 cup Bagel, 1/2 Cherry jam, 1 tbsp Margarine, 1 tsp	**Breakfast** Fat-free milk, 1 cup Cheerios, 2 cups Bagel, 1 Cherry jam, 2 tsp Margarine, 1 tsp Bran muffins, 2	**Breakfast** Fat-free milk, 1 cup Cheerios, 2 cups Orange, 1 Bran muffins, 2	**Breakfast** Fat-reduced milk, 1 cup Cheerios, 2 cups Bran muffins, 2 Orange, 1
			Snack Chopped dates, 3/4 cup	**Snack** Low-fat yogurt, 1 cup Chopped dates, 1 cup
Lunch Chicken breast (roasted), 2 oz Figs, 1 Fat-free milk, 1/2 cup Banana, 1	**Lunch** Chicken breast (roasted), 2 oz Wheat bread, 2 slices Mayonnaise, 1 tsp Raisins, 1/4 cup Cranberry juice, 1 1/2 cups Banana, 1	**Lunch** Chicken breast (roasted), 2 oz Wheat bread, 2 slices Provolone cheese, 1 oz Mayonnaise, 1 tsp Raisins, 1/3 cup Cranberry juice, 1 1/2 cups Low-fat fruit yogurt, 1 cup	**Lunch** Romaine lettuce, 1 cup Garbanzo beans, 1 cup Grated carrots, 1/2 cup French dressing, 2 tbsp Macaroni and cheese, 3 cups Apple juice, 1 cup	**Lunch** Chicken enchilada, 1 Romaine lettuce, 1 cup Garbanzo beans, 1 cup Shredded carrots, 3/4 cup Chopped celery, 1/2 cup Seasoned croutons, 1 oz French dressing, 2 tbsp Wheat bread, 2 slices Margarine, 1 tbsp Apple juice, 1 cup
Snack Oatmeal-raisin cookie, 1 Low-fat fruit yogurt, 1 cup	**Snack** Oatmeal-raisin cookies, 3 Low-fat fruit yogurt, 1 cup	**Snack** Banana, 1 Oatmeal-raisin cookies, 3	**Snack** Wheat bread, 2 slices Margarine, 1 tsp Jam, 2 tbsp	**Snack** Banana, 1 Bagel, 1 Cream cheese, 1 tbsp
Dinner Spaghetti w/ meatballs, 1 cup Romaine lettuce, 1 cup Italian dressing, 2 tsp Green beans, 1/2 cup Cranberry juice, 1 1/2 cups	**Dinner** Broiled beef sirloin, 3 oz Romaine lettuce, 1 cup Italian dressing, 2 tsp Green beans, 1 cup Fat-free milk, 1/2 cup	**Dinner** Broiled beef sirloin, 3 oz Romaine lettuce, 1 cup Garbanzo beans, 1 cup Italian dressing, 2 tsp Spinach pasta noodles, 1 1/2 cups Margarine, 1 tsp Green beans, 1 cup Fat-free milk, 1/2 cup	**Dinner** Skinless turkey breast, 2 oz Mashed potatoes, 2 cups Peas and onions, 1 cup Banana, 1 Fat-free milk, 1 cup	**Dinner** Beef sirloin, 5 oz Mashed potatoes, 2 cups Spinach pasta noodles, 1 1/2 cups Grated parmesan cheese, 2 tbsp Green beans, 1 cup Oatmeal-raisin cookies, 3 Fat-reduced milk, 1 cup
			Snack Pasta, 1 cup cooked Margarine, 2 tsp Parmesan cheese, 2 tbsp Cranberry juice, 1 cup	**Snack** Air-popped popcorn, 4 cups Raisins, 1/3 cup Cranberry juice, 2 cups
18% protein (68 grams) 64% carbohydrate (240 grams) 19% fat (32 grams)	17% protein (85 grams) 63% carbohydrate (315 grams) 20% fat (44 grams)	17% protein (128 grams) 62% carbohydrate (465 grams) 21% fat (70 grams)	14% protein (140 grams) 61% carbohydrate (610 grams) 26% fat (116 grams)	14% protein (175 grams) 63% carbohydrate (813 grams) 24% fat (136 grams)

*Daily Food Plans are available online for diets supplying 1000 to 3200 kcal/day (see www.ChooseMyPlate.gov). Additional servings from each food group have been added to supply increased calories while maintaining healthy proportions of protein, carbohydrate, and fat.

Besides the total amount of carbohydrates, the *quality* of carbohydrates can certainly influence mental and physical performance, as well. Sports nutritionists emphasize the difference between a high-carbohydrate meal and a high-carbohydrate/high-fat meal. Before endurance events, such as marathons or triathlons, some athletes seek to increase their carbohydrate reserves by eating foods such as potato chips, French fries, banana cream pie, and

TABLE 14-4 ■ Carbohydrate-Rich Foods

Starches—15 Grams Carbohydrate per Serving (80 kcal)	
One Serving	
Dry breakfast cereal*, 1/2–3/4 cup	Baked potato, 1/4 large
Cooked breakfast cereal, 1/2 cup	Bagel, 1/4 (or 4 ounces)
Cooked grits, 1/2 cup	English muffin, 1/2
Cooked rice, 1/3 cup	Bread, 1 slice
Cooked pasta, 1/3 cup	Pretzels, 3/4 ounce
Baked beans, 1/3 cup	Saltine crackers, 6
Cooked corn, 1/2 cup	Pancake, 4-inch diameter, 1
Cooked dry beans, 1/2 cup	Taco shells, 2 (add 45 kcal)

Vegetables—5 Grams Carbohydrate per Serving (25 kcal)
One Serving
Cooked vegetables, 1/2 cup
Raw vegetables, 1 cup
Vegetable juice, 1/2 cup
Examples: carrots, green beans, broccoli, cauliflower, onions, spinach, tomatoes, and vegetable juice

Fruits—15 Grams Carbohydrate per Serving (60 kcal)	
One Serving	
Canned fruit or berries, 1/2 cup	Grapes (small), 17
Fruit juice, 1/2 cup	Grapefruit, 1/2
Figs (dried), 1 1/2	Dates, 3
Apple or orange, 1 small	Peach, 1
Apricots (dried), 8	Watermelon cubes, 1 1/4 cups
Banana, 1 small	

Milk—12 Grams Carbohydrate per Serving	
One Serving	Soymilk, 1 cup
Milk, 1 cup	
Plain low-fat yogurt, 2/3 cup	

Sweets—15 Grams Carbohydrate per Serving (variable calories)	
One Serving	Ice cream, 1/2 cup
Cake, 2-inch square	Sherbet, 1/2 cup
Cookies, 2 small	

*The carbohydrate content of dry cereal varies widely. Check the labels of the ones you choose and adjust the serving size accordingly.

Modified from *Choose Your Foods: Food Lists for Diabetes* by the American Diabetes Association and Academy of Nutrition and Dietetics, 2014.

▲ Fruits provide starches and natural sugars to maximize glycogen stores. © Ingram Publishing/SuperStock

pastries. Although such foods provide carbohydrate, they also contain a lot of fat. Better high-carbohydrate food choices include pasta, rice, potatoes, bread, fruit and fruit juices, and various breakfast cereals (check the label for carbohydrate content) (Table 14-4). Sports drinks appropriate for carbohydrate loading, such as Gatorade® Endurance Carb Energy Drink and Twinlab® UltraFuel, can also help. Consuming a moderate (rather than high) amount of fiber during the final day of training is a good precaution to reduce the chances of bloating and intestinal gas during the next day's event.

FAT

A diet containing up to 35% of calories from fat is generally recommended for athletes. Rich sources of monounsaturated fat, such as canola oil, should be emphasized, and saturated fat and *trans* fat intake should be limited.

PROTEIN

For athletes, the American College of Sports Medicine, the Academy of Nutrition and Dietetics, and the Dietitians of Canada recommend protein intake within the range of 1.2 to 2.0 grams of protein per kilogram of body weight. This is considerably higher than the RDA of 0.8 gram per kilogram of body weight recommended by the Food and Nutrition Board for all adults. Sports nutrition experts contend that the RDAs have been set to prevent deficiency among the general population, not to optimize physical performance among athletes (see Further Reading 2 and 11).

What are some reasons why athletes require more protein than sedentary adults?

- The overall calorie needs of athletes are increased to meet the demands of physical activity, so more amino acids will be metabolized as fuel. For endurance athletes, in particular, protein may provide up to 15% of overall energy needs.
- Athletes, most notably those involved in strength training, need additional amino acids for repair of damaged muscle tissue and synthesis of new muscle protein.
- Beyond their use as fuel or building blocks, certain amino acids also act as chemical signals that regulate protein synthesis and other metabolic processes.

The optimal protein intake for an athlete will vary based on the athlete's activity and level of fitness. Athletes who are just beginning a strength-training program are likely to need the most protein to supply the building blocks for synthesis of new muscle tissue. Once the desired muscle mass is achieved, daily protein intake need not exceed 1.2 grams per kilogram of body weight. Some strength-training athletes tend to aim for excessive protein intakes, sometimes as high as 3 or 4 grams of protein per kilogram of body weight. To date, there is little evidence that protein intake above 2.0 grams per kilogram of body weight will benefit the athlete. Protein intakes above this amount result in an increased use of amino acids for energy needs; no further increase in muscle protein synthesis is seen.

Unless an athlete follows a low-calorie diet, the recommended range of 1.2 to 2.0 grams of protein per kilogram of body weight can be met by eating a variety of foods (review Table 14-3). To illustrate, a 117-pound (53-kilogram) woman performing moderate-intensity endurance activity can consume 58 grams of protein (53 × 1.1) during a single day by including 3 ounces of chicken (a chicken breast), 3 ounces of beef (a small, lean hamburger), and two glasses of milk in her diet. Similarly, a 170-pound (77-kilogram) man who aims to gain muscle mass through strength training needs to consume only 6 ounces of chicken (a large chicken breast), 1/2 cup of cooked beans, a 6-ounce can of tuna, and three glasses of milk to achieve an intake of 154 grams of protein (77 × 2.0) in a day. For both athletes, these calculations do not include the protein present in grains or vegetables they will also eat. By simply meeting their calorie needs, many athletes consume more protein than is required.

Despite marketing claims, protein supplements are usually an expensive and unnecessary part of a fitness plan. However, many athletes choose to use protein powders (e.g., whey, casein, or soy) as a lean and convenient way to add protein to their diet. Whey protein is a popular product, especially among strength-trained athletes. Whey is an easily digested, high-quality protein derived from cow's milk. It is particularly rich in leucine, an essential branched-chain amino acid that has been shown to stimulate gains in muscle mass during strength training (see Further Reading 2). Except in cases of milk protein allergies and kidney disease, whey protein is safe to use at the doses recommended on product labels. However, these supplements tend to be expensive. It may be more economical to rely on food sources, such as low-fat or fat-free dairy products.

Consuming excessive amounts of protein has drawbacks. As noted in Section 6.7, it increases calcium loss somewhat in the urine. It also leads to increased urine production, which could compromise body hydration. Excess animal protein also may lead to kidney stones in people with a history of this or other kidney problems. Last but not least, a dietary pattern that is so focused on protein may leave the athlete short on carbohydrates, leading to fatigue and poor athletic performance.

Is there an optimal dose of protein? Researchers suggest a dose of 20 to 25 grams of protein per meal is ideal to promote muscle synthesis (see Further Reading 11). Rather than simply focusing on total protein intake, athletes should be sure to consume foods that provide 20 to 25 grams of high-quality protein per meal at three or more meals spaced throughout the day.

ASK THE RDN   ## No-Meat Athlete

Dear RDN: *For a variety of reasons, I am considering switching to a vegan diet. However, I am a freestyler on the college women's swimming and diving team, and I want to make sure that a vegan diet would not affect my athletic performance. Can a "no-meat athlete" compete?*

A well-planned plant-based diet can absolutely support optimal athletic performance (see Further Reading 19)! From better weight management to reduced risk for chronic diseases, vegan diets offer many health benefits. However, some nutrient needs may be difficult to meet with a plant-based diet. Because you are an athlete, I am most concerned about protein, iron, calcium, and vitamin B-12.

Protein intakes of vegan athletes, especially young women, are often low. You will need more than the RDA for protein because first, you are an athlete, and second, the quality of plant proteins is lower than that of animal proteins. Protein recommendations for vegetarian and vegan athletes are 1.3 to 1.8 grams per kilogram of body weight. If you consume adequate kilocalories, you can meet your protein needs without protein or amino-acid supplements, but the *quality* of your protein matters. Be sure to consume a variety of plant proteins (legumes, grains, nuts) throughout the day to obtain all of the essential amino acids.

Iron delivers oxygen to exercising muscles and helps to convert food fuel into ATP—two processes that impact athletic performance. Iron needs can be difficult to meet even with omnivorous diets, so iron intake deserves special attention. Remember that plant (nonheme) sources of iron are not as well absorbed as animal (heme) sources, but foods with vitamin C can boost absorption of nonheme iron. Have your iron status checked periodically. If your iron stores are low, a supplement can help. Discuss supplementation with your clinician or dietitian.

Lean female athletes place themselves at risk for early osteoporosis if their diets are poor in calcium (and vitamin D). A vegan diet eliminates animal products, including dairy foods, which are excellent sources of these bone-building nutrients.

A deficiency of vitamin B-12 could also affect red blood cell health (see Section 13.4) and possibly nerve function. Unlike iron and calcium, there are no plant-based alternatives for vitamin B-12. Use of fortified foods and/or dietary supplements will be crucial to meeting your vitamin B-12 needs.

One more concern is, this highly restrictive dietary change—even though it seems like a healthful choice—could promote disordered eating behaviors. Swimmers often hold themselves to unrealistic standards for lean physical appearance, but lower body fat does not automatically translate to better performance. As you move toward a plant-based diet, make sure that your overall energy intake is adequate to support your needs for competitive training. If your weight drops too low, it could significantly affect your athletic performance and long-term bone health.

Start slowly and follow these general recommendations: Begin your day with a bowl of fortified breakfast cereal. Check the label for brands of cereal that provide at least 20% of the DV for iron and vitamin B-12, such as Cheerios® (45% DV for iron, 25% DV for B-12), Raisin Bran® (60% DV for iron, 40% DV for B-12), or Total® (100% DV for both iron and B-12). Top your cereal with almond milk (or a similar dairy alternative) that provides at least one-third of the DV for calcium. Also include calcium-fortified dairy alternatives as a substitute whenever you would have chosen dairy products (see Section 11.11). Enjoy a glass of calcium-fortified orange juice with breakfast to enhance absorption of iron from your cereal. Throughout the day, be sure to choose plentiful and varied sources of plant proteins, including legumes, nuts, seeds, and grains. Try soy and quinoa, two versatile plant proteins that contain all essential amino acids. A dietary supplement, such as a one-a-day multivitamin and mineral supplement, would be a good backup plan to close any remaining nutrient gaps, especially for vitamin B-12. Lastly, monitor changes in your weight and performance. If your calorie intake is too low, consider incorporating more nuts, nut butters, avocados, and hummus into your meals and snacks, as these are energy-dense sources of healthy fats.

These are just a few basic ideas to help you remain healthy and compete at your highest level. To tailor your food intake to your specific needs, seek the expert advice of your team's Registered Dietitian Nutritionist or an RDN at your university health center.

To your record-breaking success!

Angela Collene, MS, RDN, LD (author)

▲ Do strength-trained athletes need to ingest tuna, chicken, and lean beef at every meal to build muscle? Patrik Baboumian is a strongman competitor and former bodybuilder who follows a vegan diet. The plant-based protein sources that built his 250-pound physique include beans, peas, lentils, nuts, seeds, and protein shakes made with soy protein powder. Baboumian was a world record-holder for the log lift in his weight class and was named Germany's strongest man. © David Cooper/ Toronto Star via Getty Images

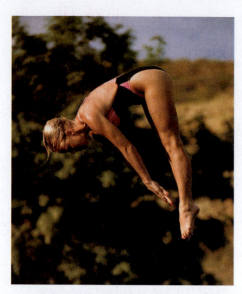

▲ Weight-restricted athletes especially should make sure they are consuming enough protein and other essential nutrients.

© PhotoLink/Getty Images

VITAMINS AND MINERALS

Compared to the needs of sedentary adults, vitamin and mineral needs are the same or slightly higher for athletes. At this time, there are not enough data to support separate DRIs specific to athletes for any of the micronutrients, but research continues. Athletes usually have high calorie intakes, so they tend to consume plenty of vitamins and minerals. An exception is athletes consuming low-calorie diets (1200 kcal or less), as seen with some female athletes participating in events in which maintaining a low body weight is crucial. These diets may not meet B vitamin and other micronutrient needs. Vegetarian athletes are also a concern. In these cases, consuming fortified foods, such as ready-to-eat breakfast cereals, or a balanced multivitamin and mineral supplement is recommended.

B Vitamins Support Energy Metabolism and Red Blood Cell Health As you learned in Section 12.1, coenzyme forms of B vitamins facilitate chemical reactions that generate ATP from carbohydrates, proteins, and fats. Some B vitamins are involved in biosynthetic reactions, such as synthesis of glycogen from glucose, as well as reactions that metabolize amino acids. Compared to the metabolism of sedentary adults, the higher volume of energy metabolism of athletes will increase demands for these coenzymes. Although no separate DRIs have been set, athletes may need more than the current RDA for some B vitamins, such as riboflavin and vitamin B-6.

Furthermore, physical performance is highly dependent on the availability of oxygen to exercising muscles. Folate, vitamin B-6, and vitamin B-12 are involved in the formation of healthy red blood cells, which transport oxygen to all body tissues (see Chapter 13).

As you can imagine, an inadequate supply of B vitamins could impair an athlete's physical performance. Certainly, deficiency symptoms such as muscle weakness, nervous system dysfunction, and anemia are not compatible with participation in competitive sports! In reality, deficiencies of B vitamins are not very common. As athletes consume greater quantities of food to meet their increased calorie needs, they typically consume enough B vitamins from food sources to support energy metabolism and red blood cell health. Taking more than the RDA for B vitamins is not likely to enhance performance.

On the other hand, for a person who is deficient in one or more of the B vitamins, supplementation could improve athletic performance. At-risk populations include vegan or senior athletes (vitamin B-12), female athletes of childbearing age (folate), and any athlete who restricts dietary intake to control body weight (a variety of micronutrients). In these cases, fortified foods or a balanced multivitamin and mineral supplement would be beneficial to overall health and athletic performance (see Further Reading 12).

Antioxidant Nutrients May Prevent Oxidative Damage Exercise leads to increased production of free radicals. The presence of some free radicals in muscle tissue is actually beneficial for muscle contraction and adaptation to exercise. However, excessive free radicals can lead to fatigue and cell damage.

Athletes' needs for antioxidants such as vitamin E and vitamin C may be somewhat greater because of the potential protection these nutrients provide. However, there is evidence that antioxidant systems in the body increase in activity as exercise training progresses. The use of large doses of vitamin E and vitamin C requires more study and is not currently an accepted part of the dietary guidance for athletes. Experts suggest consuming a diet containing foods rich in antioxidants, such as fruits, vegetables, whole-grain breads and cereals, and vegetable oils (see Further Reading 12).

Recall from Section 8.5 that nutrients in dietary supplements should not exceed any Upper Levels set over the long term. As well, men should be cautious about any use of supplements containing iron.

Iron Deficiency Impairs Performance Iron is involved in red blood cell production, oxygen transport, and energy production, so a deficiency of this mineral can noticeably detract from optimal athletic performance. Some of the consequences of iron deficiency include weakness, fatigue, and decreased work capacity. The potential causes for iron deficiency in athletes vary (see Further Reading 19). As in the general population, female athletes are most susceptible to low iron status due to monthly menstrual losses. Special diets, such as low-calorie and vegetarian (especially vegan) diets, are likely to be low in iron. Distance runners should pay special attention to iron intake because their intense workouts may lead to gastrointestinal bleeding.

A less threatening concern is *sports anemia.* At the start of an endurance training regimen, plasma volume expands, but the synthesis of additional red blood cells is slower to increase. This results in dilution of the blood; even if iron stores are adequate, blood iron tests may appear low. Sports anemia is not detrimental to performance, but it is hard to differentiate between sports anemia and true anemia. If iron status is low and not replenished, iron-deficiency anemia can markedly impair endurance performance.

Although true iron-deficiency anemia (a depressed blood hemoglobin level) is not that common among athletes, some studies suggest that iron deficiency *without* anemia may have a negative impact on physical activity and performance. Recall from Section 13.5 that iron deficiency occurs long before anemia is detected clinically. As body stores of iron are depleted, body processes that use iron, such as energy-yielding reactions, are impaired.

It is a good idea for athletes (especially adult women) to have their iron status checked at the beginning of a training season and at least once midseason. Current evidence suggests that as many as half of female athletes are iron deficient. To identify iron deficiency without anemia among athletes, many experts advocate serum ferritin testing. Ferritin is an iron transport protein; low serum ferritin levels indicate low iron stores even before red blood cell health is affected.

Any blood test indicating low iron status—sports anemia or not—warrants follow-up. A physician will need to determine the cause of iron depletion: is it due to poor dietary intake, heavy menstrual losses, or a serious medical condition, such as internal bleeding? Whatever the cause, once depleted, iron stores can take months to replenish. Dietary sources are not enough to correct iron-deficiency anemia; supplementation (under physician supervision) is required. Athletes must be especially careful to meet iron needs because preventing iron deficiency is a lot simpler than treating it.

Knowing that iron is required for red blood cell synthesis, athletes may be tempted to self-prescribe iron supplements in an attempt to boost the oxygen-carrying capacity of the blood. However, indiscriminate use of iron supplements for people with normal hemoglobin and serum ferritin levels is NOT advised (see Further Reading 6). Research does not support a benefit of iron supplementation on athletic performance for athletes with normal iron status. Furthermore, liver damage and increased rates of heart disease and some forms of cancer are possible consequences of iron toxicity. A safer alternative would be to have iron status checked periodically. In addition, monitor dietary patterns to become aware of usual iron intakes. If dietary iron intake is low, incorporate more food sources of heme iron and pair nonheme sources with vitamin C to enhance absorption. Beyond using a balanced multivitamin and mineral supplement, the decision to use an iron supplement is best left to a physician.

Calcium Intake Is Important, Especially in Women Athletes, especially women trying to lose weight by restricting their intake of dairy products, can have marginal or low dietary intakes of calcium. This practice compromises optimal bone health. Of still greater concern are women athletes who have stopped menstruating because their arduous training and low body fat interferes with the normal secretion of reproductive hormones. Disturbing evidence shows that female athletes who do not menstruate regularly have spinal bones far less dense than those of both nonathletes and female athletes who menstruate regularly. They are more likely to suffer **stress fractures** during training and will be susceptible to bone injuries throughout life. The negative impacts of low dietary calcium intake and irregular menses in female athletes outweigh the benefits of weight-bearing exercise on bone density. Increasing energy intake to restore body weight and body fat stores is important to correct hormonal imbalances and prevent further bone loss. This topic is discussed further in Section 15.6, with respect to the female athlete triad, and in Section 11.9, where osteoporosis was reviewed in detail.

Female athletes whose menstrual cycles become irregular should consult a physician to determine the cause. Decreasing the amount of training or increasing energy intake and body weight often restores regular menstrual cycles. If irregular menstrual cycles persist,

"Blood doping" is the injection of red blood cells, naturally containing iron, to enhance aerobic capacity. This is an illegal practice under Olympic guidelines.

stress fracture A fracture that occurs from repeated jarring of a bone. Common sites include bones of the foot.

severe bone loss (much of which is not reversible) and osteoporosis can result. Extra calcium in the diet does not necessarily compensate for these damaging effects of menstrual irregularities, but inadequate dietary calcium can make matters worse.

FLUID

Fluid needs for an average adult are about 9 cups per day for women and 13 cups per day for men. Athletes generally need even more water to regulate body temperature. Heat production in contracting muscles can rise 15 to 20 times above that of resting muscles. Unless this heat is quickly dissipated, heat exhaustion, heat cramps, and potentially fatal heatstroke may ensue.

Fluid and electrolyte needs vary widely, based on differences in genetics, body mass, environmental conditions, level of training, and event duration. Because fluid needs are highly individualized and dynamic, it is not appropriate to make general recommendations for fluid replacement (see Further Reading 12). Rather, an athlete should consume enough fluid to prevent short-term (i.e., fluid-related) changes in body weight. The American College of Sports Medicine recommends losing *no more than 2%* of body weight during exercise, especially in hot weather. A football player wearing equipment in hot weather can lose this much within 30 minutes! However, it is important to remember this advice even when sweating can go unnoticed, such as when swimming or during the winter.

To determine fluid needs, the athlete should first calculate 2% of his or her body weight. Next, it is useful to know the body's hourly sweat rate, which can be calculated by comparing weight loss during exercise to the amount of fluid consumed during exercise. This will require some self-monitoring of pre- and post-workout weight and fluid intake during workouts. For reference, sweat rates during prolonged exercise can range from 3 to 8 cups (750 to 2000 milliliters) per hour. If weight change cannot be monitored, urine color is another measure of hydration status (see Fig. 9-8). Urine color should be no more yellow than lemonade.

Note that thirst is a late sign of dehydration. An athlete who drinks only when thirsty may take 48 hours to replenish fluid losses. After several days of training, an athlete relying only on thirst can build up a fluid debt that will impair performance. The following fluid-replacement approach can meet an athlete's fluid needs in most cases.

- Freely drink beverages (e.g., water, diluted fruit juice, and sports drinks) during the 24-hour period before an event, even if not particularly thirsty.
- Drink 5 to 7 milliliters per kilogram of body weight (about 1.5 to 2 cups for a 150-pound male) of water or sports drink at least 4 hours before exercise. This allows time for both adequate hydration and excretion of excess fluid.
- During events lasting more than 30 minutes, athletes should consume fluid to prevent dehydration (i.e., losses of >2% body weight). Research in marathon runners suggests about 1.5 to 3.5 cups (400 to 800 milliliters) per hour to prevent dehydration. Football players wearing equipment for two-a-day practices during the heat of August may need even more than 800 milliliters per hour to prevent dehydration. The best plan is to determine individual rate of fluid losses during training and plan accordingly. In many cases, athletes, especially children and teenagers, need to be reminded to consume fluids during exercise.
- Within 4 to 6 hours after exercise, about 2 to 3 cups of fluid should be consumed for every pound lost. It is important that weight be restored before the next exercise period. Skipping fluids before or during events will almost certainly impair performance.

Sports Drinks   Is it better to rehydrate with water or a sports drink during a workout? For sports that require less than 60 minutes of exertion or when total weight loss is less than 5 to 6 pounds, the primary concern is replacing the water lost in sweat, because losses of carbohydrate stores and electrolytes (sodium, chloride, potassium, and other minerals) are not usually very great. (Sweat is about 99% water and only 1% electrolytes and other substances.) When exercise extends beyond 60 minutes, electrolyte (especially sodium) and carbohydrate replacement becomes increasingly important.

Use of sports drinks (Fig. 14-9) during long bouts of exercise—especially in hot weather—offers several advantages for athletes:

- *Water* increases blood volume to allow for efficient cooling and transport of fuels and waste products to and from cells.
- *Carbohydrates* supply glucose to muscles as they become depleted of glycogen and also add flavor, which encourages athletes to drink.
- *Electrolytes* in sports drinks help to maintain blood volume, enhance the absorption of water and carbohydrate from the intestine, and stimulate thirst.

Overall, the decision to use a sports drink hinges primarily on the duration of the activity. As the projected duration of continuous activity approaches 60 minutes or longer, the advantages of sports drinks over plain water clearly emerge. However, athletes should experiment with sports drinks during practice, instead of trying them for the first time during competition. Also, both athletes and nonathletes should recognize that sports drinks can be a source of excess calories that may result in undesired weight gain (see Newsworthy Nutrition).

"Energy" Drinks The popularity of caffeine-containing energy drinks has surged in recent years. Some studies show that caffeine improves athletic performance during endurance events (e.g., cycling) or sports that require a high level of mental alertness (e.g., archery). However, excessive caffeine consumption can lead to shakiness, nervousness, anxiety, nausea, and insomnia. In addition, the diuretic effect of caffeine, although mild, may not support optimal hydration, particularly for athletes who are not accustomed to caffeine (see Further Reading 7). Compare the caffeine and kilocalorie contents of several top-selling energy drinks (Table 14-5).

Heat-Related Illness As environmental temperature rises above 95 °F (35 °C), virtually all body heat is lost through the evaporation of sweat from the skin. As humidity rises, especially above 75%, evaporation slows and sweating is insufficient to cool the body. The result is rapid fatigue, increased work for the heart, and difficulty with prolonged exertion. Heat-related injuries—heat exhaustion, heat cramps, and heatstroke—can be deadly (Table 14-6). To decrease the risk of developing heat-related injuries, watch for rapid body-weight changes (2% or more of body weight), replace lost fluids, and avoid exercising under extremely hot, humid conditions.

FIGURE 14-9 ▲ Sports drinks for fluid and electrolyte replacement typically contain a form of simple carbohydrate plus sodium and potassium. The various sugars in this product total 14 grams per 1-cup (240-milliliter) serving. Sports drinks typically contain about 6% to 8% sugar. This provides ample glucose and other monosaccharides to fuel working muscles, and it is well tolerated. Drinks with a sugar content above 10%, such as soft drinks or fruit juices, may cause gastrointestinal distress and are not recommended.

Newsworthy Nutrition

Sports Drinks Cause Weight Gain Among Adolescents and Young Adults

Sales of sugar-sweetened soda pop continue to decline, yet sales of other sweetened beverages, such as sports drinks, are increasing. Although the value of sports drinks (e.g., Gatorade®, Powerade®) is well documented for replenishing fluids during physical activity lasting more than 1 hour, the contribution of excess sugar intake to obesity remains a concern. The aim of this prospective study was to determine the associations between sports drinks and body mass index (BMI) gains among adolescents and young adults. Over 7500 U.S. youth, age 9 to 16, were followed from 2004 to 2011. Servings per day of beverages were assessed using a food frequency questionnaire. Intake of sports drinks predicted larger increases in BMI among all youth. In addition, boys who increased their intake over the 2- to 3-year interval gained significantly more weight than their peers during the same time interval. These results suggest that, although there is less sugar per ounce in sugar-sweetened sports drinks than in soda pop, sports beverages still contain sugar and energy that appear to promote increases in BMI for both adolescents and young adults.

Source: Field AE and others: Association of sports drinks with weight gain among adolescents and young Adults. *Obesity* 22:2238, 2014.

▲ Dehydration, which can lead to illness and death, is a problem that must be avoided during physical activity in hot, humid environments. © Eyewire/Getty Images

TABLE 14-5 ■ Caffeine, Kilocalorie, and Sugar Content of Popular Energy Drinks

Beverage	Container Size (fl oz)	Caffeine (mg)	Energy (kcal)	Sugars (g)
5-Hour Energy®	1.93	215*	4	0
Amp Energy®	16	142	220	58
Monster Energy®	16	160	200	54
NOS® PowerSho®t	16	260	210	54
Red Bull®	8.4	80	110	27
Red Bull Sugarfree	8.4	80	10	0
Rockstar®	16	160	280	62

*Determined by independent lab analysis reported by *Consumer Reports,* December 2012. Caffeine content is not specified by the manufacturer but rather as part of a total amount of "energy blend." The labels state that this product has approximately the same amount of caffeine as a strong cup of coffee (typical range: 80–175 milligrams).

TABLE 14-6 ■ Heat-Related Illnesses

Heat-Related Illness	Symptoms	Recommended Treatment
Heat exhaustion is the first stage of heat-related illness that occurs because of depletion of blood volume from fluid loss by the body.	• Profuse sweating • Headache • Dizziness • Nausea • Muscle weakness • Visual disturbances • Flushed skin • Hyperthermia • Heat cramps (see next)	• Move to cool environment • Remove excess clothing • Cool the skin with ice packs or cold water • Replenish lost fluids and electrolytes
Heat cramps are a frequent complication of heat exhaustion. They usually occur in people who have experienced large sweat losses from exercising for several hours in a hot climate and have consumed a large volume of water without replacing electrolytes.	• Painful skeletal muscle cramps	• Replenish lost fluids and electrolytes
Heatstroke can occur when internal body temperature reaches 104° F. Sweating generally ceases if left untreated, and blood circulation is greatly reduced. Nervous system damage may ensue, and death results in 10% of cases.	• Hyperthermia • Hot, dry skin • Nausea • Confusion • Irritability • Poor coordination • Fainting • Seizures • Coma	• Cool the skin with ice packs or cold water *SEEK PROFESSIONAL MEDICAL ATTENTION*

Water Intoxication It is also possible for some athletes to drink so much water that they develop water intoxication (hyponatremia). Recall from Section 9.2 that hyponatremia causes cardiovascular and neurological problems and can lead to death. Endurance athletes (especially novices) may compete at relatively low exercise intensities for prolonged periods and therefore may not sweat as much as predicted. Drinking less fluid, choosing a sports drink containing sodium (usually in the form of sodium chloride), and avoiding weight gain during the activity can help prevent this problem. (A drop in blood sodium can occur in both hot and cold weather.)

> **carbohydrate loading** A process in which a high-carbohydrate diet is consumed for 6 days before an athletic event while tapering exercise duration in an attempt to increase muscle glycogen stores.

✔ CONCEPT CHECK 14.4

1. What does it mean to "cut weight" before a competition? How may this affect physical performance?

2. Greta, a point guard on the women's basketball team, complains of chronic fatigue. Describe three nutritional concerns you would investigate.

3. During one day of preseason training for football, David loses 7 pounds as a result of sweat losses. How much fluid should he drink to rehydrate after practice?

14.5 Specialized Advice for Endurance, Strength, and Power Athletes

In Section 14.4, you learned about ways in which nutrient needs can be universally affected by participation in sports. The definition of sports, however, is broad and each athlete is unique. Endurance athletes, who need to fuel activity that lasts several hours, should take a different approach to nutrition than strength and power athletes, who focus on gains in muscle mass. In this section, we present specific nutrition strategies for endurance, strength, and power athletes.

ENDURANCE ATHLETES: STRATEGIES TO DELAY OR PREVENT FATIGUE

The overarching goal for endurance athletes is to consume adequate carbohydrates and fluids. *Before* the event, endurance athletes should focus on maximizing muscle and liver glycogen stores, which will later be used to fuel muscles and maintain blood glucose. *During* an event, the goal is to prevent dehydration and glycogen depletion, as both of these conditions lead to fatigue and detract from physical performance. *After* an event, muscle glycogen stores need to be replenished, damaged muscle tissue must be repaired, and hydration should be restored.

Maximize Glycogen Stores Before the Event For athletes who compete in continuous, intense aerobic events lasting more than 90 minutes (or in shorter events taking place more than once within a 24-hour period), a **carbohydrate-loading** regimen can help to maximize the amount of energy stored in the form of muscle glycogen for the event. In one possible regimen, during the week prior to the event, the athlete gradually reduces the intensity and duration of exercise ("tapering") while simultaneously increasing the percentage of total calories supplied by carbohydrates. Shorter carbohydrate-loading regimens (e.g., 1 or 2 days before an event) may also be effective.

For example, consider the carbohydrate-loading schedule of a 25-year-old man preparing for a marathon. His typical calorie needs are about 3500 kcal per day. Six days before competition, he completes a final, hard workout of 60 minutes. On that day, carbohydrates contribute 45% to 50% of his total calorie intake. As he goes through the rest of the week, the duration of his workouts decreases to 40 minutes and then to about 20 minutes by the end of the week. Meanwhile, he increases the amount of carbohydrate in his diet to reach 70% to 80% of total calorie intake as the week continues (Table 14-7). Total calorie intake

TABLE 14-7 ■ Carbohydrate-Loading Regimen

Days Before Competition	6	5	4	3	2	1
Exercise time (minutes)	60	40	40	20	20	Rest
Carbohydrate (grams)	450	450	450	600	600	600

▲ Carbohydrate loading is appropriate only for endurance activities such as a long-distance race. © Corbis-All Rights Reserved

should decrease as exercise time decreases throughout the week. On the final day before competition, he rests while maintaining the high carbohydrate intake.

This carbohydrate-loading technique usually increases muscle glycogen stores by 50% to 85% over typical conditions (i.e., when dietary carbohydrate constitutes only about 50% of total calorie intake). A potential disadvantage of carbohydrate loading is that additional water (about 3 grams) is incorporated into the muscles along with each gram of glycogen. Although the additional water aids in maintaining hydration, for some individuals this additional water weight and related muscle stiffness detract from their sports performance.

Athletes considering a carbohydrate-loading regimen should try it during training (and well before an important competition) to experience its effects on performance. They can then determine whether it is worth the effort. Currently, expert advice is shifting away from such regimented carbohydrate loading in favor of supplying carbohydrates during the event (along with a daily diet high in carbohydrate).

Even if an endurance athlete chooses not to practice a strict carbohydrate-loading regimen, a meal should be eaten 1 to 4 hours before an endurance event to top off muscle and liver glycogen stores, prevent hunger during the event, and provide extra fluid. A pre-event meal should consist primarily of carbohydrate, contain little fat or fiber, and include a moderate amount of protein (Table 14-8). The longer the period before an event, the larger the meal can be, because there will be more time available for digestion (see box). Anything consumed within 1 hour before an event should be blended or be liquid to promote rapid stomach emptying. Examples are low-fat smoothies and sports drinks.

Carbohydrate-rich food choices for a pre-event meal include spaghetti, muffins, bagels, pancakes with fresh fruit topping, oatmeal with fruit, a baked potato topped with a small amount of sour cream, toasted bread with jam, bananas, or low-sugar breakfast cereals with reduced-fat or fat-free milk. Liquid meal-replacement formulas, such as Carnation® Instant Breakfast, also can be used. Foods especially rich in fiber can be eaten the previous day to help empty the colon before an event, but they should not be eaten the night before or on the morning of the event. Avoid fatty or fried foods, such as sausage, bacon, sauces, and gravies. Some foods (e.g., dairy products) may cause gastrointestinal upset. Athletes should experiment with the size, timing, and composition of pre-event meals during training to determine what will be tolerated.

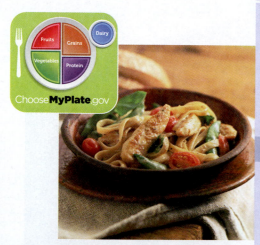

▲ Pre-event meals may require a higher proportion of grains than suggested by MyPlate to boost carbohydrate content. Choose starchy vegetables and grain-based snacks to help top off glycogen stores. How does this pasta meal compare to MyPlate?

© Getty Images/Jonelle Weaver

TABLE 14-8 ■ Convenient High-Carbohydrate Pre-Event Meals

Breakfast	
Cheerios®, ¾ cup Reduced-fat milk, 1 cup Blueberry muffin, 1 Orange juice, 4 ounces	450 kcal 92 grams (82%) carbohydrate
or	
Low-fat fruit yogurt, 1 cup Plain bagel, ½ Apple juice, 4 ounces Peanut butter (for bagel), 1 tbsp	482 kcal 84 grams (68%) carbohydrate
Lunch or Dinner	
Broiled pork chop, 3 ounces White rice, 1 ½ cups Steamed zucchini, 1 cup Chocolate milk, 1 cup Jello®, ½ cup	839 kcal 120 grams (57%) carbohydrate
or	
Spaghetti noodles, 2 cups Spaghetti sauce, 1 cup Reduced-fat milk, 1 ½ cups Green beans, 1 cup	761 kcal 129 grams (66%) carbohydrate

With regard to the timing of pre-activity meals, a general guide is to allow 4 hours for a big meal (about 1200 kcal), 3 hours for a moderate meal (about 800 to 900 kcal), 2 hours for a light meal (about 400 to 600 kcal), and an hour or less for a snack (about 300 kcal).

Emerging Research on Fat Adaptation Traditionally, high-carbohydrate diets have been the nutrition norm for endurance athletes. However, an alternative approach in training known as fat adaptation is becoming more popular among endurance athletes.

Of all the energy-yielding nutrients, carbohydrates are utilized most rapidly to fuel exercising muscles. When athletes consume a high-carbohydrate diet or practice carbohydrate loading before an endurance event, they ensure that muscle and liver glycogen will be available to muscles throughout the race. Even after carbohydrate loading, however, the total amount of energy available from muscle glycogen is limited to about 2500 kcal.

In comparison, the supply of energy from triglycerides stored in the muscle and adipose tissue is virtually limitless. Recall from Figure 14-8 that, depending on intensity, about half of the energy for endurance events comes from fat. The metabolism of fat for energy occurs more slowly, but it provides more than twice as many kilocalories per gram as carbohydrates or protein.

With fat adaptation, rather than following a traditional high-carbohydrate diet (about 65% of kilocalories from carbohydrates and only about 20% from fat) during the days leading up to an event, endurance athletes replace much of the carbohydrates with fat. For example, a high-fat training diet might consist of just 25% of kilocalories from carbohydrate with a whopping 60% of kilocalories from fat. The rationale is that high-carbohydrate diets, especially those with many simple sugars and refined grains, boost insulin secretion, which inhibits the breakdown of fat. By lowering carbohydrates and increasing the fat content of the diet, the cells will adapt to greater use of fat for fuel. If the athlete uses more fat for fuel during an endurance event, muscle glycogen might be spared, so that those stored carbohydrates would be available for a burst of speed at the end of the race (see Further Reading 10).

Research comparing the effects of high-carbohydrate or high-fat training diets on athletic performance has yielded mixed results. A possible explanation is that the muscles of "fat-adapted" athletes are able to break down more fat for fuel during exercise at low or moderate intensities, but the low carbohydrate intake depletes glycogen stores, so higher-intensity activity is impaired.

A compromise between these two approaches might be the best strategy. Some studies indicate that several weeks on a high-fat diet followed by 2 or 3 days of carbohydrate loading just before the event may enhance the ability of muscles to use fat for fuel, yet still facilitate adequate glycogen storage to fuel the sprint to the finish line.

At this time, there is not enough research evidence to support a recommendation for high-fat diets for endurance athletes. Evidence *does* clearly support a performance-enhancing effect of carbohydrate ingestion before and during physical activity. This will continue to be an area of active research, so stay on the lookout for more information on fat adaptation.

Replenish Fuel During the Event We have already established the importance of consuming adequate fluids during endurance exercise. For sporting events longer than 60 minutes, consumption of carbohydrate during activity can also improve athletic performance. Prolonged exercise depletes muscle glycogen stores and may transiently lower blood glucose, leading to physical and mental fatigue. One way to avoid "hitting the wall" is to maintain normal blood glucose concentrations by carbohydrate feedings during exercise. During short events (e.g., 30 minutes or so), carbohydrate intake during exercise is not as important because the muscles do not take up much blood glucose during short-term exercise, relying instead primarily on their glycogen stores for fuel.

A general guideline for endurance events is to consume 30 to 60 grams of carbohydrate per hour. A current trend in sports nutrition is to use multiple sources of carbohydrates (e.g., glucose, fructose, and maltodextrin) with different routes and rates of absorption to maximize the supply of glucose to cells and lessen the risk of gastrointestinal distress (see Further Reading 2 and 10).

Some experts suggest that consuming protein with carbohydrate during exercise provides added benefit. In particular, branched-chain amino acids, which can be used for fuel, are thought to delay fatigue by supplying energy and altering the production of certain neurotransmitters (see Further Reading 2). This is an area of ongoing research, but there is not enough evidence at this time to support a clear recommendation for ingesting protein during

General Guide for Approximate Pre-Event Carbohydrate Intake

Hours Before	Grams per Kilogram Body Weight	For a 70-Kilogram Person
1	1	70
2	2	140
3	3	210
4	4	280

exercise. Some products formulated for consumption during exercise do contain amino acids, so you can try various formulations to see what works best for you.

What about fat? Compared to carbohydrates, fat is more slowly digested, absorbed, and metabolized. Thus, although fat serves as fuel during prolonged aerobic activity, consumption of fat during activity is not likely to improve athletic performance and is likely to cause gastrointestinal distress.

Sports drinks are a good source of carbohydrate calories during endurance events. Sports drinks, described in detail in the Section 14.4, usually contain about 14 grams of carbohydrate per 8-oz serving. They supply the necessary fluid, electrolytes, and carbohydrates to keep an athlete performing at his or her best.

As an alternative to sports drinks, some athletes use carbohydrate gels or chews. Gels and chews are formulated with one or more sugars or starches to rapidly supply about 25 grams of carbohydrate per serving (Table 14-9). In addition, they provide electrolytes to replenish those lost in sweat. Some of these products also may contain certain amino acids, vitamins, caffeine (see Section 14.6), or herbal ingredients. An advantage of gels compared to energy bars or sports drinks is they are convenient to carry.

Popular energy bars (e.g., PowerBar) typically provide about 180 to 250 kcal and anywhere from 2 to 45 grams of carbohydrate. The wide range of carbohydrate content in energy bars is due to a variety of marketing trends in the sports supplement industry. Overall, endurance athletes should choose a bar with about 40 grams of carbohydrate and no more than 10 grams of protein, 4 grams of fat, and 5 grams of fiber. The bars are fortified with vitamins and minerals in amounts ranging from about 25% to 100% of typical human needs. Outside of sporting events, some people use energy bars as a quick and convenient meal or snack.

Check the label on these products to gauge the amount of gel or bar that provides 30 to 60 grams of carbohydrate per hour. In addition, remember that any carbohydrate-containing food must be accompanied by fluid to ensure adequate hydration.

At minimum, one serving of any of these will cost at least $1, and some brands with all natural or organic ingredients cost as much as $5. Are sports drinks, energy bars, and gels worth the price? It depends how much you are willing to pay for convenient packaging. Critics suggest that these products are essentially the nutritional equivalent of a cup of low-fat yogurt and piece of fruit (see Table 14-3). For an athlete on a tight budget, a small bag of graham crackers or jelly beans could just as easily provide a quick shot of glucose during a race. With a little bit of time and an Internet connection, you can even find recipes to make your own sports drinks and energy bars at home for a fraction of the cost of name-brand products.

There is evidence that the ergogenic effect of carbohydrate ingestion during exercise is due not only to the increased availability of fuel but also to changes in chemical signals that relay information about carbohydrate ingestion from the gastrointestinal tract to the brain. Some studies among athletes participating in events lasting less than 1 hour suggest that simply rinsing the mouth with a carbohydrate-containing fluid can decrease fatigue and enhance performance without risking gastrointestinal distress.

TABLE 14-9 ■ Energy and Macronutrient Content of Popular Energy Bars, Gels, and Chews

Energy Bars	Serving (oz)	Energy (kcal)	Carbohydrates (g)	Fiber (g)	Protein (g)	Fat (g)
Clif® Bar (chocolate chip)	2.4	240	44	5	10	4.5
Kashi® (chewy trail mix)	1.23	140	20	4	6	5
KIND® (peanut butter dark chocolate)	1.41	200	17	2.5	7	13
Luna® (nutz over chocolate)	1.69	180	25	4	9	6
PowerBar® (peanut butter)	2.13	240	44	1	9	4
Slim-Fast® (dark chocolate sea salt)	1.59	190	20	5	10	10
Energy Gels & Chews						
Clif Shot (vanilla)	1.1	100	24	0	0	0
GU™ Energy Gel (lemon sublime)	1.1	100	25	0	0	0
Jelly Belly Sport Beans® (berry)	1.0	100	24	0	0	0
PowerBar® Gel (strawberry banana)	1.44	110	27	0	0	0

Overall, choosing energy bars is preferable to choosing candy bars and packaged desserts. When used in athletic situations, these bars can be handy. Better yet, however, is to eat a variety of wholesome foods; these offer more health-protective compounds. This is also a much less expensive choice, especially for day-to-day snacking. An additional concern is that micronutrient toxicity might occur if numerous bars are eaten in a day, as many are highly fortified. Vitamin A and iron are two nutrients of special concern in this regard.

After Exercise, Replenish Glycogen and Fluid After prolonged aerobic exercise, muscle and liver glycogen stores will be depleted. An athlete's need to pay special attention to nutrition during recovery from exercise depends on the type of workout completed and the timing of the next workout. For example, multiple events in the same day will require rapid restoration of glycogen stores. However, if an athlete will be able to rest for 1 or 2 days before the next exercise session, immediate consumption of a post-workout meal is not as crucial.

To rapidly restore glycogen stores, carbohydrate-rich foods providing 1 to 1.5 grams of carbohydrate per kilogram body weight should be consumed within 30 minutes after extended (endurance) exercise. Immediately after exercise is when glycogen synthesis is greatest because the muscles are insulin-sensitive at this point. This process should then be repeated every 2 hours for the next 4 to 6 hours. Foods with a high glycemic index, such as fruit, fruit juice, bread, short-grain white rice, or a sports drink, contribute to rapid restoration of glycogen stores. Recall that Table 4-3 gives the glycemic index of various foods.

Although carbohydrate intake is the most important factor for replenishing glycogen after endurance exercise, adding an appropriate amount of high-quality protein during recovery can be helpful for stimulating glycogen synthesis and repairing damaged muscle tissue. Read more about recovery meals in the next section on nutrition strategies for strength and power athletes.

Fluid and electrolyte (i.e., sodium and potassium) intake is another essential component of recovery for an endurance athlete, especially if two workouts a day are performed or if the environment is hot and humid. Specialized recovery drinks containing carbohydrates, amino acids, and electrolytes are available, but if food and fluid intake is sufficient to restore weight loss, it generally will also supply enough electrolytes to meet needs during recovery from endurance activities.

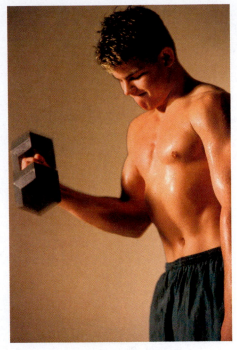

▲ A special nutrition issue that concerns strength-trained athletes is muscle dysmorphia, informally called "bigorexia." Section 15.6 will touch upon this form of body dysmorphic disorder in which individuals see themselves as being too thin, even though they are more muscular than average. People who suffer from muscle dysmorphia may practice disordered eating behaviors or use steroids to achieve high levels of muscularity. © Ingram Publishing

STRENGTH AND POWER ATHLETES: STRATEGIES TO ENHANCE MUSCLE GAIN

Strength training—improving the maximal force that can be exerted by the muscle—should be part of any well-rounded fitness program. Resistance exercises may utilize free weights, specialized weight machines, or the weight of one's own body. A workout typically includes 8 to 12 different exercises that target all the major muscle groups of the body. Most of the people you see lifting weights in the gym are probably performing several sets of 8 to 10 repetitions each, lifting about 50% of the maximum weight they could lift (1 RM). This type of workout improves muscular *endurance,* which is an important part of muscular fitness for overall health. However, to truly build muscular *strength,* athletes need to work against greater resistance (around 80% of 1 RM) over just a few repetitions (2 to 5 repetitions). For a few athletes, such as those who participate in weight-lifting or body-building competitions, muscular strength is the focus of training.

Muscular power combines strength with speed, improving the ability to apply force quickly. Examples of power sports include middle-distance running, gridiron football, rowing, and swimming. In reality, many sports and everyday activities involve muscular power: jumping for a rebound in basketball, delivering a roundhouse kick to an opponent in martial arts, or driving the ball down the fairway in a round of golf are examples of muscular power in sports.

For strength and power athletes, a few changes are needed to the general nutrition advice for athletes. First, calorie needs will be high due to the additional lean mass and high-volume training routines of these athletes. Recall that the primary types of fuel for strength and power moves are phosphocreatine (PCr) and carbohydrates for the brief bursts of activity, with fat providing energy during the resting stages. Very little protein is used as fuel during resistance exercises (review Fig. 14-8). Second, there will be some extra emphasis on protein intake in the recovery phase (see Further Readings 16 and 18).

Strength and power athletes tend to be extremely focused on consuming adequate protein to support muscle protein synthesis. Strength-training athletes in the early phases of training have the highest estimated protein needs of any athletes. Once desired muscle mass has

Many power athletes utilize a training technique called **periodization,** in which physical stresses on the body change throughout the year:

- Early in the training season, athletes work on building aerobic endurance.

- After gains in aerobic capacity have been achieved, the focus shifts to building strength, power, and sport-specific skills.

- During the competitive season, daily workouts are scaled back, but activity is intense and of long duration on game days.

- In the off-season, athletes continue to work out to stay in shape, but the volume is certainly lower than it was in season.

Athletes taking part in periodized training will use the full spectrum of energy systems we have discussed. Nutrition recommendations should also be periodized to match such dynamic training plans.

periodization Cycling the volume, intensity, and activities of workouts throughout the training season.

▲ Chocolate milk is the go-to recovery drink for many athletes. This 2-cup serving of low-fat chocolate milk is a tasty vehicle for 52 grams of carbohydrate and 16 grams of protein.

© Foodcollection/Getty Images

been achieved, protein requirements for maintenance of muscular strength decrease slightly. Meeting these recommendations for protein intake optimizes muscle protein synthesis, but consuming more than the recommended range of protein intake does not appear to offer advantage. Recall that excess amino acids are used as fuel or stored as fat; they do not directly translate into increased muscular strength.

Before and During Strength and Power Training, Focus on Calories, Carbohydrates, and Fluids Adequate hydration supports optimal athletic performance; strength and power athletes are no exception. Checking urine color or urine specific gravity is a good indication of fluid status. If the athlete is poorly hydrated before an event, water or a sports drink will be sufficient to restore hydration.

Similar to nutrition strategies for endurance athletes, adequate carbohydrate ingestion in the days leading up to and hours immediately before exercise has been shown to enhance performance for strength and power events, too. Athletes who perform many repetitions with moderate resistance will use more of their muscle glycogen stores than athletes who perform fewer repetitions with high resistance. Overall, research has shown that consuming 4 to 7 grams of carbohydrates per kilogram of body weight per day is appropriate for strength and power training. The optimal rate of carbohydrate ingestion before and during resistance activities has not yet been established, but some research indicates that 1 to 4 grams of carbohydrate per kilogram of body weight in a pre-event meal or beverage will enhance work capacity during resistance workouts.

In strength and power sports, many athletes also use creatine supplements to increase levels of phosphocreatine in muscles. Recall that phosphocreatine is used to resupply ATP during short, intense bursts of activity. When phosphocreatine stores are increased, muscle glycogen may be preserved (see Further Reading 16). Section 14.6 provides more information on creatine and other ergogenic aids.

Focus on achieving adequate hydration and maximizing muscle glycogen before activities, because there may not be an opportunity to replenish fluids and carbohydrates during strength or power competitions. During extended training sessions, however, supplying fluids and carbohydrates will enhance both physical and mental performance.

While a few sports nutrition experts advocate ingesting protein before or during a resistance workout in an effort to promote muscle protein synthesis, the bulk of evidence points to emphasizing protein in the recovery meal.

For athletes (and adults in general), fat intake should fall into the range of 20% to 35% of overall calorie intake. Dietary surveys show that usual fat intake of resistance-trained athletes is slightly higher than recommended, probably because too many of their choices of protein-rich foods (e.g., meats and dairy products) are also rich sources of fat. If fat intake is above 35% of total calories, replacing the excess fat with carbohydrates would have a favorable effect on protein balance. This is because insulin, secreted in response to glucose in the blood, triggers uptake of amino acids by cells, which provides materials for protein synthesis within the cells.

After Strength and Power Activities, Consuming Carbohydrates and Protein Promotes Recovery Those first few hours after resistance exercise, according to many researchers, are the best time to provide carbohydrates and protein to replenish muscle glycogen and promote muscle repair and synthesis. Right after exercise, the cells are insulin sensitive, so they rapidly take up glucose from the blood and store it as glycogen. General ACSM guidelines are to consume 1.0 to 1.5 grams of carbohydrate per kilogram of body weight to restore muscle glycogen. To promote muscle protein synthesis along with glycogen restoration, many sports nutrition experts recommend intakes at the upper end of that range (e.g., 1.2 to 1.5 grams of carbohydrates per kilogram of body weight) shortly after exercise (see Further Reading 16). The presence of certain amino acids further stimulates insulin secretion to enhance the uptake of glucose and synthesis of glycogen.

To promote gains in muscle mass, most sports nutrition experts recommend at least 20 grams of high-quality protein within the first 1 or 2 hours after exercise to maximize protein synthesis. Novice strength-training athletes who are seeking to gain muscle mass have

TABLE 14-10 ■ Sample Recovery Meals

Option 1
Bagel, 1 regular
Deli turkey, 1 ounce
Swiss cheese, 1 ounce
Fat-free milk, 1 cup
509 kcal, 71 grams carbohydrate, 33 grams protein, and 10 grams fat

Option 2
Low-fat flavored Greek yogurt, 16 ounces
Banana, 1 medium
533 kcal, 86 grams carbohydrate, 31 grams protein, and 8 grams fat

Option 3
Gatorade Recover Post-Game Recovery Beverage, 1 (8 fluid ounce) carton
Gatorade Recover Protein Shake, 1 (11 fluid ounce) carton
380 kcal, 65 grams carbohydrate, 28 grams protein, and 1.5 grams fat

▲ Elite athletes are subject to all the same nutritional challenges as the general public: overreliance on convenience foods, abundance of nutrition misinformation, temptations to eat out of boredom or for emotional comfort. Furthermore, they must adapt to the seasonal demands of their sport and maintain exhausting training and travel schedules. In her role as a sports dietitian for the United States Olympic Committee, Jennifer Gibson, M.Sc., R.D.N., CSSD, carefully tailored nutrition recommendations for each of her athletes based on nutritional status, sport, season, position, and body composition goals. © Jennifer Gibson

the highest requirements for protein. With advanced training, the rate of protein turnover during exercise decreases. Therefore, well-trained strength athletes require less protein to repair and maintain muscles than their untrained counterparts. Some amino acids (e.g., leucine) may stimulate the metabolic pathways that lead to synthesis of muscle protein. The process of muscle protein synthesis not only requires amino acids as building blocks, of course, but also depends on carbohydrate as a source of energy.

Overall, recovery from resistance exercise requires a combination (3:1 ratio) of carbohydrates and high-quality protein. For a 154-pound (70-kilogram) athlete, this corresponds to about 70 grams of carbohydrate and 25 grams of protein in each 2-hour interval. Table 14-10 describes sample meals of this composition.

CONCLUDING REMARKS

Nutritional strategies have the potential to optimize athletic performance. Here, we have presented several generalized guidelines to plan nutritionally adequate diets that optimize energy stores, ensure hydration, and give athletes a competitive edge. We have stressed the importance of carbohydrates and fluids before, during, and after exercise, as well as protein for muscle recovery. Above all, recognize that each athlete is unique. Remember that genetics can impact nutrition requirements. Each type of exercise demands its own set of energy sources. Sports vary in training regimens, duration, and opportunities to acquire nourishment before, during, and between events. Even within a particular sport, each player's position has its own physical demands, which can alter nutritional needs (see Further Reading 8). Finally, personal taste preferences and gastrointestinal tolerance will dictate adherence to any nutrition plan. When working with athletes, start with your solid foundation of knowledge about nutrient needs, but be attentive to individual concerns, be adaptable, and always continue to learn.

✓ **CONCEPT CHECK 14.5**

1. Which nutrient(s) should be emphasized in a pre-event meal for an endurance athlete? Provide an example of a suitable pre-event meal for a long-distance cyclist.

2. What is carbohydrate loading? List three sports for which carbohydrate loading could enhance performance.

3. Why is a combination of carbohydrate and protein recommended for recovery after resistance exercise? When should a recovery meal be provided? Suggest a suitable recovery meal.

For more information on sports nutrition, check out the following websites:
Gatorade Sports Science Institute
www.gssiweb.com
The Physician and Sportsmedicine
http://www.tandfonline.com/toc/ipsm20/current
American College of Sports Medicine
www.acsm.org
CDC's Division of Nutrition, Physical Activity, and Obesity
www.cdc.gov/nccdphp/dnpao
American Council on Exercise
www.acefitness.org

CASE STUDY   Planning a Training Diet

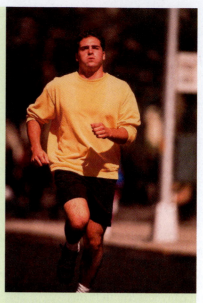

Michael is training for a 10K run coming up in 3 weeks. He has read a lot about sports nutrition and especially about the importance of eating a high-carbohydrate diet while in training. He also has been struggling to keep his weight in a range that he feels contributes to better speed and endurance. Consequently, he is also trying to eat as little fat as possible. Unfortunately, over the past week, his workouts in the afternoon have not met his expectations. His run times are slower, and he shows signs of fatigue after just 20 minutes into his training program.

His breakfast yesterday was a large bagel, a small amount of cream cheese, and orange juice. For lunch, he had a small salad with fat-free dressing, a large plate of pasta with marinara sauce and broccoli, and a diet soft drink. For dinner, he had a small broiled chicken breast, a cup of rice, some carrots, and iced tea. Later, he snacked on fat-free pretzels.

Answer the following questions, and check your responses at the end of this chapter.

1. Is the high-carbohydrate diet a good idea during Michael's training?
2. Are there any important components missing in Michael's diet? Are missing components contributing to his fatigue?
3. Describe some changes that should be made in Michael's diet, including specific foods that should be emphasized.
4. How should fluid needs be met during workouts?
5. Should Michael focus on fueling his body before, during, or after workouts?

© Comstock Images

Ergogenic Aids and Athletic Performance

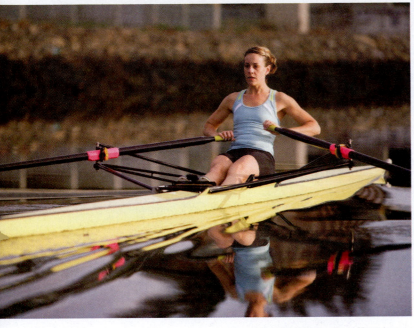

© Ty Milford/Aurora Open/Getty Images

TABLE 14-11 ■ Potentially Useful Ergogenic Aids

Substance/Practice	Purported Use
Beetroot juice	Enhance endurance performance by improving oxygen consumption (see Further Reading 10)
Beta-alanine	Increase muscle carnosine, a protein that neutralizes acidic compounds that contribute to muscle fatigue during high-intensity exercise (see Further Reading 20)
Caffeine	Increase vigilance and mental alertness; improve endurance performance (see Further Reading 17)
Creatine	Increase lean mass; improve short-term intense exercise performance; aid muscle recovery (see Further Readings 4 and 14)
Sodium bicarbonate (baking soda)	Neutralize acidic compounds that contribute to muscle fatigue (see Further Reading 14)

Extreme diet manipulation to improve athletic performance is not a recent innovation. Today's athletes are as likely as their predecessors to experiment with any substance that promises a competitive advantage. In 2014, the U.S. sports nutrition supplement market reached $5.9 billion, accounting for 6.2% of the $36.7 billion market. Bee pollen, medium-chain triglycerides, chromium picolinate, carnitine, and ginseng are just some of the likely ineffective substances used by athletes in hopes of gaining an **ergogenic** (work-producing) edge.

Based on what is known at this time, today's athletes can benefit from scientific evidence documenting the ergogenic properties of a few dietary substances. These ergogenic aids include sufficient water and electrolytes, adequate carbohydrates, and a balanced and varied dietary pattern consistent with MyPlate. Protein and amino-acid supplements are NOT needed as the vast majority of athletes can easily meet their protein needs from whole foods, as Table 14-3 demonstrates. In general, nutrient supplements should only be used to meet a specific dietary shortcoming, such as an inadequate iron intake. Beyond the proven benefits of the nutrition strategies presented in this chapter, Table 14-11 provides a short list of well-studied, safe, and potentially useful ergogenic aids.

Dietary supplements rumored to enhance athletic performance require careful evaluation. Overall, there is little scientific evidence to support the effectiveness of many substances that are touted as performance-enhancing aids. Of these, many are useless, and some are dangerous enough to promote organ damage (Table 14-12). The liver and kidneys are particularly susceptible to damage because these organs help detoxify harmful compounds

ergogenic Work-producing. An ergogenic aid is a mechanical, nutritional, psychological, pharmacological, or physiological substance or treatment intended to directly improve exercise performance.

National Collegiate Athletic Association (NCAA) and Nutrition Supplements

The NCAA's Committee on Competitive Safeguards and Medical Aspects of Sports has developed lists of permissible and nonpermissible nutritional supplements for athletic departments to provide to student athletes. The NCAA has issued a warning advising students to discuss their use of *any* dietary supplement with their team medical staff to avoid unknowingly ingesting banned substances. Following are a few key examples:

Permissible Supplements
- Vitamins and minerals
- "Energy" bars (if no more than 30% protein)
- Electrolyte replacement drinks such as Gatorade or Powerade
- Calorie replacement drinks such as Ensure or Boost

Nonpermissible Supplements
- Amino acids (including amino-acid chelates)
- CLA (conjugated linoleic acid)
- Chondroitin (unless for medical condition)
- Creatine/compounds containing creatine
- Ginkgo biloba
- Ginseng
- Glucosamine (unless for medical condition)
- Green tea
- Melatonin
- Protein powders
- St. John's wort
- Weight gainers

For a complete explanation of NCAA's rules regarding dietary supplements, see www.ncaa.org.

TABLE 14-12 ■ Dangerous or Illegal Substances and Practices

Substance/Practice	Purported Use	Risks
Anabolic steroids (e.g., testosterone, androstenedione, and tetrahydrogestrinone)	Increase muscle mass and strength	Liver cysts; increased risk of cardiovascular disease, hypertension, and reproductive dysfunction; depression, sleep disturbances, mood swings ("roid rage") *Illegal in the United States unless prescribed Banned by IOC*
Blood doping	Enhances aerobic capacity by increasing red blood cells	Blood thickening that strains the heart *Banned by IOC*
Ephedrine (stimulant)	Increases muscle strength and power, promotes mental alertness, weight loss	Heart palpitations, anxiety, and death *Banned by IOC* *Banned by NCAA*
Gamma hydroxybutyric acid (GHB)	Steroid alternative for bodybuilding	Vomiting, dizziness, tremors, seizures, and death *Illegal to produce or sell in the United States*
Growth hormone	Increases muscle mass and fat metabolism	Uncontrolled growth of the heart and other internal organs; death *Banned by IOC*

(see Further Reading 9). Athletes should be skeptical of any substance until its ergogenic effect is scientifically validated. FDA has a limited ability to regulate these dietary supplements (review Section 8.5), and the manufacturing processes for dietary supplements are not as tightly regulated by FDA as they are for prescription drugs (see Further Reading 12).

Some supplements may contain substances that will cause athletes to test "positive" for various banned substances. This was demonstrated in the 2008 Summer Olympics, when swimmer Jessica Hardy tested positive for a banned substance that she inadvertently consumed as part of a dietary supplement. Studies consistently show that many supplements do not contain the substance and/or the amount listed on the label. Not only must

athletes determine whether there is evidence that a dietary supplement is safe and effective, but they must also question if the dietary supplement contains what it is supposed to contain.

Even substances whose ergogenic effects have been supported by systematic scientific studies should be used with extreme caution, as the testing conditions may not match those of the intended use. Caution should be exercised when it comes to using the appropriate dose of supplements or using multiple types of supplements concurrently (see Further Reading 1).

Rather than waiting for a magic bullet to enhance performance, athletes are advised to concentrate their efforts on improving their training routines and sport techniques, while adhering to a well-balanced dietary pattern as described in this chapter.

Summary (Numbers refer to numbered sections in the chapter.)

14.1 A gradual increase in regular physical activity is recommended for all healthy persons. Benefits include improvements in cardiovascular health, gastrointestinal function, blood glucose regulation, and sleep; reduced risk of certain cancers; and enhanced muscle and bone strength.

14.2 The Physical Activity Guidelines for Americans advise adults to do at least 150 minutes of moderate-intensity or 75 minutes of

vigorous-intensity aerobic physical activity per week. In addition, adults should perform muscle-strengthening activities and flexibility exercises at least twice per week. Workouts should allow time for warm-up exercises to increase blood flow and warm the muscles and then end with cooldown exercises, including stretching.

14.3 Human metabolic pathways extract chemical energy from carbohydrate, fat, and protein to yield ATP. Phosphocreatine is high-energy compound that can be used to resupply ATP during short, intense activities. The mix of macronutrients used for fuel depends on the intensity and duration of activity: short-term, intense exercises primarily use carbohydrate for fuel, whereas low- or moderate-intensity endurance exercises use more fat for fuel. Protein makes a minor contribution as a fuel source.

14.4 To support physical activity, athletes require 5 to 8 kcal per minute of activity above energy needs for a sedentary person. Monitoring weight changes over time is a good way to assess the adequacy of energy intake. Athletes should obtain energy from a varied diet that includes sources of carbohydrates (6 to 10 grams of carbohydrate per kilogram of body weight; usually 60% of total energy), protein (1.2 to 2.0 grams of protein per kilogram, depending on the type of training), and fat (up to 35% of energy, focusing on vegetable oils instead of solid fats). The increased overall food intake of athletes typically furnishes adequate vitamins and minerals. Some micronutrients of concern are iron and calcium, especially for women. Athletes should drink fluid before, during (to minimize loss of body weight), and after

exercise (2 to 3 cups per pound lost). Sports drinks help replace fluid, electrolytes, and carbohydrates lost during workouts that last beyond 60 minutes.

14.5 Endurance athletes can delay or prevent fatigue by consuming enough fluids, electrolytes, and carbohydrates before, during, and after events. In addition, protein in the post-exercise period will aid muscle recovery. In addition to these strategies to maintain hydration and muscle glycogen stores, athletes who train to develop strength or power should place special emphasis on protein during the recovery period.

14.6 Athletes can benefit from ergogenic properties of sufficient water, electrolytes, and carbohydrates, and a balanced and varied diet consistent with the 2015–2020 Dietary Guidelines and MyPlate. Under some circumstances, creatine, HMB, and caffeine are useful for enhancing athletic performance. Protein and amino-acid supplements are not necessary because athletes almost always meet protein needs from foods.

Check Your Knowledge (Answers are available at the end of this question set.)

1. An energy-rich compound, phosphocreatine (PCr), is found in _____ tissue.
   a. adipose
   b. muscle
   c. liver
   d. kidney

2. A fitness program should include
   a. aerobic exercises 5 days per week.
   b. strength-training exercises 2 to 3 days per week.
   c. stretching exercises 2 to 3 days per week.
   d. all of these.

3. During muscle-building regimens, athletes should consume _____ grams of protein per kilogram body weight.
   a. 0.5 to 0.7
   b. 0.8
   c. 1.5 to 2
   d. 2 to 2.5

4. Which of these foods is the best choice for carbohydrate loading before endurance events?
   a. Potato chips
   b. French fries
   c. All-Bran® (high-fiber) cereal
   d. Rice

5. As the body adapts to regular exercise, the "training effect" results in
   a. decreased blood flow to muscles.
   b. increased lactic-acid production.
   c. decreased muscle triglyceride content.
   d. decreased resting heart rate.

6. A physically active lifestyle leads to
   a. increased bone strength.
   b. decreased risk of colon cancer.
   c. reduced anxiety and depression.
   d. all of these.

7. How many cups of fluid are required to replace each pound of weight lost during an athletic event or workout?
   a. 0.5 to 0.75 cup
   b. 1 to 1.5 cups
   c. 2 to 3 cups
   d. 4 to 5 cups

8. The benefit of a "sports" drink is to provide
   a. water to hydrate.
   b. electrolytes to enhance water absorption in the intestine and maintain blood volume.
   c. carbohydrate for energy.
   d. all of these.

9. Compared to anaerobic glucose metabolism, aerobic glucose metabolism produces more
   a. lactic acid.
   b. ATP.
   c. phosphocreatine.
   d. fatty acids.

10. Caffeine is used as an ergogenic aid by some athletes because it is thought to
    a. decrease fatigue.
    b. decrease the buildup of lactic acid.
    c. serve as an energy source.
    d. increase muscle mass and strength.

Answer Key: 1. b (LO 14.3), 2. d (LO 14.2), 3. c (LO 14.6), 4. d (LO 14.8), 5. d (LO 14.5), 6. d (LO 14.1), 7. c (LO 14.7), 8. d (LO 14.7), 9. b (LO 14.7), 10. a (LO 14.9)

Study Questions (Numbers refer to Learning Outcomes)

1. How does greater physical fitness contribute to better overall health? Explain the process. **(LO 14.1)**

2. You have set a goal to increase muscle mass and decrease body fat. Plan a weekly fitness regimen using the FITT principle. **(LO 14.2)**

3. How are carbohydrates, fat, and protein used to supply energy during a 100-meter sprint? During a weightlifting session? During a 3-mile walk? **(LO 14.3)**

4. What is the difference between anaerobic and aerobic exercise? Explain why aerobic metabolism is increased by a regular exercise routine. **(LO 14.4)**

5. Is fat from adipose tissue used as an energy source during exercise? If so, when? **(LO 14.5)**

6. What are some typical measures used to assess whether an athlete's calorie intake is adequate? **(LO 14.6)**

7. List five nutrients of specific concern for athletes and the appropriate food sources from which these nutrients can be obtained. **(LO 14.6)**

8. You plan to participate in a half-marathon. Plan your menu for the day of the event, being sure to include appropriate levels of macronutrients and fluids before, during, and after the athletic event. **(LO 14.8)**

9. Your neighbor is planning to run a 5-kilometer race. Summarize for her what you have learned about fluid intake before, during, and after the event. **(LO 14.7)**

10. Should competitive athletes take amino-acid supplements? Why or why not? **(LO 14.9)**

What the Dietitian Chose

In this chapter, you have learned that it's important to replenish carbohydrates, fluids, and electrolytes for optimal performance during endurance events, like this half-marathon. General guidelines are to consume ½ to 1 ½ cups of fluid every 15 minutes and 30 to 60 grams of carbohydrate per hour. Choosing a sports nutrition product is something you should do during training. With a few weeks to go, you have time to experiment with a product that can help you avoid "hitting the wall."

The PowerBar ProteinPlus® energy bar provides 300 kcal, 6 grams of fat, 39 grams of carbohydrate, and 23 grams of protein. This might be a tasty and convenient meal replacement during your busy weeks of training. Alternatively, it could serve as a recovery meal to help replenish your muscle glycogen stores after the race. However, during the race, its high fat and protein content would slow digestion, possibly leading to abdominal cramps. Furthermore, this product would not contribute to fluid replenishment.

The Essential Amino Energy™ drink provides 2 grams of carbohydrate and 5 grams of essential amino acids in free form, including branched-chain amino acids. The drink may help meet fluid needs, but the carbohydrate content is not sufficient to maintain blood glucose during the race. It is true that BCAAs are utilized for fuel during endurance activities and that they can enhance muscle building during weight training, but there is no consistent evidence that supplying BCAAs during endurance exercise enhances performance.

A sports drink, such as Powerade®, is superior to water for events lasting more than 60 minutes. The carbohydrates help to supply energy to the brain and muscles. The added flavor encourages consumption. The electrolytes replace those lost in sweating, increase fluid absorption, and stimulate thirst. A 32-ounce bottle of Powerade (4 servings) contains a total of 200 kcal and 56 grams of carbohydrate in 4 cups of

© Stockbyte/Getty Images

fluid. One bottle of Powerade per hour while you compete would meet your fluid and carbohydrate needs but may be inconvenient to tote while running.

The energy gel is small enough to take along during the race. The label shows 110 kcal, 1.5 grams of fat, 22 grams of carbohydrate, 12 grams of sugar, and 100 milligrams of caffeine. A Clif Shot® Turbo during the race could help replenish blood glucose and electrolytes, but it definitely won't meet your fluid requirements while racing. However, there will be water available at numerous stops along the course.

Some energy gels are caffeine free, but this one contains as much caffeine as a strong cup of coffee. Research shows that caffeine can decrease feelings of fatigue and increase mental alertness among people who are not habitual caffeine consumers. On the other hand, negative effects of excessive caffeine can include dehydration, heart palpitations, and gastrointestinal discomfort, so moderation is necessary.

In summary, both the Powerade and the Clif Shot Turbo would replenish carbohydrates and electrolytes. The Powerade would also fulfill your fluid needs, whereas you'd need to grab water along the course if you choose the energy gel. The energy gel has the advantage of being light and portable, plus the caffeine may have an ergogenic effect. Give both the Powerade and the Clif Shot Turbo energy gel a trial run during your training sessions and see which one helps you most.

CASE STUDY SOLUTION Planning a Training Diet

1. Michael is correct in following a high-carbohydrate diet.
2. In his effort to minimize his fat intake, he is probably not consuming enough calories, protein, iron, and calcium to support his training routine. He has fallen into the bagel, pasta, and pretzel routine that sports nutritionists warn is not conducive to peak performance. Low protein, iron, and overall calories may contribute to fatigue.
3. Michael's performance would improve if he also had a source of protein at each meal. He could include milk with breakfast and possibly some low-fat yogurt or low-fat cheese at lunch. He should have a snack that provides carbohydrates and protein before his workout, such as half of a sandwich with fruit and some water. The sandwich and fruit will help provide him with fuel to support his vigorous training. In the evenings, he could add some reduced-fat cheese or hummus to his snack of pretzels to improve protein intake.
4. During his workouts, he could consume a sports drink to meet fluid needs and supply some carbohydrate, or he could consume water, along with a few graham crackers or other high-carbohydrate food.
5. Overall, it is important for Michael to fuel his body before, during, and after workouts. Before and during exercise, carbohydrates and fluid will improve athletic performance. After exercise, carbohydrates coupled with protein will enhance muscle recovery.

Further Readings

1. Buell JL and others: National Athletic Trainers' Association Position Statement: Evaluation of dietary supplements for performance nutrition. *Journal of Athletic Training* 48:124, 2013.

2. Burke LM and others: BJSM reviews: A-Z of nutritional supplements: Dietary supplements, sports nutrition foods and ergogenic aids for health and performance—Part 4. *British Journal of Sports Medicine* 43:1088, 2009.

3. Castell LM and others: BJSM review: A-Z of nutritional supplements: Dietary supplements, sports nutrition foods and ergogenic aids for health and performance—Part 5. *British Journal of Sports Medicine* 44:77, 2010.

4. Cooper R and others: Creatine supplementation with specific view to exercise/sports performance: An update. *Journal of the International Society of Sports Nutrition* 9:33, 2012.

5. Garber CE and others: American College of Sports Medicine Position Stand: Quantity and quality of exercise for developing and maintaining cardiorespiratory, musculoskeletal, and neuromotor fitness in apparently healthy adults: Guidance for prescribing exercise. *Medicine and Science in Sports and Exercise* 43:1334, 2011.

6. Goodman C and others: A to Z of nutritional supplements: Dietary supplements, sports nutrition foods and ergogenic aids for health and performance—Part 21. *British Journal of Sports Medicine* 45:677, 2011.

7. Higgins JP and others: Energy beverages: Content and safety. *Mayo Clinic Proceedings* 85:1033, 2010.

8. Holway FE, Spriet LL: Sport-specific nutrition: Practical strategies for team sports. *Journal of Sports Sciences* 29:S115, 2011.

9. Navarro VJ and others: Liver injury from herbals and dietary supplements in the U.S. Drug-Induced Liver Injury Network. *Hepatology,* 2014.

10. Ormsbee MJ and others: Pre-exercise nutrition: The role of macronutrients, modified starches and supplements on metabolism and endurance performance. *Nutrients* 6:1782, 2014.

11. Phillips SM and Van Loon LJC: Dietary protein for athletes: From requirements to optimum adaptation. *Journal of Sports Sciences* 29:S29, 2011.

12. Rosenbloom C, Rosbruck M. Popular dietary supplements used in sports. *Nutrition Today* 43:60, 2008.

13. Rosenfeld V, Wattenberg C: Weight loss in wrestling: Current state of the science. Updated 2014. Available at http://www.scandpg.org/nutrition-info/nutrition-for-collegiate-sports-and-athletics/articles/

14. Sahlin K: Muscle energetics during explosive activities and potential effects of nutrition and training. *Sports Medicine* 44:S167, 2014.

15. Sawka MN and others: American College of Sports Medicine Position Stand: Exercise and fluid replacement. *Medicine and Science in Sports and Exercise* 39:377, 2007.

16. Slater G, Phillips SM: Nutrition guidelines for strength sports: Sprinting, weightlifting, throwing events, and bodybuilding. *Journal of Sports Sciences* 29:S67, 2011.

17. Spriet LL: Exercise and sport performance with low doses of caffeine. *Sports Medicine* 44:S175, 2014.

18. Stellingwerff T, Maughan RJ, Burke LM: Nutrition for power sports: Middle-distance running, track cycling, rowing, canoeing/kayaking, and swimming. *Journal of Sports Sciences* 29:S79, 2011.

19. Thomas DT and others: Position of the Academy of Nutrition and Dietetics, Dietitians of Canada, and the American College of Sports Medicine: Nutrition and athletic performance. *Journal of the Academy of Nutrition and Dietetics* 116:501, 2016.

20. Trexler ET and others: International Society of Sports Nutrition position stand: Beta-alanine. *Journal of the International Society of Sports Nutrition* 12:30, 2015.

 To get the most out of your study of nutrition, go to McGraw-Hill's online resources: Connect www.mcgrawhillconnect.com, where you will find NutritionCalc Plus, LearnSmart, and many other dynamic tools.

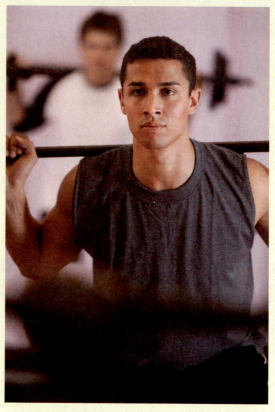

Rate Your Plate

I. Evaluating Protein Intake—A Case Study

Mark is a college student who has been lifting weights at the student recreation center. The trainer at the center recommended a protein drink to help Mark build muscle mass. Answer the following questions about Mark's current food intake and determine whether a protein drink is needed to supplement Mark's diet.

The following is a tally of yesterday's intake.

Breakfast	Frosted Mini-Wheats® cereal, 2 ounces 1% milk, 1 ½ cups Orange juice, chilled, 6 ounces Hard boiled eggs, 2 Brewed coffee, 1 cup
Lunch	Double hamburger with condiments, 1 French fries, 30 Cola, 12 ounces
Afternoon snack	Greek yogurt with honey, 1 cup Medium apple, 1
Dinner	Frozen lasagna w/meat, 2 pieces 1% milk, 1 cup Looseleaf lettuce, chopped, 1 cup Creamy Italian salad dressing, 2 tsp Medium tomato, ½ Whole raw carrot, 1
Evening snack	Low-fat vanilla ice cream, 1 cup Hot fudge chocolate topping, 2 tsp

© Comstock Images/Jupiterimages

1. Evaluate Mark's diet using NutritionCalc Plus. Is he meeting the minimum recommendations of MyPlate's Daily Food Plan for his calorie needs?

_____

2. Mark's weight has been stable at 70 kilograms (154 pounds). Determine his protein needs based on the RDA (0.8 gram per kilogram).
   a. Mark's estimated protein RDA: _____
   b. What are the maximum recommendations for protein intake for strength-training athletes?

   _____
   c. Calculate the maximum protein recommendation for Mark. _____

   _____

3. An analysis of the total calorie and protein content of Mark's current diet is 3400 kcal, 145 grams of protein (17% of total calories supplied by protein). This diet is representative of the food choices and amounts of food that Mark chooses on a regular basis.
   a. What is the difference between Mark's estimated protein needs as an athlete (from question 2) and the amount of protein that his current diet provides? _____
   b. Is his current protein intake inadequate, adequate, or excessive? _____

4. Mark takes his trainer's advice and goes to the supermarket to purchase a protein drink to add to his diet. Four products are available; they contain the following label information.

	Amino Fuel®	Joe Weider's® Sugar-Free 90% Plus Protein	Joe Weider's Dynamic Muscle Builder	Victory Super Mega Mass® 2000
Serving size	3 tbsp	3 tbsp	3 tbsp	¼ scoop
Kcal	104	110	103	104
Protein (grams)	15	24	10	5

The trainer recommends adding the supplement to Mark's diet two times a day. Mark chooses the Muscle Builder protein drink.

a. How much protein would be added to Mark's diet daily from two servings of the supplement alone (prior to mixing it with a beverage)?

b. Mark mixes the powder with the milk he already consumes at breakfast and dinner. How much protein total would Mark now consume in 1 day? (Add the protein amount from the nutrition analysis to the value from question 4a.)

c. What is the difference between Mark's estimated protein needs as an athlete and his total intake?

5. What is your conclusion—does Mark need the protein supplement?

© BananaStock/PunchStock

Student Learning Outcomes

Chapter 15 is designed to allow you to:

15.1 Contrast healthy attitudes toward uses of food with behavior patterns that could lead to unhealthy uses of food.

15.2 Describe current hypotheses about the origins of eating disorders.

15.3 List physical and mental characteristics of anorexia nervosa, and outline current best practices for its treatment.

15.4 List physical and mental characteristics of bulimia nervosa, and outline current best practices for its treatment.

15.5 Enumerate physical and mental characteristics of binge-eating disorder, and outline current best practices for its treatment.

Chapter 15
Eating Disorders

Many of us occasionally eat until we're stuffed and uncomfortable, such as at Thanksgiving dinner. Faced with savory and tempting foods, we find that we cannot easily stop eating. Usually we forgive ourselves, vowing not to overeat the next time. Nevertheless, many of us have problems controlling our food intake and body weight. The combination of too many instances of simple overeating, and too little physical activity eventually leads to progressive weight gain.

The obesity epidemic tends to upstage all other nutrition-related problems. However, the consequences of eating disorders are just as serious as obesity; indeed, if left untreated, eating disorders can be fatal. What is most alarming about these disorders—anorexia nervosa, bulimia nervosa, and binge-eating disorder—is the increasing number of cases reported each year.

It is widely accepted that eating disorders arise as a result of interactions between brain biology and environmental influences. Successful treatment of eating disorders, therefore, is complex and must go beyond nutritional therapy. Keep in mind that eating disorders are not restricted to any socioeconomic class or ethnicity. They can also strike at any age in either females or males. Let us examine the causes, effects, and treatments of these conditions in detail because eating disorders touch many of our lives.

15.6 Describe other forms of eating disorders, including night eating syndrome and the female athlete triad.

15.7 Describe methods to reduce the development of eating disorders, including the use of warning signs to identify early cases.

▲ Maintaining an ultraslim body type is an all-too-common goal in today's culture. The media and the fashion world bombard us with body images that are unrealistic for most people. © Lars A. Niki

endorphins Natural body tranquilizers that may be involved in the feeding response and function in pain reduction.

disordered eating Mild and short-term changes in eating patterns that occur in relation to a stressful event, an illness, or a desire to modify one's diet for a variety of health and personal appearance reasons.

15.1 From Ordered to Disordered Eating Habits

Eating—a completely instinctive behavior for animals—serves an extraordinary number of psychological, social, and cultural purposes for humans. Eating practices may take on religious meanings; signify bonds within families and ethnic groups; and provide a means to express hostility, affection, prestige, or class values. Within the family, supplying, preparing, and even withholding food may be a means of expressing love, hatred, or power.

We are bombarded daily with our society's portrayal of the "ideal" body. Dieting is promoted to achieve this ideal body—eternally young and admired. Television programs, billboard and Internet advertisements, videogames, magazines, and movies suggest that an ultraslim body will bring happiness, love, and ultimate success. This fantasy notion is contradictory to the fact that the rate of obesity in our society increases with each passing year. In response to this social pressure, some of us take an extreme approach: the pathological pursuit of weight control or weight loss.

Early in life, we develop images of "acceptable" and "unacceptable" body types. Of the attributes that constitute attractiveness, many people view body weight as the most important, partly because we can control our weight somewhat. Fatness is the most dreaded deviation from our cultural ideals of body image, the one most derided and shunned. In a study about weight bias conducted by researchers at Yale University, nearly half of survey respondents said they would rather give up 1 year of life than live with obesity.

It is difficult to resist comparing ourselves to the "ideal" body, but not everyone can look like a fashion model. For some people, the disparity between their own body image and the perceived ideal may be enough to trigger an eating disorder.

FOOD: MORE THAN JUST A SOURCE OF NUTRIENTS

From birth, we link food with personal and emotional experiences. As infants, we associate milk with security and warmth, so the breast or bottle becomes a source of comfort and food. As noted in Section 1.1, even when older, most people continue to derive comfort and great pleasure from food. This is both a biological and a psychological phenomenon. Indeed, eating can stimulate the release of certain neurotransmitters (e.g., serotonin) and *natural opioids* (including **endorphins**), which produce a sense of calm and euphoria in the human body. Thus, in times of great stress, some people turn to food for its naturally calming, drug-like effect.

Food is also used as a reward or a bribe. You have probably heard or spoken something similar to the following comments:

- You can have your dessert if you eat five more bites of your vegetables.
- You cannot play until you clean your plate.
- I will eat the broccoli if you let me watch TV.
- If you love me, you will eat your dinner.

On the surface, using food as a reward or bribe seems harmless. Eventually, however, this practice may encourage both caregivers and children to use food to achieve goals other than satisfying hunger and nutrient needs. Food may then become much more than a source of nutrients. Regularly using food as a bargaining chip can contribute to abnormal eating patterns. Carried to the extreme, these patterns can lead to **disordered eating.**

Disordered eating refers to short-term, mild changes in eating patterns that occur in response to a stressful event, an illness, or even a desire to modify the diet for a variety of health and personal appearance reasons. The problem may be no more than a bad habit, a style of eating adapted from friends or family members, or an aspect of preparing for athletic competition. While disordered eating can lead to weight fluctuations or nutrient deficiencies, it rarely requires in-depth professional attention. If, however, disordered eating becomes sustained or distressing, starts to interfere with everyday activities, or is linked to physiological changes, then it may require professional intervention.

ORIGINS OF EATING DISORDERS

Given the common practice of dieting in North America, it can sometimes be difficult to draw a definitive line between disordered eating and an **eating disorder.** Indeed, many eating disorders start with a simple diet. Eating disorders then go on to involve physiological changes associated with food restriction, binge eating, purging, and fluctuations in weight. They also involve a number of emotional and cognitive changes that affect the way a person perceives and experiences his or her body, such as feelings of distress or extreme concern about body shape or weight. Eating disorders are not due to a failure of will or behavior; rather, they are real, treatable medical illnesses in which certain maladaptive patterns of eating take on a life of their own.

People who suffer from eating disorders can experience a wide range of health complications, including heart conditions and kidney failure, which may even lead to death. Recognition of eating disorders as important and treatable diseases, therefore, is critical. The three main types of eating disorders are **anorexia nervosa, bulimia nervosa,** and **binge-eating disorder.** Although it is convenient to label patients with a clear-cut diagnosis, the various types of eating disorders have more similarities than distinctions, particularly in their underlying biological and psychological processes.

Specific criteria from the recently revised *Diagnostic and Statistical Manual of Mental Disorders, 5th Edition (DSM-5)* are used by clinicians to diagnose eating disorders. As you read about the different eating disorders in this chapter, look for the relevant diagnostic criteria in Tables 15-1, 15-2, and 15-3. Keep in mind that individuals may exhibit a few symptoms of eating disorders but not enough to warrant a formal diagnosis. These people may be classified as having "subthreshold" eating disorders. Also, some people show characteristics of more than one eating disorder or may migrate from one disorder to another over time. Indeed, about half of women diagnosed as having anorexia nervosa eventually develop bulimic symptoms. Still, appreciating the differences between the disorders helps us to understand the various approaches to prevention and treatment.

Over the years, researchers have theorized that dysfunctional family interactions, especially between parents and adolescents, precipitate eating disorders. While unhealthy family relationships may lead to emotional distress, there is little scientific evidence that family functioning is a primary cause for eating disorders. In fact, insinuating that the family has caused a person's eating disorder leads to feelings of guilt and shame within the family that may actually hinder efforts at treatment (see Further Reading 8).

Scientists now recognize that genes bear much of the blame for eating disorders (see Further Reading 7). Twin studies have shown that when one of a set of identical twins (i.e., who have identical DNA) has an eating disorder, it is more likely that the other twin will also have an eating disorder—more likely than in sets of fraternal twins. Genetic factors account for an estimated 50% to 83% of the overall risk for developing an eating disorder.

A variety of genes could be involved in the development of eating disorders, including those responsible for the expression of hormones and neurotransmitters involved in weight regulation and eating behaviors (review Section 7.4). In about 80% of cases, eating disorders co-occur with other psychological disorders, such as anxiety disorders, major depression, and substance abuse disorders. It appears that genes influence the brain biology that determines how we perceive ourselves and respond to food stimuli or stress. In response to environmental triggers, some individuals may resort to self-destructive coping mechanisms, including disordered eating.

Because stressful life events may precipitate an eating disorder in genetically predisposed individuals, there is a strong association between eating disorders and a history of abuse. In fact, a history of physical and sexual abuse is about twice as common among people with eating disorders compared to the population as a whole (see Further Reading 13).

eating disorder Severe alterations in eating patterns linked to physiological changes. The alterations are associated with food restriction, binge eating, inappropriate compensatory behaviors, and fluctuations in weight. They also involve a number of emotional and cognitive changes that affect the way a person perceives and experiences his or her body.

anorexia nervosa An eating disorder characterized by extreme restriction of energy intake relative to requirements leading to significantly low body weight.

bulimia nervosa An eating disorder characterized by recurrent episodes of binge eating followed by inappropriate compensatory behaviors to prevent weight gain.

binge-eating disorder An eating disorder characterized by recurrent episodes of binge eating that are associated with marked distress and lack of control over behavior, but not followed by inappropriate compensatory behaviors to prevent weight gain.

Progression from Ordered to Disordered Eating

Attention to hunger and satiety signals; limitation of calorie intake to restore weight to a healthful level

↓

Some disordered eating habits begin as weight loss is attempted, such as very restricted eating

↓

Clinically evident eating disorder recognized

epigenetics Heritable changes in gene function that are independent of DNA sequence. For example, malnutrition during pregnancy may modify gene expression in the fetus and affect long-term body weight regulation in the offspring.

Other stressful life events, such as wartime military service, the death of a loved one, or constant social pressures to achieve thinness, are potential triggers for eating disorders.

In addition to genetics, researchers are studying **epigenetics** (heritable changes in gene expression that do not involve changes to the underlying DNA sequence), as it relates to the development of eating disorders (see Further Reading 3). Some studies suggest that maternal stress or hormone levels during pregnancy can predict the future development of an eating disorder in their children (see Further Reading 20).

Overall, genes may set the stage for development of an eating disorder, but environmental factors also play a role. Identifying genes linked to eating disorders eventually could help in tailoring prevention and treatment efforts for at-risk individuals. However, the psychiatric counseling that is part of current therapy will still be of value.

THE CHANGING FACE OF EATING DISORDERS

If you were asked to paint a picture of a person with an eating disorder, who would you depict? The predominant stereotype is that eating disorders only affect young, white females of middle or upper socioeconomic status. However, the face of eating disorders is changing.

When it comes to anorexia and bulimia, women do outnumber men by about 9 to 1. Perhaps social pressures can account for part of this disparity: in the media, women are held to standards of unnatural thinness, whereas the image conveyed for men is big and muscular. However, men are affected by eating disorders as well. Among men, exercise status and sexual orientation are factors that particularly influence development of anorexia and bulimia. Male athletes are more prone than nonathletes to develop these eating disorders, especially those who participate in sports that require weight classes (e.g., boxers, wrestlers, and jockeys) or where judging is partly based on aesthetics (e.g., ice skating, diving, or dancing) (see Further Reading 14). With reference to sexual orientation, the prevalence of eating disorders in gay men is two to three times that in heterosexual men (see Further Reading 10). With the release of *DSM-5* in 2013, binge-eating disorder is now recognized as a distinct eating disorder. While men make up less than 10% of cases of anorexia and bulimia, they account for about 40% of cases of binge-eating disorder.

Eating disorders typically develop during adolescence or young adulthood. Adolescence is a period of turbulent sexual and social tensions. At this time of life, teenagers establish their own identities. While declaring independence, they seek acceptance and support from peers and parents and react strongly to how they think others perceive them. At the same time, their bodies are changing, and much of the change is beyond their control. This is a time when extreme dieting practices may take root. It is alarming that eating disorders are being diagnosed at earlier ages (see Further Reading 4). Note that calorie restriction is not always evidenced as weight loss; stunting (failure to grow in height) and delayed sexual maturation also could be signs of eating disorders among children and adolescents.

▼ Individuals who participate in sports with weight classes, such as wrestling, may practice disordered eating behaviors in order to gain a competitive advantage over other athletes in a lower weight class. © Rubberball/ Getty Images

While much of the focus has been on youth, middle-aged and older adults are not immune to the devastating effects of eating disorders. In North America, aging baby boomers are the largest demographic group. Although eating disorders rarely make their first appearance late in adulthood, it may not be until later in adulthood that people who have suffered from eating disorders for years finally seek treatment. Furthermore, some recovered adults may relapse into former disordered eating practices. Research reveals that disordered eating behaviors and dissatisfaction with body weight and shape are quite common among older women. In one study, binge eating was reported by 3.5% of a community-based sample of women over age 50; purging behaviors, such as excessive exercise, were employed by 7.8% of the women (see Further Reading 9). Negative body image can have a dramatic impact on self-esteem and overall quality of life at any age.

Until recently, most researchers have reported that eating disorders primarily affect middle- and upper-class Caucasian women. Now, studies show greater similarities in the rates of body dissatisfaction and disordered eating behaviors across ethnic and cultural groups. Perhaps minorities with eating disorders have been less likely to seek help in the past due to fear of shame or stigma, lack of resources, or language barriers. It seems more likely, however, that health care workers have been less likely to diagnose non-Caucasians as having eating disorders. Previously, it seemed that non-Caucasian cultures were more accepting of larger body shapes, but mainstream pressures for thinness now cut across cultural lines.

Do you know someone who is at risk for an eating disorder? If so, suggest that the person seek a professional evaluation because the sooner treatment begins, the better the chances for recovery. However, do not try to diagnose eating disorders in your friends or family members. Only a professional can exclude other possible diseases and correctly diagnose an eating disorder. Once an eating disorder is diagnosed, immediate treatment is advisable. As a friend, the best you can do is to encourage an affected person to seek professional help. Such help is commonly available at student health centers and student guidance/counseling facilities on college campuses.

Our passion for thinness may have its roots in the Victorian era of the nineteenth century, which specialized in denying "unpleasant" physical realities, such as appetite and sexual desire. Flappers of the 1920s set the standard for the twentieth- and twenty-first-century trend for thinness. Since 1922, the BMI values of Miss America winners have steadily decreased; during the last three decades, most winners had a BMI in the "underweight" range (less than 18.5).

✓ CONCEPT CHECK 15.1

1. Differentiate between disordered eating and an eating disorder.
2. Describe how genetics and environment interact in the development of eating disorders.
3. Why are eating disorders more common among adolescents than other age groups?

15.2 Anorexia Nervosa

Anorexia nervosa is an eating disorder characterized by extreme weight loss, an irrational fear of weight gain, and a distorted body image. These three criteria are outlined in Table 15-1 and described in detail in this section. Anorexia nervosa affects an estimated 0.8% of American women.

First, people with anorexia nervosa severely restrict energy intake relative to requirements. The term *anorexia* implies a loss of appetite; however, a denial of one's appetite more accurately describes the behavior of people with anorexia nervosa. Low energy intake leads to a body weight that is significantly less than expected when compared to others of the same age, sex, stage of physical development, and activity level. While low body weight (i.e., less than 85% of expected body weight for a given age and sex or BMI of less than 17) may indicate anorexia nervosa, a variety of other medical conditions could also result in low body weight. The next two diagnostic criteria set anorexia nervosa apart from other problems related to poor food intake or low body weight.

The second key criterion for diagnosis of anorexia nervosa involves an intense fear of gaining weight or becoming obese. Some individuals with eating disorders may deny a fear of weight gain, so persistent behaviors that interfere with weight gain are also included in this criterion. To be diagnosed with anorexia nervosa, an individual must have experienced

TABLE 15-1 ■ Diagnostic Criteria for Anorexia Nervosa

A. Extreme dietary restriction that leads to significantly low body weight
B. Overwhelming distress about weight gain (or avoidance of behaviors that may lead to weight gain) despite having a low body weight
C. Disturbed perception of one's own body weight or shape, overemphasis on body weight or shape in determining self-worth, or failure to recognize the dangers of extremely low body weight

Source: Adapted from *Diagnostic and Statistical Manual for Mental Disorders,* 5th edition. Copyright 2013 by the American Psychiatric Association.

▲ For people with eating disorders, the difference between the real and desired body images may be too difficult to accept. See the website womenshealth.gov/body-image.
© Steve Niedorf Photography/Stone/Getty Images

fear of weight gain or practiced behaviors to prevent weight gain at least 75% of the days in the last 3 months.

Third, as depicted in the photo, individuals with anorexia nervosa have a distorted body image. The term *nervosa* refers to an attitude of disgust with one's body. These individuals irrationally believe they are fat, even though others constantly comment on their thin physique. Some people with anorexia realize they are thin but continue to be haunted by certain areas of their bodies that they believe to be fat (such as thighs, buttocks, and stomach). Even though extremely low body weight results in severe health effects, as described later in this section, people with anorexia do not acknowledge the problem. They may persist in efforts at weight loss and try to thwart efforts of family members and medical professionals to increase their body weight to a healthy level.

Note that there are two subtypes of anorexia nervosa: a restricting type and a binge-eating/purging type. All individuals with anorexia nervosa severely restrict their calorie intake to achieve or maintain a low body weight. Men and women with the binge-eating/purging type of anorexia nervosa also engage in episodes of binge-eating and/or compensatory behaviors to rid the body of calories. The difference between bulimia nervosa and anorexia nervosa of the binge-eating/purging subtype is that individuals with anorexia nervosa have low body weight (e.g., BMI <17), while individuals with bulimia tend to have normal or high BMI.

COMMON BEHAVIORS OF ANOREXIA NERVOSA

Individuals who develop anorexia share some common traits. Take a young woman, for example, who is described by parents and teachers as responsible, meticulous, and obedient. She holds herself to high standards of performance and appearance. She is competitive and perfectionistic. At home, she may not allow clutter in her bedroom. Clinicians note that after a physical examination, she folds her examination gown very carefully and cleans up the examination room before leaving. As mentioned, both genetic and environmental factors contribute to both our self-perception and our responses to stress. These obsessive personality traits—rigidity and perfectionism—are related to the same brain biology that predicts development of eating disorders.

Anorexia nervosa may begin as a simple attempt to lose weight. A comment from a well-meaning friend, relative, or coach suggesting that the person seems to be gaining weight or is too fat may be all that is needed. The stress of having to maintain a certain weight to look attractive or perform better can also lead to disordered eating. Abusive experiences, a difficult breakup, or the stress of leaving home for college are examples of triggers for extreme dieting. Changing one's appearance might be viewed as a way to avoid future conflict or ensure success in a new situation.

Still, losing weight does not help people deal with anger, grief, anxiety, or depression. If these psychological issues are not resolved, individuals may intensify efforts to lose weight "to look even better," rather than work through unresolved psychological concerns. At first, dieting becomes the life focus. Such persons may derive a sense of achievement from their "success" at controlling body weight or perceive improvements in other areas of their life. What began as a diet leads to very abnormal self-perceptions and eating habits, such as cutting a pea in half before eating it.

Extreme dieting is the most important predictor of an eating disorder. (Adolescents expressing concern about their weight should be advised to focus on exercise, which does not appear to impart a risk for subsequent problems.) Once dieting begins, a person developing anorexia nervosa does not stop. As the disorder progresses, the range of foods eaten may narrow; the list of "safe foods" shortens, whereas the list of "unsafe foods" gets longer. Abnormal habits include hiding and storing food or spreading food around a plate to make it look as if much has been eaten. A person with anorexia nervosa may cook a large meal and watch others eat it while refusing to eat anything, or may insist on having different meals from the rest of the family. Frequent weighing—multiple times per day—is common (see Further Reading 24).

As mentioned, among some people with anorexia nervosa, disordered eating behaviors may eventually include bingeing on large amounts of food in a short time and/or inappropriate behaviors to compensate for the large number of calories consumed. Covered further in

▲ Extreme dietary rules severely limit nutritional intake among people with anorexia nervosa. © Stockbyte/PunchStock

Section 15.3, compensatory behaviors (sometimes called purging) include vomiting, using laxatives or diuretics, and excessive exercise. Thus, people with anorexia nervosa may exist in a state of continuous semistarvation or may alternate between periods of starvation and periods of bingeing and purging.

A state of semistarvation can cause depression, irritability, and hostility. People with anorexia may be excessively critical of themselves and usually withdraw from family and friends. Despite a strong drive for perfection, performance in school, sports, and work begins to deteriorate. (See Section 15.8 for a glimpse of the inner turmoil of a woman with anorexia nervosa.)

Ultimately, a person with anorexia nervosa eats very little food; 300 to 600 kcal daily is not unusual. In place of food, the person may consume up to 20 cans of diet soft drinks and chew many pieces of sugarless gum each day.

> A disturbing Internet trend is the attempt to promote eating disorders as a way of life. Some individuals with eating disorders have personified their illness into a role model named "Ana," who tells them what to eat and mocks them when they don't lose weight. Similarly, pro-"Mia" sites provide tips and encouragement for people with bulimia (e.g., how to induce vomiting and cover up evidence of compensatory behaviors). Pro-Ana and pro-Mia websites reject the serious health risks of eating disorders and instead dispense unsafe "thinspiration" to vulnerable individuals (see Further Reading 1).

PHYSICAL EFFECTS OF ANOREXIA NERVOSA

The state of semistarvation disturbs many body systems as it forces the body to conserve energy stores as much as possible (Fig. 15-1). Many of the following complications can be

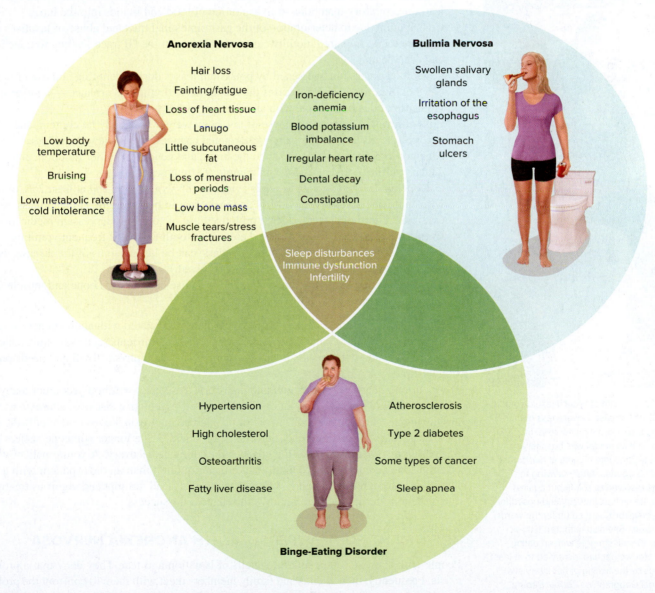

Anorexia Nervosa

- Hair loss
- Fainting/fatigue
- Loss of heart tissue
- Lanugo
- Little subcutaneous fat
- Loss of menstrual periods
- Low bone mass
- Muscle tears/stress fractures
- Low body temperature
- Bruising
- Low metabolic rate/cold intolerance

Bulimia Nervosa

- Swollen salivary glands
- Irritation of the esophagus
- Stomach ulcers

(Anorexia ∩ Bulimia)
- Iron-deficiency anemia
- Blood potassium imbalance
- Irregular heart rate
- Dental decay
- Constipation

(Center)
- Sleep disturbances
- Immune dysfunction
- Infertility

Binge-Eating Disorder

- Hypertension
- High cholesterol
- Osteoarthritis
- Fatty liver disease
- Atherosclerosis
- Type 2 diabetes
- Some types of cancer
- Sleep apnea

FIGURE 15-1 ▲ Physical effects of eating disorders. Although this figure contains many potential consequences, it is not an exhaustive list. Some of these physical effects can also serve as warning signs that a problem exists.

lanugo Downlike hair that appears after a person has lost much body fat through semistarvation. The hair stands erect and traps air, acting as insulation for the body to compensate for the relative lack of body fat, which usually functions as insulation.

▲ In 2010, the death of French fashion model Isabelle Caro increased awareness of the serious nature of anorexia nervosa. In 2006, the 5-foot, 4-inch model was hospitalized when she slipped into a coma at her lowest weight of 55 pounds. After surviving the coma, she resolved to speak out against dieting in the fashion industry and posed for a controversial billboard ad under the words "No Anorexia." She also authored a book about her 15-year struggle with an eating disorder. Her weight had increased to at least 80 pounds by the filming of her interview for National Geographic's *Taboo: Beauty* documentary, but she died, at age 28, before it aired. © Ernesto Ruscio/Getty Images

reversed by returning to a healthy weight, provided the duration of the semistarvation has not been too long (see Further Reading 17).

- Lowered body temperature and cold intolerance from loss of insulating fat layer
- Slowed metabolic rate from decreased synthesis of thyroid hormones
- Decreased heart rate as metabolism slows, leading to premature fatigue, fainting, and an overwhelming need for sleep (Other changes in heart function may occur as well, including loss of heart tissue, irregular heart rhythm, and low blood pressure.)
- Iron-deficiency anemia, which leads to further weakness
- Rough, dry, scaly, cracked, and/or cold skin, which may show multiple bruises because of the loss of the protective fat layer normally present under the skin
- Low white blood cell count, which increases the risk of infection—one cause of death in people with anorexia nervosa
- Abnormal feeling of fullness or bloating, which can last for several hours after eating
- Loss of hair from the head
- Appearance of **lanugo**—downy hairs on the body that trap air to partially counteract heat loss that occurs with loss of fat tissue
- Impaired swallowing ability due to loss of muscle tissue in the pharynx, which could lead to respiratory infections from aspiration of food and liquids into the lungs
- Constipation due to deterioration of the gastrointestinal tract and abuse of laxatives (In extreme cases, impaired motility can cause rupture of the GI tract, leading to infection and even death.)
- Low blood potassium, worsened by potassium losses during vomiting and use of some types of diuretics, which increases the risk of heart rhythm disturbances—another leading cause of death in people with anorexia nervosa
- Loss of menstrual periods because of low body weight, low body fat content, and the stress of the disease; accompanying hormonal changes contribute to bone loss
- Changes in brain size, blood flow to the brain, and neurotransmitter function, all of which contribute to depression and complicate treatment attempts
- Osteopenia or osteoporosis, which is evident in 85% of women and at least 25% of men with anorexia nervosa (Bone loss is due to decreased body weight and lean mass, several related hormonal changes, and prolonged use of some antidepressant medications.)
- Eventual loss of teeth caused by acid erosion of tooth enamel if frequent vomiting occurs (Tooth loss, along with low bone mass, can be lasting signs of the disease, even if other physical and mental problems are resolved.)
- Muscle tears and stress fractures in athletes because of decreased bone and muscle mass
- Sleep disturbances and depression

Many of the psychological and physical problems associated with anorexia nervosa arise from insufficient calorie intake, as well as deficiencies of nutrients such as thiamin, calcium, and iron. A person with this disorder is psychologically and physically ill and needs professional help.

About one-quarter of those with anorexia nervosa recover within 6 years, but many will struggle with the disease throughout life. Among all psychiatric diseases, anorexia nervosa has the highest mortality rate: 2% to 5% of people with anorexia nervosa eventually die from the disease—from heart ailments, infections, or suicide. The longer someone suffers from this eating disorder, the poorer the chances for complete recovery. A young patient with a brief episode and a supportive family has a better outlook than an older patient with a long history of disordered eating and no family support. Overall, prompt and vigorous treatment, and close long-term follow-up improve the chances for success.

TREATMENT FOR THE PERSON WITH ANOREXIA NERVOSA

People with anorexia often sink into shells of isolation and fear. They deny that a problem exists. Frequently, their friends and family members meet with them to confront the problem in a loving way. This is called an *intervention*. They present evidence of the problem and encourage immediate treatment.

Treatment requires a multidisciplinary team of experienced physicians, registered dietitian nutritionists, psychologists, and other health professionals working together. An ideal setting is an eating disorders clinic in a medical center. Outpatient therapy generally begins first. This may be extended to 3 to 5 days per week. Day hospitalization (6 to 12 hours per day) is another option. Total hospitalization is necessary once a person falls below 75% of expected weight, experiences acute medical problems, and/or exhibits severe psychological problems or suicidal risk. Still, even in the most skilled hands at the finest facilities, efforts may fail. This tells us that the prevention of anorexia nervosa is of utmost importance (see Further Reading 24).

The health care team must gain the cooperation and trust of the person with anorexia and work together to restore body weight, correct medical complications, and treat mental illness. However, the individual who has been barely existing in a state of semistarvation cannot focus on much besides food. Dreams and even morbid thoughts about food will interfere with therapy until the person regains sufficient weight. Currently, the average time for recovery from anorexia nervosa is 7 years. Many insurance companies cover only a fraction of the estimated $150,000 cost of treatment.

Nutrition Therapy The ultimate goal of nutrition therapy is to restore body weight to a healthy range. The patient must increase oral food intake and gain enough weight to raise the metabolic rate to normal and reverse as many physical signs of the disease as possible. The refeeding plan is designed first to minimize or stop any further weight loss. Then, the focus shifts to restoring appropriate food habits. After this, the expectation can be switched to slowly gaining weight; 2 to 3 pounds per week is appropriate. Tube and/or intravenous (IV) feeding is used only if immediate renourishment is required, as this can frighten the person and cause him or her to distrust medical staff.

Persons with anorexia nervosa need considerable reassurance during the refeeding process because of uncomfortable and unfamiliar effects—such as bloating and increased body temperature. These symptoms occur because of starvation-related changes in GI tract function and will usually resolve over time, but they can be frightening for the person recovering from anorexia. Rapid changes in electrolytes and minerals in the blood associated with refeeding—especially potassium, phosphorus, and magnesium—can be dangerous. Therefore, monitoring blood levels of these minerals is of critical importance during the process of incorporating more food into the diet.

In addition to helping the person with anorexia nervosa reach and maintain adequate nutritional status, the registered dietitian nutritionist provides accurate nutrition information throughout the treatment, promotes a healthy attitude toward food, and helps the person learn to eat in response to natural hunger and satiety cues. The focus then turns to identifying healthy and adequate food choices that promote weight gain to achieve and maintain a clinically estimated weight-range goal: a BMI of 20 or more for adults or BMI-for-age between the 25th and 85th percentile for children (see Section 19.1). For children and adolescents, additional energy needs for growth must be considered.

As noted, nutrient deficiencies are commonly seen in patients with anorexia nervosa. As treatment progresses, the health care team will work with the patient to fully restore nutritional status. A multivitamin and mineral supplement will be added, as well as enough calcium to raise intake to about 1500 milligrams per day. Bone loss will not likely be completely restored, even if nutrition is adequate. Particularly in adolescent patients, a critical time for accrual of bone mass or gains in height may have been missed. However, supplementation with calcium and vitamin D is still necessary to prevent further bone loss.

Excessive physical activity prevents weight gain, so professionals must help people with anorexia nervosa to regulate their activity. At many treatment centers, moderate bed rest is used in the early stages of treatment to help promote weight gain.

Experienced professional help is the key for effectively treating anorexia nervosa (see Further Reading 18). Persons with anorexia may be on the verge of suicide and starvation, and may be very resistant to therapy. Surrendering control over eating can be scary and frustrating. They may try to hide weight loss by wearing many layers of clothes, putting coins in their pockets, and drinking numerous glasses of water before stepping on the scale.

Links exist between disordered eating behaviors and substance abuse, particularly alcohol abuse. Some people may use food restriction or purging to offset the calories consumed during drinking binges. Popularly called "drunkorexia," this practice can lead to severe nutrient deficiencies and dehydration.

Psychological Therapy Once the immediate physical problems of anorexia nervosa are addressed, the focus of treatment shifts to the underlying emotional problems that preceded the eating disorder. If therapists can discover the psychological conflicts that triggered the disorder, they can develop more effective treatment strategies. Education about the medical consequences of semistarvation is also helpful. A key aspect of psychological treatment is showing affected individuals how to regain control of other facets of their lives and cope with difficult situations. As eating evolves into a normal routine, they can turn to previously neglected activities.

Family-based therapy (usually 6 to 12 months) is the preferred method of psychological treatment for anorexia nervosa among *adolescents* (see Further Reading 25). Importantly, family-based therapy for anorexia nervosa absolves parents of blame for the eating disorder. Early treatment focuses on ways the family can help the person with anorexia achieve a healthy body weight. Eventually, responsibility for eating and weight control will be transferred back to the patient. Beyond eating behaviors, family-based therapy for anorexia nervosa also helps the patient to establish healthy relationships with parents and other family members.

At this time, there is little evidence to support one particular type of psychological therapy over another for *adults* with anorexia nervosa. Therapists may use **cognitive behavioral therapy,** which involves helping the person confront and change irrational beliefs about body image, eating, relationships, and weight. However, after subsisting in a starved state for months or years, the brain chemistry of a person with anorexia nervosa is so altered that attempts at cognitive restructuring are usually not effective in the early stages of illness. Underlying issues that may have triggered the eating disorder, such as sexual abuse, also must be identified and addressed by the therapist. Guided self-help groups for people with

cognitive behavioral therapy
Psychological therapy in which the person's assumptions about dieting, body weight, and related issues are confronted. New ways of thinking are explored and then practiced by the person. In this way, an individual can learn new ways to control disordered eating behaviors and related life stress.

CASE STUDY Eating Disorders—Steps to Recovery

© Ted Foxx/Alamy

At age 16, Sarah suddenly became self-conscious about her body when her peers teased her about being overweight. She began exercising to an aerobics video for an hour each day and found that she had success in losing weight; this was the beginning of her obsession to be thin. Next, Sarah turned to eating less food to lose even more weight and began eliminating certain foods from her diet, such as candy and meat. She increased her water and vegetable intake and chewed sugarless gum to curb her appetite. Once she began dieting, it was impossible for her to stop. She enjoyed having a high degree of self-control over her body. Still, Sarah was literally obsessed with food, even staring at others while they were eating a meal. She occasionally cooked large meals and then refused to eat all but a few bites. By the time Sarah was 19 years old and 5 feet 6 inches tall, her weight had dropped from 150 to 105 pounds. Her family was concerned about her weight status, demanding that she go to a physician for an evaluation. Sarah was not happy about this idea because she worried the doctors would force her to eat and gain back unwanted weight, but she believed that her family would stop pestering her if she went. Sarah did not think she had a problem; she thought she was still grotesquely overweight. She did notice, however, that she always felt cold and was concerned that she had not menstruated in a year.

Answer the following questions and check your responses at the end of this chapter.

1. Sarah appears to have an eating disorder. Which eating disorder best describes her behavior?
2. List the behaviors that Sarah developed between ages 16 and 19 that are signs of the development of this eating disorder.
3. What physical symptoms of this disorder does Sarah have (review Fig. 15-1)?
4. Outline the therapies you think the physician will prescribe for Sarah. Where could she go for the therapy she needs? Which types of professionals would be involved?
5. Do you think Sarah has developed any vitamin or mineral deficiencies? Which ones would be most likely? How could these deficiencies be best treated?
6. What is the likelihood that she will fully recover from her condition?

eating disorders, as well as their families and friends, represent additional nonthreatening first steps into treatment.

Pharmacological Therapy There are no FDA-approved medications specifically for the treatment of anorexia nervosa. Rather, food is the treatment of choice for people with this disorder. Generally, medications are not effective in managing the primary symptoms of anorexia nervosa. Fluoxetine (Prozac®) and related medications may stabilize recovery once 85% of expected body weight has been attained. These medications work by prolonging serotonin activity in the brain, which in turn regulates mood and feelings of satiety. A variety of other pharmacological agents, such as olanzapine (Zyprexa®), may have some role in treating mood changes, anxiety, or psychotic symptoms associated with anorexia nervosa, but they have limited value unless weight gain is also achieved (see Further Reading 25).

With professional help, many people with anorexia nervosa can lead normal lives. Although they may not be totally cured, recovering individuals no longer depend on unusual eating habits to cope with daily problems. They recover a sense of normalcy in their lives. Longer follow-up—sometimes several years—is associated with better outcomes. Recovery rates are around 20% to 30% for short-term therapy but increase to 70% to 80% with 8 years of follow-up. No universal approach exists, because each case is unique. Establishing a strong relationship with either a therapist or another supportive person is especially important to recovery. Once people with anorexia nervosa feel understood and accepted by others, they can begin to build a sense of self and exercise some autonomy. As they learn alternative coping mechanisms, individuals with anorexia nervosa can relinquish dysfunctional relationships with food and instead develop healthy personal relationships.

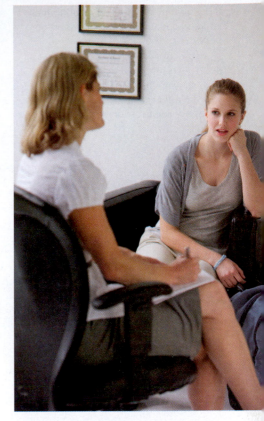

▲ Early treatment for an eating disorder, such as anorexia nervosa, improves chances of success. © Tetra Images/Getty Images

✓ CONCEPT CHECK 15.2

1. Identify the three diagnostic criteria for anorexia nervosa.
2. List five physical effects of anorexia nervosa.
3. Describe elements of nutritional, psychological, and pharmacological therapy for anorexia nervosa.

15.3 Bulimia Nervosa

Literally translated, *bulimia* means ravenous (oxlike) hunger. This eating disorder is characterized by recurrent episodes of binge eating followed by some type of compensatory behavior to prevent weight gain (see Table 15-2). Also, as with anorexia nervosa, individuals with bulimia nervosa overvalue body weight and shape.

TABLE 15-2 ■ Diagnostic Criteria for Bulimia Nervosa

A. Repeated binge eating, characterized by: 1. Eating a large amount of food in a short period of time (e.g., within 2 hours) 2. Experiencing a loss of control over eating during binges
B. Repeated use of unsafe means of preventing weight gain (e.g., self-induced vomiting; inappropriate use of laxatives, diuretics, enemas, or other medications; fasting; or excessive exercise)
C. Binge-compensate cycles occur at least one time per week for 3 months
D. Undue influence of body weight or shape on self-evaluation
E. Behaviors are distinct from the binge-eating/purging subtype of anorexia nervosa

Source: Adapted from *Diagnostic and Statistical Manual for Mental Disorders*, 5th edition. Copyright 2013 by the American Psychiatric Association.

binge eating Consuming an abnormally large amount of food within a short time period (e.g., 2 hours).

compensatory behaviors Actions taken to rid the body of excess calories and/or to alleviate guilt or anxiety associated with a binge; examples include vomiting, misuse of laxatives, or excessive exercise.

Binge eating is defined as consuming an abnormally large amount of food within a short time period (e.g., 2 hours). These binges are characterized by a lack of control over the food consumed. **Compensatory behaviors** (also known as purging) used to rid the body of excess calories consumed during a binge may include vomiting; misuse of laxatives, diuretics, or enemas; or excessive exercise. For a diagnosis of bulimia nervosa, binge eating followed by inappropriate compensatory behaviors must take place at least four times per month over a period of 3 months or more.

It is likely that many people with bulimic behavior are never diagnosed. People with bulimia nervosa lead secret lives, hiding their abnormal eating habits. Moreover, it can be difficult to recognize the disorder based on appearance, because people with bulimia nervosa are usually at or slightly above normal weight. By rough estimate, among North American women, approximately 2.6% will develop bulimia nervosa by the age of 20. An estimated 4% of college-age women have bulimia nervosa. About 10% of cases occur in men. However, most diagnoses of bulimia nervosa rely on self-reports, so the disorder may be much more widespread than commonly thought.

COMMON BEHAVIORS OF BULIMIA NERVOSA

Bulimia nervosa involves episodes of binge eating followed by various means to rid the body of excess calories. Susceptible people often have genetic factors and lifestyle patterns that predispose them to becoming overweight, and many try frequent weight-reduction diets as teenagers. The person with bulimia nervosa may think of food constantly; however, unlike the person with anorexia nervosa, who turns away from food when faced with problems, the person with bulimia nervosa turns toward food in critical situations. Also, unlike those with anorexia nervosa, people with bulimia nervosa recognize their behavior as abnormal.

Individuals with bulimia nervosa tend to be impulsive, which may be expressed in behaviors such as stealing, increased sexual activity, drug and alcohol abuse (see Newsworthy Nutrition), self-mutilation, or attempted suicide. Some experts have suggested that part of the problem may actually arise from an inability to control responses to impulse and desire. Approximately half of the people with bulimia nervosa have major depression. Lingering effects of child abuse may be one reason for these feelings. Many people with bulimia nervosa report that they have been sexually abused. They appear competent to outsiders, while they actually feel out of control, ashamed, and frustrated.

For intake to qualify as a binge, an atypically large amount of food must be consumed in a short time and the person must exhibit a lack of control over the behavior. Among sufferers of bulimia nervosa, bingeing often alternates with attempts to rigidly restrict food intake. Elaborate food rules are common, such as avoiding all sweets. Thus, eating just one cookie or doughnut may cause individuals with this disorder to feel as though they have broken a rule. At that point, in the mind of a person with bulimia, the objectionable food must be eliminated. Usually this leads to further overeating, partly because it is easier to regurgitate a large amount of food than a small amount.

Binge-compensate cycles may be practiced daily, weekly, or across longer intervals. A specific time often is set aside. Most binge eating occurs at night, when other people are less likely to interrupt, and usually lasts from 30 minutes to 2 hours. A binge can be triggered by stress, boredom, loneliness, depression, or any combination thereof. It often follows a period of strict dieting and thus can be linked to intense hunger. The binge is not at all like normal eating; once begun, it seems to propel itself. The person not only loses control but generally does not even taste or enjoy food during a binge. This separates the practice from overeating.

Most commonly, individuals with bulimia consume cakes, cookies, ice cream, and other high-carbohydrate convenience foods during binges, because these foods can be purged relatively easily and comfortably by vomiting. In a single binge, foods supplying 3000 kcal or more may be eaten. Compensatory behaviors follow in hopes that no weight will be gained; however, even when vomiting follows the binge, 33% to 75% of the calories taken in are still absorbed, inevitably causing some weight gain. When laxatives or enemas are used, about 90% of the calories are absorbed, as laxatives act in the large intestine, beyond the point of

Bingeing and purging (via vomiting) was evident in pre-Christian Roman times but was practiced in a group setting. The eating disorder bulimia nervosa is generally practiced in private. It was first described in the medical literature in 1979.

▲ Excessive exercise can be one component of bulimia if it is used as a way to offset the calorie intake from a binge. Exercise is considered excessive when it is done at inappropriate times or settings, or when a person does it despite injury or other medical complications. © Comstock Images

most nutrient absorption. The belief that purging soon after bingeing will prevent excessive calorie absorption and weight gain is a misconception.

At the onset of bulimia nervosa, sufferers often induce vomiting by placing their fingers deep into the mouth. They may bite down on these fingers inadvertently, resulting in bite marks and scars around the knuckles, a characteristic sign of this disorder. Once the disease is established, however, a person may be able to vomit simply by contracting the abdominal muscles. Vomiting may also occur spontaneously.

Another way a person with bulimia may attempt to compensate for a binge is by engaging in excessive exercise to expend a large amount of calories. In this practice, referred to as "debting," individuals try to estimate the amount of calories eaten during a binge and then exercise to counteract the excess.

People with bulimia nervosa are not proud of their behavior. After a binge, they usually feel guilty and depressed. Over time, they experience low self-esteem, feel hopeless about their situation, and are caught in a vicious cycle of obsession (Fig. 15-2). Compulsive lying, shoplifting to obtain food, and drug abuse can further intensify these feelings. A person discovered in the act of bingeing by a friend or family member may order the intruder to "get out" and "go away." Sufferers gradually distance themselves from others, spending more time preoccupied by and engaging in bingeing and compensating.

Because individuals with bulimia nervosa attempt to hide their behaviors, it may be difficult to identify them early in the disease process, when treatment is likely to be most effective. An early warning sign of bulimia is frequent trips to the bathroom during or after meals. To cover the sounds of vomiting, these individuals may run the bathroom fan or turn on the shower. Despite efforts to disguise the behavior with air fresheners, mouthwash, or breath mints, there may be a lingering odor of vomit. Be suspicious of packages or receipts for laxatives, diuretics, diet pills, or enemas. People who use exercise to compensate for binges are usually preoccupied with their workout schedule or might seem extremely stressed when they are unable to exercise. If you suspect someone is falling victim to bulimia nervosa, encourage the individual to get professional help. Early intervention can prevent some of the serious physical health effects described next.

FIGURE 15-2 ▲ Bulimia nervosa's vicious cycle of obsession. © Peter Dazeley/ Getty Images

PHYSICAL EFFECTS OF BULIMIA NERVOSA

Repeated vomiting is a physically destructive method of purging. Indeed, the majority of health problems associated with bulimia nervosa, as noted here, arise from vomiting (see Further Reading 18):

- Repeated exposure of teeth to stomach acid causes demineralization (Fig. 15-3), making the teeth painful and sensitive to heat, cold, and acids. Eventually, the teeth may decay severely, erode away from fillings, and fall out. Dental professionals are sometimes the first health professionals to notice signs of bulimia nervosa.
- Blood potassium can drop significantly with regular vomiting or the use of certain diuretics. This can disturb the heart's rhythm and even produce sudden death.
- Salivary glands may swell as a result of infection and irritation from persistent vomiting.
- Ulcers, bleeding, and perforations may develop in the stomach or esophagus.
- Constipation may result as a complication of frequent laxative use.
- Syrup of ipecac, formerly used as a home remedy to induce vomiting in cases of accidental poisoning, has been abused by people with bulimia nervosa. Major health agencies (e.g., the American Academy of Pediatrics) now advise against its use, and most pharmacies no longer sell it because ipecac is now known to be toxic to the heart, liver, and kidneys.

FIGURE 15-3 ▲ Dental erosion resulting from frequent episodes of self-induced vomiting by a patient with bulimia nervosa. Courtesy of Carl M. Allen, DDS, MSD

▲ Developing regular eating habits helps a person with bulimia nervosa to stop the binge-purge cycle. © Royalty-Free/Corbis

The mortality rate for patients with bulimia nervosa is estimated around 0.4%. Patients with anorexia are about five times more likely to die from their disease than those with bulimia nervosa. Nonetheless, bulimia is a serious and potentially debilitating disorder that can lead to death, usually from suicide, cardiac arrest, or overwhelming infections.

TREATMENT FOR THE PERSON WITH BULIMIA NERVOSA

Therapy for bulimia nervosa, as for anorexia nervosa, requires a team of experienced clinicians (see Further Reading 23). Individuals with bulimia nervosa are less likely than those with anorexia nervosa to enter treatment in a state of semistarvation. However, if a person with bulimia nervosa has lost significant weight, this must be treated before psychological treatment begins. Although clinicians have yet to agree on the best therapy for bulimia nervosa, they generally agree that treatment should last at least 16 weeks. Hospitalization may be indicated in cases of extreme laxative abuse, regular vomiting, substance abuse, and depression, especially if physical harm is evident.

Nutritional Therapy Nutritional counseling by a registered dietitian nutritionist has two main goals: reestablishing regular eating habits and correcting misconceptions about food.

In general, the focus is not on stopping bingeing and purging per se, but on developing regular eating habits. Once this is achieved, the binge-purge cycle should start to break down. Initially, the registered dietitian nutritionist must help the person to decrease the amount of food in a binge. This will decrease the risk of esophageal tears from related purging by vomiting. A decrease in the frequency of this type of purging will also decrease damage to the teeth. Next, to develop a normal eating pattern, some specialists encourage their patients to develop daily meal plans and keep a food diary in which they record food intake, internal sensations of hunger, environmental factors that precipitate binges, and thoughts and feelings that accompany binge-compensate cycles.

Avoiding binge foods and not constantly stepping on a scale may be recommended early in treatment. Setting time limits for the completion of meals and snacks can also be

Newsworthy Nutrition

Substance Use Among Adolescents With Eating Disorders

Previous research suggests a relationship between eating disorders and substance use. Between 2001 and 2012, researchers collected data from 290 adolescents (ages 12 to 18) with eating disorders who sought treatment at the University of Chicago Medical Center. Analyses showed that 24.6% of adolescents with anorexia nervosa and 48.7% of adolescents with bulimia nervosa had used substances. Alcohol was most commonly used, followed by cannabis, tobacco, and other illicit drugs. Binge drinking was reported by 27.5% of those who used alcohol. Substance use in this cohort was lower than use reported for the general population of adolescents, but this may be due to underreporting or the relatively young sample. It is notable that substance use was twice as common among adolescents with bulimia compared to anorexia. As hypothesized, the authors found that frequency of binge-purge cycles was directly related to substance use among adolescents with bulimia nervosa. The authors pointed out that the impulsive and risky nature of alcohol, tobacco, and other drug use is consistent with some behavioral traits of bulimia nervosa, which may be related to disruptions in neuroendocrine pathways. It is imperative to identify these behaviors early because the coexistence of eating disorders with substance use greatly increases health risks for adolescents.

Source: Mann AP and others: Factors associated with substance use in adolescents with eating disorders. *Journal of Adolescent Health* 55:182, 2014.

important for people with eating disorders. Many individuals with bulimia eat quickly and have trouble interpreting satiety cues. Suggesting that they put their utensil down after each bite is a behavioral technique that a therapist might try during recovery for bulimia. (In comparison, many people with anorexia eat in an excessively slow manner—for example, taking 1 hour to eat a muffin cut into tiny, bite-size pieces.)

Providing accurate information about bulimia nervosa and its consequences can help affected individuals to recognize the need to change the behavior. Over the long term, individuals are discouraged from following strict rules about dieting, because this mimics the typical obsessive attitudes associated with bulimia nervosa. Rather, they must learn to honor internal hunger and satiety cues and to choose a variety of foods from each food group.

Psychological Therapy The primary aim of psychotherapy is to improve people's self-acceptance and to help them be less concerned about body weight. Cognitive behavioral therapy is generally used. Psychotherapy helps correct the all-or-none mentality that is typical of people with bulimia nervosa: "If I eat one cookie, I'm a failure and might as well binge." The premise of this psychotherapy is that if abnormal attitudes and beliefs can be altered, normal eating will follow. In addition, the therapist guides the person in establishing food habits that will minimize bingeing: to avoid fasting, to eat regular meals, and to use alternative methods—other than eating—to cope with stressful situations. Another goal of therapy is to help the person with bulimia to accept some depression and self-doubt as normal. Group therapy can be useful to foster strong social support.

The binge-purge cycle can create an initial state of euphoria in the person. Giving up this euphoria has been equated to giving up an addiction.

Pharmacological Therapy Although pharmacological agents should not be used as the sole treatment for bulimia nervosa, studies indicate that some medications may be beneficial in conjunction with other therapies. Fluoxetine (Prozac®) is the only antidepressant that has been approved by FDA for use in the treatment of bulimia nervosa (in combination with psychological therapy). It can help to increase feelings of satiety after eating and thereby reduce the frequency of binges. (Women of childbearing age should be cautious because fluoxetine has been linked to increased rates of miscarriages and other complications of pregnancy.) Physicians also may prescribe other similar forms of antidepressants, other classes of psychiatric medications, or certain antiseizure medications (e.g., topiramate [Topamax®]).

People with bulimia nervosa must recognize that they have a serious disorder that can have grave medical complications if not treated. Relapse is likely, so therapy should be long term. As seen with anorexia, earlier intervention and longer duration of treatment are associated with better outcomes. After just 1 year of therapy, about one-fourth of patients with bulimia nervosa experience recovery, but most will require many years of therapy. Those with bulimia nervosa need professional help because of their depression and high risk for suicide. About 50% of people with bulimia nervosa recover completely from the disorder. Others continue to struggle with it to varying degrees for a lifetime. Such a difficult course of treatment underscores the need for prevention.

✓ CONCEPT CHECK 15.3

1. Describe the eating behaviors of bulimia nervosa. What triggers them? What distinguishes them from simple overeating at a holiday meal?

2. What is a compensatory behavior? List at least three examples of inappropriate compensatory behaviors.

3. Describe at least three physical effects of bulimia nervosa.

4. Outline the basic components of nutritional therapy for people with bulimia nervosa. How do psychological and pharmacological therapies contribute to recovery?

Up to 25% of college-age women exhibit some degree of binge eating. Such behavior may have a negative impact on physical appearance, health, social life, and academics.

15.4 Binge-Eating Disorder

First officially described in 1994, binge-eating disorder is a growing, complex, and serious problem. With the 2013 publication of *DSM-5,* binge-eating disorder is now recognized as a distinct eating disorder alongside anorexia nervosa and bulimia nervosa. Its inclusion as an official diagnosis will improve the availability of treatments and success of outcomes for people who suffer from the disorder.

Generally, binge-eating disorder can be defined as binge-eating episodes not accompanied by compensatory behaviors (as seen in bulimia nervosa) at least one time per week, on average, for at least 3 months. The diagnostic criteria for binge-eating disorder are listed in Table 15-3.

While anorexia and bulimia disproportionately affect females, about 40% of people with binge-eating disorder are males. For adults, the lifetime prevalence of binge-eating disorder is estimated to be about 3.5% for women and about 2.0% for men. Among the general U.S. population, about 4 million have this disorder. However, many more people in the general population are likely to have less severe forms of the disorder that do not meet all the criteria described in Table 15-3. The number of cases of binge-eating disorder is far greater than that of either anorexia nervosa or bulimia nervosa. This disorder is most common among the severely obese and those with a long history of frequent restrictive dieting, although obesity is not a criterion for having binge-eating disorder. Compared to anorexia and bulimia, binge-eating disorder tends to be diagnosed later in life, usually in the late 40s or early 50s.

Like anorexia and bulimia, binge-eating disorder seems to arise when a person with a genetic predisposition for the disorder is stressed by an environmental trigger, such as emotional stress. Individuals with binge-eating disorder may have disruptions in neurotransmitter function or altered activity in the part of the brain that responds to rewarding stimuli. There is a strong association between binge-eating disorder and other psychological disorders, especially anxiety, depression, and addiction (see Further Readings 3 and 10).

COMMON BEHAVIORS OF BINGE-EATING DISORDER

As described, a binge refers to the uncontrolled consumption of an unusually large amount of food within a discrete period of time. A binge can include any food, but most often consists of foods that carry the social stigma of "junk" or "bad" foods—ice cream, cookies, sweets, potato chips, and similar snack foods. During binges, food is eaten without regard to biological need and often in a recurrent, ritualized fashion. Unlike those with bulimia nervosa, people with binge-eating disorder do not attempt to purge the excess calories.

▲ Binge-eating disorder is seen in both men and women. © Ryan McVay/Getty Images

TABLE 15-3 ■ **Diagnostic Criteria for Binge-Eating Disorder**

A. Recurrent binge eating, characterized by:
   1. Eating a large amount of food in a short period of time (e.g., within 2 hours)
   2. Experiencing a loss of control over eating during binges

B. Episodes of binge-eating are associated with at least three of the following:
   1. Rapid rate of eating
   2. Continuing to eat beyond feelings of fullness
   3. Overeating in the absence of hunger
   4. Eating alone to avoid embarrassment
   5. Feelings of self-disgust, depression, or guilt after overeating

C. Extreme distress about binge eating

D. Binges occur at least one time per week for 3 months

E. Behaviors are distinct from bulimia nervosa and anorexia nervosa

Source: Adapted from *Diagnostic and Statistical Manual for Mental Disorders, 5th edition.* Copyright 2013 by the American Psychiatric Association.

Binge eating is usually triggered by negative emotions, such as stress, anxiety, loneliness, grief, or anger (see Further Reading 21). In fact, almost half of those with severe binge-eating disorder exhibit clinical depression. Often, people with binge-eating disorder have not learned to express or appropriately deal with their feelings, so they turn to food to cope with stress or meet emotional needs. Those who regularly practice binge eating may grow up nurturing others instead of themselves, avoiding their own feelings and taking little time for themselves. Unfortunately, unresolved conflicts and unmet emotional needs will resurface. To make matters worse, binge eating itself brings added feelings of guilt, embarrassment, and shame.

Typically, binge eaters isolate themselves and eat large quantities of a favorite food. For example, a person might find comfort in consuming large quantities of food—such as a whole pizza in one sitting—when an emotional setback occurs. Other people with this disorder eat food continually over an extended period, called grazing. For instance, someone with a stressful or frustrating job might come home every night and graze until bedtime.

Many people with binge-eating disorder have struggled to lose weight throughout their lives. As noted in Section 7.8, overly restrictive diets can lead to hunger and a sense of deprivation that triggers binge eating. People with binge-eating disorder tend to perceive themselves as hungry more often than normal. During periods when little food is eaten, they get very hungry and obsessive about food. Restricting favorite foods, such as chocolate, leads to feelings of deprivation. When these individuals finally give themselves permission to eat a forbidden food or loosen up a rigid meal plan, they feel driven to eat in a compulsive, uncontrolled way. People with binge-eating disorder usually began this cycle of strict dieting alternating with binge eating during adolescence or in their early twenties and have had little success with traditional weight-control programs.

PHYSICAL EFFECTS OF BINGE-EATING DISORDER

Although obesity is not among the criteria for diagnosis of binge-eating disorder, about 70% of those with the disorder are obese. The physical effects of the disorder reflect the comorbid conditions of obesity, which were extensively described in Table 7-2. The most deadly physical effects are listed here:

- Hypertension from excess body weight and high sodium intake
- Elevated cholesterol levels, which contribute to atherosclerosis (Binge eating may have a more severe effect on blood lipids than simply overeating by grazing throughout the day because large meals are linked to high insulin and high triglycerides.)
- Cardiovascular disease, which contributes to deaths from heart attacks and strokes
- Type 2 diabetes, which is strongly linked to obesity (An estimated one in five women with type 2 diabetes exhibits binge-eating behaviors.)

TREATMENT FOR THE PERSON WITH BINGE-EATING DISORDER

Approximately 30% of participants in organized weight-control programs have binge-eating disorder. This means registered dietitian nutritionists and others who lead weight management programs may be the first to identify binge-eating disorder among their clients. As with anorexia and bulimia, binge-eating disorder truly is a psychological problem with nutritional consequences. The success of traditional weight-loss therapies for people with binge-eating disorder has been poor because these approaches fail to address the underlying psychological causes of the disorder. True, people with binge-eating disorder will likely benefit from increased nutrition knowledge, but unless they find a way to manage or overcome negative emotions that underlie eating behaviors, the success of attempts to improve food choices and incorporate physical activity into the lifestyle will be short lived. Thus, first addressing the psychological needs of individuals with binge-eating disorder is essential to successful treatment.

The primary goal of treatment for people with binge-eating disorder is to decrease and eventually eliminate episodes of binge eating. Losing excess body weight, alleviating

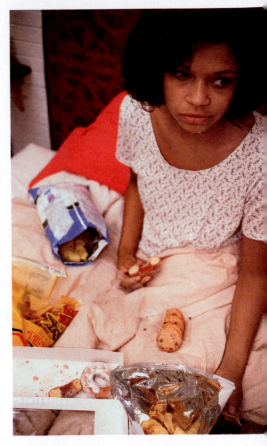

▲ Some experts describe binge-eating disorder as an addiction to food, involving psychological dependence. The person becomes attached to the behavior and is driven to continue it, senses only limited control over it, and persists at it despite negative consequences. © Jack Star/PhotoLink/Getty Images

Mindfulness meditation is another strategy being studied to address the psychological issues that lead to bingeing. Mindful eating programs train a person to become aware of, accept, and acknowledge the daily experiences that can be triggers for binge eating but not to respond with emotional eating. Early studies show beneficial effects on body weight, stress, and symptoms of depression (review the discussion of mindful eating in Section 7.8 and see Further Reading 22).

comorbid conditions of obesity, and improving psychological disturbances are secondary goals of therapy (see Further Reading 3).

Psychological Therapy Similar to treatments for bulimia nervosa, there is growing evidence that cognitive behavioral therapy techniques are useful for overcoming binge-eating disorder. Many people with binge-eating disorder may experience difficulty in identifying personal emotional needs and expressing emotions. This problem is a common predisposing factor in binge eating, so communication issues should be addressed during treatment. Binge eaters often must be helped to recognize their buried emotions in anxiety-producing situations and then encouraged to share them with their therapist or therapy group. Learning simple but appropriate phrases to say to oneself can help stop bingeing when the desire is strong. Even if negative situations cannot be changed, people must learn how to adapt to and bear with them effectively—not through self-destructive binge-eating behaviors.

Cognitive behavioral therapy can be delivered in many forms. One-on-one sessions with a therapist and group therapy are the most common methods. Self-help groups such as Overeaters Anonymous® can also help. Their treatment philosophy, which parallels that of Alcoholics Anonymous®, is to create an environment of encouragement and accountability to overcome this eating disorder. Recently, even web-based adaptations of cognitive behavioral therapy have proved to be useful.

Although psychological therapy has been valuable for correcting binge-eating behavior, it is not always successful at inducing weight loss among a population of overweight and obese individuals who may have one or more other health issues related to obesity. Thus, nutrition therapy is an important part of treatment for binge-eating disorder (see Further Reading 2).

Nutrition Therapy Once effective coping mechanisms are learned, the registered dietitian nutritionist can educate the patient on developing normal eating patterns and making healthful food choices. First, those with binge-eating disorder must learn to eat in response to hunger—a biological signal—rather than in response to emotional needs or external factors (such as the time of day, boredom, or the simple presence of food). Counselors often direct binge eaters to record their perceptions of physical hunger throughout the day and at the beginning and end of every meal. These people must learn to respond to a prescribed amount of fullness at each meal.

Individuals recovering from binge-eating disorder should initially avoid weight-loss diets because feelings of food deprivation can trigger binge eating. Even if exposure to favorite binge foods is limited in the early stages of treatment, many experts feel that learning to eat all foods—but in moderation—is an effective long-term goal for people with binge-eating disorder. This practice can prevent the feelings of desperation and deprivation that come from limiting particular foods.

Pharmacological Therapy Psychological and nutritional therapies are useful tools to treat binge-eating disorder, but they are not 100% effective. Thus, there is growing interest in drug therapy (see Further Reading 3). As of 2015, the first drug to be approved for treatment of binge-eating disorder is lisdexamfetamine dimesylate (Vyvanse®), a stimulant that has been used to treat attention-deficit hyperactivity disorder. Some antidepressants (e.g., fluoxetine [Prozac®] and duloxetine [Cymbalta®]) and antiseizure medications (e.g., topamirate [Topamax®]) have also demonstrated some success in reducing binge eating. Despite their usefulness for reducing binge eating, these medications still may not induce significant weight loss. Orlistat (Xenical®) and phentermine (Adipex-P®), discussed in Section 7.9, can assist with weight-loss efforts after binge eating is under control. The newest weight-loss medication, lorcaserin (Belviq®), has yet to be extensively tested for treatment of binge-eating disorder.

Given the similarities between binge eating and other addictive behaviors, medications used to treat substance abuse (e.g., naltrexone) are being studied for use among patients with binge-eating disorder. Another novel therapy that requires additional research is a glutamate-modulating agent called Namenda®, which is used in patients with Alzheimer's disease.

ASK THE RDN Intermittent Fasting

Dear RDN: I have had bad luck with traditional diets, but I've heard rave reviews of the "Fast Diet." Is an intermittent fasting program a good way to lose weight and keep it off?

There are three basic methods of intermittent fasting: whole-day fasting, alternate-day fasting, and time-restricted feeding. The definition of "fasting" can vary from one plan to the next; some plans allow only calorie-free beverages and sugar-free gum during fasts, whereas other plans recommend reducing energy intake to 20% to 25% of your usual intake (i.e., a modified fast) on fast days. Plans also differ in recommendations for food choices during feeding phases; some prescribe specific calorie and nutrient goals, while others promote *ad libitum* food intake during feeding phases. Proponents of intermittent fasting recommend that a person experiment to find the method that best fits his or her lifestyle.

With whole-day fasting, like the "Fast Diet," you would eat normally on most days of the week, but undertake a complete or modified fast 1 or 2 days each week. With alternate-day fasting, days of normal eating alternate with complete or modified fasts. For time-restricted feeding protocols, you would delay the first meal of the day to achieve a fast of 14 to 20 hours (including overnight), but an *ad libitum* feeding period would be allowed for the remaining hours of the day.

Besides weight loss, purported benefits of intermittent fasting include improved insulin sensitivity, enhanced ability to use fat for energy, decreased triglyceride levels, and reduced inflammation—changes that may potentially decrease risks for chronic diseases and lead to a longer life. Much of the research to date, however, has been conducted in animals, with few controlled studies in humans.

Reviews of current (although sparse) studies of the effects of intermittent fasting suggest that it may be a reasonable alternative to the traditional weight-loss method of moderate daily calorie restriction for some people (see Further Reading 9, 23, 25, and 31). Weight loss and improvements in metabolic effects are similar with these two weight-loss methods. However, intermittent fasting is not a good fit for everyone. If you struggle with blood sugar control (e.g., hypoglycemia or diabetes) or are pregnant, you should not attempt intermittent fasting. Quite predictably, some side effects of any fasting regimen include hunger, headaches, fatigue, and irritability. Some critics of intermittent fasting point out that underfeeding in this way could lead to nutrient deficiencies. We, as registered dietitian nutritionists, can help you choose nutrient-dense foods during the feeding phases of any of these dietary patterns. Also, there is some concern that prolonged fasting may decrease your metabolic rate, which would make long-term weight maintenance very difficult (recall Ask the RDN in Chapter 12). Because we have limited data on the long-term safety of intermittent fasting, it is not clear how much fasting is too much. Fasting too frequently may result in malnutrition, reduced immune function, organ damage, or eating disorders.

Wait—*eating disorders*?

Take a step back and look at the basic dietary patterns advocated here. Much like the dietary patterns of individuals with anorexia nervosa, intermittent fasting programs involve calorie counting and extended periods of hunger. For some plans, foods are classified as "safe" or "off limits," which promotes an unhealthy, dichotomous view of foods and ties eating into emotions such as guilt, shame, and fear. Intermittent fasting programs that advise fasting (deprivation) followed by several hours or days of eating *ad libitum* (indulgence) may foster binge eating. Participants may feel as if they've failed themselves and others when they have trouble adhering to a strict regimen. For a person who already exhibits anxiety, depression, or obsessive traits, intermittent fasting may be a gateway to pathological dieting and eating disorders.

Although intermittent fasting may be a reasonable alternative to daily moderate calorie restriction for some people, more research is needed to determine which protocol is best and if mental and physical health are affected over the long term. If you are determined to try intermittent fasting, continue to seek the advice of a registered dietitian nutritionist to ensure that your dietary pattern still meets your nutritional needs. Importantly, if you tend to obsess about food and body weight or you already have problems with depression or anxiety, steer clear of this dietary pattern. Recall what you learned in Section 15.1: eating disorders often begin with a simple diet. If efforts to control weight begin to interfere with daily activities and are linked to physiological and emotional changes, professional help will be needed to treat an eating disorder.

Fueling, not fasting,

Angela Collene, MS, RDN, LD, Author

Overall, people who have binge-eating disorder are usually unsuccessful in controlling it on their own. Furthermore, unrecognized binge-eating disorder will undermine the success of weight-loss therapies among many overweight and obese individuals who do seek professional help. By asking questions about eating patterns, feelings of loss of control over eating behaviors, and feelings of guilt after eating, health professionals can screen weight-loss clients for binge-eating disorder and refer affected individuals to appropriate treatments.

✓ CONCEPT CHECK 15.4

1. What differentiates binge-eating disorder from bulimia nervosa?
2. List at least three health effects that may result from binge-eating disorder.
3. Why do people with binge-eating disorder have little success in traditional weight-loss programs?

15.5 Other Eating Disorders

Besides those already covered, there are several lesser-known types of eating disorders. Some of these, such as **pica** (discussed next), rumination disorder, and avoidant/restrictive food intake disorder (discussed in Section 19.4), are distinct eating disorders with their own sets of diagnostic criteria. In *DSM-5,* the category of Other Specified Feeding or Eating Disorders (OSFED) encompasses several disorders that do not meet all of the criteria for diagnosis of anorexia, bulimia, or binge-eating disorder. These include several categories of subthreshold eating disorders, **purging disorder,** and **night eating syndrome.**

PICA

Pica, which will be mentioned again in Section 18.5 as it relates to pregnancy, is a disorder in which a person persistently eats nonnutritive, nonfood substances over a period of at least 1 month. A few examples of nonfood substances ingested by people with pica are clay, dirt, ice, chalk, or wood. Pica could lead to some serious health consequences, including microbial infections, poisoning from toxins present in the nonfood material, gastrointestinal blockages, or nutrient deficiencies (in cases when nonfood substances displace nutritive foods in the diet). Pica tends to co-occur with other mental disorders, such as autism or obsessive-compulsive disorder.

OTHER SPECIFIED FEEDING OR EATING DISORDERS

Subthreshold Eating Disorders Individuals who meet some but not all of the criteria for diagnosis with anorexia nervosa, bulimia nervosa, or binge-eating disorder may fall into one of five subthreshold classifications. For example, **atypical anorexia nervosa** describes a person who meets most of the criteria for diagnosis of anorexia nervosa but whose weight is still within a normal range. This could occur if an overweight person has just begun severely restricting calories. Despite significant weight loss, BMI may still fall within the healthy range of 18.5 to 24.9. Other diagnoses in this category include cases of bulimia nervosa or binge-eating disorder in which episodes of binge-eating occur less than once per week (**bulimia nervosa of low frequency** or **binge-eating disorder of low frequency**) or have taken place for less than 3 months (**bulimia nervosa of limited duration** or **binge-eating disorder of limited duration**).

Purging Disorder Purging disorder is the name given to the behavior of people who repeatedly purge (i.e., vomit) to promote weight loss even in the absence of binge-eating (see Further Reading 15). This disorder is related to body dissatisfaction, anxiety, and

---

pica The practice of eating nonfood items, such as dirt, laundry starch, or clay.

purging disorder An eating disorder characterized by repeated purging (e.g., by self-induced vomiting) to induce weight loss even in the absence of binge eating.

night eating syndrome Eating a lot of food in the late evening and nocturnal awakenings with ingestion of food.

atypical anorexia nervosa A subthreshold eating disorder in which a person meets most of the criteria for diagnosis of anorexia nervosa, except weight is within a normal range.

bulimia nervosa of low frequency A form of other specified feeding or eating disorders in which a person meets all of the criteria for diagnosis of bulimia nervosa—except the frequency of binge-compensate cycles is less than once per week.

binge-eating disorder of low frequency A form of other specified feeding or eating disorders in which a person meets all of the criteria for diagnosis of binge-eating disorder—except the frequency of binges is less than once per week.

bulimia nervosa of limited duration A form of other specified feeding or eating disorders in which a person meets all of the criteria for diagnosis of bulimia nervosa—except the duration of the disordered eating behavior is less than 3 months.

binge-eating disorder of limited duration A form of other specified feeding or eating disorders in which a person meets all of the criteria for diagnosis of binge-eating disorder—except the duration of the disordered eating behavior is less than 3 months.

depression. The physical effects of purging disorder are the same as those of bulimia nervosa and include dental problems, mouth sores, damage to the esophagus, constipation, dehydration, electrolyte imbalances, and overall malnutrition.

Night Eating Syndrome Night eating syndrome is characterized by recurrent episodes of night eating, manifested by eating after awakening from sleep or by excessive food consumption after the evening meal. With night eating syndrome, the person is fully aware of and able to recall the behavior, which results in marked distress. Although night eating syndrome was first observed among obese patients, it also occurs among nonobese people. It has been estimated to occur in 1.5% of the general population and in 8.9% of patients treated in obesity clinics; it tends to co-occur with other eating disorders. Some typical signs and symptoms of night eating syndrome include:

▲ Night eating syndrome is characterized by waking at least once during the night and needing to eat to be able to fall asleep again. © BananaStock/PunchStock

- Not feeling hungry in the morning and delaying the first meal until several hours after waking
- Overeating in the evening with more than 25% of daily food intake consumed after dinner
- Difficulty falling asleep and a need to eat something to help fall asleep faster
- Waking at least once during the night with a need to eat to be able to fall asleep again
- When eating produces feelings of guilt and shame
- Feeling depressed, especially at night

Research shows that the circadian rhythm (your body's 24-hour clock) of food intake appears to be disturbed in night eating syndrome. Studies have also shown that night eating syndrome is prevalent among outpatients with sleep apnea, restless leg syndrome, or some psychiatric conditions. Behavioral changes, such as establishing and monitoring the sleep-wake schedule and performing regular exercise, can help. Symptoms are significantly improved with use of the antidepressant sertraline (Zoloft®).

☑ **CONCEPT CHECK 15.5**

1. List three ways pica could harm health.
2. Describe three different cases in which a person would be diagnosed with subthreshold eating disorders.
3. How is purging disorder similar to bulimia nervosa? How do these two disorders differ?
4. List three characteristics of night eating syndrome.

15.6 Additional Disordered Eating Patterns

There is a growing number of other patterns of disordered eating that have not yet been classified by *DSM-5* but are worthy of mention. Some of the patterns mentioned in this section, such as **female athlete triad,** have been the subject of much research. Others have been discussed mainly in popular media, yet health practitioners report encountering them regularly. Continued research is required to establish a set of diagnostic criteria, describe the course of the disorder, and establish evidence-based treatments.

female athlete triad A condition characterized by disordered eating, lack of menstrual periods (amenorrhea), and osteoporosis.

FEMALE ATHLETE TRIAD

Mentioned in Section 14.4, females participating in appearance-based and endurance sports are at heightened risk of developing eating disorders. One study of college-age female athletes found that 15% of swimmers, 62% of gymnasts, and 32% of varsity athletes exhibited disordered eating patterns.

FIGURE 15-4 ▲ The female athlete triad occurs when the athlete has low energy availability (with or without an eating disorder), lack of menstrual periods, and osteoporosis. Stress fractures and chronic fatigue also occur. This triad often is seen in appearance-related sports, such as gymnastics. Long-term health is at risk; thus, prevention and early treatment are crucial. © Royalty-Free/Corbis

The tragic case of Christy Henrich illustrates why anyone at risk for the female athlete triad should seek professional help. As a young teenager, Christy weighed 95 pounds and was 4 feet 11 inches tall. She showed promise as a gymnast but was told that she was too fat to excel in gymnastics. Christy continued her training but often starved herself, some days consuming just an apple and frequently purging by vomiting. Christy's eating disorder eventually rendered her too weak to compete. She was hospitalized after her weight had dropped to 47 pounds. She died, just after her 22nd birthday, from the effects of long-term semistarvation.

Food restriction and stress can precipitate irregular menstruation among female athletes. When body fat is low, estrogen production decreases. Remember from Section 11.2, estrogen stimulates osteoblasts (bone-forming cells). In this way, low body fat impairs bone health. Some of these young women have bone mass measurements equivalent to those of 50- to 60-year-olds. This increases the risk for bone fractures during sports and general activities.

The American College of Sports Medicine (ACSM) has named this syndrome "female athlete triad" because it consists of three parts: low energy availability (whether intentional or unintentional), lack of menstrual periods, and osteoporosis (Fig. 15-4). Many coaches, trainers, and even some health professionals mistakenly believe that loss of menstrual periods is a normal consequence of a high level of physical activity. To combat misinformation, the ACSM has issued a plea to teachers, coaches, health professionals, and parents to educate female athletes about the triad and its health consequences (see Further Reading 22).

Those exhibiting symptoms of the female athlete triad should seek treatment from a multidisciplinary team of health professionals. Involving the coach or trainer in therapy is usually a key factor in the success of the treatment plan. Suggestions for treatment are as follows:

- Reduce preoccupation with food, weight, and body fat.
- Gradually increase meals and snacks to an appropriate amount.
- Achieve an appropriate weight for height.
- Establish regular menstrual periods.
- Decrease training time and/or intensity by 10% to 20%.

Increasing caloric intake will increase body weight and body fat. Estrogen production then increases and should stabilize bone mass. During therapy, a physician may prescribe a multivitamin and mineral supplement as well as calcium supplements as needed to maintain a daily calcium intake of 1200 to 1500 milligrams. Even with intervention, however, much of the bone loss that has already occurred is irreversible.

MUSCLE DYSMORPHIA

Muscle dysmorphia has gained attention as a psychological condition with many similarities to other eating disorders (see Further Reading 21). First identified among male bodybuilders in the 1990s, muscle dysmorphia was initially termed "reverse anorexia." Men (and some women) with this disorder perceive themselves as *too thin,* rather than too fat, and are preoccupied with strict weightlifting and diet regimens to achieve a high level of muscularity. Among high school and college-aged men, in particular, body dissatisfaction may lead to disordered eating and exercise practices.

In muscle dysmorphia, numerous hours are devoted to working out at the gym; planning and eating low-carbohydrate, high-protein meals; and keeping meticulous records of exercise, body measurements, and food intake. The dietary practices (e.g., high-volume eating, protein intakes of up to 5 grams per kilogram) and use of unproven ergogenic aids or anabolic steroids can result in physical impairment. Such exercise and eating routines also interfere with social, occupational, and recreational activities. People with muscle dysmorphia may avoid social contact, eating in restaurants, and being seen without clothes because of distress over appearing too thin. Considering its many similarities with anorexia nervosa and a tendency for people with muscle dysmorphia to cross over to other forms of eating disorders over time, some experts support recognition of muscle dysmorphia as an eating disorder.

DIABULIMIA

Adolescents with diabetes are at heightened risk of eating disorders (see Further Readings 5 and 15. As you learned in Chapter 4, when insulin is absent or when cells are insulin resistant, cells are unable to use glucose for energy. Weight loss occurs because carbohydrate calories essentially are wasted. After a person starts insulin or insulin-sensitizing therapy, cells are able to utilize glucose and store fat, so weight gain is a common side effect. About one of three teens with type 1 diabetes admits to intentionally skipping doses of insulin to induce weight loss. This practice, so-called "diabulimia," can lead to severe hyperglycemia and its myriad consequences, which include eye damage, kidney damage, diabetic coma, or death. On the other hand, about one of five teens with type 1 diabetes uses overdoses of insulin to compensate for episodes of binge eating, a practice that could lead to dangerously low levels of blood sugar. Among adolescents with type 2 diabetes, up to 25% show signs of binge-eating disorder. For youth with diabetes, evidence of poor blood sugar control, frequently missed clinic visits, and the presence of depression can be warning signs of eating disorders.

ORTHOREXIA

As you have learned about nutrition in this course, you may have changed some of your own food choices. Obviously, a focus on healthy eating can help with weight management and prevention of disease, but when strict food rules begin to interfere with everyday life, they can be pathological. Some people worry excessively about the availability of food they permit themselves to eat, such as low-fat, sugar-free, or organic food choices. Although not currently classified as an eating disorder, orthorexia describes an emerging condition in which healthful eating becomes an obsession (see Further Readings 6). The term comes from Greek words meaning "straight or proper appetite." Unlike cases of anorexia or bulimia, orthorexia does not usually originate in the drive for thinness. Rather, a need for perfection or purity lies at the heart of orthorexia. Such extreme dietary perfectionism may be related to obsessive-compulsive disorder.

▲ Orthorexia describes a condition in which a person is unduly concerned with eating only healthful foods. © McGraw-Hill Education/Andrew Resek, photographer

✓ CONCEPT CHECK 15.6

1. List the three components of the female athlete triad.
2. How is muscle dysmorphia similar to anorexia nervosa? How is it different?
3. What is diabulimia? List some of the harmful physical effects of such practices.
4. How would you distinguish between healthy eating and orthorexia?

15.7 Prevention of Eating Disorders

A key to developing and maintaining healthful eating behavior is to realize that some concern about diet, health, and weight is normal. It is also normal to experience variation in what we eat, how we feel, and even how much we weigh. For example, it is common to experience some minimal weight change (up to 2 to 3 pounds) throughout the day and even more over the course of a week. A large weight fluctuation or ongoing weight gain or weight loss is more likely to indicate a problem. If you notice a large change in your eating habits, how you feel, or your body weight, it is a good idea to consult your physician. Treating physical and emotional problems early helps lead you to peace of mind and good health.

With a view on society as a whole, many people begin to form opinions about food, nutrition, health, weight, and body image prior to or during puberty. Parents, friends, and professionals working with young adults should consider the following advice for preventing eating disorders:

- Discourage restrictive dieting and meal skipping. Fasting is also discouraged (except for religious occasions).
- Provide information about normal changes that occur during puberty.
- Correct misconceptions about nutrition, healthy body weight, and approaches to weight loss.
- Carefully phrase any weight-related recommendations and comments.

- Do not overemphasize numbers on a scale. Instead, teach the basics of proper nutrition and regular physical activity in school and at home.
- Encourage normal expression of disruptive emotions.
- Encourage children to eat only when they are hungry.
- Provide adolescents with an appropriate, but not unlimited, degree of independence, choice, responsibility, and self-accountability for their actions.
- Increase self-acceptance and appreciation of the power and pleasure emerging from one's body.
- Enhance tolerance for diversity in body weight and shape.
- Build respectful environments and supportive relationships.
- Encourage coaches to be sensitive to weight and body-image issues among athletes.
- Emphasize that thinness is not necessarily associated with better athletic performance.
- Support programs for eating disorder screening and prevention at high schools and colleges.

Our society as a whole can benefit from a fresh focus on nutritious food practices and a healthful outlook toward food and body weight. Not only is treatment of eating disorders far more difficult than prevention, but these disorders also have devastating effects on the entire family. For this reason, caregivers and health care professionals must emphasize the importance of an overall healthful dietary pattern that focuses on moderation, as opposed to restriction and perfection.

Overall, the challenge facing many North Americans is achieving a healthy body weight without excessive dieting. A growing number of health professionals support a nondiet approach to weight management. This means adopting and maintaining sensible eating habits, a physically active lifestyle, and realistic and positive attitudes and emotions while practicing creative ways to handle stress. Certain cultural ideals of beauty can trigger eating disorders; changing these values might reduce the pressures predisposing some people to various types of disordered eating behavior. The "size acceptance" approach, discussed in Section 7.4, fights discrimination against overweight and obese people and asserts that each person should be free to find his or her natural weight. Women who combine careers and motherhood are saying that they have more important things to worry about. Some trend-setters in the fashion industry are tolerating more curves. We cannot change the genes that predispose people to eating disorders (at least not yet!), but we can make a difference in the environmental triggers that set these devastating disorders in motion.

These websites provide further information on eating disorders:

- Academy for Eating Disorders, www.aedweb.org
- The National Eating Disorders Association, www.nationaleatingdisorders.org
- National Institute of Mental Health's concise review of eating disorders, www.nimh.nih.gov/health/publications/eating-disorders/eating-disorders.pdf

✓ CONCEPT CHECK 15.7

1. Why is prevention of eating disorders so important?
2. Imagine you are a coach for a high school girls' softball team. What could you do to foster an environment that prevents eating disorders among this group of adolescent girls?

Eating Disorder Reflections

© Ted Foxx/Alamy

Reflections From A Woman with Anorexia Nervosa

It was the spring of my freshman year of high school, and I had just turned 15 years old. I was determined to land a leading role in the upcoming high school musical, *West Side Story*. I thought I should lose some weight to appear more attractive to the student director Shawn, so I decided to give up "junk" food. The next day, my friend Sandra looked at my lunch, spread out neatly on a napkin before me, and squawked, "Dill pickles?! Who brings dill pickles for lunch in a zip-lock baggie?" The other girls at the table fell into a fit of hysterics. "Casting for *West Side Story* is coming up," I said, "and I gave up 'junk' food to try to lose a few extra pounds." One of my friends thought it would be funny to give me one M&M—just to smell. Aren't they funny? So I put it in a little Tupperware container and kept it in my backpack as a reminder. Every once in a while, I did smell it.

For the next few weeks, there were times when I would find myself cracking open the refrigerator door and just staring at what

I knew to be a deliciously crunchy, crisp, and cold Kit Kat bar in the dairy bin. I didn't eat it though. At the mall with my friends, Bridgette and Nora wanted to stop and get a cinnamon bun. They chided me, but I didn't budge. The cinnamon bun smelled so good. But as I sat opposite them in the food court and watched them overdramatize its ooey-gooey goodness, I felt a sense of pride that I could make a decision and stick with it. I could see that they were jealous of my willpower.

When Easter came around, I took a look at the contents of the Easter basket my mom insisted on preparing and turned up my nose at it. I had proven to myself that I could resist temptation . . . why stop now?

After the musical, I started running with my friend, Laura. She was getting in shape for the next season of field hockey. After school, we met in the locker room, changed out of our school clothes, and out we went. The running helped. Every morning, just after going to the bathroom and before getting any breakfast, I would pop onto the scale in my mom's bathroom. One hundred and fifteen pounds and still going. At 5 feet 7 inches, that wasn't too bad.

Cheese and butter had made it to the "no" list by the time I was 16 and down to 105 pounds. Fat-free was my mantra. For my 16th birthday, my friends threw a little surprise party for me. Nora, knowing I would put up a fight, made me a cake. "It's your birthday! You can have a piece of cake!" I politely said no, that I would cut it for everyone else, but I really didn't want any. They pestered me, and Nora started to feel offended, so finally I took a few bites, so she wouldn't burst into tears. It had been so long since I'd had so much sugar. I felt bloated and sick. I ate nothing for the rest of the day, and only six saltines, an apple, and two stalks of celery the next day. Those foods were on the "yes" list. Salads also were okay but only with salt and vinegar. I told my parents that the dissections in biology class had given me a distaste for meat, but really, I just didn't want all those calories. For a while, I craved food day and night, but slowly, I was getting better and better at holding my ground.

By my senior year, I was skipping lunches altogether, opting instead to hang out in the library and read over my AP bio text. "Where were you at lunch today?" Bridgette would ask later. "Oh, I had some reading to do. The AP exam is going to be tough." At 100 pounds, I was getting closer to finding out what "tough" really meant.

Even though Laura moved out of state, I didn't give up on exercising. Now, my mom's stair stepper in the basement was my favorite. I'd take my biology notes, prop them up in front of me, and step-step-step until I had burned 400 kcal. I felt so efficient knowing that I could multitask. Sometimes I'd exercise twice a day. As senior year wore on, though, it got harder and harder to get up in the morning and put on my tennis shoes. And then one morning, in the shower, I just collapsed under the stream of hot water.

I ended up in this hospital bed with an IV in my arm. At 92 pounds, my body was starving. As it turns out, if you don't give your body enough fuel, you start to cannibalize yourself, in a sense. My body had been so hungry, my muscles had been wasting away, and the episode in the shower was due to a problem with my heart. It's a problem I have created . . . not my parents or my distant group of friends . . . only me. My mom was there, next to me, caressing the arm with the IV tube, putting her whole life on hold because of me. Isn't this what I'd wanted—to be in control of my own destiny?

Where do I go from here?

Thoughts of a Bulimic Woman

From Hall L, Cohn L: *Bulimia—A Guide to Recovery.* Gurze Books: Carlsbad, CA, 1992. Reprinted with permission.

I am wide awake and immediately out of bed. I think back to the night before, when I made a new list of what I wanted to get done and how I wanted to be. My husband is not far behind me on his way into the bathroom to get ready for work. Maybe I can sneak onto the scale to see what I weigh this morning before he notices me. I am already in my private world. I feel overjoyed when the scale says that I stayed the same weight as I was the night before, and I can feel that slightly hungry feeling. Maybe it will stop today; maybe today everything will change. What were the projects I was going to get done?

We eat the same breakfast, except that I take no butter on my toast, no cream in my coffee, and never take seconds (until Doug gets out the door). Today I am going to be really good, and that means eating certain predetermined portions of food and not taking one more bite than I think I am allowed. I am very careful to see that I don't take more than Doug. I judge myself by his body. I can feel the tension building. I wish Doug would hurry up and leave so I can get going!

As soon as he shuts the door, I try to get involved with one of the myriad responsibilities on my list. I hate them all! I just want to crawl into a hole. I don't want to do anything. I'd rather eat. I am alone; I am nervous; I am no good; I always do everything wrong anyway; I am not in control; and I can't make it through the day, I know it. It has been the same for so long. I remember the starchy cereal I ate for breakfast. I am into the bathroom and onto the scale. It measures the same, but I don't want to stay the same! I want to be thinner! I look into the mirror. I think my thighs are ugly and deformed looking. I see a lumpy, clumsy, pear-shaped wimp. There is always something wrong with what I see. I feel frustrated, trapped in this body, and I don't know what to do about it.

I float to the refrigerator knowing exactly what is there. I begin with last night's brownies. I always begin with the sweets. At first, I try to make it look like nothing is missing, but my appetite is huge and I resolve to make another batch of brownies. I know there is half of a bag of cookies in the bathroom, thrown out the night

▲ Bulimic episodes add to the despair felt in this disorder. © Royalty-Free/Corbis

before, and I polish them off immediately. I take some milk so my vomiting will be smoother. I like the full feeling I get after downing a big glass. I get out six pieces of bread and toast one side of each in the broiler, turn them over and load them with pats of butter, and put them under the broiler again until they are bubbling. I take all six pieces on a plate to the television and go back for a bowl of cereal and a banana to have along with them. Before the last piece of toast is finished, I am already preparing the next batch of six more pieces. Maybe another brownie or five and a couple of large bowls full of ice cream, yogurt, or cottage cheese.

My stomach is stretched into a huge ball below my rib cage. I know I'll have to go into the bathroom soon, but I want to postpone it. I am in never-never land. I am waiting, feeling the pressure, pacing the floor in and out of the rooms. Time is passing. Time is passing. It is getting to be time. I wander aimlessly through each of the rooms again, tidying, making the whole house neat and put back together. I finally make the turn into the bathroom. I brace my feet, pull my hair back and stick my finger down my throat, stroking twice, and get up a huge pile of food. Three times, four times, and another pile of food. I can see everything come back. I am so glad to see those brownies because they are so fattening. The rhythm of the emptying is broken and my head is beginning to hurt. I stand up feeling dizzy, empty, and weak. The whole episode has taken about an hour.

Summary (Numbers refer to numbered sections in the chapter.)

15.1 Disordered eating encompasses mild and short-term changes in eating patterns that occur as a result of life stress, illness, or a desire to change body weight. When carried to the extreme, disordered eating may progress to an eating disorder, in which severe changes in eating patterns have lasting and detrimental effects. Current research on the origins of eating disorders indicates that genetic factors dictate brain biology, which affects how certain individuals perceive their bodies and respond to life stresses. Thus, a person who is genetically predisposed to eating disorders may use disordered eating behaviors to cope with feelings of depression, anger, or guilt. The three main types of eating disorders are anorexia nervosa, bulimia nervosa, and binge-eating disorder.

15.2 Anorexia nervosa is characterized by extreme weight loss (e.g., BMI of less than 17), a distorted body image, and an irrational fear of weight gain and obesity. Weight loss is achieved primarily by restricting food intake. Physical consequences include a profound decrease in body weight and body fat, heart irregularities, iron-deficiency anemia, impaired immunity, digestive dysfunction, and loss of menstrual periods. Treatment of anorexia nervosa includes increasing food intake to support gradual weight gain. Family-based psychological counseling can help anorexic individuals establish healthy eating behaviors and body image.

15.3 Similar to anorexia nervosa, bulimia is characterized by overvalu-ation of body weight and shape. However, the disordered eating patterns of bulimic individuals involve recurrent binge eating followed by compensatory behaviors. Binge-eating is consuming an abnormally large amount of food within a short time period. A person with bulimia nervosa has lack of control over bingeing behaviors and feels extremely distressed after a binge. Inappropriate compensatory behaviors used to rid the body of excess calories include vomiting or misusing laxatives, diuretics, or enemas. Alternately, fasting and excessive exercise may be used. Vomiting as a means of purging is especially destructive to the body; it can cause severe tooth decay, stomach ulcers, irritation of the esophagus, low blood potassium, and other problems. Treatment of buli-mia nervosa includes psychological and nutritional counseling. Prozac® is the only FDA-approved medication for treatment of bulimia nervosa, but other antidepressants and antiseizure medications are sometimes prescribed.

15.4 Binge-eating disorder is the most widespread eating disorder. It tends to be diagnosed in middle age and affects men and women nearly equally. It is characterized by recurrent episodes of bingeing, which cause marked distress, but are not followed by compensatory behaviors. About 70% of people with binge-eating disorder are obese. The health effects that stem from binge-eating disorder are comorbid conditions of obesity, including hypertension, high blood cholesterol, cardiovascular disease, and type 2 diabetes. Treatment involves cognitive behavioral therapy and nutrition counseling. Vyvanse® is the only FDA-approved drug for treatment of binge-eating disorder. Antidepressants and other medications may also be useful.

15.5 Pica is an eating disorder in which a person persistently ingests nonnutritive, nonfood items such as clay, dirt, or ice. Subthreshold eating disorders (e.g., atypical anorexia nervosa, bulimia nervosa of low frequency or limited duration, or binge-eating disorder of low frequency or limited duration) capture those individuals who meet some but not all of the criteria for diagnosis of anorexia nervosa, bulimia nervosa, or binge-eating disorder. People with purging disorder practice purging behaviors to achieve weight loss, but they do not exhibit the binge-eating behaviors typical of bulimia nervosa. Individuals with night eating syndrome consume more than 25% of daily food intake after dinner, may have difficulty falling asleep without eating, and wake up at least once during the night to consume food.

15.6 Several additional disordered eating patterns that are not classified as eating disorders include the female athlete triad, muscle dysmorphia, diabulimia, and orthorexia. The female athlete triad consists of disordered eating, loss of menstrual periods, and osteoporosis. Muscle dysmorphia could be described as "reverse anorexia"; a person views oneself as less muscular than desired, and resorts to patterns of disordered eating and obsessive exercise to achieve a muscular body shape. Diabulimia refers to the misuse of diabetes medication to regulate body weight. Some type 1 diabetic patients will skip doses of insulin to induce weight loss but then suffer the consequences of hyperglycemia. Alternatively, overdoses of insulin or glucose-lowering medications could be used to counter the effects of a binge. This practice could result in hypoglycemia. Orthorexia refers to an obsession with healthy eating such that overly restrictive food choices interfere with other aspects of life, such as social interactions.

15.7 Prevention of eating disorders is crucial because treatments are expensive, lengthy, and not 100% effective. Encouraging healthy attitudes about eating and exercise from a young age will aid in preventing the development of eating disorders. Those who work closely with children and young adults should encourage acceptance of diversity in body sizes and carefully phrase comments about body weight. Helping children to develop healthy ways to cope with emotions is also important.

15.8 Anorexia nervosa and bulimia nervosa are both biologically based disorders that are characterized by undue influence of body weight or shape on one's self-evaluation. The coping mechanisms (i.e., extreme dietary restriction versus binge-compensate cycles) used by people with these disorders can vary greatly.

Check Your Knowledge (Answers are available at the end of this question set.)

1. For 3 weeks leading up to her friend's wedding, Teresa skipped meals and restricted her food intake to 800 kcal per day so that she could fit into her bridesmaid dress. After the wedding, she resumed eating 2200 kcal per day. This is an example of
   a. disordered eating.
   c. size acceptance.
   b. an eating disorder.
   d. muscle dysmorphia.

2. Factors that could contribute to the development of eating disorders include
   a. genetics.
   c. sexual abuse.
   b. social pressures to be thin.
   d. all of these.

3. Anorexia nervosa can be defined as
   a. compulsive eating.
   c. denial of appetite.
   b. hyperactivity.
   d. purging.

4. The most likely long-term health consequence of anorexia nervosa is
   a. fractures resulting from bone loss.
   b. atherosclerotic heart disease.
   c. esophageal ulcers.
   d. cancer.

5. Bulimia is most frequently first recognized by a
   a. dietitian.
   c. dentist.
   b. physician.
   d. physical therapist.

6. The *most life-threatening* health risk from frequent vomiting due to bulimia nervosa is
   a. a drop in blood potassium.
   c. weight gain.
   b. constipation.
   d. swollen salivary glands.

7. Binge-eating disorder can be characterized as
   a. bingeing accompanied by purging.
   b. secretive eating.
   c. eating to avoid feeling and dealing with emotional pain.
   d. the early phase of bulimia nervosa.

8. Night eating syndrome is characterized by
   a. eating dinner but no breakfast or lunch.
   b. the need to eat to fall asleep.
   c. waking at night to purge by vomiting.
   d. consuming all of the daily calories at night.

9. Female athlete triad consists of
   a. anorexia nervosa, lack of family support, and overtraining.
   b. disordered eating, overtraining, and lack of menstrual periods.
   c. osteoporosis, lack of menstrual periods, and low energy availability.
   d. osteoporosis, lack of sleep, and low energy availability.

10. If you were assigned to speak to a group of middle school 4-H students about healthy eating, which message would be best?
    a. Ask children to sort various snack ideas into "good" or "bad" groups.
    b. Illustrate how many minutes of exercise are needed to burn the calories in various snacks.
    c. Advise kids to restrict favorite treats (e.g., ice cream), except as a reward for reaching a goal, such as getting a good grade on a test.
    d. Emphasize that children should eat when they are hungry and stop eating when they are full.

Answer Key: 1. a (LO 15.1), 2. d (LO 15.2), 3. c (LO 15.3), 4. a (LO 15.3), 5. c (LO 15.4), 6. a (LO 15.4), 7. c (LO 15.5), 8. b (LO 15.6), 9. c (LO 15.6), 10. d (LO 15.7)

Study Questions (Numbers refer to Learning Outcomes)

1. What are the typical characteristics of a person with anorexia nervosa? What may influence a person to begin rigid, self-imposed dietary patterns? **(LO 15.3)**

2. List the detrimental physical effects of bulimia nervosa. Describe important goals of the psychological and nutrition therapy used to treat patients with bulimia nervosa. **(LO 15.4)**

3. What medications are currently used in the treatment of anorexia nervosa, bulimia nervosa, and binge-eating disorder? **(LOs 15.3–15.5)**

4. Explain the role of excessive exercise in eating disorders. **(LO 15.1)**

5. How might parents or other role models contribute to the development of an eating disorder? Suggest an attitude that a parent or an adult friend of yours displayed that may not have been conducive to developing a healthy relationship with food. **(LO 15.7)**

6. Based on your knowledge of good nutrition and sound dietary habits, answer the following questions:
   a. How can repeated bingeing and purging lead to significant nutrient deficiencies?

   b. How can significant nutrient deficiencies contribute to major health problems in later life?
   c. A friend asks you, the nutrition expert, if it is okay to "cleanse" the body by eating only grapefruit for a week. What is your response? **(LO 15.1)**

7. Provide an example of the way society contributes to development of eating disorders. **(LO 15.2)**

8. List the three components of the female athlete triad. What is the major health risk associated with loss of menstrual periods in the female athlete? **(LO 15.6)**

9. How does binge-eating disorder differ from bulimia nervosa? Describe factors that contribute to the development of binge-eating disorder. **(LO 15.5)**

10. Provide two recommendations to reduce the problem of eating disorders in our society. **(LO 15.7)**

What the Dietitian Chose

It can be uncomfortable to confront a friend about an unhealthy behavior. You may worry about compromising your friendship. The eating and excessive exercise behaviors you have witnessed may be short-term disordered eating and may pass in a few weeks. On the other hand, they might just be the tip of the iceberg. Ignoring her behavior will not make it go away. As you have learned in this chapter, eating disorders can have serious consequences, and the earlier they are treated, the better the outcome. If you feel unable to address your concerns one on one with your roommate, you can seek help from a resident assistant in your dorm, a school counselor, or a nurse in the student health center. You will not be betraying your friendship; you will be showing how much you care about her by taking action.

Diagnosing an eating disorder is a complex task. People with eating disorders may deny the problem, hide their behaviors, and be irrational and uncooperative with those who try to help them. Do not try to diagnose your friend, but do try to keep the lines of communication open. Tell her what you have observed and ask her how you can help. She may open up to you and be glad she is not alone in her struggle. Then again, she may get angry and withdraw from you. Try to share what you know about eating disorders without lecturing or admonishing her. Also, be aware that your friend is going through a difficult emotional struggle that has probably been years in the making. Do not assume you know what she is going through.

Discussing healthy weight-management techniques with your roommate is not likely to help her if she has fallen prey to an eating disorder. She is already critical of her appearance and weight; your advice, although well intended and backed by the nutrition

© Don Mason/Blend Images LLC

knowledge you have picked up in this course, may be construed as judgmental. Eating disorders are not about food. It is important to be supportive but not critical. Taking the focus off food and body weight is important. Do not try to force her to eat or slow down on her exercise. If you can help get your roommate to seek professional treatment, psychiatric counseling will help to address her unhealthy relationship with food; eventually, nutrition counseling will help her to establish better eating habits.

Get prepared before you confront your roommate. Find out what information and resources are available on campus so you can share them with her. Recognize that you are not going to cure her disorder—she needs professional help. You can be supportive and patient as she deals with her inner turmoil. Listen and offer to go with her to seek care. Someday, you may be a health professional who is able to diagnose and counsel victims of eating disorders. For now, leave it to a qualified professional.

CASE STUDY SOLUTION — Eating Disorders—Steps to Recovery

1. Sarah has the characteristics to be diagnosed with anorexia nervosa: she restricts food intake to maintain a weight below 85% of that expected (BMI = 17), has a distorted view of her appearance, and fears weight gain.

2. Sarah's disordered eating habits began when she became self-conscious about her body when her peers teased her about being overweight. She began exercising each day and was successful at losing weight. Her disordered eating then began with restricting her food intake more. She enjoyed the self-control she had over her body.

3. The case study specifically mentions that Sarah's menstrual periods have ceased and she is intolerant to cold temperatures.

4. Her treatment will most likely involve outpatient therapy. A team of health professionals, consisting of a physician, registered dietitian, and psychologist, would provide therapy. She will need to reduce her physical activity and consume enough calories (e.g., 1000 to 1600 kcal per day initially) to promote weight gain. Her food intake will be increased by increments of about 100 to 200 kcal every few days until an acceptable rate of weight gain is achieved. The goal is to achieve a BMI that falls within

the normal range (e.g., 20). Family-based psychological therapy will help Sarah to correct misperceptions about food and body image and develop healthy coping strategies. After her body weight has stabilized, antidepressant medications may assist her recovery.

5. Several nutrient deficiencies are likely. Those with the most salient health effects are deficiencies of calcium and iron. The physician would likely prescribe a multivitamin and mineral supplement, along with an additional supplement of calcium as needed to make sure intake is in the range of 1200 to 1500 milligrams per day. Additional iron may be needed if Sarah is anemic. This overall practice will correct vitamin and mineral deficiencies. The calcium in particular will contribute to bone maintenance.

6. Sarah's outlook for recovery is not good unless she realizes she has a problem. Even if she is willing to accept the therapy and counseling, relapse is common. Sarah's disordered eating habits have been in place for about 3 years, so her problem is deeply rooted. The chances of recovery are greater if intervention is early in the course of the disease and if follow-up is continued for several years.

Further Readings

1. Borzekowski DLG and others: e-Ana and e-Mia: A content analysis of pro-eating disorder websites. *American Journal of Public Health* 100:1526, 2010.

2. Brownley KA and others: Pharmacological approaches to the management of binge eating disorder. *Drugs* 75:9, 2015.

3. Campbell IC and others: Eating disorders, gene-environment interactions, and epigenetics. *Neuroscience and Behavioral Reviews* 35:784, 2011.

4. Campbell K and Peebles R: Eating disorders in children and adolescents: State of the art review. *Pediatrics* 134:582, 2014.

5. Colton PA and others: Eating disorders in girls and women with type 1 diabetes: A longitudinal study of prevalence, onset, remission, and recurrence. *Diabetes Care* 38:1212, 2015.

6. Getz L: Understanding orthorexia—when healthful eating becomes an obsession. *Today's Dietitian* 16:18, 2014.

7. Klump K and others: Academy for Eating Disorders position paper: Eating disorders are serious mental illnesses. *International Journal of Eating Disorders* 42:97, 2009.

8. Le Grange D and others: Academy of Eating Disorders position paper: The role of the family in eating disorders. *International Journal of Eating Disorders* 43:1, 2010.

9. Luca A, Luca M, Calandra C: Eating disorders in late-life. *Aging and Disease* 6:48, 2015.

10. Matthews-Ewald MR, Zullig KJ, Ward RM: Sexual orientation and disordered eating behaviors among self-identified male and female college students. *Eating Behaviors* 15:441, 2014.

11. Mehler PS, Brown C: Anorexia nervosa—medical complications. *Journal of Eating Disorders* 3:11, 2015.

12. Mehler PS, Rylander M: Bulimia nervosa—medical complications. *Journal of Eating Disorders* 3:12, 2015.

13. Mitchison D, Hay P: The epidemiology of eating disorders: Genetic, environmental, and societal factors. *Clinical Epidemiology* 6:89, 2014.

14. Mitchison D, Mond J: Epidemiology of eating disorders, eating disordered behaviour, and body image disturbance in males: A narrative review. *Journal of Eating Disorders* 3:20, 2015.

15. Orenstein BW: Intermittent fasting: The key to long-term weight loss? *Today's Dietitian* 26(12):40, 2014.

16. Murray SB, Anderson LK: Deconstructing "atypical" eating disorders: An overview of emerging eating disorder phenotypes. *Current Psychiatry Reports* 17:86, 2015.

17. Nattiv A and others: American College of Sports Medicine position stand: The female athlete triad. *Medicine & Science in Sports & Exercise* 39:1867, 2007.

18. Ozier AD, Henry BW: Position of the American Dietetic Association: Nutrition intervention in the treatment of eating disorders. *Journal of the American Dietetic Association* 111:1236, 2011.

19. Patterson RE and others: Intermittent fasting and human metabolic health. *Journal of the Academy of Nutrition and Dietetics* 115:1203, 2015.

20. Rivera HM, Christiansen KJ, Sullivan EL: The role of maternal obesity in the risk of neuropsychiatric disorders. *Frontiers in Neuroscience* 9, 2015.

21. Seher CL: Binge-eating disorder—learning about this condition can help RDs counsel patients more effectively. *Today's Dietitian* 14:34, 2012.

22. Sojcher R and others: Evidence and potential mechanisms for mindfulness practices and energy psychology for obesity and binge-eating disorder. *Explore* 8:271, 2012.

23. Waterhous T and others: Practice paper of the American Dietetic Association: Nutrition intervention in the treatment of eating disorders. *Journal of the American Dietetic Association* 111:1261, 2011.

24. Yeo M, Hughes E: Eating disorders: Early identification in general practice. *Australian Family Physician* 40:108, 2011.

25. Zipfel S and others: Anorexia nervosa: Etiology, assessment, and treatment. *Lancet Psychiatry* 2:1099, 2015.

Rate Your Plate

I. Assessing Risk of Developing an Eating Disorder

British investigators have developed a five-question screening tool called the SCOFF Questionnaire for recognizing eating disorders:*

1. Do you make yourself **Sick** because you feel full?

2. Do you lose **Control** over how much you eat?

3. Have you lost more than **One** stone (about 13 pounds) recently?

4. Do you believe yourself to be **Fat** when others say you are thin?

5. Does **Food** dominate your life?

Two or more positive responses suggest an eating disorder.

1. After completing this questionnaire, do you feel that you might have an eating disorder or the potential to develop one?

   _____

   _____

© Digital Vision/PunchStock

2. Do you think any of your friends might have an eating disorder?

   _____

   _____

3. What counseling and education resources exist in your area or on your campus to help with a potential eating disorder?

   _____

   _____

4. If a friend has an eating disorder, what do you think is the best way to assist him or her in getting help?

   _____

   _____

*Morgan JF and others: The SCOFF Questionnaire, *British Medical Journal* 319:1467, 1999.

II. Helping Prevent Eating Disorders

You have been asked to speak to a junior high school class about eating disorders. What are four major points that you would make to help prevent disordered eating in this population?

1. _____
2. _____
3. _____
4. _____

Here are points you may consider:

1. Extreme thinness is oversold in the media. Extremely low weight (i.e., BMI of less than 17.5) is generally not healthy.

2. Self-induced vomiting is dangerous. Damage to the teeth, stomach, and esophagus often results.

3. Loss of menstrual periods is a sign of illness. It is important to see a physician about this. Bone deterioration is a common result.

4. The treatment of eating disorders in early phases aids success. These diseases are difficult to treat once firmly established.

© Nicholas Pitt/Digital Vision/Getty Images RF

Student Learning Outcomes

Chapter 16 is designed to allow you to:

16.1 Define and characterize the terms *hunger*, *malnutrition*, and *undernutrition*.

16.2 Examine undernutrition in the United States and highlight several programs established to combat this problem.

16.3 Examine undernutrition in the developing world and evaluate the major obstacles that hinder a solution.

16.4 Outline some possible solutions to undernutrition in the developing world.

16.5 Evaluate the consequences of undernutrition during critical periods in a person's life.

Undernutrition Throughout the World

What Would You Choose?

"You'd better clean your plate! There are starving children in Africa who would love to eat that dinner!" Mom was right: we often overlook the fact that we live in an affluent nation with access to plentiful food and clean water, whereas something as simple as clean drinking water is merely a dream in many developing nations. In fact, the problems of hunger and food insecurity exist in your own community. It is probably not feasible (or sanitary) to send your leftover green beans overseas, but there are some simple steps you can take to support local, national, and international agencies seeking to provide clean water and nutritious food for people in need. After considering the benefits of direct aid versus empowering others to help themselves, what would you choose to help reduce world hunger?

a Organize a group of friends to prepare and hand out peanut butter and jelly sandwiches to homeless people.

b Donate $10 per month to an international aid organization that supplies food to starving children in Africa.

c Participate in a 5K run/walk event that raises funds and awareness to combat world hunger.

d Buy locally grown fruits and vegetables at your community's farmers market.

Think about your choice as you read Chapter 16, then see What the Dietitian Chose at the end of the chapter.

Today, nearly one in seven people worldwide is chronically undernourished—too hungry to lead a productive, active life. The problems of poverty and undernutrition are widespread—even though there is enough food available to sufficiently feed all of us. Some progress has been made in decreasing the amount of poverty.

Within the developing world, over 900 million people are malnourished, with Asia having the largest number. This level of malnutrition is the main cause of lowered resistance to disease, infection, and death, with children under 5 years being the most susceptible.

This chapter examines the problem of undernutrition, the conditions that create it, and some solutions that are in progress. If we are to eradicate undernutrition, we all have to understand the problem. We must begin to assume responsibility today, not tomorrow, to work on solutions to hunger close to home and in faraway nations. It is important to recognize that many political, economic, and social factors worldwide, such as rising food prices, war, environmental catastrophes, and the global threat of AIDS, contribute to the hunger problem. The United Nations Millennium Development Goals (MDGs) are eight goals that address poverty, hunger, disease, illiteracy, environmental degradation, and discrimination against women. A global action plan was adopted in 2010. Progress toward each goal are presented in this chapter. So, why must we act today to stem this tide of undernutrition? This chapter provides some answers.

food insecure The state of being without reliable access to a sufficient quantity of affordable, nutritious food.

nutrition security Secure access to a nutritious diet coupled with a sanitary environment and adequate health services and care.

▲ Malnutrition is associated with overpopulation in some developing countries. © Getty Images

16.1 World Hunger: A Crisis of Nutrition Security

Uncertainty regarding the source of one's next meal remains a daily experience for close to 1 billion people around the world. This situation is troubling, considering that agriculture worldwide produces more than enough food to meet the energy requirements of each of the planet's 7 billion people. Even with this abundance, 805 million people—1 out of every 9 people on Earth—were still unable to access enough food in 2014 to lead active, healthy lives. Hence, these individuals were **food insecure.** This statistic comes from the United Nations Food and Agriculture Organization (FAO), which measures undernutrition around the world. Availability, access, utilization, and stability are the four pillars of food security, which exists when people have physical, social, and economic access to sufficient, safe, and nutritious food to meet their dietary needs and food preferences for an active and healthy life.

Food security is actually a component of a larger concept called **nutrition security.** The FAO defines nutrition security as secure access to an appropriately nutritious diet (i.e., protein, carbohydrate, fat, vitamins, minerals, and water), coupled with a sanitary environment and adequate health services and care, in order to ensure a healthy and active life for all household members (see Further Reading 11). The combined term *food and nutrition security* can be used to emphasize both food and health requirements (see Further Reading 1).

The serious problems of food insecurity and malnutrition exist in virtually every nation in the world (Fig. 16-1). They are most common in regions of the developing world, with Asia and the Pacific having the largest number (520 million), along with sub-Saharan Africa (214 million), and Latin America and the Caribbean (37 million). Nearly all people suffering from food insecurity, hunger, or malnutrition are poor. There has been global interest in poverty and hunger for decades, and new development goals have been set forth by the United Nations (UN). In 2010, the UN Millennium Development Goals (MDGs) of 2000 were reaffirmed and a global action plan adopted. The MDGs are eight goals that address

FIGURE 16-1 ▶ Undernutrition in 2012–2014 by region (in millions). Regions have differed in their rates of progress toward reducing hunger. South-Eastern Asia, Eastern Asia, Latin America, and the Caribbean have seen the greatest decline, whereas the rates have increased in Western Asia and sub-Saharan Africa.

Source: FAO.

Total = 805 million

Caucasus and Central Asia **10**

Developed regions **15**

Oceania **1**

Western Asia **19**

Northern Africa **13**

Latin America and the Caribbean **37**

South-Eastern Asia **64**

Southern Asia **276**

Eastern Asia **161**

Sub-Saharan Africa **214**

poverty, hunger, disease, illiteracy, environmental degradation, and discrimination against women. To date, with concerted efforts at the global, regional, national, and local levels, the MDGs have saved the lives of millions and improved living conditions for countless more. The MDGs, targeted outcomes, and progress are listed in Table 16-1 and will be discussed throughout this chapter (see Further Reading 17).

TABLE 16-1 ■ Millennium Development Goals and Progress

Millennium Development Goals	MDG Targets	MDG Progress
Goal 1: Eradicate extreme poverty and hunger	• Halve, between 1990 and 2015, the proportion of people whose income is less than $1.25 a day • Achieve full and productive employment and decent work for all, including women and young people • Halve, between 1990 and 2015, the proportion of people who suffer from hunger	• Extreme poverty has declined significantly over the last two decades. In 1990, nearly half of the population in the developing world lived on less than $1.25 a day; that proportion dropped to 14% in 2015. • Globally, the number of people living in extreme poverty has declined by more than half, falling from 1.9 billion in 1990 to 836 million in 2015. Most progress has occurred since 2000. • The number of people in the working middle class (i.e., living on more than $4 a day) has almost tripled between 1991 and 2015. This group now makes up half the workforce in the developing regions, up from just 18% in 1991. • The proportion of undernourished people in developing regions has fallen by almost half since 1990, from 23.3% in 1990–1992 to 12.9% in 2014–2016.
Goal 2: Achieve universal primary education	• Ensure that, by 2015, children everywhere, boys and girls alike, will be able to complete a full course of primary schooling	• The primary school net enrollment rate in developing regions has reached 91% in 2015, up from 83% in 2000. • The number of out-of-school children of primary school age worldwide has fallen by almost half, to an estimated 57 million in 2015, down from 100 million in 2000. • Sub-Saharan Africa has had the best record of improvement in primary education of any region since the MDGs were established. The region achieved a 20 percentage point increase in the net enrollment rate from 2000 to 2015, compared to a gain of 8 percentage points between 1990 and 2000. • The literacy rate among youth aged 15 to 24 has increased globally from 83% to 91% between 1990 and 2015. The gap between women and men has narrowed.
Goal 3: Promote gender equality and empower women	• Eliminate gender disparity in primary and secondary education, preferably by 2005, and in all levels of education no later than 2015	• Many more girls are now in school compared to 15 years ago. The developing regions as a whole have achieved the target to eliminate gender disparity in primary, secondary and tertiary education. • In Southern Asia, only 74 girls were enrolled in primary school for every 100 boys in 1990. Today, 103 girls are enrolled for every 100 boys. • Women now make up 41% of paid workers outside the agricultural sector, an increase from 35% in 1990. • Between 1991 and 2015, the proportion of women in vulnerable employment as a share of total female employment has declined 13 percentage points. In contrast, **vulnerable employment** among men fell by 9 percentage points. • Women have gained ground in parliamentary representation in nearly 90% of the 174 countries with data over the past 20 years. The average proportion of women in parliament has nearly doubled during the same period. Yet, still only one in five members are women.
Goal 4: Reduce child mortality	• Reduce by two-thirds, between 1990 and 2015, the under-5 mortality rate	• The global under-5 mortality rate has declined by more than half, dropping from 90 to 43 deaths per 1,000 live births between 1990 and 2015. • Despite population growth in the developing regions, the number of deaths of children under 5 has declined from 12.7 million in 1990 to almost 6 million in 2015 globally. • Measles vaccination helped prevent nearly 15.6 million deaths between 2000 and 2013. The number of globally reported measles cases declined by 67% for the same period. • About 84% of children worldwide received at least one dose of measles-containing vaccine in 2013, up from 73% in 2000.

TABLE 16-1 ■ *(continued)*

Millennium Development Goals	MDG Targets	MDG Progress
Goal 5: Improve maternal health	• Reduce by three quarters, between 1990 and 2015, the maternal mortality ratio (number of women who die during pregnancy and childbirth, per 100,000 live births) • Achieve universal access to reproductive health	• Since 1990, the maternal mortality ratio has declined by 45% worldwide, with most reduction occurring since 2000. • In Southern Asia, the maternal mortality ratio declined by 64% between 1990 and 2013, and in sub-Saharan Africa it fell by 49%. • More than 71% of births were assisted by skilled health personnel globally in 2014, an increase from 59% in 1990. • In Northern Africa, the proportion of pregnant women who received four or more antenatal visits increased from 50% in 1990 to 89% in 2014. • Contraceptive prevalence among women aged 15 to 49, married or in a union, increased from 55% in 1990 worldwide to 64% in 2015.
Goal 6: Combat HIV/AIDS, malaria, and other diseases	• Have halted, by 2015, and begun to reverse the spread of HIV/AIDS • Achieve, by 2010, universal access to treatment for HIV/AIDS for all those who need it • Have halted, by 2015, and begun to reverse the incidence of malaria and other major diseases	• New HIV infections fell by approximately 40% between 2000 and 2013, from an estimated 3.5 million cases to 2.1 million. • By June 2014, 13.6 million people living with HIV were receiving antiretroviral therapy (ART) globally, an immense increase from just 800,000 in 2003. ART averted 7.6 million deaths from AIDS between 1995 and 2013. • Over 6.2 million malaria deaths have been averted between 2000 and 2015, primarily of children under 5 years of age in sub-Saharan Africa. The global malaria incidence rate has fallen by an estimated 37% and the mortality rate by 58%. • More than 900 million insecticide-treated mosquito nets were delivered to malaria-endemic countries in sub-Saharan Africa between 2004 and 2014. • Between 2000 and 2013, tuberculosis prevention, diagnosis, and treatment interventions saved an estimated 37 million lives. The tuberculosis mortality rate fell by 45% and the prevalence rate by 41% between 1990 and 2013.
Goal 7: Ensure environmental sustainability	• Integrate the principles of sustainable development into country policies and programs and reverse the loss of environmental resources • Reduce biodiversity loss, achieving, by 2010, a significant reduction in the rate of loss • Halve, by 2015, the proportion of people without sustainable access to safe drinking water • Achieve, by 2020, a significant improvement in the lives of at least 100 million slum dwellers	• Ozone-depleting substances have been virtually eliminated since 1990, and the ozone layer is expected to recover by the middle of this century. • Terrestrial and marine protected areas in many regions have increased substantially since 1990. In Latin America and the Caribbean, coverage of terrestrial protected areas rose from 8.8% to 23.4% between 1990 and 2014. • In 2015, 91% of the global population is using an improved drinking water source, compared to 76% in 1990. • Of the 2.6 billion people who have gained access to improved drinking water since 1990, 1.9 billion gained access to piped drinking water on premises. Over half of the global population (58%) now enjoys this higher level of service. • Globally, 147 countries have met the drinking water target, 95 countries have met the sanitation target, and 77 countries have met both. • Worldwide, 2.1 billion people have gained access to improved sanitation. The proportion of people practicing open defecation has fallen almost by half since 1990. • The proportion of urban population living in slums in the developing regions fell from approximately 39.4% in 2000 to 29.7% in 2014.
Goal 8: Global partnership for development	• Develop further an open, rule-based, predictable, nondiscriminatory trading and financial system • Address the special needs of the least developed countries • Address the special needs of landlocked countries and small island developing states • Deal comprehensively with the debt problems of developing countries • In cooperation with pharmaceutical companies, provide access to affordable essential drugs in developing countries • In cooperation with the private sector, make available benefits of new technologies, especially information and communications	• Official development assistance from developed countries increased by 66% in real terms between 2000 and 2014, reaching $135.2 billion. • In 2014, Denmark, Luxembourg, Norway, Sweden, and the United Kingdom continued to exceed the United Nations official development assistance target of 0.7% of gross national income. • In 2014, 79% of imports from developing to developed countries were admitted duty free, up from 65% in 2000. • The proportion of external debt service to export revenue in developing countries fell from 12% in 2000 to 3% in 2013. • As of 2015, 95% of the world's population is covered by a mobile-cellular signal. • The number of mobile-cellular subscriptions has grown almost tenfold in the last 15 years, from 738 million in 2000 to over 7 billion in 2015. • Internet penetration has grown from just over 6% of the world's population in 2000 to 43% in 2015. As a result, 3.2 billion people are linked to a global network of content and applications.

HUNGER

We will begin our look at the problem of world hunger and malnutrition by defining some key terms. The physiological state that results when not enough food is eaten to meet energy needs is **hunger.** It also describes an uneasiness, discomfort, weakness, or pain caused by lack of food. The medical and societal costs of the undernutrition that can result from hunger are high rates of preterm births, mental disabilities, inadequate growth and development, poor academic performance, decreased work output, and chronic disease. Although malnutrition does occur in North America, it is typically not a result of extreme poverty over a large segment of the population. Instead, there are often specific causes, such as an eating disorder, alcoholism, inadequate care in skilled nursing facilities (nursing homes), or homelessness. There is also some degree of moderate malnutrition in some of the poorer segments of North American society (i.e., those earning less than the current poverty level). Fortunately, there are resources such as food pantries and food stamps, though sometimes there are bureaucratic obstacles to getting these resources to the people who actually need them. In addition, there is **food insecurity,** which describes a state of anxiety about running out of food or running out of money to buy more food. In 2014, 14% of households in the United States (over 48 millions households) reported experiencing food insecurity.

Around the world, poverty is a primary cause of malnutrition. In the United States, child poverty reached a record high level in 2014, with 15.3 million children (20% of all children under the age of 18) in families living below the federal poverty level. Poverty is defined as a family of four having an income less than of $24,250 per year in 2015 (see current poverty guidelines). Research, however, estimates that families need an income of about twice that level to cover basic expenses. Living in poverty impairs a child's ability to learn and contributes to inadequate growth, behavioral problems, and poor health. The risks of poverty are greatest for young children. Fortunately, the United States does offer food assistance programs for low-income families; therefore, most children in the United States that utilize these services are shielded from hunger.

MALNUTRITION AND MICRONUTRIENT DEFICIENCIES

A condition of impaired development or function caused by either a chronic deficiency or excess in caloric and/or nutrient intake is **malnutrition.** When food supplies are low and the population is large, **undernutrition** is common, leading to nutritional deficiency diseases, such as **goiter** (from an iodine deficiency) and **xerophthalmia** (from poor vitamin A intake). However, when the food supply is ample or overabundant, incorrect food choices coupled with an excessive intake can lead to overnutrition and obesity and its related chronic diseases, such as type 2 diabetes.

Undernutrition is the most common form of malnutrition among the poor in both developing and developed countries. Undernutrition is also the primary cause of specific nutrient deficiencies that can result in muscle wasting, blindness, scurvy, pellagra, beriberi, anemia, rickets, goiter, and a host of other problems (Table 16-2).

The most critical micronutrients missing from diets worldwide (Fig. 16-2) are iron, vitamin A, iodine, zinc, and various B vitamins (e.g., folate), as well as selenium and vitamin C (see Further Readings 5 and 6). About 1 billion people, mostly in the developing world, are affected by iron deficiency. The same is true for zinc deficiencies. With poor iron status, cognitive development will likely be impaired, particularly if prolonged deficiency occurs during early infancy. An estimated 50 million people worldwide also suffer brain damage from preventable maternal iodine deficiency. In addition, new studies from the United Kingdom and Australia suggest that pregnant women who do not consume enough iodine may put their children at risk of lower intelligence and reading ability (refer to Section 12.8, and see Newsworthy Nutrition later in this section).

It is estimated that in vitamin A–deficient areas, a large percentage of those who are deficient are pregnant women; and at least 250 million preschool children are vitamin A deficient. Although severe vitamin A deficiency, which causes blindness, is on the decline, up to 500,000 preschool-age children are still blinded by it each year, with half of them

vulnerable employment Employment status groups that are less likely to have formal work arrangements, and are therefore more likely to lack decent working conditions, adequate social security, and "voice" through effective representation by trade unions and similar organizations. Vulnerable employment is often characterized by inadequate earnings, low productivity, and difficult conditions of work that undermine workers' fundamental rights.

hunger The primarily physiological (internal) drive to find and eat food.

food insecurity A condition of anxiety regarding running out of either food or money to buy more food.

malnutrition Failing health that results from longstanding dietary practices that do not coincide with nutritional needs.

undernutrition Failing health that results from a longstanding dietary intake that is not enough to meet nutritional needs.

goiter An enlargement of the thyroid gland; this is often caused by insufficient iodine in the diet.

xerophthalmia Hardening of the cornea and drying of the surface of the eye, which can result in blindness.

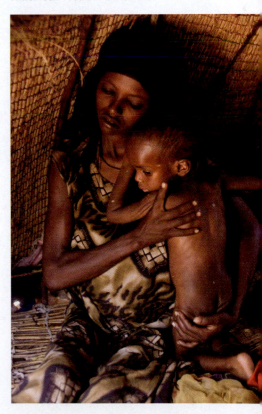

▲ Minimal intakes of protein and zinc limit the growth of children worldwide. About 25% of children in developing countries show evidence of inadequate growth and development. © Mike Goldwater/Alamy

TABLE 16-2 ■ Nutrient-Deficiency Diseases That Commonly Accompany Undernutrition

Disease and Key Nutrient Involved*	Typical Effects of Deficiency	Sources of Deficient Nutrient	Target Populations for Interventions
Xerophthalmia Vitamin A	Blindness from chronic eye infections, dryness, restricted growth, and keratinization of epithelial tissues	Fortified milk, sweet potatoes, spinach, greens, carrots, cantaloupe, and apricots	Asia and Africa
Rickets Vitamin D	Poorly calcified bones, bowed legs, and other bone deformities	Fortified milk, fish oils, and sun exposure	Asia, Africa, and parts of the world where religious dress prevent women and children from receiving adequate sun exposure; older adults in developed nations
Beriberi Thiamin	Nerve degeneration, altered muscle coordination, and cardiovascular problems	Sunflower seeds, pork, whole and enriched grains, and dried beans	Victims of famine in Africa and alcoholics worldwide
Ariboflavinosis Riboflavin	Inflammation of oral cavity; nervous system disorders	Milk, mushrooms, spinach, liver, and enriched grains	Victims of famine in Africa
Pellagra Niacin	Diarrhea, dermatitis, dementia, and death	Mushrooms, bran, tuna, chicken, beef, peanuts, and whole and enriched grains	Victims of famine in Africa and survivors of war-torn Eastern Europe
Megaloblastic anemia Folate	Enlarged red blood cells, fatigue, and weakness	Green leafy vegetables, legumes, oranges, and liver	Asia and Africa
Scurvy Vitamin C	Delayed wound healing, internal bleeding, and abnormal formation of bones and teeth	Citrus fruits, strawberries, broccoli, and tomatoes	Victims of famine in Africa
Iron-deficiency anemia Iron	Reduced work output, retarded growth, and increased health risk in pregnancy	Meats, seafood, broccoli, peas, bran, whole grains, and enriched products	Worldwide
Goiter Iodine	Enlarged thyroid gland in teenagers and adults, possible mental retardation, and congenital hypothyroidism	Iodized salt and saltwater fish	South America, Eastern Europe, and Africa

*Although the nutrients are listed separately to illustrate the important role of each one, often two or more nutrition-deficiency diseases are found in an undernourished person in the developing world.

The Irish potato famine of 1840 to 1850 caused an estimated 2 million deaths and resulted in nearly as many people emigrating to other countries, such as the United States and Canada. More than 3 million people may have perished in the great famine of 1943 in Bengal, India. China suffered a famine from 1959 to 1961 with mortality ranging from 20 to 43 million. In 1974, another 1.5 million starved in the country of Bangladesh.

likely to die within 12 months of losing their sight. The United Nations Children's Fund (UNICEF) reports that the lives of one in three children could be saved annually in the developing world if vitamin A supplements were provided a few times each year. The annual cost per child is 3 to 6 cents.

Of the 7.1 billion people in the world, about 2 billion may experience episodes of food shortages and be affected by some form of micronutrient malnutrition. Death and disease from infections, particularly those causing acute and prolonged diarrhea or respiratory disease, increase dramatically when the infections occur during a state of sustained undernutrition. Chronic undernutrition leaves many people in the developing world in a chronic state of depressed immunity, in turn greatly increasing the risk of death, especially during childhood.

Newsworthy Nutrition

Maternal iodine (iodide) deficiency could lead to lower educational outcomes

The hypothesis of this study was that children born to mothers with mild iodine deficiency during pregnancy will have poorer educational outcomes in primary school than peers whose mothers did not have iodine deficiency during pregnancy. The study was a longitudinal design with follow-up when the children were 9 years old. The study participants were children born in Australia between 1999 and 2001. The mild iodine deficiency during pregnancy was followed with the children subsequently growing up in an iodine-adequate environment. Children whose mothers had mild iodine deficiency had reductions of 10.0% in spelling, 7.6% in grammar, and 5.7% in English-literacy performance compared with children whose mothers were not iodine deficient. The authors conclude that even mild iodine deficiency during pregnancy can have long-term adverse impacts on fetal brain development that will affect cognition and are not improved by iodine sufficiency during childhood.

Source: Hynes KL and others: Mild iodine deficiency during pregnancy is associated with reduced educational outcomes in the offspring: 9-Year follow-up of the gestational iodine cohort. *Journal of Clinical Endocrinology and Metabolism* 98(5):1954, 2013.

FIGURE 16-2 ▲ Critical micronutrient deficiencies worldwide.

Protein-calorie malnutrition (PCM) is a form of undernutrition caused by an extremely deficient intake of calories or protein and is generally accompanied by illness. The dramatic results of PCM—**kwashiorkor** and **marasmus**—were described in Section 6.8. This chapter focuses on the more subtle effects of a chronic lack of food.

FAMINE

The extreme form of chronic hunger is **famine.** Periods of famine are characterized by large-scale loss of life, climate change, social disruption, economic chaos, and worldwide conflict. As a result of these extreme events, the affected community experiences a downward spiral characterized by human distress; sales of land, livestock, and other farm assets; mass migration; division and impoverishment of the poorest families; crime; and humanitarian crises, as recently seen in Libya and Somalia with 90% of their population affected by violence and insecurity. In the midst of all this, undernutrition rates soar; infectious diseases, such as cholera, spread; and many people die.

Special efforts are needed to eradicate the fundamental causes of famine. These causes vary by region and decade, but the most common cause of famine is crop failure. The most obvious reasons are extreme weather conditions such as floods or drought, war, and civil strife. War deserves a special focus and will be specifically addressed in Section 16.3.

GENERAL EFFECTS OF SEMISTARVATION

In the initial stages, the results of undernutrition from semistarvation are often so mild that physical symptoms are absent and blood tests do not usually detect these slight metabolic changes. Even in the absence of detectable symptoms, however, undernourishment may affect the ability to work, learn, reproduce, and recover from illnesses or injuries. Recall from Section 2.5 that as tissues continue to be depleted of nutrients, blood tests eventually detect biochemical changes, such as a drop in blood hemoglobin concentration. Physical symptoms, such as body weakness or fatigue, tend to follow with further depletion. Finally, the full-blown symptoms of the deficiency are recognizable, such as when blindness accompanies a vitamin A deficiency.

protein-calorie malnutrition (PCM) A condition resulting from regularly consuming insufficient amounts of calories and protein. The deficiency eventually results in body wasting, primarily of lean tissue, and an increased susceptibility to infections. Also known as *protein-energy malnutrition (PEM)*.

kwashiorkor A disease occurring primarily in young children who have an existing disease and consume a marginal amount of calories and insufficient protein in relation to needs. The child generally suffers from infections and exhibits edema, poor growth, weakness, and an increased susceptibility to further illness.

marasmus A disease resulting from consuming a grossly insufficient amount of protein and calories; one of the diseases classed as protein-calorie malnutrition. Victims have little or no fat stores, little muscle mass, and poor strength. Death from infections is common.

famine An extreme shortage of food, which leads to massive starvation in a population; often associated with crop failures, war, and political unrest.

The effects of hunger are diverse, widespread, and devastating:

- Reduced energy and strength
- Diminished concentration
- Impaired ability to learn
- Lowered productivity
- Worsening of chronic health conditions
- Increased susceptibility to infectious diseases
- Deterioration of mood
- Slowed recovery from illness and injury
- Decreased birth weights
- Decreased growth in infants and children

Historical Research on Undernutrition

In the 1940s, a group of researchers led by Dr. Ansel Keys examined the general effects of undernutrition on adults. Previously healthy men were fed a diet averaging about 1800 kcal daily for 6 months. During this time, the men lost an average of 24% of their body weight. After about 3 months, the participants complained of fatigue, muscle soreness, irritability, intolerance to cold, and hunger pains. They exhibited a lack of ambition, self-discipline, concentration, and were often moody, apathetic, and depressed. Their heart rate and muscle tone decreased and they developed edema. When the men were permitted to eat normally again, feelings of recurrent hunger and fatigue persisted, even after 12 weeks of rehabilitation. Full recovery required about 8 months. This study helps us understand the general state of undernourished adults worldwide.

Source: Keys, A: Will you starve that they be better fed? *Brochure*, May 27, 1944.

When a few people in a population develop a severe deficiency, this may represent only the "tip of the iceberg." Typically, a much greater number of individuals in that area may be suffering milder degrees of undernutrition. These deficiencies should not, therefore, be dismissed as trivial, especially in the developing world. In many low- and even middle-income countries, it is typical for a combination of micronutrient deficiencies to occur together. These are caused by any number of factors, including diets of poor nutritional quality related to seasonal variation in food availability, low bioavailability of nutrients from plant sources, cultural food practices, and poverty. It is becoming clear that combined deficiencies of specific vitamins and minerals (especially iron and zinc) can significantly reduce work performance, even in the absence of obvious physical symptoms. This resulting state of ill health, in turn, diminishes the ability of individuals, communities, and even whole countries to perform at peak levels of physical and mental capacity (Fig. 16-3). Because nutritional requirements are high during periods of rapid growth, pregnant women, infants, and children are especially vulnerable to the effects of undernutrition. Studies of pregnant women and children in developing countries have proven the negative impact of micronutrient deficiencies on birth size, length of gestation, growth, and intellectual development (see Newsworthy Nutrition in this section).

Strategies to address the multiple nutrient deficiencies in developing countries have included supplementation and fortification of ready-to-use foods and beverages. Although supplementation has been the most widely practiced intervention, public health experts believe that fortification of a commonly consumed food could be a single, cost-effective intervention strategy that would target a larger population. Studies of micronutrient supplementation during pregnancy have shown an increase in birth weight and a reduction in low birth weights but no impact on preterm births or perinatal mortality. In children, micronutrient supplementation with three or more nutrients has resulted in increases in height and weight (see Further Reading 5).

Added to their lack of nourishment, the inhabitants of poverty-stricken countries must also contend with recurrent infections, poor sanitation, extreme weather conditions, and regular exposure to infectious diseases. Deficiencies of micronutrients, especially iron and zinc, can lead to reduced immune function and thereby increase the risk of diseases, such as diarrhea and pneumonia.

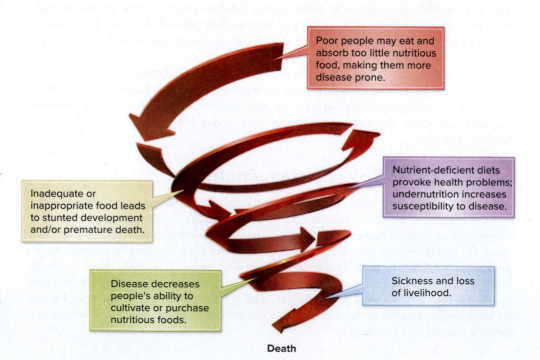

Poor people may eat and absorb too little nutritious food, making them more disease prone.

Nutrient-deficient diets provoke health problems; undernutrition increases susceptibility to disease.

Sickness and loss of livelihood.

Disease decreases people's ability to cultivate or purchase nutritious foods.

Inadequate or inappropriate food leads to stunted development and/or premature death.

Death

FIGURE 16-3 ▶ The downward spiral of poverty and illness can ultimately end in death (based on World Food Programme graphic).

✓ **CONCEPT CHECK 16.1**

1. What are the characteristics of hunger?
2. What is the definition of food insecurity?
3. Define the term *nutrition security*.
4. What are the health results of chronic hunger?
5. What is the primary cause of undernutrition?
6. At which stages of the life cycle is undernutrition especially damaging?
7. What are the effects of chronic undernutrition?

16.2 Undernutrition in the United States

In 2014, roughly 44.7 million (14.8%) people in the United States were living at or below the poverty level, estimated at about $23,850 annually for a family of four (see Further Reading 8). For the fourth consecutive year, the number of people in poverty at the national level was not statistically different from the previous year's estimates. For most groups, the number of people in poverty either decreased or did not show a statistically significant change. The poverty rate for children under age 18 was 21.1%, 13.5% for those aged 18 to 64, and 10.0% for people aged 65 and older. In 2012, the percentage of the population living in food-insecure households in Canada is lower (one in eight persons or 4 million total) than in the United States (one in six persons). According to 2014 U.S. Census data, the highest rates of poverty were found among Blacks (26%), followed by Hispanics (of any race, 24%), Asians at 12%, and Whites at 10% (see Further Reading 15).

The poor often face difficult choices when deciding between purchasing food and other essentials. According to the *Hunger in America 2014 Study,* 57% of households report choosing between purchasing food and housing costs, 69% between food and utilities, 66% between food and medicine, and 67% between food and access to transportation. While housing and utility costs, medical care, and transportation fares are nonnegotiable, a person can always eat less. Food is one of the few flexible items in a poor person's budget. The short-term consequences of eating less may be less dramatic than getting evicted, but the long-term cumulative effects are significant.

▲ Poverty aggravates the problem of hunger in the United States. © PhotoLink/Photodisc/Getty Images

HELPING THE HUNGRY IN THE UNITED STATES

Until the twentieth century, individuals and a wide variety of charitable, often church-related organizations provided most of the help to poor, undernourished people in the United States. Early programs rarely distributed direct cash payments to poor people because these were thought to reduce recipients' motivation to improve their circumstances or change behaviors, such as excessive drinking, that contributed to their poverty. Beginning in the early 1900s, the involvement of local, county, and state governments in providing assistance to the poor has steadily increased.

Low-Income People and Families After observing extensive hunger and poverty during his presidential campaign in the 1960s, President John F. Kennedy revitalized the Food Stamp Program, which had begun two decades earlier, and expanded commodity distribution programs. In October 2008, the name of the Food Stamp Program was changed to the Supplemental Nutrition Assistance Program (SNAP) (Table 16-3). The new name reflects the program's focus on nutrition and putting healthy food within reach for low-income households. SNAP helps low-income people and families buy food they need for good health. The program allows recipients to use an electronic benefit transfer (EBT) card to purchase food and garden seeds—but not tobacco, cleaning items, alcoholic beverages, and nonedible products—at stores authorized to accept them. In 2015, the maximum dollar

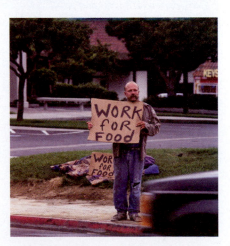

▲ This man is hoping to find work to fill his basic need of food. There are many federal food assistance programs for those in need. © PhotoLink/Getty Images

TABLE 16-3 ■ Some Federally Subsidized Programs That Supply Food for People in the United States

Program	Eligibility	Description
Supplemental Nutrition Assistance Program (formerly Food Stamp Program)*	Low-income families	Electronic benefit transfer (debit) cards are given to purchase food at grocery stores; the amount is based on size of household and income.
The Emergency Food Assistance Program (TEFAP)*	Low-income families	Provides nutrition assistance to needy Americans through distribution of USDA food commodities.
Commodity Supplemental Food Program	Certain low-income populations, such as pregnant women, children up to the age of 6 years, and seniors	USDA surplus foods are distributed by county agencies; not found in all states; may be based on nutritional risk.
Special Supplemental Nutrition Program for Women, Infants, and Children (WIC)*	Low-income pregnant/lactating women, infants, and children less than 5 years at nutritional risk	Coupons are given to purchase milk, cheese, fruit juice, cereal, infant formula, and other specific food items at grocery stores; includes nutrition education component. Includes new Farmers' Market Nutrition Program (FMNP).
National School Lunch Program*	Low-income children of school age	Free or reduced-price lunch is distributed by the school; meal follows USDA pattern based on MyPlate; cost for the child depends on family income. For students who do not participate in the lunch program, special milk program may be available.
School Breakfast Program	Low-income children of school age	Free or reduced-price breakfast is distributed by the school; meal follows USDA pattern; and cost for the child depends on family income.
Child and Adult Care Food Program	Children enrolled in organized child-care programs and seniors in adult-care programs; income guidelines are the same as those for the National School Lunch Program	Reimbursement is given for meals supplied to children at the site; meals must follow USDA guidelines based on MyPlate.
Congregate Meals for the Elderly	Age 60 or over (no income guidelines)	Free noon meal is furnished at a site; meal follows specific pattern based on one-third of nutrient needs.
Home-Delivered Meals	Age 60 or over, homebound	Noon meal is delivered at no cost or for a donation at least 5 days a week. Sometimes additional meals for later consumption are delivered at the same time; often referred to as "Meals on Wheels."
Summer Food Service Program	Residence in a low-income neighborhood or participation in a program	Free, nutritious meals and snacks are given to children in a low-income area at a central site, such as a school or a community center during long school vacations.
Food Distribution Program on Indian Reservations*	Low-income American Indian and non-Indian households on reservations; members of federally recognized tribes	Alternative to Supplemental Nutrition Assistance Program, distributes monthly food packages; includes nutrition education component.
Fresh Fruit and Vegetable Program	Low-income elementary schools	Provides free fresh fruits and vegetables to increase their consumption and combat childhood obesity.

*Benefits increased through the American Recovery and Reinvestment Act of 2009.

amount of SNAP benefits a household of four can receive each month was $649, depending on their income and expenses. Over 45.4 million Americans—about one in seven adults—participated in this program in September 2015. Despite some improvements in economic conditions, the need for food assistance remains relatively high in the United States.

School Breakfast and Lunch Programs The U.S. Congress established the School Breakfast Program in 1965 as politicians became aware of the number of hungry children coming to school. School breakfast and lunch programs still enable low-income students—14.1 million for breakfast and 30.5 million for lunch in 2015—to receive meals free or at reduced cost if certain income guidelines are met. The basis of eligibility for free and reduced-price meals can be determined by categorical, direct, community, or income-based eligibility.

Senior Nutrition Services The Older Americans Act (OAA) authorizes the elderly nutrition services program to reduce hunger and food insecurity among older individuals, promote socialization of older individuals, promote the health and well-being of older individuals, and delay adverse health conditions for older individuals. Over 11 million (one in five) older adults are served annually by OAA programs. The 2016 budget proposes an increase of $138 million for the OAA, including a $60 million increase for the congregate and home-delivered meals programs.

▲ Food insecurity is part of the North American landscape. A "safety net" of programs exists, but it is porous. USDA

Women, Infants, and Children In 1972, the Special Supplemental Nutrition Program for Women, Infants, and Children (WIC) was authorized. This program provides food vouchers and nutrition education to low-income, nutritionally at-risk pregnant and lactating women and their young children. It served 8.3 million women and children each month in 2014. Read more about child and adolescent nutrition assistance programs in Further Reading 3.

Sometimes, severe undernutrition due to involuntary hunger does occur in the United States. More often, though, Americans experience periodic episodes of hunger and food insecurity. Unemployment, medical and housing expenses, and even occasional holiday shopping can cause a household to be hungry or food insecure.

Government food assistance programs are like a "safety net": they are strong, yet porous. These programs were originally known as "welfare," and were designed to provide short-term relief for Americans suffering financial hardship. Now, many low- and middle-income U.S. households rely on food pantries and federal assistance chronically and for the majority of their nutritional needs. Feeding America® estimates that one in seven Americans—that is, 46 million people—relied on food pantries and emergency meal service programs to feed themselves and their families in 2014. Statistics show that most people requesting emergency food assistance are members of families (i.e., children and their parents). This is not surprising considering that households with children report a higher rate of food insecurity than households without children, and the rate is even higher for households with children headed by single parents.

The American Recovery and Reinvestment Act, also known as the "stimulus package," was signed in 2009 in an effort to increase a variety of federal benefits and services, including those offered by the federal food and nutrition programs committing over $830 billion between 2009 and 2019 (see Table 16-3). The enhancement of these programs helped those workers and families hardest hit by the economic crisis. Privately funded programs have also stepped in to add to state and federal efforts to combat hunger and related food insecurity in the United States. There are more than 150,000 charitable food providers (such as food banks and food pantries) helping to address this problem.

Undernutrition in North America is a much more subtle problem than in developing countries. To the untrained eye, undernourished children may just seem skinny, when, in fact, their growth is being stunted by insufficient nutrients. More likely, though, children from food-insecure households are prone to be overweight. This may be the result of considerable reliance on convenience foods that provide excessive saturated fat and sugar. The availability of cooking facilities also affects nutrient intake among the poor. Without adequate cooking facilities, people may buy expensive convenience foods that require no preparation. These are typically highly processed snack foods, which provide calories but are often lacking in nutrients.

SOCIOECONOMIC FACTORS RELATED TO UNDERNUTRITION

In the United States, persistent hunger and food insecurity are largely associated with two interrelated conditions: poverty and homelessness. Thus, the economic, social, and political changes that lead to an increase in the number of poor or homeless people also tend to intensify the problem of undernutrition.

▲ Food pantries and soup kitchens are important sources of nutrients for a growing number of people in the United States. Consider volunteering some of your time to a local program. © Brand X Pictures/PunchStock

Poverty Poverty is determined in the United States using poverty thresholds that are issued each year by the Census Bureau. Persons are designated as poor if they have income less than that deemed sufficient to purchase the basic needs of food, shelter, clothing, and other essentials. Poverty, however, is complex and does not mean the same thing to all people. Poverty can usually be characterized as *situational* or *generational*. Households can fall into situational poverty as the result of dire or unexpected circumstances, such as the head of the household getting laid off from a job or a family member needing expensive medical treatment. Some have linked situational poverty to the seven D's: divorce, death, disease, downsizing, disablement, disasters, and debt. Situational poverty may affect entire communities as a result of economic downturns and may be alleviated by temporary social service programs. In contrast, generational poverty refers to a culture of persistent poverty passed from parents to children, with two or more generations living in poverty. Generational poverty is more complex because the cultures and traditions of previous generations are passed on to future generations and often include an undervaluation of the benefits of education and a lack of self-efficacy when it comes to changing one's economic circumstances.

A major driving force behind poverty is underemployment. This relationship increased significantly with the economic recession that caused unemployment to soar between December 2007 and September 2009, when 7.6 million jobs were lost across all major private-sector industries. The impact of unemployment was enhanced because many states cut their welfare assistance, resulting in more people living in poverty and in need of food assistance, at risk of homelessness, and without sufficient health care. Fortunately, the economy has more recently experienced some recovery. After cresting at 10% in October 2009, the unemployment rate has declined as the labor market has grown slowly and steadily. In December 2015, the number of unemployed persons was 7.9 million, resulting in an unemployment rate of 5.0%.

Access to Healthy Food Access to affordable and nutritious foods from supermarkets, grocery stores, or other retailers is also a challenge to many Americans, making it harder for them to eat a balanced, nutrient-dense diet (see Further Reading 7). In 2011, 23.5 million Americans, including 6.5 million children, lived in low-income areas without access to stores that were likely to sell affordable healthy foods such as fresh fruits and vegetables. These impoverished areas with little access to healthy foods have been named **food deserts.** The USDA originally defined a food desert as a low-income area where a significant number of residents (33% or 500 people, whichever was less), lived far from a supermarket. "Far" was more than a mile in an urban area or more than 10 miles in a rural area. In a new tool called the Food Access Research Atlas, low-income census tracts where a substantial number or share of people are far from supermarkets can be viewed and mapped. New measures include accessibility to sources of healthy food, as measured by distance to a store or by the number of stores in an area; individual-level resources that may affect accessibility, such as family income or vehicle availability; and neighborhood-level indicators of resources, such as the average income of the neighborhood and the availability of public transportation (see Further Reading 10).

The Let's Move! initiative has improved the availability of nutritious and affordable food from grocery stores, small retailers, corner markets, and farmers markets in communities with limited access. In 2011, several national retail stores, as well as some regional companies, agreed to bring more nutritious and fresh food to underserved communities by opening or expanding more than 1500 stores. These changes were aimed at serving about 9.5 million people and creating tens of thousands of jobs. These retailers still have some work to do, however. Although stores like Walmart, Kroger, Costco, Target, and Safeway opened more than 10,000 new locations between 2011 and the first quarter of 2015, an Associated Press analysis found that only a little over 250 new supermarkets cropped up in the expansive food deserts.

The Healthy Food Financing Initiative (HFFI), a component of the Let's Move! program, provides government financing for developing and equipping grocery stores, small retailers, corner stores, and farmers markets selling healthy food in low-income communities. In addition, this initiative provides employment and business opportunities in underserved areas. Farmers markets are gaining attention as a simple and local approach in impacting hunger and health. Many farmers markets now participate in senior programs, WIC, SNAP, and the SNAP Double Dollar program, where shoppers using their SNAP EBT card will receive matching funds for SNAP purchases at that market.

food deserts Urban neighborhoods and rural towns without ready access to fresh, healthy, and affordable food.

▲ The Healthy Food Financing Initiative was established to bring grocery stores, corner stores, and farmers markets to underserved communities in America so that children and their families can have access to healthy foods. © Donald Iain Smith/Getty Images

Homelessness The growing shortage of affordable rental housing and a simultaneous increase in poverty are the two trends largely responsible for the rise in homelessness over the past 25 years. In 2009, data from major cities indicated increases of homelessness by as much as 20% since the foreclosure crisis began in 2007. The homelessness created by the gap between the number of affordable housing units and the number of people needing them impacts the health and well-being of all individuals. Homeless children are most vulnerable and are twice as likely to experience hunger compared to children with a home.

Over 578,420 people experienced homelessness—meaning they were sleeping outside or in an emergency shelter or transitional housing program on any given night in 2014. Families most commonly become homeless as a result of an unexpected financial crisis that prevents them from retaining their housing. Events similar to those that cause situational poverty—a medical emergency, death in the family, loss of a job—can lead to homelessness. People in poverty must make difficult choices when limited resources cover only some necessities such as housing, food, child care, health care, and education. Because housing absorbs a high percentage of income, it is often sacrificed. The National Alliance to End Homelessness indicates that most homeless families are able to quickly rebound from homelessness, requiring only short-term public assistance before returning to independence and stability.

As the recession gripped America from 2007 to 2010, the number of people using shelters or transitional housing in suburban and rural areas increased 57% while the use of shelters in urban areas decreased. Regrettably, veterans make up over 8% of the homeless population, often due to war-related disabilities that affect their ability to work. In 2014, communities across America identified almost 50,000 homeless veterans during point-in-time counts.

Chronic homelessness is defined as involving either long-term and/or repeated occurrences of homelessness combined with physical and/or mental disability. Based on a single night in 2015, there were approximately 83,170 adults in America experiencing chronic homelessness. Compared to the demographic characteristics of the overall population of homeless people, chronically homeless individuals are more likely to be older, male, non-white, and experiencing long-term unemployment. These individuals account for 15% of the homeless population and are most likely to live in shelters and consume the majority of the homeless assistance resources. Without access to health care, they may cycle through emergency departments and inpatient beds, detox programs, jails, prisons, and psychiatric institutions, all at high public expense. Fortunately, progress has been made in addressing chronic homelessness in the last decade, resulting in a 22% decline in this population.

▲ Three-quarters, or about 75,000, of the chronically homeless are older men. © Jack Star/PhotoLink/Getty Images

POSSIBLE SOLUTIONS TO POVERTY AND HUNGER IN THE UNITED STATES

For many years, government-funded food assistance programs have helped to alleviate some problems of undernutrition in the United States (see Further Reading 2). An increasing number of people who are experiencing poverty are accessing the Supplemental Nutrition Assistance Program benefits and other federal assistance programs. As a result of the American Recovery and Reinvestment Act of 2009, more federal funds were infused into assistance programs, but these additional funds have recently begun to expire.

Obtaining adequate food to not only survive, but thrive, is a tremendous challenge, especially when homeless people are forced to live outside. Although many people assume that food pantries and soup kitchens are abundant and accessible for every needy person, there are many barriers to accessing these resources. The majority of food pantries are staffed by volunteers and dependent on food donations. They often have very limited hours of operation, require appointments well in advance, often require proof of residence, and limit the amount of food clients can take home per month. Homeless people often lack proper identification and proof of residence, do not have cooking facilities and equipment needed for food preparation, and do not have adequate storage to prevent foodborne illnesses and practice safe food-handling procedures. Food availability through soup kitchens is limited in most cities and absent in most rural areas.

An additional challenge is that a growing number of cities—31 across the nation so far—have taken strides to restrict or ban the act of food-sharing with the homeless. These laws

Two objectives of *Healthy People 2020* are to eliminate very low food security among children from 1.3% of households in 2008 to 0.2% in 2020 and to reduce hunger by reducing food insecurity from 14.6% of households in 2008 to 6% in 2020.

are troubling, considering that most cities do not have adequate food resources to meet the needs of their poor and homeless. Advocacy groups have raised questions about individual rights and freedoms and have successfully challenged these practices in court cases. Advocates and food providers appear eager to work with cities and other government agencies to help address the problems of hunger and homelessness by improving access to federal food benefits and other food resources. State governments have also begun moving to protect the right of individuals and groups to share food with others. New Jersey recently passed a law that strengthens the state's Good Samaritan law by allowing "universities to donate food to charitable organizations without fear of lawsuit[s]."

Through these recent efforts, lack of access to healthy food is now recognized as a solvable problem. The HFFI, a partnership between the U.S. Departments of Treasury, Agriculture, and Health and Human Services, is a multiyear initiative that engages the private sector and aims to eliminate food deserts across the country within 7 years. As mentioned, the HFFI attracts investment in underserved communities by providing financing tools such as low-cost loans, grants, tax credits, and technical assistance to healthy food retailers. The HFFI appears to be an effective and sustainable solution to the limited access to healthy foods. Its impact can be far reaching in terms of improving the nutritional status and overall health of families and children and reducing health disparities while creating jobs and stimulating the local economy in low-income areas.

Despite the highest motivation, the outlook is bleak for many people who attempt to gain independence from assistance programs. Teen pregnancy may have cut short the education or vocational training of one or both parents, thwarting efforts to earn adequate income. Often, the expense of reliable and safe child care far exceeds the meager income from a minimum-wage job. Those that secure a part-time or entry-level position often lose benefits that are based upon income. Illness of either the parents or children may prevent adults from holding steady employment. Poor communication skills, inability to relocate, and a lack of economic reserves also complicate financial independence. Regardless of how wasteful government assistance appears to some people, welfare benefits will probably be maintained until there is widespread systematic changes.

✓ CONCEPT CHECK 16.2

1. What are the primary food assistance programs established in the United States during the 1960s?

2. What factors influence the presence of poverty, homelessness, and undernutrition?

3. What programs have been launched recently to provide long-term solutions to hunger?

16.3 Undernutrition in the Developing World

Undernutrition in the developing world is also tied to poverty, and any true solution must address this issue. However, these countries have a multitude of problems so complex and interrelated that they cannot be treated separately. Programs that have proved helpful in the United States (and throughout the rest of North America) are only a starting point in this context. The major obstacles challenging those seeking a solution are illustrated in Figure 16-4 and require individual consideration.

FOOD/POPULATION RATIO

The world has over 7.3 billion inhabitants. Population growth exceeds economic growth in much of the developing world, and as a result, poverty is on the rise globally. This disrupts the balance in the food:population ratio, tipping it toward food shortages. If we want to ensure a decent life for a widening segment of humanity, many experts suggest that the growth in the earth's most vulnerable populations should slow.

▲ This young Maasai woman, with her baby on her back, lives in Kenya, which is in a region with low contraceptive rates and the highest rates of maternal death.

© Britta Kasholm-Tengve/Getty Images

FIGURE 16-4 ◄ Many factors contribute to undernutrition in the developing world. Any solutions to the problem must take these multifaceted factors into consideration.

According to 2015 statistics from the Food and Agriculture Organization (FAO), there are 795 million hungry people in the world and 98% reside in developing countries. More than three-quarters of all hungry people live in rural areas of Africa and Asia and remain totally dependent on local agriculture for all of their food needs. Unfortunately, major food and health disparities continue to exist between developed and developing countries, among the rich and the poor, and even within the family unit (i.e., males may be fed before females).

Economists estimate that world food production will continue to increase more rapidly than the world population, allowing the food:population ratio to increase through the year 2020. This will come at a high cost in terms of the water, fertilizer, and chemicals (pesticides, fungicides, fertilizer) needed to allow for adequate food production. In the short term, the primary problem is not related to production, but instead related to the supply chain—both distribution and use. This reality is even more dire in poverty-stricken areas of developing nations. Unfortunately, many vulnerable people do not have the income to purchase their own farmland or the means to purchase food from nonlocal sources.

Most viable farmland in the world is already in use, and because of poor farming practices or competing land-use demands, the number of farmable acres is decreasing annually. For these reasons, *sustainable* world food output—an amount that does not deplete the earth's resources—is now running well behind food consumption. This discrepancy suggests that food production in less-developed countries will not keep up with population growth and will soon lag behind.

Family planning can contribute to the reduction of poverty and hunger, and *decrease* the number of maternal and childhood deaths. On a daily basis, approximately 800 women die from preventable causes related to pregnancy and childbirth; 99% of these occur in developing countries. In addition, more than 220 million women in developing countries lack access to modern contraception. Global organizations, such as Population Services International, are working to (1) empower women and couples in developing countries to lead healthier lives by increasing access to family planning and maternal health products and services; and (2) address policy, financing, delivery, and sociocultural barriers to women who desire access to such information, services, and supplies. Although strides have been made, the **global maternal mortality ratio** declined by only 3.1% per year, still well under the MDG goal of a 5.5% decline.

Promoting breastfeeding also contributes to infant health and birth control. Women who do not breastfeed generally begin to ovulate again within a month or so after childbirth. Although it is not a completely reliable method of contraception, exclusively breastfeeding an infant may delay ovulation after childbirth, thereby lowering the likelihood of fertilization for approximately 6 months. When childbirth is more widely spaced, not only do fewer total births occur, but the mother has a longer period in which to physically

global maternal mortality ratio The number of maternal deaths per 100,000 live births.

▲ Women in developing countries are forced to spend large parts of their day fetching water. © 68/Ocean/Corbis

human immunodeficiency virus (HIV)
The virus that leads to acquired immune deficiency syndrome (AIDS).

recover from pregnancy, and the infant receives feeding priority for a longer time. One possible exception to the healthful nature of breastfeeding occurs, however, when mothers are infected with the **human immunodeficiency virus (HIV).** The risk of transferring the virus through human milk is about 10%. Depending on the circumstances, this risk may outweigh the benefits of breastfeeding.

Increasing per capita income and improving education, especially for women in developing nations, are considered to be the most successful long-term solutions to excessive population growth. Global fertility is projected to decline to 2.5 children per woman birthed in 2010-2015 to 2.4 in 2025–2030. Additional reductions are projected for the least developed countries, from 4.3 in 2010–2015 to 3.5 in 2025–2030. Yet even with these positive shifts, slower-than-projected fertility declines would still result in much higher population totals in subsequent time periods. The major concern remains whether there are enough resources worldwide to raise per capita income and provide enough education to slow total population growth.

WAR AND POLITICAL/CIVIL UNREST

The Millennium Summit of the United Nations in September 2000 resulted in the Millennium Declaration that included the resolution to "spare no effort to free our peoples from the scourge of war." Against that background stands the reality that worldwide military spending was $1776 billion in 2014. The five major contributors to military expenditures are the United States, China, Russia, Saudi Arabia, and France. In contrast, the 2015–2016 United Nations Peacekeeping operations budget is only $8.3 billion—less than half of 1% of all global military expenditures.

Aside from the economic impact of military spending, civil disruptions and wars continue to set back the progress of addressing poverty and contribute to massive undernutrition. Globally, 1 in every 122 humans is now either a refugee, internally displaced, or seeking political or religious asylum. In 2014, almost 14 million people became newly displaced—quadrupling from the previous year. The main reason for the acceleration has been the recent war in Syria, the world's largest driver of displacement.

In 2014, over 11 million people were uprooted by violence, mainly as war refugees in Syria, Afghanistan, and Somalia. These war-torn areas contribute to the 20 million refugees worldwide. In Madaya alone (a region of Syria), over 40,000 refugees are facing starvation. Millions of deaths are anticipated and at least that many more displaced refugees. While war continues to rage, health, education, and public services continue to decline for affected populations. All the while, poverty increases.

As noted, war-related famine affects millions of people, mainly in South Asia and sub-Saharan Africa, and now the Middle East. To assess hunger, the International Food Policy Research Institute (IFPRI) annually calculates the Global Hunger Index (GHI), a tool designed to measure and track hunger worldwide. The GHI uses a multidimensional approach to assess hunger that includes population undernourishment, child wasting, child stunting, and child mortality. Since 2000, Rwanda, Angola, and Ethiopia had the largest declines in hunger, yet despite their improvements, the hunger levels in these countries remain serious. Eight countries, mainly in Africa, suffer from levels of hunger that are alarming. To date, GHI scores have not been calculated for Somalia due to data constraints, yet it is clearly considered one of the most food-insecure countries in the world.

Sadly, food has become a weapon in many wars. At the local level, fields are often mined and water wells purposefully contaminated. Even when food is readily available and accessible, political divisions may impede its distribution to the point that undernutrition will plague countries for years. Especially during emergencies, programs designed to aid the hungry have been undermined by unstable administrations, corruption, and political influence. During this chaos, relief agencies may be caught between warring factions and those attempting to alleviate suffering. The UN World Food Programme (WFP) recently reported that although 2.5 million people are in dire need of emergency food in Syria, they could only reach 1.5 million due to hostile ground conflicts and unsafe conditions. Similarly, Saudi Arabia implemented a full-scale naval blockade when it announced its recent

▲ This mother, holding her 27-month-old malnourished child at a camp for internally displaced persons in North Darfur, Sudan, is dependent on assistance from relief organizations that are often not welcome in the war-torn country. USAID war against Yemen. This continues to prove devastating given Yemen imports over 90% of its food.

During the 1960s and 1970s, the problem of undernutrition in developing countries was perceived as a technical one: how to produce enough food for the growing world population. The problem is now seen as largely political: how to achieve cooperation among and within nations, so that gains in food production and infrastructure are not weapons of war. The best answer may lie in a combination of approaches: finding technical solutions to address chronic hunger and poverty, and resolving political crises that push developing nations into a state of acute hunger and chaos.

AGRICULTURE AND THE RAPID DEPLETION OF NATURAL RESOURCES

As we continue to deplete the earth's resources, population control grows increasingly critical. Agriculture production is approaching its limits in many areas worldwide. Environmentally unsustainable farming methods have been undermining food production, especially in developing countries. In addition, climate change is increasingly linked to hunger and poverty. Climatic change patterns, characterized by drought, flooding, and severe storms, require significant alterations in farming practices.

The **green revolution** was a phenomenon that began in the 1960s when crop yields rose dramatically in some countries, such as the Philippines, India, and Mexico. The increased use of fertilizers, irrigation, and the development of superior crops through careful plant breeding made this boost in agricultural production possible. The green revolution was intended as a stopgap measure until world leaders could control population growth. Many of the technologies associated with the green revolution have now achieved their potential. Additional gains in productivity have been a challenge to accomplish because of the lack or loss of productive farmland.

The movement toward practices in **sustainable agriculture** and the development of new crops through food **biotechnology** have begun to improve crop yields on the shrinking amount of farmable land. Crops that are pest or chemical resistant or biofortified have been produced as a result of biotechnology. Controversy still surrounds the use of this technology, and more research is warranted on the effects of these crops on human health and the environment (see Section 16.4 on use of biotechnology).

The world's fertile farmland is increasingly threatened by increased erosion, salinization, desertification, and deforestation. Other areas of the world remain uncultivated or ungrazed because they are too rocky, steep, infertile, dry, wet, or inaccessible to sustain farming. Agriculture is the largest user of freshwater resources. Nearly all global irrigation water is being used, and groundwater supplies are becoming depleted at rapid rates. The eventual water shortage is projected to increase war and civil unrest in arid areas of the world, such as Northern Africa and the Middle East. China, which has more than 20% of the world's irrigated land, is also plagued with a growing scarcity of fresh water. In the future, billions of people are expected to face ongoing water shortages.

In recent years, the amount of fish caught worldwide has leveled off as fish consumption has increased. Fish, once considered the poor person's protein, is quickly becoming depleted in our oceans. Fish farming simply cannot compensate for the degree of reduction in wild fish populations. Coastal fisheries in West Africa are overexploited and in the past 30 years, stocks have declined by 50%. Yet 400 million people in Southeast Asia and Africa must depend on fish for their protein and nutritional needs.

We can only exploit the earth's resources so far. If the world population continues to expand at its current rate, we face the potential threats of serious famine and death. A profound change is needed if we are to nourish an estimated 9 billion inhabitants of Planet Earth by 2050. The Food and Agriculture Organization (FAO) *State of Food Insecurity in the World 2015* report calls for global sustainability support and practices. Agricultural systems should sustain the environment while providing adequate, healthy food. If food production is to keep up with the expanding population, immediate action is needed to protect the earth's already deteriorated environment from further destruction (see Further Reading 11).

green revolution Refers to increases in crop yields that accompanied the introduction of new agricultural technologies in less-developed countries, beginning in the 1960s. The key technologies were high-yielding, disease-resistant strains of rice, wheat, and corn; greater use of fertilizer and water; and improved cultivation practices.

sustainable agriculture Agricultural system that provides a secure living for farm families; maintains the natural environment and resources; supports the rural community; and offers respect and fair treatment to all involved, from farm workers to consumers to the animals raised for food.

biotechnology A collection of processes that involves the use of biological systems for altering and, ideally, improving the characteristics of plants, animals, and other forms of life.

(a)

© Ohio State University Extension, outreach arm of the College of Food, Agricultural, and Environmental Sciences

(b)

▲ Rich agricultural resources in North America, as seen in these wheat fields, contrast with gardens being tended by a farmer on a floating island in Myanmar (formerly Burma).

© Getty Images

INADEQUATE SHELTER AND SANITATION

When people die from undernutrition, other factors such as inadequate shelter and sanitation almost always contribute. No one can survive very long without clean water, nor can we stay healthy for any length of time without proper sanitation and shelter. Regrettably, many more people suffer from the effects of poor sanitation and an unreliable water supply in developing countries than are affected by war and political/civil unrest. Without water, sanitation, and hygiene (WASH), sustainable development remains impossible.

The tremendous movement of individuals to urban settings has caused a population redistribution that has challenged the capacity for shelter and sanitation. Between 1995 and 2005, urban populations of developing countries increased by an average of 1.2 million people per week (170,000 people every day). It is expected that in the next 30 years, most urban population growth will be in cities of developing countries, reaching almost 5.2 billion in 2050. Today, over half of the world's population currently live in towns and cities and by 2050, we can expect 70% of people to reside in urban areas. People go to the cities to find employment and resources the countryside can no longer provide. In developing countries, the poor make up most of the urban population, and their needs for housing and community services often exceed available governmental resources. Over 30% of current urban dwellers live in slums, totaling 1 billion people worldwide.

Most poverty-stricken urban residents live in overcrowded, self-made shelters, which lack a safe and adequate water supply and are only partially served by public utilities. The WHO/UNICEF Joint Monitoring Programme for Water Supply and Sanitation (JMP) has estimated that as of 2015, 2.4 billion people lacked improved sanitation facilities, and 663 million people still use unsafe drinking water sources. The shantytowns and ghettos of the developing world are often worse than the rural areas the people left behind. The urban poor need cash to purchase food, so they often subsist on diets even more meager than the homegrown rural fare. Making matters worse, haphazard shelters often lack facilities to protect food from spoilage or damage by insects and rodents. This inability to protect food supplies in some developing countries leads to the loss of as much as 40% of all perishable foods.

The shift from rural to urban life takes its greatest toll on infants and children. WHO/UNICEF reports that inadequate access to safe water and sanitation services, combined with poor hygiene practices, kills and sickens thousands of children every day. For example, more than half of the 5.9 million deaths of children (under age 5 years) that occurred in developing countries in 2015 could have been prevented by improving the standards of environmental hygiene. Contributing to this issue is the fact that infants are often weaned early from breast milk to infant formula, partly because the mother must find employment. Mothers may also be influenced by advertisements depicting images of sophisticated, formula-feeding women. Unfortunately, because infant formulas are relatively expensive, poor parents may try to conserve the formula by either overdiluting the mixture or using too little to meet the infant's needs. The water supply may not be safe, so the prepared formula is also likely to be contaminated with bacteria. Human milk, in contrast, is much more hygienic, readily available, and nutritious. It also provides infants with immunity to some ailments. In most situations, breastfeeding should be promoted as the safest and most nutritious choice for infant feeding.

Poor sanitation also creates a critical public health problem and, along with undernutrition, particularly raises the risk of infection. Inadequate sanitation is another example of the inferior infrastructure in the developing world. Human urine and feces are two of the most dangerous substances encountered in routine daily living. In addition, rotting garbage and associated insect and rodent infestations are potent sources of disease-causing organisms commonly seen in urban areas of the developing world. The inability to dispose of the massive numbers of dead people (and animals) resulting from civil wars causes additional sanitation problems. In some developing countries, diarrheal diseases account for as many as one-third of all deaths in children younger than 5 years of age. Additional repercussions of poor sanitation are that children are denied access to education because their schools lack private and decent sanitation facilities.

Fortunately, organizations such as UNICEF are working in more than 100 countries across the globe to improve water supplies and sanitation facilities in schools and communities

Blood loss caused by intestinal and bloodborne parasite infections is a common cause of anemia among poor populations, especially when people do not wear shoes. Parasites, such as hookworms, can easily penetrate the soles of the feet and legs and enter the bloodstream. Although hookworm disease has been largely eradicated in the United States and other industrialized nations through improved sanitation, it continues to plague more than one-eighth of the world's population, mostly in tropical regions.

▲ Inadequate sanitation facilities and the consumption of contaminated water cause the majority of all diseases. WHO/UNICEF estimated that as of 2015, 2.4 billion people lack improved sanitation facilities, and 663 million people still use unsafe drinking water sources. © Dr. Parvinder Sethi

and to promote safe hygiene practices. The UNICEF WASH programs are designed to support the Millennium Development Goal for water and sanitation, which was to halve, by 2015, the proportion of people without sustainable access to safe water and basic sanitation. Although they met their goal for safe drinking water, there is more work to do. Over 663 million people still lack access to safe water. Read more about the sanitation crisis in Further Reading 18.

THE IMPACT OF AIDS WORLDWIDE

Nutrition security is impacted greatly in developing counties by the high prevalence of HIV infection and AIDS. HIV/AIDS impairs absorption of nutrients, increases nutrient requirements, and decreases the capacity to work. About 37 million people around the world were known to be infected with HIV or had gone on to develop AIDS from the infection at the end of 2014. The epidemic varies considerably among countries and regions. Sub-Saharan Africa continues to be most severely affected, with 25.8 million (nearly 5% of its adults) living with HIV. African cases account for almost 70% of the global total of new HIV infections (see Further Reading 12).

An individual can be infected with HIV through contact with bodily fluids including blood, semen, vaginal secretions, and human milk. Thus, the virus can be transmitted through sexual contact, through blood-to-blood contact, and from a mother to an infant during pregnancy, delivery, or breastfeeding. The virus has a very limited ability to exist outside the body. Read more about HIV and breastfeeding in Newsworthy Nutrition and Further Reading 14. Once infected with HIV, the individual is said to be HIV positive. If untreated, the viral disease progresses over the next few years, and the individual develops opportunistic infections with symptoms such as diarrhea, lung disease, weight loss, and a form of cancer. Once the individual has developed these symptoms, that person is said to have AIDS. Without treatment, an individual will likely die from AIDS within 4 to 5 years.

Global efforts at preventing HIV infection have begun to have significant effects. One of the Millennium Development Goals was to combat HIV/AIDS, malaria, and other diseases with a target to halt and begin to reverse the spread of HIV/AIDS by 2015. The HIV epidemic worldwide has stabilized, and the rate of new HIV infections has decreased in several countries (see Further Reading 12). It is encouraging that between 2000 and 2015, new HIV infections have decreased by 35%. Globally, the number of adults and children newly infected with HIV in 2014 (2 million) was significantly lower than in 2000 (3.1 million).

Every day, 230 people per hour contract HIV. AIDS leads to millions of deaths worldwide and creates orphans in many countries. Although its death toll has declined worldwide since 2001, AIDS killed 1.2 million adults and children in 2014. In 2015, approximately 37 million people were living with HIV/AIDS and 2.6 million were children (under 15 years of age). Most (88%) live in sub-Saharan Africa and were infected by their HIV-positive mothers during pregnancy, childbirth, or breastfeeding.

One of the specific targets of the UNAIDS Political Declaration on HIV/AIDS is to eliminate new infections among children and substantially reduce the number of mothers dying from AIDS-related causes. Reductions in the number of children newly infected with HIV have begun. In 2013, there were 240,000 new cases of HIV infection in children, which was a 58% decline since 2002, the year when the highest number (580,000) of children became newly infected with HIV. Furthermore, two-thirds of the total drop in new HIV infections between 2009 and 2011 was in newborns. Progress, however, has not been universal. Again, more than 90% of the children who acquired HIV live in sub-Saharan Africa. Several countries have seen only modest declines in the number of children newly infected with HIV, and the Middle East and North Africa is the only region that has seen no reduction in the number of newly infected children (Table 16-4). Reductions in the number of adults that are newly infected with HIV, as well as the direct use of preventive antiretroviral medications, appear to be the reason for the declines in the number of children acquiring HIV. Antiretroviral therapy is now credited for preventing more than 7.6 million deaths since 1995.

North America also has an AIDS problem. In the United States, it is estimated that more than 1.2 million people are infected with HIV, with one in eight (12.8%) unaware of their

▲ A particularly sad consequence of AIDS in Africa is the number of AIDS orphans—children whose parents have both died of AIDS. AIDS orphans then become responsible for the care of their siblings and other family members. © Royalty-Free/Corbis

TABLE 16-4 ■ **Regional Statistics for Adults and Children Living with HIV for 2001 and 2013. Arrows Indicate Increases or Decreases Between 2001 and 2013.**

Region		Adults and Children Living with HIV	Adults and Children Newly Infected with HIV
Sub-Saharan Africa	2013	24.7 million ↑	1.5 million ↓
	2001	20.9 million	2.4 million
Middle East and North Africa	2013	230,000 ↑	25,000 ↓
	2001	210,000	27,000
Asia and the Pacific	2013	4.8 million ↑	350,000 ↓
	2001	4.1 million	449,000
Latin America	2013	1.6 million ↑	94,000 ↑
	2001	1.2 million	93,000
Caribbean	2013	250,000 ↑	12,000 ↓
	2001	240,000	22,000
Eastern Europe and Central Asia	2013	1.1 million ↑	110,000 ↓
	2001	970,000	130,000
Western and Central Europe and North America	2013	2.3 million ↑	88,000 ↑
	2001	1.7 million	79,000
Global	2013	35.0 million ↑	2.1 million ↓
	2001	29.4 million	3.2 million

Source: UNAIDS Report on the Global AIDS Epidemic, 2014.

infections. It is estimated that 13,712 people with AIDS died in 2012 and that about 658,507 people in the United States have died from the disease since it surfaced in the early 1980s. Over 50,000 new cases of HIV infection are reported in the United States annually. HIV affects a large percentage of blacks in the United States, and gay and bisexual men are most seriously affected by HIV. Overall, from 2008 through 2011, the annual estimated number and rate of diagnoses of HIV infection remained stable in the United States.

Toward Universal Treatment Although no vaccine is available to prevent AIDS, the latest antiretroviral drugs can significantly slow the progression of the disease. Providing AIDS drugs to pregnant women is also an effective preventive measure. In pregnant women, a goal of therapy is prevention of perinatal HIV transmission and to maximize viral suppression to reduce the transmission of HIV to the fetus and newborn. Adverse effects have been noted during pregnancy so clinicians should follow the current Perinatal ART guidelines. However, there are many barriers to the use of these drugs, especially in the developing world. For example, the latest therapies require taking a drug cocktail of over 10 pills each day. A few missed doses can significantly reduce the effectiveness of the drugs and result in faster disease progression. Another barrier is economic: a typical drug regimen can cost over $10,000 per year, not including unforeseen hospital stays.

Fortunately, drug companies and governments have worked successfully to lower the cost of AIDS drugs for developing nations. Most countries that aspire to expand access to treatment set a goal of providing antiretroviral treatment to around 80% of those in need. It is estimated that 10.5 million people are currently on the life-saving antiretroviral therapy. Although this is an 22-fold increase over the past 14 years, global treatment is still reaching only 40% of those that need it, meaning there are still millions of people waiting to be treated. Progress to the goal of ensuring access to HIV treatment has been slower for children than for adults. As of 2014, just 32% of HIV-infected children had access to antiretroviral therapy. The international community must remain committed to achieving this goal.

Nutrition and AIDS Although adequate nutrition cannot prevent or cure HIV infection or AIDS, nutritional status can affect the progression of the disease. A focus on eliminating or

Newsworthy Nutrition

Should HIV-positive women choose breastfeeding for their infants?

Exclusive breastfeeding is recommended for infants of HIV-positive women during the first months of life if available replacement feeding methods are not acceptable, feasible, affordable, sustainable, or safe for their circumstances. This study of South African HIV-positive women found that exclusive breastfeeding was successful when the women had a strong belief in the benefits of breastfeeding, a supportive home environment, when they could recall key messages on mother-to-child transmission risks and mixed feeding, and could resist pressure from the family to introduce other fluids.

Source: Doherty T and others: A longitudinal qualitative study of infant-feeding decision making and practices among HIV-positive women in South Africa. *Journal of Nutrition* 136:2421, 2006.

reducing malnutrition can significantly slow disease progression and severity, and improve longevity. A dietary pattern adequate in energy, protein, and micronutrients can lessen the impact of infections associated with AIDS. Low levels of vitamins A and E can contribute to a more rapid onset of symptoms, including body wasting and fever. Maintenance of an optimal nutritional status should be an integral focus of the treatment for AIDS. Daily use of a balanced vitamin and mineral supplement has also been shown to slow health declines in people with HIV/AIDS. Nutritional counseling by a registered dietitian nutritionist (RDN) is paramount in assessing nutritional status, providing personalized education and recommendations, and monitoring outcomes. Multiple studies have documented higher energy expenditure in adults with HIV compared to healthy controls. The main goals of nutritional treatment are to achieve and maintain a healthy body weight, body composition, and lab values; minimize nutrition-related side effects and complications; improve quality of life; and expand access to nutrition services (see Further Reading 4).

✓ CONCEPT CHECK 16.3

1. Why does undernutrition continue despite adequate food resources?
2. What are some solutions to limiting population growth, especially in developing countries where birth rates are high?
3. How have war and declines in natural resources contributed to undernutrition in developing countries?
4. What effects have overpopulation and increased urbanization had on nutrition and disease risk?
5. How many people globally are currently infected with HIV?
6. How is HIV transmitted?
7. What have been the trends in terms of numbers of new cases of HIV infection since the early 2000s?

16.4 Reducing Undernutrition in the Developing World

Reducing undernutrition in the developing world is quite complex and takes considerable time to accomplish. It has been a common practice for affluent nations to supply famine areas with direct food aid; however, this is not a long-term solution. Although it reduces the number of deaths from famine, it can also reduce incentives for local production by

FIGURE 16-5 ▶ The United Nations Sustainable Development Goals: 17 goals to transform our world.

Source: United Nations/www.globalgoals.org

▲ Food security is fostered by communities raising and distributing locally grown food.

© Erin Koran

driving down food prices. In addition, the affected countries may have little or no means of transporting the food to those who need it most, and the donated foods may not be culturally acceptable. In the short run or during a crisis, there is no choice: aid must be provided because people are starving (see Further Reading 1). Still, improving the infrastructure for poor people, especially rural people, needs to be the long-term focus.

With the adoption of the Millennium Declaration (MGD) in 2000 by all United Nations member states, world leaders committed to address the many dimensions of extreme poverty and create a better life for those in need by 2015. These eight goals aimed to impact poverty and hunger with targets including halving, between 1990 and 2015, the proportion of people whose income is less than $1.25 a day and the proportion of people who suffer from hunger. Although reducing extreme poverty rates was met 5 years ahead of the 2015 target, poverty remains a significant problem, primarily in rural areas. Globally, over 800 million individuals still live in extreme poverty. In 2016, the United Nations launched the next transformative agenda to address key issues related to global health—namely, the Sustainable Development Goals. These 17 bold goals outline a 15-year agenda, adopted by world leaders, to serve as a blueprint for global health and sustainability (Fig. 16-5).

DEVELOPMENT TAILORED TO LOCAL CONDITIONS

Although world food supplies have grown faster than the population in recent years, an increase in undernutrition has resulted from a lack of food distribution and access. In addition, millions of farmers are losing access to resources they need to be self-reliant. There is a growing realization that unless economic opportunities can be created as part of a plan for sustainable development, rural residents who do not own land will flock to the overcrowded cities.

For the most part, the sustainable solutions lie in helping people meet their own needs and directing them to resources and employment opportunities, rather than giving them resources. Experience has shown that the provision of credit—along with training, food storage facilities, and marketing support—allows rural people to actively participate in their success, which benefits their families and communities.

One U.S. program, the Peace Corps, has helped to improve conditions in developing nations for over 50 years by providing education, distributing food and medical supplies, and building structures for local use. The aim of the Peace Corps is to help create independent, self-sustaining economies around the world. The MDGs became key components of the educational curriculum for Peace Corps volunteers. Becoming a Peace Corps volunteer is a meaningful way to make a difference around the world. Learn more about this program at www.peacecorps.gov.

Suitable technologies for processing, preserving, marketing, and distributing nutritious local staples also need to be encouraged, so that small farmers can flourish. Education on how to use whole foods to create healthful dietary patterns adds further benefit. Supplementing indigenous foods with nutrients that are in short supply, such as iron, various B vitamins, zinc, and iodine, also deserves consideration. One such program involves enriching rice with vitamin A in various parts of the world. Later in this section, we examine the role of biotechnology in improving nutrient quality and other characteristics of plants and animals, another positive step in lessening undernutrition. In addition, advances in water purification need to be employed.

Another MDG aims to ensure environmental sustainability, which may include promoting extensive land ownership and thus increasing the availability of food. If food resources are concentrated among a minority of people, as often happens with unequal land ownership, food is unlikely to be equally distributed unless efficient transportation systems are in place.

Raising the economic status of impoverished people by employing them is as important as expanding the food supply. If an increase in food supply is achieved without an accompanying rise in employment, there may be no long-term change in the number of undernourished people. Although food prices may fall with increased mechanization, use of fertilizers, and other modern farming technologies, these advances can also displace people from jobs, a result that may harm, rather than help, the population.

IMPROVING GENDER EQUALITY

Impoverished women are a special concern. In addition to working longer hours than men, they grow most of the food for family consumption and account for three-fourths of the labor force in the informal sector of the economy and an increasing proportion in the formal sector. Of the 3 billion people in the world living on less than $2 a day, 70% are women. Clearly, economic opportunities for women and education regarding family planning must be augmented.

Empowerment of women is critical to improve the level of nutrition security, increase the production and distribution of food and other agricultural products, and enhance living conditions in general. The **gender and development (GAD) approach** works toward improving the status of women through the active participation of both men and women. Using this approach, one specific target of the MDGs was to eliminate gender disparity in all levels of education. By increasing women's access to education, information and communication technologies, economic resources, and governance, the GAD approach reduces poverty, promotes development, achieves gender equality, protects women's human rights, and eliminates violence against women. Although paid women workers outside of agriculture increased from 35% in 1990 to 41% in 2015, women continue to experience significant gaps in terms of poverty, labor market and wages, and participation in private and public decision making. There is still plenty of room for improvement.

SUSTAINABLE AGRICULTURE

Over the years, changes in agricultural practices have had many positive results on the availability of food around the world. Along with the positive effects on farming, however, there have been significant negative impacts. Most significant among these are the depletion of topsoil, contamination of groundwater, decline of family farms, neglect of living and working conditions for farm laborers, increasing costs of production, and lack of integration of economic and social conditions in rural communities.

The concept of **sustainable development** has been embraced as economic growth that will reduce poverty while, at the same time, protect the environment and preserve natural capital. The United Nations cites economic development, social development, and environmental protection as the "reinforcing pillars" of sustainable development. The role of the agriculture industry in promoting practices that contribute to environmental and social issues has been at the center of discussions of sustainable development. As a result, interest in alternative farming practices has grown and a movement toward **sustainable agriculture** has emerged. Sustainable agriculture describes farming systems that can indefinitely maintain their productivity and usefulness to society. Sustainable agriculture flows directly from the MDG and the newly released (2016) Sustainable Development Goals. The targets depend on integration of several goals, including environmental health, economic profitability, and

▲ This school teacher and her students are in a classroom in a village in Senegal, Africa. Eliminating gender disparity by including more girls at all levels of education was a target of the Millennium Development Goals. © Author's Image/PunchStock

gender and development (GAD) approach Understanding the roles and responsibilities of both men and women in the process of sustainable development.

sustainable development Economic growth that will simultaneously reduce poverty, protect the environment, and preserve natural capital.

sustainable agriculture Agricultural system that provides a secure living for farm families; maintains the natural environment and resources; supports the rural community; and offers respect and fair treatment to all involved, from farm workers to consumers to the animals raised for food.

social and economic equity. It addresses many environmental and social concerns and offers innovative and economically viable opportunities for many in the food system, including growers, laborers, consumers, and policymakers. Sustainable agriculture is gaining support and acceptance from conventional farmers in many countries.

Sustainable agriculture involves maintaining or enhancing the land and natural resources for use long into the future. In addition, the social responsibilities of human resources, including working and living conditions of laborers, the needs of rural communities, and consumer health and safety, must be considered both in the present and in the future. The potential of sustainability is best understood when the consequences of farming practices on both human communities and the environment are considered. Farmers around the globe are transitioning to sustainable agriculture by taking small realistic steps based on their personal goals and family economics. Reaching the goal of worldwide sustainable agriculture requires participation by all stakeholders, including farmers, laborers, retailers, consumers, researchers, and policymakers, as articulated by the MDG for global partnership for development.

BIOTECHNOLOGY

The ability of humans to modify natural resources has enabled us to improve the production and yield of many important foods. Traditional **biotechnology** is almost as old as agriculture. The first farmer to improve stocks by selectively breeding the best bull with the best cows was implementing biotechnology. The first baker to use yeast to make bread rise took advantage of biotechnology.

By the 1930s, biotechnology made possible the selective breeding of improved plant hybrids. As a result, corn production in the United States quickly doubled. Through similar methods, agricultural wheat was crossed with wild grasses to confer more desirable properties, such as greater yield, increased resistance to mildew and bacterial diseases, and tolerance to salt or adverse climatic conditions. Another type of biotechnology uses hormones rather than breeding. In the last decade, Canadian salmon have been treated with a hormone that allows them to mature three times faster than normal—without changing the fish in any other way. In general terms, biotechnology can be understood as the use of living things—plants, animals, bacteria—to manufacture novel products.

THE NEW BIOTECHNOLOGY

The new biotechnology used in agriculture includes several methods that directly modify products. It differs from traditional methods because it directly changes some of the genetic material (DNA) of organisms to improve characteristics. Cross-breeding of plants or animals is no longer the only tool. Development of **genetic engineering** began in the 1970s. The field now features a wide range of cell and subcell techniques for the synthesis and placement of genetic material into organisms (Fig. 16-6).

This process of **recombinant DNA technology** allows access to a wider gene pool, and it permits faster and more accurate production of new and more useful microbial, plant, and animal species. In comparison, conventional breeding is inefficient and has inconsistent results; biotechnology uses genetic material more precisely. Scientists select the traits they desire and genetically engineer or introduce the gene that produces that trait into plants or animals (now called a **genetically modified organism [GMO]** or **transgenic organism**). Genetic engineering has not replaced conventional breeding practices; both work together.

Biotechnology has been used to enhance crops in several categories. The primary category is the addition of a unique characteristic, called an *input trait,* to a crop. These enhanced input traits include herbicide (weed killer) tolerance, insect and virus protection, and tolerance to environmental

biotechnology A collection of processes that involves the use of biological systems for altering and, ideally, improving the characteristics of plants, animals, and other forms of life.

genetic engineering Manipulation of the genetic makeup of any organism with recombinant DNA technology.

recombinant DNA technology A test tube technology that rearranges DNA sequences in an organism by cutting the DNA, adding or deleting a DNA sequence, and rejoining DNA molecules with a series of enzymes.

genetically modified organism (GMO) Any organism created by genetic engineering.

transgenic organism Organism that contains genes originally present in another organism.

DNA of the host plant, corn

Gene from bacteria (Bt gene) that produces a protein toxic to the European corn borer

Bt gene inserted into DNA of corn plant. Now the corn plant is genetically modified. It makes the Bt toxin and so is resistant to the European corn borer.

FIGURE 16-6 ▲ Biotechnology involves various techniques for transferring foreign DNA into an organism. In this diagram, a sample of DNA is cleaved out of a larger DNA fragment and inserted into the DNA of a host cell. Thus, the host cell contains new genetic information, with the potential of providing the cell with new capabilities. For corn, this could mean resistance to the European corn borer, a plant predator that feeds on corn and attacks hundreds of crops. The corn plant is now referred to as a genetically modified organism (GMO). In another application, bacteria can be engineered to produce the human form of the hormone insulin.

stressors such as drought. Other categories are value-added *output traits,* such as plant oils with increased levels of omega-3 fatty acids, and crops that produce pharmaceuticals. Scientists have engineered plants that grow with the use of less pesticides and new forms of potatoes that can be stored longer without preservatives. In addition, biotechnology allows scientists to create fruits and grains with greater amounts of nutrients such as beta-carotene (e.g., "golden rice") and vitamins E and C. Biotechnology is being used cautiously and conservatively, so the benefits are subtle. The ultimate benefits, however, could be significant in developing countries given the technology and access.

Few consumers in the United States realize that over 90% of corn and 93% of soybeans produced in the United States have been genetically engineered to either resist certain insects, thereby reducing pesticide use, and/or survive when sprayed with herbicides that kill surrounding weeds. Papaya and sugar beet plants have been genetically engineered for viral resistance. Corn has been genetically altered by inserting a gene from the bacterium *Bacillus thuringiensis,* usually referred to as the Bt gene, into the corn DNA (see Fig. 16-6). The gene allows the corn plant to make a protein lethal to predator caterpillars that destroy the crop. The Bt protein in the corn is present in low concentrations with no effect on humans; it is digested along with the other proteins in corn. In fact, for many years, organic farmers have used the Bt bacteria directly on plants to destroy pests without changing the DNA of the plant.

The FDA is confident that approved varieties of genetically engineered foods are safe to consume. Food manufacturers, therefore, are not required to disclose the genetically modified ingredient content on food labels. FDA does not believe labeling of GMO products is needed because they pose no health risk. However, some consumers remain concerned about possible, unforeseen effects of manipulating the food supply. Currently, North America has a voluntary, independent verification process for identification of non-GMO products. The Non-GMO Project is a nonprofit organization focused on expanding the non-GMO food supply, educating and informing consumers, and providing non-GMO food choices. The non-GMO verification seal (http://www.nongmoproject.org) is an assurance that a product has been produced according to consensus-based best practices for GMO avoidance.

Recently, the debate about whether products containing GMOs are dangerous to human health has resurfaced. Grass-roots coalitions have been active, and GMO labeling bills or referenda have been introduced in about 20 states. In 2013, Connecticut became the first state to pass a law requiring GMO labeling of packaged foods. A bill has also been introduced at the federal level that would direct the FDA to "clearly label" genetically engineered foods. Some legislators recommend that the United States should follow the 64 other nations, including those of the European Union, that require GMO labeling of packaged foods. Discussions are also occurring about the "probable impacts" of having varied labeling requirements passed by states rather than having a federal standard. The companies that supply seeds for genetically engineered crops to farmers are frequent targets of protests against GMOs. Their argument against requiring labels on genetically engineered foods is that this type of labeling would imply that those foods are unsafe.

Public response to use of biotechnology has been mixed. Even the scientific community has conflicting opinions about this technology, with supporters as convinced about the benefits as opponents are of the risks. The biggest debate in the United States surrounds the potential environmental hazards of introducing genes from one species to another. Some challengers even question the reduction in pesticide use that accompanies the cultivation of genetically modified crops. Although the use of genetically modified crops may reduce the need for environmentally harmful activities, such as spraying crops with pesticides, critics point out that seeds produced with additional insecticide, such as the Bt protein, may lead to rapid insect resistance because the insecticides are continuously emitted. Use of traditional pesticides involves prudent application, in part to avoid insect resistance. In addition, accidental release of genetically modified animals, such as fish, may go on to harm wild varieties.

Although the risks of biotechnology may appear to be momentarily negligible, they may be cumulative and therefore of concern in the long run. The FDA carefully examines all products developed using this technology and will enforce labeling of potential allergens

▲ Both traditional plant breeding and biotechnology have produced high-yielding and disease-resistant plant varieties, including new varieties of corn. © Kent Knudson/PhotoLink/Getty Images

that may be newly present in food altered by biotechnology. The public has long been opposed to processes perceived as harmful to the environment, such as producing unnatural products. Skepticism surrounds unnatural products, as exemplified by Western Europe's ban of hormones used in beef and milk production, and of almost all genetically modified foods.

A 2014 global analysis of over 145 studies of biotechnology crops over the past 20 years confirmed the significant benefits of biotech crops. The study found that on average, GMO technology has reduced chemical pesticide use by 37%, increased crop yield by 22%, and increased farmer profits by 68%. This study estimated the value added to be over $133 billion for the years spanning 1996 to 2013 (see Further Reading 13).

ROLE OF THE NEW BIOTECHNOLOGY IN THE DEVELOPING WORLD

Eighteen million farmers in 28 countries planted more than 181 million biotech crops in 2014. The top four GMOs include soy, corn, rapeseed, and cotton. The United States maintained the largest growth of biotech crops with 180 million acres of corn, soybean, cotton, canola, sugarbeet, alfalfa, papaya, and squash. Brazil was second with 104 million acres. The majority of global biotech crops, over 400 million acres, were grown in 20 developing countries in 2014. Of the 18 million farmers that benefited from growing biotech crops in 2014, 16.5 million or 90% were small resource-poor farmers from developing countries. These included 7 million small farmers in China and another 7 million small farmers in India, who collectively planted a record 37 million acres of biotech crops.

Whether applications of genetic engineering will help to significantly reduce undernutrition in the developing world remains to be seen. Unless price cuts accompany the increased production, only landowners and suppliers of biotechnology will enjoy the benefits. Small farmers may benefit if they can afford to purchase the genetically modified seeds. This point deserves emphasis—the person who cannot afford to buy enough food today will still face that same predicament in the future.

As with most innovations, the more successful farmers—often those with larger farms—will adopt new biotechnology first. Because of this, the present trend toward fewer and larger farms will continue in the developing world, a movement that undermines the solution to one of the most pressing undernutrition issues. Furthermore, biotechnology does not promise dramatic increases in the production of most grains and cassava, the primary food resources in developing parts of the world.

With the introduction of drought- and pest-resistant crops, as well as self-fertilizing crops, agricultural biotechnology may help to lessen world hunger. Perhaps the most promising potential of genetically modified foods today lies within the realm of plant breeding for micronutrients. Developing countries will have a tool to treat and prevent nutrient deficiencies among their populations if they have access to farming resources to increase the micronutrient composition of crops. In addition, greater yields for indigenous plants, such as tomatoes that tolerate high soil salinity, are another hopeful outcome. Biotechnology will likely be a useful tool against the complex scourge of world undernutrition. Improved crops produced by this technology, together with political and other efforts, can contribute to success in the battle against worldwide undernutrition.

SOME CONCLUDING THOUGHTS

The economic loss from undernutrition is staggering, and the amount of human pain and suffering it causes is incalculable. With all the international relief efforts and assistance from governments and private organizations combined, we are still battling undernutrition. Read more about the progress toward the Millennium Development Goals and the lack of progress on hunger in several regions of the world, even as poverty has decreased in Further Reading 17.

Ultimately, the depletion of world resources, massive debt incurred by poorer countries, threat of danger to more prosperous countries nearby, and toll taken in human lives all affect the world economy and well-being. The resulting instability can go on to affect the developing world, as has been apparent in recent years. Life is not necessarily fair, but the aim

▲ Soybeans are a common GMO food in the marketplace. Over 90% of the soybeans grown in the United States are genetically modified. © Ohio State University Extension, outreach arm of the College of Food, Agricultural, and Environmental Sciences

of civilization should be to make it more so. The world has enough food and the technical expertise to end hunger. With world leaders affirming the UN Millenium Sustainability Goals (2016) and working to achieve its targets by 2030, we have a promising coordinated political effort that is making progress toward lasting reductions in hunger.

ASK THE RDN   Non-GMO Diet

Dear Author: Lately, my friends on social media have been discussing the hazards of genetically modified foods. Many of them promote a non-GMO lifestyle. Is this a nutritionally adequate eating pattern?

Great question! First, let me outline what science shows about their safety. Then you can make an informed decision.

Some benefits of genetic engineering in agriculture include increased crop yields, reduced food costs, diminished pesticide and chemical use, enhanced food safety and food security, and reductions in soil erosion and environmental stress. GMOs have created more tolerant crops that are able to grow where they might not otherwise flourish. Globally, the use of GMOs hold great promise for reducing the prevalence of nutrition-related deficiencies and disease. For example, vitamin A-enhanced rice, also known as "golden rice," can correct vitamin A deficiencies and blindness for millions of people.

The FDA has approved GMOs for human consumption. Health experts cite hundreds of studies, spanning two decades, to support the safety of GMOs. Despite mounting evidence, the potential for unknown consequences remains. Some individuals believe that intentionally altering nature is intrinsically incorrect or immoral. Many groups are calling for clear labeling rules so consumers can make informed decisions when purchasing foods. Yet, in order to label products, there must be a clear definition and assessment of what constitutes a GMO.

Any alterations to an organism's natural state may affect metabolism, growth, and environmental outcomes. Potential health risks to humans include the possibility of exposure to new allergens or the advent of antibiotic-resistant organisms. Environmental concerns include the rise in "superweeds" requiring stronger pesticides or the possibility that genes may migrate to other species.

Yes, a non-GMO lifestyle can include a nutritionally adequate eating pattern, but it will require some inconvenience, extra costs, and close attention to food labels. Currently, up to 80% of conventionally processed food in the United States contains some genetically modified ingredients. The main tenets of a non-GMO dietary pattern align with the Dietary Guidelines, which emphasize a plant-based eating pattern—that is, rich in fiber and low in highly processed foods. Specific tips to reduce or avoid GMO exposure include:

- Focus on produce. Most fresh fruits and vegetables are non-GMO, yet some zucchini, squash, edamame, sweet corn, and papaya from Hawaii or China are considered high risk. Look for those products labeled "organic" because organic foods cannot contain GMOs.
- Look for the non-GMO-verified seal. Until GMO labeling is required, this seal can help you find GMO-free products.
- Embrace fiber. Most nuts, seeds, grains, and beans are GMO free.
- Avoid highly processed and packaged food. GMO food ingredients such as corn, canola oil, soy, and sugar beets are often used in food processing.
- Select wild-caught seafood. Some farm-raised seafood contains GMOs.

Balancing the pros and cons,

Colleen Spees, PhD, RDN, LD, FAND (author)

CRITICAL THINKING

Stan has read about various relief efforts to help undernourished people in developing countries, especially the emergency food aid programs for famine-ravaged areas. Yet many of these efforts appear temporary, and he wonders what long-range approaches might help alleviate the problem of undernutrition. What suggestions would you give Stan about possible long-term solutions for undernutrition in developing countries?

✓ CONCEPT CHECK 16.4

1. Why is development tailored to local conditions important in combating world hunger?

2. What is the definition of sustainable agriculture?

3. What are three traits for which biotechnology is used to enhance crops?

16.5 Nutrition and Your Health
Undernutrition at Critical Life Stages

PREGNANCY

Undernutrition poses the greatest health risk during pregnancy. Every day, approximately 830 women die from preventable causes related to pregnancy and childbirth. A pregnant woman needs extra nutrients to meet both her own needs and those of her developing offspring. Nourishing the fetus may deplete maternal stores of nutrients. Maternal iron-deficiency anemia is one possible consequence of malnutrition during pregnancy (Section 18.4).

Birth rates in Africa are the highest in the world. In Niger, for example, a woman gives birth to an average of nearly eight children. Close behind are countries such as Chad, Somalia, Mali, and Nigeria where an average of six to seven children are born to each woman. Coupled with chronic undernutrition, a woman's risk of dying increases with every pregnancy and birth. This results in a strong connection between a high fertility rate and high maternal mortality rates. Although most of us consider pregnancy and childbirth as natural parts of life, for women living in developing countries and without access to health care, pregnancy and childbirth complications are among the leading causes of death. The cumulative effect of successive pregnancies does not allow the mother to recover key nutrients, such as iron and folate, lost during pregnancy and breastfeeding. Since 1990, the maternal mortality ratio has been cut nearly in half. In South Asia, maternal mortality rates have declined by 64% between 1990 and 2013, and in sub-Saharan Africa, it fell by 49%. The new Sustainable Development Goal is to reduce the global maternal mortality ratio to less than 70 per 100,000 live births by 2030.

Critical Life Stages When Undernutrition Is Particularly Devastating

Prolonged undernutrition is detrimental to many aspects of human health, resulting in increased maternal, infant, and child mortality; loss of parents (especially linked to AIDS); exploitation of women; reduced work capacity; reduced intellectual and social development; and overall human suffering, especially in a famine. It is particularly damaging during periods of growth and old age. A conceptual framework of malnutrition, developed by UNICEF, lists the immediate causes of malnutrition as inadequate dietary intake and unsatisfactory health. The underlying causes relate to families and include lack of access to food, inadequate care for women and children, and insufficient health services. Basic causes relate to human and economic resources and affect communities and nations. Effective strategies to combat malnutrition should embrace a life cycle approach. Public health programs should be complementary and comprehensive across vulnerable periods of the whole reproductive cycle (see Further Reading 16).

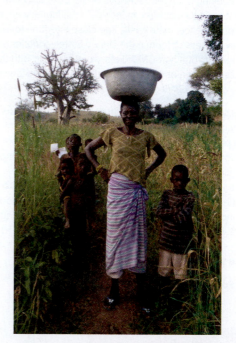

▲ This Lobi tribeswoman, standing with her six children in a grassy field in Burkina Faso, Africa, is an illustration of the typical birth rate in this region. Maternal nutrient levels become depleted with successive pregnancies followed by breastfeeding. © Lissa Harrison

FETAL AND INFANT STAGES

A fetus faces major health risks from undernutrition during gestation. To support growth and development of the brain and other body tissues, a growing fetus requires a rich supply of protein, vitamins, and minerals. When these nutrient needs are not met, the infant is often born before 37 weeks of gestation, well before the ideal 40 weeks. Preterm birth and low birth weight (5.5 pounds [2.5 kilograms] or less) contribute to 60% to 80% of all neonatal deaths. If the infant survives, abnormal growth and development can result. In extreme cases, low-birth-weight infants face 5 to 10 times the normal risk of dying before their first birthday, primarily due to complications of reduced lung development. When low birth weight is accompanied by other physical abnormalities, medical costs may exceed $200,000. Clearly, these costs can only be met in developed countries.

Worldwide, the incidence of infants born with low birth weight is 15% of all births. Much higher rates, however, occur in developing countries, with the highest rates in Pakistan (32%), India (28%), Nanru China (27%), Niger (27%), and Haiti (25%). Undernutrition is a major contributor to these high rates of low birth weight in developing countries. About 8% of infants born in the United States and 6% in Canada have low birth weights. In the United States, low birth weight accounts for more than half of all infant deaths and 75% of deaths of infants younger than 1 month. Pregnancy during the teenage years, when a girl's body is still growing, contributes to low birth weight worldwide.

CHILDHOOD

Early childhood, when growth is rapid, is another period when undernutrition is extremely risky. The greatest impact of undernutrition occurs in the first 1000 days of life: from conception to a child's second birthday. Irreversible damage is the result if optimal nutrition is not available at critical timepoints in development. The central nervous system—including the brain—is highly vulnerable because of rapid growth through early childhood. After the preschool years, brain growth and development slow dramatically. Nutritional deprivation, especially in early infancy, can lead to permanent brain impairment. Without an effective intervention, it is projected that ongoing undernutrition could leave more than 1 billion children with mental impairments by 2020.

In general, impoverished children are at the greatest risk for nutrient deficiencies and subsequent consequences. The WHO reports that nearly 165 million suffer from stunted growth. Iron-deficiency anemia is also more common among low-income children. This deficiency can lead to fatigue, reduced stamina, stunted growth, impaired motor development, and learning problems. Undernutrition in childhood can also weaken immune function and increase the risk of infection when nutrients such as protein, vitamin A, and zinc are low in a diet. Clearly, undernutrition and illness have a cyclical relationship. Not only does undernutrition lead to illness, but illness, particularly diarrheal and other infectious diseases, increases undernutrition. For this reason, millions of these children in developing countries are dying from the combination of malnutrition and infection. Conversely, when missing nutrients, such as vitamin A and zinc, are restored to a children's diet, improvements in health are evident.

Reducing the under-5 child mortality rate by two-thirds between 1990 and 2015 was the MDG goal. Improvement is evident in a narrowing of the gap in child mortality. Death rates have already been reduced from 90 to 43 per 1000 live births from 1990 to 2015. Despite this progress, 6 million children under 5 years of age died in 2015. Furthermore, the progress made in recent decades has been unequally distributed across regions and countries and within countries. India (21%) and Nigeria (13%) account for one-third of all under-5 deaths. These statistics indicate that undernutrition is one of the most important challenges to overcome, because it is estimated to be an underlying cause in as many as 45% of the preventable deaths among children under age 5. One of the 2016 Sustainable Development Goals is to end preventable deaths of newborns and children under 5 years of age, with all countries aiming to reduce neonatal mortality to at least as low as 12 per 1000 live births and under-5 mortality to at least as low as 25 per 1000 live births by 2030.

LATER YEARS

The WHO predicts a significant increase in the number of people age 65 years or older from an estimate of 524 million in 2010 to almost 1.5 billion in 2050. Most of this increase in global aging will be in developing countries. Older adults, especially older women living alone in poverty, are at risk for undernutrition. All older adults require nutrient-dense foods in amounts dependent on their current health and degree of physical activity. Many older adults have fixed incomes and incur significant medical costs over time, so food often becomes a low-priority item. In addition, depression, social isolation, and declining physical and mental health can compound the problem of undernutrition in older adults.

▲ This senior Lobi tribeswoman in Burkina Faso, Africa, with an ivory piercing in her upper lip, reminds us that the population of people aged 65 years or older will increase exponentially in developing countries. © Lissa Harrison

© Digital Vision/PunchStock

CASE STUDY Undernutrition During Childhood

Jamal traveled to the Philippines with his church group last summer. During their stay, they helped build shelters in a village where, a few weeks before, a storm had destroyed several houses. Jamal noticed that many of the children were very short, much shorter than the children in his neighborhood in the United States. His group worked in a remote, low-elevation area where the storm and subsequent flooding had caused the most damage. On several occasions, he noticed young mothers crouched on curbs or in doorways, holding their children. These children rarely moved; they appeared pale and listless. In contrast to the children Jamal's group had met at a church in the capital city, most of the children in this village were not active and lively. One evening, a nurse from the local clinic came to speak to Jamal's group. She said that many children in this area do not get enough to eat and that health problems were rampant. She considered the recent storm a blessing in disguise, hoping it would spur the Philippine government to send supplies to the village, particularly food and medicines. Jamal was shocked by such a degree of suffering. He wonders why children in the Philippines can be starving to death while so many children in his hometown in the United States have more food than they need.

Answer the following questions, and check your responses at the end of this chapter.

1. Which nutrients are likely to be deficient in the diets of these children?
2. Which nutrient deficiencies contribute to poor growth or "stunting" of growth?
3. Which nutrient deficiencies may be reducing immune defenses?
4. Are these children likely to be consuming adequate calories? What effect does consumption of inadequate calories have on growth?
5. Why might the recent storm be a blessing for this small village?
6. List some reasons why the children in Jamal's neighborhood at home are more likely to be overweight.

Summary (Numbers refer to numbered sections in the chapter.)

16.1 Poverty is commonly linked to chronic or periodic undernutrition. Malnutrition can occur when the food supply is either scarce or abundant. The resulting deficiency conditions and degenerative diseases contribute to poor health.

Undernutrition is the most common form of malnutrition in developing countries. It results from inadequate intake, absorption, or use of nutrients or food energy. Many deficiency conditions consequently appear, and infectious diseases thrive because the immune system cannot function properly.

Undernutrition diminishes both physical and mental capabilities. In poor countries, this is worsened by recurrent infections, unsanitary conditions, extreme weather, inadequate shelter, and exposure to diseases.

16.2 In North America, famine is not seen, but food insecurity and undernutrition remain problems, due in large part to poverty. Single parents and their children are likely to live in poverty. Soup kitchens, food stamps, the school lunch and breakfast programs, and the Special Supplemental Nutrition Program for Women, Infants, and Children (WIC) have focused on improving the nutritional health of poor and at-risk people. When adequately funded, these programs have proved effective in reducing undernutrition.

16.3 Multiple factors contribute to the problem of undernutrition in the developing world. In densely populated countries, food resources, as well as the means for distributing food, may be inadequate.

Environmentally unsustainable farming methods hamper future efforts to grow food. Limited water availability hinders food production. Natural disasters, urbanization, war, and disease all contribute to the major problem of undernutrition.

16.4 Proposed solutions to world undernutrition must consider multiple interacting factors, many thoroughly embedded in cultural traditions. Family planning efforts, for example, may not succeed until life expectancy increases. Through education, efforts should be made to upgrade farming methods, improve crops, limit pregnancies, encourage breastfeeding when it is safe to do so, and improve sanitation and hygiene.

Direct food aid is only a short-term solution. In what may appear to be a step backward, many experts recommend more sustainable subsistence-level farming. Small-scale industrial development is another way to create meaningful employment and purchasing power for vast numbers of the rural poor. Various biotechnology applications may also prove beneficial. Since the year 2000, the United Nations member states have combined efforts to achieve goals related to eliminating poverty and hunger.

16.5 The greatest risk of undernutrition occurs during critical periods of growth and development: gestation, infancy, and childhood. Low birth weight is a leading cause of infant deaths worldwide. Many developmental problems are caused by nutritional deprivation during critical periods of brain growth. People in their later years are also at great risk.

Check Your Knowledge (Answers are available at the end of this question set.)

1. There are an estimated _____ chronically undernourished people in the world.
   - a. 14 million
   - b. 1 billion
   - c. 3 billion
   - d. 6 billion

2. The number one killer of children in developing countries is
   - a. xerophthalmia.
   - b. iron-deficiency anemia.
   - c. iodine deficiency.
   - d. diarrhea.

3. The human organism is particularly susceptible to the effects of undernutrition during
   - a. pregnancy.
   - b. infancy.
   - c. childhood.
   - d. all of these stages.

4. All of the following are barriers to solving undernutrition in the developing world *except*
   - a. external debt.
   - b. poor infrastructure.
   - c. a lack of manpower.
   - d. expanding population.

5. Many of the child deaths each year in developing countries could be prevented if
   - a. technology were improved.
   - b. doctors were more specialized.
   - c. mothers would learn more about nutrition.
   - d. sanitation and hygiene were improved.

6. The Supplemental Nutrition Assistance Program (SNAP) allows
   - a. low-income families to buy surplus food at government stores with government-issued electronic benefit transfer cards.
   - b. low-income people to purchase food, cleaning supplies, alcoholic beverages, and anything else sold in supermarkets with electronic benefit transfer cards.
   - c. low-income people to turn in government-issued electronic benefit transfer cards for cash to buy food.
   - d. low-income people to purchase food and seeds with government-issued electronic benefit transfer cards.

7. A long-term solution to world hunger is
   - a. the green revolution.
   - b. cash crops.
   - c. jobs and self-sufficiency.
   - d. government and private aid.

8. Bt corn has been genetically modified to make
   - a. the bacterium *Bacillus thuringiensis*.
   - b. a protein toxic to caterpillars that can destroy the corn plant.
   - c. a sugar that makes the corn sweeter.
   - d. a fat that makes corn oil healthier.

9. Genetically modified soybeans make up approximately _____% of the soybeans grown in the United States.
   - a. 25
   - b. 50
   - c. 75
   - d. 90

10. FDA requires the statement "contains genetically modified ingredients" on the label of all foods containing genetically modified ingredients.
    - a. True
    - b. False

Answer Key: 1. b (LO 16.1), 2. d (LO 16.3), 3. d (LO 16.5), 4. c (LO 16.3), 5. d (LO 16.3), 6. d (LO 16.2), 7. c (LO 16.4), 8. b (LO 16.4), 9. d (LO 16.4), 10. b (LO 16.4)

Study Questions (Numbers refer to Learning Outcomes)

1. Describe the difference between malnutrition and undernutrition. **(LO 16.1)**

2. Describe, in a short paragraph, any evidence of undernutrition that you saw while you were growing up, in person or on television. What are or were the likely roots of these problems? **(LO 16.1)**

3. What do you believe are the major factors contributing to undernutrition in affluent nations, such as the United States? What are some possible solutions to this problem? **(LO 16.2)**

4. List three long-term consequences of undernutrition during fetal development or infancy. **(LO 16.5)**

5. What federal programs are available to address the problem of undernutrition in the United States? **(LO 16.2)**

6. Outline how war and civil unrest in developing countries have worsened problems of chronic hunger over the past few years. **(LO 16.3)**

7. How important is population control in addressing the problem of world hunger now and in the future? Support your answer with three main points. **(LO 16.3)**

8. Why is solving the problem of undernutrition a key factor in the ability of developing countries to reach their full potential? **(LO 16.3)**

9. Name three nutrients often lacking in the diets of undernourished people. What effects can be expected with each deficiency? **(LO 16.1)**

10. Describe how sustainable agriculture and biotechnology can improve food availability worldwide. **(LO 16.4)**

What the Dietitian Chose

The correct response for the question posed at the beginning of this chapter is *all of the above!* Do what comes naturally to you—whether it is donating your spare change or volunteering your spare time—to move thought into action against local and global hunger. Indeed, the need is great and opportunities to get involved abound.

As you learned in this chapter, there are basically two ways to address the problem of hunger: providing direct food aid and empowering others to help themselves. Providing direct aid (e.g., donating money) is a short-term solution—one that necessarily fills an immediate gap between resources and requirements. In the long run, however, solving the problem of hunger will take bottom-up changes that enable struggling communities to provide their own food and clean water.

It may be easier and more comfortable to visualize the hunger problem in a faraway place, such as in a developing country. In reality, however, poverty and hunger lurk in your own community. You can help local efforts by donating nonperishable items to local food pantries, volunteering at summer food service programs for school-age children, or simply by shopping for locally grown foods direct from farmers in your neighborhood.

In your quest to get involved, look for organizations whose focus is to help set up sustainable solutions in communities: empowering local citizens to grow their own food, maintaining their own clean water supplies, or building their own local economies:

- Action Against Hunger: www.actionagainsthunger.org
- The Alliance to End Hunger: www.alliancetoendhunger.org
- Blood: Water Mission: www.bloodwater.org

▲ Volunteer your time at a local food pantry or soup kitchen. Check out http://www.serve.gov/site-page/help-end-hunger to find a volunteer opportunity near you. © Getty Images

- Bread for the World: www.bread.org
- The Hunger Project: www.thp.org
- The International Food Policy Research Institute: www.ifpri.org
- MAZON: A Jewish Response to Hunger: http://mazon.org
- Stop Hunger Now: www.stophungernow.org

There are many creative ideas for raising funds and awareness to end world hunger. Check out the Rate Your Plate section at the end of this chapter for more ideas and put your own talents and passions to work for a good cause!

CASE STUDY SOLUTION   Undernutrition During Childhood

1. Based on the reports that the children do not get enough to eat and the outward signs of the children's health, it is likely that protein, vitamin A, iron, iodine, and zinc are deficient in the diets of these children.

2. Protein, vitamin A, iron, iodine, and zinc deficiencies contribute to poor and stunted growth because of their essential functions in the body. One or more of these deficiencies is likely present in many children in the village.

3. Protein, vitamin A, iron, iodine, and zinc deficiencies may also contribute to depressed immune function, which can cause diarrhea and illness. These deficiencies make these children particularly vulnerable.

4. The dietary intakes of these children are likely to be marginal in caloric content. A low calorie intake in addition to protein and micronutrient deficiencies further compromises growth and overall health during childhood. Recall from Chapter 6 that protein-calorie malnutrition (PCM) is a form of undernutrition caused by an extremely deficient intake of calories or protein and is often accompanied by illness.

5. The recent storm will hopefully cause the Philippine government to send food and medicines to the village, which will be a short-term solution to some of the residents' nutrition and health needs.

6. Poverty and undernutrition occur at much lower rates in the United States and other developed countries. In Chapter 19, you will learn about the rising prevalence of childhood overweight and obesity in developed nations. As we discussed in Chapter 7, maintaining a healthy weight requires the proper balance of calories in and calories out. It is important to realize, however, that undernutrition (e.g., micronutrient deficiencies) can exist alongside overnutrition (e.g., excess calories).

Further Readings

1. Academy of Nutrition and Dietetics: Position of the Academy of Nutrition and Dietetics: Nutrition security in developing nations: Sustainable food, water, and health. *Journal of the Academy of Nutrition and Dietetics* 113:581, 2013.

2. American Dietetic Association: Position of the American Dietetic Association: Food insecurity in the United States. *Journal of the American Dietetic Association* 110:1368, 2010.

3. American Dietetic Association: Position of the American Dietetic Association: Child and adolescent nutrition assistance programs. *Journal of the American Dietetic Association* 110:791, 2010.

4. American Dietetic Association: Position of the Academy of Nutrition and Dietetics: Nutrition intervention and human immunodeficiency virus infection. *Journal of the American Dietetic Association* 110:1105, 2010.

5. Bhutta ZA and others: Meeting the challenges of micronutrient malnutrition in the developing world. *British Medical Bulletin* 106(1):7, 2013.

6. Christian P, Tielsch JM: Evidence for multiple micronutrient effects based on randomized controlled trials and meta-analyses in developing countries. *Journal of Nutrition* 142:173S, 2012.

7. Dammann KW, Smith C: Race, homelessness, and other environmental factors associated with the food-purchasing behavior of low-income women. *Journal of the American Dietetic Association* 110:1351, 2010.

8. DeNavas-Walt C, Proctor BD: *Income and poverty in the United States: 2014 current population reports.* Washington, DC: United States Census Bureau, September 2015.

9. Panel on Treatment of HIV-Infected Pregnant Women and Prevention of Perinatal Transmission. Recommendations for use of antiretroviral drugs in pregnant HIV-1-infected women for maternal health and interventions to reduce perinatal HIV transmission in the United States. https://aidsinfo.nih.gov/contentfiles/lvguidelines/PerinatalGL.pdf. Accessed January 13, 2016.

10. Economic Research Service, U.S. Department of Agriculture: Food access research atlas. March 11, 2015. http://www.ers.usda.gov/data-products/food-access-research-atlas.aspx. Accessed December 15, 2015.

11. Food and Agriculture Organization, International Fund for Agricultural Development, and World Food Programme: *The state of food insecurity in the world 2015. Strengthening the enabling environment for food security and nutrition.* Rome, Italy: FAO, 2015.

12. Joint United Nations Programme on HIV/AIDS (UNAIDS) and World Health Organization. UNAIDS report on the global AIDS epidemic 2015. http://www.unaids.org/en/resources/documents/2015/GARPR_2015_guidelines. Accessed January 13, 2016.

13. Klumper W, Qaim M: A meta-analysis of the impacts of genetically modified crops. *PLoS One*160:9, 2014.

14. Kuhn L and others: Breastfeeding and AIDS in the developing world. *Current Opinion in Pediatrics* 21:83, 2009.

15. Dietitians of Canada. Food insecurity in Canada 2015. http://www.dietitians.ca/Dietitians-Views/Food-Security/Individual-and-Household-Food-Insecurity.aspx. Accessed January 13, 2016.

16. Stoltzfus RJ: Iron interventions for women and children in low-income countries. *Journal of Nutrition* 141:756S, 2011.

17. United Nations: *The Millennium Development Goals report 2015.* New York: United Nations, 2015.

18. United Nations Children's Fund: Water, sanitation, and hygiene. www.unicef.org/wash/. Accessed December 15, 2015.

I. Fighting World Undernutrition on a Personal Level

If you want to do something about world and domestic undernutrition, consider the following activities. It is a noble act to try to make a difference, even if you can take only one small step. As with any change in behavior, do not try to do too many things at once. Try one or two activities that represent your commitment to solving this problem.

1. Volunteer at a local soup kitchen, homeless shelter, or food pantry for a time (once a week for 1 month, for example). What insights did you gain?

2. Coordinate the efforts of a campus organization to donate money to an antihunger agency such as the following:

Antihunger Agencies	Web Address	Description
Bread for the World	www.bread.org	Bread for the World is a nationwide Christian citizens' movement seeking justice for the world's hungry people by lobbying our nation's decision makers.
CARE USA	www.care.org	CARE is one of the world's largest private international relief and development organizations, with the goal of saving lives, building opportunities, and bringing hope to people in need.
Catholic Relief Services	www.crs.org	This Catholic Charities organization started Food for All, a worldwide campaign to combat hunger.
EarthSave International	www.earthsave.org	This nonprofit agency seeks to improve the health of underserved populations, especially related to hunger and obesity.
Feeding America	www.feedingamerica.org	Feeding America, the largest domestic hunger-relief organization, shows you how to help online and has information about the latest updates.
UN Food and Agriculture Organization	www.fao.org	The Food and Agriculture Organization of the United Nations has worked to alleviate poverty and hunger by promoting agricultural development, improved nutrition, and the pursuit of food security. This website will keep you up-to-date on recent issues and provides an extensive list of publications related to food security.
Oxfam America	www.oxfamamerica.org	Oxfam works with people in more than 90 countries to create lasting solutions for hunger, poverty, and injustice.
Save the Children Foundation	www.savethechildren.org	Someone somewhere dies of hunger every 3.6 seconds. You can help stop the clock: go to and click on Donate Free Food to send a meal to someone in need. This site is affiliated with the UN World Food Programme, which tracks the number of clicks and then sends a bill to one of its corporate or nonprofit sponsors.
UN World Food Programme	www.wfp.org	The world's largest humanitarian agency fighting hunger worldwide.

3. Get on a hunger relief organization's mailing list, read its newsletters for information on upcoming fundraisers and other activities, and become involved.

4. Utilize your love of good food and healthy cooking to organize a local meal for the hungry or a benefit dinner to raise money for local food pantries. Resources to set up projects may be available from mission organizations. For example, with Blood: Water Mission's Lemon: Aid Project, students or families can use something as simple as the sale of a refreshing drink to fund potable drinking water in rural communities in Africa.

5. Participate in food drives organized by local community agencies by contributing food or services. Food-drive organizers may need volunteers to transport the donations to a food pantry. Pay attention to events around World Food Day, October 16.

6. Point, click, and fight hunger. Internet users can find information on hunger at several sites, including those listed throughout this chapter.

II. Joining the Battle Against Undernutrition

Imagine that you recently spent your summer vacation in a developing country and saw evidence of undernutrition and hunger. Then imagine that you are now asking a large corporation to support your efforts to ease hunger and suffering in this area. Develop a two-paragraph statement outlining why addressing hunger issues in this area is important. Include how the corporation could specifically assist and support you.

© Lifesize/Getty Images

Student Learning Outcomes

Chapter 17 is designed to allow you to:

17.1 List some types and common sources of viruses, bacteria, fungi, and parasites that can make their way into food.

17.2 Compare and contrast food preservation methods.

17.3 Understand the foodborne illnesses caused by bacteria, viruses, and parasites.

17.4 Describe the main reasons for using chemical additives in foods, the general classes of additives, and the functions of each class.

17.5 Identify sources of toxic environmental contaminants in food and the consequences of their ingestion.

Chapter 17
Safety of Our Food Supply

The first Food and Drug Act in the United States was passed over 110 years ago, in 1906, as a result of public pressure to improve food preparation standards. Today, warnings about the safety of food and water appear everywhere. While we are told to eat more fruits, vegetables, fish, and poultry and to drink more water, we are also warned that these may contain dangerous substances. Therefore, we still must ask, "How safe is our food and water?"

Scientists and health authorities agree that North Americans enjoy a relatively safe food supply, especially if foods are stored and prepared properly. Although tremendous progress has been made regarding food safety, microorganisms and certain chemicals in foods can still pose a health risk. As always, the nutritional and health benefits of food must be balanced against any food-related hazards. This chapter focuses on these hazards: how real they are and how you can minimize their effect on your life. You bear some responsibility for this; government agencies and industry can only do so much. The Dietary Guidelines encourage us to prepare and store foods safely. Which foods pose the greatest risk for foodborne illness? Is any food safe after being stored in the refrigerator for 6 months? Are food additives and pesticides an even greater day-to-day concern? This chapter provides some answers.

17.6 Understand the reasons behind pesticide use, the possible long-term health complications, and the safety limits set for their use.

17.7 Understand the effects of conventional and sustainable agriculture on our food choices.

17.8 Describe the procedures that can be used to limit the risk of foodborne illness.

17.1 Food Safety: Setting the Stage

During the early stages of urbanization in North America, contaminated water and food, especially milk, were responsible for large outbreaks of devastating human diseases. These experiences led to the development of procedures for purifying water, treating sewage, and **pasteurizing** milk. Since that time, safe water and milk have become more universally available, yet not always accessible. The greatest health risk from food today is contamination of a variety of foods by **viruses** and **bacteria** and, to a lesser extent, by various forms of **fungi** and **parasites.** These microorganisms can all cause **foodborne illness.** The Centers for Disease Control estimate that foodborne illness affects about one in six Americans each year. We generally have a safe food supply, but there are occasional instances of foodborne illnesses, such as those listed in Table 17-1.

This list of examples of foodborne illness outbreaks confirms that microbial contamination is still a concern today. In fact, it is the cause of most incidents of foodborne illness. North Americans are also concerned about health risks from chemicals such as food additives in foods. On a day-to-day basis, however, food additives cause only about 4% of all cases of foodborne illness in North America. Microbial contamination of food is by far the more important issue for our short-term health, so it will be discussed first. This chapter will then cover chemical food-safety hazards, including the use and safety of food additives, and discuss the risks of pesticides in foods.

EFFECTS OF FOODBORNE ILLNESS

According to the U.S. Centers for Disease Control and Prevention, foodborne illness causes 48 million illnesses, 128,000 hospitalizations, and 3000 deaths in the United States each year (see Further Readings 11 and 16). Some people are particularly susceptible to foodborne illness, including:

- Infants and children
- Older adults
- Those with liver disease, diabetes, HIV infection (and AIDS), or cancer
- Postsurgical patients
- Pregnant women
- People taking immunosuppressant agents (e.g., transplant patients)

Some bouts of foodborne illness, especially when coupled with ongoing health problems, are lengthy and lead to food allergies, seizures, blood poisoning (from **toxins** or microorganisms in the bloodstream), or other illnesses. Foodborne illnesses often result from the unsafe handling of food at home, so we each bear some responsibility for preventing them (see Further Readings 5, 7 and 12). You cannot usually tell that a particular food contains harmful microorganisms by taste, smell, or sight; therefore, you might not even suspect that food has caused your distress. In fact, your last case of diarrhea may have been caused by foodborne illness.

In response to the significant public health burden of foodborne illness that is largely preventable, the FDA Food Safety Modernization Act was signed into law by President Barack Obama in 2011. This law has strengthened the food-safety system, enabling FDA to better protect public health. It allows FDA to focus on prevention of food-safety problems before they occur. The law also provides new tools for inspection and compliance and for holding imported foods to the same standards as domestic foods. The law is summarized in the Academy of Nutrition and Dietetics Position Paper on Food and Water Safety (see Further Reading 1). As a result of this legislation, the National Integrated Food Safety Initiative supports multistate, multi-institutional, multidisciplinary, and multifunctional food safety research, extension, and education activities. The law also directed FDA to build a national food-safety system that is integrated and in partnership with state and local authorities. Several government agencies are at work on problems regarding food safety (Table 17-2). Of course, the work of these agencies does not substitute for individual safety efforts.

---

pasteurizing The process of heating food products to kill pathogenic microorganisms and reduce the total number of bacteria.

virus The smallest known type of infectious agent, many of which cause disease in humans. A virus is essentially a piece of genetic material surrounded by a coat of protein. They do not metabolize, grow, or move by themselves. They reproduce only with the aid of a living cellular host.

bacteria Single-cell microorganisms; some produce poisonous substances, which cause illness in humans. Bacteria can be carried by water, animals, and people. They survive on skin, clothes, and hair, and thrive in foods at room temperature. Some can live without oxygen and survive by means of spore formation.

fungi Simple parasitic life forms, including molds, mildews, yeasts, and mushrooms. They live on dead or decaying organic matter. Fungi can grow as single cells, like yeast, or as a multicellular colony, as seen with molds.

parasite An organism that lives in or on another organism and derives nourishment from it.

foodborne illness Sickness caused by the ingestion of food containing harmful substances.

toxins Poisonous compounds produced by an organism that can cause disease.

aril Clear, ruby-colored fruit or seed pod that surrounds a tiny, crisp seed inside a pomegranate.

TABLE 17-1 ■ Examples of Recent Foodborne Illness Outbreaks

Viruses

- **Norovirus:** In December 2015, at least 120 Boston College students were sickened by norovirus after eating at a Boston Chipotle® restaurant. Also in 2015, there were 12 outbreaks linked to norovirus on international cruise ships reported to the Vessel Sanitation Program. These outbreaks occurred on six different cruise lines, affecting 1406 passengers and 130 crew members. The largest outbreak occurred on a Royal Caribbean® ship in January 2015, when 198 of 1948 passengers (10%) and 9 crew members became ill on the *Grandeur of the Seas.*

- **Hepatitis A:** In 2013, 162 people were sickened and 71 were hospitalized in 10 states by pomegranate **arils** in Townsend Farms® Organic Antioxidant Blend of frozen berries contaminated with hepatitis A and sold at Costco Warehouse® stores. In 2003, over 500 adults in the United States contracted hepatitis A after eating raw green onions in a Mexican restaurant. These were contaminated during growth in Mexico and not properly washed by food service workers.

Bacteria

- **Salmonella:** In 2015, 838 people from 38 states were infected with strains of *Salmonella Poona.* The outbreak was linked to cucumbers imported from Mexico and resulted in 165 hospitalizations and four deaths. In 2008–2009, two outbreaks of salmonella cost the food industry millions of dollars. One outbreak was traced to imported jalapeno and serrano peppers from a Mexican farm and led to 282 hospitalizations and two deaths. The other outbreak, traced to peanut butter from a processing plant in Georgia, may have caused at least eight deaths.

- **Shigella:** In October 2015, 190 people developed shigellosis after eating at Mariscos restaurant in San Jose, California. At least 11 of the *Shigella* victims were treated in hospital intensive care units. In 2001, a large multiple-restaurant outbreak of infection with *Shigella* was traced to tomatoes. A total of 886 restaurant patrons became ill. The illness was linked to bruised and overripe tomatoes that were purchased and served on a salad bar.

- **Listeria:** In January 2016, packaged salads produced at a Dole® facility in Ohio were linked to one death in Michigan and 12 people hospitalized in six states. In 2015, Blue Bell Creameries® products were implicated in an outbreak of listeriosis in 10 people from four states. All 10 victims were hospitalized. Five of the people contracted listeriosis while hospitalized for unrelated problems sometime between January 2014 and January 2015. While in the hospital, all had consumed milkshakes made with the "Scoops" Blue Bell ice cream product. Three of these people died as a result of their *Listeria* infection. In 2011, 147 persons in 28 states were infected with *Listeria* from cantaloupes. Most of those affected were older than 60 years; 143 were hospitalized and 33 died.

- **Escherichia coli:** *E. coli* O157:H7 has caused several multistate outbreaks in the United States in the past few years. In 2015, rotisserie chicken salad made and sold in Costco Wholesale stores was the likely source of an outbreak of *E. coli* O157:H7 that affected 19 people in seven states; 5 people were hospitalized and two developed kidney failure. Also in 2015, a common meal item or ingredient served at Chipotle Mexican Grill restaurants in nine states was the likely source of an outbreak of *E. coli* O157:H7. Of the 53 people infected, 20 were hospitalized. In 2009, prepackaged Nestle Toll House® refrigerated cookie dough was associated with an outbreak of *E. coli* O157:H7 in 30 states with 72 persons infected, 34 persons hospitalized, and 10 developing kidney failure.

Most patients reported eating the cookie dough products raw. The FDA and CDC continue to warn consumers not to eat raw dough for cookies or other baked goods because of the possible contamination with *Salmonella* or *E. coli* bacteria. In a more widespread outbreak in 2006, 199 persons (22 were children under 5 years) in 26 states were infected with *E. coli* O157:H7 from fresh spinach. Of these, 102 were hospitalized, 31 developed kidney failure, and 3 died. The world's deadliest outbreak of *E. coli* occurred during the summer of 2011 with 3332 persons infected, more than 600 in intensive care, and a death toll of 36. The outbreak occurred mainly in Germany and involved the rare antibiotic-resistant *E.coli* O104:H4 strain from vegetable sprouts from a small, organic farm. The largest *E. coli* O157:H7 outbreak in the United States on record affected 781 persons attending the Washington County Fair in upstate New York in 1999. The bacterium was found in infected well water, killed a 79-year-old man and a 4-year-old girl, and caused 10 other children to undergo kidney dialysis.

- **Clostridium botulinum:** In April 2015, the largest botulism outbreak in the United States in nearly 40 years occurred among 77 persons who ate a church potluck meal in Fairfield County, Ohio. Consumption of homemade potato salad prepared with improperly home-canned potatoes was implicated as the vehicle for botulism. Of the 29 patients, 25 received botulinum antitoxin and 11 required endotracheal intubation and mechanical ventilation; one patient died of respiratory failure shortly after arriving at the emergency department (see Further Reading 8).

- **Vibrio:** In 2015, the number of *Vibrio vulnificus* cases in Florida was 42, higher than any year since 2008. The death toll was 13, the highest since 2011. The majority of the illnesses were linked to eating raw oysters.

- **Bacillus cereus:** In August 2012, an outbreak of *B. cereus* at a Belgian kindergarten, tied to food leftovers, involved 20 toddlers who suffered vomiting within 30 minutes after lunch. All cases recovered within a few hours. In August 2003, five children of a family in Belgium became sick with *B. cereus* food poisoning after eating pasta salad. One child died of liver failure and other complications 13 hours after the meal.

- **Campylobacter:** In March 2015, raw milk produced by Claravale Farm® of San Benito County, California, tested positive for *Campylobacter* and was implicated in illnesses in six northern California residents diagnosed with campylobacteriosis.

Parasites

- **Cryptosporidium:** In August 2014, 11 persons in Idaho contracted cryptosporidiosis from drinking raw goat milk. One patient was hospitalized.

Toxins

- **Ciguatera:** In November 2015, six persons in Florida contracted Ciguatera fish poisoning after eating black grouper originating from Mexico. Five of the persons shared a meal of black grouper heads. All became ill with nausea, vomiting, abdominal cramps, and diarrhea within hours of eating the fish. Other symptoms were muscle pain and weakness, dizziness, and numbness. Ciguatera fish poisoning is a foodborne illness acquired by eating predatory reef fish that have accumulated naturally occurring ciguatoxins found in several algae.

TABLE 17-2 ■ **Agencies Responsible for Monitoring the U.S. Food Supply***

Agency	Responsibilities
United States Department of Agriculture (USDA) Food Safety and Inspection Service (FSIS) www.fsis.usda.gov	• FSIS is the public health agency in the USDA responsible for ensuring that the nation's commercial supply of meat, poultry, and egg products is safe, wholesome, and correctly labeled and packaged.
Food and Drug Administration (FDA) www.fda.gov or call 1-800-FDA-4010 For the FDA Center for Food Safety and Applied Nutrition (CFSAN) information, call 1-888-SAFEFOOD (1-888-723-3366)	• Protects consumers against impure, unsafe, and fraudulently labeled products • Sets standards for specific foods • FDA Center for Food Safety and Applied Nutrition (CFSAN) regulates foods other than the meat, poultry, and egg products regulated by FSIS.
Centers for Disease Control and Prevention (CDC) www.cdc.gov	• Leads federal efforts to gather data on foodborne illnesses, investigate foodborne illnesses and outbreaks, and monitor the effectiveness of prevention and control efforts in reducing foodborne illnesses • Plays a key role in building state and local health department capacity to support foodborne disease surveillance and outbreak response
Environmental Protection Agency (EPA) www.epa.gov	• Regulates pesticides • Establishes water quality standards
National Marine Fisheries Service or NOAA Fisheries www.nmfs.noaa.gov	• Domestic and international conservation and management of living marine resources • Voluntary seafood inspection program; can use official mark to show federal inspection
Bureau of Alcohol, Tobacco, Firearms and Explosives (ATF) www.atf.gov	• Enforces laws on alcoholic beverages
State and local governments www.FoodSafety.gov	• Regulates milk safety • Monitors food industry within their borders • Inspection of food-related establishments

*Government agencies responsible for monitoring food safety in Canada and the specific laws followed can be found at http://www.inspection.gc.ca/.

WHY IS FOODBORNE ILLNESS SO COMMON?

Foodborne illness is carried or transmitted to people by food. Most foodborne illnesses are transmitted through food in which microorganisms are able to grow rapidly. These foods are generally moist, rich in protein, and have a neutral or slightly acidic pH. Unfortunately, this describes many of the foods we eat every day, such as meats, eggs, and dairy products.

Our food industry tries whenever possible to prolong the shelf life of food products; however, a longer shelf life allows more time for bacteria in foods to multiply. Some bacteria even grow at refrigeration temperatures. Partially cooked—and some fully cooked—products pose a particular risk because refrigerated storage may only slow, not prevent, bacterial growth. The risk of contracting foodborne illness also is high because of consumer trends. These include: (1) a greater consumer interest in eating raw or undercooked animal products; (2) more people taking medication that suppresses their ability to combat foodborne infectious agents; and (3) the continuing increase in the number of older adults in the population.

The risk of illness from foodborne microorganisms increases as more of our foods are prepared in kitchens outside the home. With the high number of two-income families, many people look for convenient and easy-to-prepare foods. Supermarkets have become an alternative to cooking at home by offering a variety of prepared foods from the meat departments, salad bars, and bakeries. Supermarkets offer entrées that can be served immediately or reheated. The foods are usually prepared in central kitchens or processing plants and shipped to individual stores. Recall the outbreak of *E. coli* O157:H7 food poisoning from rotisserie chicken salad made and sold in Costco Wholesale stores (see Table 17-1).

This centralization of food production by the food processing and restaurant industry enhances the risk of foodborne illness. If a food product is contaminated in a central processing plant, consumers over a wide area can suffer foodborne illness. For example, in 1994, a contaminated ice cream mix used in a Schwan® ice cream plant in Minnesota resulted in 224,000 suspected cases of *Salmonella* bacterial infections. The contamination was caused by a contractor's truck that delivered the ice cream pre-mix to Schwan's in a truck that had carried raw, unpasteurized eggs and had not been properly washed between loads. In 1992 and 1993, 4 children died and 732 became ill in Washington and surrounding Western states after eating at any one of 73 Jack in the Box® fast-food restaurants. The source of the problem was undercooked hamburger contaminated with the bacterium *E. coli* 0157:H7. Because restaurants are inspected by health departments only about every 6 months, we must rely on each restaurant to handle foods safely.

Greater consumption of ready-to-eat foods imported from foreign countries is another cause of increased foodborne illness in North America. In the past, food imports were mostly raw products processed here under strict sanitation standards. Now, however, we import more ready-to-eat processed foods—such as berries from Guatemala and shellfish from Asia—some of which are contaminated. U.S. authorities are reexamining inspection procedures for these imports. For example, a 2012 outbreak of *Listeria* was caused by contaminated ricotta cheese imported from Italy.

The use of antibiotics in animal feeds is also increasing the impact of outbreaks and the severity of cases of foodborne illness (recall the outbreak of *E. coli* in German sprouts described in Table 17-1). The FDA 2014 Annual Report on Antimicrobials in Food-Producing Animals showed 16,000 tons of antibiotics approved for use in livestock were sold and distributed in the United States in 2014—a 4% increase from 2013 and a 22% rise from 2009. It is good to know that animals pass the antibiotics through their systems before they are slaughtered and animal products to be used for human consumption are tested for antibiotics. The real danger from such widespread use of antibiotics is that it encourages the development of antibiotic-resistant strains of bacteria. In other words, the animals may be a reservoir of pathogens that can grow even when exposed to typical antibiotic medicines. This issue of resistant bacteria in food-producing animals is a particular concern to the CDC and is receiving considerable attention by scientists in the field. The CDC encourages the judicious use of antibiotics in humans and animals because both uses contribute to the emergence, persistence, and spread of resistant bacteria.

Finally, more cases of foodborne disease are reported now because scientists are more aware of the roles of various players in the process. Every decade, the list of microorganisms suspected of causing foodborne illness lengthens. In addition, health care providers are more likely to suspect foodborne contaminants as a cause of illness. Furthermore, we now know that besides serving as a good growth medium for some microorganisms, food, especially seafood, also is a carrier for many microorganisms as well. The FDA's Center for Food Safety and Applied Nutrition is an excellent source of information about food safety.

▲ Restaurants that choose to serve raw or undercooked foods of animal origin, such as eggs or meats, are required to have a consumer advisory on the menu warning customers of the health risks of ordering such foods. © Fuse/Getty Images

▲ Food contaminated in a central plant can result in illness in people across the nation. In the case of juices, pasteurization is an effective method of reducing the risk of foodborne illness. © Ohio State University Extension, outreach arm of the College of Food, Agricultural, and Environmental Sciences

✓ CONCEPT CHECK 17.1

1. What are the annual rates of hospitalizations and deaths as a result of foodborne illnesses in the United States ?

2. What lifestyle changes have made foodborne illness so common today?

3. What agencies are responsible for monitoring the safety of our food supply?

17.2 Food Preservation—Past, Present, and Future

For centuries, salt, sugar, smoke, fermentation, and drying have been used to preserve food. Ancient Romans used sulfites to disinfect wine containers and preserve wine. In the age of exploration, European adventurers traveling to the New World salted their meat to preserve it. Most preserving methods work on the principle of decreasing water content. Bacteria need abundant stores of water to grow; yeasts and molds can grow with less water, but some is still necessary. Adding sugar or salt binds water and so decreases the water available to these microbes. The process of drying evaporates free water.

Decreasing the water content of some high-moisture foods, however, would cause them to lose essential characteristics. To preserve such foods as cucumbers, cabbage, milk and grape juice, fermentation has been an ancient alternative to produce pickles, sauerkraut, yogurt, and wine, respectively. Selected bacteria or yeast are used to ferment or pickle foods. The fermenting bacteria or yeast make acids and alcohol, which minimize the growth of other bacteria and yeast.

Today, we can add pasteurization, sterilization, refrigeration, freezing, canning, chemical preservation, and food **irradiation** to the list of food preservation techniques. Two specific methods of food sterilization are **aseptic processing,** which simultaneously sterilizes the food and package separately before the food enters the package, and **ultra-high temperature (UHT) processing,** which sterilizes food by heating it above 275 °F (135 °C) for 1 to 2 seconds. Liquid foods, such as fruit juices, are especially easy to process in this manner. With aseptic packaging and UHT processing, boxes of sterile milk, smoothies, and juices can remain unrefrigerated on supermarket shelves, free of microbial growth, for many years.

Food irradiation is a preservation technique that could dramatically improve food safety because it takes minimal doses of radiation to control pathogens such as *E. coli* O157:H7 and *Salmonella.* In 1997, FDA approved the use of irradiation for pathogen control in raw red meat to reduce risk of *E. coli* and other infectious microorganisms. Other additions to the approved list are eggs (still in the shell) and seeds. Irradiation also extends the shelf life of other meats, spices, dry vegetable seasonings, and fresh fruits and vegetables. The **radiation** energy used does not make the food radioactive. The energy essentially passes through the food, as in microwave cooking, and no radioactive residues are left behind. The irradiation controls growth of insects, bacteria, fungi, and parasites in foods because the energy is strong enough to break chemical bonds, destroy cell walls and cell membranes, break down DNA, and link proteins together.

Irradiated food, except for dried seasonings, must be labeled with the international food irradiation symbol, the Radura, and a statement that the product has been treated by irradiation. Foods treated in this way are safe in the opinion of FDA and many other health authorities, including the American Medical Association, World Health Association, and the International Atomic Energy Agency. Although the demand for irradiated foods is still low in the United States, other countries, including Canada, Japan, Italy, and Mexico, all use food irradiation technology widely. Certain consumer groups continually try to block its use in the United States, claiming that irradiation diminishes the nutritional value of food and that it can lead to the formation of harmful compounds, such as carcinogens. The safety of irradiated food has been evaluated and confirmed by FDA for over 30 years. It has also been shown that irradiation does not compromise nutritional quality or noticeably change the taste, texture, or appearance of food. Harmful compounds are not found in irradiated food at any higher level than in foods that are not irradiated. Keep in mind that even when foods, especially meats, have been irradiated, it is still important to follow basic food-safety procedures, as later contamination during food preparation is possible.

irradiation A process in which radiation energy is applied to foods, creating compounds (free radicals) within the food that destroy cell membranes, break down DNA, link proteins together, limit enzyme activity, and alter a variety of other proteins and cell functions of microorganisms that can lead to food spoilage. This process does not make the food radioactive.

aseptic processing A method by which food and container are separately and simultaneously sterilized; it allows manufacturers to produce boxes of milk that can be stored at room temperature.

ultra-high temperature (UHT) processing Method of sterilizing food by heating it above 275 °F (135 °C) for 1 to 2 seconds. Also called *ultra-heat treatment*.

radiation Literally, energy that is emitted from a center in all directions. Various forms of radiation energy include X rays and ultra-violet rays from the sun.

▲ The Radura® international label denotes prior irradiation of the food product.
Source: USDA

✓ CONCEPT CHECK 17.2

1. What food preservation techniques have been used for centuries?

2. What is the UHT technique and what types of foods are preserved with this process?

3. Why is irradiation considered a safe technique to preserve food?

17.3 Foodborne Illness Caused by Microorganisms

Most cases of foodborne illness are caused by specific viruses, bacteria, and other fungi. Prions—proteins involved in maintaining nerve cell function—can also turn infectious and lead to diseases such as bovine spongiform encephalopathy, better known as mad cow disease.

BACTERIA

Bacteria are single-cell organisms found in the food we eat, the water we drink, and the air we breathe. Many types of bacteria cause foodborne illness, including *Bacillus, Campylobacter, Clostridium, Escherichia, Listeria, Vibrio, Salmonella,* and *Staphylococcus* (Table 17-3). Bacteria are everywhere: each teaspoon of soil contains about 2 billion bacteria. Luckily, only a small number of all bacteria pose a threat.

▲ An electron micrograph of *Escherichia coli* bacteria, strain O157:H7, magnified 6836x. Although most strains of *E. coli* are harmless and live in the intestines of healthy humans and animals, this strain produces a toxin that causes severe illness. The first recognized outbreak of illness from *E. coli* O157:H7 occurred in 1982 from contaminated hamburgers and caused bloody diarrhea. Since then, most infections have been linked to eating undercooked ground beef. © CDC/Janice Haney Carr

TABLE 17-3 ■ **Bacterial Causes of Foodborne Illness**

Bacteria	Typical Food Sources	Illness	Additional Information
***Salmonella* species** © Photodisc/Getty Images	Raw and undercooked meats, poultry, eggs, and fish; produce, especially raw sprouts; peanut butter; unpasteurized milk	**Onset:** 12–72 hours **Symptoms:** nausea, fever, headache, abdominal cramps, diarrhea, and vomiting; can be fatal in infants, the elderly, and those with impaired immune systems **Duration:** 4–7 days	Estimated 1 million infections per year; bacteria live in the intestines of animals and humans; food is contaminated by infected water and feces; about 2000 strains of *Salmonella* bacteria can cause disease, but 3 strains account for almost 50% of cases; *Salmonella enteritidis* infects the ovaries of healthy hens and contaminates eggs; almost 20% of cases are from eating undercooked eggs or egg-containing dishes; reptiles, such as turtles, also spread the disease
Campylobacter jejuni © I. Rozenbaum/F. Cirou/Photo Alto	Raw and undercooked meat and poultry (more than half of raw poultry in the United States is contaminated), unpasteurized milk, and contaminated water	**Onset:** 2–5 days **Symptoms:** muscle pain, abdominal cramping, diarrhea (sometimes bloody), and fever **Duration:** 2–7 days	Estimated 845,000 infections/year; produces a toxin that destroys intestinal mucosal surfaces; can cause Guillain-Barré syndrome, a rare neurological disorder that causes paralysis
***Escherichia coli* (O157:H7, O104:H4, and other strains)** © CDC/Janice Haney Carr	Undercooked ground beef; produce (e.g., lettuce, spinach, and sprouts); unpasteurized juice and milk	**Onset:** 1–8 days **Symptoms:** bloody diarrhea and abdominal cramps; in children under age 5 and the elderly, hemolytic uremic syndrome (HUS) is a serious complication; red blood cells are destroyed and kidneys fail; can be fatal **Duration:** 5–10 days	Leading cause of bloody diarrhea in the United States; estimated 100,000 illnesses/year; lives in the intestine of healthy cattle; cattle and cattle manure are chief sources; illness caused by the powerful Shiga toxin made by the bacteria (so called because toxin is virtually identical to that produced by *Shigella dysenteria* toxin); petting zoos, lakes, and swimming pools can contain pathogenic *E. coli*

TABLE 17-3 ■ *(continued)*

Bacteria	Typical Food Sources	Illness	Additional Information
***Shigella* species** © Comstock Images/PictureQuest	Fecal/oral transmission; water supplies, produce, and other foods contaminated by infected food handlers with poor hygiene	**Onset:** 1–3 days **Symptoms:** abdominal cramps, fever, and diarrhea (often bloody) **Duration:** 5–7 days	Estimated 448,000 cases/year in U.S.; humans and primates are the only sources; common in day care centers and custodial institutions from poor hygiene; traveler's diarrhea often caused by *Shigella dysenteriae*
Staphylococcus aureus © Michael Lamotte/Cole Group/Getty Images	Ham, poultry, egg salads, cream-filled pastries, custards, and whipped cream	**Onset:** 1–6 hours **Symptoms:** diarrhea, vomiting, nausea, and abdominal cramps **Duration:** 1–3 days	Estimated 241,148 cases per year; bacteria live on skin and within nasal passages of up to 25% of people; can be passed to foods; multiplies rapidly when contaminated foods are held for extended time at room temperature; illness caused by a heat-resistant toxin that cannot be destroyed by cooking
Clostridium perfringens © Ingram Publishing/SuperStock	Beef, poultry, and gravy	**Onset:** 8–24 hours **Symptoms:** abdominal pain and diarrhea, usually mild; can be more serious in elderly or ill persons **Duration:** 1 day or less	Estimated 1 million cases/year; anaerobic bacteria widespread in soil and water; multiplies rapidly in prepared foods, such as meats, casseroles, and gravies, held for extended time at room temperature
Listeria monocytogenes © Digital Vision/Getty Images	Unpasteurized milk and soft cheeses, raw meats, uncooked vegetables, ready-to-eat deli meats and hotdogs, and refrigerated smoked fish	**Onset:** 9–48 hours for early symptoms, 14–42 days for severe symptoms **Symptoms:** fever, muscle aches, headache, vomiting; can spread to nervous system, resulting in stiff neck, confusion, loss of balance, or convulsion; can cause premature birth and stillbirth **Duration:** days to weeks	Estimated 1600 cases with 255 fatalities per year; widespread in soil and water and can be carried in healthy animals; grows at refrigeration temperatures; about one-third of cases occur during pregnancy; high-risk persons should avoid uncooked deli meats, soft cheeses (e.g., feta, Brie, and Camembert), blue-veined cheeses, Mexican-style cheeses (e.g., queso blanco made from unpasteurized milk), refrigerated meat spreads or pates, uncooked refrigerated smoked fish
Clostridium botulinum © Kari Marttila/Alamy	Improperly home-canned vegetables, meats, and fish; improperly canned commercial foods; herb-infused oils; bottled garlic; potatoes baked in foil and held at room temperature; honey	**Onset:** 18–36 hours but can be 6 hours to 10 days **Symptoms:** neurological symptoms—double and blurred vision, drooping eyelids, slurred speech, difficulty swallowing, muscle weakness, and paralysis of face, arms, respiratory muscles, trunk, and legs; can be fatal **Duration:** days to weeks	Estimated 100 cases/year; caused by a neurotoxin; *C. botulinum* grows only in the absence of air in non-acidic foods; incorrect home canning causes most botulism, but in 2007, commercially canned chili sauce caused an outbreak; honey can contain botulism spores and should not be given to infants younger than 1 year of age

TABLE 17-3 ■ *(continued)*

Bacteria	Typical Food Sources	Illness	Additional Information
Vibrio © Rozenbaum/F. Cirou/Photo Alto	*V. parahemolyticus:* raw and undercooked shellfish, especially oysters	**Onset:** 24 hours **Symptoms:** watery diarrhea, nausea, vomiting, fever, chills **Duration:** 3 days	Found in coastal waters; more infections in summer; number of infections hard to determine because it is difficult to isolate in the laboratory
	V. vulnificus: raw and undercooked shellfish, especially oysters	**Onset:** 1–2 days **Symptoms:** vomiting, diarrhea, and abdominal pain; in more severe cases, bloodstream infection with fever, chills, decreased blood pressure, and blistering skin lesions **Duration:** 3 or more days	Estimated 95 cases/year; found in coastal waters; more infections in summer; those with impaired immune systems and liver disease at higher risk of infection; fatality rate of 50% with bloodstream infection
	V. cholerae: contaminated water and food, human carriers	**Onset:** 2–3 days **Symptoms:** severe, dehydrating diarrhea, and vomiting; dehydration, cardiovascular collapse, and death can occur	Occurs mainly in countries without adequate water purification and sewage treatment
Yersinia enterocolitica © Foodcollection	Raw or undercooked pork, particularly pork intestines (chitterlings); tofu; water; unpasteurized milk	**Onset:** 4–7 days **Symptoms:** fever, abdominal pain, and diarrhea (often bloody) **Duration:** lasts 1–3 weeks or longer	Yersinosis most common in children under age 5 years; relatively rare; bacteria live mainly in pigs but can be found in other animals

Bacteria can cause foodborne illness in three ways:

1. **Foodborne infection:** foodborne bacteria directly invade the intestinal wall
2. **Toxin-mediated infection:** foodborne bacteria produce a harmful toxin as they colonize the GI tract
3. **Foodborne intoxication:** bacteria secrete a toxin into food before it is eaten, which causes harm to humans after the food is ingested

The main way to distinguish an infectious route from an intoxication is time: if symptoms appear in 4 hours or less, it is an intoxication. *Salmonella,* for example, causes an infection because the bacteria cause the illness. *Clostridium botulinum, Staphylococcus aureus,* and *Bacillus cereus* produce toxins and therefore cause illness from intoxication. In addition, whereas most strains of *E. coli* are harmless, *E. coli* O157:H7 and O104:H4 produce a toxin that can cause severe illness, including severe bloody diarrhea and **hemolytic uremic syndrome (HUS).**

Bacterial foodborne illnesses typically cause gastrointestinal symptoms such as vomiting, diarrhea, and abdominal cramps. *Salmonella, Listeria, E. coli* O157:H7 and O104:H4, and *Campylobacter* are the bacterial foodborne illnesses of particular interest because they are the ones most often associated with death. *E. coli* O157:H7 and O104:H4 have caused deaths when HUS has developed. Listeriosis is of particular concern for pregnant women because they are about 20 times more likely to get this infection than other healthy adults, and listeriosis can cause spontaneous abortion or stillbirth because the *Listeria* bacteria can cross the placenta and infect the fetus. Of the 1651 cases of listeriosis in the United States from 2009 through 2011, 292 were fatal.

foodborne infection Occurs when a person eats food containing harmful microorganisms, which then grow in the intestinal tract and cause illness.

toxin-mediated infection Occurs when a person eats food containing harmful bacteria. While in the intestinal tract, the bacteria produce toxins that cause illness.

foodborne intoxication Results when a person eats food containing toxins that cause illness.

hemolytic uremic syndrome (HUS) Disease characterized by anemia caused by destruction of red blood cells (hemolytic), acute kidney failure (uremic), and a low platelet count.

°C	°F	
121	250	Temperature range for canning low-acid foods (kills spores).
116	240	A pressure-canner is required to reach these temperatures.
100	212	
		Temperature range for destroying bacteria (but not their spores), parasitic worms, and protozoa.
74	165	
		Temperature range for holding thoroughly cooked food; prevents growth of bacteria but does not necessarily destroy them.
60	140	
52	125	
		DANGER ZONE
		Bacteria grow quickly; do not store within this temperature range for more than 1 to 2 hours.
15	60	
4	40	Recommended refrigerator temperature; still, some bacteria can grow.
0	32	
−18	0	Freezing; bacteria cannot grow, but many will survive; growth can resume on thawing.

FIGURE 17-1 ▲ Effects of temperature on microbes that cause foodborne illness.

anaerobic Not requiring oxygen.

Effects of Temperature: The Danger Zone To proliferate, bacteria require nutrients, water, and warmth. Most grow best in *danger zone* temperatures of 40 to 140 °F (48 to 60 °C) (Fig. 17-1). Pathogenic bacteria typically do not multiply when food is held at temperatures above 140 °F (60 °C) or stored at safe refrigeration temperatures, 32 to 40 °F (0 to 4.4 °C). One important exception is *Listeria* bacteria, which can multiply at refrigeration temperatures. Also note that high temperatures can kill toxin-producing bacteria, but any toxin produced in the food will not be inactivated by high temperatures. Most pathogenic bacteria also require oxygen for growth, but *Clostridium botulinum* and *Clostridium perfringens* grow only in **anaerobic** (oxygen-free) environments, such as those found in tightly sealed cans and jars. Food acidity can affect bacterial growth, too. Although most bacteria do not grow well in acidic environments, some, such as disease-causing *E. coli,* can grow in acidic foods, such as fruit juice.

VIRUSES

Viruses, like bacteria, are widely dispersed in nature. Unlike bacteria, however, viruses can reproduce only after invading body cells, such as those that line the intestines. Experts speculate that about 70% of foodborne illness cases go undiagnosed because they result from viral causes, and there is no easy way to test for these pathogens. Table 17-4 describes the two most common viral causes of foodborne illness, Norovirus and Hepatitis A, along with typical food sources and symptoms of the illnesses they cause.

Norovirus is the number one pathogen contributing to domestically acquired foodborne illnessses. In 2014, there were 286 reported

TABLE 17-4 ■ **Viral Causes of Foodborne Illness**

Viruses	Typical Food Sources	Illness	Additional Information
Norovirus (Norwalk and Norwalk-like viruses), human rotavirus	Foods prepared by infected food handlers; shellfish from contaminated waters; vegetables and fruits contaminated during growing, harvesting, and processing (see Further Reading 11)	**Onset:** 1–2 days **Symptoms:** "stomach flu"—severe diarrhea, nausea, vomiting, stomach cramping, low-grade fever, chills, and muscle aches **Duration:** 1–2 days or longer	Estimated to cause over 20 million cases of gastroenteritis, 70,000 hospitalizations, and 800 deaths per year. Viruses found in stool and vomit of infected persons; food handlers can contaminate foods or work surfaces; Noroviruses are very infectious—as few as 10–100 particles can lead to infection; workers with norovirus symptoms should not work until 2 or 3 days after they feel better.
Hepatitis A virus	Foods prepared by infected food handlers, especially uncooked foods or those handled after cooking, such as sandwiches, pastries, and salads; shellfish from contaminated waters; vegetables and fruits contaminated during growing, harvesting, and processing	**Onset:** 15–50 days **Symptoms:** anorexia, diarrhea, fever, jaundice, dark urine, and fatigue; may cause liver damage and death **Duration:** several weeks up to 6 months	Infected food handlers contaminate food and transmit the disease to dozens of persons; children and young adults are most susceptible; a vaccine is available, decreasing the number of infections dramatically; immunoglobulin given within 1 week to those exposed to hepatitis A virus can also decrease infection.

FIGURE 17-2 ▲ Settings of Norovirus outbreaks from food contamination in the United States in 2009–2012

Source: *CDC National Outbreak Reporting System, 2009–2012.*

Norovirus outbreaks that caused 5553 illnesses, 65 hospitalizations, and 3 deaths. It causes an illness commonly misdiagnosed as the "stomach flu." Norovirus infection has a sudden onset and usually a short duration of only 1 to 2 days. Noroviruses cause almost all (over 90%) of the highly publicized diarrheal disease outbreaks on cruise ships. They are hardy and survive freezing, relatively high temperatures, and chlorination up to 10 parts per million. The most commonly reported Norovirus outbreaks are at long-term care facilities (Fig. 17-2).

PARASITES

Parasites live in or on another organism, known as the host, from which they absorb nutrients. Humans may serve as hosts to parasites. These tiny ravagers rob millions of people around the globe of their health and, in some cases, their lives. Those hardest hit live in tropical countries where poor sanitation fosters the growth of parasites.

The more than 80 foodborne parasites known to affect humans include mainly **protozoa** (one-celled animals), such as *Cryptosporidium* and *Cyclospora,* and **helminths,** such as tapeworms and the roundworm *Trichinella spiralis.* Table 17-5 describes common parasites and typical food sources and symptoms of the illnesses they cause. Parasitic infections spread via person-to-person contact and contaminated food, water, and soil.

▲ Raw shellfish, especially bivalves (e.g., oysters and clams), present a particular risk related to foodborne viral disease. These animals filter feed, a process that concentrates viruses, bacteria, and toxins present in the water as it is filtered for food. Adequate cooking of shellfish will kill viruses and bacteria, but toxins may not be affected. It is important to buy shellfish from reliable sources that have harvested these foods from safe areas. © Image Source/Corbis

protozoa One-celled animals that are more complex than bacteria. Disease-causing protozoa can be spread through food and water.

helminth Parasitic worm that can contaminate food, water, feces, animals, and other substances.

TABLE 17-5 ■ Parasitic Causes of Foodborne Illness

Parasite	Typical Food Sources	Illness	Additional Information
Trichinella spiralis	Pork, wild game	**Onset:** weeks to months **Symptoms:** GI symptoms followed by muscle weakness, fluid retention in the face, fever, and flulike symptoms	The number of trichinosis infections has decreased greatly because pigs are now less likely to harbor this parasite; cooking pork to 160 °F (72 °C) will kill trichinella, as will freezing it for 3 days at −4 °F (−20 °C).

© Foodcollection

TABLE 17-5 ■ (continued)

Parasite	Typical Food Sources	Illness	Additional Information
Anisakis © Image Source/Corbis	Raw or undercooked fish	**Onset:** 12 hours or less **Symptoms:** violent stomach pain, nausea, and vomiting	Caused by eating the larvae of roundworms; the infection is more common where raw fish is routinely consumed
Tapeworms © Image Source/Corbis	Raw beef, pork, and fish	**Symptoms:** Abdominal discomfort and diarrhea	Tapeworm larvae can get into the muscles of their hosts and cause infection when raw or undercooked meat from an infected animal is eaten.
Toxoplasma gondii © Tetra Images/Alamy	Raw or undercooked meat, unwashed fruits and vegetables	**Onset:** 5–20 days **Symptoms:** most people are asymptomatic; those with symptoms have fever, headache, sore muscles, and diarrhea; can be fatal to the fetus of pregnant women	Parasite is spread to humans from animals, including cats, the main reservoir of the disease; humans acquire the disease from ingesting contaminated meat or from fecal contamination from handling cat litter.
Cyclospora cayetanensis © Don Farrall/Getty Images	Water, contaminated food	**Onset:** 1 week **Symptoms:** watery diarrhea, vomiting, muscle aches, fatigue, anorexia, and weight loss **Duration:** 10–12 weeks	Most common in tropical and subtropical areas, but since 1990, about a dozen outbreaks, affecting 3600 people, have occurred in the United States and Canada.
Cryptosporidium © John A. Rizzo/Getty Images	Water, contaminated food	**Onset:** 2–10 days **Symptoms:** watery diarrhea, abdominal pain, fever, nausea, vomiting, and weight loss; those with impaired immune systems become more ill **Duration:** I–2 weeks in otherwise healthy people	Outbreaks occur worldwide; the largest U.S. outbreak was in 1993 in Milwaukee, with more than 443,000 persons affected; also is causing an increasing number of outbreaks in U.S. water parks, community swimming pools, and spas.

1. What is the temperature "danger zone"?
2. What type of microorganisms pose the greatest risk for foodborne illness?
3. What is the setting for the most Norovirus outbreaks?

17.4 Food Additives

By the time you see a food item on the market shelf, it usually contains substances added to make it taste better, increase its nutrient content or shelf life, or make it easier to process. Other substances may have accidentally found their way into the foods you buy. All of these extraneous substances are known as **additives,** and, although some may be beneficial, others, such as sulfites, may be harmful for some people. All purposefully added substances must be evaluated by FDA.

Food additives are classified into two types: **intentional food additives** (directly added to foods) and **incidental food additives** (indirectly added as contaminants). Both types of agents are regulated by FDA in the United States. Currently, more than 2800 different substances are intentionally added to foods. As many as 10,000 other substances enter foods as contaminants. This includes substances that may reasonably be expected to enter food through surface contact with processing equipment or packaging materials.

additives Substances added to foods, either intentionally or incidentally.

intentional food additives Additives knowingly (directly) incorporated into food products by manufacturers.

incidental food additives Additives that appear in food products indirectly, from environmental contamination of food ingredients or during the manufacturing process.

WHY ARE FOOD ADDITIVES USED?

Most additives are used to limit food spoilage. Common food additives serve the general function of **preservatives,** which can extend the shelf life of some foods. For example, antioxidants (e.g., vitamin E and sulfites) prevent discoloration caused by exposure to oxygen and enzymes. Antimicrobial additives (e.g., potassium sorbate) retard the growth of microbes in food products. Table 17-6 describes common food additives in detail.

Additives are also used to reduce food spoilage caused by the activity of some enzymes that leads to undesirable changes in color and flavor in foods. This type of food spoilage

preservatives Compounds that extend the shelf life of foods by inhibiting microbial growth or minimizing the destructive effect of oxygen and metals.

TABLE 17-6 ■ Types of Food Additives—Sources and Related Health Concerns

Food Additive Class	Attributes	Health Risks
Acidic or alkaline agents, such as citric acid, calcium lactate, and sodium hydroxide	Acids impart a tart taste to foods; inhibit mold growth; lessen discoloration and rancidity; and reduce the risk of botulism in naturally low-acid vegetables. Alkaline agents improve flavor by neutralizing acids produced during fermentation.	No known health risks when used properly
Alternative low-calorie sweeteners (see Table 4-2)	Sweeten foods without adding more than a few calories	Moderate use of these alternative sweeteners is considered safe (except for use of aspartame by people with the disease PKU)
Anticaking agents, such as calcium silicate	Absorb moisture to keep table salt and powdered food products free flowing	No known health risks when used properly
Antimicrobial agents, such as salt and sodium benzoate	Inhibit mold and fungal growth	Salt increases the risk of developing hypertension, especially in sodium-sensitive individuals; no known health risks from other agents when used properly
Antioxidants, such as BHA (butylated hydroxyanisole), BHT (butylated hydroxytoluene), vitamin E, vitamin C, and sulfites	Delay food discolorations from oxygen exposure; reduce rancidity from the breakdown of fats; maintain the color of deli meats; prevent the formation of cancer-causing nitrosamines	Sulfites can cause an allergic reaction in about 1 in every 100 people. Symptoms include difficulty breathing, wheezing, hives, diarrhea, abdominal pain, cramps, and dizziness. Salad bars, dried fruit, and wine are typical sources of sulfites.

TABLE 17-6 ■ (continued)

Food Additive Class	Attributes	Health Risks
Color additives, such as tartrazine	Make foods more visually appealing	Tartrazine (FD&C yellow number 5) can cause allergic symptoms such as hives and nasal discharge, especially in people allergic to aspirin. FDA requires all forms of synthetic colors used in a food to be listed on its label.
Curing and pickling agents, such as salt, nitrates, and nitrites	Nitrates and nitrites act as preservatives, especially to prevent the growth of *Clostridium botulinium;* often used in conjunction with salt	Salt increases the risk of developing hypertension, especially in sodium-sensitive individuals. Nitrate and nitrite consumption has been associated with synthesis of nitrosamines. Some nitrosamines are cancer-causing agents. The American Institute for Cancer Research (AICR) and World Health Organization (WHO) recommends avoiding processed meats to lower colorectal cancer risk based on evidence that regular consumption of even small amounts of processed meats increase colorectal cancer risk.
Emulsifiers, such as monoglycerides and lecithins	Suspend fat in water to improve uniformity, smoothness, and body of foods, such as baked goods, ice cream, and mayonnaise	No known health risks when used properly
Fat replacements, such as maltodextrins, emulsifiers, fiber, modified food starch, and engineered fats (see Section 5.3)	Limit calorie content of foods by reducing some of the fat content	Generally no known health risks when used properly; possible loss of fat-soluble vitamins and GI side effects if used in excess
Flavor and flavoring agents, such as natural and artificial flavors, sugar, and corn syrup	Impart more or improve flavor of foods	Sugar and corn syrup can increase risk for dental caries. Generally no known health risks for flavoring agents when used properly; possible weight gain and its comorbid conditions from excess calories.
Flavor enhancers, such as monosodium glutamate (MSG) and salt	Help bring out the natural flavor of foods, such as meats	Some people (especially infants) are sensitive to the glutamate in MSG and after exposure experience flushing, chest pain, facial pressure, dizziness, sweating, rapid heart rate, nausea, vomiting, increase in blood pressure, and headache. Affected individuals should look for the word *glutamate* on food labels, especially on labels for isolated protein, yeast extract, bouillon, and soup stock.
Humectants, such as glycerol, propylene glycol, and sorbitol	Retain more moisture, texture, and fresh flavor in foods such as candies, shredded coconut, and marshmallows	No known health risk when used properly
Leavening agents, such as yeast, baking powder, and baking soda	Introduce carbon dioxide into food products	No known health risk when used properly
Maturing and bleaching agents, such as bromates, peroxides, and ammonium chloride	Shorten the time needed for maturation of flour to become usable for baking products	No known health risk when used properly
Nutrient supplements, such as vitamin A, vitamin D, and iodine	Enhance the nutrient content of foods such as margarine, milk, and ready-to-eat breakfast cereals	No known health risk if intake from such supplemental sources combined with other natural food sources of a nutrient does not exceed the Upper Level set for a particular nutrient
Stabilizers and thickeners, such as pectins, gums, gelatins, and agars	Impart a smooth texture and uniform color and flavor to candies, frozen desserts, chocolate milk, and beverages containing alternative sweeteners; prevent evaporation and deterioration of flavorings used in cakes, puddings, and gelatin mixes	No known health risk when used properly
Sequestrants, such as EDTA and citric acid	Bind free ions to prevent them from causing rancidity in products containing fat	No known health risk when used properly

occurs when enzymes in a food react to oxygen—for example, when apple and peach slices darken or turn rust color as they are exposed to air. Antioxidants are a type of preservative that slows the action of oxygen-requiring enzymes on food surfaces. These preservatives include vitamins E and C and a variety of sulfites.

Without the use of some food additives, it would be impossible to produce massive quantities of foods and safely distribute them nationwide or worldwide, as is now done. Despite consumer concerns about the safety of food additives, many have been extensively studied and proven safe when FDA guidelines for their use are followed.

THE GRAS LIST

The Federal Food, Drug, and Cosmetic Act requires that any substance that is intentionally added to food is subject to review and approval by FDA before it is used, unless the substance is generally recognized by qualified experts as having been adequately shown to be safe under the conditions of its intended use. In 1958, all food additives used in the United States and considered safe at that time were put on a **generally recognized as safe (GRAS)** list. The U.S. Congress established the GRAS list because it believed manufacturers did not need to prove the safety of substances that had been used for a long time and were already generally recognized as safe.

A substance can be removed from the GRAS list if the FDA can prove that it does *not* belong on the list. A few substances, such as cyclamates, failed the review process and were removed from the list. Red dye #3 was removed because it is linked to cancer. Many chemicals on the GRAS list have not yet been rigorously tested, primarily because of expense and because they have long histories of use without evidence of toxicity or their chemical characteristics do not suggest that they are potential health hazards. Substances may be added to the GRAS list if there are enough data to establish that the substance is safe under the conditions of its intended use.

The American Heart Association (AHA) and other experts have recently questioned the appropriateness of the GRAS listing for salt. They have suggested that sodium, one of the two components of salt, "has negative health consequences" and therefore does not meet the "safe" requirement of the GRAS. The AHA would like to see FDA amend the GRAS listing for sodium chloride in an effort to reduce sodium content in processed foods (see Further Reading 6).

In a broader sense, the AHA and others are concerned that food manufacturers can make their own GRAS determinations, not needing to seek premarket approval from the FDA to use an additive in that way. The AHA would like to see improvements in the documentation of GRAS determinations and notification to the FDA. In 2010, the U.S. Government Accountability Office (GAO) published the report, "FDA Should Strengthen Its Oversight of Food Ingredients Determined to Be Generally Recognized as Safe (GRAS)" (see Further Reading 17) that supported the concerns of the AHA.

ARE SYNTHETIC CHEMICALS ALWAYS HARMFUL?

Although human endeavors contribute some toxins to foods, such as synthetic pesticides and industrial chemicals, nature's poisons (see Section 17.5) are often even more potent and widespread. Nothing about a natural product makes it inherently safer than a synthetic product. Many synthetic products are laboratory copies of chemicals that also occur in nature. Some cancer researchers estimate that we ingest at least 10,000 times more (by weight) natural toxins produced by plants than we do synthetic pesticide residues. Plants produce these toxins to protect themselves from predators and disease-causing organisms. Some of these plant toxins are the beneficial phytochemicals we have already discussed (see Section 8.4). This comparison does not make synthetic chemicals any less toxic, but it does put them in perspective.

Lastly, toxicity is related to dosage. Consider vitamin E, often added to food to prevent rancidity of fats. This chemical is safe when used within certain limits. However, high doses have been associated with health problems, such as interfering with vitamin K activity in the body (review Section 13.2). Thus, even well-known, commonly used chemicals can be toxic in some circumstances and at some concentrations.

▲ Emulsifiers improve the texture of foods such as ice cream, baked goods, and cookies. © Royalty-Free/Corbis

sequestrants Compounds that bind free metal ions. By so doing, they reduce the ability of ions to cause rancidity in foods containing fat.

generally recognized as safe (GRAS) A list of food additives that in 1958 were considered safe for consumption. Manufacturers were allowed to continue to use these additives, without special clearance, when needed for food products. FDA bears responsibility for proving they are not safe, and can remove unsafe products from the list.

Sugar, salt, corn syrup, and citric acid constitute 98% of all additives (by weight) used in food processing.

▲ Color additives make some foods more desirable. © Jules Frazier/Getty Images

Delaney Clause A clause to the 1958 Food Additives Amendment of the Pure Food and Drug Act in the United States that prevents the intentional (direct) addition to foods of a compound shown to cause cancer in laboratory animals or humans.

Some important terms used by toxicologists:

toxicology Scientific study of harmful substances

safety Relative certainty that a substance will not cause injury

hazard Chance that injury will result from use of a substance

toxicity Capacity of a substance to produce injury or illness at some dosage

toxicology Scientific study of harmful substances.

safety Relative certainty that a substance will not cause injury.

hazard Chance that injury will result from use of a substance.

toxicity Capacity of a substance to produce injury or illness at some dosage.

TESTS OF FOOD ADDITIVES FOR SAFETY

Food additives are tested by FDA for safety on at least two animal species, usually rats and mice. Scientists determine the highest dose of the additive that produces no *observable effects* in the animals. These doses are proportionately much higher than humans ever encounter. The maximum dosage that produced no observable effects is then divided by at least 100 to establish a margin of safety for human use. This 100-fold margin is used because it is assumed that we are at least 10 times more sensitive to food additives than laboratory animals and that any one person might be 10 times more sensitive than another. This broad margin essentially ensures that the food additive in question will cause no harmful health effects in humans.

One important exception applies to the procedure for testing intentional food additives: if an additive is shown to cause cancer, even though only in high doses, no margin of safety is allowed. The food additive cannot be used because it would violate the **Delaney Clause** in the 1958 Food Additives Amendment. This clause prohibits intentionally adding to foods a compound introduced after 1958 that causes cancer at any level of exposure. Evidence for cancer could come from either laboratory animal or human studies. A few exceptions to this clause, including the curing and pickling agents nitrites and nitrates, are allowed.

Incidental food additives are another matter. FDA cannot ban various industrial chemicals, pesticide residues, and mold toxins from foods, even though some of these contaminants can cause cancer. These products are not purposely added to foods. FDA sets an acceptable level for these substances. An incidental substance found in a food cannot contribute to more than one cancer case during the lifetimes of 1 million people. If a higher risk exists, the amount of the compound in a food must be reduced until the guideline is met.

In general, if you consume a variety of foods in moderation, the chances of food additives jeopardizing your health are minimal. Pay attention to your body. If you suspect an intolerance or a sensitivity, consult your physician for further evaluation. Remember that in the short run, you are more likely to suffer from foodborne illness due to the microbial contamination of food than from consuming additives.

APPROVAL FOR A NEW FOOD ADDITIVE

Before a new food additive can be added to foods, FDA must approve its use. Besides rigorously testing an additive to establish its safety margins, manufacturers must give FDA information that (1) identifies the new additive; (2) gives its chemical composition; (3) states how it is manufactured; and (4) specifies laboratory methods used to measure its presence in the food supply at the amount of intended use.

Manufacturers must also offer proof that the additive will accomplish its intended purpose in a food, that it is safe, and that it is to be used in no higher amount than needed. Additives cannot be used to hide defective food ingredients, such as rancid oils; to deceive customers; or replace good manufacturing practices. A manufacturer must establish that the ingredient is necessary for producing a specific food product.

Despite these guidelines, many activists and public health watchdogs are not satisfied with FDA procedures for regulating and monitoring the safety of food additives. These groups have urged FDA and food manufacturers to stop the use of various chemicals until their safety can be more fully determined. A major incentive to these requests is the fact that many of the chemicals used in the United States are illegal to use as food additives in the countries of the European Union and others such as Brazil, Canada, India, and Japan.

If you are bewildered or concerned about all the additives in your diet, you can easily avoid most of them by consuming unprocessed whole foods. However, no evidence shows that this will necessarily make you healthier, nor can you avoid all additives, because some, such as pesticides, are used even on whole foods. It amounts to a personal decision. Do you have confidence that FDA and food manufacturers are adequately protecting your health and welfare, or do you want to take more personal control by minimizing your intake of compounds not naturally found in foods? Read about some "clean eating" strategies in the following Ask the RDN.

ASK THE RDN ## The *Eat-Clean® Diet*

Dear Author: *I have recently decided to "clean up my act" and avoid preservatives, artificial sweeteners, and other additives in my food. There is a* Clean Eating *magazine and an Eat-Clean Diet. Is the* Eat-Clean Diet *nutritionally sound or is it just another fad diet?*

"Clean" has become a popular term to describe some trendy lifestyle practices such as "clean eating" and "cleansing" (see Further Reading 9). The *Eat-Clean Diet* by Tosca Reno has been around since 2007 and has expanded into a lucrative business model that sells many versions of her popular eating and fitness plan, as well as some very pricey "raw food kits."

Reno describes her program as "a diet plan of unprocessed, whole foods like fruits, vegetables, whole grains, and lean meats, and void of artificial ingredients, preservatives, 'chemically charged foods,' sugars, saturated fat, and *trans* fat." She claims that the diet "allows you to eat more, weigh less, and become the healthiest you can be." Other promises include decreased hunger; a 3-pound-per-week weight loss; increased energy; healthier teeth and gums; and skin that glows.

The specific principles include:

- Eat six small (i.e., 200 to 300 kcal) meals per day.
- Never miss a meal and eat breakfast within an hour of wakening.
- Eat lean protein (20 to 21 grams) and complex carbohydrates at every meal.
- Consume fresh fruits and vegetables.
- Control portions.
- Drink 2 to 3 liters of water (about 8 to 13 cups) every day.
- Consume 2 or 3 servings of healthy fats every day.

Do these recommendations sound familiar? They should because they are right in step with the eating patterns we have already recommended, including the Dietary Guidelines for Americans, the DASH Diet, and the Mediterranean diet. Thus, the key concepts embodied in the *Eat-Clean Diet* are not unique. Its tips for successful weight loss are basic to other credible plans: portion control; emphases on lean proteins, healthy fats, and minimally processed foods of plant origin; and plenty of water. Like any sound weight-loss program, the *Eat Clean Diet* also encourages a routine of strength training and cardiovascular exercise.

Putting the "clean" in the *Eat Clean Diet* comes down to stripping away:

1. Foods with chemical additives like food dyes and sodium nitrite
2. Foods with preservatives
3. Artificial sweeteners
4. Sugary beverages, such as soda and juice
5. Highly processed foods, especially white flour and sugar
6. Artificial foods, such as processed cheese slices
7. Saturated fats and *trans* fats
8. Alcohol
9. "Anti-foods" (e.g., calorie-dense foods with no nutritional value)
10. Food that comes in a box or bag
11. Foods with more than one to three unpronounceable ingredients

Some of this advice is overly restrictive and may even contradict scientific evidence. For example, it is not necessary to totally eliminate saturated fats and small amounts are typically unavoidable in a varied eating pattern. Also, there is evidence that small amounts of alcohol can provide cardiovascular benefits. In addition, Reno recommends several dietary supplements—advice that seems to counter the "clean" diet mantra to avoid all unnatural chemicals.

Clean eating can be achieved simply by being mindful of your food's origins. As nutrition experts, we encourage a "farm-to-table" mindset. Simply stated, clean eating focuses on choosing foods as close to their original or natural form as possible. Think in terms of whole foods that have been minimally processed, if at all. This is why whole grains and fresh fruits and vegetables are on the top of the "clean" foods list. Remember that there is a large body of evidence that a plant-based diet—including whole grains, fruits, and vegetables—promotes good health and prevents disease.

▲ Your choice to consume fresh rather than processed foods will lower your intake of food additives. For most people, however, food additives are not a threat to health.
© Rob Melnychuk/Getty Images

Also, remember that "processing" is a broad term that might refer to something as minimal as adding salt or peeling a potato (see Further Reading 3). Cooking is another type of processing that alters the original form of a food. At the extreme is "ultra-processing," when ingredients are manipulated in a manufacturing or laboratory setting to produce a highly processed food, such as a diet soft drink. Minimally processed foods can certainly remain in your eating plan, but ultra or highly processed foods should be avoided because they are likely to contain artificial ingredients and highly refined components. Unfortunately, many highly processed foods are deceptively marketed as being "healthy" or "nutritious" because they have been enriched or fortified with a selection of nutrients. Reading labels is the only method to ensure you are aware of the ingredients in a food or beverage.

Here is a simpler guide to "clean eating." When shopping or dining out, reach for:

Unprocessed foods:
- Fresh fruits and vegetables
- Dried beans
- Nuts and seeds
- Farm-fresh eggs

Minimally processed foods :
- Unrefined grains: whole-wheat bread and pasta, popcorn, steel-cut oatmeal, quinoa, and brown rice
- Frozen fruits and vegetables without sauces or additives
- Unprocessed lean meats: wild or pastured
- Hormone-free dairy
- Plant oils
- For packaged foods, choose minimally processed foods with few ingredients (should be recognizable whole foods or spices).
- Focus on the perimeter of the grocery store, for whole foods such as produce, meats, and dairy.
- A mix of raw and cooked foods. While cooking can lead to the loss of some nutrients, especially water-soluble vitamins, cooking enhances the absorption of fat-soluble vitamins and carotenoids, and makes many foods safer to eat. Choose quick cooking methods such as steaming or stir-frying to preserve nutrients and the natural state of the food.
- Control portion size to stay within your calorie needs.

Keeping it clean and simple,

Anne M. Smith, PhD, RDN, LD (author)

✔ CONCEPT CHECK 17.4

1. What are some of the functions of the additives used in food?
2. What is the difference between intentional and incidental additives?
3. How do scientists determine safe limits for the amount of additives that are allowed in foods?
4. What is the purpose of the Delaney Clause?

17.5 Natural Substances in Foods That Can Cause Illness

Foods contain a variety of naturally occurring substances that can cause illness. Table 17-7 shows some of the more important examples and the problems they can cause.

People have coexisted for centuries with these naturally occurring substances and have learned to avoid some of them and limit intake of others. They pose little health risk because

TABLE 17-7 ■ **Examples of Natural Substances in Foods That Can Cause Illness**

Substance	Source	Effect
Safrole	Sassafras, mace, and nutmeg	Causes cancer when consumed in high doses
Solanine	Potato shoots and throughout the potato when it has been stressed by exposure to light or pests and indicated by green spots on potato skins	Inhibits the action of neurotransmitters
Mushroom toxins	Some species of mushrooms such as the jack-o'-lantern	Stomach upset, dizziness, hallucinations, and other neurological symptoms. More lethal varieties can cause liver and kidney failure, coma, and even death. FDA regulates commercially grown and harvested mushrooms. No systematic controls on individual gatherers harvesting wild species, except in Illinois and Michigan.
Avidin	Raw egg whites (cooking destroys avidin)	Binds the vitamin biotin in a way that prevents its absorption, so a biotin deficiency may ultimately develop over the long term
Thiaminase	Raw fish, clams, and mussels	Destroys the vitamin thiamin
Tetrodotoxin	Puffer fish	Causes respiratory paralysis
Oxalic acid	Spinach, strawberries, sesame seeds	Binds calcium and iron in the foods and so limits absorption of these nutrients
Senna or comfrey	Herbal teas	Diarrhea and liver damage

we have developed cooking and food preparation methods to limit the potency of harmful substances, such as thiaminase. Spices are used in such small amounts that health risks do not result. Farmers know potatoes must be stored in the dark, so that solanine will not synthesize. Nevertheless, it is important to understand that some potentially harmful chemicals in foods occur naturally.

IS CAFFEINE A CAUSE FOR CONCERN?

Why all the controversy over a cup of coffee? Researchers have spent a great deal of time on the study of caffeine, the substance of greatest concern in the favorite beverage of so many. Caffeine is a stimulant found as a natural or added ingredient in many beverages and chocolate. On average, we consume 75% of our caffeine intake as coffee, 15% as tea, 10% as soft drinks, and 2% as chocolate (Table 17-8). (For teenagers and young adults, this ratio is often relatively higher for soft drinks and lower for coffee.)

Caffeine is not often consumed by itself. With the popularity of trendy coffee shops that serve everything from mocha java to flavored lattes, it is difficult to separate caffeine intake from cream, sugar, alternative sweeteners, and flavorings. Although a 6-ounce cup of black coffee contains just 7 kcal, adding cream and sugar increases the kilocalorie count significantly. Adding half-and-half will give you an extra 46 kcal; liquid nondairy creamer adds 48 kcal; and 1 teaspoon of sugar adds about 23 kcal. So what is the conscientious coffee drinker to think? Let us explore the myths and facts of caffeine intake.

Caffeine does not accumulate in the body and is normally excreted within several hours following consumption. Caffeine can cause anxiety, increased heart rate, insomnia, increased urination (possibly resulting in dehydration), diarrhea, and gastrointestinal upset in high doses. Those already suffering from ulcers or heartburn may experience irritation due to increased acid production and because caffeine relaxes sphincter muscles in the esophagus. Those who have anxiety or panic attacks may find that caffeine worsens their symptoms. Some people need little caffeine to feel such effects, and the threshold for children is likely even lower than that for adults.

Withdrawal symptoms are also real. Former coffee drinkers may experience headache, nausea, and depression for a short time after discontinuing use. These symptoms can be

▲ Many varieties of wild mushrooms, such as this jack-o'-lantern variety, contain deadly toxins. © AwakenedEye/Getty Images

The proposed Food Labeling Modernization Act of 2015 would require food manufacturers to clearly label caffeine content of foods and beverages.

TABLE 17-8 ■ Caffeine Content of Common Sources

Item	Milligrams of Caffeine	
	Typical	**Range***
Coffee (8 fl oz)		
Regular, brewed, drip method	85	65–120
Regular, brewed, percolator	75	60–85
Decaffeinated, brewed	3	2–4
Espresso (1 fl oz serving)	40	30–50
Teas (8 fl oz)		
Brewed, black tea	40	20–90
Brewed, green tea	20	8–30
Iced	25	9–50
Instant	28	24–31
Soft drinks (8 fl oz)	24	20–40
Coca-Cola®	23	
Mountain Dew®	36	
"Energy drinks" such as Red Bull® (8.3 fl oz)	80	0–80
Chocolate-flavored beverages (8 fl oz)		
Cocoa beverage	6	3–32
Chocolate milk beverage	5	2–7
Chocolate foods (1 oz)		
Milk chocolate	6	1–15
Dark chocolate, semisweet	20	5–35
Baker's® chocolate	26	26
Chocolate-flavored syrup	4	4

*For the coffee and tea products, the range varies due to brewing method, plant variety, brand of product, and so on.

For a more extensive list of caffeine content of food and drugs, visit www.cspinet.org/new/cafchart.htm.

▲ A cup of tea typically contains half the amount of caffeine as coffee. © John A. Rizzo/ Getty Images

▲ Coffee is a common source of caffeine for many adults. © Royalty-Free/Corbis

expected to peak at 20 to 48 hours following the last intake of caffeine. Symptoms hold true even for those trying to quit as little as a cup of coffee per day. Slow tapering of use over a few days is recommended to avoid these problems.

Are there more serious consequences of consuming caffeine regularly? It has been hypothesized that caffeine consumption can lead to certain types of cancer, such as pancreatic and bladder cancers. The association of caffeine with cancer, however, has not been supported in recent literature. In fact, regular coffee consumption has been linked to a decreased risk of colon and liver cancer (see Further Reading 14).

Negative press has dwindled with regard to a link between cardiovascular disease and moderate coffee consumption. Heavy use does increase blood pressure for a short period of time. Coffee consumption also has been linked to increased LDL-cholesterol and triglycerides in the blood. This association was found to be caused by cafestol and kahweol, two oils in ground coffee. However, filtered and instant coffees do not contain the harmful oils. It is prudent, though, to limit the amount of coffee in general, especially from French coffee presses and from espresso, as these beverages are not filtered.

Women are thought to be at higher risk for a variety of deleterious effects with caffeine consumption, including miscarriages, osteoporosis, and birth defects in their offspring. Heavy caffeine use does mildly increase the amount of calcium excreted in urine. For this reason, it is important that heavy coffee drinkers check their diets for adequate calcium sources. Some studies show a higher likelihood for miscarriages in women consuming more than 500 milligrams of caffeine per day (about five 8-ounce cups of coffee). The position of the American College of Obstetricians and Gynecologists is that moderate caffeine intake, less than 200 milligrams a day, won't increase the risk of miscarriage, preterm birth, or birth defects (see Section 18.8 and Further Reading 2).

In contrast to these potential harmful effects of caffeine, coffee consumption has been linked to reducing the risk of developing basal cell carcinoma, depression, and cardiovascular disease. Swedish scientists recently found that women ages 40 to 83 who consumed more than a cup of coffee per day for 10 years had a 22% to 25% lower risk of stroke. Coffee consumption has also been shown to decrease a person's risk of type 2 diabetes and Parkinson's disease. Though some women attest to the idea that caffeine improves premenstrual symptoms, no study proves this theory. Some older formulations of weight-loss drugs contained caffeine, under the assumption that it made the drugs more effective. FDA has since banned this use as it was found to be ineffective. Some newer research findings suggest caffeine may reduce the risk of developing headaches, cirrhosis of the liver, some forms of kidney stones, gallstones, some nerve-related diseases, and type 2 diabetes.

Though the debate over caffeine will likely continue as long as North Americans drink coffee, research does not support many old misconceptions about caffeine. These studies are reinforcing the idea of moderation. A prudent dose of caffeine is 200 to 300 milligrams (about 2 to 3 cups of regular, brewed coffee) per day. Review Table 17-3 concerning the caffeine content of typical sources.

✔ CONCEPT CHECK 17.5

1. What are some examples of naturally occurring substances that can cause illness?
2. What is the typical caffeine content of 8-ounce cups of coffee and tea?
3. What are some of the negative effects of caffeine on the body?
4. Coffee consumption has been linked to a decreased risk of which disorders?

17.6 Environmental Contaminants in Food

A variety of environmental contaminants can be found in foods. Aside from pesticide residues, other potential contaminants that deserve attention are listed in Table 17-9. A general program to minimize exposure to environmental contaminants includes knowing which foods pose greater risks and consuming a wide variety of foods in moderation.

Lead Poisoning in Flint, Michigan

In December 2015, a state of emergency was declared in Flint, Michigan, when it was discovered that the proportion of infants and children with above-average levels of lead in their blood had nearly doubled since 2014 when the city switched from treated Lake Huron water (via Detroit) to using the Flint River as its water source. The Flint River water was deemed corrosive, causing lead to leach from aging pipes, which resulted in extremely high levels of lead. Lead contamination of the water supply is the suspected cause of extremely high blood lead levels and a variety of serious health problems in 6000 to 12,000 city residents. Flint officials have sought federal support to deal with the "irreversible" effects of lead exposure on the city's children. It is predicted that future needs will include an increase in special education and mental health services.

TABLE 17-9 ■ Potential Environmental Contaminants in Our Food Supply

Chemical Substance	Sources	Toxic Effects	Preventive Measures
Acrylamide	Fried foods rich in carbohydrate cooked at high temperatures for extended periods, such as French fries and potato chips	Known carcinogen for laboratory animals; relationship between acrylamide ingestion and development of cancer in humans has not been proven	Limit intake of deep-fat fried foods rich in carbohydrate.
Bisphenol A (BPA)	Leaching of BPA from plastic food and beverage packages	Reproductive and developmental defects in animals	Use BPA-free bottles and cups. Consensus among regulatory agencies in the U.S. and Canada is that current levels of BPA exposure are not harmful, even for infants. To prevent exposure to BPA do not microwave plastic containers, avoid plastic packaging with recycle codes 3 or 7, and reduce use of canned foods. Read more about BPA in Section 9.2 and Section 19.3.
Cadmium	Plants grown in soil rich in cadmium Clams, shellfish, tobacco smoke Occupational exposure in some cases	Kidney disease Liver disease Prostate cancer (debatable) Bone deformities Lung disease (when inhaled)	Consume a wide variety of foods, including seafood sources.

TABLE 17-9 ■ (continued)

Chemical Substance	Sources	Toxic Effects	Preventive Measures
Dioxin	Trash-burning incinerators Bottom-feeding fish from the Great Lakes Fat from animals exposed to dioxin via water or soil	Abnormal reproduction and fetal/infant development Immune suppression Cancer (only clearly shown in laboratory animals)	Pay attention to warnings of dioxin risks from local fish and limit intake as suggested. Consume a variety of fish from diverse water sources.
Lead	Contaminated water supply (see box, Lead Poisoning in Flint, Michigan) Lead-based paint chips and dust in older homes Occupational exposure (e.g., radiator repair) Lead caps on wine bottles Fruit juices and pickled vegetables stored in galvanized or tin containers or leaded glass Some solder used in joining copper pipes in older homes Mexican pottery dishes Some imported herbal remedies Leaded glass containers	Anemia Kidney disease Nervous system damage (tiredness and changes in behavior are symptoms) Reduced learning capacity in childhood (even from mild lead exposure)	Avoid paint chips and related dust in older homes; see information about programs to reduce lead-based paint hazards in homes at www.hud.gov/offices/lead. Meet iron and calcium needs to reduce lead absorption. Wipe the inside and outside neck of wine bottles before use if the bottle has a lead cap. Store fruit juices and pickled vegetables in glass or plastic or waxed paper containers. Let water run 1 minute or so if off for more than 2 hours, and use only cold water for cooking; do not soften drinking water. Do not store alcoholic beverages in leaded glass containers.
Mercury	Swordfish, shark, king mackerel, and tilefish. Fresh and canned albacore tuna is also a possible source (light chunk tuna is very low in mercury.)	Reduced fetal/child development and birth defects; toxic to nervous system	Consume affected food no more than once per week (no more than two times per week for albacore tuna). Pregnant and breastfeeding women as well as young children should avoid these species of fish, but some albacore tuna consumption is fine. Two to three fish meals per week is appropriate for pregnant (and nursing) women if different types of fish are eaten. Read more about mercury later in this section, in Environmental Contaminants in Fish.
Polychlorinated biphenyls (PCBs)	Fish from the Great Lakes and Hudson River Valley (e.g., coho salmon) Farmed salmon are a possible source	Cancer has been shown in laboratory animals Potential for liver, immune, and reproductive disorders	Pay attention to warnings of PCB contamination from local fish and limit intake as suggested on the fishing license or on state advisories. Choose a variety of fish from diverse water sources. Read more about PCBs later in this section, in Environmental Contaminants in Fish.
Urethane	Alcoholic beverages such as sherry, bourbon, sake, and fruit brandies	Cancer in laboratory animals	Avoid generous amounts of typical sources.

PESTICIDES IN FOOD

Pesticides used in food production produce both beneficial and unwanted effects. Most health authorities believe that the benefits outweigh the risks. Pesticides help ensure a safe and adequate food supply and help make foods available at reasonable cost. Nevertheless, consumers have come to assume that "synthetic" is dangerous and "organic" is safe. Some researchers believe that this sentiment is grounded in fear and fueled by unbalanced reports. Other scientists say concern about pesticides is valid and overdue.

Most concern about pesticide residues in food appropriately focuses on long-term rather than acute toxicity, because the amounts of residue present, if any, are extremely small.

These low concentrations found in foods are not known to produce adverse effects in the short term, although harm has been caused by the high amounts that occasionally result from accidents or misuse. For humans, pesticides pose a danger mainly in their cumulative effects, so their threats to health are difficult to determine. However, problems of the contamination of underground water supplies and destruction of wildlife habitats indicate that North Americans would probably be better off by reducing the use of pesticides. The U.S. federal government and many farmers are working toward that end. Section 16.4 discussed the latest use of biotechnology to reduce pesticide use.

WHAT IS A PESTICIDE?

Federal law defines a pesticide as any substance or mixture of substances intended to prevent, destroy, repel, or mitigate any pest. The built-in toxic properties of pesticides lead to the possibility that other, nontarget organisms, including humans, might also be harmed. The term *pesticide* tends to be used as a generic reference to many types of products, including insecticides (to kill insects), herbicides (to kill weeds), rodenticides (to kill rodents), and fungicides (to control fungi, mold, and mildew). A pesticide product may be chemical or bacterial, natural or synthetic.

For agriculture, EPA allows about 10,000 pesticides to be used, containing some 300 active ingredients. The latest EPA report on pesticide use in the United States indicates that 877 million pounds of agricultural pesticide were used in 2007, down slightly from 948 million pounds in 2000. This is 22% of the estimated 5.2 billion pounds of pesticides used worldwide. Herbicides are the most widely used type of pesticide in the United States.

Once a pesticide is applied, it can turn up in a number of unintended and unwanted places. It may be carried in the air and dust by wind currents, remain in soil attached to soil particles, be taken up by organisms in the soil, decompose to other compounds, be taken up by plant roots, enter groundwater, or invade aquatic habitats. Each is a route to the food chain; some are more direct than others.

WHY USE PESTICIDES?

The primary reason for using pesticides is economic: the use of agricultural chemicals increases production and lowers the cost of food, at least in the short run. Many farmers believe that it would be impossible to stay in business without pesticides, which help protect farmers from ruinous losses. It is estimated that for every $1 that is spent on pesticides to increase crop yields, $4 are saved in crops. Farmers also rely more on pesticides to produce cosmetically attractive fruits and vegetables. Consumer demands have changed over the years. At one time, we would not have thought twice about buying an apple with a worm hole. Today, consumers find worm holes and other imperfections less acceptable.

On the practical side, pesticides can protect against the rotting and decay of fresh fruits and vegetables. Also, food grown without pesticides can contain naturally occurring organisms that produce carcinogens at concentrations far above current standards for pesticide residues. For example, fungicides help prevent the carcinogen aflatoxin (caused by growth of a fungus) from forming on some crops. Thus, although some pesticides may do little more than improve the appearance of food products, others help keep foods fresher and safer to eat.

REGULATION OF PESTICIDES

The responsibility for ensuring that residues of pesticides in foods are below amounts that pose a danger to health is shared by FDA, EPA, and the Food Safety and Inspection Service (FSIS) of the USDA in the United States. Table 17-2 listed the roles of various food protection agencies. FDA is responsible for enforcing pesticide tolerances in all foods except meat, poultry, and certain egg products, which are monitored by USDA. A newly proposed pesticide is exhaustively tested, perhaps over 10 years or more, before it is approved for use.

▲ There are risks and benefits associated with pesticide use. The greatest short-term risk is in rural communities, where exposure is more direct. These crops are being dusted from the air with pesticide. © Royalty-Free/Corbis

One of the problems with pesticides is they create new pests because they destroy the predators (spiders, wasps, and beetles) that naturally keep most plant-feeding insect populations in check. The brown plant hopper, which has plagued Indonesian rice fields, was not a serious problem before heavy pesticide use began to kill its predators in the early 1970s. In the United States, such major pests as spider mites and the cotton bollworm were merely nuisances until pesticides decimated their predators.

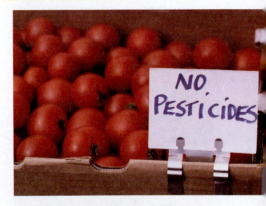

▲ Fruits and vegetables grown without use of synthetic pesticides are available and may bear an "organic" label (see Table 2-10 for rules regarding use of the term "organic" on food labels). These products generally are more expensive than conventional produce. Consumers need to decide if the potential benefits of the products are worth the extra cost. © Nancy R. Cohen/Getty Images

▲ FDA's yearly evaluation of a **market basket** of typical foods shows that pesticide content is minimal in most foods. © C Squared Studios/ Getty Images

market basket Food the FDA buys, prepares, and analyzes as part of the ongoing Total Diet Study (TDS), which monitors levels of about 800 contaminants and nutrients in the average U.S. diet; the number varies slightly from year to year. About 280 kinds of foods and beverages from representative areas of the country are included four times a year.

EPA must decide that the pesticide causes no unreasonable adverse effects on people and the environment and that benefits of use outweigh the risks of using it. FDA tests thousands of raw products each year for pesticide residues. (A pesticide is considered illegal in this case if it is not approved for use on the crop in question or if the amount used exceeds the allowed tolerance.)

HOW SAFE ARE PESTICIDES?

Dangers from exposure to pesticides through food depend on how potent the chemical toxin is, how concentrated it is in the food, how much and how frequently it is eaten, and the consumer's resistance or susceptibility to the substance. Accumulating information links pesticide use to increased cancer rates in farm communities. For rural counties in the United States, the incidence of lymph, genital, brain, and digestive tract cancers increases with higher-than-average pesticide use. Respiratory cancer cases increase with greater insecticide use. In tests using laboratory animals, scientists have found that some of the chemicals present in pesticide residues cause birth defects, sterility, tumors, organ damage, and injury to the central nervous system. Some pesticides persist in the environment for years.

Still, some researchers argue that the cancer risk from pesticide residues is hundreds of times less than the risk from eating such common foods as peanut butter, brown mustard, and basil. Plants manufacture toxic substances to defend themselves against insects, birds, and grazing animals (including humans). When plants are stressed or damaged, they produce even more of these toxins. Because of this, many foods contain naturally occurring chemicals considered toxic, and some are even carcinogenic.

The USDA Pesticide Data Program (PDP) collects data on pesticide residues in food, particularly foods most likely consumed by infants and children. For samples collected in 2014, less than 1% of domestic and about 3% of imported samples had residues over tolerance. These findings are consistent with previous studies over the past 10 years. They indicate that, in general, pesticide residues in food are below EPA tolerances, confirming the safety of the food supply relative to pesticide residues. Visit the EPA website (https://www3.epa.gov) for more information about pesticides and food.

PERSONAL ACTION

Every year, the Environmental Working Group (EWG) publishes a *Shopper's Guide to Pesticides in Produce™*. The EWG is an environmental health research and advocacy organization whose mission is to serve as a watchdog to help Americans get factual information so they can make healthier choices and enjoy a cleaner environment. One of its goals is to help ensure that food products are free of harmful chemicals. Its *Shopper's Guide* includes a list of fruits and vegetables called "The Dirty Dozen™" because they are most likely to contain the highest amounts of pesticide residue (Table 17-10). In 2015, apples topped the list, followed by peaches, nectarines, strawberries, grapes, and celery. The Dirty Dozen Plus category includes crops that did not meet traditional Dirty Dozen criteria but were commonly contaminated with pesticides exceptionally toxic to the nervous system.

The *Shopper's Guide* also features a list of fruits and vegetables called "The Clean 15" because they are least likely to contain pesticide residues. To avoid pesticide exposure, consumers are encouraged to choose organic produce when buying anything on "The Dirty Dozen" list. In addition, the EWG says that buying nonorganic produce from the "The Clean 15" group is relatively safe. The EWG reminds consumers that "the health benefits of a diet rich in fruits and vegetables outweigh the risks of pesticide exposure."

FDA and other scientific organizations believe that the hazards of pesticides are comparatively low and in the short run are less dangerous than the hazards of foodborne illness created in our kitchens. We can encourage farmers to use fewer pesticides to reduce exposure to our foods and water supplies, but we will have to settle for produce that is not perfect in appearance or that has been grown with the aid of biotechnology. Additional advice for limiting exposure to pesticides is found in Table 17.11.

▲ This fruit salad is a healthy choice because cantaloupe, pineapple, and kiwi are some of the fruits found on the Clean 15 list. © MIXA/ Getty Images

TABLE 17.10 ■ The 2015 Dirty Dozen Fruits and Vegetables to Avoid (Unless Organically Grown) and the Clean 15 That Are Relatively Safe

Dirty Dozen	Clean 15
1. Apples	1. Avocados
2. Peaches	2. Sweet corn
3. Nectarines	3. Pineapples
4. Strawberries	4. Cabbage
5. Grapes	5. Sweet peas (frozen)
6. Celery	6. Onions
7. Spinach	7. Asparagus
8. Sweet bell peppers	8. Mangos
9. Cucumbers	9. Papayas
10. Cherry tomatoes	10. Kiwi
11. Snap peas (imported)	11. Eggplant
12. Potatoes	12. Grapefruit
Dirty Dozen Plus	13. Cantaloupe (domestic)
Hot peppers	14. Cauliflower
Kale/collard greens	15. Sweet potatoes

Source: Environmental Working Group, 2015 *Shopper's Guide to Pesticides.*

© Comstock Images/PictureQuest

TABLE 17.11 ■ What You Can Do to Reduce Exposure to Pesticides

WASH: Wash and scrub all fresh fruits and vegetables thoroughly under running water to remove bacteria and soil. Running water has an abrasive effect that soaking does not have. This will help remove bacteria and traces of chemicals from the surface of fruits and vegetables and dirt from crevices. Special antibacterial washing products are not necessary.

PEEL AND TRIM: Peel fruits and vegetables when possible to reduce dirt, bacteria, and pesticides. Discard outer leaves of leafy vegetables. Trim fat from meat and skin from poultry and fish because some pesticide residues collect in fat.

SELECT A VARIETY: Eat a variety of foods from a variety of sources, to provide a better mix of nutrients and reduce your likelihood of exposure to a single pesticide.

CHOOSE ORGANIC: Some consumers are looking to organically grown and produced foods as a way to reduce exposure to synthetic pesticides. If cost is an issue, then choose organic for most of the dirty dozen.

USE INSECT REPELLENTS SAFELY: Read the label for pesticide safety information and apply insect repellents safely. See www.epa.gov/pesticides/factsheets/pest_ti.htm for more pesticide safety tips.

Source: United States Environmental Protection Agency

ENVIRONMENTAL CONTAMINANTS IN FISH

The presence of the environmental contaminants mercury and polychlorinated biphenyls (PCBs) in fish has caused some confusion regarding the risks and benefits of fish consumption. In our previous discussion of the benefits of omega-3 fatty acids (see Section 5.7), it was recommended that we include cold-water fatty fish, such as salmon or tuna, in our diet about twice a week. Conversely, you may have heard recommendations to eat less fish

▲ This wild Alaskan salmon on organic green beans is a top choice among types of fish based on its high nutritional value and low mercury levels. © Digital Vision/Getty Images

because they are a source of environmental contaminants. Balancing the benefits and risks of consuming fish is tricky, and not all experts agree (see Further Reading 10). For example, advice from FDA and EPA indicates that salmon is safe to eat, even during pregnancy, because it is low in mercury. In contrast, the Environmental Defense Fund (EDF) advocacy group recommends that all adults, not just pregnant women, limit consumption of wild salmon (except Alaskan) to only one serving per month and farmed salmon to no more than two servings a month (based on PCB contamination).

Mercury and PCBs are by-products of industrial processes and accumulate in fish tissue. PCBs were banned from use in 1979, but environmental levels have been decreasing very slowly and therefore still persist in our food supply, especially seafood. The contaminants become more concentrated in bigger fish as they eat smaller, contaminated fish. Fish are of primary concern because they are the only predators we eat regularly. The Institute of Medicine (IOM), Food and Agriculture Organization (FAO), FDA, and EPA have issued similar guidelines for fish consumption. These groups advise pregnant women to eat up to 12 ounces of low-mercury fish per week and to avoid the four highest-mercury fish, which are swordfish, shark, tilefish, and king mackerel. For other adults, the basic recommendation is to "eat fish" but do not always eat the same type so you are not exposed to the same contaminants over and over.

As a nation, Americans do not eat enough fish to cause concern about high intakes of environmental contaminants. On average, we consume only about 4 ounces of seafood per week. Around 80% of that is shrimp, canned tuna, salmon, and white fish, which are relatively low in environmental contaminants. Most Americans would benefit from eating more fish—a rich source of omega-3 fatty acids. Research shows that the risk of dying from heart disease is about 50% greater among people who do not eat fish compared to those who eat one or two servings of fatty fish each week. Overall, it appears that the benefits of consuming fish twice per week outweigh the potential risks discussed in this section. Pregnant women should follow the FDA/EPA guidelines, and the rest of us should eat a variety of types of fish, focusing on the smaller, fatty fish at the bottom of the food chain.

✓ CONCEPT CHECK 17.6

1. What is a pesticide?
2. What are the benefits of pesticide use?
3. What agencies regulate the use of pesticides?
4. What foods are on the "Dirty Dozen" list?
5. What environmental contaminants can be found in fish, and which fish are most likely to contain these toxins?

17.7 Food Production Choices

Agriculture—the production of food and livestock—has supplied humans with food for millennia. At one time, nearly everyone was involved in food production. Today, only about one in three people around the globe (less than 1% in the United States) is now involved in farming. Approximately 570 million farms, primarily run by individuals, produce about 80% of the world's food. Numerous advances in agricultural sciences are affecting our food supply; of particular note are organic food production and sustainable agriculture. Many of these new developments in agriculture are aimed at reducing the overall **carbon footprint** (carbon dioxide and methane emissions) generated from the farm to the fork.

ORGANIC FOODS

The term **organic food** refers to the way agricultural products are produced. Organic production relies on farming practices such as **biological pest management,** composting,

carbon footprint The greenhouse gas emissions caused by an organization, event, product, or individual.

organic food Food grown without use of pesticides, synthetic fertilizers, sewage sludge, genetically modified organisms, antibiotics, hormones, or ionizing radiation.

biological pest management Control of agricultural pests by using natural predators, parasites, or pathogens. For example, ladybugs can be used to control an aphid infestation.

manure applications, and crop rotation to maintain healthy soil, water, crops, and animals. Synthetic pesticides, fertilizers, and hormones; antibiotics; sewage sludge (used as fertilizer); genetic engineering; and irradiation are not permitted in the production of organic foods. However, many synthetic substances and natural pesticides may be used in organic crop production (see U.S. Organic Regulations at https://www.ams.usda.gov/grades-standards/organic-standards for more information). Additionally, organic meat, poultry, eggs, and dairy products must come from animals allowed to graze outdoors and consume only organic feed.

Organic foods are increasingly available in supermarkets, specialty stores, farmers markets, and restaurants (see Further Reading 13). Consumers can select organic fruits, vegetables, grains, dairy products, meats, eggs, and many processed foods, including sauces and condiments, breakfast cereals, cookies, and snack chips. Interest in personal and environmental health has contributed to the increasing availability and sales of organic foods. According to the Organic Trade Association, U.S. sales of organic foods exceeded $39 billion in 2014. This reflects an increase of 11% over the previous year. Canada's organic market has also tripled since 2006, reaching $3.7 billion in 2012. Despite this rapid growth, only 4.2% of foods sold are organic. Organic foods, because they often cost more to grow and produce, are typically more expensive than comparable conventional foods.

The Organic Foods Production Act of 1990 established standards for the production of foods that bear the USDA Organic seal. Foods labeled and marketed as organic must be grown on farms that are certified by the USDA as following all of the rules established in the 1990 act. Products labeled "100% organic" may only contain organically produced ingredients and processing aids, excluding water and salt. No other ingredients or additives are permitted. Foods made from multiple ingredients (e.g., breakfast cereal) can be labeled as *organic* if at least 95% of their ingredients (by weight) meet organic standards. The term *made with organic ingredients* can be used if at least 70% of the ingredients are organic. Small organic producers and farmers with sales less than $5000 per year are exempt from the certification regulation. Some farmers use organic production methods but choose not to be USDA certified. Their foods cannot be labeled as organic, but many of these farmers market and sell to those seeking organic foods.

There has been an increase in USDA support and funding for research, cost-share assistance, and other organic food programs since 2002, when national organic standards were implemented. The organic food market grew exponentially in 2009, when the USDA offered $50 million in new funding to encourage greater production of organic food in the United States. With the additional financial support for farmers and ranchers, the number of certified organic operations in the United States increased to 19,474 in 2014, out of a global total of 27,814. Because most stores now offer organic products, consumers have the opportunity to compare products and prices. Increased availability and use of coupons, the proliferation of private label and store brands, and better-value products offered by major organic brands all have contributed to increased sales.

Organic Foods and Health Consumers may choose to eat organic foods to reduce their synthetic pesticide exposure, to protect the environment, and out of the belief that they will improve the overall nutritional quality of their diets. Organic produce typically carries fewer pesticide residues than conventional produce; however, the residues on both organic and nonorganic produce are tested annually by the USDA and remain below government safety thresholds. Cautious consumers may consider organic as a wise choice for vulnerable populations (e.g., young children, seniors) and opt for organic foods to encourage environmentally friendly **sustainable agriculture** practices.

In terms of nutritional quality, a large study examined 50 years' worth of scientific evidence about the nutrient content of organic and conventional foods. The researchers concluded that organic and conventional foods are not significantly different in their nutrient content or nutritional value (see Further Reading 15). At this point, it is not possible to recommend organic foods over conventional foods based on nutrient content: both can meet nutritional needs. A healthy dose of common sense also is important; an "organic" label does not change a less healthy food into a more healthy food. For example, organic potato chips have the same calorie and fat content as conventional potato chips.

sustainable agriculture Agricultural system that provides a secure living for farm families; maintains the natural environment and resources; supports the rural community; and offers respect and fair treatment to all involved, from farm workers to consumers to the animals raised for food.

▲ The USDA organic seal identifies organic foods grown on USDA-certified organic farms. Source: USDA

▲ USDA organic products have strict production and labeling requirements. Organic products must be (1) produced without excluded methods, (e.g., genetic engineering, ionizing radiation, or sewage sludge); (2) produced using allowed substances; and (3) overseen by a USDA National Organic Program—authorized certifying agent, following all USDA organic regulations. © C Squared Studios/Getty Images

Newsworthy Nutrition

German organic sprouts cause deadly *E. coli* outbreak

The world's deadliest outbreak of *Escherichia coli* occurred during the summer of 2011. The outbreak occurred mainly in Germany and involved a rare strain of *E. coli*, known as O104:H4, which causes bleeding in the GI tract. In June 2011, 3950 persons had been infected, more than 600 were in intensive care, and the death toll from the outbreak reached 53. Several hundred also contracted its potentially fatal kidney complication, known as hemolytic uremic syndrome. This German case-control study concluded that the *E. coli* infection was caused by tainted vegetable sprouts from a small, rather traditional organic sprout farm. The sprout seeds were mostly imported from overseas, and the *E. coli* bacteria were antibiotic resistant. Experts say these types of outbreaks are becoming more common due to large-scale industrial farming and the widespread use of antibiotics.

Source: Buchholz U and others: German outbreak of *Escherichia coli* O104:H4 associated with sprouts. *New England Journal of Medicine* 365:1763, 2011.

One concern raised about organic foods is that food safety may be jeopardized because animal manures used for fertilizers may contaminate food with pathogens. Although a major outbreak of foodborne illness was linked to organically grown sprouts in Europe (see Newsworthy Nutrition), research does not show that certified organic food has higher contamination with bacterial pathogens. To avoid exposure to potential pathogens, consumers should wash or scrub all produce—organic and conventional—under running water. This safe food handling practice is critical for individuals with depressed immune systems.

Unlike the term *organic,* the term *natural* is not regulated by any federal agency. Products labeled as "natural" are generally those derived from natural ingredients, such as a plant source, which retain their native properties in the finished product. Meat or poultry labeled "natural" is expected to be minimally processed and contain no artificial flavoring, coloring, chemical preservative, or other artificial or synthetic ingredients. Also understand that many "natural" products are detrimental to health. Manure and arsenic are natural products, yet harmful if ingested. Unfortunately, few regulations are in place to ensure adherence to the policies, and there is debate over what constitutes "minimally processed." Although all organic products fit this definition of natural, not all natural products are necessarily organic. Legislation has recently been proposed (the Food Labeling Modernization Act of 2015) that seeks to define and regulate use of the term "natural" on food labels.

SUSTAINABLE AGRICULTURE

Conventional agriculture focuses on maximizing production through the use of large acreages, powerful machines, chemicals to control pests, and synthetic fertilizers to boost growth. In contrast, sustainable agriculture is an integrated system of plant and animal production that will, over the long term, satisfy human food needs, enhance environmental quality, efficiently use nonrenewable resources, sustain the economic viability of farm operations, and enhance the quality of life for farmers and society as a whole. A culture of sustainability has emerged, including a clear trend for sustainable food choices manufactured in an environmentally responsible way.

The United Nations Sustainable Development Goals (SDGs) include a goal aimed at promoting sustainable agriculture (see Section 16.4). Successful sustainable practices, such as crop rotation, intercropping (growing two or more crops in proximity), and steppe farming (also known as terrace farming), have increased productivity in countries such as South America. Crop rotation protects the soil by reducing nutrient depletion of the soil. Intercropping encourages plants to thrive in varying soil characteristics. Steppe farming increases productivity by enabling planting on hillsides by terracing slopes to hold water for a long duration and retain the top soil more effectively.

Lifestyle of Health and Sustainability (LOHAS) describes a growing demographic group focused on sustainable living. An increasing number of today's college students are joining this market segment and developing behaviors associated with social responsibility. These consumers are driving changes in many areas, including the food industry. The food industry has responded with a move toward "green" initiatives that should be sustainable for the long term. Slow Food USA is an example of a nonprofit group dedicated to creating a framework for a deeper environmental connection to our food and aiming to inspire and empower Americans to build a food system that is sustainable, healthy, and delicious.

Sustainable Seafood In 2010, the Dietary Guidelines recommended 8 ounces of seafood per week for adults. The Scientific Report of the 2015 Dietary Guidelines Advisory Committee reported that less than 10% of the U.S. population, across all age groups, met this recommendation. The challenge of increasing fish consumption, while also being wary of environmental contaminants in seafood, was discussed in Section 17.6. Seafood choices become even more complex when we consider the issue of overfishing and protecting endangered species of fish (see Further Reading 4). An "overfished" species is a population whose survival is jeopardized due to harvesting at a rate that exceeds the replenishing of stock. The good news is that fish production, whether farmed or wild caught, has a lower environmental cost compared to the production of meats. Fewer greenhouse gases are emitted, fewer chemicals and antibiotics are used, and fewer pounds of protein in feed are used than in beef, pork, or poultry production.

Fortunately, the United States has rigorous standards and closely monitors its fishing and aquaculture (fish farming) operations. The National Oceanic and Atmospheric Administration (NOAA) Fisheries establishes strict fishing catch levels in U.S. waters; enforces these catch limits on fishing vessels, docks, and ports; and oversees, monitors, and enforces the standards for U.S. aquaculture. As a result, when we buy U.S. wild-caught or farmed fish, we are making a sustainable choice. Look for the words "U.S. seafood product" on fish labels to ensure the fish or shellfish has been sustainably harvested.

The sustainable solution, however, is not that simple at the fish market or restaurant. This challenge persists because the vast majority (90%) of the seafood we eat in the United States comes from international sources. About half of this seafood is from Southeast Asia and a significant portion of it is caught by American fishermen, exported overseas for processing, and then imported back to the United States. Americans have a limited seafood palate, with only 10 species making up 90% of the seafood we eat. Fortunately, four of the most popular fish—shrimp, salmon, tilapia, and pangasius—are largely raised by certified and sustainable aquaculture operations. For example, salmon must be farmed to supply two-thirds of the 350 million tons of salmon that Americans consume annually. While many consumers perceive that wild-caught fish are the more environmentally friendly variety, many unregulated wild-caught fishing harvests have reached their peak capacity and are threatening future global seafood supplies. While sustainable seafood sourcing remains complex, consumers need to know that both farmed and wild-caught fish can be healthy, sustainable, and economical choices.

LOCALLY GROWN FOODS

With people everywhere more interested in the origins of their food, more grocery store shelves are devoted to "locally grown" products. Consumers are demanding increased transparency with the food supply, and local food helps answer questions about where food comes from and how it was grown. Retailers are using the "locally grown" label to respond to consumer desires for fresh, safe products that also support small, local farmers and help the environment. Local products typically provide fresher options, do not have the added costs of long transportation, and thus use less fossil fuel. Food service establishments are also placing greater emphasis on supporting local producers, encouraging a farm-to-fork approach.

Until recently, farmers markets were the typical way consumers had access to locally grown, farm-fresh produce. Farmers markets are also an integral part of the way that urban communities are linked to farms and continue to gain popularity. In 2014, there were 8284 farmers markets operating throughout the United States, nearly double what was available just 5 years ago.

Acceptable Fish

Groups such as the Natural Resources Defense Council (www.nrdc.org) and Seafood Watch (www.seafoodwatch.org) regularly update lists of acceptable fish.

▲ The locavore movement is based on the assumption that local products are more nutritious and taste better and encourages consumers to buy from farmers markets or produce their own food. © Lars A. Niki

locavore Someone who eats food grown or produced locally or within a certain radius such as 50, 100, or 500 miles.

The interest in "local" foods has become such a phenomenon that the term *locavore* was the 2007 Word of the Year in the *New Oxford American Dictionary*. A **locavore** is defined as someone who eats food grown or produced locally or within a certain radius from home, such as 50, 100, or 150 miles. The locavore movement has gained prominence due to food-safety concerns by consumers and the search for local, sustainable foods. It also encourages consumers to buy from farmers markets or produce their own food, with the argument that fresh, local products are more nutritious and taste better.

There is no evidence, however, that locally grown products are safer. Although many small producers have proper food-safety practices, they often lack the expensive food-safety audits that are more common among big producers. Food-safety auditors evaluate evidence of insects on produce, sanitation practices, and similar food-safety criteria. Undetected foodborne illness outbreaks are more likely with "local" products delivered in small quantities and sold in a small area. Local products are not necessarily pesticide free and may not be cheaper, given that smaller growers lack the economic advantages of bigger growers. The outbreak of foodborne illness linked to a local organic farm was discussed in the Newsworthy Nutrition.

Unlike organic products, there are no regulations specifying the meaning of "locally grown." Whole Foods Market, Inc. is the biggest retailer of natural and organic food and the most recognized for buying and selling locally grown produce. Whole Foods considers "local" to be anything produced within 7 hours of one of its stores, with most local producers located within 200 miles of a store. Walmart, the world's largest retailer, has also become a large buyer of locally grown fruits and vegetables and considers anything "local" if it is grown in the same state as it is sold. Searchable databases and mapping resources such as MarketMaker (https://foodmarketmaker.com) are available to connect growers with buyers, restaurants with distributors, and consumers with local farmers markets. These tools make it easier for people to find and sell locally grown foods. Positive attitudes toward organic, local, and sustainable food production practices are on the rise and appear to be increasing the conversations around dietary patterns and quality. For example, a study of college students in Minnesota showed that college students who put a high importance on alternative food production methods had a higher quality diet. They consumed more fruits and vegetables and dietary fiber, fewer added sugars and sugar-sweetened drinks, and less fat.

community supported agriculture (CSA) Partnership between local food producers and community members. Farmers offer a share of foods to individuals, families, or companies that have pledged support to the CSA either financially and/or by working for the CSA.

▲ Farmers participating in community supported agriculture (CSA) offer another avenue for exposing customers to locally grown foods. © Iconotec.com

Visit www.localharvest.org to find farmers markets, family farms, and other sources of sustainably grown food in your area.

Look up www.farmtoschool.org to find a Farm to School Program near you.

COMMUNITY SUPPORTED AGRICULTURE

Consumers are not only taking comfort in knowing where their food comes from but also becoming interested in community connections with local and regional farmers. Stemming from the interest in locally grown food, there is growing national support for local food collaboratives and community supported agriculture. **Community supported agriculture (CSA)** programs involve a partnership between local food producers and consumers. During each growing season, CSA farmers offer a share of foods to individuals, families, or companies that have pledged support to the CSA either financially and/or by working for the CSA.

Another example of a farm-community partnership is the National Farm to School Network, a nonprofit effort to connect farmers with nearby school (K–12) cafeterias. The objectives of this program are to serve healthy meals in school cafeterias; improve student nutrition; provide agriculture, health, and nutrition education opportunities; and support local and regional farmers. Between 1997 and 2012, this program grew from only 6 local programs to 40,328 in all 50 states, resulting in 12,429 schools incorporating the local bounty into their menus. Administrators of the program have found that if kids can meet the farmer who actually grew the food, they are much more likely to eat it.

✓ **CONCEPT CHECK 17.7**

1. What are the basic requirements for foods to be labeled as organic?
2. What is the definition of sustainable agriculture?
3. What is the locavore movement, and what are its advantages?
4. What is a community supported agriculture (CSA) program?

17.8 Nutrition and Your Health
Preventing Foodborne Illness

© White Rock/Getty Images

You can greatly reduce the risk of foodborne illness by following some important rules (see Further Readings 7 and 12). It is a long list because many risky habits need to be addressed.

Purchasing Food

- When shopping, select frozen foods and perishable foods such as meat, poultry, or fish last. Always have these products put in separate plastic bags, so that drippings do not contaminate other foods in the shopping cart. Do not let groceries sit in a warm car; this allows bacteria to grow. Get the perishable foods such as meat, eggs, and dairy products home and promptly refrigerate or freeze them.
- Do not buy or use food from damaged containers that leak, bulge, or are severely dented or from jars that are cracked or have loose or bulging lids. Do not taste or use food that has a foul odor or spurts liquid when the can is opened; the deadly *Clostridium botulinum* toxin may be present.
- Purchase only pasteurized milk and cheese (check the label). This is especially important for pregnant women because highly toxic bacteria and viruses that can harm the fetus thrive in unpasteurized milk.
- Purchase only the amount of produce needed for a week's time. The longer you keep fruits and vegetables, the more time is available for bacteria to grow.
- When purchasing precut produce or bagged salad greens, avoid those that look slimy, brownish, or dry; these are signs of improper holding temperatures.
- Observe sell-by and expiration dates on food labels and do not buy products that are near or past these dates.
- Follow food recalls because a Class I recall means that there is a "reasonable probability" that consuming the food will cause serious health consequences or death.

Preparing Food

- Thoroughly wash your hands for 20 to 30 seconds with hot, soapy water before and after handling food. This practice is especially important when handling raw meat, fish, poultry, and eggs; after using the bathroom; after playing with pets; or after changing diapers.
- Make sure counters, cutting boards, dishes, and other equipment are thoroughly sanitized and rinsed before use. Be especially careful to use hot, soapy water to wash surfaces and equipment that come in contact with raw meat, fish, poultry, and eggs as soon as possible to remove *Salmonella* bacteria that may be present. Otherwise, bacteria on the surfaces will infect the next foods that come in contact with the surface, a process called **cross-contamination.** In addition, replace sponges and wash kitchen towels frequently. (Microwaving sponges for 30 to 60 seconds also helps rid them of live bacteria.)
- If possible, cut foods to be eaten raw on a clean cutting board reserved for that purpose. Then clean this cutting board using hot, soapy water. If the same board must be used for both meat and other foods, cut any potentially contaminated items, such as meat, last. After cutting the meat, wash the cutting board thoroughly. The FDA recommends cutting boards with unmarred surfaces made of easy-to-clean, nonporous materials such as plastic, marble, or glass. Wooden boards should be made of a nonabsorbent hardwood, such as oak, maple, or bamboo, and have no obvious seams or cracks. Recently, bamboo has become popular for cutting boards because its dense wood resists knife scarring and water penetration, leaving bacteria without a place to multiply. Keep a separate wooden cutting board for chopping produce and slicing bread to prevent cross-contamination. Many foods are served raw, so any bacteria clinging to them are not destroyed. Furthermore, the FDA recommends that all cutting boards be replaced when they become streaked with hard-to-clean grooves or cuts, which may harbor bacteria. In addition, cutting boards should be sanitized once a week in a dilute bleach solution. Flood the board with the solution, let it sit for a few minutes, then rinse thoroughly.

cross-contamination Process by which bacteria or other microorganisms are unintentionally transferred from one substance or object to another, with harmful effect.

- Ignore the 5-second rule of picking up food that has fallen on the floor because food picks up bacteria immediately upon contact.
- When thawing foods, do so in the refrigerator, under cold potable running water, or in a microwave oven. Also, cook foods immediately after thawing under cold water or in the microwave. Never let frozen foods thaw unrefrigerated all day or night. Also, marinate food in the refrigerator.
- Avoid coughing or sneezing over foods, even when you are healthy. Cover cuts on hands with a sterile bandage. This helps stop *Staphylococcus* bacteria from entering food.
- Carefully wash fresh fruit and vegetables under running water to remove dirt and bacteria clinging to the surface, using a vegetable brush if the skin is to be eaten. People have become ill from *Salmonella* introduced from melons used in making a fruit salad and from oranges used for fresh-squeezed orange juice. The bacteria were on the outside of the melons and oranges.
- Completely remove moldy portions of food or do not eat the food. If a food is covered in mold, discard the food. Mold growth is prevented by properly storing food at cold

▲ Washing hands thoroughly (for at least 20 to 30 seconds) with hot water and soap should be the first step in food preparation. The four Fs of food contamination are fingers, foods, feces, and flies. Handwashing especially combats the finger and fecal routes. Courtesy of USDA, HHS and the Ad Council

A tool used by the food service industry in the battle against foodborne illness is Hazard Analysis Critical Control Point (HACCP). By applying the principles of HACCP, food handlers critically analyze how they approach food preparation and what conditions may exist that might allow pathogenic microorganisms to enter and thrive in the food system. Once specific hazards and critical control points (potential problems) are identified, preventive measures can be used to reduce specific sources of contamination.

The USDA simplified the rules of foodborne illness prevention into four actions as part of its food-safety program (check out www.foodsafety.gov):

1. **Clean.** Wash hands and surfaces often.
2. **Separate.** Don't cross-contaminate.
3. **Cook.** Cook to proper temperatures.
4. **Chill.** Refrigerate promptly.

The Dietary Guidelines for Americans also stress the importance of these four actions.

▲ Food safety logo of USDA.

The World Health Organization's Golden Rules for Safe Food Preparation:

1. Choose foods processed for safety.
2. Cook food thoroughly.
3. Eat cooked foods immediately.
4. Store cooked foods carefully.
5. Reheat cooked foods thoroughly.
6. Avoid contact between raw and cooked foods.
7. Wash hands repeatedly.
8. Keep all kitchen surfaces meticulously clean.
9. Protect foods from insects, rodents, and other animals.
10. Use pure water.

temperatures and using the food promptly. Also discard soft foods with high moisture content such as bread, yogurt, soft cheeses, and deli meats if there are spots of mold on them. It is safe to trim off any moldy spots of dense foods such as hard cheeses or firm fruits and vegetables.
- Use refrigerated ground meat and patties in 1 to 2 days and frozen meat and patties within 3 to 4 months.

Cooking Food

- Cook food thoroughly and use a bimetallic thermometer to check for doneness, especially for fresh beef and fish (145 °F [63 °C]), pork (145 °F [63 °C]), and poultry (165 °F [74 °C]) (Fig. 17-3). Eggs should be cooked until the yolk and white are hard. The FDA does not recommend that eggs be prepared sunny-side up. Alfalfa sprouts and other types of sprouts should be cooked until they are steaming. Cooking is by far the most reliable way to destroy foodborne viruses and bacteria, such as Norovirus and toxic strains of *E. coli*. Freezing only temporarily halts viral and bacterial growth.
- A general precaution is to not eat raw animal products. As noted, many restaurants now include an advisory on menus stating that an increased risk of foodborne illness is associated

- For outdoor cooking, cook food completely at the picnic site, with no partial cooking in advance.

Storing and Reheating Cooked Food

- Keep foods out of the "danger zone" (see Fig. 17-1) by keeping hot foods hot and cold foods cold. Hold food below 40 °F (4 °C) or above 140 °F (60 °C). Foodborne microorganisms thrive in more moderate temperatures (60 to 110 °F [16 to 43 °C]). Some microorganisms can even grow in the refrigerator. Again, do not leave cooked or refrigerated foods, such as meats and salads, at room temperature for more than 2 hours (or 1 hour in hot weather) because that gives microorganisms an opportunity to grow. Store dry food at 60 to 70 °F (16 to 21 °C).
- Reheat leftovers to 165 °F (74 °C); reheat gravy to a rolling boil to kill *Clostridium perfringens* bacteria, which may be present. Merely reheating to a good eating temperature is not sufficient to kill harmful bacteria.
- Store peeled or cut-up produce, such as melon balls, in the refrigerator.

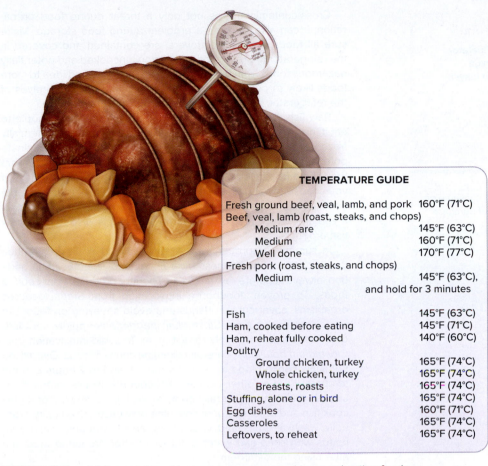

TEMPERATURE GUIDE

Fresh ground beef, veal, lamb, and pork	160°F (71°C)
Beef, veal, lamb (roast, steaks, and chops)	
Medium rare	145°F (63°C)
Medium	160°F (71°C)
Well done	170°F (77°C)
Fresh pork (roast, steaks, and chops)	
Medium	145°F (63°C), and hold for 3 minutes
Fish	145°F (63°C)
Ham, cooked before eating	145°F (71°C)
Ham, reheat fully cooked	140°F (60°C)
Poultry	
Ground chicken, turkey	165°F (74°C)
Whole chicken, turkey	165°F (74°C)
Breasts, roasts	165°F (74°C)
Stuffing, alone or in bird	165°F (74°C)
Egg dishes	160°F (71°C)
Casseroles	165°F (74°C)
Leftovers, to reheat	165°F (74°C)

FIGURE 17-3 ▲ Minimum internal temperatures when cooking or reheating foods.

Source: USDA Food Safety and Inspection Service, Safe Minimum Internal Temperature Chart, www.fsis.usda.gov

with eating undercooked eggs. As long as restaurants provide this warning on their menus, however, they are allowed to cook eggs to any temperature requested by the consumer. FDA warns us not to consume homemade ice cream, eggnog, and mayonnaise if made with unpasteurized, raw eggs because of the risk of *Salmonella* foodborne illness. The pasteurization of eggs or egg products kills *Salmonella* bacteria. Consuming raw seafood, especially oysters, also poses a risk of foodborne illness. Properly cooked seafood should flake easily and/or be opaque or dull and firm. If it is translucent or shiny, it is not done.

- Cook stuffing separately from poultry (or stuff immediately before cooking, and then transfer the stuffing to a clean bowl immediately after cooking). Make sure the stuffing reaches 165 °F (74 °C). *Salmonella* is the major concern with poultry.
- Once a food is cooked, consume it right away, or cool it to 40 °F (4 °C) within 2 hours. If it is not to be eaten immediately, in hot weather (80 °F and above) make sure that this cooling is done within 1 hour. Do this by separating the food into as many shallow pans as needed to provide a large surface area for cooling. Be careful not to recontaminate cooked food by contact with raw meat or juices from hands, cutting boards, or other dirty utensils.
- Serve meat, poultry, and fish on a clean plate—never the same plate used to hold the raw product. For example, when grilling hamburgers, do not put cooked items on the same plate used to carry the raw product out to the grill.

- Keep leftovers in the refrigerator only for the recommended length of time (Fig. 17-4).
- Make sure the refrigerator stays below 40 °F (4 °C). Either use a refrigerator thermometer or keep it as cold as possible without freezing milk and lettuce.
- When the power goes out, keep the freezer and refrigerator doors closed as much as possible. Food can stay cold in an unopened refrigerator for about 4 hours; after 4 hours without power, discard perishable foods such as milk, meat,

▲ Sushi, like all raw fish or meat dishes, is a high-risk food. For maximum protection from foodborne illness, animal foods should be cooked thoroughly before eating. © Foodcollection

When in doubt, throw it out!

Food	Refrigerator Storage Time (days)
Meats	
Cooked ground beef/turkey	3–4
Deli meat	2–3
Cooked pork	3–4
Cooked poultry	3–4
Cooked beef, bison, lamb	3–4
Seafood	
Raw (e.g. sushi/sashimi)	Must consume on day of purchase
Cooked	2
Other Entrees	
Pizza	1–2
Pasta/rice	1–2
Casserole	3–4
Soups and Chili	
Chili with meat	2–3
Chili without meat	3–4
Soup/stew	3–4
Side Dishes	
Fresh salad	1–2
Fresh vegetables	1–2
Pasta or potato salad	2–3
Deviled egg	2–3
Hard boiled egg	7
Potato (any style)	3–4
Cooked vegetables	3–4
Dessert	
Cream pie	2–3
Fruit pie	2–3
Pastries	7
Cake	7
Cheesecake	7

FIGURE 17-4 ▲ Length of time to keep leftovers in the refrigerator. Visit www.homefoodsafety.org for more tips on keeping your food safe.

leftovers, and deli meats. Unopened freezers will keep food frozen for 2 days if full and 1 day if half full. Meat, poultry, and seafood can be refrozen if the freezer has not risen above 40 °F.

Cross-contamination is not only a threat during food preparation; it can also become a problem during food storage. Make sure all foods, including leftovers, are contained and covered in the refrigerator to prevent drippings from uncooked and potentially hazardous foods from tainting other foods. It is a good idea to store foods likely to pose risk of foodborne illness on lower shelves of the refrigerator, beneath other foods to be eaten raw.

Raw fish dishes, such as sushi, can be safe for most people to eat if they are made with very fresh fish that has been commercially frozen and then thawed. The freezing is important to eliminate potential health risks from parasites. The FDA recommends that the fish be frozen to an internal temperature of −10 °F for 7 days. If you choose to eat uncooked fish, purchase the fish from reputable establishments that have high standards for quality and sanitation. If you are at high risk for foodborne illness, it is wise to avoid raw fish products.

In summary, thoroughly cook all meat and poultry to reduce the risk of foodborne illness from *E. coli* and *Salmonella*. In addition, always separate raw meats and poultry products from cooked foods. To prevent foodborne intoxication from *Staphylococcus* organisms, cover cuts on hands and avoid sneezing on foods. To avoid intoxication from *Clostridium perfringens,* rapidly cool leftover foods and thoroughly reheat them. To avoid intoxication from *Clostridium botulinum,* carefully examine canned foods. Overall, do not allow cooked food to stand for more than 1 to 2 hours at room temperature. For other causes of foodborne illness, precautions already mentioned generally apply as well. In addition, thoroughly cook fish and other seafood; consume only pasteurized dairy products; wash all fruits and vegetables; and thoroughly wash your hands with soap and water before and after preparing food and after using the bathroom.

To reduce the risk of bacteria surviving during microwave cooking:

- Cover food with glass or ceramic when possible to decrease evaporation and heat the surface.
- Stir and rotate food at least once or twice for even cooking. Then, allow microwaved food to stand, covered, after heating is completed to help cook the exterior and equalize the temperature throughout.
- Use the oven temperature probe or a meat thermometer to check that food is done. Insert it at several spots.
- If thawing meat in the microwave, use the oven's defrost setting. Ice crystals in frozen foods are not heated well by the microwave oven and can create cold spots, which later cook more slowly.

CASE STUDY Preventing Foodbourne Illness at Gatherings

Nicole attended a gathering of her coworkers on a warm Saturday in July. The theme of the party was international dining. Nicole and her husband brought an Argentinian dish, potato and beef empanadas. They followed the recipe and cooking time carefully, removing the dish from the oven at 1 P.M. and keeping it warm by wrapping the pan in a towel. They traveled in their car to the party and set the dish out on the buffet table at 3 P.M. Dinner was to be served at 4 P.M. However, the guests were enjoying themselves so much lounging around the host's pool and drinking ginger beer (also on the menu) that no one began to eat until 6 P.M. Nicole made sure she sampled the empanadas that she and her husband made, but her husband did not. She also had some salad, garlic bread, and a sweet dessert made with coconut.

© Digital Vision

The couple returned home at 11 P.M. and went to bed. At about 2 A.M., Nicole knew something was wrong. She had severe abdominal pain and had to make a dash to the bathroom. She spent most of the next 3 hours in the bathroom with severe diarrhea. By dawn, the diarrhea subsided and she started to feel better. After a few cups of tea and a light breakfast, she was feeling like herself by noon.

Answer the following questions and check your responses at the end of the chapter.

1. Based on her symptoms, what type of foodborne illness did Nicole contract?
2. Why is the beef the most likely vehicle for this type of foodborne illness?
3. Why is consuming food at large gatherings risky?
4. What precautions for avoiding foodborne illness were ignored by Nicole and the rest of the people at the party?
5. How could this scenario be rewritten to substantially reduce the risk of foodborne illness?

Summary (Numbers refer to numbered sections in the chapter.)

17.1 Infants, children, older adults, postsurgical patients, immunosuppressed individuals, and pregnant women are most susceptible to foodborne illness. The risk of foodborne illness has increased as more of our foods are prepared outside of the home.

17.2 In the past, salt, sugar, smoke, fermentation, and drying were used to protect against foodborne illness. Today, careful cooking, pasteurization, irradiation, attention to food temperature, and thorough handwashing provide additional insurance.

17.3 Viruses, bacteria, and other microorganisms in food pose the greatest risk for foodborne illness. Major causes of foodborne illness are Norovirus and the bacteria *Campylobacter jejuni*, *Salmonella*, *Staphylococcus aureus*, and *Clostridium perfringens*. In addition, such bacteria as *Clostridium botulinum*, *Listeria monocytogenes*, and *Escherichia coli* have been found to cause illness.

17.4 Food additives are used primarily to extend shelf life by preventing microbial growth and the destruction of food components by oxygen, metals, and other substances. Food additives are classified as those intentionally added to foods and those that incidentally appear in foods. An intentional additive is limited to no more than one-one-hundredth of the greatest amount that causes no observed symptoms in animals. Under its jurisdiction in the United States, the Delaney Clause allows FDA to ban the use of any intentional food additive that causes cancer.

17.5 Toxic substances occur naturally in a variety of foods, such as green potatoes, raw fish, mushrooms, and raw egg whites. Cooking foods limits their toxic effects in some cases; others are best to avoid altogether, such as toxic mushroom species and the green parts of potatoes.

17.6 A variety of environmental contaminants and pesticide residues can be found in foods. It is helpful to know which foods pose the greatest risks and act accordingly to reduce exposure, such as washing fruits and vegetables before use.

17.7 While conventional agriculture emphasizes large yields and low costs, the more recent trend toward sustainability considers the long-term environmental impact of agricultural practices. Consumers are driving up demand for organic and locally grown products.

17.8 Safe food handling can be summed up in four easy steps: (1) *clean* hands and surfaces often; (2) *separate* raw and ready-to-eat foods to prevent cross-contamination; (3) *cook* (and reheat) potentially hazardous foods thoroughly, measuring temperature with a food thermometer; and (4) *chill* foods by refrigerating promptly after eating. Two of these practices focus on food temperature; foods should not be held in the "danger zone" (40 to 140 °F) for more than 2 hours.

Check Your Knowledge (Answers are available at the end of this question set.)

1. Nitrite prevents the growth of
   a. *Clostridium botulinum.*
   b. *Escherichia coli.*
   c. *Staphylococcus aureus.*
   d. yeasts.

2. Substances used to preserve foods by lowering the pH are
   a. smoke and irradiation.
   b. baking powder and soda.
   c. salt and sugar.
   d. vinegar and citric acid.

3. Food additives widely used for many years without apparent ill effects are on the ____ list.
   a. FDA
   b. GRAS
   c. USDA
   d. Delaney

4. The foodborne illness organism often associated with small cuts and boils is
   a. *Listeria.*
   b. *Staphylococcus.*
   c. *C. botulinum.*
   d. *Salmonella.*

5. *Salmonella* bacteria are usually spread via
   a. raw meats, poultry, and eggs.
   b. pickled vegetables.
   c. home-canned vegetables.
   d. raw vegetables.

6. It is unwise to thaw meats or poultry
   a. in a microwave oven.
   b. in the refrigerator.
   c. under cool running water.
   d. at room temperature.

7. Milk that can remain on supermarket shelves, free of microbial growth, for many years has been processed by which of the following methods?
   a. Use of humectants
   b. Using antibiotics in animal feed
   c. Use of sequestrants
   d. Aseptic processing

8. Those at greatest risk for foodborne illness include
   a. pregnant women.
   b. infants and children.
   c. immunosuppressed individuals.
   d. all of these individuals.

9. Pasteurization involves the
   a. exposure of food to high temperatures for short periods to destroy harmful microorganisms.
   b. exposure of food to heat to inactivate enzymes that cause undesirable effects in foods during storage.
   c. fortification of foods with vitamins A and D.
   d. use of irradiation to destroy certain pathogens in foods.

10. Food can be kept for long periods by adding salt or sugar because these substances
    a. make the food too acidic for spoilage to occur.
    b. bind to water, thereby making it unavailable to the microorganisms.
    c. effectively kill microorganisms.
    d. dissolve the cell walls in plant foods.

Answer Key: 1. a (LO 17.4), 2. d (LO 17.2), 3. b (LO 17.4), 4. b (LO 17.1), 5. a (LO 17.1), 6. d (LO 17.8), 7. d (LO 17.2), 8. d (LO 17.3), 9. a (LO 17.2), 10. b (LO 17.4)

Study Questions (Numbers refer to Learning Outcomes)

1. What three trends in food purchasing and production have led to a greater number of cases of foodborne illness? (**LO 17.1**)

2. Which types of foods are most likely to be involved in foodborne illness? Why are they targets for contamination? (**LO 17.2**)

3. Identify three major classes of microorganisms responsible for foodborne illness. (**LO 17.3**)

4. Define the term *food additive* and give examples of four intentional food additives. What are their specific functions in foods? What is their relationship to the GRAS list? (**LO 17.4**)

5. Describe the federal process that governs the use of food additives, including the Delaney Clause.(**LO 17.4**)

6. Put into perspective the benefits and risks of using additives in food. Point out an easy way to reduce the consumption of food additives.

Do you think this is worth the effort in terms of maintaining health? Why or why not? (**LO 17.4**)

7. Name some substances that occur naturally in foods but may cause illness. (**LO 17.5**)

8. Describe four recommendations for reducing the risk of ill effects from environmental contaminants. (**LO 17.6**)

9. Describe some of the advances in agricultural science that are positively affecting our food supply. (**LO 17.7**)

10. List four techniques other than thorough cooking that are important in preventing foodborne illness. (**LO 17.8**)

What the Dietitian Chose

Exposure to environmental stressors may cause plants to produce more phytochemicals that have a positive impact on human health. However, current research is insufficient to recommend organic over conventional produce on the basis of nutrient content. The dietitian would choose canned and frozen fruits and vegetables, which have greater nutrient content compared to fresh or organic products that are harvested early and often purchased several days or weeks later. The ideal situation would be to grow our own produce or purchase it at a farmer's market, allowing us to consume it very close to harvest. Recall from Section 8.1, maximal nutrient content coincides with the peak of ripeness. Thus, produce will have its highest vitamin and phytochemical content if it is harvested at peak ripeness.

Products labeled organic must comply with standards regarding use of fertilizers, pesticides, hormones, antibiotics, genetic engineering, and irradiation. Organic food producers may use natural preservatives. Buying fresh or frozen produce and preparing meals at home are the best ways to avoid excessive preservative intake.

Organic produce is no less likely to be contaminated with microorganisms than conventionally grown foods. Although manure is used as organic fertilizer, statistics show similar levels of foodborne illness organisms from either type of food. It is still important to follow food-safety advice, such as washing all fresh produce before eating it.

▲ Exposure to pesticides is lower from organic foods although conventional foods remain well below the USDA pesticide residue limits. © Ingram Publishing

CASE STUDY SOLUTION   Preventing Foodborne Illness at Gatherings

1. Nicole likely contracted *Clostridium perfringens,* based on the fact that she had diarrhea but did not vomit and the symptoms occurred about 8 hours after consuming the contaminated food (review Table 17-3).

2. Spores of *Clostridium perfringens* are typically present in meat. Thorough cooking will kill any of the live bacteria present, but the product may still contain spores. These can later develop into bacteria if the food is kept in a warm setting for a few hours. The beef in the empanadas was likely the bearer of the spores, and they likely germinated and produced a toxin as the beef sat in the car and on the buffet table.

3. Consuming food at large gatherings is risky for several reasons. First, foods for these events are typically cooked ahead of time and not consumed right away. Unfortunately, the foods end up remaining in the "danger zone" between 40 and 140 °F. Hot foods should be kept hot and cold foods cold, but proper refrigeration or heating equipment is not always available at these events. In addition, many people handle foods and serving utensils at large gatherings. It is important for everyone handling food or serving utensils to thoroughly wash their hands before and after handling food and to avoid coughing or sneezing over foods. Also, when returning to the buffet table, always use a clean plate to avoid cross-contamination. Finally, the focus at these events is usually on having fun and socializing and not on food safety.

4. The main precaution that was ignored was keeping the food out of the "danger zone." Overall, it is risky to leave perishable items such as meat, fish, poultry, eggs, and dairy products at room temperature for more than 1 to 2 hours.

5. Ideally, the cooked food should have remained at room temperature for no longer than 1 hour. Thus, soon after Nicole and her husband took it out of the oven, it should have been separated into a few smaller pans to speed cooling and then refrigerated because they knew that it was not going to be served within 1 to 2 hours. Before leaving, they could have recombined the dish into one clean pan. Once they arrived at the party, the dish should have been refrigerated again and then thoroughly reheated when it was time to eat.

Further Readings

1. Academy of Nutrition and Dietetics: Position of the Academy of Nutrition and Dietetics: Food and water safety. *Journal of the Academy of Nutrition and Dietetics* 114:1819, 2014. http://www.eatrightpro.org/resource/practice/position-and-practice-papers/position-papers/food-and-water-safety

2. Committee on Obstetric Practice: Moderate caffeine consumption during pregnancy. Committee Opinion No. 462. American College of Obstetricians and Gynecologists. *Obstetrics and Gynecology* 116:467, 2010.

3. Dennett C: Processed foods: Problem or panacea? *Today's Dietitian* 17(8):40, 2015.

4. Geiger S: Eating seafood sustainably. *Today's Dietitian* 14(6):38, 2012.

5. Glover L: How to avoid foodborne illness. *U.S. News & World Report,* August 2015. http://health.usnews.com/health-news/health-wellness/articles/2015/08/26/how-to-avoid-foodborne-illness

6. Institute of Medicine Report: *Strategies to reduce sodium intake in the United States.* Consensus Report. April 20, 2010. www.iom.edu/Reports/2010/Strategies-to-Reduce-Sodium-Intake-in-the-United-states.aspx

7. Kosa KM and others: Most Americans are not prepared to ensure food safety during power outages and other emergencies. *Food Protection Trends* 31:428, 2011.

8. McCarty CL: Notes from the field: Large outbreak of botulism associated with a church potluck meal—Ohio, 2015. *CDC Morbidity and Mortality Weekly Report* 64(29):802, 2015.

9. Novella S: The clean eating delusion. *Science-Based Medicine,* January 20, 2016. https://www.sciencebasedmedicine.org/the-clean-eating-delusion/

10. Oken E and others: Which fish should I eat? Perspectives influencing fish consumption choices. *Environmental Health Perspectives* 120:790, 2012.

11. Scallan E and others: Foodborne illness acquired in the United States—Major pathogens. *Emerging Infectious Diseases* 17:7, 2011.

12. Schardt D: Safe at home: How to keep your kitchen from making you sick. *Nutrition Action Healthletter,* p. 3, November 2011.

13. Schardt D: Going organic: What's the payoff? *Nutrition Action Healthletter,* p. 1, October 2012.

14. Setiawan VW: Association of coffee intake with reduced incidence of liver cancer and death from chronic liver disease in the US Multiethnic Cohort. *Gastroenterology* 148(1):118, 2015.

15. Smith-Spangler C and others: Are organic foods safer or healthier than conventional alternatives?: A systematic review. *Annals of Internal Medicine* 157:348, 2012.

16. US Centers for Disease Control and Prevention: *CDC estimates of foodborne illness in the United States.* January 8, 2014. www.cdc.gov/foodborneburden. Accessed January 16, 2015.

17. US Government Accountability Office Report to Congressional Requesters. *FDA should strengthen its oversight of food ingredients determined to be generally recognized as safe (GRAS).* GAO-10-246: February 3, 2010. Publicly released: March 5, 2010.

To get the most out of your study of nutrition, go to McGraw-Hill's online resources: Connect www.mcgrawhillconnect.com, where you will find NutritionCalc Plus, LearnSmart, and many other dynamic tools.

Rate Your Plate

I. Take a Closer Look at Food Additives

Evaluate a food label of a convenience food item (e.g., frozen entrée, ready-to-eat baked good) either in the supermarket or one you have available.

1. Write out the list of ingredients.

2. Identify the ingredients that you think may be food additives.

3. Based on the information available in this chapter, what are the functions of these food additives?

4. How might this food product differ without these ingredients?

© Digital Vision/Getty Images

II. Take a Closer Look at Organic Foods

Visit one or more supermarkets to see what organic foods are available. Note your findings in the chart.

	Available	Not Available
Meat		
Poultry		
Milk		
Eggs		
Cheese		
Lettuce		
Apples		
Bananas		
Broccoli		
Other produce		
Breakfast cereal		
Snack chips		
Crackers		
Bread		
Pasta		

© Harrison Eastwood/Getty Images

Do you currently purchase organic foods? Why or why not?

© Getty Images

Student Learning Outcomes

18.1 Describe how nutrition affects fertility.

18.2 Summarize the physiological changes of pregnancy, how they affect the nutrient requirements of a woman, and list nutrients that may need to be supplemented during pregnancy.

18.3 Define "success" in terms of positive health outcomes during pregnancy and identify lifestyle factors that promote a successful pregnancy for both the mother and the infant.

18.4 Specify optimal ranges of weight gain during pregnancy for women with low, healthy, or high prepregnancy BMI.

18.5 Outline guidelines for exercise during pregnancy.

Chapter 18
Nutrition During Pregnancy and Breastfeeding

What Would You Choose?

As a pregnant vegetarian, which of the following meals would you choose as the best source of iron?

a Spinach salad with hard-boiled eggs and a whole-wheat roll

b Lean hamburger with cheese, lettuce, and tomato, and roasted red potatoes

c Bean and cheese soft taco and stewed tomatoes

d Kellogg's® Smart Start® cereal, fat-free milk, and orange juice

Think about your choice as you read Chapter 18, then see What the Dietitian Chose at the end of the chapter.

The responsibility of nourishing and protecting a child is exhilarating and, at the same time, intimidating. Parents' desire to produce a healthy baby can arouse interest in nutrition and health information. They usually want to do everything possible to maximize their chances of having a healthy newborn.

Despite these intentions, the infant mortality rate in North America is higher than that seen in many other industrialized nations. In Canada, about 5 of every 1000 infants per year die before their first birthday, whereas in the United States, it is almost 6 infants. These are alarming statistics for two countries that have such a high per capita expenditure for health care compared to many other countries in the world. Comparatively, the rate of infant mortality in Sweden is less than 3 of every 1000 infants. In addition, in the United States, about 11% of pregnant women receive inadequate prenatal care.

Some aspects of fetal and newborn health are beyond our control. Still, conscious decisions about social, health, environmental, and nutritional factors during pregnancy significantly affect the baby's future. Choosing to breastfeed the infant adds further benefits. Let us examine how eating well during pregnancy and breastfeeding can help a baby to have a healthy start in life.

18.6 Describe the discomforts and complications of pregnancy that may be reduced by improving dietary patterns.

18.7 Summarize the physiological processes involved in breastfeeding and how breastfeeding affects the nutritional requirements of a woman.

18.8 Design an adequate, balanced meal plan for a pregnant or breastfeeding woman based on MyPlate.

18.9 List several advantages of breastfeeding for both the mother and the infant.

18.10 Relate nutritional status of the parents to the risk of birth defects in the child.

18.1 Nutrition and Fertility

"Surprise, we're pregnant!" Considering the fact that only about half of all pregnancies are planned, a positive pregnancy test can be shocking news. Even when planned, women often do not suspect they are pregnant during the first few weeks after conception. They may not seek medical attention until 2 to 3 months after conception. Without fanfare, though, the **embryo** grows and develops daily. As you will learn in this chapter, the mother's nutritional status will affect the health of her baby before and long after birth. For that reason, the health and nutrition habits of a woman who is trying to become pregnant—or has the potential to become pregnant—are vitally important.

For up to 15% of couples who are planning for pregnancy, however, that pregnancy test shows a negative result month after month. **Infertility** refers to the inability of a couple to conceive after 1 year of unprotected intercourse. There are numerous possible causes for male and female infertility, many of which are outside the couple's control. In some cases, however, nutrition and lifestyle changes can improve a couple's chances of conceiving a child.

The nutritional status of both the mother- and the father-to-be can affect the likelihood of conception (see Further Reading 17). Some of the nutritional factors discussed in this chapter will affect the hormone levels involved in reproduction. Others directly affect the viability of the egg or the sperm. Thus far, research clearly supports a link between body fat and fertility, and some evidence points to roles of certain dietary fats, carbohydrates, antioxidant nutrients, B vitamins, zinc, and iron.

ENERGY BALANCE

Recall from Section 7.1 that energy balance is the relationship between energy in and energy out. **Positive energy balance** describes a situation in which the amount of calories consumed exceeds the amount of calories required to support basic body processes and physical activity. Sustained over time, positive energy balance leads to gains in both lean mass and adipose tissue. **Negative energy balance** occurs when calorie intake falls short of calorie needs. Prolonged negative energy balance leads to loss of both lean and adipose tissue. At either extreme, prolonged energy imbalance can impair fertility.

It is important to note that adipose tissue serves as more than just a storage depot for energy; it also produces estrogen and other hormones and cellular signaling molecules with widespread effects. For example, leptin, a hormone produced primarily by adipose tissue, affects appetite, metabolic rate, immune function, growth, and reproduction.

Reproductive function is costly in terms of energy. Synthesis of reproductive hormones, maintenance of normal menstrual cycles, pregnancy, and breastfeeding require calories. With negative energy balance, little energy is available to maintain normal reproductive function. Consequently, many underweight women experience **amenorrhea,** a sign of impaired ovulation. Some causes of low energy availability are undernutrition that stems from poverty (see Section 16.5), an eating disorder (see Section 15.2), or high levels of athletic training (see Section 14.4). During World War II, for example, a famine in Holland drastically cut the calorie intake of women to about 1000 kcal per day. Many women became amenorrheic, and birth rates declined by about 50% during that time period. Studies in female athletes indicate that energy intake of at least 30 kcal per kilogram of lean mass is needed for normal reproductive function among women. For men, low body fat can decrease sex drive and sperm count.

On the opposite end of the spectrum, prolonged positive energy balance also decreases fertility. The extra adipose tissue affects the availability of reproductive hormones and induces insulin resistance. For women, these endocrine changes impair the success of ovulation and implantation. In fact, excess body fat is thought to cause about 25% of problems with ovulation that lead to infertility. Among men, excess body fat increases estrogen levels and decreases testosterone. Also, extra fat tissue increases the temperature of the testicular area. The changes in hormones and temperature result in lower sperm production.

embryo In humans, the developing offspring in utero from about the beginning of the third week to the end of the eighth week after conception.

infertility Inability of a couple to conceive after 1 year of unprotected intercourse.

positive energy balance The state in which energy intake is greater than energy expended, generally resulting in weight gain.

negative energy balance The state in which energy intake is less than energy expended, resulting in weight loss.

amenorrhea Absence of menstrual periods in a woman of reproductive age.

Excess body fat also increases oxidative stress, which damages DNA in both the egg and the sperm. For overweight or obese adults, studies show that losing just 5% to 10% of body weight can increase the chances of conception.

HORMONAL BALANCE

As we discuss the ways energy imbalances influence fertility, it is important to mention **polycystic ovary syndrome (PCOS).** PCOS, characterized by many tiny cysts that surround the ovaries like a strand of pearls, is the leading cause of female infertility. Two main hormonal alterations are typical of PCOS: high testosterone and high insulin. All women secrete some testosterone, but women with PCOS secrete more than normal. The high levels of male hormones lead to some of the signs and symptoms of PCOS: excess hair growth on the face, acne, and a tendency to deposit fat around the waist. Insulin resistance is a common feature of the syndrome. Thus, women with PCOS are at higher risk for diabetes (see Section 4.7), high blood pressure (see Section 9.9), and cardiovascular disease (see Section 5.8). Importantly for our discussion here, women with PCOS have irregular or absent periods, difficulty becoming pregnant, and higher-than-average rates of miscarriage.

Many dietary and lifestyle changes have been studied to see how they can alter the course of PCOS. To date, evidence most clearly indicates that weight loss is important to improve metabolic and fertility issues among overweight women with PCOS. If an overweight woman with PCOS loses just 5% of her body weight, regardless of diet composition, her chances of conception improve. Daily physical activity, known to improve insulin sensitivity, is a key component of any weight management strategy (see Section 7.7).

In addition to managing body weight, the quality and quantity of carbohydrates may make a difference in controlling PCOS and improving fertility. Some experts recommend reducing carbohydrate intake to the lower end of the range recommended by the Food and Nutrition Board (about 45% of total kcal) and choosing low glycemic-index carbohydrates. For example, women with PCOS are urged to choose whole grains instead of refined grains and whole fruits and vegetables rather than juices, and to steer clear of sugar-sweetened beverages. There are claims that following a low-carbohydrate diet (less than 45% of total kcal) is useful for women with PCOS, but these claims are not well supported by research. Severely restricting carbohydrate choices could limit the intake of important nutrients, such as B vitamins.

KEY NUTRIENTS

Vitamins Routine intake of a daily multivitamin and mineral supplement has been linked to improved fertility in many studies. There are a variety of micronutrients that may contribute, but folic acid tops the list for both men and women. As you learned in Section 13.3, folate is involved in DNA synthesis and the metabolism of homocysteine. For no other cells is proper DNA synthesis so important as for the egg and sperm, which transmit genetic information from one generation to the next! Foods such as leafy green vegetables, strawberries, and orange juice are sources of natural folate. The synthetic form, folic acid, can be found in dietary supplements and fortified foods, such as ready-to-eat breakfast cereals.

The chemical reactions of metabolism produce free radicals (molecules with unpaired electrons) that can damage cell membranes and DNA. The body has some antioxidant mechanisms that limit the activity of free radicals, but when the production of free radicals exceeds the antioxidant capacity of the body, oxidative damage to cells is likely. Free radicals can damage egg and (especially) sperm cells and can affect how well a fertilized egg implants and matures. Research studies show that dietary patterns rich in antioxidant nutrients—vitamin E, vitamin C, selenium, zinc, beta-carotene, and some other plant pigments—are linked to improved fertility for both men and women. Foods of plant origin, including brightly colored fruits and vegetables, whole grains, and plant oils, are rich sources of antioxidant nutrients.

Minerals Iron and zinc are two minerals that have been linked to fertility. Zinc appears to be especially important for male fertility. Not only is it involved as a cofactor in antioxidant reactions that could protect sperm from oxidative damage, but zinc is also required for

▲ Several studies show a link between a low glycemic-index eating pattern and improved fertility for women with PCOS. © McGraw-Hill Education/Jill Braaten, photographer

polycystic ovary syndrome (PCOS) A condition of hormonal imbalance (e.g., elevated testosterone and insulin) in a woman that can lead to infertility, weight gain in the abdominal region, excessive growth of body hair, and acne.

normal sexual maturation (recall the photo of the zinc-deficient teenager in Figure 10-15) and production of sperm and reproductive hormones. Men with poor zinc status may have poor sperm quality (e.g., low sperm production, impaired sperm motility, and/or damaged DNA). Studies have shown that zinc supplements can improve sperm quality in men who are deficient in zinc.

For women, iron and zinc are needed for normal ovulation. Data from a large observational study of nurses showed that use of iron supplements before conception was linked to improved ovulatory function and therefore better fertility. Interestingly, in this study, higher intakes of nonheme iron (from plant sources) were specifically related to improved fertility (see Ask the RDN).

When trying to conceive, should you switch to decaf? There has been some concern that caffeine could decrease fertility, but the evidence is mixed. In some studies, intake of more than 4 cups of coffee (about 500 mg caffeine) has been linked to decreased fertility, but most studies show no clear link between moderate caffeine intake and fertility.

Dietary Fat As recommended for the general population of healthy adults, men and women who are trying to conceive should try to limit sources of saturated and *trans* fats. For women, a diet rich in saturated and *trans* fat promotes insulin resistance and impairs ovulation. For men, high intakes of saturated and *trans* fat are linked to poor sperm quality. Instead of consuming the typical American fare of pizza and fast foods, men and women should emphasize plant oils and fish oils, which provide more unsaturated fats. Among men experiencing infertility, boosting intakes of omega-3 fatty acids, the type of polyunsaturated fatty acids found in fish oils and walnuts, can improve sperm quality.

ALCOHOL

While trying to conceive, it is safest to avoid alcohol. Most studies show that higher intakes of alcohol (i.e., more than one or two drinks per day) are related to lower rates of conception. Alcohol can decrease levels of estrogen and testosterone and can therefore disrupt the normal cycles of ovulation and sperm production. In Section 18.8, you will learn about the devastating effects of alcohol on the developing babies in utero. Given the fact that many women do not realize they are pregnant until several weeks after conception, it is best to avoid alcohol while trying to conceive.

ASK THE RDN   The Fertility diet

Dear RDN: My husband and I have been trying to conceive for 2 years. We have an appointment to see a fertility specialist, but I recently found The Fertility Diet. Is this a good resource for couples who are trying to get pregnant?

The Fertility Diet, written in 2007 by scientists from the Harvard School of Public Health, sums up findings from the Nurses' Health Study II regarding relationships between diet, lifestyle, and pregnancy success. Based on extensive data collected from 18,555 women who were trying to conceive during the study, the authors boiled down their conclusions into 10 recommendations:

1. Avoid *trans* fats.
2. Use more unsaturated fats.
3. Eat more vegetable protein.
4. Choose "low and slow" carbohydrates (e.g., whole grains, foods with low glycemic index).
5. Temporarily trade in low-fat and fat-free dairy products for full-fat versions.
6. Use a daily multivitamin and mineral supplement that contains folic acid.
7. Ensure adequate iron intake from sources other than red meats.
8. Choose water for hydration; coffee, tea, and alcohol can be used in moderation, but sugar-sweetened beverages should be avoided.
9. Lose 5% to 10% of body weight (if overweight).
10. Incorporate moderate exercise.

With the exception of tip #5, all of these recommendations are in line with current dietary advice for Americans from major health authorities, including the 2015–2020 Dietary Guidelines.

For women who are trying to get pregnant, in particular, these recommendations are in agreement with the latest research on diet and fertility covered in this section.

What about #5? Grab an ice cream scoop? Public health messages have been telling us to choose low-fat and fat-free dairy foods for decades. Why might women seeking to become pregnant benefit from drinking whole milk and eating ice cream? The authors hypothesize that dairy fat, which does contain many hormones from lactating and sometimes pregnant cows, may influence the woman's hormone levels in a way that improves fertility. This is an intriguing hypothesis, but one that certainly warrants further investigation. Notably, in their chapter on dairy choices, the authors also point out that dairy products may not be the best way for Americans to obtain calcium, in general. Instead, they advocate plant sources of calcium, dietary supplements, and a daily dose of sunshine to support bone health.

In addition to the tips offered in *The Fertility Diet,* I would also encourage you to find ways to include at least five servings per day of fruits and vegetables. These foods have much to offer in terms of the micronutrients that are needed to support a healthy pregnancy, and can also help with blood glucose control and weight management.

Research demonstrates that insulin resistance underlies many cases of infertility. Dietary changes that improve insulin sensitivity—losing excess body fat, choosing healthy fats, avoiding dramatic rises and falls in blood sugar throughout the day—can optimize a woman's chances of ovulating normally and becoming pregnant. Furthermore, adequate intake of several key micronutrients—iron and folic acid—are vital for growth and development of the fetus.

Keep in mind that the Nurses' Health Study (like most research on diet and fertility) is an observational study. Even though these dietary patterns are associated with improved fertility, they have not been tested as part of a controlled experiment. Also, the authors provide the rationale for these dietary and lifestyle strategies to counter ovulatory infertility only; dietary changes are less likely to help women with infertility due to structural abnormalities or other health conditions. In other words, neither *The Fertility Diet* nor any other diet or lifestyle change can guarantee a healthy pregnancy; however, this chapter does offer the best of what we know to enhance your chances of success.

In sum, *The Fertility Diet* provides excellent nutrition advice, backed by the Nurses' Health Study and many other research studies, that can be adopted by the whole family. The authors have a knack for explaining complex scientific concepts in terms nonscientists can understand. Furthermore, the book includes practical advice, meal plans, and recipes to help women translate science into food choices.

Wishing you pink or blue,

Angela Collene, MS, RDN, LD (author)

✓ CONCEPT CHECK 18.1

1. How is energy balance related to fertility?
2. What is polycystic ovary syndrome? What hormonal changes are involved in PCOS, and how do they affect fertility?
3. List three nutrients that have been linked to fertility.

18.2 Prenatal Growth and Development

The length of a normal pregnancy is 38 to 42 weeks, measured from the first day of the woman's last menstrual period. For purposes of discussion, the duration of pregnancy is commonly divided into three periods, called **trimesters.** For 8 weeks after conception, a human embryo develops from a fertilized **ovum** into a **fetus.**

Until birth, the mother nourishes the fetus via a **placenta,** an organ that forms in her uterus to accommodate the growth and development of the fetus (Fig. 18-1). The role of the placenta is to exchange nutrients, oxygen, and other gases between the mother and fetus and

trimesters Three 13- to 14-week periods into which the normal pregnancy (on average, 40 weeks) is divided somewhat arbitrarily for purposes of discussion and analysis. Development of the offspring, however, is continuous throughout pregnancy, with no specific physiological markers demarcating the transition from one trimester to the next.

ovum The egg cell from which a fetus eventually develops if the egg is fertilized by a sperm cell.

fetus The developing life form from about the beginning of the ninth week after conception until birth.

placenta An organ that forms in the uterus in pregnant women. Through this organ, oxygen and nutrients from the mother's blood are transferred to the fetus, and fetal wastes are removed. The placenta also releases hormones that maintain the state of pregnancy.

FIGURE 18-1 ▶ The fetus in relationship to the placenta. The placenta is the organ through which nourishment flows to the fetus.

- Amniotic fluid
- Umbilical cord (fetal circulation)
- Placenta (supplies nutrients and oxygen from maternal circulation)
- Uterus

to eliminate waste products. This occurs through a network of capillaries that bring the fetal blood close to the maternal blood supply, but the two blood supplies do not mix.

EARLY GROWTH—THE FIRST TRIMESTER IS A CRITICAL TIME

zygote The fertilized ovum; the cell resulting from the union of an egg cell (ovum) and sperm until it divides.

In the formation of the human organism, egg and sperm unite to produce the **zygote** (Fig. 18-2). From this point, the reproductive process occurs rapidly:

- Within 30 hours: zygote divides in half to form two cells.
- Within 4 days: cell number climbs to 128 cells.
- At 14 days: the group of cells is called an embryo.
- Within 35 days: heart is beating, embryo is 1/30 of an inch (8 millimeters) long, eyes and limb buds are clearly visible.
- At 8 weeks: the embryo is known as a fetus.
- At 13 weeks (end of first trimester): most organs are formed, and the fetus can move.

Growth begins in the first trimester with a rapid increase in cell number. This type of growth dominates embryonic and early fetal development. The newly formed cells then begin to grow larger. Further growth is a mix of increases in cell number and cell size. By the end of 13 weeks—the first trimester—most organs are formed and the fetus can move (see Fig. 18-2).

spontaneous abortion Cessation of pregnancy and expulsion of the embryo or nonviable fetus prior to 20 weeks' gestation. This is the result of natural causes, such as a genetic defect or developmental problem; also called *miscarriage*.

As the embryo or fetus develops, nutritional deficiencies, toxicities, and other harmful environmental exposures have the potential to damage organ systems. For example, adverse reactions to medications, high intakes of vitamin A, exposure to radiation, or trauma can alter or arrest the current phase of fetal development, and the effects may last a lifetime (review Fig. 18-2). The most critical time for these potential problems is during the first trimester. Most **spontaneous abortions**—premature terminations of pregnancy that occur naturally—happen at this time. About one-half or more pregnancies end in this way, often so early that a woman does not even realize she was pregnant. (An additional 15% to 20% are lost before normal delivery.) Early spontaneous abortions usually result from a genetic defect or fatal error in fetal development. Smoking (any form of nicotine or marijuana), alcohol abuse, use of aspirin and NSAIDs, and illicit drug use raise the risk for spontaneous abortion.

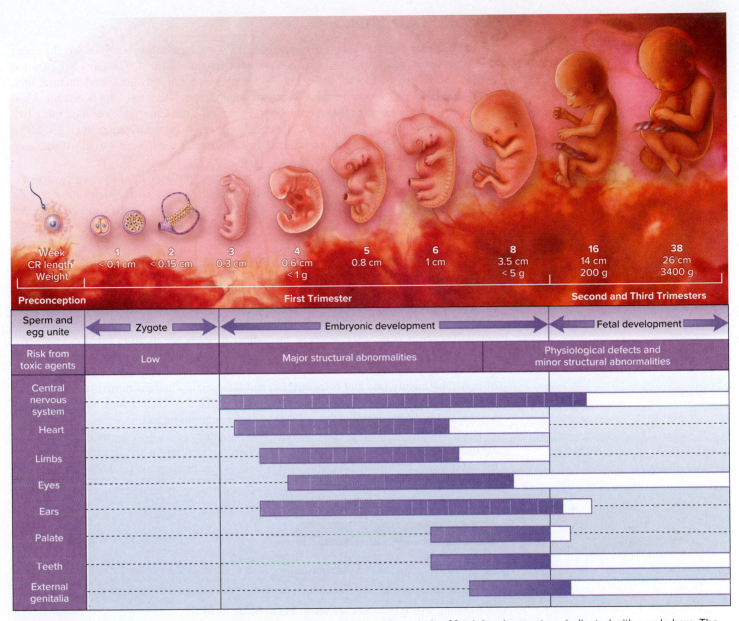

Week	1	2	3	4	5	6	8	16	38
CR length*	< 0.1 cm	< 0.15 cm	0.3 cm	0.6 cm	0.8 cm	1 cm	3.5 cm	14 cm	26 cm
Weight				< 1 g			< 5 g	200 g	3400 g

	Preconception	First Trimester	Second and Third Trimesters
Sperm and egg unite	← Zygote →	← Embryonic development →	← Fetal development →
Risk from toxic agents	Low	Major structural abnormalities	Physiological defects and minor structural abnormalities
Central nervous system			
Heart			
Limbs			
Eyes			
Ears			
Palate			
Teeth			
External genitalia			

FIGURE 18-2 ▲ Harmful effects of toxic agents during pregnancy. Vulnerable periods of fetal development are indicated with purple bars. The purple shading indicates the time of greatest risk to the organ. The most serious damage to the fetus from exposure to toxins is likely to occur during the first 8 weeks after conception, two-thirds of the way through the first trimester. As the white bars in the chart show, however, damage to vital parts of the body—including the eyes, brain, and genitals—can also occur during the later months of pregnancy.

A woman should avoid substances that may harm the developing fetus, especially during the first trimester. This holds true, as well, for the time when a woman is trying to become pregnant. As previously mentioned, she is unlikely to be aware of her pregnancy for at least a few weeks. In addition, the fetus develops so rapidly during the first trimester that, if an essential nutrient is not available, the fetus may be affected even before evidence of the nutrient deficiency appears in the mother.

For this reason, the *quality*—rather than the *quantity*—of the woman's nutritional intake is most important during the first trimester. In other words, the mother should consume the same amount of calories as she did before she became pregnant, but she should focus on choosing more nutrient-dense foods. Although some women lose their appetite and feel nauseated during the first trimester, they should be careful to meet nutrient needs as much as possible.

gestation The period of intrauterine development of offspring, from conception to birth; in humans, normal gestation is 38 to 42 weeks.

SECOND TRIMESTER

By the beginning of the second trimester (i.e., 13 weeks' **gestation**), a fetus weighs about 1 ounce. Arms, hands, fingers, legs, feet, and toes are fully formed. The fetus has ears and begins to form tooth sockets in its jawbone. Organs continue to grow and mature, and, with a stethoscope or Doppler instrument, physicians can detect the fetal heartbeat. Most bones are distinctly evident through the body. Eventually, the fetus begins to look more like an infant. It may suck its thumb and kick strongly enough to be felt by the mother. As shown in Figure 18-2, the fetus can still be affected by exposure to toxins, but not to the degree seen in the first trimester.

During the second trimester, the mother's breast weight typically increases by approximately 30% due to the development of milk-producing cells and the deposition of 2 to 4 pounds of fat for **lactation.** This stored fat serves as a reservoir for the extra calories that will be needed to produce breast milk.

lactation The period of milk secretion following pregnancy; typically called *breastfeeding*.

THIRD TRIMESTER

By the beginning of the third trimester, a fetus weighs about 2 to 3 pounds. The third trimester is a crucial time for fetal growth. The fetus will double in length and increase its weight by three to four times. The fetus takes higher priority than the mother with regard to iron and will severely deplete the stores of the mother if she is not meeting her iron needs. An infant born after only about 26 weeks of gestation has a good chance of surviving if cared for in a nursery for high-risk newborns. However, the infant will not have acquired the stores of minerals (mainly iron and calcium), fat, and fat-soluble vitamins normally accumulated during the last month of gestation. This and other medical problems, such as a poor ability to suck and swallow, complicate nutritional care for preterm infants.

By full term, the fetus usually weighs 7 to 9 pounds (3 to 4 kilograms) and is about 20 inches (50 centimeters) long. Soft spots (fontanels) on top of the head indicate where the skull bones are growing together. These bones close by the time the baby reaches 12 to 18 months of age.

> ✓ **CONCEPT CHECK 18.2**
>
> 1. What is the role of the placenta?
> 2. Describe how risks for fetal malformations vary throughout pregnancy.
> 3. During which trimester are most organs being formed?
> 4. During which trimester does fetal size increase the most?

18.3 Success in Pregnancy

The goal of pregnancy is to achieve optimal health for both the baby and the mother. For the mother, a successful pregnancy is one in which her physical and emotional health is protected so that she can return to her prepregnancy health status. For the infant, two widely accepted criteria are (1) a gestation period longer than 37 weeks; and (2) a birth weight greater than 5.5 pounds (2.5 kilograms). Sufficient lung development, likely to have occurred by 37 weeks of gestation, is critical to the survival of a newborn. The longer the gestation (up to 42 weeks), the greater the ultimate birth weight and maturation state, leading to fewer medical problems and better quality of life for the infant.

As you read this chapter, you will notice frequent references to lifelong effects of maternal nutrition, physical activity, and other lifestyle practices on the child. This is called the *developmental origins of health and disease hypothesis,* or more simply, the **fetal origins hypothesis.** Emerging evidence links prenatal influences, such as famines, fasting, exposure

fetal origins hypothesis A theory that links nutritional and other environmental insults that occur during gestation to the future health of the offspring.

to alcohol, environmental pollution, and even stress to the child's risks for disease later in life (see Newsworthy Nutrition in Section 18.4). As we learn more about how environmental factors shape the ways our genes are expressed, it becomes increasingly evident that many aspects of our physical and mental health are programmed while we are yet in utero. What's more, these epigenetic changes may be passed down from generation to generation.

Overall, a successful pregnancy is the outcome of many complex gene-environment interactions. The decisions a mother and father make today can affect the health of their child for years to come. Although a mother's decisions, practices, and precautions during pregnancy contribute to the health of her fetus during all three trimesters, she cannot guarantee her fetus good health because some genetic and environmental factors are beyond her control. She and others involved in the pregnancy should not hold an unrealistic illusion of total control.

Low-birth-weight (LBW) infants are those weighing less than 5.5 pounds (2.5 kilograms) at birth. In the United States, 1 of 12 newborns is born LBW. Most commonly, LBW is associated with **preterm** birth. Medical costs during the first year of life for LBW infants are higher than those for normal-weight infants. In fact, hospital-related costs of caring for a preterm and/or LBW infant are more than $55,000 for the first year of life in the United States. For comparison, average medical costs during the first year of life for a healthy, full-term infant are around $5,000. Overall, preterm births cost employers more than $12 billion in excess health care costs each year. (See the March of Dimes website at www.marchofdimes.org for additional information on preterm birth.)

Full-term and preterm infants who weigh less than the expected weight for their duration of gestation as a result of insufficient growth are described as **small for gestational age (SGA).** Thus, a full-term infant weighing less than 5.5 pounds at birth is SGA but not preterm, whereas a preterm infant born at 30 weeks' gestation is probably LBW without being SGA. Infants who are SGA are more likely than normal-weight infants to have medical complications, including problems with blood glucose control, temperature regulation, growth, and development in the early weeks after birth.

PRENATAL CARE AND COUNSELING

Adequate prenatal care is a primary determinant of success in pregnancy. Ideally, women should receive examinations and counseling *before* becoming pregnant and continue regular prenatal care throughout pregnancy. If prenatal care is inadequate, delayed, or absent, untreated maternal nutritional deficiencies can deprive a developing fetus of needed nutrients. In addition, untreated health conditions, such as anemia, AIDS, hypertension, or diabetes, must be carefully addressed to minimize complications during pregnancy. Treating ongoing infections will also decrease risks of fetal damage. Without prenatal care, a woman is three times more likely to deliver a LBW baby—one who will be 40 times more likely to die during the first 4 weeks of life than a normal-birth-weight infant. Although the ideal time to start prenatal care is before conception, about 20% of women in the United States receive *no* prenatal care throughout the first trimester—a critical time to positively influence the outcome of pregnancy. One goal of *Healthy People 2020* is to increase by 10% the number of women who receive prenatal care beginning in the first trimester.

Food habits cannot be predicted from income, education, or lifestyle. Although some women already have good dietary habits, most can benefit from nutritional advice. All should be reminded of habits that may harm the growing fetus, such as severe dieting or fasting. By focusing on appropriate prenatal care, nutrient intake, and healthy habits, parents give their fetus—and later, their infant—the best chance of thriving. Overall, the chances of producing a healthy baby are maximized with education, an adequate diet, and early and consistent prenatal medical care.

▲ A healthy newborn. At birth, a baby usually weighs about 7.5 pounds and is 20 inches long. © Don Bayley/Getty Images

low birth weight (LBW) Referring to any infant weighing less than 2.5 kilograms (5.5 pounds) at birth; most commonly results from preterm birth.

preterm An infant born before 37 weeks of gestation; also referred to as *premature*.

small for gestational age (SGA) Referring to infants who weigh less than the expected weight for their length of gestation. This corresponds to less than 2.5 kilograms (5.5 pounds) in a full-term newborn. A preterm infant who is also SGA will most likely develop some medical complications.

A goal of *Healthy People 2020* is to reduce low birth weight by 5% and preterm births by 10%. Currently, about 8% of live births are of low birth weight and about 12% are preterm.

▲ To ensure optimal health and rapid treatment of medical conditions that develop during pregnancy, a pregnant woman should consult with her health care provider on a regular basis. Ideally, this consultation should begin before she becomes pregnant. © Blend Images

Women with acquired immune deficiency syndrome (AIDS) may pass HIV to the fetus during pregnancy or delivery. About one in three infected newborns will develop AIDS symptoms and die within just a few years. Studies show that these odds of mother-to-child transmission can be cut significantly if the woman begins taking highly active antiretroviral therapy (HAART) and receiving routine obstetrical care. Before HAART was available, up to 45% of babies born to mothers with the AIDS virus were infected. Now, transmission is less than 2%. Thus, screening pregnant women for AIDS and providing HAART to those with AIDS are advocated by many experts. One target of the United Nations' recently released Sustainable Development Goals is to end the epidemic of AIDS by 2030.

EFFECTS OF MATERNAL AGE

The age of the mother is another factor that determines pregnancy outcome. The ideal age for pregnancy is between 20 and 35 years of age. Outside that age range—at either extreme—complications are more likely to arise. The rates of teen pregnancy have declined since 1990; still, approximately 273,000 babies are born to teen mothers in the United States each year—the highest of any industrialized country. Teen pregnancy increases risk for negative outcomes for both mother and child (Table 18-1) and costs taxpayers an estimated $9.4 billion each year.

Pregnant teens frequently exhibit a variety of risk factors that can complicate pregnancy and pose risk to the fetus (see Further Reading 13). For instance, teenagers are more likely than adult women to be underweight at the start of pregnancy and to gain too little weight during pregnancy. In addition, their bodies lack the physical maturity needed to carry a fetus safely. Even with prenatal care—and 7% of teenage mothers receive none at all—10% of children born to teenage mothers are of low birth weight and 14.5% are preterm.

Advanced maternal age also poses special risks for pregnancy. The likelihood of LBW and preterm delivery increases modestly, but progressively, with maternal age beyond 35 years. Given close monitoring, however, a woman older than 35 years has an excellent chance of producing a healthy infant.

CLOSELY SPACED AND MULTIPLE BIRTHS

Siblings born in succession to a mother with less than a year between birth and subsequent conception are more likely to be born LBW than those spaced farther apart. The risks of LBW, preterm birth, or SGA are 30% to 40% higher for infants conceived less than 6 months following a birth compared to those conceived 18 to 23 months following a birth. These poor outcomes are probably related to insufficient time to rebuild nutrient stores depleted by the previous pregnancy. Similarly, multiple births (i.e., twins) increase the risk for preterm birth.

EXPOSURE TO TOXIC CHEMICALS

Figure 18-2 depicts how and when toxic agents can harm the developing fetus. In preparation for and during pregnancy, the mother should undoubtedly eliminate alcohol, tobacco, and illicit drugs (e.g., marijuana and cocaine). During organ development, exposure to these toxic chemicals can cause malformations. The adverse effects of fetal exposure to alcohol during gestation are discussed in Section 18.8. Smoking is linked to preterm birth and appears to increase the risk of birth defects, sudden infant death, childhood cancer, and disabilities.

Illicit drug use is particularly harmful during pregnancy. Many chemicals in recreational drugs cross the placenta and affect the fetus, whose detoxification systems are immature. Marijuana, the most common recreational drug used during the reproductive years, can result in reduced blood flow to the uterus and placenta, leading to poor fetal growth. Risks of low birth weight and preterm birth are increased for infants whose mothers used marijuana during pregnancy. Use of psychoactive drugs, such as cocaine and methamphetamines, restricts fetal growth and brain development, the effects of which may plague the child for a lifetime.

TABLE 18-1 ■ **Effects of Teenage Pregnancy on Mother and Child**

For Mother	For Child
↑ Depression and other mental health problems	↓ Birth weight
↑ Use of illicit drugs and alcohol	↑ Premature birth
↑ Poverty and reliance on public assistance	↑ Infant mortality
↓ Graduation rates from high school and college	↑ Hospital admissions during childhood
↑ Single parenthood	↓ Academic performance
	↓ Nutritional status
	↑ Rates of imprisonment during adulthood

Even prescribed and common over-the-counter medications could have harmful effects on the developing fetus. Problem drugs include aspirin (especially when used chronically or heavily), hormone ointments, nose drops and related "cold" medications, rectal suppositories, weight-control pills, antidepressants, and medications prescribed for preexisting illnesses. Some herbal therapies also have the potential to damage the fetus. Lower doses and/or safer alternatives should be substituted when a woman is planning to or has become pregnant.

In addition to these toxic chemicals, health hazards in the mother's environment, including job-related hazards and exposure to X-rays, should be minimized.

FOOD SAFETY

Any foodborne illness during any stage of life is a concern. One type of foodborne illness that poses particular danger for pregnant women is caused by the bacterium *Listeria monocytogenes* (review Section 17.3). Infection with this microorganism typically causes mild flulike symptoms, such as fever, headache, and vomiting, about 7 to 30 days after exposure. However, pregnant women, newborn infants, and people with depressed immune function may suffer more severe symptoms, including spontaneous abortion and serious blood infections. In these high-risk groups, 25% of infections may be fatal. Unpasteurized milk, soft cheeses made from raw milk (e.g., brie, Camembert, feta, and blue cheeses), and some raw vegetables (e.g., cabbage and sprouts) can be sources of *Listeria* organisms, so it is especially important that pregnant women (and other people at high risk for infection) avoid these products. Experts advise consuming only pasteurized milk products and cooking meat, poultry, and seafood thoroughly to kill *Listeria* and other foodborne organisms. It is unsafe in pregnancy to eat any raw meats or other raw animal products, uncooked hot dogs, or undercooked poultry. These food safety recommendations are included in the 2015–2020 Dietary Guidelines for Americans, Appendix 14.

The USDA warns pregnant women to thoroughly cook (e.g., microwave) all ready-to-eat meats, including hot dogs and cold cuts, until they are steaming to reduce risk of *Listeria* infections.

PREPREGNANCY BMI

Women should aim to achieve a healthy body weight prior to becoming pregnant. Infants born to women who begin pregnancy substantially above or below a healthy weight are more likely to experience problems than those born to women who begin pregnancy at a normal weight. For instance, babies born to obese women are at increased risk of birth defects, death in the first few weeks after birth, and obesity in childhood. Many obese pregnant women experience high blood pressure, diabetes, and more difficult deliveries.

At the other extreme, women who begin pregnancy underweight (BMI under 18.5) are more likely to have infants who are low birth weight and premature compared to women at a normal weight. These differences may be because underweight women tend to have lighter placentas and lower nutrient stores, especially iron, than heavier women, which could negatively affect fetal growth and development. An underweight woman can improve her nutrient stores and pregnancy outcome by gaining weight before pregnancy or gaining extra weight during pregnancy.

NUTRITIONAL STATUS

Is attention to good nutrition worth the effort? Yes! Much research suggests that an adequate vitamin and mineral intake at least 8 weeks before conception and throughout pregnancy can improve outcomes of pregnancy (see Further Reading 14). Extra nutrients and calories support fetal growth and development, of course, but also undergird the synthesis of maternal tissues. Her uterus and breasts grow, the placenta develops, her total blood volume increases, the heart and kidneys work harder, and stores of body fat increase. In particular, meeting folate needs (400 micrograms of synthetic folic acid per day) helps to prevent birth defects such as neural tube defects (see Section 18.8) and decrease the risk of preterm delivery. Low intakes of calcium and iron or excessive intakes of vitamin A also are causes for concern during pregnancy.

▲ In the United States, low-income pregnant women and their children benefit from the nutritional and medical attention provided by the WIC program. © UpperCut Images/Getty Images

Although it is difficult to predict the degree to which poor nutrition will affect each pregnancy, a daily diet containing only 1000 kcal has been shown to greatly restrict fetal growth and development. Increased maternal and infant death rates seen in famine-stricken areas of Africa provide further evidence.

Genetic background can explain little of the observed differences in birth weight between developed and developing countries. Both environmental factors and nutritional factors are important. The worse the nutritional status of the mother at the beginning of pregnancy, the more valuable a healthy prenatal diet and/or use of prenatal supplements are in improving the course and outcome of her pregnancy.

NUTRITION ASSISTANCE FOR LOW-INCOME FAMILIES

Poverty impacts pregnancy in many ways. Families of low socioeconomic status tend to receive inadequate health care. A lack of education, limited access to health care, or scant financial resources may contribute to poor health practices, such as dietary patterns that fail to meet the mother's increased nutrient requirements.

Several U.S. government programs provide high-quality health care and foods to reduce infant mortality. These government-subsidized programs are designed to alleviate the negative impact of poverty, insufficient education, and inadequate nutrient intake on pregnancy outcomes. An example of such a program is the Special Supplemental Nutrition Program for Women, Infants, and Children (WIC). This program offers health assessments and vouchers for foods that supply high-quality protein, calcium, iron, and vitamins A and C to pregnant women, infants, and children (up to age 5 years) from low-income populations. The WIC program is available in all areas of the United States and has a staff trained to promote healthy behaviors during pregnancy. More than 8 million women, infants, and young children are benefiting from this program, yet many eligible pregnant women are not participating.

✓ CONCEPT CHECK 18.3

1. In one or two sentences, how would you define success in pregnancy?
2. Define the terms *preterm, low birth weight,* and *small for gestational age.*
3. How is maternal age related to the outcome of pregnancy?
4. Is attention to good nutrition during pregnancy worth the effort? Why or why not?

18.4 Increased Nutrient Needs to Support Pregnancy

Pregnancy is a time of increased nutrient requirements. There are some general principles that are true for most women with regard to increased nutrient needs. However, recognize that each expectant mom will benefit from individualized counseling tailored to her unique nutritional and health needs.

CALORIE NEEDS

To support the growth and development of the fetus, pregnant women need to increase their calorie intake. Calorie needs during the first trimester are essentially the same as for nonpregnant women. However, during the second and third trimesters, it is necessary for a pregnant woman to consume approximately 350 to 450 kcal more per day than her prepregnancy needs (the upper end of the range is needed in the third trimester).

Rather than seeing this as an opportunity to fill up on sugary desserts or fat-filled snacks, pregnant women should consume these extra calories in the form of nutrient-dense foods.

For example, throughout the day, about six whole-wheat crackers, 1 ounce of cheese, and ½ cup of fat-free milk would supply the extra calories (and also some calcium). Although she "eats for two," the pregnant woman must not double her normal calorie intake. The "eating for two" concept refers more appropriately to increased needs for several vitamins and minerals. Micronutrient needs are increased by up to 50% during pregnancy, whereas calorie needs during the second and third trimesters represent only about a 20% increase.

If a woman is physically active during her pregnancy, she may need to increase her calorie intake by even more than the estimated 350 to 450 kcal per day. Her greater body weight requires more calories for activity. Many women find that they are inactive during the later months, partly because of their increased size, so an extra 350 to 450 kcal in their daily diets is usually enough.

STAYING ACTIVE DURING PREGNANCY

Even though pregnancy is not the time to begin an intense fitness regimen, women can generally take part in most low- or moderate-intensity activities during pregnancy. In fact, the American College of Obstetrics and Gynecology recommends that pregnant women perform at least 30 minutes per day of moderate-intensity physical activity. Walking, cycling, swimming, or light aerobics for at least 150 minutes per week is generally advised. Such exercise may prevent pregnancy complications and promote an easier delivery (see Further Reading 4). Some research indicates that regular physical activity during pregnancy lowers a woman's risk of developing gestational diabetes by 50% and preeclampsia by 40%. These disorders of pregnancy are discussed further in Section 18.6. Figure 18-3 illustrates the broad range of benefits of exercise during pregnancy for both the mother and the baby. Indeed, preliminary research indicates that exercising during pregnancy could lower the risk for obesity in the child later in life.

Women who were highly active prior to pregnancy can maintain their activities as long as they remain healthy and review plans with their health care providers (see Further Reading 4). Adequate fluid intake before, during, and after physical activity is of heightened importance to regulate body temperature, because heat stress can be harmful to the developing fetus. Activities with inherent risk of falls or abdominal trauma—downhill skiing, horseback riding, and contact sports (e.g., soccer and basketball)—can potentially harm the fetus and should be avoided. In addition, pregnant women should avoid activities that

Why Exercise During Pregnancy?

Benefits for Mother	Benefits for Baby
Prevents excessive weight gain during pregnancy	**During Gestation**
Improved cardiovascular function	Decreased resting heart rate
Lower risk for gestational diabetes	Healthier placenta
Lower risk for gestational hypertension	Increased amniotic fluid
Reduced bone loss associated with pregnancy	Possible improvements in brain development
Less edema in the legs and feet	Longer gestation
Better sleep	**After Gestation**
Decreased back pain	Lower birth weight
Improved satisfaction with body image	Leaner BMI during childhood

FIGURE 18-3 ◄ Benefits of exercise during pregnancy for the mother and baby. Photo © Tanya Constantine/Blend Images LLC

require excess straining (e.g., heavy weightlifting) or exposure to extremes in air pressure (e.g., SCUBA diving).

Women with high-risk pregnancies, such as those experiencing premature labor contractions, may need to restrict physical activity. To ensure optimal health for both herself and her infant, a pregnant woman should first consult her primary care provider about physical activity and possible limitations.

OPTIMAL WEIGHT GAIN

Healthy prepregnancy weight and appropriate weight gain during pregnancy are excellent predictors of pregnancy outcome (see Further Readings 7, 10, and 11). The mother's diet should allow for approximately 2 to 4 pounds (0.9 to 1.8 kilograms) of weight gain during the first trimester and then a subsequent weight gain of 0.8 to 1 pound (0.4 to 0.5 kilogram) weekly during the second and third trimesters (Fig. 18-4). A healthy goal for total weight gain for a woman of normal weight (based on BMI; Table 18-2) averages about 25 to 35 pounds (11.5 to 16 kilograms). Women of normal prepregnancy BMI carrying twins should aim to gain within the range of 37 to 54 pounds, whereas overweight or obese women pregnant with twins should gain less (31 to 50 pounds or 25 to 42 pounds, respectively).

For women who begin pregnancy with a low BMI, the goal for total weight gain increases to 28 to 40 pounds (12.5 to 18 kilograms). The goal decreases to 15 to 25 pounds (7 to 11.5 kilograms) for overweight women. Target weight gain for obese women is 11 to 20 pounds (5 to 9 kilograms). Figure 18-4 shows why the typical recommendation begins at 25 pounds.

A weight gain of between 25 and 35 pounds for a woman starting pregnancy at normal weight has repeatedly been shown to yield optimal health for both mother and fetus if gestation lasts at least 38 weeks. The weight gain should yield a birth weight of 7.5 pounds (3.5 kilograms). Although some extra weight gain during pregnancy is usually not harmful (about 5 to 10 pounds), it can set the stage for a pattern of weight gain during the childbearing years if the mother does not return to her approximate prepregnancy weight after delivery.

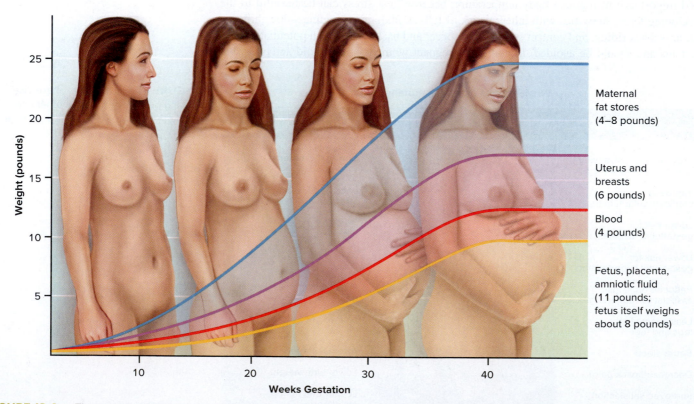

Maternal fat stores (4–8 pounds)

Uterus and breasts (6 pounds)

Blood (4 pounds)

Fetus, placenta, amniotic fluid (11 pounds; fetus itself weighs about 8 pounds)

FIGURE 18-4 ▲ The components of weight gain in pregnancy. A weight gain of 25 to 35 pounds is recommended for most women. The various components total about 25 pounds.

TABLE 18-2 ■ Recommended Weight Gain in Pregnancy Based on Prepregnancy Body Mass Index (BMI)

Prepregnancy BMI Category	Total Weight Gain*	
	(pounds)	(kilograms)
Low (BMI less than 18.5)	28 to 40	12.5 to 18
Normal (BMI 18.5 to 24.9)	25 to 35	11.5 to 16
High (BMI 25.0 to 29.9)	15 to 25	7 to 11.5
Obese (BMI greater than 30.0)	11 to 20	5 to 9

*The listed values are for pregnancies with one fetus. For women of normal BMI carrying twins, the range is 37 to 54 pounds (17 to 24.5 kilograms), or less for heavier women.

Source: Data from *Weight Gain During Pregnancy: Reexamining the Guidelines,* Copyright 2009 by the Institute of Medicine and National Research Council of the National Academies. National Academies Press, Washington, DC.

Overweight and obesity do contribute to complications during pregnancy. Excess maternal body weight increases risk for diabetes, hypertension, blood clots, and spontaneous abortions during pregnancy. After childbirth, lasting effects of excess gestational weight gain include increased BMI, central body fat distribution, and elevated blood pressure. For the baby, there is a greater chance of birth defects and macrosomia, in which the fetus grows larger than average in utero. Larger infants contribute to a greater need for surgical delivery (i.e., Cesarean sections) among overweight and obese mothers. Over the long term, excessive maternal weight gain during pregnancy has been linked to increased risk for obesity and metabolic syndrome in the child.

Gestational weight gain is a key issue in prenatal care and a concern of many mothers-to-be. Even after the 2009 release of the weight gain guidelines summarized in Table 18-2, many women report receiving *no* guidance regarding weight gain from health care providers before or during pregnancy. Considering the extensive consequences of either inadequate or excessive weight gain during gestation, health professionals should take a more active role in educating pregnant mothers about what weight changes to expect, the consequences of too little or too much weight gain, and how to make corrections if the weight gain trajectory veers off course (see Further Reading 5). Weight gain during pregnancy should generally follow the pattern in Figure 18-4. Weekly monitoring of weight changes, especially on a chart that shows expected weight gains, can help a pregnant woman to assess how much to adjust her food intake and physical activity.

Realistic information about increased calorie requirements should be provided. Pregnant women need to understand that "eating for two" is more about increasing diet quality (i.e., choosing nutrient-dense foods) than diet quantity. Furthermore, as you learned in Section 7.8, successful weight management strategies involve a behavioral component; some women need to learn skills, such as self-monitoring of weight, dietary intake, and physical activity. Online tools (e.g., USDA's SuperTracker) and smartphone apps (e.g., Sprout Pregnancy™) offer specialized tools to make self-monitoring tasks simple and social.

If a woman deviates from the desirable pattern, she should make appropriate adjustments, but weight loss during pregnancy is never advised. For example, if a woman begins to gain too much weight during her pregnancy, she should not lose weight to get back on track. Even if a woman gains 35 pounds in the first 7 months of pregnancy, she must still gain more during the last 2 months. She should, however, slow the increase in weight to parallel the rise on the prenatal weight gain chart. In other words, the sources of the unnecessary calories should be found and minimized. Alternately, if a woman has not gained the desired weight by a given point in pregnancy, she should not gain the needed weight rapidly. Instead, she should slowly gain a little more weight than the typical pattern to meet the goal by the end of the pregnancy. A registered dietitian nutritionist can help make any needed adjustments.

During pregnancy, women in North America are more likely to gain excess weight and make poor food choices than to eat too little.

▲ Appropriate weight gain during pregnancy improves outcomes for both the mother and the baby. © John Slater/Getty Images

▲ During pregnancy, the Adequate Intake for total water increases 0.3 liter (1 ¼ cups) above prepregnancy needs to 3 liters (about 12 ½ cups) per day. For breastfeeding, consume 3.8 liters (16 cups) daily. © Getty Images

Newsworthy Nutrition

Mothers' weight gain during pregnancy is linked to cognitive development of children

The Avon Longitudinal Study of Parents and Children (ALSPAC) includes 13,617 mother-offspring pairs in the United Kingdom who have been followed from pregnancy, through childbirth, and now into the offspring's young adulthood. In this analysis of gestational weight gain, children of mothers who gained less than recommended weight during pregnancy had lower School Entry Assessment scores at 4 years of age and lower performance on final examinations at 16 years of age. This study highlights the importance of adhering to the 2009 Institute of Medicine recommendations for gestational weight gain. Appropriate weight gain during pregnancy improves multiple aspects of health for both the mother and the child.

Source: Gage SH and others: Associations of maternal weight gain in pregnancy with offspring cognition in childhood and adolescence: Findings from the Avon Longitudinal Study of Parents and Children. *American Journal of Epidemiology* 177:402, 2013.

PROTEIN, CARBOHYDRATE, AND LIPID NEEDS

The RDA for protein increases by an additional 25 grams per day during pregnancy (Fig. 18-5). All women should check to make sure they are eating enough protein as well as enough calories (so that protein can be spared for synthesis of new tissue). However, many women already consume protein in excess of their needs and therefore do not need to focus specifically on increasing protein intake. Small changes are usually all that is necessary. For example, simply adding a cup of fat-free milk to the diet adds 90 nutrient-dense kilocalories and 8 grams of protein.

The RDA for carbohydrate increases to 175 grams daily, primarily to prevent ketosis. Ketone bodies, a by-product of metabolism of fat for energy, are thought to be poorly used by the fetal brain, implying possible slowing of fetal brain development. Carbohydrate intakes of most women, pregnant or not, already exceed the RDA (see Fig. 18-5).

Fat intake should increase proportionally with calorie intake during pregnancy to maintain around 20% to 35% of total calories from fat. Pregnancy is not a time for a low-fat diet, as lipids are a source of extra calories and essential fatty acids needed during pregnancy. Recommendations for the types of lipids during pregnancy are generally the same as for nonpregnant adults: saturated fat should contribute no more than 10% of total calories and *trans* fat should be avoided.

During pregnancy, it is particularly important to make sure to consume adequate essential fatty acids—linoleic acid (omega-6) and alpha-linolenic acid (omega-3). As you learned in Section 5.6, essential fatty acids cannot be synthesized in the body and must be consumed in the diet. For the developing fetus, essential fatty acids are required for growth, brain development, and eye development. Recommendations are slightly increased by pregnancy to 13 grams per day of omega-6 fatty acids and 1.4 grams per day of omega-3 fatty acids. These needs can be met by consuming 2 to 4 tablespoons per day of plant oils. Consumption within the range of 8 to 12 ounces per week of fish is recommended for meeting needs for essential fatty acids in the diet (see Further Reading 19). Some women may have difficulty incorporating the recommended amount of fish into their diets. Fish oil supplements are a good alternative, but consumers should choose brands that have been distilled to remove environmental contaminants. (See Section 18.8 for a discussion of mercury in fish.)

VITAMIN NEEDS

Vitamin needs increase from prepregnancy RDAs/AIs by up to 30% for most of the B vitamins and even greater for vitamin B-6 (45%) and folate (50%) (Fig. 18-6). Vitamin A needs only increase by 10%, so a specific focus on this vitamin is not needed. And remember, excess amounts of vitamin A are harmful to the developing fetus.

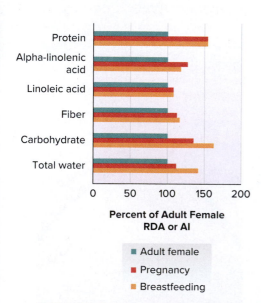

Percent of Adult Female RDA or AI

■ Adult female
■ Pregnancy
■ Breastfeeding

FIGURE 18-5 ▲ Relative macronutrient and water requirements for pregnancy and breastfeeding. Note that there is no RDA or AI for total fat; needs are based on 20% to 35% of overall energy intake.

The extra amounts of vitamin B-6 and other B vitamins (except folate) needed in the diet are easily met via wise food choices, such as a serving of a typical ready-to-eat breakfast cereal and some lean animal protein sources. Folate needs, however, often merit specific diet planning and possible vitamin supplementation. The synthesis of DNA, and therefore cell division, requires folate, so this nutrient is especially crucial during pregnancy. Ultimately, both fetal and maternal growth depend on an ample supply of folate. Red blood cell formation, which requires folate, increases during pregnancy. Serious folate-related anemia therefore can result if folate intake is inadequate. The RDA for folate increases during pregnancy to 600 micrograms DFE per day (review Section 13.3 for calculation of DFE). This is a critical goal in the nutritional care of a pregnant woman. Increasing folate intakes to meet 600 micrograms DFE per day for a pregnant woman can be achieved through dietary sources, a supplemental source of folic acid, or a combination of both. Choosing a diet rich in synthetic folic acid, such as from ready-to-eat breakfast cereals or meal replacement bars (look for approximately 50% to 100% of the Daily Value), is especially helpful in meeting folate needs. Recall from Section 13.3 that synthetic folic acid is much more easily absorbed than the various forms of folate found naturally in foods (see Further Reading 14).

Emerging evidence indicates that low maternal levels of vitamin D during pregnancy affect multiple health parameters in the offspring. About 54% of black women and 42% of white women have insufficient blood levels of the active form of vitamin D, even though many take a daily supplement containing 400 IU of vitamin D. Aside from its well-known roles in bone health and the incidence of rickets, poor vitamin D status is implicated in serious complications of pregnancy, including higher rates of diabetes and hypertension that occur during pregnancy and poor growth of the fetus (see Further Reading 22). Vitamin D's role in immune regulation is illustrated by higher rates of respiratory infections and mother-to-child transmission of HIV when its status is deficient. Because of the ability of vitamin D to modulate gene expression, vitamin D status is critically important during early fetal development through infancy. Diseases that develop later in childhood or adulthood, such as type 1 diabetes, multiple sclerosis, asthma, schizophrenia, and certain types of cancer, are associated with low vitamin D status during gestation. The RDA for pregnant women is 15 micrograms (600 IU) of vitamin D daily (the same as for nonpregnant women), but many experts advocate increasing this recommendation to 25 micrograms (1000 IU) or more (see Further Reading 6). Currently, there is no recommendation for universal vitamin D screening or supplementation, but the American College of Obstetricians and Gynecologists advises that for deficient individuals, 1000 to 2000 IU per day is a safe level of supplemental vitamin D during pregnancy.

MINERAL NEEDS

Mineral needs generally increase during pregnancy, especially the requirements for iodine, iron, and zinc (Fig. 18-7; see Further Reading 9). (Calcium needs do not increase but still may deserve special attention because many women find it difficult to meet their calcium needs in general.)

Pregnant women need extra iodine (RDA of 220 micrograms per day) to support thyroid hormone synthesis (for the mother and the developing fetus) and fetal brain development. If a mother is deficient in iodine during pregnancy, she may develop a goiter (see Section 12.8), and her child may suffer from a devastating birth defect called **congenital hypothyroidism** (formerly called *cretinism*). Section 18.8 provides further information on this and other nutrition-related birth defects. Typical iodine intakes are plentiful if the woman uses iodized salt.

The extra iron (RDA of 27 milligrams per day) is needed to synthesize a greater amount of hemoglobin during pregnancy and to provide iron stores for the fetus. About 2% of women begin pregnancy with clinically diagnosed iron-deficiency anemia, but an estimated one-third of pregnant women have poor iron stores, so heavy demands for iron during pregnancy cannot be met. The consequences of iron-deficiency anemia—especially during the first trimester—can be severe. Negative outcomes include preterm delivery, LBW infants, and increased risk for fetal death in the first weeks after birth.

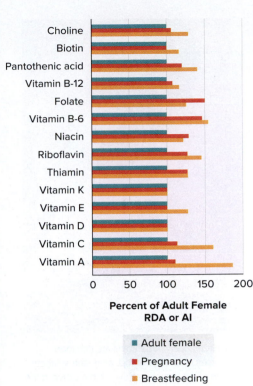

FIGURE 18-6 ▲ Relative vitamin requirements for pregnancy and breastfeeding.

congenital hypothyroidism A birth defect that impairs thyroid hormone synthesis. If untreated, this can lead to mental retardation and stunting of growth.

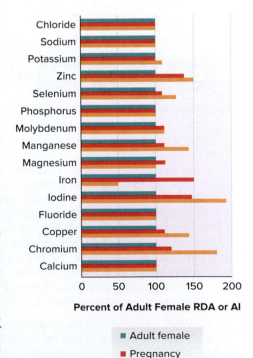

FIGURE 18-7 ▲ Relative mineral requirements for pregnancy and breastfeeding.

▲ Green, leafy vegetables are rich food sources of folate, but folic acid—the synthetic form of the vitamin—is even more active in the body than the natural form. *Healthy People 2020* includes a goal of increasing by 10% the proportion of women of childbearing potential who consume at least 400 micrograms of folic acid per day. Currently, about 23% of women of childbearing age consume adequate folic acid from fortified foods or dietary supplements. © Brand X Pictures/Jupiterimages

Women often need a supplemental source of iron, especially if they do not consume iron-fortified foods, such as highly fortified breakfast cereals containing close to 100% of the Daily Value for iron (18 milligrams). The American College of Obstetricians and Gynecologists recommends screening for iron deficiency for all pregnant women and provision of iron supplements for women who are deficient. In addition, most prenatal supplements contain iron. A potential pitfall is that iron supplements can decrease appetite and can cause nausea and constipation. To alleviate these problems, it may be helpful to take these supplements between meals or just before going to bed. Milk, coffee, or tea should not be consumed with an iron supplement because these beverages have compounds that interfere with iron absorption. Eating foods rich in vitamin C along with nonheme iron-containing foods and iron supplements helps increase iron absorption from those sources. Pregnant women who are not anemic may wait until the second trimester, when pregnancy-related nausea generally lessens, to start prenatal supplements if gastrointestinal side effects are a problem.

The RDA for zinc increases from 8 to 11 milligrams per day during pregnancy. Zinc is involved in many enzyme functions and protein synthesis. Zinc deficiency during pregnancy has been linked to preterm and LBW births. The zinc intakes of pregnant women in the United States are generally adequate, but low-income women and those who follow vegan or vegetarian diets are more susceptible to poor zinc status. Also, because iron and zinc compete for absorption, high levels of iron supplementation during pregnancy may impair zinc absorption. Incorporating lean animal proteins or a fortified ready-to-eat breakfast cereal in the diet is a good way to obtain enough extra zinc during pregnancy.

USE OF PRENATAL VITAMIN AND MINERAL SUPPLEMENTS

With the exceptions of folate, iron, and vitamin D, the vitamin and mineral intakes of pregnant women in developed countries are generally adequate (see Further Reading 2). Research evidence supports routine supplementation with folic acid and iron during pregnancy. Beyond these two nutrients, some studies indicate that use of a multivitamin and mineral supplement is advantageous for reducing the number of LBW and SGA births. More research is needed to know if prenatal supplements are effective for reducing many other

---

CASE STUDY EATING FOR TWO

Lily and her husband have just found out that Lily is pregnant with their first child. She is 25 years old, weighs 135 pounds, and is 67 inches tall. Lily has been reading everything she can find on pregnancy because she knows that her health is important to the success of her pregnancy.

Lily knows she should avoid alcohol, especially because alcohol is potentially toxic to the growing fetus. Lily is not a smoker, does not take any medications, and limits her coffee intake to 4 cups a day and soft drink intake to 3 colas per day. Based on her reading, she has decided to breastfeed her infant and has already inquired about childbirth classes. She has modified her diet to include some extra protein, along with more fruits and vegetables. She has also started taking an over-the-counter vitamin and mineral supplement. Lily has always kept in good shape, and she is admittedly worried about gaining too much weight during pregnancy. Recently, she started a running program 5 days a week, and she plans to continue running throughout her pregnancy.

Answer the following questions, and check your responses at the end of this chapter.

© Hill Street Studios/Blend Images LLC

1. What recommendations do you have regarding Lily's use of dietary supplements?
2. What is Lily doing to prevent neural tube defects? What else could she do?
3. What recommendations would you make regarding Lily's caffeine consumption?
4. Should Lily include fish as a source of protein in her diet? Why or why not?
5. Constipation is a common complaint during pregnancy. What suggestions do you have to help Lily avoid this health concern?
6. What information would you share with Lily about appropriate weight gain during pregnancy?

pregnancy complications. To date, there is not enough evidence to recommend prenatal multivitamin and mineral supplements for all pregnant women, but they are prescribed routinely by most health care providers. Some supplements formulated for pregnancy are sold over the counter, while others are dispensed by prescription because of the high synthetic folic acid content (1000 micrograms), which could pose problems for others, such as older people (see Chapter 16). These supplements are high in iron (27 milligrams per pill). There is no evidence that use of such supplements causes significant health problems in pregnancy, with the possible exception of combined amounts of supplementary and dietary vitamin A (see Section 18.8).

Instances when prenatal supplements may especially contribute to a successful pregnancy are those involving women living in poverty, teenagers, women with an inadequate diet, women carrying multiple fetuses, women who smoke or use alcohol or illegal drugs, and vegans. In other cases, healthy diets can provide the needed nutrients. When choosing a multivitamin, rely on brands that display the USP symbol on their label, signifying that the supplement meets the content, quality, purity, and safety standards of the United States Pharmacopeial Convention (see Section 8.5). Of course, avoid megadoses of any nutrient. Skip supplements containing herbs, enzymes, and amino acids. Many of these ingredients have not been evaluated for safety during pregnancy or breastfeeding and may be toxic to the fetus. Furthermore, discard supplements that are past the expiration date, as some ingredients lose potency over time.

✓ CONCEPT CHECK 18.4

1. Patrice required 2200 kcal per day before she became pregnant. How many kilocalories will she need each day during her first, second, and third trimesters?

2. What is optimal weight gain during pregnancy for a woman who begins pregnancy at a healthy BMI? How does this differ for a woman who begins pregnancy underweight? Overweight? Obese?

3. List several nutrients that may need to be supplemented in the diet of a pregnant woman and the reason for each.

18.5 Eating Patterns for Pregnant Women

One dietary approach to support a successful pregnancy is based on MyPlate. For an active 24-year-old woman, about 2200 kcal is recommended during the first trimester (the same as recommended for such a woman when not pregnant). The plan should include:

- 3 cups of calcium-rich foods from the dairy group. Specifically, choices from the dairy group should include low-fat or fat-free versions of milk, yogurt, and cheese. These foods are good sources of protein, calcium, and vitamin D. For those who cannot tolerate dairy products, soymilk, other dairy alternatives, and calcium-fortified foods can be useful to meet nutrient needs.
- 6 ounce-equivalents from the protein group. Foods from the protein group help to provide the extra iron and zinc needed during pregnancy. Within the protein foods group, most people would benefit from selecting plant-based sources more often.
- 3 cups from the vegetables group. One cup of vegetables should be a green vegetable or other rich source of folate.
- 2 cups from the fruits group. One cup of fruit each day should be a good vitamin C source.
- 7 ounce-equivalents from the grains group. Choices from the grains group should focus on whole-grain and enriched foods. One ounce of a whole-grain, ready-to-eat breakfast cereal significantly contributes to meeting many vitamin and mineral needs.
- 6 teaspoons of vegetable oil. Plant oils provide essential fatty acids, yet they are low in saturated fatty acids.

Moms-to-be can personalize MyPlate for each trimester at www.choosemyplate.gov/moms-pregnancy-breastfeeding.

- By selecting nutrient-dense foods from the food groups, the dietary pattern should be moderate in sodium (no more than 2300 milligrams per day), saturated fat (limit to 24 grams per day), and added sugars (limit to 55 grams per day).

In the second and third trimesters, about 2600 kcal is recommended for this woman. The plan should now include:

- 3 cups of calcium-rich foods from the dairy group or use of calcium-fortified foods
- 6 ½ ounce-equivalents from the protein group
- 3 ½ cups from the vegetables group
- 2 cups from the fruits group
- 9 ounce-equivalents from the grains group
- 8 teaspoons of vegetable oil
- By selecting nutrient-dense foods from the food groups, the dietary pattern should be moderate in sodium (no more than 2300 milligrams per day), saturated fat (limit to 29 grams per day), and added sugars (limit to 65 grams per day).

Table 18-3 illustrates one daily menu based on the 2600-kcal plan for pregnancy for women in the second or third trimesters. This menu meets the extra nutrient needs associated

TABLE 18-3 ■ **Sample 2600-kcal Daily Menu That Meets the Nutritional Needs of Most Pregnant and Breastfeeding Women***

	Vitamin B-6	Folate	Iron	Zinc	Calcium
Breakfast					
1 cup Kellogg's® Smart Start® cereal	✓	✓	✓	✓	✓
1 cup orange juice		✓			
1 cup fat-free milk	✓				✓
Snack					
2 tbsp peanut butter	✓	✓	✓	✓	
2 stalks of celery		✓			
1 slice whole-wheat toast		✓	✓	✓	
1 cup plain low-fat yogurt	✓				✓
½ cup strawberries		✓			
Lunch					
2 cups spinach and fruit salad with 2 tbsp oil and vinegar dressing		✓			✓
2 slices whole-wheat toast		✓	✓	✓	
1 ½ ounces provolone cheese	✓				✓
Snack					
5 whole-wheat crackers		✓	✓	✓	
1 cup grape juice					
Dinner					
2 bean burritos	✓	✓	✓	✓	✓
1 cup cooked broccoli		✓			✓
1 tsp soft margarine					
Unsweetened iced tea					
Snack					
Granola bar (2 ounces)					
½ banana	✓	✓	✓	✓	

*This diet meets nutrient needs for pregnancy and breastfeeding. Lack of a check (√) indicates a poor source of the nutrient. The vitamin- and mineral-fortified breakfast cereal used in this example makes an important contribution to meeting nutrient needs. Fluids can be added as desired. Total intake of fluids, such as water, should be 10 cups per day for pregnant women or about 13 cups per day for breastfeeding women.

with pregnancy. Women who need to consume more than this—and some do for various reasons—should incorporate additional fruits, vegetables, and whole-grain breads and cereals, not poor nutrient sources such as desserts and sugared soft drinks.

It is a common myth that women instinctively know what to eat during pregnancy. Cravings during the last two trimesters are often related to hormonal changes in the mother or family traditions. Such "instinct" cannot be trusted, however, based on observations that some women crave nonfood items (called **pica**) such as laundry starch, chalk, cigarette ashes, and soil (clay). This practice can be extremely harmful to the mother and the fetus. Following the nutrition advice of respected health professionals, such as registered dietitian nutritionists, is much more reliable than relying on cravings to meet nutrient needs.

PREGNANT VEGETARIANS

Women who are either **lactoovovegetarians** or **lactovegetarians** generally do not face special difficulties in meeting their nutritional needs during pregnancy. Like nonvegetarian women, they should be concerned primarily with meeting vitamin B-6, iron, folate, and zinc needs.

On the other hand, for a vegan, careful diet planning during preconception and pregnancy is crucial to ensure sufficient protein, vitamin D (particularly in the absence of sufficient sun exposure), vitamin B-6, iron, calcium, zinc, and especially a supplemental source of vitamin B-12. The basic vegan diet described in Section 6.9 should be modified to include more whole grains, beans, nuts, and seeds to supply the necessary extra amounts of some of these nutrients. As mentioned, use of a prenatal multivitamin and mineral supplement also is generally advocated to help fill micronutrient gaps. However, although these are high in iron, this is not true for calcium (200 milligrams per pill). If iron and calcium supplements are used, they should not be taken together to avoid possible competition for absorption.

▲ How does this lunch of spinach and fruit salad and whole-wheat toast compare to MyPlate? Is iced tea a good beverage choice? Why or why not? © Getty Images/Jonelle Weaver

pica The practice of eating nonfood items, such as dirt, laundry starch, or clay.

lactoovovegetarian A person who consumes plant products, dairy products, and eggs.

lactovegetarian A person who consumes plant products and dairy products.

✓ CONCEPT CHECK 18.5

1. List three nutrients of special concern for a pregnant woman who practices a vegan lifestyle.

2. Modify the sample 2600-kcal daily menu in Table 18-3 so that it would be suitable for a pregnant vegan woman.

3. Michaela tells you about her pregnancy craving for ice cream. She says she has been eating one or two ice cream bars after lunch every day and usually stops for a milkshake at a fast-food restaurant on her way home from work. What nutrition information would you share with her?

18.6 Physiological Changes of Concern During Pregnancy

During pregnancy, fetal needs for oxygen and nutrients as well as excretion of waste products increase the burden on the mother's lungs, heart, and kidneys. Although a mother's digestive and metabolic systems work efficiently, some discomfort accompanies the changes her body undergoes to accommodate the fetus.

HEARTBURN, CONSTIPATION, AND HEMORRHOIDS

Hormones (such as progesterone) produced by the placenta relax smooth muscles in the uterus and the gastrointestinal tract. This often causes heartburn as stomach acid refluxes into the esophagus (review Section 3.12). When this occurs, the woman should avoid lying down after eating, eat less fat so that foods pass more quickly from the stomach into the small intestine, and avoid spicy foods, which can worsen symptoms. She should also consume most liquids between (rather than with) meals to limit the volume of stomach contents and thus relieve some of the pressure that encourages reflux. Women with more severe cases may temporarily need antacids or related medications.

The hormone-induced relaxation of muscles in the GI tract may also lead to constipation. This is especially likely to develop late in pregnancy, when the fetus competes with the GI tract for space in the abdominal cavity. To alleviate constipation, a woman should focus on consuming adequate fluid and fiber and should perform regular exercise. The AI for fiber in pregnancy is 28 grams, slightly more than for the nonpregnant woman. Fluid needs are 10 cups per day. The extra iron in prenatal supplements may also contribute to constipation. If this is the case, a clinician can reevaluate the woman's needs for supplemental iron. Alleviating constipation can also help to prevent hemorrhoids, which affect about one-third of pregnant women.

EDEMA

Placental hormones cause various body tissues to retain fluid during pregnancy. Blood volume also greatly expands during pregnancy. The extra fluid normally causes some swelling (edema). There is no reason to restrict salt severely or use diuretics to limit mild edema. However, the edema may limit physical activity late in pregnancy and occasionally requires a woman to elevate her feet or wear compression stockings to control the symptoms. Overall, edema is only a mild nuisance unless it is accompanied by hypertension and the appearance of extra protein in the urine (see Hypertensive Disorders of Pregnancy later in this section).

NAUSEA AND VOMITING OF PREGNANCY

About 70% to 85% of pregnant women experience nausea during the early stages of pregnancy. Nausea and vomiting of pregnancy are probably related to changes in GI motility induced by pregnancy-related hormones. Although commonly called "morning sickness," pregnancy-related nausea may occur at any time and persist all day. It is often the first signal to a woman that she is pregnant.

To help control mild nausea, pregnant women can try the following: avoiding nauseating foods, such as fried or greasy foods; cooking with good ventilation to dissipate nauseating smells; eating saltine crackers or dry cereal before getting out of bed; avoiding large fluid intakes early in the morning; and eating smaller, more frequent meals. The iron in prenatal supplements triggers nausea in some women, so changing the type of supplement used or postponing use until the second trimester may provide relief in some cases. If a woman thinks her morning sickness is related to her prenatal supplement, she should discuss switching to another supplement with her primary care provider.

There is evidence that the following practices may also be useful for the prevention and treatment of nausea and vomiting of pregnancy; however, a pregnant woman should consult her primary care provider before trying any of these remedies:

- History of use of a balanced multivitamin and mineral supplement at the time of conception
- Use of megadoses of vitamin B-6 (10 to 25 milligrams taken three to four times a day), especially coupled with the antihistamine doxylamine (10 milligrams) with each dose
- Ginger may also be helpful (350 milligrams taken three times per day)

Usually, nausea is mild and stops after the first trimester. However, in up to 3% of pregnancies, nausea and vomiting are prolonged and severe enough to cause weight loss, dehydration, and dangerous electrolyte imbalances. In these cases, the preceding practices offer little relief; medical attention is needed to protect the health of the mother and her growing baby.

ANEMIA

To supply fetal needs, the mother's blood volume expands to approximately 150% of normal. The number of red blood cells, however, increases by only 20% to 30%, and this occurs

▲ A few saltine crackers upon waking or between meals can help lessen pregnancy-related nausea. © Royalty-Free/Corbis

more gradually. As a result, a pregnant woman has a lower ratio of red blood cells to total blood volume in her system. This hemodilution is known as **physiological anemia.** It is a normal response to pregnancy, rather than the result of inadequate nutrient intake.

However, if iron stores and/or dietary iron intake are not sufficient to meet her increased needs, the pregnant woman may develop iron-deficiency anemia. The Dietary Guidelines for Americans identify iron as a nutrient of public health concern because several population groups, including pregnant women, are likely to have low intakes of this nutrient. Iron-deficiency anemia requires medical attention at any stage of the life cycle, but consequences for the fetus are especially severe (see Section 18.4). Lean meats, beans, and fortified grains are nutrient-dense sources of iron that should be emphasized to prevent anemia during pregnancy (review Section 13.5). Importantly, once anemia has developed, dietary supplements will be needed to replete iron status; dietary changes alone are not sufficient to correct iron deficiency.

physiological anemia The normal increase in blood volume in pregnancy that dilutes the concentration of red blood cells, resulting in anemia; also called *hemodilution*.

GESTATIONAL DIABETES

Hormones synthesized by the placenta decrease the efficiency of insulin. This leads to a mild increase in blood glucose, which helps supply calories to the fetus. If the rise in blood glucose becomes excessive, this leads to **gestational diabetes,** often beginning between weeks 20 and 28, particularly in women who have a family history of diabetes or who are obese. Other risk factors include maternal age over 35 and gestational diabetes in a prior pregnancy.

In North America, gestational diabetes develops in as many as 9% of pregnancies (estimates vary based on the diagnostic criteria). Today, pregnant women with risk factors for type 2 diabetes (e.g., obesity, family history) should be screened for undiagnosed type 2 diabetes at the first prenatal visit. Pregnant women without type 2 diabetes should be screened for diabetes between 24 and 28 weeks using an oral glucose tolerance test (i.e., checking for elevated blood glucose concentration 1 to 2 hours after consuming a dose of glucose; see Further Reading 18). If gestational diabetes is detected, a special diet that distributes carbohydrates throughout the day needs to be implemented. Carbohydrate choices should be mostly whole, unprocessed grains, vegetables, fruits, and beans, which have a lower impact on blood glucose than refined grains or foods with lots of added sugars. Sometimes insulin injections or oral medications are also needed. Regular physical activity also helps to control blood glucose (see Further Reading 1).

The primary risk of uncontrolled diabetes during pregnancy is that the fetus can grow quite large. This is a result of the oversupply of glucose from maternal circulation coupled with an increased production of insulin by the fetus, which allows fetal tissues to take up an increased amount of building materials for growth. The mother may require a Cesarean section if the fetus is too large for a vaginal delivery. Another threat is that the infant may have low blood glucose at birth, because of the tendency to produce extra insulin that began during gestation. Other concerns are the potential for early delivery, low iron stores, and increased risk of birth trauma and malformations.

Although gestational diabetes often disappears after the infant's birth, it increases the mother's risk of developing diabetes later in life, especially if she fails to maintain a healthy body weight. Uncontrolled blood sugar during gestation may have some long-term repercussions for the child, as well. Studies show that infants of mothers with gestational diabetes may also have higher risks of developing obesity, metabolic syndrome, and type 2 diabetes as they grow to adulthood. For all these reasons, proper control of blood glucose during pregancy is extremely important.

gestational diabetes A high blood glucose concentration that develops during pregnancy and returns to normal after birth; one cause is the placental production of hormones that antagonize the regulation of blood glucose by insulin.

HYPERTENSIVE DISORDERS OF PREGNANCY

Hypertension (blood pressure greater than 140/90 mmHg) occurs in about 6% to 8% of pregnancies in the United States. Sometimes, women enter pregnancy with chronic hypertension. However, when hypertension first appears after 20 weeks of gestation, it is termed **gestational hypertension** (formerly called *pregnancy-induced hypertension*).

gestational hypertension Blood pressure greater than 140/90 mmHg that is first diagnosed after 20 weeks of gestation. This may evolve into preeclampsia or eclampsia.

preeclampsia A form of gestational hypertension characterized by protein in the urine.

eclampsia A severe form of gestational hypertension characterized by protein in the urine and seizures (formerly called *toxemia*).

About half of women with gestational hypertension eventually develop **preeclampsia** (mild form) or **eclampsia** (severe form). Early symptoms include a rise in blood pressure, excess protein in the urine, edema, changes in blood clotting, headache, and visual disturbances. Very severe effects, including convulsions, can occur in the second and third trimesters. If not controlled, eclampsia eventually damages the liver and kidneys, and the mother and fetus may die.

The causes for hypertensive disorders of pregnancy are not well understood but likely involve interactions among genetics, certain environmental or lifestyle influences, and abnormal function of the placenta. The populations most at risk for these disorders are women under age 17 or over age 35, overweight or obese women, and those who have had multiple-birth pregnancies. A family history of gestational hypertension in the mother's or father's side of the family, diabetes, African-American race, and a woman's first pregnancy also raise risk.

Gestational hypertension resolves once the pregnancy ends, making delivery the most reliable treatment for the mother. However, if eclampsia develops before the fetus is ready to be born, medical intervention is necessary. Bed rest and administration of magnesium sulfate are the most effective treatment methods. Magnesium likely acts to relax blood vessels and so leads to a reduction in blood pressure. There is good evidence that adequate intakes of calcium and vitamin D are involved in reducing incidence of gestational hypertension. There is interest in the use of antioxidants to prevent or treat gestational hypertension, but results of a recent trial showed that vitamin C and E supplementation during pregnancy is not effective in preventing the disorder. Several other treatments, such as various antiseizure and antihypertensive medications, fish oils, and selenium, are under study (see Further Reading 23).

✓ **CONCEPT CHECK 18.6**

1. What diet and lifestyle strategies would you suggest to a pregnant woman who complains of morning sickness?
2. Define gestational diabetes. What are the potential consequences of this disorder for the mother and baby?
3. Differentiate between chronic hypertension and gestational hypertension. Define preeclampsia and eclampsia.

18.7 Breastfeeding

Breastfeeding the new infant complements the attention given to diet during pregnancy. The Academy of Nutrition and Dietetics (AND) and the American Academy of Pediatrics (AAP) recommend breastfeeding exclusively for the first 6 months, with the continued combination of breastfeeding and infant foods until 1 year (see Further Readings 12 and 15). The World Health Organization goes beyond that to recommend breastfeeding (with appropriate solid food introduction; see Section 19.3) for at least 2 years. Still, surveys show that only about 70% of North American mothers breastfeed their infants in the hospital, and at 4 and 6 months, only 33% and 20%, respectively, are still breastfeeding their infants. The number falls to 18% at 1 year of age. These statistics refer to Caucasian women; minority women are even less likely to be breastfeeding at these time intervals.

Women who choose to breastfeed usually find it an enjoyable, special time in their lives that strengthens the bond with their new infant. Although bottle feeding with an infant formula is also safe for infants, as discussed in Section 19.2, it cannot replicate all of the benefits derived from breastfeeding. If a woman does not breastfeed her child, milk production ceases within a few days after birth.

▲ Breastfeeding is the preferred way to feed a young infant. © Diane McDonald/Getty Images

PLANNING TO BREASTFEED

Almost all women are physically capable of breastfeeding their children (see the later section "Medical Conditions Precluding Breastfeeding" for exceptions). In most cases, problems encountered in breastfeeding are due to a lack of knowledge or support. Anatomical problems in breasts, such as inverted nipples, can be corrected during pregnancy. Breast size generally increases during pregnancy and is no indication of success in breastfeeding. Most women notice a dramatic increase in the size and weight of their breasts by the third or fourth day of breastfeeding. If these changes do not occur, a woman needs to seek advice from her clinician or a lactation consultant.

Breastfed infants must be followed closely by caregivers over the first few days of life to ensure that feeding and weight gain are proceeding normally. Monitoring is especially important with a mother's first child because the mother will be inexperienced with the technique of breastfeeding. The infant is at risk of dehydration and blood clots if feeding does not proceed smoothly.

First-time mothers who plan to breastfeed should learn as much as they can about the process early in their pregnancy. Although it is the most natural way to feed a newborn child, the technique does not always come naturally. Gathering information on breastfeeding, what obstacles to anticipate, and how to respond to such obstacles will help new mothers and their babies to succeed with breastfeeding. It also helps to have an experienced friend, family member, or a professional lactation consultant to call for advice when questions arise.

HUMAN MILK PRODUCTION

During pregnancy, breast weight increases by 1 to 2 pounds due to the action of placental hormones that stimulate the formation of milk-producing cells. Milk will be produced in the **lobules** (Fig. 18-8). A cluster of lobules forms a lobe. Tiny ducts lead from each lobe to the nipple, where milk is ejected from the breast.

Most of the protein found in human milk is synthesized by breast tissue. Some proteins also enter the milk directly from the mother's bloodstream. These proteins include immune factors (e.g., antibodies) and enzymes. Some of the fats in human milk come from the mother's diet; other fats are synthesized by breast tissue. The sugar galactose is synthesized in the breast, whereas glucose enters from the mother's bloodstream. Together, these sugars form lactose, the main carbohydrate in human milk.

Lactation is regulated by two hormones: prolactin and oxytocin. **Prolactin** is the hormone that stimulates milk production in the lobules of the breast. As milk is produced between feedings, it is stored in the lobules. An important brain-breast connection—commonly called the **let-down reflex**—is necessary to release the milk stored in the lobules. This reflex occurs in response to the infant suckling at the breast. Stimulation of the nerves in the nipple area signals the pituitary gland to release **oxytocin,** which allows the lobules to contract and let down (release) stored milk (Fig. 18-9). The milk then travels via ducts to the nipple. The mother may feel a tingling sensation shortly before milk flow begins. Throughout the feeding, the suckling of the infant further stimulates prolactin release from the pituitary gland, so milk synthesis within the lobules continues. The more the infant suckles, the more milk is produced. Because of this, even twins (and triplets) can be breastfed adequately.

If the let-down reflex does not operate, little milk is available to the infant. The infant gets frustrated, which then frustrates the mother. The let-down reflex is easily inhibited by

---

Healthy People 2020 goals for breastfeeding:

- 82% of women breastfeeding their infants at time of hospital discharge
- 60% breastfeeding for 6 months
- 34% still breastfeeding at 1 year

lobules Saclike structures in the breast that store milk; also called *alveoli*.

prolactin A hormone secreted by the pituitary gland that stimulates the synthesis of milk in the breast.

In the United States, although 70% of women initiate breastfeeding after birth, only about one-third of mothers are still breastfeeding their infants at 6 months of age. What if more women chose to breastfeed their infants? A recent analysis estimated the potential public health impact of near universal breastfeeding. By reducing the risk of problems like gastrointestinal and respiratory infections, researchers projected that 823,000 infants deaths and 20,000 cases of breast cancer could be prevented per year (see Further Reading 20).

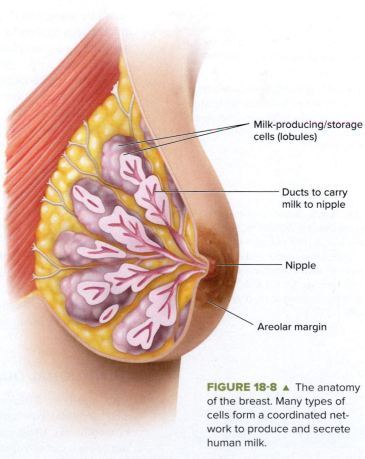

- Milk-producing/storage cells (lobules)
- Ducts to carry milk to nipple
- Nipple
- Areolar margin

FIGURE 18-8 ▲ The anatomy of the breast. Many types of cells form a coordinated network to produce and secrete human milk.

1 Suckling stimulates nerves in the nipple and areola that transmit impulses to the hypothalamus.

2 In response, the hypothalamus stimulates the posterior pituitary to release oxytocin and the anterior pituitary to release prolactin.

3 Oxytocin stimulates lobules in the breast to let down (release) milk from storage. Prolactin stimulates additional milk production.

Hypothalamus

Spinal cord

Posterior pituitary

Anterior pituitary

3a Oxytocin (milk letdown) **3b** Prolactin (milk production)

Mammary gland

FIGURE 18-9 ▲ Let-down reflex. Suckling sets into motion the sequence of events that lead to milk let-down, the flow of milk into ducts of the breast.

let-down reflex A reflex stimulated by infant suckling that causes the release (ejection) of milk from milk ducts in the mother's breasts; also called *milk ejection reflex*.

oxytocin A hormone secreted by the pituitary gland. It causes contraction of the musclelike cells surrounding the ducts of the breasts and the smooth muscle of the uterus.

Disposable diapers can absorb so much urine that it is difficult to judge when they are wet. A strip of paper towel laid inside a disposable diaper makes a good wetness indicator. Alternatively, cloth diapers may be used for a day or two to assess whether nursing is supplying sufficient milk.

nervous tension, a lack of confidence, and fatigue. Mothers should be especially aware of the link between tension and a weak let-down reflex. They need to find a relaxed environment where they can breastfeed.

After a few weeks, the let-down reflex becomes automatic. Milk ejection can be triggered just by thinking about her infant or seeing or hearing another one cry. At first, however, the process can be a bit bewildering. A mother cannot measure the amount of milk the infant takes in, so she may fear that she is not adequately nourishing the infant.

As a general rule, a well-nourished breastfed infant should (1) have three to five wet diapers per day by 3 to 5 days of age and four to six wet diapers per day thereafter; (2) show a normal pattern of weight gain; and (3) pass at least one or two stools per day that look like lumpy mustard. In addition, softening of the breast during the feeding indicates that enough milk is being consumed. Parents who sense their infant is not consuming enough milk should consult their primary care provider immediately because dehydration can develop rapidly. Losing more than 7% of birth weight indicates a feeding problem that requires intervention.

It generally takes 2 to 3 weeks to fully establish the feeding routine: Infant and mother begin to feel comfortable, the milk supply meets infant demand, and initial nipple soreness disappears. Establishing the breastfeeding routine requires patience, but the rewards are great. The adjustments are easier if supplemental formula feedings are not introduced until breastfeeding is well established, after at least 3 to 4 weeks. Then it is fine if a supplemental bottle or two of infant formula per day is needed, but supplemental feedings will decrease milk production.

NUTRITIONAL QUALITIES OF HUMAN MILK

Human milk is different in composition from cow's milk. Unless altered (i.e., to make infant formula), cow's milk should never be used in infant feeding until the infant is at least 12 months old. Unaltered cow's milk is too high in minerals and protein and does not contain enough carbohydrate to meet infant needs. In addition, the major protein in cow's milk is harder for an infant to digest than the major proteins in human milk. The proteins in cow's milk may also spur allergies in some infants. Finally, certain compounds in human milk presently under study show other possible benefits for the infant.

Colostrum At the end of pregnancy, the first fluid made by the human breast is **colostrum.** This thick, yellowish fluid may leak from the breast during late pregnancy and is produced in earnest for a few days after birth. Colostrum contains antibodies, immune system cells, and growth factors, some of which pass intact through the infant's immature GI tract into the bloodstream. The first few months of life are the only time when we can readily absorb whole proteins across the GI tract. These immune factors and cells protect the infant from some GI tract diseases and other infectious disorders, compensating for the infant's immature immune system during the first few months of life.

One component of colostrum, the **lactobacillus bifidus factor,** encourages the growth of *Lactobacillus bifidus* bacteria. These beneficial bacteria limit the growth of potentially toxic bacteria in the intestine. Overall, breastfeeding promotes the intestinal health of the breastfed infant in this way.

colostrum The first fluid secreted by the breast during late pregnancy and the first few days after birth. This thick fluid is rich in immune factors and protein.

Lactobacillus bifidus factor A protective factor secreted in the colostrum that encourages growth of beneficial bacteria in the newborn's intestines.

Mature Milk Human milk composition gradually changes until it achieves the normal composition of mature milk several days after delivery. Human milk looks very different from cow's milk. (Table 19-3 provides a direct comparison.) Human milk is thin and almost watery in appearance and often has a slightly bluish tinge. Its nutritional qualities, however, are impressive.

Human milk's proteins form a soft, light curd in the infant's stomach and are easy to digest. Some human milk proteins bind iron, reducing the growth of some bacteria that can cause diarrhea. Still other proteins offer the important immune protection already noted.

The lipids in human breast milk are high in linoleic acid and cholesterol, which are needed for brain development. Breast milk also contains long-chain omega-3 fatty acids, such as docosahexaenoic acid (DHA). This polyunsaturated fatty acid is used for the synthesis of tissues in the central nervous system, especially in the brain and in the retina of the eye.

The fat composition of human milk changes during each feeding. The consistency of milk released initially (*fore milk*) resembles that of skim milk. It later has a greater fat content, similar to whole milk. Finally, the milk released after 10 to 20 minutes (*hind milk*) is essentially like cream. Babies need to nurse long enough (e.g., a total of 20 or more minutes) to get the calories in the rich hind milk to be satisfied between feedings and to grow well. The overall calorie content of human milk is about the same as that of infant formulas (67 kcal per 100 milliliters).

Human milk composition also allows for adequate fluid status of the infant, provided the baby is exclusively breastfed. Caregivers often wonder if the infant needs additional water if stressed by hot weather, diarrhea, vomiting, or fever. The AAP advises against supplemental water or juice during the first 6 months of life. The practice may unnecessarily introduce pathogens or allergens. Excessive water can lead to brain disorders, low blood sodium, and other problems. Thus, before 6 months of age, supplemental water and juice should be given only with a clinician's guidance.

Human Milk for Preterm Infants Can a mother breastfeed her preterm infant? In some cases, human milk is the most desirable form of nourishment, depending on infant weight and length of gestation. Feeding of human milk to preterm infants has been linked to lower infant mortality, decreased risk of infections, reduced stays in the neonatal intensive care unit, fewer hospital readmissions, better growth, and improved brain development (see Further Reading 15).

Breastfeeding a preterm infant, however, demands great maternal dedication. Preterm infants sometimes have a weak or uncoordinated suck and swallow reflex, so it may be necessary to express milk from the breast and feed the infant through a tube until the infant's feeding ability develops. Fortification of the milk with such nutrients as calcium, phosphorus, sodium, and protein is often necessary to meet the needs of a rapidly growing preterm infant. In some cases, special feeding problems may prevent the use of human milk or necessitate supplementing it with specialized formula. Sometimes total parenteral nutrition

▲ If human milk is used to feed the preterm infant, fortification of the milk with certain nutrients is often needed. © Royalty-Free/ Corbis

▲ Eating 8 to 12 ounces (2 to 3 servings) of fish per week will help breastfeeding women ensure that their infants receive ample omega-3 fatty acids. It is important, however, to avoid those fish likely to be contaminated with mercury (swordfish, shark, king mackeral, and tile fish). For more information about mercury in seafood, see Further Reading 19.
© Royalty-Free/Corbis

Most substances that the mother ingests are secreted into her milk. For this reason, she should avoid alcohol, limit intake of caffeine, and check all medications with a pediatrician. Some mothers believe that certain foods, such as garlic and chocolate, flavor the breast milk and upset the infant. If a woman notices a connection between a food she eats and the infant's subsequent fussiness, she could consider avoiding that food. However, she might experiment again with it later, as infants become fussy for other reasons. Some researchers propose that the passage of flavors from the mother's diet into her milk affords an opportunity for the infant to learn about the flavor of the foods of its family long before solids are introduced. These researchers suspect that bottle-fed infants are missing significant sensory experiences that, until recent times in human history, were common to all infants.

atopic disease A condition involving an inappropriate immune response to environmental allergens; examples include asthma, eczema, and seasonal allergies.

(intravenous feeding) is the only option. Working as a team, the pediatrician, neonatal nurses, and registered dietitian nutritionist must guide the parents in this decision.

EATING PATTERN FOR WOMEN WHO BREASTFEED

Nutrient needs for a breastfeeding mother change to some extent from those of the pregnant woman in the second and third trimester (see the DRI summary tables in Appendix G). Needs for folate and iron decrease while needs for calories, vitamins A, E, and C, riboflavin, copper, chromium, iodide, manganese, selenium, and zinc increase. Still, these increased needs of the breastfeeding mother will be met by the general diet plan proposed for a woman in the latter stages of pregnancy. Recall that each day of this diet plan includes at least:

- 3 cups of calcium-rich foods such as from the dairy group or use of calcium-fortified foods to make up for any gap between calcium intake and need
- 6 ½ ounce-equivalents from the protein group
- 3 ½ cups from the vegetables group
- 2 cups from the fruits group
- 9 ounce-equivalents from the grains group
- 8 teaspoons of vegetable oil

Table 18-3 provided a menu for such a plan. As in pregnancy, a serving of a highly fortified ready-to-eat breakfast cereal (or use of a balanced multivitamin and mineral supplement) is advised to help meet extra nutrient needs. And, as mentioned for pregnant women, breastfeeding mothers should consume 8 to 12 ounces of low-mercury fish per week (or 1 gram per day of omega-3 fatty acids from a fish oil supplement) because the omega-3 fatty acids present in fish are secreted into breast milk and are likely to be important for development of the infant's nervous system.

Milk production requires approximately 800 kcal every day. The estimated energy requirement during lactation is an extra 400 to 500 kcal daily above prepregnancy recommendations. The difference between that needed for milk production and the recommended intake—about 300 kcal—should allow for a gradual loss of the extra body fat accumulated during pregnancy, especially if breastfeeding is continued for 6 months or more and the woman performs some physical activity. This shows just one of the natural benefits of following pregnancy with at least several months of breastfeeding.

After giving birth, women are often eager to shed the excess "baby fat." Breastfeeding, however, is no time for crash diets. A gradual weight loss of 1 to 4 pounds per month by the nursing mother is appropriate. At significantly greater rates of weight loss—when calories are restricted to less than about 1500 kcal per day—milk output decreases. A reasonable approach for a breastfeeding mother is to eat a balanced diet that supplies at least 1800 kcal per day; has moderate fat content; and includes a variety of dairy products, fruits, vegetables, and whole grains.

To promote the best possible feeding experience for the infant, there are several other dietary factors to consider. Hydration is especially important during breastfeeding; the woman should drink fluids every time her infant nurses. Drinking about 13 cups of fluids per day encourages ample milk production. Poor health habits, such as smoking cigarettes or drinking more than two alcoholic beverages a day, can decrease milk output. (Even less alcohol can have a deleterious effect on milk output in some women.) To avoid exposure to harmful levels of mercury, precautions concerning fish likely to contain mercury should extend past pregnancy for the breastfeeding mother. There is no evidence that maternal diet restrictions (e.g., peanuts, eggs, and fish) during pregnancy or breastfeeding prevent food allergies in infants. The AAP recommends exclusive breastfeeding and delaying introduction of solid foods until 4 to 6 months of age as the best approaches for preventing **atopic diseases** (see Further Reading 8).

BREASTFEEDING TODAY

The vast majority of women are capable of breastfeeding and their infants would benefit from it (see Table 18-4 and Further Reading 15). Nonetheless, some circumstances may

TABLE 18-4 ■ Advantages of Breastfeeding

For Infant
• Bacteriologically safe
• Always fresh and ready to go
• Provides antibodies and substances that contribute to maturation of the immune system
• Contributes to maturation of gastrointestinal tract via *Lactobacillus bifidus* factor
• Decreases risk of infections, such as diarrhea, respiratory disease, and ear infections
• Reduces risk of food allergies and intolerances, as well as some other allergies
• Reduces risk of celiac disease and inflammatory bowel diseases
• Establishes habit of eating in moderation, linked to 15% to 30% lower risk of obesity and 40% lower risk of type 2 diabetes later in life
• Contributes to proper development of jaws and teeth for better speech development
• May enhance nervous system development and eventual learning ability
• Decreases risk of childhood leukemia and lymphoma

For Mother
• Contributes to earlier recovery from pregnancy due to the action of hormones that promote a quicker return of the uterus to its prepregnancy state
• Decreases risk of several chronic diseases later in life, including hypertension, cardiovascular disease, and diabetes
• Decreases the risk of ovarian and premenopausal breast cancer
• Potential for quicker return to prepregnancy weight
• Potential for delayed ovulation, thus reducing chances of pregnancy in the short term

make breastfeeding impractical or undesirable for a woman. Mothers who do not want to breastfeed their infants should not feel pressured to do so. Breastfeeding provides advantages, but none so great that a woman who decides to bottle feed should feel she is compromising her infant's well-being.

Advantages of Breastfeeding Human milk is tailored to meet infant nutrient needs for the first 4 to 6 months of life. In some cases, however, infant dietary supplements, used under a pediatrician's guidance, are recommended.

- The AAP recommends *all* infants, including exclusively breastfed infants, be given 400 IU of vitamin D per day, beginning shortly after birth and continuing until the infant consumes that much from food [e.g., at least 2 cups (0.5 liter) of infant formula per day]. Some sun exposure also helps in meeting vitamin D needs.
- Iron supplements are generally necessary for infants who were preterm, LBW, have blood disorders, or who were born with low iron stores.
- The AAP does not advise fluoride supplements before 6 months of age. After 6 months, the pediatrician or dentist may recommend supplemental fluoride if the infant's exposure to fluoride from drinking water, foods, and oral hygiene products is insufficient.
- Vitamin B-12 supplements are recommended for the breastfed infant whose mother is a complete vegetarian (vegan).

Fewer Infections. Due in part to the antibodies in human milk, breastfeeding reduces the infant's overall risk of developing infections. Breastfed infants also have fewer ear infections (otitis media) because they do not sleep with a bottle in their mouth. Experts strongly discourage allowing an infant to sleep with a bottle in the mouth; milk can pool in the mouth, throat, and inner ear, creating a growth medium for bacteria, which can lead to ear infections and dental caries. By reducing these common ailments, parents can decrease discomfort for the infant, avoid related trips to the doctor, and prevent possible hearing loss.

Lower Risk of Diseases. Research now links breastfeeding with reduced risks for many diseases. Breastfed infants may learn to self-regulate food intake and avoid overeating, which may explain the connection to lowered risk for obesity and type 2 diabetes among adults who were breastfed as infants. The immunologic benefits of breastfeeding seem to be involved in lowered rates of type 1 diabetes, celiac disease, and inflammatory bowel diseases. Reductions in risks of childhood leukemia and lymphoma have also been observed.

Fewer Allergies and Intolerances. Breastfeeding also reduces the chances of some allergies, especially in allergy-prone infants (see Section 19.7). The key time to attain this benefit from breastfeeding is during the first 4 to 6 months of an infant's life. A longer commitment is best, but breastfeeding for even a few weeks is beneficial. Infants are also better able to tolerate human milk than formulas. Formulas sometimes must be switched several times until caregivers find the best one for the infant.

Convenience and Cost. Breastfeeding frees the mother from the time and expense involved in buying and preparing formula and washing bottles. Human milk is ready to go and sterile. This allows the mother to spend more time with her baby.

Possible Barriers to Breastfeeding Widespread misinformation, the mother's need to return to a job, and social reticence serve as barriers to breastfeeding.

Misinformation. The major barriers to breastfeeding stem from misinformation, such as the idea that one's breasts are too small, and the lack of role models. One positive note has been the widespread increase in the availability of lactation consultants over the past several years. First-time mothers who are interested in breastfeeding can find invaluable support from lactation consultants or by talking to women who have experienced it successfully. In almost every community, a group called La Leche League offers classes in breastfeeding and advises women who have problems with it (800-LALECHE or www.lalecheleague.org).

Return to an Outside Job. Working outside the home can complicate plans to breastfeed. One possibility after a month or two of breastfeeding is for the mother to express and save her own milk. She can use a breast pump or manually express milk into a sterile plastic bottle or nursing bag (used in a disposable bottle system). Federal legislation passed in 2010 requires employers to provide reasonable breaks and a private space (other than a bathroom) for breastfeeding mothers to pump milk.

Storing expressed human milk requires careful sanitation and rapid chilling. It can be stored in the refrigerator for 3 to 5 days or be frozen for 3 to 6 months. Thawed milk should be used within 24 hours.

There is a knack to learning how to express milk, but the freedom can be worth it, because it allows others to feed the infant the mother's milk. A schedule of expressing milk and using supplemental formula feedings is most successful if begun after 1 to 2 months of exclusive breastfeeding. After 1 month or so, the baby is well adapted to breastfeeding and probably feels enough emotional security and other benefits from nursing to feed both ways.

Some women can juggle both a job and breastfeeding, but others find it too cumbersome and decide to formula-feed. A compromise—balancing some breastfeedings, perhaps early morning and night, with infant formula feedings during the day—is possible. However, too many supplemental infant formula feedings decrease milk production.

Social Concerns. Another barrier for some women is embarrassment about nursing a child in public. Historically, our society has stressed modesty and has discouraged public displays of breasts—even for as good a cause as nourishing babies. In the United States, no state or territory has a law prohibiting breastfeeding. However, indecent exposure (including the exposure of women's breasts) has long been a common law or statutory offense. Now, 49 states, the District of Columbia, and the Virgin Islands have specific laws that protect a

▲ Breast milk can be expressed by the mother using a manual, battery-operated, or electric (shown) breast pump. In 2010, President Barack Obama signed an amendment to the Fair Labor Standards Act that requires most U.S. employers to allow break time and a private setting for breastfeeding mothers to express milk. © 2008 Medela AG.

woman's right to breastfeed in any location. Women who feel reluctant should be reassured that they do have social support and that breastfeeding can be done discreetly.

Medical Conditions Precluding Breastfeeding. Breastfeeding may be ruled out by certain medical conditions in either the infant or the mother. For example, breastfeeding is contraindicated for infants with galactosemia, an inherited disorder in which the body cannot break down galactose. Recall from Section 4.2 that lactose, the main carbohydrate in human breast milk, is made of glucose and galactose. When galactose is not properly broken down, its byproducts can damage body organs.

Certain medications, which pass into the milk and adversely affect the nursing infant, are best avoided while breastfeeding. In addition, a woman in North America or other developed region of the world who has a serious chronic disease (such as tuberculosis, AIDS, or HIV-positive status) or who is being treated with chemotherapy medications should not breastfeed.

Cosmetic Alterations to the Breast. Nipple piercings should have no impact on a woman's ability to breastfeed, but the jewelry should be removed before each feeding. Repeated removal and reinsertion of the jewelry may be inconvenient and irritating, so it may be best to leave the jewelry out for the entire period of breastfeeding. Breast tattoos will not impair breastfeeding, either. However, getting a new nipple piercing or breast tattoo while breastfeeding is not advised due to the pain of healing and possibility of infection. Past breast augmentation or reduction surgeries may impair a woman's ability to breastfeed if milk-producing tissue was damaged during the surgery.

Environmental Contaminants in Human Milk There is some legitimate concern over the levels of various environmental contaminants in human milk. However, the benefits of human milk are well established, and the risks from environmental contaminants are still largely theoretical. A few measures a woman could take to counteract some known contaminants are to (1) consume a variety of foods within each food group; (2) avoid freshwater fish from polluted waters; (3) carefully wash and peel fruits and vegetables (or choose organically raised produce, which has lower levels of pesticides than conventional produce); and (4) remove the fatty edges of meat, as pesticides concentrate in fat. In addition, a woman should not try to lose weight rapidly while nursing (more than 0.75 to 1 pound per week) because contaminants stored in her fat tissue might then enter her bloodstream and affect her milk. If a woman questions whether her milk is safe, especially if she has lived in an area known to have a high concentration of toxic wastes or environmental pollutants, she should consult her local health department.

Phenylketonuria (PKU), a disorder of phenylalanine metabolism described in Section 6.1, was once thought to be a contraindication for breastfeeding. However, infants with PKU can enjoy the benefits of part-time breastfeeding in combination with specialized phenylalanine-free infant formulas.

✓ CONCEPT CHECK 18.7

1. What do AND and AAP recommend for duration of breastfeeding?

2. Describe the physiological processes of milk production and letdown. Be sure to mention the hormones involved in these processes.

3. List three advantages of breastfeeding for the mother and three advantages for the infant.

4. Identify three micronutrients that may need to be supplemented in the diets of breast-fed infants and give the rationale for each.

5. Describe three potential barriers to breastfeeding and suggest ways to overcome them.

18.8 Nutrition and Your Health
Preventing Birth Defects

© Floortje/Getty Images

Eating well for a healthy pregnancy not only supplies materials for fetal growth and development but also helps to direct the amazing process of building a new life. Considering the complexity of the human body and its more than 20,000 genes, it is not surprising that abnormalities of structure, function, or metabolism are sometimes present at birth. Birth defects impact 1 of every 33 babies born in the United States. In some cases, they are so severe that a baby cannot survive or thrive. Defects in embryonic or fetal development are the presumed cause of many spontaneous abortions and are at the root of about 20% of infant deaths before 1 year of age. However, many babies with birth defects can go on to live healthy and productive lives.

A wide range of physical or mental disabilities result from birth defects. Heart defects are present in approximately 1 of every 100 to 200 newborn babies, accounting for a large proportion of infant deaths. Cleft lip and/or cleft palate are malformations of the lip or roof of the mouth and occur in approximately 1 in 700 to 1000 births. Neural tube defects are malformations of the brain or spinal cord that occur during embryonic development. Examples include spina bifida, in which all or part of the spinal cord is exposed, and anencephaly, in which some or all of the brain is missing (Fig. 18-10). Babies born with spina bifida can survive to adulthood but in many cases have disabilities, such as paralysis, incontinence, and cognitive disorders. Babies born with anencephaly die soon after birth. Neural tube defects occur in 1 in 1000 births. Down syndrome, a

condition in which an extra chromosome leads to mental retardation and other physical alterations, occurs in about 1 in 800 births. Other common birth defects include musculoskeletal defects, gastrointestinal defects, and metabolic disorders.

What causes a birth defect? About 15% to 25% of birth defects are known to be genetic (i.e., inherited or spontaneous mutations of the genetic code). Another 10% are due to environmental influences (e.g., exposure to **teratogens**). The specific cause of the remaining 65% to 75% of birth defects is unknown. Although the etiology of birth defects is multifactorial and many elements are beyond human control, good nutrition practices can positively influence the outcome of pregnancy.

Folic Acid

During the 1980s, researchers in the United Kingdom noticed a relationship between poor dietary habits and a high rate of neural tube defects among children of impoverished women. Subsequent intervention studies demonstrated that administration of a multivitamin supplement during the periconceptional period—the months before conception and during early pregnancy—reduced the recurrence of these birth defects. The specific link between dietary folic acid and neural tube defects was tested and confirmed in several follow-up studies. As you learned in Section 13.3, folate plays a leading role in the synthesis of DNA and the metabolism of amino acids. The rapid cell growth of pregnancy increases needs for folate during pregnancy to 600 micrograms DFE per day. Some women, for genetic reasons, may have an even higher requirement. Adequate folic acid in the periconceptional period decreases the risk of neural tube defects by about 70% and has also been associated with decreased risk of cleft lip/palate, heart defects, and Down syndrome.

In 1998, FDA mandated fortification of grain products to provide 140 micrograms of folic acid per 100 grams of grain consumed. In Canada, the level of fortification is 150 micrograms of folate per 100 grams of grain consumed. In general, this increases the average consumption of dietary folic acid by 100 micrograms per day.

Adequate folate status is crucial for all women of childbearing age because the neural tube closes within the first 28 days of pregnancy, a time when many women are unaware they are pregnant. A well-planned diet can meet the RDA for folic acid, but the U.S. Public Health Service, March of Dimes, and Dietary Guidelines for Americans recommend that all women of childbearing

In North America, maternal death as a result of childbirth is uncommon—only about 14 deaths in every 100,000 live births. The infant mortality rate, however, is much higher: for each 100,000 live births, about 600 infants die within the first year. The infant death rate among African-Americans is more than double the rates among whites and Hispanics in the United States.

teratogen A compound (natural or synthetic) that may cause or increase the risk of a birth defect. Exposure to a teratogen does not always lead to a birth defect; its effects on the fetus depend on the dose, timing, and duration of exposure.

FIGURE 18-10 ▶ Spina bifida is one type of neural tube defect. Very early in fetal development, a ridge of neural-like tissue forms along the back of the embryo. As the fetus develops, this ridge develops into both the spinal cord and nerves at the lower end and the brain at the upper end. At the same time, the bones that make up the back gradually surround the spinal cord on all sides. In spina bifida, the backbones do not form a complete ring to protect the spinal cord. Deficient folate status in the mother during the beginning of pregnancy, especially in combination with a genetic abnormality in folate metabolism, greatly increases the risk of neural tube defects.

age take a daily multivitamin and mineral supplement that contains 400 micrograms of folic acid. Women who have already had a child with a neural tube defect are advised to consume megadoses of folic acid—4000 micrograms per day. They are to begin supplementation at least 1 month before any future pregnancy. This must be done under strict physician supervision.

Iodine

Low iodine status during the first trimester of pregnancy—a critical period of brain development—may lead to congenital hypothyroidism (formerly called *cretinism*: see Further Reading 24). If left untreated, consequences (which may vary in severity) include mental retardation, stunting of growth, impaired hearing and speech, and infertility. Some other physical features are evident in Figure 18-11. When the defect is identified early (by newborn screening tests), these harmful effects can be prevented by treatment with thyroid hormones. With use of iodized salt, however, congenital hypothyroidism due to iodine deficiencies is rare.

Antioxidants

A case can be made for antioxidants in the prevention of birth defects as well. Free radicals are constantly generated within the body as a result of normal metabolic processes. An abundance of free radicals results in damage of cells and their DNA, which can lead to gene mutations or tissue malformations. Some research points to free radicals as a source of damage during embryo development and organogenesis. Antioxidant systems within the body act to minimize the damage caused by free radicals, and researchers hypothesize that dietary sources of antioxidants may aid in the prevention of birth defects. At this time, there is insufficient evidence to support supplementation of individual nutrients that participate in antioxidant systems—vitamin E, vitamin C, selenium, zinc, and copper—for the prevention of birth defects. However, use of a balanced multivitamin and mineral supplement while consuming a diet rich in whole grains, legumes, and a variety of fruits and vegetables will provide enough of these nutrients to meet current recommendations.

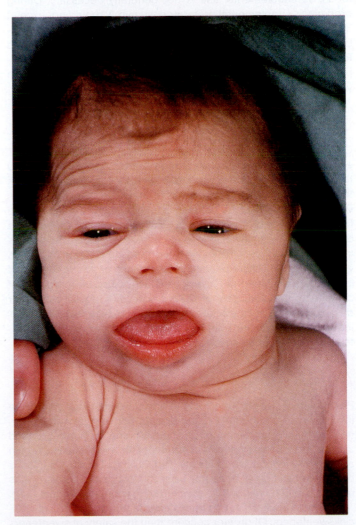

FIGURE 18-11 ▲ Child with congenital hypothyroidism due to maternal iodine deficiency. This birth defect leads to mental retardation, stunting of growth, and other physical defects, such as large tongue, enlarged head, and puffy eyes. © Medical-on-Line/Alamy

Vitamin A

While the needs for most vitamins and minerals increase by about 30% during pregnancy, the requirement for vitamin A increases by only 10%. Studies have shown the teratogenic potential of vitamin A in doses as low as approximately 3000 micrograms RAE per day. This is just over three times the RDA of 770 micrograms RAE per day for pregnant adult women.

Fetal abnormalities resulting from vitamin A toxicity primarily include facial and cardiac defects, but a wide range of defects have been reported. It is rare that food sources of vitamin A would lead to toxicity. Recall from Section 10.3 that preformed vitamin A is found in liver, fish, fish oils, fortified milk and yogurt, and eggs. Carotenoids, found in fruits and vegetables, are precursors of vitamin A that are converted into vitamin A in the small intestine, liver, and kidneys. However, the efficiency of absorption of carotenoids decreases as intake increases. Vitamin A excesses typically arise from high-dose dietary supplements rather than food sources.

Typical North American diets supply adequate vitamin A from foods, so supplemental use is not generally necessary. During pregnancy, supplemental preformed vitamin A should not exceed 3000 micrograms RAE per day (15,000 IU per day). Most multivitamins and prenatal vitamins supply less than 1500 micrograms RAE per day. A balanced diet and prudent use of dietary supplements are actions that can sidestep potential problems with vitamin A toxicity.

Caffeine

Caffeine has been scrutinized for its safety during pregnancy, especially for any link with rate of birth defects. Caffeine decreases the mother's absorption of iron and may reduce blood flow through the placenta. In addition, the fetus is unable to detoxify caffeine. Research shows that as caffeine intake increases, so does the risk of miscarriage or delivering a LBW infant. Heavy caffeine use during pregnancy may also lead to caffeine withdrawal symptoms in the newborn. These risks are reported with caffeine intakes in excess of 500 milligrams, or the equivalent of about 5 cups of coffee per day. Moderate use of caffeine (up to 200 milligrams of caffeine, or the equivalent of 12 fluid ounces of regular coffee per day), however, is not associated with risk for birth defects. Accounting for caffeine intake from tea, over-the-counter medicines containing caffeine, and chocolate is also important.

Aspartame

Phenylalanine, a component of the artificial sweetener aspartame (NutraSweet® and Equal®), is a cause for concern for some pregnant women. High amounts of phenylalanine in maternal blood disrupt fetal brain development if the mother has a disease known as *phenylketonuria* (see Obesity and Chronic Health Conditions below). If the mother does not have this condition, however, it is unlikely that the baby will be affected by moderate aspartame use.

For most adults, diet soft drinks are the primary source of artificial sweeteners. Of greater concern than the safety of sweeteners during pregnancy is the quality of foods and beverages consumed. A high intake of diet soft drinks may crowd out healthier beverages, such as water and low-fat milk.

Obesity and Chronic Health Conditions

Even before becoming pregnant, women of childbearing age should have regular medical checkups to keep an eye on any health conditions that already exist or to identify any developing health problems. In some cases, the condition itself increases risk for birth defects. Obesity, high blood pressure, and uncontrolled diabetes are common health problems known to increase the risk for birth defects, including neural tube defects. In other cases, medications used to control illnesses may pose a risk to the developing fetus. Other health issues, such as seizure disorders and metabolic disorders, could also affect fetal development. A preconception visit with a health professional can help to sort out and make plans to minimize such risks. Once a woman has become pregnant, early and regular prenatal care can aid in the success of a pregnancy.

Women with diabetes are two to three times more likely to give birth to a baby with birth defects compared to women with normal glucose metabolism. Examples of birth defects common in this group include malformations of the spine, legs, and blood vessels of the heart. Some experts speculate that the mechanism by which diabetes increases birth defects is via excessive free radicals, which lead to oxidative damage of DNA during early gestation. Careful control of blood glucose drastically lowers risk for women with diabetes. Optimal blood glucose control can be achieved through a combination of dietary modifications and medications. Given that diabetes is on the rise among women of childbearing age, this elevated rate of birth defects has become an area of heightened concern.

Another health condition for which maternal nutritional control is of utmost importance is PKU. Recall from Section 6.1 that PKU is an error of metabolism in which the liver lacks the ability to process phenylalanine, leading to an accumulation of this amino acid and its metabolites in body tissues. Babies born to women who have phenylketonuria that is not controlled by diet are at heightened risk for brain defects, such as microcephaly and mental retardation (see Further Reading 3).

Alcohol

Conclusive evidence shows that repeated consumption of four or more alcoholic drinks at one sitting harms the fetus (see Further Reading 21). Such binge drinking is especially perilous during the first 12 weeks of pregnancy, as this is when critical early developmental events take place in utero. Experts have not determined a safe level of alcohol intake during pregnancy. Until a safe level can be established, women are advised not to drink any alcohol—from beverages, foods, or medications (check the label)—during pregnancy or when there is a chance of conception. The embryo (and, at later stages, the fetus) has no means of detoxifying alcohol.

Women with chronic alcoholism produce children with a variety of physical and intellectual problems collectively called **fetal alcohol spectrum disorders (FASDs).** The most severe of these disorders is **fetal alcohol syndrome (FAS).** A diagnosis of FAS is

fetal alcohol spectrum disorders (FASDs) A group of irreversible physical and mental abnormalities in the infant that result from the mother's consuming alcohol during pregnancy.

fetal alcohol syndrome (FAS) Severe form of FASD that involves abnormal facial features and problems with development of the nervous system and overall growth as a result of maternal alcohol consumption during pregnancy.

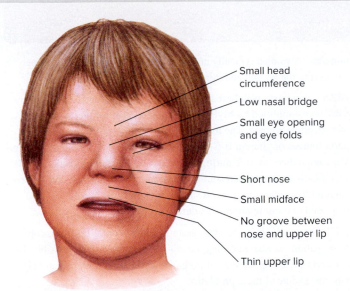

Small head circumference

Low nasal bridge

Small eye opening and eye folds

Short nose

Small midface

No groove between nose and upper lip

Thin upper lip

FIGURE 18-12 ▲ Fetal alcohol syndrome. The facial features shown are typical of affected children. Additional abnormalities in the brain and other internal organs accompany fetal alcohol syndrome but are not immediately apparent from simply looking at the child. Milder forms of alcohol-induced changes from a lower alcohol exposure to the fetus are known as alcohol-related neurodevelopmental disorders (ARNDs) and alcohol-related birth defects (ARBDs).

based mainly on poor fetal and infant growth, physical deformities (especially of facial features), and mental retardation (Fig. 18-12). Irritability, hyperactivity, short attention span, and limited hand-eye coordination are other symptoms of FAS. Defects in vision, hearing, and mental processing may also develop over time. Other FASDs consist of some but not all of the defects of FAS. **Alcohol-related neurodevelopmental disorders (ARNDs)** include behavior and learning problems resulting from exposure to alcohol in utero. **Alcohol-related birth defects (ARBDs)** typically include malformations of the heart, kidneys, bones, and/or ears.

Exactly how alcohol causes these defects is not known. One line of research suggests that alcohol, or products of the metabolism of alcohol (e.g., acetaldehyde), cause faulty movement of cells in the brain during early stages of nerve cell development or block the action of certain brain neurotransmitters. In addition, inadequate nutrient intake, reduced nutrient and oxygen transfer across the placenta, cigarette smoking commonly associated with alcohol intake, drug use, and possibly other factors contribute to the overall result.

All major health authorities recommend that alcoholic beverages not be consumed by pregnant women. For more information about fetal alcohol syndrome, visit the website www.cdc.gov/ncbddd/fasd/.

alcohol-related neurodevelopmental disorders (ARNDs) One or more abnormalities of the central nervous system (e.g., small head size, impaired motor skills, hearing loss, or poor hand-eye coordination) related to confirmed alcohol exposure during gestation.

alcohol-related birth defects (ARBDs) One or more birth defects (e.g., malformations of the heart, bones, kidneys, eyes, or ears) related to confirmed alcohol exposure during gestation.

Environmental Contaminants

There is little evidence to link birth defects with the amounts of pesticides, herbicides, or other contaminants in foods or public water supplies in North America. However, evaluating such a link can be methodologically difficult, and many would argue that regulations concerning contaminants in the food and water supply are too permissive. Thus, it seems prudent to take measures to decrease intake of pesticides and other contaminants wherever possible. For fruits and vegetables, peeling, removing outer leaves, and/or thoroughly rinsing and scrubbing with a brush under running water will remove the majority of contaminants. In animal products, toxins are most likely to accumulate in fatty tissues. Therefore, removing skin, discarding drippings, and trimming visible fat will decrease exposure from meat, poultry, and fish.

For fish, mercury is of particular concern because it can harm the nervous system of the fetus. Thus, FDA warns pregnant women to avoid swordfish, shark, king mackerel, and tile fish because of possible high mercury contamination. Largemouth bass are also implicated. In general, intake of other fish and shellfish should not exceed 12 ounces per week. Canned albacore tuna is a potential mercury source, so it should not be consumed in amounts exceeding 6 ounces per week (see Further Reading 19). Most experts agree that the benefits of consuming fish far outweigh the potential risks of environmental contaminants (see Further Reading 16). As a rule of thumb, consuming a *variety* of foods minimizes risk of exposure to any one contaminant from the food supply.

In Summary

Although many risk factors for birth defects are beyond our control, a woman of childbearing potential can make some wise nutrition choices to improve her chances of having a healthy baby without birth defects. A varied and balanced diet, such as the food plan for pregnant women described in this chapter, along with a daily multivitamin and mineral supplement with 400 micrograms of folic acid will ensure adequate nutrient status. It is estimated that daily use of a multivitamin and mineral supplement containing folic acid will decrease the rate of all birth defects by 50%. Discuss use of any other dietary supplements with a primary care provider or registered dietitian nutritionist to be sure that the fetus will not be exposed to toxic levels of vitamin A or other dangerous food components. Early and consistent prenatal care can help control obesity and any chronic health conditions that may complicate a pregnancy. Also, avoiding alcohol during pregnancy will eliminate any risk for fetal alcohol spectrum disorders.

Although it seems that advice for a healthy pregnancy is always directed at the mother, fathers-to-be are not off the hook! Health is a family affair, so encouraging healthy eating habits and avoiding smoking and alcohol are important for fathers, too. As you read in the beginning of this chapter, the genetics of the baby are certainly an outcome of both parents. Indeed, inadequate supplies of zinc, folate, antioxidants, and omega-3 fatty acids affect the quality of sperm. Overall, the periconceptional period is a time for good nutrition and careful lifestyle practices for mothers- and fathers-to-be.

A goal of *Healthy People 2020* is 98.3% abstinence from alcohol, cigarettes, and illicit drugs by pregnant women, a 10% improvement over current statistics.

Summary (Numbers refer to numbered sections in the chapter.)

18.1 Energy imbalances can adversely affect fertility by altering hormone levels and promoting oxidative damage. Polycystic ovary syndrome, which tends to co-occur with upper-body obesity, is an condition of hormonal imbalance that causes infertility. Other than managing body weight, nutritional factors that may improve male and/or female fertility include low glycemic index carbohydrates, unsaturated fats, antioxidants, folate, iron, and zinc.

18.2 Pregnancy is arbitrarily divided into three trimesters of 13 to 14 weeks each. The first trimester is characterized by a rapid increase in cell number as the zygote grows to be an embryo, then a fetus. During the first trimester, the growing organism is most susceptible to damage from exposure to toxic agents or nutrient deficiencies. By the start of the second trimester, the organs and limbs have formed and will continue to grow and develop. The third trimester is marked by rapid fetal growth and storage of nutrients in preparation for life outside the womb.

18.3 A successful pregnancy results in optimal health for both the infant and the mother. Pregnancy success is defined as (1) gestation longer than 37 weeks; and (2) birth weight greater than 5.5 pounds (2.5 kilograms). Factors that predict pregnancy success include early and regular prenatal care, maternal age within the range of 20 to 35 years, and adequate nutrition. Factors that contribute to poor pregnancy outcome include inadequate prenatal care, obesity, underweight, teenage pregnancy, smoking, alcohol consumption, use of certain prescription medications and all illicit drugs, inadequate nutrition, heavy caffeine use, and various infections, such as listeriosis.

18.4 For women with a healthy prepregnancy BMI (18.5 to 24.9), total weight gain should be within the range of 25 to 35 pounds. Underweight women and those carrying multiple fetuses should gain more; overweight and obese women should gain less. During the first trimester, although she need not increase diet quantity, the woman should focus on diet quality to meet increased requirements for protein, carbohydrate, essential fatty acids, fiber, water, and many vitamins and minerals. A woman typically needs an additional 350 to 450 kcal per day during the second and third trimesters.

18.5 Following a plan based on the Dietary Guidelines for Americans as exemplified by MyPlate is recommended for pregnant and breastfeeding women. The mother-to-be should especially emphasize good sources of vitamin B-6, folate, vitamin D, iron, zinc, and calcium. Vegetarian diets are safe during pregnancy, but vegan mothers should specifically seek out good sources of vitamin B-12 and vitamin D. Prenatal multivitamin and mineral supplements are useful for meeting increased nutrient requirements during pregnancy.

18.6 Gestational hypertension, gestational diabetes, heartburn, constipation, nausea, vomiting, edema, and anemia are all possible discomforts and complications of pregnancy. Nutrition therapy can help minimize some of these problems.

18.7 Almost all women are physically able to breastfeed their infants. The nutritional composition of human milk is different from that of unaltered cow's milk and is much more desirable for the infant.

For the infant, the advantages of breastfeeding over formula feeding are numerous, including fewer infections, reduced risk of allergies and food intolerances, and lower rates of obesity and type 2 diabetes throughout life. Benefits for the mother include reduced risk of certain cancers, earlier recovery from pregnancy, and faster return to prepregnancy weight. For mothers who choose not to breastfeed or in medical situations that contraindicate breastfeeding (e.g., galactosemia), infants can be adequately nourished with formula.

18.8 There are several steps pregnant women can take to help prevent birth defects. Achieve a healthy body weight before pregnancy and strive to gain weight within the ranges recommended by the Institute of Medicine. Adequate intakes of folic acid, iodine, and antioxidant nutrients are essential for prevention of many types of birth defects. Excesses of vitamin A and caffeine should be avoided. There is no safe level of alcohol intake known during pregnancy. Dietary control of diseases (e.g., diabetes and PKU) will also protect the fetus.

Check Your Knowledge (Answers are available at the end of this question set.)

1. Which of the following nutrition interventions is most likely to improve fertility?
   a. Taking a vitamin E supplement
   b. Losing excess body fat
   c. Consuming a low-carbohydrate diet
   d. Taking an iron supplement

2. Increased carbohydrate needs during pregnancy are set to
   a. prevent ketosis.
   b. alleviate nausea.
   c. prevent gestational hypertension.
   d. supply adequate folate.

3. An infant born at 38 weeks' gestation weighing 5 pounds can be described as
   a. preterm.   c. SGA.
   b. LBW.   d. LBW and SGA.

4. If a woman is 5 feet 2 inches tall and weighs 150 pounds before becoming pregnant, how much weight should she gain during pregnancy?
   a. 28 to 40 pounds (12.5 to 18 kilograms)
   b. 25 to 35 pounds (11.5 to 16 kilograms)
   c. 15 to 25 pounds (7 to 11.5 kilograms)
   d. As little as possible

5. Benefits of exercise during pregnancy include
   a. preventing excessive gestational weight gain.
   b. improved sleep.
   c. lower risk for gestational diabetes.
   d. all of these.

6. Which of the following may help to alleviate nausea during pregnancy?
   a. Postponing meals until the afternoon
   b. Drinking large amounts of water
   c. Postponing use of iron supplements until the second trimester
   d. All of these

7. Physiologically, milk production requires _____ kcal per day.
   a. 300   c. 800
   b. 500   d. 1000

8. An eating pattern for a woman in the third trimester of pregnancy differs from her prepregnancy diet in that
   a. fluid needs are higher.
   b. additional solid fats and added sugars are allowed.
   c. there are more servings from the grains group.
   d. all of these apply.

9. Advantages of breastfeeding include
   a. decreased ear infections in the infant.
   b. decreased diarrheal diseases in the infant.
   c. decreased risk of breast cancer for the mother.
   d. all of these.

10. Consuming a single cup of coffee per day is associated with
    a. spontaneous abortion.   c. birth defects.
    b. LBW.   d. none of these.

Answer Key: 1. b (LO 18.1), 2. a (LO 18.2), 3. d (LO 18.3), 4. c (LO 18.4), 5. d (LO 18.5), 6. c (LO 18.6), 7. c (LO 18.7), 8. d (LO 18.8), 9. d (LO 18.9), 10. d (LO 18.10)

Study Questions (Numbers refer to Learning Outcomes)

1. Provide three key pieces of nutrition advice for parents seeking to maximize their chances of conceiving. Why did you identify those specific factors? **(LO 18.1)**

2. Identify four key nutrients for which intake should be significantly increased during pregnancy. **(LO 18.2)**

3. Why does teenage pregnancy receive so much attention these days? At what age do you think pregnancy is ideal? Why? **(LO 18.3)**

4. Outline current weight-gain recommendations for pregnancy. What is the basis for these recommendations? **(LO 18.4)**

5. Suggest several safe exercises for a pregnant woman. **(LO 18.5)**

6. What nutrition advice would you give to a friend who suffers from morning sickness? **(LO 18.6)**

7. Describe the physiological mechanisms that stimulate human milk production and release. How can knowing about these help mothers breastfeed successfully? **(LO 18.7)**

8. Describe a day's diet based on the Dietary Guidelines as exemplified by MyPlate that meets the increased nutrient needs of pregnancy. **(LO 18.8)**

9. Give three reasons a woman should give serious consideration to breastfeeding her infant. **(LO 18.9)**

10. Describe the importance of folic acid for conception and fetal development. **(LO 18.10)**

What the Dietitian Chose

The spinach salad meal with hard-boiled egg and whole-wheat roll provides only about 2 grams of iron. It is a healthy, nutrient-dense choice that provides some protein but does not make a significant contribution to meeting iron needs.

A hamburger is a source of iron—this meal would provide about 4.5 milligrams of iron—but it would not be a choice for a person who follows a vegetarian diet.

The bean and cheese taco option provides just as much iron (4.5 milligrams) as the hamburger meal and would be appropriate for a vegetarian. Even though the nonheme iron in beans is not as well absorbed as the heme iron in beef, the 20 milligrams of vitamin C in the stewed tomatoes will enhance iron absorption.

All of these meals, however, pale in comparison to the iron contribution of the fortified, ready-to-eat breakfast cereal. One cup of Kellogg's Smart Start cereal provides 18 milligrams of iron and the 72 milligrams of vitamin C in 1 cup of orange juice will enhance iron absorption. In one easy meal, any pregnant woman could obtain more than half of the 27-milligram RDA for iron during pregnancy.

© Digital Vision/PunchStock

CASE STUDY SOLUTION   Eating For Two

1. Lily's use of an over-the-counter vitamin and mineral supplement provides ample synthetic folic acid and can help fill some gaps between dietary intakes and requirements for various nutrients. Still, she should discuss this supplement use with her primary care provider or registered dietitian nutritionist and would eventually benefit more from a prenatal supplement, as this will have more iron than the over-the-counter supplement. She should be sure not to exceed 100% of the Daily Value for preformed vitamin A because toxicities of this vitamin could cause birth defects. Lily is wise to avoid use of herbal supplements during pregnancy unless her health care provider approves of them.

2. Folate deficiency is known to be linked to neural tube defects. The synthetic folic acid in vitamin and mineral supplements is well absorbed and will certainly help to meet her needs for this nutrient. Consuming more fruits and vegetables—especially green leafy vegetables—is also a wise choice. A fortified, ready-to-eat breakfast cereal also contributes to vitamin and mineral intake. Her primary care provider may prescribe a prenatal supplement instead of the over-the-counter supplement.

3. Many experts would say that she is consuming too much caffeine and would be wise to cut down coffee and caffeine-containing soft drinks to a total of two servings or fewer per day.

4. If Lily likes fish, she could include two servings of fish per week in her diet plan for pregnancy and breastfeeding. Fish are a good source of protein and supply healthy fats,

including omega-3 fatty acids, linked to brain and eye development in the fetus. However, Lily should avoid some types of fish that may have high mercury content, which can harm the nervous system of the developing fetus. Fish that typically have high levels of mercury include swordfish, shark, king mackerel, and tile fish.

5. The additional fruits and vegetables Lily is consuming will provide some fiber to help prevent constipation. Other ideas to increase her fiber intake include consuming a variety of whole grains and incorporating beans and legumes into her diet plan. Lily should also increase her fluid intake and be sure to maintain regular exercise, such as walking.

6. Lily expressed concern about her weight gain during pregnancy. Research clearly shows that adequate weight gain during pregnancy is critical for growth and development of the fetus. Inadequate weight gain contributes to risk for delivering a low-birth-weight or small-for-gestational-age baby. On the other hand, excessive weight gain during pregnancy can present problems as well. Excessive weight gain may promote long-term health problems and complicate the pregnancy with gestational diabetes or large-for-gestational age babies. At her prepregnancy weight and height, Lily's BMI (21) is within the normal range, so she should aim to gain 25 to 35 pounds during the entire pregnancy. During the second and third trimesters, consuming an extra 350 to 450 kcal per day of nutrient-dense foods will help her to meet this goal. Regular, moderate exercise is also recommended throughout pregnancy. However, pregnancy is not a time to begin a vigorous exercise routine. Walking or riding a stationary bike are good activities to regulate weight gain. Lily should be reassured that her choice to breastfeed her baby will help her to lose those extra pounds after the baby is born.

Further Readings

1. American Diabetes Association: Standards of Medical Care in Diabetes—2016. *Diabetes Care* 39:S1, 2016.

2. Blumfield ML and others: Micronutrient intakes during pregnancy in developed countries: Systematic review and meta-analysis. *Nutrition Reviews* 71:118, 2013.

3. Committee on Genetics: Policy Statement: Maternal phenylketonuria. *Pediatrics* 122:445, 2008. Reaffirmed January 2013.

4. Committee on Obstetric Practice: *Committee Opinion #650: Physical activity and exercise during pregnancy and the postpartum period,* December 2015. https://www.acog.org/-/media/Committee-Opinions/Committee-on-Obstetric-Practice/co650.pdf?dmc=1&ts=20160120T2059531109. Accessed January 20, 2016.

5. Deierlein AL, Siega-Riz AM: How can we assist women in managing gestational weight gain? *Women's Health* 8:603, 2012.

6. Dror DK, Allen LH: Vitamin D inadequacy in pregnancy: Biology, outcomes, and interventions. *Nutrition Reviews* 68:464, 2010.

7. Fraser A and others: Associations of gestational weight gain with maternal body mass index, waist circumference, and blood pressure measured 16 years after pregnancy: The Avon Longitudinal Study of Parents and Children (ALSPAC). *American Journal of Clinical Nutrition* 93:1285, 2011.

8. Greer FR and others: Effects of early nutritional interventions on the development of atopic disease in infants and children: The role of maternal dietary restriction, breastfeeding, timing of introduction of complementary foods, and hydrolyzed formulas. *Pediatrics* 121:183, 2008.

9. Grieger JA, Clifton VL: A review of the impact of dietary intakes in human pregnancy on infant birthweight. *Nutrients* 7:153, 2015.

10. Han Z and others: Maternal underweight and the risk of preterm birth and low birth weight: A systematic review and meta-analysis. *International Journal of Epidemiology* 40:65, 2011.

11. Institute of Medicine and National Research Council: *Weight gain during pregnancy: Reexamining the guidelines.* Washington, DC: National Academies Press, 2009.

12. Lessen R, Kavanagh K: Position of the Academy of Nutrition and Dietetics: Promoting and supporting breastfeeding. *Journal of the Academy of Nutrition and Dietetics* 115:444, 2015.

13. March of Dimes Foundation: *Teenage pregnancy,* July 2012. http://www.marchofdimes.org/materials/teenage-pregnancy.pdf. Accessed January 22, 2016.

14. Proctor SB, Campbell CG: Position of the Academy of Nutrition and Dietetics: Nutrition and lifestyle for a healthy pregnancy outcome. *Journal of the Academy of Nutrition and Dietetics* 114:1099, 2014.

15. Section on Breastfeeding: Policy Statement: Breastfeeding and the use of human milk. *Pediatrics* 129:e827, 2012.

16. Starling P and others: Fish intake during pregnancy and fetal neurodevelopment—a systematic review of the evidence. *Nutrients* 7:2001, 2015.

17. Swinney B: Eating to fuel fertility. *Today's Dietitian* 15:38, 2013.

18. Toiba R: Gestational diabetes. *Today's Dietitian* 15:48, 2013.

19. U.S. Food and Drug Administration and U.S. Environmental Protection Agency: *Fish: What pregnant women and parents should know,* June 2014. http://www.fda.gov/downloads/Food/FoodborneIllnessContaminants/Metals/UCM400358.pdf. Accessed January 20, 2016.

20. Victora CG and others: Breastfeeding in the 21st century: Epidemiology, mechanisms, and lifelong effect. *The Lancet* 387:475, 2016.

21. Viteri OA and others: Fetal anomalies and long-term effects associated with substance abuse in pregnancy: A literature review. *American Journal of Perinatology* 32:405, 2015.

22. Wei S and others: Maternal vitamin D status and adverse pregnancy outcomes: A systematic review and meta-analysis. *Journal of Maternal-Fetal and Neonatal Medicine* 26:889, 2013.

23. Xu H and others: Role of nutrition in the risk of preeclampsia. *Nutrition Reviews* 67:639, 2009.

24. Zimmerman MB: Iodine deficiency in pregnancy and the effects of maternal iodine supplementation on the offspring: A review. *American Journal of Clinical Nutrition* 89:668S, 2009.

 To get the most out of your study of nutrition, go to McGraw-Hill's online resources: Connect www.mcgrawhillconnect.com, where you will find NutritionCalc Plus, LearnSmart, and many other dynamic tools.

Putting Your Knowledge About Nutrition and Pregnancy to Work

A college friend, Gayle, tells you that she is newly pregnant. You are aware that she usually likes to eat the following foods for her meals:

Breakfast

Skips this meal, or eats a granola bar Coffee

Lunch

Sweetened yogurt, 1 cup
Small bagel with cream cheese
Occasional piece of fruit
Regular caffeinated soda, 12 ounces

Snack

Chocolate candy bar

Dinner

2 slices of pizza, macaroni and cheese, or 2 eggs with 2 slices
   of toast
Seldom eats a salad or vegetable
Regular caffeinated soda, 12 ounces

© Andersen Ross/Getty Images

Snacks

Pretzels or chips, 1 ounce
Regular caffeinated soda, 12 ounces

1. Using the NutritionCalc Plus software, evaluate Gayle's usual diet for protein, carbohydrate, folate, vitamin B-6, iron, and zinc. How does her intake compare with the recommended amounts for pregnancy?

   _____

   _____

   _____

2. Now redesign her diet, making sure that her intake meets pregnancy needs for protein, carbohydrate, folate, vitamin B-6, and zinc. (Hint: Fortified foods, such as breakfast cereal, are generally nutrient-rich foods, which can more easily help meet one's needs.) Increase the iron content as well, but it still may be below the RDA for pregnancy.

   _____

   _____

   _____

© BananaStock/PunchStock

Student Learning Outcomes

Chapter 19 is designed to allow you to:

19.1 Describe the extent to which nutrition affects growth and physiological development from infancy through adolescence.

19.2 List specific nutrients often found to be lacking in the diets of infants, toddlers, preschoolers, and teenagers and make recommendations to remedy the problems.

19.3 Identify dietary strategies to meet the basic nutritional needs for normal growth and development for an infant and discuss some do's and don'ts associated with infant feeding.

19.4 Outline several challenges parents might face in dealing with eating habits during childhood and adolescence.

19.5 Describe the long-term effects of childhood obesity and suggest ways to prevent or treat the problem.

19.6 Identify common food allergens and suggest several practices that may reduce the risk of developing a food allergy.

Chapter 19

Nutrition from Infancy Through Adolescence

What Would You Choose?

Your brother and his wife have asked you to care for your 18-month-old niece, Lila, while they enjoy a weekend get-away at the lake to celebrate their anniversary. Before they drop her off, you make a trip to the grocery store to pick up some kid-friendly foods. Lila does not have any food allergies, but your brother warned you that she has developed some "picky" eating behaviors. Which of the following snack foods would you choose for your little houseguest?

a Reduced-fat popcorn

b Raw baby carrots with ranch dressing

c Fat-free light yogurt

d Whole-grain crackers with sliced cheddar cheese

Think about your choice as you read this chapter, then see What the Dietitian Chose at the end of the chapter.

Children born in North America have access to some of the best health care in the world. Even so, the numbers of children and teenagers with obesity and type 2 diabetes are on the rise. Kids spend more time in their computer chairs and less time in active play. Soft drinks and energy drinks have replaced much of the milk that children and teenagers previously consumed daily. Consumption of fruits, vegetables, and whole grains—although these are abundantly available—consistently falls short of recommendations. Evidently, there is room for improvement in the dietary patterns of most American children. How can we influence healthy eating behaviors?

Education designed to change nutrition habits should start early and involve the family. During infancy and early childhood, the family controls food intake, informs food preferences, and models eating behaviors. Family mealtimes help children to establish healthy eating habits and aid in the prevention of childhood obesity. As children grow older, family meals are a time to teach children communication skills and improve self-esteem. Dietary habits and social skills learned early in life will equip children as they reach school age, when peer and media influences take on heightened importance. This chapter examines the dynamic nutritional needs of the growing years—all the way from infancy through adolescence.

19.1 Assessing Growth

During infancy, future eating patterns and attitudes toward foods begin to take shape. If parents and other caregivers model good nutrition and are flexible, they can lead a child into lifelong healthful food habits. A family environment that encourages healthy eating will provide the nutrients needed to optimize physical growth and development. However, these advantages do not guarantee that a child will thrive.

Children also need specific attention focused on them; they need to grow in a stimulating environment, and they need a sense of security. For example, children hospitalized for growth failure gain weight more quickly when tactile stimulation, such as holding and rocking the infant, accompanies needed nutrients.

THE GROWING INFANT

All babies seem to do is eat and sleep. There is a good reason for this. An infant's birth weight doubles in the first 4 to 6 months and triples within the first year. Never again is growth so rapid. Such rapid growth requires a lot of nourishment and sleep. After the first year, growth is slower; it takes 5 more years to double the weight seen at 1 year. An infant also increases in length in the first year by 50% and then continues to gain height through the teen years. These gains are not necessarily continuous; spurts of rapid growth alternate with periods of relatively little change. Height is typically maximized by age 19, although continued growth may occur in the early twenties, especially for boys. Head size in proportion to total height shrinks from one-fourth to one-eighth during the climb from infancy to adulthood.

The human body needs a lot more food to support growth and development than it does to merely maintain its size once growth ceases. When nutrients are missing at critical phases of this process, growth and development may slow or even stop. Adequate amounts of kilocalories, protein, calcium, iron, and zinc are particularly important during these years. In developing nations, about one-third of the children under 5 years of age are short and underweight for their ages. Poor nutrition—called **undernutrition**—is at the heart of the problem. Undernourished children are smaller versions of nutritionally fit children. In poorer countries, when breastfeeding ceases, children are often fed a high-carbohydrate, low-protein diet (see Section 16.5). This diet supports some growth but does not allow children to attain their full genetic and developmental potential. Undernutrition occurs in North America, as well, but **overnutrition** is much more prevalent.

undernutrition Failing health that results from a longstanding dietary intake that is not enough to meet nutritional needs.

overnutrition A state in which nutritional intake greatly exceeds the body's needs.

EFFECT OF UNDERNUTRITION ON GROWTH

As with the fetus in utero, the long-term effects of nutritional problems in infancy and childhood depend on the severity, timing, and duration of the nutritional insult to cellular processes.

The single best indicator of a child's nutritional status is growth: gains in weight are a good reflection of growth in the short term, whereas gains in height are an indicator of growth over the long term. An inadequate dietary pattern during a critical stage of infancy or childhood hampers the cell division that should occur at that stage. Mild zinc deficiencies among North American children, for example, have been linked to diminished growth. Altering dietary patterns after exposure to early childhood nutrient deficiencies will not compensate for losses in physical or mental development, however, because the hormonal and other conditions needed for growth will not likely be present. In addition, gains in height are no longer possible after the skeleton reaches maturation. This happens as growth plates at the ends of the bones fuse, which begins around 14 years of age in girls and 15 years of age in boys. The final stages of this process end at about age 19 in girls and age 20 in boys. Furthermore, muscles can increase in diameter later in life, but their linear growth is limited by the length of the bone.

For these reasons, a 15-year-old Central American girl who is 4 feet 8 inches tall cannot attain the adult height of a typical North American girl simply by eating better. Girls experience their peak rate of growth right before the onset of menstrual periods. Once the time for growth ceases (in women, this is about 5 years after they start menstruating), a sufficient nutrient intake helps maintain health and weight but cannot make up for lost growth in height.

USING GROWTH CHARTS

Health professionals assess a child's pattern of growth by plotting measurements of height and weight on growth charts (Fig. 19-1). The charts contain **percentile** divisions, which represent the typical measurements for 90% to 96% of children. A percentile represents the rank of the person among 100 peers matched for age and gender. If a young boy, for example, is at the 90th percentile of height-for-age, he is shorter than 10% and taller than 89% of children his age. A child at the 50th percentile is considered average. Fifty of 100 children will be taller than this child; 49 will be shorter.

A variety of growth charts for boys and girls are available from the Centers for Disease Control and Prevention (CDC) website (see Fig. 19-1). For children from birth to age 2, use the growth charts developed by the World Health Organization (WHO) in 2006

percentile Classification of a measurement of a unit into divisions of 100 units.

Children under 2 to 3 years of age are measured lying on their backs with knees unflexed, so the term *length* is used rather than *height* or *stature*.

(a)   (b)

FIGURE 19-1 ▲ Growth charts for assessment of children in the growing years. The growth of a young girl and a boy are plotted to show how the charts are used in health care settings. For children from birth to age 2, CDC recommends using growth charts developed by WHO in 2006. For ages 2 to 20, use the CDC growth charts, developed by the National Center for Health Statistics and CDC in 2000. (a) Length-for-age and weight-for-age plotted for a young girl (Ella). A certain length (height) and weight correspond to a percentile value (i.e., a ranking of the individual among 100 peers). Ella has been tracking around the 50th percentile for length throughout the first 2 years of her life; her weight, which started out near the 50th percentile, is now between the 75th and 90th percentiles. (b) BMI-for-age plotted for a young boy (Logan) up to age 10. While Logan's BMI-for-age was around the 50th percentile when he was a preschooler, by age 10, he is above the 85th percentile. He would be classified as overweight according to his BMI-for-age.

Sources: (a) Centers for Disease Control and Prevention, based on WHO Child Growth Standards (2009); (b) Centers for Disease Control and Prevention (2000).

▲ Brain growth is faster in infancy than in any other stage of life. An infant's head needs to be large (about one-quarter of body length) to allow for such growth. By the time she reaches adulthood, this girl's head will only be about one-eighth of her height. © Pixtal/AGE Fotostock

to assess length-for-age, weight-for-age, weight-for-length, and head-circumference-for-age measurements. WHO growth charts are based on data collected from children from various regions of the world who were raised *under conditions for optimal growth and development*. This means that they were breastfed as infants; had caregivers who followed recommended infant and child feeding practices set forth by WHO; had adequate health care; had mothers who did not use alcohol during pregnancy; and were not exposed to tobacco before or after birth. In contrast, older growth charts for young children were based on data from primarily white children who were mostly formula-fed during infancy. The WHO growth standards emphasize that breastfeeding is the biological norm for infant nutrition.

For children from ages 2 to 20, growth charts developed by the National Center for Health Statistics are available to assess weight-for-age and stature-for-age. However, the preferred growth chart for children and adolescents is body mass index (BMI)-for-age. For adults, BMI has fixed cutoff points (e.g., a BMI of 25 for an adult is considered overweight). Please note, as Figure 19-1 shows, this is not true for children; BMI reference ranges are both gender and age specific.

In addition to taking measurements of weight and length, a health professional measures the infant's head circumference. Tracking head circumference-for-age on a growth chart (also available from CDC) is a means of assessing brain growth. The brain grows faster during the first year than at any other time of life. Unusual head circumference measurements can alert the health care team to a genetic disorder. A small head circumference could also be a result of malnutrition, infection, impaired mental development, or maternal substance abuse during pregnancy. An abnormally large measurement may be a sign of a tumor or fluid on the brain. Variations in head circumference may be due to harmless familial traits, but extreme deviations from the norm or rapid changes in percentiles over time warrant further investigation.

Infants and children should have their growth assessed during regular health check-ups. It takes 1 to 3 years for the genetic potential (in terms of percentile ranking on growth charts) of infant growth to be established. By 3 years of age, a child's measurements, such as length (height) for age, should track consistently along an established percentile. If the child's growth does not keep up with his or her length-for-age percentile, the physician needs to investigate whether a medical or nutritional problem is affecting growth. Likewise, when a child's BMI-for-age approaches the highest percentiles, caregivers should be concerned. A child between the 85th and 95th percentiles for BMI-for-age is considered overweight. At or above the 95th percentile, a child is considered obese (Table 19-1).

The growth charts available from the CDC are intended for healthy children; they may not be appropriate for children born at very low birth weight or who have special health care needs. Preterm infants tend to be smaller than full-term infants in the early months but typically catch up in growth within 2 or 3 years. Catch-up growth requires that the child move up in percentiles. Specialized growth charts have been developed for children with special health care needs that affect growth and development, such as Down syndrome.

TABLE 19-1 ■ Weight Status Classifications for Children, Ages 2 to 20

Weight Status Classification	BMI-for-Age Percentile
Underweight	<5th percentile
Healthy weight	5th to 85th percentile
Overweight	85th to 95th percentile
Obese	≥95th percentile

Source: Centers for Disease Control and Prevention.

GROWTH IN BODY FAT

Since 1970, researchers have speculated that overfeeding during infancy may increase the number of adipose tissue cells. Today, we know that the number of adipose cells can also increase as adulthood obesity develops. If energy intake is limited during infancy to minimize the number of adipose cells, the growth of other organ systems may also be severely restricted, especially brain and nervous system development. In addition, most overweight infants become normal-weight preschoolers without dietary restrictions. For these reasons, it is unwise for an infant's dietary pattern to be restrictive—especially fat intake. After the first 12 months, fat intake can range from 30% to 40% of total kilocalories for ages 1 to 3 years and 25% to 35% of total kilocalories for older children and teenagers.

FAILURE TO THRIVE

About 5% to 10% of infants or children do not grow as expected. An infant may fail to reach important milestones, such as doubling birth weight by 6 months of age. On growth charts, weight-for-age may track below the fifth percentile. This condition of inadequate growth is termed **failure to thrive** (see Further Reading 5).

In some cases, failure to thrive has a specific medical cause. Physical problems that may limit energy intake include poor oral cavity development or problems with breastfeeding (e.g., poor latch-on skills). Even if a child consumes enough food and beverages, growth may still falter if there are physical problems, such as celiac disease, which limit nutrient absorption. Lastly, some medical conditions, such as heart or lung disorders, lead to greatly increased kilocalorie requirements.

However, about 80% of infants or children who fail to thrive have no apparent disease; environmental or social problems are at the root of their undernutrition. Poverty is the biggest environmental risk factor for undernutrition leading to failure to thrive. Needing to stretch food dollars, caregivers may overdilute formula—a detrimental practice that fills the child up without providing adequate kilocalories. Sometimes the cause is poor infant-parent interaction, including situations of abuse or neglect. Either too little or too much concern over child feedings can lead to nutrition problems. Most poor interactions, however, arise from the parents' inexperience with infant feeding rather than from intentional negligence.

Whatever the cause, the consequences of failure to thrive are serious and far reaching. Possible outcomes include poor physical growth, impaired mental development, and behavioral problems. When health professionals encounter an infant failing to thrive, the true causes need to be identified and then treated. If a lack of financial resources is at the root of the problem, appropriate referrals to social services should be made. Counseling about proper nutrition and the importance of healthy parent-child interactions can help to get a child's growth back on track.

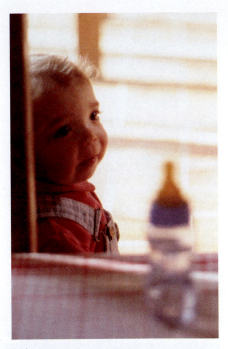

▲ Children older than 2 years are less likely to experience failure to thrive because they can often get food for themselves. Younger children, for the most part, are limited to what caregivers provide. © PhotoAlto/PictureQuest

failure to thrive Condition of inadequate growth during infancy or early childhood caused by poor nutritional intake, inefficient nutrient absorption, or excessive energy expenditure; commonly defined as weight-for-age below the fifth percentile on multiple occasions or weight declining two or more major percentile lines on a standardized growth chart.

✔ CONCEPT CHECK 19.1

1. How do health care providers assess the growth of infants and children?
2. Define childhood overweight and obesity in terms of BMI-for-age.
3. If a female adolescent is short for her age due to a brief period of undernutrition between ages 10 to 12, can she catch up in growth after proper nutrition is restored? Why or why not?
4. What is failure to thrive? List some possible causes.

19.2 Infant Nutritional Needs

Infants' nutritional needs vary as they grow. For the first 4 to 6 months of life, human milk or infant formula supplies needed nutrients. Age-appropriate solid foods should be added to the infant's diet after 4 to 6 months of age. Even after solid foods are added, the basis of an infant's diet for the first year is still human milk or infant formula. Because of the critical importance of adequate nutrition in infancy and the difficulties encountered in feeding some infants, there is more discussion in this chapter on this developmental period than on the later periods of childhood.

ENERGY

Due to rapid growth and a high metabolic rate, the energy requirements per pound of body weight for an infant are the highest of any life stage (Table 19-2). For example, a 6-month-old infant requires two to four times more kilocalories per pound of body weight than an adult.

Healthy 6-month-old infant

$$\frac{700 \text{ kcal}}{15 \text{ pounds}} = 47 \frac{\text{kcal}}{\text{pound}}$$

Healthy 20-year-old woman

$$\frac{2200 \text{ kcal}}{135 \text{ pounds}} = 16 \frac{\text{kcal}}{\text{pound}}$$

Infants need a concentrated source of kilocalories to meet these high demands. Exclusive feeding of either human milk or infant formula is ideal for the first 6 months of life; both are high in fat and supply about 640 kcal/quart (670 kcal/liter; Table 19-3). After 4 to 6 months of age, supplementing the diet with developmentally appropriate solid foods provides additional kilocalories, nutrients, and variety for the developing infant.

CARBOHYDRATE

Carbohydrate needs in infancy are 60 grams per day at 0 to 6 months and 95 grams per day at 7 to 12 months. These needs are based on the typical intakes of human milk by breastfed infants and their eventual intake of solid

TABLE 19-2 ■ Estimated Energy Requirements of Infants and Toddlers

Age	EER Equation
0 to 3 months	(89 kcal × weight in kilograms) + 75
4 to 6 months	(89 kcal × weight in kilograms) − 44
7 to 12 months	(89 kcal × weight in kilograms) − 78
13 to 35 months	(89 kcal × weight in kilograms) − 80

TABLE 19-3 ■ Composition of Human and Cow's Milk and Infant Formulas (per Liter)[a]

	Energy (kcal)	Protein (grams)	Fat (grams)	Carbohydrate (grams)	Minerals[b] (grams)
Milk					
Human milk	670[c]	11	45	70	2
Cow's milk, whole[d]	670	36	36	49	7
Cow's milk, fat free[d]	360	36	1	51	7
Casein/Whey-Based Formulas					
Similac®	680	14	36	71	3
Enfamil®	670	15	37	69	3
Good Start®	670	16	34	73	3
Soybean Protein-Based Formulas					
ProSobee®	670	20	35	67	4
Isomil®	680	16	36	68	4
Transition Formulas/Beverages[e]					
Similac Go and Grow®	630	17	34	68	3
EnfaGrow® Next Step®	480	32	10	64	6

[a]At 3 months of age, infants typically consume 0.75 to 1 liter of human milk or formula per day.

[b]Calcium, phosphorus, and other minerals.

[c]Rough estimate; ranges from 650 to 700 kcal per liter.

[d]Not appropriate for infant feeding, based primarily on high protein and mineral content.

foods. These carbohydrate goals are easily satisfied by usual eating patterns of infants who are consuming a developmentally appropriate diet.

Do infants need fiber? There are no set AIs for fiber for infants and children younger than 2 years of age. For the first 6 months of life, breast milk or formula, which contains no fiber, is adequate nutrition. As solid foods are introduced, include some fruits, vegetables, and whole grains. Some experts recommend working up to about 5 grams of fiber per day by 1 year of age. Keep in mind that too much fiber can limit nutrient absorption because it binds to some minerals and speeds the passage of food through the GI tract. Let the child's bowel habits be your guide. If the child is constipated, try increasing fiber and fluid intakes. On the other hand, if the child is uncomfortably gassy or is having many soft bowel movements per day, decrease the amount of fiber in the diet.

PROTEIN

Daily protein needs in infancy are about 9 grams per day for younger infants and about 11 grams per day for older infants. These recommendations are based on the typical consumption of human milk by breastfed infants for 0 to 6 months and then on the increased protein needs for growth for older infants. About half of total protein intake should come from essential (indispensable) amino acids. As with carbohydrate, protein needs are easily satisfied by either human milk or infant formula. However, as you learned in Section 6.5, protein metabolism generates waste products that must be excreted by the kidneys. Dietary patterns that are excessive in protein may stress the infant's immature kidneys, so protein intake should not greatly exceed these recommendations.

In North America, infant protein deficiency is unlikely, except in cases of inappropriate formula preparation, such as when an infant's formula is excessively diluted with water. Protein deficiency may also be induced by elimination diets used to detect food **allergies.** As foods are eliminated from the diet, infants may not be offered enough protein to compensate for that supplied by the suspected food allergen (see Section 19.7).

allergy A hypersensitive immune response that occurs when immune bodies produced by us react with a protein we sense as foreign (an antigen).

FAT

Infants need about 30 grams of fat per day. Essential fatty acids should make up about 15% of total fat intake (about 5 grams per day). Both recommendations are again based on the typical consumption of human milk by breastfed infants and the eventual intake of solid foods. Fats are an important part of the infant's dietary pattern because they are vital to the development of the nervous system. Also, fats are a concentrated source of energy (9 kcal per gram). The stomach capacity of an infant is limited, so a concentrated source of kilocalories is necessary to meet overall energy requirements. Thus, restriction of fat intake is not advised for infants or children under age 2 (Fig. 19-2).

Arachidonic acid (ARA) and docosahexaenoic acid (DHA) are two long-chain fatty acids that have important roles in infant development. The nervous system, especially the brain and eyes, depends on these fatty acids for proper development. During the last trimester, DHA and ARA provided by the mother accumulate in the brain and retinas of the eyes in the fetus. Breastfed infants continue to acquire these fatty acids from human milk, especially if their mothers are regularly eating fish. Since 2002, infant formula manufacturers have been adding ARA and DHA to their products to match the average fatty acid composition of human milk. Such infant formulas are particularly useful for feeding preterm infants.

VITAMINS OF SPECIAL INTEREST

All of the essential vitamins play important roles in infant growth and development, but three vitamins—K, D, and B-12—are of special interest for infants because levels tend to be low and the consequences of deficiency are dire.

In Section 13.2, you learned about the role of vitamin K in blood clotting. Newborn infants have low levels of vitamin K because (1) limited amounts of this vitamin are transferred from the mother to the fetus during gestation; (2) breastmilk is not particularly high

FIGURE 19-2 ▶ The labels on infant foods, like those on adult foods, contain a Nutrition Facts panel; however, the information provided on infant food labels differs from that on adult food labels, especially with respect to total fat, saturated fat, and cholesterol content (see Fig. 2-13 for a comparison). Some cereal brands are fortified with various other micronutrients.

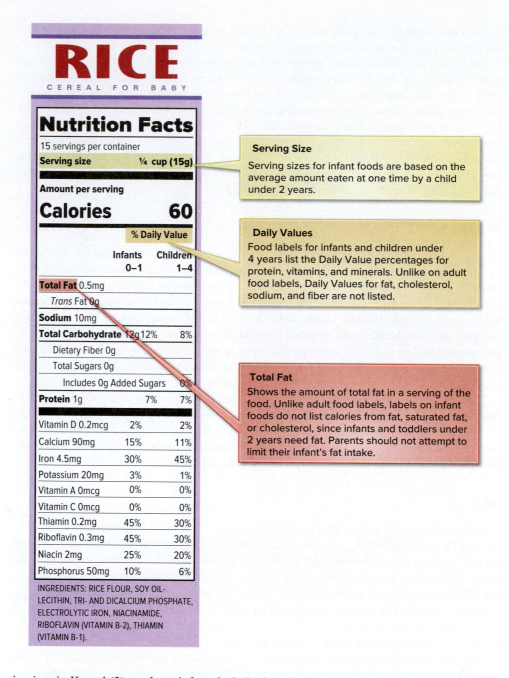

Serving Size
Serving sizes for infant foods are based on the average amount eaten at one time by a child under 2 years.

Daily Values
Food labels for infants and children under 4 years list the Daily Value percentages for protein, vitamins, and minerals. Unlike on adult food labels, Daily Values for fat, cholesterol, sodium, and fiber are not listed.

Total Fat
Shows the amount of total fat in a serving of the food. Unlike adult food labels, labels on infant foods do not list calories from fat, saturated fat, or cholesterol, since infants and toddlers under 2 years need fat. Parents should not attempt to limit their infant's fat intake.

in vitamin K; and (3) newborn infants lack the intestinal bacteria that synthesize vitamin K. Infant vitamin K deficiency can lead to a rare but potentially fatal bleeding problem. To prevent hemorrhage, vitamin K is routinely given by injection to all infants at birth.

For bone health, immune function, and chronic disease prevention, the American Academy of Pediatrics recommends that all infants and children consume 400 IU vitamin D per day starting soon after birth (review Section 11.5). Supplemental vitamin D is necessary for all breastfed infants, as well as for formula-fed infants who consume less than 1 quart (approximately 1 liter) of formula per day (see Further Reading 21). However, no further benefits are seen beyond 400 IU per day and toxicity is possible if intake exceeds 1000 IU per day. Any use of supplemental vitamin D can be discontinued when dietary sources provide at least 400 IU of vitamin D per day.

For breastfed infants whose mothers are total vegetarians (vegans), a supplemental source of vitamin B-12 is vitally important to prevent anemia, failure to thrive, and irreversible damage to the nervous system. Recall from Section 13.4 that vitamin B-12 is only found in foods of animal origin. Infant formula does contain vitamin B-12, but the breast milk of a mother who avoids all animal products will be deficient in vitamin B-12.

MINERALS OF SPECIAL INTEREST

Two minerals of special interest in the diets of infants are iron and fluoride. Infants also need adequate amounts of zinc (see Section 10.7) and iodine (see Section 12.8) to support growth. However, when human milk and infant formula are provided in quantities to meet kilocalorie needs, zinc and iodine requirements are generally met.

Infants are born with some internal stores of iron. However, if food sources of iron are not part of the infant's dietary pattern, body iron stores will be depleted by about 6 months of age. If the mother was iron deficient during the pregnancy, these iron stores will be exhausted even sooner. As you will recall from Section 13.7, iron-deficiency anemia can lead to poor mental development in infants. Several studies indicate that iron-deficiency anemia during infancy, even if corrected, has a lasting impact in terms of cognition, motor development, and behavior later in life.

To maintain a desirable iron status, the American Academy of Pediatrics recommends that formula-fed infants should be given an iron-fortified formula from birth. Years ago, low-iron formulas were prescribed for infants with gastrointestinal distress; however, current evidence shows that they do not improve GI symptoms but rather place an infant at risk for iron deficiency. Low-iron infant formulas are still available, but their use is strongly discouraged.

Breast milk is lower in iron than fortified infant formulas, but the form of iron in breast milk is much more bioavailable than the form in infant formula. Even so, by about 6 months of age, breastfed infants need solid foods to supply extra iron. This need for iron is a major consideration in the decision to introduce solid foods. Liquid iron supplements are rarely needed, except for preterm or LBW infants, those with blood disorders, or those born with inadequate stores of iron (i.e., due to maternal iron deficiency during pregnancy; see Further Reading 19).

Breast milk is a poor source of fluoride and formula manufacturers use fluoride-free water in formula preparation, so intake of this mineral during the first 6 months of life is low. However, fluoride supplementation is not advised before 6 months of age. After 6 months, the pediatrician or dentist may recommend fluoride supplements to aid in tooth development if fluoride supplied by tap water, foods, and toothpaste is inadequate.

WATER

An infant needs about 3 cups (700 to 800 milliliters) of water per day to regulate body temperature and transport oxygen, nutrients, and wastes throughout the body. For the vast majority of infants, human milk or formula supply enough water to keep the infant well hydrated.

In infants, dehydration can occur rapidly and have devastating consequences. In the first few days after birth, improper feeding techniques can leave an infant deprived of water and nutrients. In addition, protracted episodes of vomiting or diarrhea can quickly deplete an infant of fluid and electrolytes.

To identify dehydration, look for these signs:

- More than 6 hours without a wet diaper
- Dark-yellow or strong-smelling urine
- Unusually tired and fussy
- Dry mouth and lips
- Absence of tears when crying
- Eyes and soft spot on the head appear sunken
- Cold and splotchy hands and feet

Severe dehydration can result in rapid loss of kidney function and warrants medical intervention. In some cases, hospitalization and intravenous rehydration may be necessary. Most of the time, dehydration can be corrected with special fluid-replacement formulas containing electrolytes, such as sodium and potassium. These oral rehydration solutions (e.g., Pedialyte®) are available in supermarkets and pharmacies to treat mild to moderate dehydration. A health care provider should guide any use of these products.

Caregivers often wonder if breast milk or formula is sufficient to keep an infant hydrated, especially in hot weather. They may be tempted to give an infant supplemental water or fruit juice. In some stores, bottled water products marketed specifically for infants may be

The American Dental Association does not recommend fluoridated bottled water for use by infants because it heightens risk for enamel **fluorosis** during early tooth development.

fluorosis Discoloration of tooth enamel sometimes accompanied with pitting due to consuming a large amount of fluoride for an excessive period.

hyponatremia Dangerously low blood sodium level.

placed alongside infant formulas and electrolyte-replacement solutions, giving the mistaken impression that bottled water products are an appropriate feeding supplement or substitute for fluid replacement for infants. Even in hot weather, the American Academy of Pediatrics does not recommend supplemental water or juice during the first 6 months. Excess water can cause **hyponatremia** in infants. It is important to remember that excessive fluid can be harmful, especially to the brain.

Overall, it is best to rely exclusively on breast milk or infant formula to meet infant fluid needs up to 6 months of age, unless a health care provider suggests otherwise. In sum, extremes in fluid intake—either too little or too much—can lead to health problems.

✓ CONCEPT CHECK 19.2

1. Using the EER equations listed in Table 19-2, calculate the kilocalorie needs of a healthy 4-month-old infant who weighs 15 pounds (6.8 kilograms).

2. Review Table 19-3. Why is unaltered cow's milk NOT recommended for infant feeding?

3. Do infants require any supplemental vitamins or minerals? If so, which ones? What is the rationale for their use?

4. You are planning a family trip to the zoo on a hot summer day. How can you keep your 3-month-old baby from becoming dehydrated?

19.3 Guidelines for Infant Feeding

Oral nutrition for infants comes in two forms: human breast milk or infant formula. As you learned in Section 18.7, breastfeeding is the preferred method of infant feeding (review Table 18-4). Besides its benefits for immune development, improved mother-infant bonding, and lower long-term risk for chronic diseases, breast milk offers optimal nutrition that is uniquely suited for human infants. For mothers who do not breastfeed, whether due to necessity or preference, infant formula is a workable substitute. In fact, formula manufacturers model their products on human milk. In areas of the world with safe water supplies, formula feeding is a safe and nutritionally adequate alternative to breastfeeding.

BREAST MILK IS THE BEST MILK

Human milk is uniquely suited to meet the nutritional needs of human infants. Table 19-3 gives the composition of human milk, but recognize that these numbers are just estimates. Maternal diet and nutritional status may impact the composition of breast milk, particularly for fatty acids and some micronutrients. In addition, the true composition of human milk changes over time as the infant matures and even within a feeding.

Breast milk provides up to 55% of total kilocalories as fat. Fat is a dense source of kilocalories, so it helps to meet the high energy needs of the growing infant even though the infant cannot consume a large volume of milk at one time. Interestingly, the fat content of breast milk changes within each feeding. When the baby first latches on and begins suckling, the consistency of breast milk is thin and watery; the infant takes in necessary carbohydrates, protein, vitamins, and minerals. As the feeding goes on, the fat content of the milk increases to fulfill kilocalorie needs and satisfy the infant's hunger for a few hours. The specific types of fat in human milk are ideal for infants, too. The short- and medium-chain fatty acids in breast milk are easily digested. Some of the fatty acids—ARA and DHA—are essential for proper brain and eye development. If the mother's diet is rich in these fats, her milk will be a better source of them for her infant, as well.

Carbohydrates provide about 35% to 40% of the kilocalories in human milk. The main carbohydrate in human milk is lactose, a disaccharide that tastes sweet and is easily digested in the human infant's digestive tract. Although lactase production tends to decline later in

▲ Breastfeeding takes some skill and patience on the part of the mother, especially in the first few weeks, but the physical and emotional benefits are worth the effort. © Getty Images

life, lactose intolerance is quite rare among infants (review Section 4.4). Human milk also contains some oligosaccharides that have a **prebiotic** effect on the community of beneficial microorganisms in the infant's gut. A healthy microbial population in the GI tract influences development of the infant's immune system.

Protein supplies less than 10% of the total kilocalories in human milk. The kidneys of the newborn infant are still immature, so they can be stressed by high protein intakes. The proteins that are present in human milk are easily digested and unlikely to trigger food allergies. These proteins do more than supply kilocalories and building blocks for tissue synthesis. They also promote the proper development of the immune system and enhance nutrient absorption.

For the most part, the micronutrient needs of the infant can be met by human milk. A notable exception, described in Section 19.2, is vitamin D. Recall that the American Academy of Pediatrics recommends 400 IU per day of supplemental vitamin D for all infants (breastfed and formula-fed) until their dietary intake supplies this amount. For breastfed infants of mothers who follow a vegan diet, have had bariatric surgery, or have pernicious anemia, vitamin B-12 supplements are recommended. Last, if an infant has depleted iron stores (e.g., preterm birth or mother was deficient in iron during pregnancy), iron supplementation may be warranted.

Breastfeeding during infancy impacts future feeding behaviors, as well. Interesting research shows that the flavors of the mother's diet are transferred into her milk. This can positively affect the infant's acceptance of a variety of solid foods later in life. Breastfeeding also reinforces the natural ability of the infant or child to self-regulate food intake. The infant has to do some work to get milk from the mother's breast, so it is unlikely that the infant will override satiety cues and overeat from the breast. Much research supports the hypothesis that breastfed infants learn to eat based on internal cues of hunger and satiety, leading to better body weight management and lower risk for cardiovascular diseases and type 2 diabetes throughout life.

FORMULA FEEDING FOR INFANTS

Young infants cannot tolerate unaltered cow's milk because of its high protein and mineral content. Cow's milk is perfect for the growth needs of calves, but not for human infants! Thus, cow's milk must be altered by formula manufacturers to be safe for infant feeding. Altered forms of cow's milk, known as infant formulas, must conform to strict federal guidelines for nutrient composition and quality.

Formulas generally contain lactose and/or sucrose for carbohydrate, heat-treated proteins from cow's milk, and vegetable oils for fat (review Table 19-3). Soy protein–based formulas are available for vegan infants or those who cannot tolerate lactose or the types of proteins found in cow's milk. Infants with milk protein allergies are often sensitive to soy as well, so the best choice for infants with allergies is a **hydrolyzed protein formula.** In this type of formula, the proteins have been broken down into small polypeptides and amino acids. A variety of other specialized formulas are also available for specific medical conditions. In any case, it is important to use an iron-fortified formula unless a pediatrician recommends otherwise.

Some transition formulas/beverages have been introduced for older infants and toddlers (review Table 19-3). A few of these products are intended for use after 6 months of age if the infant is consuming solid foods, but most are intended for use only by toddlers (i.e., age 12 months and older). These transition products are lower in fat than human milk or standard infant formulas; their iron content is higher than that of cow's milk; and their overall mineral content is generally more like that of human milk than cow's milk. According to the manufacturers, the advantages of these transition formulas/beverages over standard formulas for older infants and toddlers include reduced cost and better flavor. Parents should consult their primary care provider with regard to the use of these products.

Infant formula comes in several different forms. Some infant formulas come in ready-to-feed, liquid form. These can be simply poured into a clean bottle and fed to the infant without further preparation. Powdered and concentrated fluid formula preparations are also

prebiotic Selectively fermented ingredient that results in specific changes in the composition and/or activity of the gastrointestinal microbiota, thus conferring benefits upon the host.

hydrolyzed protein formula Infant formula in which the proteins have been broken down into smaller peptides and amino acids to improve digestibility and reduce exposure to potential food allergens; sometimes called *predigested* or *hypoallergenic infant formula.*

Bisphenol A (BPA) is a chemical used in the production of many plastics. Human exposure to BPA, mainly through leaching of the chemical from packaging into foods and beverages, is widespread. Concern about exposure stems from animal studies that link high doses of BPA with reproductive and developmental defects and cancer. The consensus among regulatory agencies in the United States and Canada is that current levels of BPA exposure are not harmful, even for infants. Nevertheless, in response to public concern, FDA has banned the use of BPA in the manufacture of baby bottles, sippy cups, and packaging for infant formulas.

▲ FDA regulation is no longer necessary for the use of BPA-based materials in the manufacture of baby bottles because its use has been abandoned. © McGraw-Hill Education/Mark Dierker photographer

▲ Falling asleep while feeding is a sign that the infant has had enough to eat. © Steve Mason/Getty Images

commonly used. Powdered or concentrated formulas should be combined with clean, cold water, precisely following the directions on the formula label. The formula is then warmed, if desired, and fed immediately to the infant.

The following are some tips for safe preparation and storage of infant formula:

- All containers and utensils used to prepare formula should be washed with hot, soapy water and thoroughly rinsed with clean water before use. Household dishwashers are a good way to clean bottles and utensils, too. It is not necessary to boil the containers and utensils prior to use.
- Use cold water to prepare infant formula. Hot water that sits in a hot water heater or runs through pipes made with lead is more likely to accumulate contaminants than cold water (see Section 17.6). For homes with older plumbing systems, it is prudent to let cold tap water run for 1 to 2 minutes before filling a bottle or cup.
- If well water will be used to make infant formula, it should be tested regularly for contaminants, such as naturally occurring nitrates, which can lead to a severe form of anemia (especially among babies younger than 1 year).
- If microbial contamination of well water or municipal tap water is a concern, water should be brought to a rolling boil (for 1 minute) and then cooled to room temperature (for up to 30 minutes) before use in formula preparation. Caregivers should pay close attention to local water advisories. Some pediatricians recommend boiling (then cooling) the water to be used in formula preparation for infants up to 6 months of age, regardless of reports about water safety.
- American Dental Association does not recommend that formula be mixed with bottled "nursery water," which can be found alongside infant formula in most supermarkets, to limit risk of tooth discoloration from high fluoride levels.
- To warm a bottle of formula, run hot water over it or place it briefly in a pan of simmering water. Infant formulas should not be heated in a microwave oven because hot spots may develop, which can burn the infant's mouth and esophagus.
- Refrigerating prepared formula for 1 day is safe. However, formula left over from a feeding should be discarded because it will be contaminated by bacteria and enzymes from the infant's saliva.

FEEDING TECHNIQUE

Infants swallow a lot of air as they ingest either formula or human milk. To alleviate discomfort, it is important to burp an infant during feeding (every 1 to 2 ounces) and again at the end of the feeding. Spitting up a bit of milk is normal at this time.

Formula intake and feeding frequency may vary considerably from one infant to another and also from one day to the next. In general, a formula-fed infant should consume about 2 1/2 fluid ounces (75 milliliters) of formula per pound of body weight each day (see Table 19-4), up to about 32 fluid ounces (960 milliliters) in one day. In most cases, however, the infant's appetite is a better guide than any standardized recommendations. When the infant begins acting full, bottle feeding should be stopped, even if some milk is left in the bottle. Common signals that an infant has had enough include turning the head away, being inattentive, falling asleep, or becoming playful. Breastfeeding infants usually have had

TABLE 19-4 ■ Typical Formula Intake of Infants

Age	Amount per Feeding	Frequency
<1 month	2 to 3 fluid ounces (60 to 90 ml)	Every 3 to 4 hours
1 to 6 months	4 to 6 fluid ounces (120 to 180 ml)	Every 4 to 6 hours
6 to 12 months	6 to 8 fluid ounces (180 to 240 ml)*	Every 4 to 6 hours

Source: Data from American Academy of Pediatrics: *Caring for your baby and young child: Birth to age 5*. 6th ed. New York: Bantam Books, 2014.

*With introduction of age-appropriate solid foods

enough to eat after about 20 minutes. Although it is difficult to tell how much milk breastfed infants are getting, they also give signs when full.

By carefully observing and responding appropriately to the cues of the bottle-feeding or breastfeeding infant, caregivers can be assured that the infant's kilocalorie needs are being met and can (1) foster a climate of trust and responsiveness; and (2) help a child develop a habit of respecting internal cues of hunger and satiety.

EXPANDING THE INFANT'S MEALTIME CHOICES

By about 6 months of age, the infant is ready to start eating "table food." Initially, table foods add to—rather than replace—human milk or formula. In the first attempts to introduce solid foods, just getting the food into the infant's mouth may be a challenge. By the end of the first year, though, the infant should be eating a variety of protein sources, vegetables, fruits, and grains so that the diet begins to reflect a balanced pattern (Table 19-5). Throughout the process of expanding the infant's mealtime choices, the caregiver must proceed slowly and respond to the infant's cues that he or she is hungry or has had enough to eat. Feeding habits developed through early exposures to food will set the stage for healthy eating to last a lifetime.

Recognizing the Infant's Readiness for Solid Foods Parents may believe that the early addition of solid foods will help an infant sleep through the night. Actually, this achievement is a developmental milestone, and the type of food consumed by the infant is of little relevance to a good night's sleep. Before 4 to 6 months of age, infants are not physically mature enough to consume much solid food. Only occasionally does a rapidly growing infant need solid foods to meet kilocalorie and nutrient needs before 6 months of age.

▲ Iron-fortified rice cereal is recommended as the first solid food to be fed to infants.
© E. Dygas/Getty Images

TABLE 19-5 ■ Sample Daily Menu for a 1-Year-Old Child*

Breakfast	Snack
1 to 2 tbsp unsweetened applesauce	½ ounce cheddar cheese
¼ cup Cheerios®	4 whole-wheat crackers
½ cup whole milk	½ cup whole milk
Snack	**Dinner**
½ hard-cooked egg	1 ounce roasted turkey (finely diced)
½ slice whole-wheat toast with ½ tsp butter	1 to 2 tbsp mashed potatoes with ½ tsp butter
½ cup mandarin orange segments	1 to 2 tbsp cooked carrots (cut in strips, not coins)
½ cup water	½ cup whole milk
Lunch	**Snack**
1 ounce roasted chicken, minced	½ banana
1 to 2 tbsp rice with ½ tsp butter	2 oatmeal cookies (no raisins)
1 to 2 tbsp cooked peas	½ cup whole milk
½ cup whole milk	

Nutritional Analysis	
Total energy (kcal)	1100
% energy from	
Carbohydrate	40%
Protein	19%
Fat	41%

*This diet is just a start. A 1-year-old may need more or less food. In those cases, serving sizes should be adjusted. The milk can be fed by cup; some can be put into a bottle if the child has not been fully weaned from the bottle.

How does the caregiver know it is time to introduce solid foods? Infant size can serve as a rough indicator of readiness: reaching a weight of at least 13 pounds (6 kilograms) is a preliminary sign of readiness for solid foods. Another physiological cue is frequency of feeding, such as consuming more than 32 ounces (1 liter) of formula daily or breastfeeding more than 8 to 10 times within 24 hours. Underlying these noticeable signals are several important developmental factors:

1. *Nutritional need.* Before the infant is 6 months old, nutritional needs can generally be met with human milk and/or formula. After 6 months of age, however, many infants need additional kilocalories. In terms of individual nutrients, iron stores are exhausted by about 6 months of age. Developmentally appropriate, nutrient-dense foods will help to meet the infant's kilocalorie and iron needs.
2. *Physiological capabilities.* Before about 3 months of age, an infant's digestive tract cannot readily digest starch. Also, kidney function is limited until about 4 to 6 weeks of age. Until then, waste products from excessive amounts of dietary protein or minerals are difficult to excrete. As the infant ages, the ability to digest and metabolize a wider range of food components improves.
3. *Physical ability.* Three physical markers indicate that a child is ready for solid foods: (1) the disappearance of the extrusion reflex (thrusting the tongue forward and pushing food out of the mouth); (2) head and neck control; and (3) the ability to sit up with support. These usually occur around 4 to 6 months of age, but they vary with each infant.
4. *Allergy prevention.* A newborn infant's intestinal tract is "leaky"; whole proteins can readily be absorbed from birth until 4 to 5 months of age. If the infant is exposed too early to some types of proteins—particularly those in cow's milk and egg whites—the infant may be predisposed to future allergies and autoimmune conditions (e.g., type 1 diabetes). The best known way to minimize risk for allergies is to breastfeed the infant exclusively for the first 4 to 6 months of life (see Section 19.7).

With these considerations in mind—nutritional need, physiological and physical readiness, and allergy prevention—the American Academy of Pediatrics recommends that solid foods not be introduced until about 6 months of age and that infants receive no cow's milk before 1 year.

Foods to Match Needs and Developmental Abilities During the First Year If solid foods are introduced before 6 months of age, the primary goal of the food should be to meet iron needs. Therefore, the first solid foods should be iron-fortified cereals. Some pediatricians may recommend lean ground (strained) meats for more absorbable forms of iron. Rice is the best cereal to begin with because it is least likely to trigger allergies.

When starting solid foods, it is important to start with a teaspoon serving size of a single-ingredient food item, such as rice cereal, and increase the serving size gradually. Once the new food has been fed for about a week without adverse effects, another food can be added to the infant's diet. At first, this can be another type of cereal or perhaps a cooked and strained (or mashed) vegetable, meat, fruit, or egg yolk.

Waiting about 7 days between the introduction of each new food is important because it can take that long for evidence of an allergy or intolerance to materialize. Also, it is important to avoid introducing mixed foods until each component of the combination dish has been given separately without an adverse reaction. Signs of food allergies include diarrhea, vomiting, a rash, or wheezing. If one or more of these signs appears, the suspected problem food should be avoided for several weeks and then reintroduced in a small quantity. If the problem continues, a pediatrician should be consulted. Fortunately, many babies outgrow food allergies later in childhood.

Until 2008, parents and caregivers were advised to avoid feeding children a wide range of highly allergenic foods, including egg whites, chocolate, peanuts, tree nuts, fish, and other seafood. Now, the American Academy of Pediatrics acknowledges that there is no evidence that delaying introduction of solid foods—including these common food allergens—beyond 6 months of age is of any benefit for prevention of food allergies and other **atopic diseases** (see Further Reading 1).

atopic disease A condition involving an inappropriate immune response to environmental allergens; examples include asthma, eczema, and seasonal allergies.

Example of Typical Solid Food Progression, Starting at 6 Months of Age*

Week 1	Rice cereal
Week 2	Add strained carrots
Week 3	Add applesauce
Week 4	Add oat cereal
Week 5	Add cooked egg yolk
Week 6	Add strained chicken
Week 7	Add strained peas
Week 8	Add plums

*Extending the rice cereal step for a month or so is advised if solid food introduction begins at 4 months of age. Also, if at any point signs of allergy or intolerance develop, substitute another similar food item.

Many strained foods for infant feeding are available at the supermarket. Single-food items are more desirable than mixed dinners and desserts, which are less nutrient dense. Most brands have no added salt, but some fruit desserts contain added sugar, which is not recommended for infant feeding. Read food labels carefully to find the most nutrient-dense foods for infants.

As an alternative to store-bought baby foods, plain, unseasoned cooked foods—vegetables, fruits, and meats—can be ground up in an inexpensive baby food grinder at home. Another option is to puree a larger amount of food in a blender, freeze it in ice-cube portions, store in plastic bags, and defrost and warm as needed. Careful attention to food safety is necessary. Seasonings that may please the rest of the family should not be added to infant foods made at home. The infant does not notice the difference if salt, sugar, or spices are omitted. It is best to introduce infants to a variety of foods, so that by the end of the first year, the infant is consuming many foods—human milk or formula, meats, fruits, vegetables, and grains.

To ease early attempts at feeding solid foods, consider the following tips:

- Use a baby-sized spoon; a small spoon with a long handle is best.
- Hold the infant comfortably on the lap, as for breastfeeding or bottle feeding, but a little more upright to ease swallowing. When in this position, the infant expects food.
- Put a small dab of food on the spoon tip and gently place it on the infant's tongue.
- Convey a calm and casual approach to the infant, who needs time to get used to food.
- Expect the infant to take only two or three bites of the first meals.
- Present a new food on several consecutive days to aid an infant's acceptance of that food.

Self-feeding skills require coordination and can develop only if the infant is allowed to practice and experiment. By 6 to 7 months of age, the infant has learned to handle finger foods and transfer objects from one hand to the other with some dexterity. At about this time, teeth also begin to appear. By age 7 to 8 months, infants can push food around on a plate, play with a drinking cup, hold a bottle, and self-feed a cracker or a piece of toast. Through mastery of these manipulations, infants develop confidence and self-esteem. It is important that parents be patient and support these early self-feeding attempts, even though they appear inefficient.

At 9 to 10 months of age, the infant's desire to explore, experience, and play with foods may hinder feeding. Food is used as a means to explore the environment, and therefore, feeding time is often very messy—a bowl of macaroni may end up in the child's hair! Caregivers need to relax and take this phase of infant development in stride. By the end of the first year, finger-feeding becomes more efficient, and chewing is easier as more teeth erupt. Still, experimentation and unpredictability are to be expected.

WEANING FROM THE BREAST OR BOTTLE

Around the age of 6 months, expressed breast milk, formula, or water can be offered in a sippy cup with a wide, flat bottom. Drinking from a cup rather than from a bottle helps to prevent **early childhood caries** (Fig. 19-3). If an infant drinks continuously from a bottle, the carbohydrate-rich fluid bathes the teeth, providing an ideal growth medium for bacteria adhering to the teeth. These bacteria then make acids, which dissolve tooth enamel. To avoid dental caries, infants should not be put to bed with a bottle or placed in an infant seat with a bottle propped up.

By about 10 months of age, infants are learning to self-feed and likewise to drink independently from a cup. As children drink from a cup more frequently, fewer bottle feedings and/or breastfeedings are necessary. Infants should begin drinking from a cup by 1 year of age and should be completely weaned from a bottle by 18 months of age. The added mobility of crawling and walking should naturally lead to gradual weaning from the bottle or breast. Even so, getting a baby out of the bedtime-bottle habit can be difficult. Determined caregivers can either endure a few nights of their baby's crying or slowly wean the baby away from the bottle with either a pacifier or water (for a week or so).

▲ Repeated exposure fosters acceptance of new tastes and textures. © Corbis/PictureQuest

early childhood caries Tooth decay that results from formula or juice (and even human milk) bathing the teeth as the child sleeps with a bottle in the mouth. The upper teeth are mostly affected as the lower teeth are protected by the tongue; formerly called *nursing bottle syndrome* and *baby bottle tooth decay.*

FIGURE 19-3 ▲ Early childhood caries. An extreme example of tooth decay probably resulting from frequently putting the child to bed with a bottle. The upper teeth have decayed almost all the way to the gum line. © Paul Casamassimo, DDS, MS

▲ Infants should begin drinking from a cup by 1 year of age. Cups with lids help to prevent spills, but caregivers should allow a toddler to practice without a lid as dexterity and coordination improve. © Digital Vision/Getty Images

WHAT TO FEED AN INFANT

It can be difficult for new parents to make sense of nutrition goals for infants in the face of changing dietary recommendations from health authorities, cultural preferences, and outdated advice from friends and family. In response to various controversies surrounding infant feeding, the American Academy of Pediatrics has issued a number of statements concerning infant diets. The following guidelines are based on these statements:

- *Build to a variety of foods.* For the first 6 months of life, human milk (or infant formula) is all an infant needs. (Vitamin D supplementation is an exception.) When the infant is ready, start adding new foods, one at a time. During the first year, the goal is to teach an infant to enjoy a variety of nutritious foods. A lifetime of healthy eating habits begins with this important first step.
- *Pay attention to your infant's appetite to avoid overfeeding or underfeeding.* Feed infants when they are hungry. Never force an infant to finish an unwanted serving of food. Watch for signs that indicate hunger or fullness. This will reinforce the infant's natural capability to self-regulate food intake.
- *Infants need fat.* Although excessive intake of fat contributes to many adult health problems, it is an essential source of kilocalories for growing infants. Fat also helps the nervous system to develop.
- *Choose fruits, vegetables, and grains, but do not overdo high-fiber foods.* During the second half of the first year, infants should be fed a variety of fruits and vegetables. However, studies show that by 1 year of age, vegetable choices are dominated by white potatoes. Continuing to offer choices of colorful vegetables during late infancy and the toddler years will enhance intake of important vitamins, minerals, and phytochemicals. In terms of fiber, although many adults benefit from high-fiber diets, they are not ideal for infants. They are bulky, filling, and often low in kilocalories. The natural amounts of fiber and nutrients in fruits, vegetables, and grains are appropriate as part of a healthy infant diet.
- *Infants need sugars in moderation.* Sugars are an additional source of kilocalories for active, rapidly growing infants. Foods such as human milk, fruits, and small portions of 100% juices are natural sources of sugars and other nutrients as well. On the other hand, an excessive intake of added sugars, particularly from sugar-sweetened beverages, contributes to the epidemic of childhood obesity. Caregivers should choose infant foods that do not contain added sugars. Foods that contain artificial sweeteners should also be avoided; they do not provide the kilocalories or nutrients growing infants need.
- *Infants need sodium in moderation.* Sodium is a necessary mineral found naturally in almost all foods. As part of a healthy diet, infants need sodium for their bodies to work properly. However, average intakes of sodium among infants and toddlers are above the AI. Caregivers should delay introduction of cow's milk (a natural source of sodium) until 1 year of age and refrain from offering heavily seasoned and processed foods.
- *Choose foods containing iron, zinc, and calcium.* Infants need good sources of iron, zinc, and calcium for optimum growth throughout the first 2 years. These minerals are important for healthy blood, optimal growth, and strong bones. Many infant and toddler foods (e.g., cereal, crackers, and biter biscuits) are fortified with these minerals.

WHAT NOT TO FEED AN INFANT

The following are several foods and practices to avoid when feeding an infant:

- *Excessive infant formula or human milk.* After 6 months of age, solid foods should play an increasing role in satisfying an infant's growing appetite. Age-appropriate solid foods provide necessary kilocalories and iron, plus they help the infant to develop motor skills. About 24 to 32 ounces (¾ to 1 liter) of human milk or formula daily is ideal after 6 months, with complementary foods supplying the rest of the infant's kilocalorie needs.
- *Foods that tend to cause choking.* Foods that are round or ovoid in shape, larger than a 0.5 inch in diameter, or of a soft or sticky texture can easily get lodged in a child's

throat. These foods include hot dogs, hard or gummy candies, whole nuts, grapes, coarsely cut meats, raw carrots, popcorn, and peanut butter. Caregivers should not allow younger children to gobble snack foods during playtime and should supervise all meals.

- *Potential food allergens before 6 months of age.* Cow's milk, egg whites, peanuts, tree nuts, soy, and wheat are responsible for 90% of food allergies in childhood. If any solid foods are introduced before 6 months of age, they should be iron-fortified rice or oat cereals, pureed meats, vegetables, or fruits.

- *Cow's milk, especially low-fat or fat-free cow's milk.* The American Academy of Pediatrics strongly urges parents not to give children under age 2 fat-reduced, 1%, or fat-free milk. Before age 2, the amount of this milk needed to meet kilocalorie needs would supply too many minerals and in turn could overwhelm the kidneys' ability to excrete the excess. The lower fat intake might also harm nervous system development. Beyond 2 years, children can drink fat-reduced, 1%, or fat-free milk, because by this age they are consuming enough solid foods to meet kilocalorie and fat needs.

- *Goat's milk.* Although perceived by some to pose lower risk for food allergies, goat's milk is low in folate, iron, vitamin C, and vitamin D, and should not be used as a source of nourishment for infants.

- *Excessive fruit juice.* The fructose and sorbitol contained in some fruit juices, especially apple and pear juices, can lead to diarrhea because they are slowly absorbed. Also, if fruit juice or related drink products are replacing formula or milk in the diet, the infant may not be receiving adequate kilocalories, calcium, or other nutrients essential for proper growth. Studies have shown a link between excessive amounts of fruit juice and failure to thrive, GI tract complications, obesity, short stature, and poor dental health. Thus, these substances should be used sparingly. Limit fruit juice to 4 to 6 ounces per day for children from 6 months to 6 years of age.

- *Food safety hazards.* The immune system is still maturing during infancy and early childhood, so it is important to avoid potential sources of foodborne illness (review Chapter 17). For example, raw (unpasteurized) milk or soft cheeses (e.g., queso fresco) may be contaminated with bacteria or viruses. Meat, poultry, eggs, and seafood should be cooked to proper temperatures. In addition, honey may contain spores of *Clostridium botulinum,* which can lead to the potentially fatal foodborne illness known as *botulism.* Safe food handling starts with proper handwashing.

- *Excessive nutrient supplementation.* Intake of supplemental vitamins or minerals above 100% of the RDA or AI for age can increase risk for nutrient toxicities.

A Summary of Infant Feeding Recommendations

Breastfed Infants

- Breastfeed for 6 months or longer, if possible. Then introduce infant formula if and when breastfeeding declines or ceases. (Breast milk can also be pumped and placed in a bottle for later use.)

- Provide a vitamin D supplement (400 IU per day).

- Investigate the need for vitamin B-12, fluoride, and iron supplementation to prevent deficiencies.

Formula-Fed Infants

- Use iron-fortified infant formula for the first year of life.

- Provide a vitamin D supplement if formula intake provides less than 400 IU per day.

- Investigate the need for a fluoride supplement if the water supply is not fluoridated.

All Infants

- Add iron-fortified cereal at about 6 months of age.

- Provide a variety of basic, soft foods after 6 months of age, advancing to a varied diet.

CASE STUDY Undernutrition during Infancy

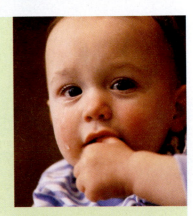

© Jules Frazier/Getty Images

Damon is a 7-month-old boy who has been taken into a clinic for a routine checkup. On examination, he was found to be moderately underweight relative to his age and body length. His pediatrician scheduled a follow-up appointment in 3 months. At the 10-month visit, Damon appeared sluggish and was even more underweight for his age and length.

A registered dietitian nutritionist interviewed Damon's 16-year-old mother to collect information on Damon's dietary intake. His intake over the previous 24 hours consisted of two 8-ounce bottles of infant formula, three 8-ounce bottles of Kool-Aid®, and a hot dog. Damon may have been fed some additional items on the nights that his mother left him with a neighbor, so that she could go out with friends for a few hours. Thus, she was not aware of all that he ate.

Answer the following questions, and check your responses at the end of this chapter.

1. Damon's mother did not specify what type of formula she gives to her child or how she prepares it. What questions would you ask about his formula?
2. What potential dangers await Damon if his growth continues to lag behind?
3. What foods should Damon's caregivers offer that are appropriate for his age and nutritional needs?
4. What problems might arise from consumption of sugary drinks from a bottle?
5. Does Damon need any vitamin or mineral supplements?

✓ CONCEPT CHECK 19.3

1. List three similarities between human milk and infant formula. List three differences.
2. Describe four ways to assess an infant's readiness for solid foods.
3. Excessive intake of added sugars is common in late infancy. Describe several ways to limit intake of added sugars in an infant's diet.
4. List three foods to avoid feeding infants during the first year of life.

Quick Guide to Child Nutrition Needs

Carbohydrates

- 130 grams per day to supply energy for the central nervous system and prevent ketosis

Protein

- 13 to 19 grams per day (ages 1 to 3)
- 34 to 52 grams per day (older children)

Fat

- 5 grams (minimum) per day of essential fatty acids
- 30% to 40% of total kcal (ages 1 to 3)
- 25% to 35% of total kcal (older children)

19.4 Toddlers and Preschool Children: Nutrition Concerns

The rapid growth rate that characterizes infancy tapers off during the toddler and preschool years. The average annual weight gain is only 4.5 to 6.6 pounds (2 to 3 kilograms) and the average annual height gain is only 3 to 4 inches (7.5 to 10 centimeters) between the ages of 2 and 5. As the growth rate tapers off, energy needs decrease and eating behaviors change. For example, among toddlers, the decreased growth rate leads to a decreased appetite, often called "picky eating."

Energy needs (relative to body weight) gradually decline from approximately 100 kcal per kilogram during infancy to about 90 kcal per kilogram for the preschooler. As you can see in Table 19-6, as the child gets older, physical activity level is a consideration when determining energy requirements.

Except in cases of poverty or homelessness (review Section 16.2), the diets of toddlers and preschoolers in the United States and Canada are adequate in calories and most nutrients. A few nutrients of particular concern among this age group are iron, calcium, and sodium (see Further Reading 13).

Iron Childhood iron-deficiency anemia is most likely to appear in children between the ages of 6 and 24 months—a time when iron stores from gestation have run out, but intake of iron from food sources may be inadequate. It can lead to decreases in both stamina and learning ability because the oxygen supply to cells decreases. Another effect is lowered resistance to disease. The targeted efforts of the Special Supplemental Nutrition Program for Women, Infants, and Children (WIC) have helped to decrease the occurrence of iron deficiency among children, but it still remains a problem for almost 16% of toddlers and about 5% of preschoolers.

The RDA for iron is 7 milligrams per day for children ages 1 to 3 and 10 milligrams per day for children ages 4 to 8. The best way to prevent iron-deficiency anemia in children is to provide foods that are adequate sources of iron. Even though some animal products are high in saturated fat and cholesterol, the high proportion of heme iron in many animal foods

TABLE 19-6 ■ Approximate Energy Needs of Toddlers and Preschoolers

Boys				Girls			
	Physical Activity				Physical Activity		
Age	Sedentary	Moderately Active	Active	Age	Sedentary	Moderately Active	Active
2	1000	1000	1000	2	1000	1000	1000
3	1000	1400	1400	3	1000	1200	1400
4	1200	1400	1600	4	1200	1400	1400
5	1200	1400	1600	5	1200	1400	1600

Source: Dietary Guidelines 2015–2020, http://health.gov/dietaryguidelines/2015/guidelines/appendix-2/

allows the iron to be more readily absorbed than is iron from plant foods. Focus on lean cuts of meat, such as ground sirloin. Fortified breakfast cereals also contribute to meeting iron (and other nutrient) needs. Consuming a source of vitamin C will aid absorption of the less readily absorbed iron in plants, fortified foods, and supplements. While dietary changes can be effective for preventing iron-deficiency anemia, supplementation will be required to correct existing anemia (review Section 13.5).

Calcium Childhood is a period of rapid bone growth and mineralization. As you learned in Section 11.1, bone mass can only accrue until the early twenties; after age 30, bone mass starts to decline. It is vital, therefore, to maximize bone mass during childhood and adolescence. The RDA for calcium for ages 1 to 3 is 700 milligrams per day. Between the ages of 4 and 8, calcium needs increase to 1000 milligrams per day. However, national surveys of food intake show that the diets of children fall short of the RDA for this important nutrient.

Milk and other dairy products are the primary source of calcium in the diets of children, but unfortunately, milk consumption has declined as intake of sweetened beverages has increased. Two cups per day of milk will help toddlers and preschoolers meet their requirements for bone-building nutrients. Children up to 2 years of age should drink whole milk because they need the extra fat for energy, but after 2 years of age, reduced-fat or fat-free milk is preferred. For children who do not consume dairy products, whether due to choice or necessity, there are alternative sources of calcium and other bone-building nutrients. Fortified beverages, such as soy milk, almond milk, or orange juice, can supply as much calcium per serving as cow's milk (see Section 11.11). Some legumes and vegetables are sources of calcium, as well, but the mineral is not as bioavailable as it is from dairy foods.

Sodium While iron and calcium intakes fall short of needs in preschool children, excessive sodium intake is a concern (see Further Reading 8). High intakes of fast foods and highly processed foods elevate sodium intakes to about 1000 milligrams per day more than preschoolers need. Caregivers can lower sodium intake by limiting salt added during cooking and at the table, by cutting back on use of highly processed foods (e.g., luncheon meats and hot dogs), by rinsing canned beans and vegetables before cooking, and by encouraging consumption of fruits, vegetables, and whole grains in place of prepackaged snacks.

Feeding skills are an important part of physical and cognitive development. Young children explore their environment through the tastes and textures of foods, develop dexterity using utensils and drinking from a cup, and begin to express their autonomy by refusing certain foods. At this time in life, children are also testing boundaries to find out what is acceptable in their little corner of the world. Messy mealtimes, food refusals, and **food jags** can be sources of tension in families. Creating a more harmonious family atmosphere at mealtime is an important way to keep these behaviors from becoming serious feeding problems (see "Understanding 'Picky Eating'" later in this section). Caregivers must understand that these are normal phases of child development but should also be consistent about setting limits for behavior at the dinner table.

Because of the preschool child's reduced appetite, planning a dietary pattern that meets nutrient needs poses a special challenge to caregivers. Nutrient density is an important consideration for this age group. Overall, parents should focus on offering a variety of healthy choices, allowing the child to exert some autonomy over the specific type of food and the amount eaten.

MyPlate is a useful, easy-to-understand tool for children. The *proportions* apply to all ages, even though the *portions* will be smaller for children. Table 19-7 gives a general food plan that conforms to MyPlate proportions and is appropriate for preschool and school-age children. Until a child is about 5 years of age, a good starting point for portion sizes in the vegetables group, fruits group, and protein group is about 1 tablespoon per year of life. The serving sizes and the number of servings per day can be increased as needed to meet the recommendations outlined in Table 19-7. The same advice does not

▲ Cow's milk is a source of bioavailable calcium and vitamin D for toddlers and preschoolers, but overreliance on milk can crowd out other nutrient-dense foods. Children who drink more than 3 cups of milk per day are likely to consume inadequate amounts of iron and fiber. © Andrew Olney/age fotostock

food jag A period of time (usually a few days or weeks) during which a person will eat only a limitied variety of foods.

▲ MyPlate Kids' Place features educational games, music, and other activities. See http://www.choosemyplate.gov/kids. Source: USDA

TABLE 19-7 ■ Food Plans for Children Based on MyPlate Daily Checklists

Food Group	Serving Size	Approximate Number of Servings[a]				
		Age 2[b]	Age 5[b]	Age 8[b]	Age 12[b, c]	Age 16[b, c]
Grains	ounce	3	5	5	6–7	6–10
Vegetables	cup	1	1.5	2	2.5–3	2.5–3.5
Fruits	cup	1	1.5	1.5	1.5–2	2–2.5
Dairy	cup	2	2.5	2.5	3	3
Protein	ounce	2	4	5	5–6	5.5–7
Limit these to:						
Sodium	milligrams	1500	1900	1900	2200	2300
Saturated fat	grams	11	16	18	20–24	22–31
Added sugar	grams	25	35	40	45–55	50–70

[a]Log on to www.chooseMyPlate.gov for other ages and other physical activity levels.

[b]Based on 30–60 minutes of physical activity per day.

[c]The lower amounts are appropriate for girls.

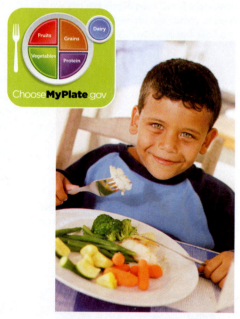

▲ How does this boy's dinner of broiled fish, broccoli, green beans, carrots, and squash compare to MyPlate? Which groups are missing? © BananaStock/PunchStock

Renowned child nutrition expert Ellyn Satter, MS, RDN, explains, "Parents are responsible for the *what, when,* and *where* of feeding; children are responsible for the *how much* and *whether* of eating."

apply to the grains or dairy groups, but consuming too much milk can leave the diet short on iron.

Luckily, normal-weight children have a built-in feeding mechanism that adjusts hunger to regulate food intake at each stage of growth. If a child is developing and growing normally and the caregiver is providing a variety of healthful foods, all can be confident of the child's well-being.

It is important to promote a healthy attitude about eating. While caregivers will want to focus on nutrient-dense foods, there is no reason to be overly restrictive about child food choices. In fact, when parents are extremely controlling about the family's food intake, children may be at risk for body dissatisfaction and disordered eating. There is room for occasional indulgences, a skipped meal or two, or once in a while "less than ideal" choices. It is eating and lifestyle patterns over the course of a month (and lifetime) that matter. Children master their eating when adults set a good example, provide opportunities to learn, give support for exploration, and limit inappropriate behavior.

In the next part of this section, we will consider some typical complaints and concerns of parents, explore the causes, and make suggestions for achieving optimal nutrition during the toddler and preschool years. Beyond these pages, USDA's MyPlate (www.ChooseMyPlate.gov) and Team Nutrition (www.fns.usda.gov/tn/team-nutrition) offer resources for planning nutritious, age-appropriate meals and snacks. Additional nutrition guidance, starting with pregnancy and extending through the preschool years, is available from the Start Healthy, Stay Healthy Resource Center at www.gerber.com.

UNDERSTANDING "PICKY EATING"

Many parents are baffled by their toddler's erratic eating behaviors. Toddlers and preschoolers tend not to eat as much or as regularly as infants. One day, a young child may pick at his food and staunchly refuse to eat his green beans, but on the next day, he might ask for a second helping. Parents often need reminding that toddlers and preschoolers cannot be expected to eat as voraciously as infants or to eat adult-size portions. Because the growth rate slows after infancy, a toddler's drive to eat is not so intense. In addition, children are sometimes more interested in playing and exploring than eating!

Youngsters also tend to be wary of new foods. One reason is that they have more taste buds, and their taste buds are more sensitive than those of adults. A general distrust of unfamiliar things is common in this age group. Thus, familiarity plays an important role in food acceptance.

Adults can encourage young children to broaden their food repertoire by repeating exposure to new food choices. It may take 10 or more exposures to a new food before a child finds it acceptable, but if adults can be patient and persevere, children will build good food habits.

Food preferences change rapidly in childhood and are influenced by food temperature, appearance, texture, and taste. The following are a few practical tips for improving acceptance of nutrient-dense foods.

- Build on what they know and accept. Pairing a new food item with a familiar one can help to foster acceptance of the new food.
- Enlist the child's aid in food selection and preparation. For example, let the child pick out the tomatoes and squash from the local farmers market.
- Serve meals on a sectioned plate. Sometimes children object to having foods mixed, as in stews and casseroles, even if they normally like the ingredients separately.
- Keep it crunchy. Certain food characteristics, such as crisp textures and mild flavors, are appealing to children. Kids who reject mushy, cooked carrots may enjoy them raw or lightly steamed. (After about age 4, children can safely eat raw vegetables without fear of choking.)
- Finger foods are fun. Preschoolers eventually develop skill with spoons and forks and can even use dull knives, but it is still a good idea to serve some finger foods, especially with healthy dips such as yogurt sauce or hummus.
- Save the best for last. If a child is prone to leave his or her chicken on the plate untouched, serve the chicken first. Hunger is the best means of getting a child to eat!

▲ Letting a child help select or prepare her food can increase the likelihood she will eat her food. © Indeed/Aflo/Getty Images

The dinner table should not become a battleground. Caregivers should avoid nagging, forcing, and bribing children to encourage eating. Using dessert as leverage to get a child to eat vegetables tends to elevate the status of dessert, while making the vegetables seem less palatable. Indirectly, such tactics reinforce picky-eating behaviors due to the added attention given to them. In addition, pressuring children to clean their plates may teach them to override their internal cues for satiety. One reasonable policy is the one-bite rule: children should take at least one bite or taste of the foods presented to them. Also, caregivers should realize that what they *do* speaks louder than what they *say;* if caregivers eat a variety of nutrient-dense foods, children will imitate their behavior.

When a child refuses to eat, it is best not to overreact. Doing so may give the child the idea that not eating is a means of getting attention or manipulating a scene. Most children do not starve themselves to any point approaching physical harm. When children refuse to eat, have them sit at the table for a while; if they still are not interested in eating, remove the food and wait until the next scheduled meal or snack. Finally, instead of giving attention to negative behaviors, focus on positive behaviors when they occur. Praise a child for trying something new. Overall, mealtime should be a relaxed, pleasant opportunity to enjoy healthful foods and good company (see Further Reading 2).

Food jags, common among preschoolers, are typically no cause for alarm. A child may switch from one specific food focus to another with equal intensity (older infants may also act this way). If the caregiver continues to offer choices, the child will soon begin to eat a wider variety of foods again, and the specific food focus will disappear as suddenly as it appeared.

Although picky eating is usually just a manifestation of slower growth and a desire for autonomy, a child's sudden loss of appetite may be a sign of underlying illness, such as an infection or gastrointestinal problem. Be alert for signs of eating disorders, as well. Extreme, self-imposed dietary restrictions could be an early sign of anorexia nervosa (review Section 15.2). Alternatively, **avoidant/restrictive food intake disorder (ARFID)** is an eating disorder primarily diagnosed among children. With this disorder, a child lacks interest in eating specific foods or all foods in general, which leads to weight loss or failure to grow as expected, as well as many nutrient deficiencies. The restricted food intake is much more severe than the picky eating or intermittent food refusal typical of childhood; children with this disorder become malnourished and may need tube feeding or intravenous feeding. It is most likely related to stress, anxiety, or depression. In some cases, the disorder may be a response to an adverse experience, such as choking or vomiting after eating a certain food.

avoidant/restrictive food intake disorder (ARFID) Eating disorder characterized by failure to meet energy or nutrient needs, resulting in significant weight loss, nutritional deficiencies, or dependence on tube or intravenous feeding; the eating disturbance is not better explained by lack of available food, a medical problem, or another eating disorder.

REDEFINE SNACKING

Parents may be concerned that frequent snacking will prevent children from eating well at mealtimes. However, children have small stomachs and need to eat every 3 to 4 hours. Sticking to three meals a day offers no special nutritional advantages; it is just a social custom.

TABLE 19-8 ■ Twenty Healthy Snack Ideas for Children

	Iron	Zinc	Calcium	Vitamin C	Fiber
Almonds (1 oz)*			✓		✓
Unsweetened applesauce (1/2 cup)				✓	✓
Bean and cheese burrito (1)	✓	✓	✓		✓
Cheese (1 oz) and whole-wheat crackers (6)	✓	✓	✓		✓
Reduced-sugar dried cranberries (1/4 cup)				✓	✓
Frozen fruit pieces (1 cup)				✓	✓
Fruit salad (1 cup)				✓	✓
Fruit smoothie with bananas and strawberries (1 cup)				✓	✓
Hard-boiled egg	✓	✓			
Hummus (2 tbsp) with bell pepper rings (1 cup)				✓	✓
Low-fat microwave popcorn (3 tbsp unpopped)*					✓
Mini-pizzas on whole-grain English muffins (2)	✓	✓	✓	✓	
Peanut butter (2 tbsp) and apple slices (1 cup)*		✓			✓
Quick breads, such as banana bread, 1 slice	✓				✓
String cheese (1 stick)		✓	✓		
Trail mix (1/4 cup)*	✓	✓			✓
Tuna salad (1/2 cup) in whole-wheat pita pocket	✓	✓			✓
Whole-grain cereal (1 cup)	✓	✓		✓	✓
Whole-wheat pasta salad with veggies (1 cup)	✓	✓			✓
Yogurt (6 oz) with granola (2 tbsp)			✓		✓

*Snack items that are best suited for children older than age 4 due to potential for choking.

▲ For children older than age 4, crunchy raw vegetables with hummus make a good afternoon snack. © Ingram Publishing/SuperStock

Instead, offering five or six small meals can help children meet their nutritional requirements more successfully than limiting them to three meals each day. If the stretch between lunch and dinner is 6 hours, an afternoon snack about 2 hours before dinner could provide some needed nutrients and may preempt a cranky attitude at the evening meal.

The location of snacking is important. Sitting calmly at the table instead of running around the house will decrease the risk for choking. Limiting distractions by turning off the television will help to prevent mindless eating. The caregiver could offer two or three nutrient-dense options and allow the child to choose one; responsibility for food choices by the child should start at an early age. Lastly, caregivers should promote handwashing and good oral hygiene just as for a meal.

When we eat is not nearly as important as *what* we eat. Perhaps families simply need to redefine snacking altogether. A snack should not be synonymous with an indulgent dessert. Rather, a snack should be a small meal of nutrient-dense foods. Let hunger—not the clock—guide the timing of meals and snacks. It is important that these snack choices be planned ahead in order to have healthy choices available (Table 19-8). Fruits and vegetables (fresh, frozen, or canned) and whole-grain breads and crackers are good snack choices. Working parents should make sure their children are provided with nutritious snacks to tide them over until dinnertime.

CHOOSE DIETARY SUPPLEMENTS CAREFULLY

Major scientific groups, such as the Academy of Nutrition and Dietetics and the American Society for Nutrition, state that multivitamin and mineral supplements are generally unnecessary for healthy children; it is better to emphasize whole foods. In fact, consuming fortified foods and supplements may lead to intakes above the UL for some nutrients, such as vitamin A and zinc. Children's supplements that are made to look like candy may result in accidental overdose, particularly of iron. Fortified, low-sugar, ready-to-eat breakfast cereals with milk are especially helpful in closing any gap between current micronutrient intake and needs, such as for folate, vitamin D, vitamin E, iron, or zinc.

For a child who is ill, has a very erratic food preference pattern or appetite, or is on a weight-loss diet, the American Academy of Pediatrics states that the child may benefit from a children's multivitamin and mineral supplement not exceeding 100% of Daily Values on the label. Still, as mentioned many times in this book, such a practice does not substitute for an otherwise healthy dietary pattern—children included. If current childhood feeding practices are to become more healthful, the focus should be on whole-grain breads and cereals, fruits, vegetables, and lean sources of protein, and low-fat milk and milk products.

REDUCE LEAD POISONING

Humans may be exposed to lead from drinking contaminated water, consuming or inhaling lead dust (e.g., from cracked and peeling lead paint), contaminated dietary supplements (e.g., calcium supplements derived from bone meal), or foods stored or prepared in lead-containing vessels. In the United States, nearly half a million children between the ages of 1 and 5 have unacceptably high blood lead levels. Young children are particularly vulnerable to lead poisoning because they are small, absorb lead quickly, spend a lot of time on the floor, and are apt to put objects in their mouths. In the short term, symptoms of lead poisoning include gastrointestinal distress, lack of appetite, irritability, fatigue, and anemia. Over the long term, devastating effects include intellectual and behavioral impairments and increased risk for several chronic diseases in adulthood.

Although it does not address the source of exposure, proper nutrition can reduce the risks of lead poisoning for children. Consuming regular meals, moderating fat intake, and ensuring adequate iron and calcium status are dietary practices known to reduce lead absorption. Adequate zinc, thiamin, and vitamin E intakes also reduce the harmful effects of absorbed lead. For lowest lead levels, only cold water should be used for drinking and preparation of formula or food. Letting cold water run from the tap for about 2 minutes after a long period of inactivity (e.g., overnight) will limit the amount of lead that has accumulated in tap water. If the public water supply contains a high concentration of lead, bottled water is a safer alternative, particularly for formula preparation. Overall, a balanced meal plan that offers a variety of whole grains, lean meats, and low-fat dairy products is especially useful for protecting children from lead poisoning.

ALLEVIATE CONSTIPATION WITH LIFESTYLE CHANGES

Constipation, a common problem among children, can be defined as hard, dry stools that are difficult to pass. Typically, a 4-year-old child has one bowel movement per day, but normal bowel habits vary widely. Therefore, the frequency of bowel movements is not as important as the consistency of stools. Pediatricians diagnose constipation after 2 or more weeks of delayed or difficult bowel movements. In rare situations, constipation can be a sign of a serious problem. If a child has a fever or vomiting along with constipation, if there is blood in the stool, or if the abdomen becomes swollen, caregivers should seek immediate medical attention.

What causes constipation? Although there could be a serious medical problem, most cases are related to lifestyle. Lack of physical activity contributes to constipation. Also, on average, children (and adults) in the United States barely obtain half of the AI for fiber. Altered bowel habits also may be a sign of a food allergy or intolerance to a food component such as cow's milk. The majority of the time, however, constipation results from the child withholding bowel movements. For children, a painful bowel movement can be so traumatic that they try to resist subsequent bowel movements. The longer they hold their stools, the harder and drier they get, leading to another painful movement. This cycle disrupts regular bowel habits, leading to distress and, if not treated, **fecal impaction.**

When presented with a constipated child, a primary care provider first has to rule out a medical cause, such as an intestinal blockage. Treatment of fecal impaction may require evacuation of the bowels (e.g., with an enema). Once bowels have been evacuated, lifestyle changes are necessary to prevent future problems. Although various types of laxatives may be prescribed by the health care provider in the short term, diet and lifestyle are the safest strategies over the long term. First, regular bowel habits must be established. For example,

Choking is a preventable hazard for young children. Some suggestions for caregivers include:

- Set a good example at the table by taking small bites and chewing foods thoroughly.
- Have children sit at the table, take their time, and focus on their food during meals and snacks.
- Avoid giving children any foods that are round, firm, sticky, or cut into large chunks, especially before molars emerge (around age 4). For toddlers and preschoolers, some examples of foods to avoid are nuts, grapes, raisins, popcorn, peanut butter, and hard pieces of raw fruits or vegetables.

Between 2014 and 2015, the water supply in the city of Flint, Michigan, became contaminated with extremely high levels of lead. Read more about the far-reaching impact of this lead exposure in Section 17.6.

fecal impaction The presence of a mass of hard, dry feces that remains in the rectum as a result of chronic constipation.

Fiber Recommendations for Children (Food and Nutrition Board)

Young Children

| 1-3 years | 19 grams/day |
| 4-8 years | 25 grams/day |

Boys

| 9-13 years | 31 grams/day |
| 14-18 years | 38 grams/day |

Girls

| 9-13 years | 26 grams/day |
| 14-18 years | 26 grams/day |

parents should set aside time for the child to use the toilet, without rushing, after each meal. Rewards, such as stickers on a chart, may be used to reinforce good habits. Increasing physical activity while cutting back on sedentary activities (e.g., watching television or playing video games) can help to promote regular bowel movements. The primary dietary interventions to alleviate constipation include eating more fiber and drinking more fluids. In the initial stages of treatment, providing certain fruit juices (e.g., prune, grape, and apple) and substituting soy milk for cow's milk may relieve constipation.

Ultimately, whole fruits (e.g., plums, peaches, and apricots) are better choices than juices because whole fruits are less concentrated sources of calories. Other foods to emphasize for fiber include vegetables, whole-grain breads and cereals, and beans. The daily fiber goals for children set by the Food and Nutrition Board vary by age (see accompanying note). Few children meet these goals. It is important to increase fluid consumption along with fiber to avoid another fecal impaction. Accompanying fluid recommendations are 4 cups (900 milliliters) per day for toddlers and about 5 cups (1200 milliliters) per day for older children.

PLAN VEGETARIAN DIETS APPROPRIATELY

Vegetarian diets can pose several risks for young children. These include the possibility of developing iron-deficiency anemia, a deficiency of vitamin B-12, and rickets from a vitamin D deficiency. During the first few years of life, children also may not consume enough calories when following a bulky vegetarian diet. These known pitfalls are easily avoided by informed diet planning (review Section 6.9). Dietary patterns for children who eat totally vegetarian fare should focus on the following:

- A variety of plant sources of protein to provide a full complement of essential amino acids (e.g., beans, nuts, and grains)
- A synthetic source of vitamin B-12 (e.g., dietary supplement or fortified breakfast cereal)
- Plenty of plant sources of iron (e.g., beans, dried fruits, and fortified grain products)
- Good sources of zinc (e.g., whole grains, beans, nuts, and seeds)
- Foods that are fortified with vitamin D (e.g., fortified orange juice), along with regular sun exposure
- Rich plant sources of calcium (e.g., fortified milk or juice), almonds, some forms of tofu, and green, leafy vegetables

PROMOTE GOOD ORAL HEALTH

A healthy dietary pattern goes a long way in reducing the risk for dental caries in young children. In addition to beginning oral hygiene when teeth start to appear and seeking early pediatric dental care, the following diet-related tips can help reduce dental problems in children:

- Drink fluoridated water (or any water) as opposed to carbohydrate-rich or acidic beverages (e.g., fruit juice, soft drinks, sports drinks, and energy drinks). If sugary or acidic beverages are consumed, it is better to drink them *with* meals rather than *between* meals. Sipping juice continuously between meals (e.g., from a sippy cup) exposes teeth to caries-promoting sugars and acids.
- Use small amounts of fluoridated toothpaste twice daily. In areas without fluoridated water, discuss fluoride needs with a dentist or pediatrician.
- Snack in moderation. Again, constant exposure of teeth to sugars and acids throughout the day (i.e., grazing) tends to promote caries.
- Make wise snack choices. We automatically think of sticky, sugary snacks as promoters of dental caries, but foods such as pretzels and popcorn provide a source of carbohydrates for oral bacteria, as well. In contrast, crunchy fruits and vegetables, such as apples or celery, can help to brush away sticky food particles. Snacking on dairy products, such as cheese, can actually buffer the acids that lead to tooth decay.
- If toddlers or preschoolers are chewing gum, sugarless gum is the best choice, as this has been shown to reduce the incidence of dental caries.

LINKS BETWEEN AUTISM AND NUTRITION

Autism spectrum disorder (ASD) is characterized by a range of problems with social interaction, verbal and nonverbal communication, and/or unusual, repetitive, or limited activities and interests. These disorders usually are diagnosed in early childhood and affect an estimated 1 in every 68 children, with higher prevalence in boys than girls. The causes for ASD are not well understood, but there is a definite genetic component.

ASD can both affect and be affected by nutritional status (see Further Reading 18). In addition to developmental and behavioral abnormalities, many children with ASD also experience GI disorders, such as constipation, diarrhea, or reflux disease. Such disorders may impair nutrient intake or absorption. Medications used to treat behavioral problems may alter appetite. Some children with ASD may have feeding problems related to developmental impairments. Also, selective eating behaviors may affect nutrient intake. Children with ASD can be very rigid with their food selections, rejecting foods or entire food groups based on sensory qualities such texture, color, and temperature. Thus, careful attention to nutrient-dense food choices is of prime importance.

There are many nutrient-based theories concerning the causes and treatment of ASD. Nutritional interventions, such as dietary restrictions or nutrient supplements, are commonly employed by families affected by ASD. A widely used nutritional intervention is the gluten-free, casein-free (GFCF) diet, which eliminates all wheat, barley, rye, and milk products (see Further Reading 12 and Ask the RDN). At this time, the American Academy of Pediatrics does not endorse any specific diet as a treatment for autism.

Other popular therapies for ASD include supplementation with probiotics, vitamins B-6 and B-12, folic acid, magnesium, trimethylglycine and dimethylglycine, melatonin, and omega-3 fatty acids. Although sparse, research on these therapies is encouraging. There is evidence of altered absorption or metabolism of nutrients among children with autism, so even with adequate nutrient intake, availability of some nutrients for metabolic processes may be low. Even though these supplements carry a low risk of adverse effects, caution is necessary to avoid overdose. Because of the rising incidence of ASD and the lack of curative treatments, nutritional interventions for ASD will continue to be an active area of research.

ASK THE RDN   Autism Diet

Dear Author: My 4-year-old son was just diagnosed with autism. He is a picky eater and often cries because his belly hurts, so I think he may have some food sensitivities. I read about an autism diet that is gluten free and casein free (GFCF). Could this diet help him feel better and treat his autism?

I can understand your frustration. A diagnosis of autism spectrum disorder can be bewildering and the lack of treatment options may leave you feeling helpless. A dietary intervention may seem like a reasonable, low-risk option.

Proponents of the GFCF diet believe that some children have a "leaky gut," which allows food proteins to be absorbed intact from the GI tract into the bloodstream and possibly reach the brain. Certain proteins may cross the blood-brain barrier and exert druglike effects, leading to the behaviors of autism spectrum disorder. They assert that by eliminating the offending food proteins, symptoms of autism may be reduced. This sounds scientifically plausible, yet there is little science to support this theory. The levels of these druglike proteins in body fluids are no higher among children with autism than normal-functioning children.

You mentioned that your son is known to be a "picky eater." Many children on the autism spectrum display selective eating behaviors; they are more sensitive than other children to colors, tastes, temperatures, and textures. Also, children with autism prefer consistent routines and may refuse new foods. There is a strong possibility that the diet itself may prove disruptive and may affect your child's social and emotional functioning. Placing your son on a restrictive diet may further limit his food choices. Eliminating gluten will entail cutting out many types of breads, pastas, bakery products, crackers, and other snack foods. Removing casein will require avoidance of milk, yogurt, cheese, butter, and many frozen desserts. By eliminating dietary sources of gluten and casein, your child is at risk for deficiencies of iron, calcium, vitamin D, and several B vitamins. Indeed, studies have shown that children with autism already have diets deficient in key nutrients. Children who follow a casein-free diet may have low bone mass or delayed bone development related to deficient intake of calcium and vitamin D. Children on a gluten-free diet have lower levels of folate and vitamin B-6, leading to elevated homocysteine. This can place them at risk for chronic disease as they age.

Clearly, the GFCF diet is not risk free. But would the risks be acceptable if the diet helps to improve symptoms? Unfortunately, there is very little evidence to support either the safety or the efficacy of the GFCF diet. The few studies that do show a positive outcome are of poor quality, meaning they were of short duration, had small numbers of subjects, poor study designs, and a high risk of bias.

Knowing that children with autism are at risk for dietary inadequacies, the best dietary strategy is to offer a variety of nutrient-dense foods at each meal. Consulting with a registered dietitian nutritionist would be helpful to assess your son's current dietary patterns and create a personalized plan to alleviate GI symptoms and ensure his nutritional needs are met. For a child with extremely limited dietary intake, multivitamin and mineral supplementation may be an option. Overall, a dietary restriction should only be used if there is evidence that your son has an allergy or intolerance to a food. If you are concerned that his GI distress may be due to a food allergy or intolerance, you should consult your primary care provider about allergy testing.

Despite the lack of evidence to support the GFCF diet for treatment of autism spectrum disorders, many parents will choose to try it anyway, hoping for positive results. There may, in fact, be a subset of children with autism who do respond to dietary treatments. If you are determined to try the GFCF diet, please seek the help of a registered dietitian nutritionist who can help you to plan meals and snacks that will still meet your son's nutrient needs while adhering to dietary restrictions.

Keeping it nutritious,

Angela Collene, MS, RDN, LD (author)

✓ CONCEPT CHECK 19.4

1. Picky eating is a common complaint among parents of preschoolers. Why is picky eating common at this age? Provide three or more suggestions to help a preschooler choose nutritious foods.

2. How often do preschoolers need to eat throughout the day? List three nutrient-dense snack ideas that would be appropriate for a 3-year-old child.

3. Should toddlers and preschoolers take a multivitamin and mineral supplement? Why or why not?

4. Explain the connections between nutrition and oral health. List three ways to reduce risk for dental caries with healthy eating habits.

5. What are some nutrition concerns of children with autism spectrum disorder?

19.5 School-Age Children: Nutrition Concerns

The dietary patterns of many school-age students can be improved, particularly with regard to fruit, vegetable, whole-grain, and beverage choices. One survey of U.S. schoolchildren revealed that on the day of the survey, 40% of the children ate no vegetables, except for potatoes or tomato sauce, and 20% ate no fruits. Less than 20% of school-age girls consume

2 tbsp apple sauce

1/2 cup brown rice

1/2 cup milk

2 tbsp peas and carrots

1 oz diced turkey

Age 2
228 kcal

1/2 sliced kiwi

6 oz low-fat yogurt

1 tbsp ranch dressing

1/2 peanut butter and jelly sandwich on whole-wheat bread

1/2 cup broccoli florets

Age 4
381 kcal

12 grapes

1 cup skim milk

3/4 cup corn

beef taco with lettuce, tomato, cheese, and sour cream

Age 8
520 kcal

1 slice Italian bread

1 apple

1 cup skim milk

1 cup tossed salad with mixed greens, tomato, carrot, cucumber and 2 tbsp ranch dressing

4-inch square piece of lasagna

Age 16
723 kcal

FIGURE 19-4 ▲ Using MyPlate to build a healthy meal for children. MyPlate is a useful tool for all Americans, ages 2 and older. MyPlate proportions apply to children as well as adults, but portion sizes and food choices vary by age.

adequate calcium. In general, the nutritional concerns and goals applicable to school-age children are the same as those discussed in relation to preschoolers. However, with the added pressures of peers, health messages from the media, and an increasing desire for independence, these goals may be harder to achieve as children grow older. MyPlate's daily food patterns, which are tailored to age, gender, height, weight, and activity level, continue to be a good basis for diet planning, with an emphasis on moderating fat and sugar intake and ensuring adequate iron, zinc, and calcium intake (Fig. 19-4). Now let us look at several nutritional issues of particular concern during the school-age years.

REVERSING TRENDS FOR OVERWEIGHT AND OBESITY

By far the most troublesome nutritional problem facing children today is the rise in childhood obesity. Since the 1970s, the incidence of childhood overweight and obesity has more

▲ Supersized portions of foods such as hamburgers and sugar-sweetened soft drinks are fueling a nation of supersized kids. © Image100/Corbis

than tripled! In the past decade, the rate of childhood obesity has stabilized, but still, about one-third of U.S. school-age children are now classified as overweight or obese. The rates of childhood obesity are highest among children from low-income families and minority populations.

In the short run, the main consequences of childhood obesity are ridicule, embarrassment, possibly depression, and short stature linked to early puberty. In the long run, significant health problems associated with obesity, such as cardiovascular disease, type 2 diabetes, hypertension, and osteoarthritis may appear in adulthood or earlier. Childhood obesity is a serious health threat because about 40% of obese children (and about 80% of obese adolescents) become obese adults.

Research points to many potential causes of childhood obesity. Recall the nature versus nurture discussion in Section 7.4. Some infants are born with a genetic predisposition to obesity. They may experience lower metabolic rates, which means they use calories more efficiently and can store fat more easily. However, studies also suggest that genetic factors account for only one-third of individual differences in body weight.

Researchers believe that, although diet is an important factor, inactivity is also a major contributor to the increase in childhood obesity. Studies show that as children age, physical activity steadily declines and screen time increases. Screen time includes time spent watching television, working at the computer, or using phones and other electronic devices. Only about one-half of children are getting the recommended 60 minutes of exercise per day. It does not help that physical education classes are now elective in many high schools. Today's generation of children now engages in 7 hours per day of screen time, on average. The American Academy of Pediatrics recommends a limit of 14 hours of screen time per week for children over age 2 (no television is recommended for children younger than 2 years). In addition, excessive snacking, overreliance on fast-food restaurants, parental neglect, advertising and other messages in the media, lack of safe areas to play, and the abundant availability of high-calorie food choices contribute to childhood obesity. Soft drinks and other sugared beverages are especially implicated.

Recall from Section 16.4, the United Nations Sustainable Development Goals call for efforts to control noncommunicable diseases, such as obesity. In 2016, WHO released their Report of the Commission on Ending Childhood Obesity (ECHO). The ECHO Report quantifies global rates of childhood obesity and recognizes the problems of an increasingly obesogenic environment. To combat the global epidemic of childhood obesity, the commission recommends promoting healthy foods and physical activity beginning before conception (for the mother), and extending all the way through childhood. To access the full report, see http://www.who.int/end-childhood-obesity/final-report/en/.

The initial approach in treating an overweight or obese child is to assess physical activity. If a child spends too much time in sedentary activities (such as watching television or playing video games), more physical activities should be encouraged. The Physical Activity Guidelines for Americans recommend 60 minutes or more of moderate to vigorous physical activity per day for children and adolescents. Learning to engage in and enjoy regular physical activity will help children to maintain a healthy body weight throughout life. An increase in physical activity will not just happen; parents and other caregivers need to plan for it. Getting the family together for a brisk walk after dinner encourages healthy habits for all involved. Age-appropriate activities for elementary school-age children include walking, dancing, jumping rope, and participation in organized sports that focus on fun rather than intense competition. For middle school–age children, more complex organized sports (e.g., soccer and basketball) are of interest, and some weight training with small weights can also be beneficial.

Moderation in calorie intake is important. High-calorie foods, such as sugar-sweetened soft drinks and whole milk, should be limited. The focus should be on more vitamin- and mineral-dense foods and healthy snacks. An emphasis on appropriate portion sizes may help youth learn to curb excessive food consumption. Making small changes, such as substituting low-fat for whole milk or fruit canned in its own juice instead of heavy syrup, can moderately cut calories without sacrificing taste or disrupting normal eating patterns. To specifically address the increased burden of overweight and obesity among minority populations, health professionals must become versed in varied cultural food preferences.

▲ To get kids involved in exercise, new physical education classes have been introduced into some schools. Lessons on rock climbing, in-line skating, and recreational jogging help to promote activity because they take the focus away from teams and competition, which often discourage and embarrass kids who lack athletic talent. © Valerie Loiseleux/Getty Images

Resorting to a weight-loss diet is usually not necessary; it is best to change dietary and physical activity patterns to allow for weight maintenance. Children have an advantage over adults in dealing with obesity: their bodies can use stored energy for growth. An overweight child who maintains his or her body weight through a growth spurt will end up with a more favorable body composition. This is one reason it is desirable to address obesity in childhood. If weight loss is necessary in younger children, it should be gradual, about 0.5 to 1 pound per week. The child should be watched closely to ensure that the rate of growth continues to be normal; calorie intake should not be so low that gains in height diminish. In some cases, medications [e.g., orlistat (Xenical)] may be prescribed by a primary care provider. For the 1% to 2% of American children who are morbidly obese, bariatric surgery is an option for weight management (see Further Reading 24).

EARLY SIGNS OF CARDIOVASCULAR DISEASE

Also paralleling the increase in childhood obesity, early signs of cardiovascular disease have become increasingly prevalent among children and adolescents. One of five American youths between the ages of 12 and 19 years has abnormal blood lipids. Therefore, lifestyle modifications to delay the progression of the disease are important throughout the lifespan. The American Academy of Pediatrics now recommends universal blood lipid screening for all children around the ages of 9 to 11. Even earlier screening is recommended for "at-risk" children who are overweight, have high blood pressure, smoke, or have diabetes; have a family history of cardiovascular disease; or whose family history is unknown. For children whose cholesterol is elevated, lifestyle approaches such as weight management through dietary modification and increased physical activity are the first line of therapy (see Further Reading 10). Following a dietary pattern that is consistent with the Dietary Guidelines and conforms to MyPlate would be appropriate for prevention of cardiovascular disease. Some high-risk children may be candidates for cholesterol-lowering medications.

TYPE 2 DIABETES AMONG YOUTH

Type 2 diabetes was once regarded as an adult condition. As reviewed in Section 4.7, it frequently occurs in overweight people over age 40. However, an alarming increase in the frequency of the disease among children (and teenagers) has been documented. This is primarily due to the rise in obesity in this age group. Up to 85% of children with the disease are overweight at diagnosis.

Starting at age 10, children who are overweight or obese and who have risk factors for type 2 diabetes should be screened for type 2 diabetes every 2 years. Besides obesity and a sedentary lifestyle, examples of risk factors include having a close relative with the disease or belonging to a nonwhite population. In 2013, the American Academy of Pediatrics released the first-ever guidelines for management of type 2 diabetes in children (see Further Reading 7). These guidelines provide recommendations for monitoring of blood glucose, use of medications, weight management, and physical activity. Dietary management strategies include a regular schedule of meals and snacks; education on appropriate portion sizes; limiting sugar-sweetened beverages, high-fat foods, snacks, and fast foods; and focusing on incorporating more fruits, vegetables, and low-fat or fat-free dairy products. For physical activity, experts advise children to engage in moderate- or vigorous-intensity physical activity for at least 60 minutes each day.

START THE DAY WITH BREAKFAST

You have heard it before: *Breakfast is the most important meal of the day.* Yet, as many as one-third of school-age children do not eat breakfast. The problem gets worse as children reach the teenage years. Children who skip breakfast are missing out on important nutrients that fuel the brain and the body. A fortified, low-sugar, ready-to-eat breakfast cereal is typically the greatest source of iron, vitamin A, and folic acid for children ages 2 to 18. Although there is controversy over the true benefit of breakfast for cognitive ability, children who eat breakfast

▲ For kids who complain about waking up early to make time for breakfast, consider preparing a portable breakfast (e.g., a sandwich bag full of dry cereal, nuts, and dried cranberries) the night before, for grab-and-go convenience the next morning. © Ingram Publishing/SuperStock

are more likely to meet their daily needs for vitamins and minerals compared to children not eating breakfast (see Further Reading 22). Also, a growing body of research shows that starting the day with breakfast reduces risk for obesity (see Newsworthy Nutrition).

Fortified, low-sugar, ready-to-eat breakfast cereals offer lots of nutrition in a tasty and convenient package. Consumption of breakfast cereal is responsible for improved intakes of vitamin A and iron. Eating breakfast in general is linked to better intakes of vitamin A, vitamin C, calcium, iron, and fiber. Note that breakfast menus need not be limited to traditional fare. A little imagination can spark the interest of even the most reluctant child. Instead of conventional breakfast foods, parents can offer leftovers from dinner, such as pizza, spaghetti, soups, yogurt topped with trail mix, chili with beans, or sandwiches. For lasting energy and satiety, combine traditional carbohydrate-rich breakfast foods with a source of protein, such as low-fat cheese, nuts, or eggs.

CHOOSE HEALTHY FATS

Dietary patterns of school-age children should include a variety of foods from each major group, not necessarily excluding any specific food because of its fat content. Overemphasis on fat-reduced diets during childhood has been linked to an increase in eating disorders and encourages an inappropriate "good food, bad food" attitude.

However, surveys of dietary intake among children show that they are consuming too much saturated fat, most of which comes from whole milk, other full-fat dairy products, and fatty meats. Furthermore, few children (or adults) meet recommendations to include two servings of fish per week to ensure adequate intake of omega-3 fats. Emphasizing low-fat dairy products (after age 2), offering broiled or baked fish, choosing leaner cuts of meat, trimming visible fat from meats, and removing the skin from poultry before serving foods will establish heart-healthy eating habits to last a lifetime. Snacks for children should include only moderate fat and sugar and emphasize fruit, vegetables, whole grain, and dairy choices. Ideas for healthy snacks are found in Table 19-8.

SELECT APPROPRIATE BEVERAGES

Maintaining proper hydration is important for children. The fluid needs of school-age children range from approximately 1 ½ to 2 ½ liters per day, depending on age and gender. However, over the past 30 years, beverage choices have shifted from water and low-fat or fat-free milk to the empty calories provided by sugar-sweetened beverages. In fact, sugar-sweetened beverages (e.g, soft drinks, flavored fruit drinks, and sports drinks) and the sweeteners added to flavored milk account for about 200 empty kcal per day for school-age children (see Further Reading 3). The 135% increase in sugar-sweetened beverage consumption has paralleled the threefold rise in childhood obesity since the 1970s. Such high intakes of sugar-laden beverages are not only contributing excess calories, but are also linked to increased levels of inflammation and worsened blood lipid profiles among children (see Further Reading 11). Even 100% fruit juices, which are perceived by many to be an important source of vitamin C and potassium for children, have been linked to obesity, fatty liver, and metabolic syndrome (see Further Reading 23).

Replacing sugar-sweetened beverages with water and choosing unflavored, low-fat, or fat-free milk instead of flavored milk would reduce sugar intake by about 10 ½ teaspoons per day and shrink overall kilocalorie intake by about 10%. Furthermore, replacing 100% fruit juices with whole fruits would supply important nutrients in a lower-calorie package for children. Overall, children should be given water and low-fat or fat-free milk as primary beverage choices. Fruit juice should be limited to 4 to 6 fluid ounces per day for young children or 8 to 12 fluid ounces per day for older children.

PROMOTE SOUND NUTRITION IN SCHOOLS

Children spend the majority of their waking hours in school, so it is a great place to learn about and practice healthy eating habits (see Further Reading 4). A strong emphasis on

▲ Excessive consumption of fruit juice is linked to obesity, unhealthy blood lipids, fat accumulation in the liver, and dental caries among children. The American Academy of Pediatrics recommends no more than 4 to 6 ounces per day for children 1 to 6 years (and 8 to 12 ounces per day for ages 7 to 18 years).
© Creatas/PunchStock

nutrition education in schools can help children understand why healthy dietary patterns will make them feel more energetic, look healthier, and work more efficiently. USDA's Team Nutrition initiative supports child nutrition programs with education materials that promote healthy food choices and physical activity.

School breakfasts and lunches provided a nutritional safety net for more than 30 million students during the 2014–2015 school year. Of those meals, 72% were provided free or at reduced prices for children from low-income families.

Most schools have included nutrition education in their health or science curricula, but until recently, these healthy nutrition messages were not consistently backed up by the food offerings in school cafeterias. In 2010, President Barack Obama signed into law the Healthy Hunger-Free Kids Act, which extended funding for the National School Lunch Program, School Breakfast Program, and several other federal nutrition programs. The law also authorized USDA to make significant changes to the nutritional quality of foods provided in schools. Public school food service programs now have to meet nutrition standards that stipulate the inclusion of fruits, vegetables, and whole grains in meals. School cafeterias offer skim or 1% milk instead of whole milk. These standards also will gradually reduce the saturated fat, *trans* fat, and sodium content of meals over the coming years.

Breakfasts and lunches prepared by school cafeterias are not the only targets of school nutrition reforms. In 2014, new standards for the quality of competitive foods sold on school campuses (e.g., from snack bars and vending machines) went into effect. These guidelines set calorie limits on snacks and restrict the levels of saturated fat, sugar, and sodium in foods that can be sold to students.

These new school nutrition regulations are based on research studies that show how changing the quality of foods offered to students at school can stem the rise in children's BMI. Students' food choices, however, depend a lot on how the food choices taste. School food service programs, although they receive some government reimbursement, often rely on cafeteria, snack bar, or vending machine sales to break even. It remains to be seen how these school nutrition reforms will influence children's eating behaviors.

If we are to reduce childhood obesity, improving nutritional awareness at school is only part of the solution. Positive nutrition influences must extend beyond the classroom and into the home. Caregivers and other adult role models need to create safe opportunities for children to be active and must practice what they preach when it comes to healthy habits at home.

✓ CONCEPT CHECK 19.5

1. Provide an example of a meal that resembles MyPlate and is appropriate for a 7-year-old child.

2. List three lifestyle changes to reduce childhood obesity. In what significant way do weight management strategies for children differ from those for adults?

3. Describe appropriate beverage choices for school-age children. What are the implications of excessively consuming sugar-sweetened beverages?

4. Tim refuses to eat breakfast before school. He doesn't like cereal, toast, or any of the other usual breakfast foods. What can Tim's parents do to ensure that he eats nutritious foods before leaving for school?

19.6 Teenage Years: Nutrition Concerns

Teenagers are on the cusp of adulthood; parents and schools may still be providing healthful food choices for them, yet they are capable of acquiring and preparing food for themselves. They pursue their independence, experience identity crises, seek peer acceptance, and worry about physical appearance. Advertisers push a vast array of products—candy, fast foods, soft drinks, and energy drinks—at the teenage market. Frequently, these foods crowd out nutrient-dense foods, thus limiting intake of calcium, iron, zinc, fat-soluble vitamins, and folate.

Teens often do not think about the long-term benefits of good health. Developmentally, they have a hard time relating today's actions to tomorrow's health outcomes. Still, positive dietary

The physical changes of puberty cause body dissatisfaction for some adolescents. Late-blooming boys may be frustrated with slow gains in height and muscularity, whereas girls can be dissatisfied with gains in fat mass, which are a normal part of development. Be alert for signs of eating disorders (see Chapter 15).

patterns do not require giving up favorite foods. In moderation, small portions of fast foods and sweet treats can fit into a healthy dietary pattern based on abundant fruits and vegetables, lean sources of protein, fat-free and reduced-fat dairy products, and whole-grain products.

One of the most salient nutritional changes among adolescents is an increase in kilocalorie intake. Most girls begin a rapid growth spurt between the ages of 10 and 13, and most boys experience rapid growth between the ages of 12 and 15. Early-maturing girls may begin their growth spurt as early as age 7 to 8, whereas early-maturing boys may begin growing by age 9 to 10. Nearly every organ and bone in the body grows during this adolescent growth spurt. Girls gain about 10 inches (25 centimeters) in height, and boys gain about 12 inches (30 centimeters). Girls tend to accumulate both lean and fat tissue, whereas boys tend to gain mostly lean tissue. This growth spurt provides about 50% of ultimate adult weight and about 15% of ultimate adult height (review Fig. 19-1).

As the growth spurt begins, teenagers begin to eat more. Physically active teenage boys, especially, seem driven to consume everything in sight! Teenage girls need 1800 to 2400 kcal per day, whereas teenage boys require 2200 to 3200 kcal per day. If teens choose nutrient-dense foods, they can take advantage of their ravenous appetites to easily satisfy their increased requirements for calcium, iron, and zinc. As discussed for younger age groups, MyPlate can serve as a guide (see Table 19-7 and Fig. 19-4). Unfortunately, teens very often meet (or exceed) their increased energy needs with empty calories rather than nutrient-dense food options. About one-third of their calories come from solid fats and added sugars.

Fruit and vegetable intake among teenagers is generally dismal; only about one-fourth of high school students regularly consume a minimum of five servings per day of fruits and vegetables. Sadly, potato chips and French fries make up more than one-third of the vegetable servings consumed by teens. Low consumption of fruits and vegetables correlates with inadequate intakes of vitamins A, C, and E, folate, magnesium, and fiber. Also, as teens (especially girls) trade their glasses of milk for bottles of soft drinks and other sugar-sweetened beverages, their intakes of calcium, phosphorus, and vitamin D fall short of recommendations. On the other hand, intakes of saturated fat, cholesterol, sodium, and sugars exceed the recommendations set by the American Heart Association, placing teens at risk for obesity and cardiovascular disease.

Childhood obesity, introduced in Section 19.5, continues to be a major nutritional problem into adolescence. Among children between the ages of 12 and 19, 17% are obese. There are gender and ethnic disparities for adolescent obesity: black females and Hispanic males are at highest risk. Overweight and obese teens are likely to become obese adults and to develop comorbid conditions, such as type 2 diabetes, hypertension, cardiovascular diseases, sleep apnea, and joint problems. If a teen is still growing, he or she has an advantage in terms of weight management; by holding body weight steady while height gains are achieved, body mass index will decrease over time. However, if a teen attains ultimate adult height and is still obese, a weight-loss regimen may be necessary. Weight loss should be gradual, perhaps 1 pound per week, and generally follow the advice in Chapter 7.

Calcium and Vitamin D Over the last 20 years, soft drinks have been replacing milk as the preferred beverage among children. (Figure 2-1 shows the stark contrast between milk and typical soft drinks with respect to calcium and other nutrients.) Intake of milk is especially poor among adolescent females, who may view dairy products as a source of unwanted calories. This trend in milk consumption begins early in childhood, but we discuss it here because the gap between needs and actual intake of bone-building nutrients is greatest during the adolescent growth spurt. Less than 10% of girls and less than 25% of boys meet recommendations for calcium intake. To make matters worse, one of five children is deficient in vitamin D. Meanwhile, the adolescent growth spurt marks a critical time for bone development. Calcium requirements for 14- to 18-year-old girls and boys are 1300 milligrams per day—higher than during any other time of life. As you learned in Section 11.11, failure to maximize bone mineralization during childhood sets the stage for development of osteoporosis later in life.

Three servings per day from the dairy group are recommended for all teenagers and young adults to meet calcium needs. If dairy products are not consumed, alternative calcium

▲ An active lifestyle coupled with a healthy dietary pattern should be part of the teen years. Both habits contribute to bone development and strength. © SW Productions/Getty Images sources need to be included. Nondairy sources of calcium include almonds, legumes, some green vegetables, and fortified foods (e.g., fruit juices, cereal, and granola bars). However, it is important to note that these alternative sources of calcium may not provide other important nutrients supplied by dairy products, such as protein and vitamins A, D, and B-12.

Iron About 10% of teenagers have low iron stores or iron-deficiency anemia. Iron-deficiency anemia is a highly undesirable condition for a teen. It can lead to fatigue and a decreased ability to concentrate and learn, such that academic and physical performance suffers. Iron-deficiency anemia sometimes appears in boys during their growth spurt, but adolescent females are at greatest risk of deficiency due to heavy menstrual flow and poor dietary intake. It is important that teenagers choose good food sources of iron, such as lean meats and fortified grain products. Teenage girls, in particular, need to eat good sources of iron (or regularly consume a balanced multivitamin and mineral supplement containing iron).

Many of the nutritional issues of adolescents—obesity, snacking, beverage choices, and skipping meals—have been adequately described with reference to younger children. Here, we present a few nutrition dilemmas that pertain especially to teenagers.

▲ The teenage years are noted for snacking. With reasonable food choices, teenagers can have healthful diets. © SW Productions/Getty Images

BREAK THE FAST-FOOD HABIT

It is convenient, casual, inexpensive, and all their friends work there. These are reasons why, on any given day, about 40% of the nation's youth eat food from a fast-food restaurant. Unfortunately, the average trip to a fast-food establishment yields about 300 extra kilocalories, 14 additional grams of fat, and 400 milligrams of sodium *in excess* of typical home-prepared meals for teenagers (see Further Reading 17).

By making some small changes in their food selections, teens can still enjoy dining out with friends without detriment to their health. When building a sandwich, opt for one layer of meat instead of double or triple patties and select grilled instead of fried meat. For deli sandwiches, choose moderate portions of lean meats, such as roasted turkey or chicken, rather than fatty slices of bologna and salami. Skip the condiments or request them on the side; the mayonnaise on a typical fast-food sandwich supplies about 100 fat-laden kcal. Each slice of cheese supplies another 80 to 100 kcal. When it comes to choosing a side dish, a small baked potato or a garden salad with reduced-fat dressing will provide fewer kilocalories and more nutrients than the typical 500-kcal large serving of fries. Kilocalories from regular soft drinks—especially when free refills are available—can quickly add up. Teens should choose reduced-fat or fat-free milk as a nutrient-dense alternative or opt for water. For pizza, choose veggie toppings instead of sausage and pepperoni. If possible, order a pizza with low-fat cheese and whole-grain crust.

When burgers are measured in pounds instead of ounces, portion control is an issue. While already large, portion sizes at fast-food establishments continue to grow. Choosing items from the kids' menu can lessen the impact of dining out on adolescent wallets and waistlines. Supersized meals, while they may seem economical, should be avoided unless they are to be divided and shared among friends. All of us can benefit from the calorie information that many restaurants have already placed on their menus in anticipation of the mandatory posting that will soon be required (see Section 1.1).

CURB CAFFEINE INTAKE

The combined demands of school, work, extracurricular activities, social commitments, and late-night screen time leave many adolescents looking for a quick pick-me-up. Commonly, they are turning to caffeine, the most widely used stimulant on the planet. Soft drinks, a common choice among youth, provide about 25 milligrams of caffeine per serving. On average, 30% of adolescents report consuming energy beverages, which typically contain between 100 and 200 milligrams of caffeine per serving. Consumption of coffee and tea, which yield about 100 milligrams of caffeine per cup, is on the rise among teens. Various foods, including chocolate and some types of candies or sports nutrition products, contain caffeine as well. Average caffeine intake from all sources is just over 100 milligrams per day among teens. Many consumers are unaware of how much caffeine they are consuming; the exact amount of caffeine is not always listed on energy drink labels because (1) it is not currently required by food labeling laws; and (2) some manufacturers (especially of energy drinks) consider it to be part of a "proprietary blend."

For children, the American Academy of Pediatrics advises limiting caffeine intake to 100 milligrams per day, if it is used at all. Some of the negative effects of caffeine at any age are gastrointestinal distress, sleep disturbances, anxiety, increased blood pressure, and irregular heartbeat. For children, in particular, there is concern that excessive caffeine intake could affect normal neurological and cardiovascular development. Furthermore, disturbances in normal sleep patterns could affect growth and learning ability. Alarmingly, there have been thousands of reports of caffeine poisoning—and even some deaths—as a result of excessive intake of energy drinks. Clearly, excessive caffeine intake has no place in the diets of children (see Further Reading 6).

CHOOSING VEGETARIAN DIETS

Teenagers, who strive to forge an identity by adopting dietary patterns different from those of their families, may choose to follow vegetarian diets. As discussed in Section 6.9, vegetarians enjoy many health benefits, including lower body weight and better control of blood glucose and cholesterol. Indeed, an increased focus on plant foods is needed among adolescents, who often miss out on their recommended daily servings of fruits and vegetables. However, teens may not know enough about a vegetarian dietary pattern to keep from developing health problems, such as iron-deficiency anemia. The bulkiness of a plant-based diet is not as much of a concern for teens as it is for younger children with smaller stomach capacity, but a strictly vegetarian diet must be monitored for adequate energy, protein, iron, vitamin B-12, calcium, and vitamin D (the latter if sun exposure is not sufficient) at any age. These nutrients are particularly important in teenagers, as their diets are often already nutrient poor.

Teens often cite concern for the humane treatment of animals as their main reason for choosing vegetarian diets, but be observant of teens who choose vegetarianism as a method of weight loss. Vegetarianism is sometimes used as a socially acceptable way to restrict the diet and, for some, can be an early sign of disordered eating.

ALCOHOL ABUSE AMONG TEENS

In Section 19.5, we discussed how the beverage choices of school-age children are in need of improvement because they provide too much sugar and not enough micronutrients. The nutrient density of beverages continues to be a problem among teenagers, but a new problem arises: alcohol abuse. Developmentally, adolescents are prone to experimentation, rebellion, and risk taking, so use of this illegal and dangerous substance is common among teenagers. Results of the national Youth Risk Behavior Survey demonstrate that approximately 20% of teenagers have tried alcohol by the age of 13. At some point throughout the teenage years, about 70% of teens report drinking alcohol at least once, and 22% report binge drinking.

It is just harmless fun, right? Wrong! The statistics show that alcohol use beginning in adolescence has severe consequences (see Further Reading 15). The adolescent's body and brain are still developing. Exposure to alcohol can decrease brain mass in the area of the brain involved in decision making, memory, and learning. This is evidenced by academic problems and poor decision making, which can lead to legal troubles, physical assault, and risky sexual behaviors. The most dangerous consequence of poor judgment is drinking and driving. About 1 in 10 teenagers admits to drinking and driving, a risky behavior that is implicated in about one-third of fatal motor vehicle accidents involving teens. Alcohol also contributes to other causes of accidental injuries and deaths, such as drowning, falls, and burns.

Adolescent alcohol abuse exacts a toll on long-term physical health, as well. Studies show that alcohol abuse beginning during adolescence is a strong predictor of alcohol abuse during adulthood. In Section 20.5, you will learn more about the effects of alcohol consumption on adults. Nutritional status can be affected because alcohol abuse is often accompanied by nutrient-poor diets. Also, weight gain from empty calories increases the risk for obesity-related diseases, such as hypertension and cardiovascular disease. These physical consequences may not surface until later in life, but it is certain that the effects of alcohol on the liver, brain, and cardiovascular system can start early.

Alcohol use by teenagers should not be viewed as a normal part of growing up. On the contrary, the physical, emotional, and intellectual consequences of underage drinking can be longstanding and devastating. Parents and other caregivers should talk to their children about the consequences of alcohol abuse, set clear rules, monitor their children's behavior, and be positive role models.

Newsworthy Nutrition

Glycemic Index of Food Choices May Influence Acne

About 80% to 90% of teens experience acne to some degree. Although it is popularly believed that nuts, chocolate, and pizza contribute to acne, scientific studies have failed to show a strong role for any of these dietary factors. Based on the results of observational research, two dietary factors stand out as possible contributors to acne: foods with high **glycemic index (GI)** and high consumption of dairy products. Both of these dietary patterns are hypothesized to increase insulin levels, which through various mechanisms lead to increased sebum production and altered skin cell growth. To date, the highest-quality evidence supports the link between glycemic index of food choices and acne among males, but research on dairy products as well as on the fatty acid content of the diet is still underway. Whether or not it improves acne, changing the diet to include more whole grains, fruits, vegetables, and legumes would have multiple health benefits.

Source: Burris J and others: Acne: The role of medical nutrition therapy. *Journal of the Academy of Nutrition and Dietetics* 113:416, 2013.

glycemic index (GI) The blood glucose response of a given food, compared to a standard (typically, glucose or white bread). Glycemic index is influenced by starch structure, fiber content, food processing, physical structure, and macronutrients in the meal such as fat.

✓ CONCEPT CHECK 19.6

1. Which two minerals are most likely to be deficient in teen diets? Exemplify two rich food sources of each of these minerals that could help teenagers meet their nutrient needs.

2. Design a meal for a teen that resembles MyPlate and can be purchased from a fast-food restaurant.

3. Are energy drinks safe for consumption by children of any age? Why or why not?

4. List three consequences of alcohol abuse that are specific to adolescents.

19.7 Nutrition and Your Health
Food Allergies and Intolerances

© Corbis Super/Alamy

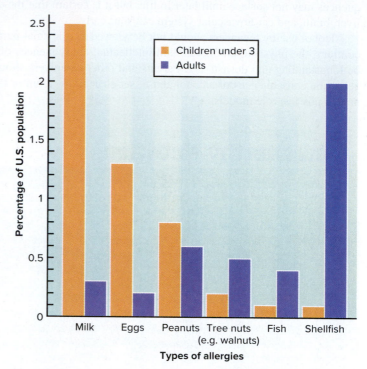

FIGURE 19-5 ▲ Types of allergies and percentage of U.S. population with those allergies.

Source: *Journal of Allergy and Clinical Immunology* (study done by Mount Sinai School of Medicine).

Food allergies are on the rise. Between 1997 and 2011, food allergies among children increased by 50%. What used to be a rare medical incident is now the cause for 92,000 childhood emergency room visits and 84 child fatalities per year. Accounting for direct medical costs, special foods, and time lost from work, food allergies cost Americans $25 billion per year. Today, food allergies affect about 8% (5.9 million) of children in the United States, one-third of whom suffer from multiple food allergies (see Further Reading 9).

Adverse reactions to foods—indicated by sneezing, coughing, nausea, vomiting, diarrhea, hives, and other rashes—are broadly classed as **food allergies** (also called hypersensitivities) or **food intolerances.** The term *food sensitivity* is ill defined, but generally refers to any symptom that is perceived to be food related. In our discussion, we group adverse food reactions into two categories. Those caused by an immune response are termed food allergies, and those not caused by an immune response are food intolerances. Let us examine each process, first allergies and then intolerances.

Food Allergies: Symptoms and Mechanisms

Allergic reactions to foods are common (Fig. 19-5) and occur more frequently in females than males. Food allergies occur most often during infancy and young adulthood.

Symptoms of food allergies may affect the following:

- **Skin:** itching, tingling*, redness, hives, and swelling
- **GI tract:** nausea, vomiting, diarrhea, intestinal gas, bloating, pain, constipation, and indigestion
- **Respiratory tract:** runny nose, wheezing, congestion, and difficulty breathing*
- **Cardiovascular system:** low blood pressure* and rapid heart rate*

These symptoms usually set in shortly after consuming the offending food protein and may last for a few seconds or a few days. The symptoms marked with an asterisk (*) are signs of a rapid and potentially fatal type of allergic response called **anaphylaxis.** This severe allergic response results in low blood pressure and respiratory distress. A person who is extremely sensitive to a food may not be able to touch the food or even be in the same room where it is being cooked without reacting to it. Although any food can trigger anaphylaxis, the most common culprits are peanuts (a legume, not a nut), tree nuts (e.g., walnuts, pecans), shellfish, milk

food allergy An adverse reaction to food that involves an immune response; also called *food hypersensitivity*.

food intolerance An adverse reaction to food that does not involve an allergic reaction.

anaphylaxis A severe allergic response that results in lowered blood pressure and respiratory distress. This can be fatal.

(look for an ingredient called casein on the label), eggs (look for the ingredient albumin on the label), soybeans, wheat, and fish. Other foods frequently identified with adverse reactions include meat and meat products, fruits, and cheese. For a small number of people, avoiding foods such as peanuts or shellfish is a matter of life and death.

Basically, allergies are an inappropriate response of the immune system. When immune cells identify a harmful foreign protein (**antigen**), they destroy it and produce antibodies to it, so that the next response to the harmful substance will be swift and effective. Almost all food allergies are caused by proteins in foods that act as antigens (also called **allergens**). In these cases, the immune system mistakes the food protein for a harmful substance and mounts an immune response, leading to symptoms such as hives, runny nose, and GI disturbances.

No one is sure why the immune system sometimes overreacts to harmless proteins. The early introduction (e.g., before 4 months of age) of solid foods to infants may trigger food allergies. The reasoning is that the infant's GI tract is immature and "leaky," allowing some undigested proteins to be absorbed into the bloodstream. This is beneficial for the absorption of immune proteins from breast milk; however, if some food proteins are introduced before the GI tract has matured, these antigens may enter the bloodstream and stimulate an immune response.

The **hygiene hypothesis** offers another interesting explanation: in our "germophobic" society, with the protection of antibiotics, hand sanitizers, and antimicrobial soaps and cleaners, our immune systems are not vigorously challenged by antigens. As a result, the immune system may become sensitized to innocuous substances, such as food proteins. Current research supports the hygiene hypothesis. Children who grow up on farms or who have pets and are thereby exposed to many antigens have fewer allergies and asthma than children who grow up in more sterile environments. Whatever the explanation, one thing is clear: food allergies are an important concern for many parents and others who work with children.

Recently, researchers have proposed a link between low levels of vitamin D and food allergies. The rise in incidence of food allergies has paralleled an increase in vitamin D deficiency. The relationship between vitamin D and food allergies may be mediated by the vitamin's role in immune function.

antigen Any substance that induces a state of sensitivity and/or resistance to microorganisms or toxic substances after a lag period; a foreign substance that stimulates a specific aspect of the immune system.

allergen A foreign protein, or antigen, that induces excess production of certain immune system antibodies; subsequent exposure to the same protein leads to allergic symptoms. Whereas all allergens are antigens, not all antigens are allergens.

hygiene hypothesis Assumption that reduced exposure to microorganisms in the environment (e.g., as a result of overuse of antibacterial soaps and antibiotics) impairs proper development of the immune system, making a person more susceptible to allergies and autoimmune diseases.

elimination diet A restrictive diet that systematically tests foods that may cause an allergic response by first eliminating them for 1 to 2 weeks and then adding them back, one at a time.

TESTING FOR A FOOD ALLERGY

The diagnosis of a food allergy can be a difficult task (see Further Reading 14). It requires the participation of a skilled clinician. To determine whether a food allergy is present, the health professional will record a detailed history of symptoms, including the time from ingestion to onset of symptoms, duration of symptoms, most recent reaction, food suspected of causing a reaction, and quantity and nature of food needed to produce a reaction. A family history of allergic diseases can also help, as allergies tend to run in families. A physical examination may reveal evidence of an allergy, such as skin diseases and asthma. Various diagnostic tests can rule out other conditions (Table 19-9).

If the patient history and physical exam suggest a food allergy, the health professional then faces the task of identifying the source of the food allergy. The first step in diagnosing a food allergy is to eliminate from the diet (for 1 to 2 weeks) all food components that appear to cause allergic symptoms. This is called an **elimination diet.** The person generally starts out eating foods to which almost no one reacts, such as rice, vegetables, noncitrus fruits, and fresh meats and poultry. If symptoms are still present, the person can more severely restrict the diet or even use special formula diets that are hypoallergenic.

Once a diet is found that causes no symptoms, foods can be added back one at a time. This type of food challenge is an option only when the culprit foods are known to pose no risk of anaphylaxis in the person. Doses of ½ to 1 teaspoon (2 ½ to 5 milliliters) are given at first. The amount is increased until the dose approximates usual intake. Any reintroduced food that causes significant symptoms to appear is identified as an allergen for the person.

Laboratory tests can also aid in diagnosis of food allergies. Skin testing involves pricking the skin with a small amount of purified food extract and observing any allergic response (e.g., a red eruption at the prick site). These types of tests are easy and safe, even for infants, but they may not clearly diagnose a food allergy.

TABLE 19-9 ■ **Diagnosing Food Allergies**

History	Include description of symptoms, time between food ingestion and onset of symptoms, duration of symptoms, most recent allergic episode, quantity of food required to produce reaction, suspected foods, and allergic diseases in other family members.
Physical examination	Look for signs of an allergic reaction (rash, itching, intestinal bloating, etc.).
Elimination diet	Remove the suspected food allergen for 1 to 2 weeks or until symptoms clear.
Food challenge	Add back small amounts of excluded foods, one at a time, as long as anaphylaxis is not a possible consequence.
Blood test	Determine the presence of antibodies in blood that bind to food antigens tested.
Skin test	Place a sample of the suspected allergen under the skin and watch for an inflammatory reaction.

A positive skin-prick test merely indicates that a person has been sensitized to a food; it cannot definitively identify if that food is the cause for the symptoms in question. Newer types of blood testing, however, have more diagnostic value. Blood tests estimate the blood concentration of antibodies that bind certain foodborne antigens.

LIVING WITH FOOD ALLERGIES

Once potential allergens are identified, dietary modifications must be made (see Further Reading 16). In some cases, small amounts of the offending food can be consumed without an observable reaction. Also, some food allergens are destroyed by heating, so cooking may eliminate the allergic response. This is effective primarily for allergies to fruits or vegetables, not for the more common allergies to milk, peanuts, or seafood. For most cases, though, complete avoidance of allergy-causing food ingredients is the safest course of action. This makes careful reading of food labels essential. The Food Allergen Labeling and Consumer Protection Act of 2006 requires manufacturers to clearly identify the presence of major food allergens (milk, eggs, fish, shellfish, peanuts, tree nuts, wheat, and soy) on food product labels. Recently proposed legislation may soon add sesame seeds to the list of food allergens that must be listed on food labels.

A major challenge when treating a person with a food allergy is to make sure that what remains in the dietary pattern can still provide essential nutrients. The small food intake of children permits less leeway in removing offending foods that may contain numerous nutrients. A registered dietitian nutritionist can help guide the diet-planning process to ensure that the remaining food choices still meet nutrient needs or to guide supplement use, if that is necessary.

Studies show that about 25% of young children with food allergies outgrow them. Parents should be made aware of this and not assume the allergy will be lifelong. Food allergies diagnosed after 3 years of age are often longer lived, but not always. It is common for children to outgrow allergies to milk, soy, or eggs, but allergies to peanuts, tree nuts, and shellfish are likely to endure. Periodic reintroduction of offending foods can be tried every 6 to 12 months or so, to see whether the allergic reaction has decreased. If no symptoms appear, tolerance to the food has developed.

Several strategies are under study to ease the dietary restrictions imposed by food allergies. One possibility includes treatment with antibodies that will increase the threshold at which an allergic response occurs. For a person with an allergy to peanuts, for example, this would alleviate some anxiety about severe reactions to trace amounts of peanuts found in foods. Similarly, immunotherapy, which exposes allergic individuals to very small but progressively larger amounts of food allergens, may help some people build up a tolerance to certain food components. Vaccines are another area of research. Also, scientists are working on genetically engineered foods that do not contain common allergens.

PREVENTING FOOD ALLERGIES

With the rising number of cases of food allergies, many new parents wonder when and how to introduce new foods during infancy and early childhood. It is evident that introducing foods other than human milk or infant formula before 4 months of age is associated with higher risk of allergic diseases. Most experts, including the American Academy of Pediatrics and the American Academy of Allergy, Asthma, and Immunology, advise waiting to introduce solid foods until 4 to 6 months of age for lowest risk of food allergies. Delaying introduction of solid foods beyond 6 months of age is not advised.

Any food can contain a potential allergen, but certain foods have been found to have high allergenic potential. The eight leading food allergens in the United States are milk, eggs, peanuts, tree nuts, fish, shellfish, wheat, and soy. The American Academy of Pediatrics and the National Institute of Allergy and Infectious Diseases no longer advise delaying the introduction of highly allergenic foods beyond 6 months of age, even for infants with a family history of food allergies (see Newsworthy Nutrition).

Until recently, allergy-prone women were advised to avoid highly allergenic foods during pregnancy and breastfeeding. Allergens can cross the placenta during pregnancy and are secreted in breast milk. However, research does not demonstrate a benefit of maternal dietary restrictions in preventing food allergies in infants.

The best course of action is to breastfeed the infant exclusively for 6 months and continue to breastfeed through 12 months with appropriate introduction of solid foods to meet the infant's nutritional needs. Human milk contains factors that play a role in the maturation of the small intestine. Formula-fed infants, especially those on cow milk-based formulas, have a greater risk for developing food allergies. There is evidence that hydrolyzed infant formulas (in which the large proteins have been broken down into smaller peptides) may be useful in allergy prevention for infants

> People with a history of serious allergic reactions and those who have asthma should carry a self-administered form of epinephrine, such as EpiPen®, to subside an episode of anaphylaxis, should it occur.

▲ In 2006, the Food Allergen Labeling and Consumer Protection Act mandated that food manufacturers make consumers aware of the presence of highly allergenic ingredients in their products. © FoodIngredients/Alamy

> Free information on food allergies is available by contacting Food Allergy Research and Education (FARE). The telephone number is (800) 929-4040; the website is www.foodallergy.org.

Newsworthy Nutrition

EARLY INTRODUCTION OF PEANUT PROTEIN REDUCES PEANUT ALLERGY

Based on a hypothesis that early introduction of food proteins in infants' diets increased risk for food allergies, pediatricians once advised parents to delay introduction of potential food allergens (e.g., 2 years for eggs and 3 years for peanuts, tree nuts, and fish). However, in the 1990s, evidence started to accumulate that delaying introduction of a variety of foods provided no benefit for preventing food allergies. For instance, Jewish children raised in the United Kingdom, where peanuts were not introduced until after 1 year of age, were 10 times more likely to develop peanut allergies than Jewish children raised in Israel, where peanut-based foods are introduced within the first year of life. The Learning Early About Peanut allergy (LEAP) trial aimed to see if early introduction of peanut protein could prevent peanut allergies among at-risk children. The randomized, controlled trial included 640 infants, between 4 and 11 months of age, who were at risk for food allergies (based on existing allergies, severe eczema, or both). Participants were divided into two groups based on previous sensitization to peanut protein (i.e., skin testing showed if the infants' immune systems had already reacted to peanut protein from dietary, skin, or respiratory exposure). Then, the infants were randomized to treatment or control groups. The treatment group received at least 6 grams of peanut protein per week in the form of a peanut-based snack food or smooth peanut butter, while the control group was advised to avoid dietary exposure to peanuts. At 5 years of age, the children were tested for peanut allergy using an oral food challenge. Among the children who were not sensitized to peanuts at baseline, peanut consumption reduced the risk of developing peanut allergy by 86.1% compared to controls. Among the children who were initially sensitized to peanut protein, treatment with peanut protein reduced the risk of developing peanut allergy by 70%. The researchers concluded that early (<11 months), sustained peanut consumption reduced peanut allergy among children at risk of food allergies.

Source: Du Toit G and others: Randomized trial of peanut consumption in infants at risk for peanut allergy. *New England Journal of Medicine* 372:803, 2015.

at risk of developing food allergies. However, hydrolyzed formulas are about three times as costly as cow milk-based formulas.

FOOD INTOLERANCES

Food intolerances are adverse reactions to foods that do not involve immunologic mechanisms. Generally, larger amounts of an offending food are required to produce the symptoms of an intolerance than to trigger allergic symptoms. Common causes of food intolerances include:

- Constituents of certain foods (e.g., red wine, tomatoes, and pineapples) that have a druglike activity, causing physiological effects such as changes in blood pressure
- Certain synthetic compounds added to foods, such as sulfites, food-coloring agents, and monosodium glutamate (MSG)
- Food contaminants, including antibiotics and other chemicals used in the production of livestock and crops, as well as insect parts not removed during processing
- Toxic contaminants, which may be ingested with improperly handled and prepared foods containing *Clostridium botulinum*, *Salmonella* bacteria, or other foodborne microorganisms (see Section 17.3)
- Deficiencies in digestive enzymes, such as lactase (review Section 4.4)

Almost everyone is sensitive to one or more of these causes of food intolerance, many of which produce GI tract symptoms. Sulfites, added to foods and beverages as antioxidants, cause flushing, spasms of the airway, and a loss of blood pressure in susceptible people. Wine, dehydrated potatoes, dried fruits, gravy, soup mixes, and restaurant salad greens commonly contain sulfites. A reaction to MSG may include an increase in blood pressure, numbness, sweating, vomiting, headache, and facial pressure. MSG is commonly found in restaurant food and many processed foods (e.g., soups). A reaction to tartrazine, a yellow food-coloring additive, includes spasm of the airway, itching, and reddening skin. Tyramine, a derivative of the amino acid tyrosine, is commonly found in "aged" foods such as cheeses and red wines. This natural food constituent can cause high blood pressure in people taking monoamine oxidase (MAO) inhibitor medications, which may be prescribed for clinical depression.

The basic treatment for food intolerances is to avoid specific offending components. However, total elimination often is not required because people generally are not as sensitive to compounds causing food intolerances as they are to allergens.

Summary (Numbers refer to numbered sections in the chapter.)

19.1 Growth is rapid during infancy; birth weight doubles in 4 to 6 months, and length increases by 50% in the first year. An adequate dietary pattern, especially in terms of calories, protein, iron, and calcium, is essential to support normal growth. Growth charts can be used to assess changes in body weight, height (or length), head circumference, and body mass index over time.

19.2 The energy needs of infants are highest per kilogram of body weight compared to any other life stage (about 100 kcal per kilogram). Fat should make up about 50% of total energy intake. DHA and ARA are important fatty acids for nervous system development. Carbohydrate needs range from 60 grams per day for younger infants to 95 grams per day for older infants. Protein needs are 9 grams per day for younger infants and 11 grams per day for older infants. Supplementation with vitamin D, iron, and fluoride may be appropriate for some infants. Adequate hydration can be maintained using only breast milk or formula; supplemental water is not recommended during the first 6 months of life.

19.3 Infant nutrient needs can be met by human milk or iron-fortified infant formula for the first 6 months of life. Most infants do not need solid foods before 6 months of age. Introduction of solid foods should be based on an infant's nutritional needs, physical abilities, and developmental readiness. Solid foods should be introduced one at a time, starting with iron-fortified infant cereals or ground meats (sources of iron). Some foods to avoid giving infants in the first year include honey, unaltered cow's milk (especially fat-reduced varieties), foods with added salt or sugar, and foods that may cause choking.

19.4 A slower growth rate results in decreased appetite among preschool children. Other common nutrition-related concerns include iron-deficiency anemia, constipation, and dental caries. With smaller portion sizes and picky eating behaviors, it is crucial to offer several small meals and snacks with a variety of nutrient-dense foods. Follow the example set forth by MyPlate, but use smaller portions (e.g., 1 tablespoon of food per year of life). For autism spectrum disorders, several nutritional interventions, including the gluten-free, casein-free diet, and some dietary supplements, are under study.

19.5 Among school-age children, excessive energy and fat intakes coupled with low levels of physical activity have led to an alarming increase in overweight, obesity, type 2 diabetes, and cardiovascular disease. Parents can provide healthful food choices and encourage at least 60 minutes of physical activity per day. When controlled early through dietary and exercise interventions, the problem of obesity may correct itself as the child continues to grow in height. Other important nutrition strategies for school-age children include starting the day with breakfast and selecting low-fat or fat-free milk or water instead of sugar-sweetened beverages. Recent changes in meal offerings through schools are aimed at curtailing the rise in childhood obesity.

19.6 During the adolescent growth spurt, both boys and girls have increased needs for iron, calcium, and overall calories. Inadequate calcium intake by teenage girls is a major concern because it can set the stage for the development of osteoporosis later in life. Adolescents need to limit their intakes of high-fat and high-sugar fast foods and snacks and use caffeine in moderation (if at all). Alcohol abuse during adolescence has many severe consequences, including impaired brain development and increased risk for liver and cardiovascular diseases in adulthood.

19.7 The most common food allergies are associated with peanuts, tree nuts, shellfish, milk, eggs, soybeans, wheat, and fish. Food allergies occur most often during infancy and young adulthood. Dietary treatment for food allergies involves complete avoidance of the food allergen.

Check Your Knowledge (Answers are available at the end of this question set.)

1. Inadequate intake of which of the following results in poor growth?
   a. Calories
   b. Iron
   c. Zinc
   d. All of these

2. Cow's milk is a nutrient-dense source of all of the following except
   a. protein.
   b. iron.
   c. calcium.
   d. zinc.

3. To ensure adequate vitamin and mineral intake for a picky eater,
   a. provide a fortified breakfast cereal.
   b. promise dessert as a reward for eating meats and vegetables.
   c. use a multivitamin and mineral supplement.
   d. avoid all of these.

4. An 11-month-old girl who weighs 19 pounds needs approximately _____ kcal per day.
   a. 690
   b. 810
   c. 845
   d. 930

5. Introduction of cow's milk should be delayed until 12 months of age because it
   a. contains too much fat.
   b. supplies too much lactose.
   c. contains too much protein.
   d. does all of these.

6. Your niece breaks out in hives and feels nauseous after eating a salad containing mango. She probably has a food
   a. sensitivity.
   b. allergy.
   c. intolerance.
   d. All of these are correct.

7. Which of the following are benefits of consuming a fortified, ready-to-eat breakfast cereal instead of skipping breakfast?
   a. Improved academic performance
   b. Meeting RDAs for iron and calcium
   c. Lower risk for childhood obesity
   d. All of these

8. A gluten-free, casein-free diet has been studied for treatment of
   a. rickets.
   b. anemia.
   c. lead poisoning.
   d. autism.

9. If moderate weight loss is needed, a school-age child should
   a. eat fewer meals.
   b. follow a low-carbohydrate eating plan.
   c. exercise for 60 minutes per day or more.
   d. avoid dairy products.

10. You are trying to introduce an apple and blueberry puree to a 7-month-old infant, but she rejects it. You should
    a. assume she doesn't like apples and blueberries.
    b. offer the food again on another day.
    c. force a spoonful into her mouth.
    d. do none of these.

Answer Key: 1. d (LO 19.1), 2. b (LO 19.2), 3. a (LO 19.2), 4. a (LO 19.3), 5. c (LO 19.3), 6. b (LO 19.6), 7. d (LO 19.4), 8. d (LO 19.4), 9. c (LO 19.5), 10. b (LO 19.3)

Study Questions (Numbers refer to Learning Outcomes)

1. List two factors that limit "catch-up" growth when a nutrient-deficient dietary pattern has been consumed throughout childhood. **(LO 19.1)**

2. A 3-month-old infant is taken to a clinic with failure to thrive. What are two possible explanations? **(LO 19.1)**

3. Which two nutrients are of particular concern in planning dietary patterns for teenagers? Why does each deserve to be singled out? **(LO 19.2)**

4. List three nutrients of concern for a child who chooses a vegetarian lifestyle. **(LO 19.2)**

5. Outline three key factors that help to determine when to introduce solid foods into an infant's dietary pattern. **(LO 19.3)**

6. Compare the guidelines for infant feeding summarized in this chapter with the Dietary Guidelines for Americans for children over age 2 and adults discussed in Chapter 2. Which guidelines are similar? Do any contradict each other? If so, why? **(LO 19.3)**

7. Describe the pros and cons of snacking. What is the basic advice for healthful snacking from childhood through the teenage years? **(LO 19.4)**

8. List three reasons why preschoolers are noted for "picky" eating. For each, describe an appropriate parent response. **(LO 19.4)**

9. What three factors are likely to contribute to obesity in a typical 10-year-old child? **(LO 19.5)**

10. List evidence-based strategies to reduce the risk of food allergies in infants. **(LO 19.6)**

What the Dietitian Chose

At 18 months of age, Lila's dietary pattern should include small portions of a variety of foods from each MyPlate food group. She should have several teeth by now, but her chewing ability is still limited. As a young child, Lila has high nutrient needs and yet has a small stomach capacity, so snacking makes an important contribution to meeting overall nutrient needs.

Reduced-fat popcorn is a healthy, low-fat snack for older children and adults. Feeding children bulky foods with low energy density, however, can lead to fullness without meeting nutritional needs. Furthermore, popcorn is a choking hazard.

Although baby carrots with ranch dressing would be a good source of beta-carotene and plant oils, toddlers are not expert chewers just yet, and large pieces of hard, crunchy foods present a choking hazard. Slicing the carrots into long, thin strips would be a better idea.

Fat-free, light yogurt is a good source of calcium and vitamin D for building healthy bones and certainly does not present a choking risk; however, infants and toddlers need the fat and sugar in dairy products to supply calories for their growing bodies. Whole-milk yogurt such as YoBaby® would be a better choice.

Whole-grain crackers with sliced cheddar cheese would be an excellent snacking option for Lila. This snack provides a healthy balance of carbohydrates, protein, and fat. Using whole-grain crackers, rather than those made with refined flour, will boost the vitamin and mineral content (review Section 4.3).

Toddlers are known for picky eating behaviors. Lila's slower pace of growth may reduce her appetite and she may be more interested in exploring the world around her than sitting down for a meal. Make sure Lila sits down to eat and supervise her while she is eating. Finally, be a good role model. If she sees you eat the healthy snacks you have offered, she will be more likely to accept them.

© Dynamic Graphics/JupiterImages

CASE STUDY SOLUTION — Undernutrition During Infancy

1. Ask if the formula is iron fortified. Also, verify that Damon's caregivers are appropriately preparing his formula by adding the correct amount of powder or concentrated liquid to water. Be sure that Damon's caregivers plan to continue giving him formula until 1 year of age.

2. The scenario described puts Damon at risk for failure to thrive, likely due to his caregivers' lack of knowledge about appropriate infant feeding practices. His dietary pattern is probably lacking in total calories as well as calcium, iron, and zinc. Inadequacies may lead to stunted growth, cognitive problems, behavioral problems, and weak bones.

3. In addition to an iron-fortified infant formula, Damon should be eating iron-fortified infant cereals, pureed fruits and vegetables, ground meats, and even some table foods that are soft and cut into small pieces. After a child reaches 6 months of age, nutrient-dense, solid foods help to meet increased nutrient demands. Processed foods, such as the hot dog described in the scenario, are usually high in sodium, fat, or sugars. Hot dogs and other foods that are round, compressible, and small in diameter are choking hazards for infants and children under age 4. These are not ideal for meeting Damon's nutritional needs. Allowing Damon to self-feed to some extent will help him to develop motor skills and build confidence.

4. Infants should not be drinking sugar-sweetened beverages such as colas or fruit-flavored drinks, as these items lack the nutrient density essential to meeting Damon's needs. If his caregivers provide juice at all, the total amount should be limited to 6 fluid ounces of 100% fruit juice. To prevent early childhood caries and develop self-feeding skills, Damon should be learning to drink from a cup rather than a bottle.

5. The combination of an appropriately prepared, iron-fortified infant formula and a variety of solid foods should provide Damon all the nutrients he needs. However, if he is anemic, he may need an iron supplement.

Further Readings

1. Abrams EM: Introducing solid foods: Age of introduction and its effect on risk of food allergy and other atopic diseases. *Canadian Family Physician* 59:721, 2013.

2. Academy of Nutrition and Dietetics: Position of the American Dietetic Association: Nutrition guidance for healthy children ages 2 to 11 years. *Journal of the Academy of Nutrition and Dietetics* 114:1257, 2014.

3. Briefel RR and others: Reducing calories and added sugars by improving children's beverage choices. *Journal of the Academy of Nutrition and Dietetics* 113:269, 2013.

4. Briggs M and others: Position of the American Dietetic Association, School Nutrition Association, and Society for Nutrition Education: Comprehensive school nutrition services. *Journal of the American Dietetic Association* 110:1738, 2010.

5. Cole SZ, Lanham JS: Failure to thrive: An update. *American Family Physician* 83:829, 2011.

6. Committee on Nutrition and the Council on Sports Medicine and Fitness: Sports drinks and energy drinks for children and adolescents: Are they appropriate? *Pediatrics* 127:1182, 2011.

7. Copeland KC and others: Management of newly diagnosed type 2 diabetes mellitus (T2DM) in children and adolescents. *Pediatrics* 131:364, 2013.

8. Ford CN and others: Trends in dietary intake among US 2–6-year-old children, 1989–2008. *Journal of the Academy of Nutrition and Dietetics* 113:35, 2013.

9. Gupta RS and others: Childhood food allergies: Current diagnosis, treatment, and management strategies. *Mayo Clinic Proceedings* 88:512, 2013.

10. Kavey RW and others: Expert panel on integrated guidelines for cardiovascular health and risk reduction in children and adolescents: Summary report. *Pediatrics* 128:S213, 2011.

11. Kosova EC and others: The relationship between sugar-sweetened beverage intake and cardiometabolic markers in young children. *Journal of the Academy of Nutrition and Dietetics* 113:219, 2013.

12. Mari-Bauset S and others: Evidence of the gluten-free and casein-free diet in autism spectrum disorders: A systematic review. *Journal of Child Neurology* 29:1718, 2014.

13. Moag-Stahlberg A: *The state of family nutrition and physical activity: Are we making progress? Report of the American Dietetic Association and American Dietetic Association Foundation,* 2011. http://www.eatright.org/foundation/fnpa.

14. National Institute of Allergy and Infectious Diseases: *Guidelines for the diagnosis and management of food allergy in the United States: Summary for patients, families, and caregivers.* May 2011. http://www.niaid.nih.gov/topics/foodAllergy/clinical/Documents/FAguidelinesPatient.pdf. Accessed January 31, 2016.

15. Office of Juvenile Justice and Delinquency Prevention: Effects and consequences of underage drinking. *Juvenile Justice Bulletin,* 2012. http://www.ojjdp.gov/pubs/237145.pdf.

16. Orenstein BW: Pediatric food allergies. *Today's Dietitian* 16:12, 2014.

17. Powell LM, Nguyen BT: Fast-food and full-service restaurant consumption among children and adolescents: Effect on energy, beverage, and nutrient intake. *JAMA Pediatrics* 167:14, 2013.

18. Privett D: Autism spectrum disorder: Research suggests good nutrition may manage symptoms. *Today's Dietitian* 15:46, 2013.

19. Short MW, Domagalski JE: Iron deficiency anemia: Evaluation and management. *American Family Physician* 87:98, 2013.

20. Thalheimer JC: Update on infant formulas. *Today's Dietitian* 26:32, 2014.

21. Wagner CL and others: Prevention of rickets and vitamin D deficiency in infants, children, and adolescents. *Pediatrics* 122(5):1142, 2008.

22. Williams PG: The benefits of breakfast cereal consumption: A systematic review of the evidence base. *Advances in Nutrition* 5:636S, 2014.

23. Wojcicki JM, Heyman MB: Reducing childhood obesity by eliminating 100% fruit juice. *American Journal of Public Health* 102:1630, 2012.

24. World Health Organization: *Report of the Commission on Ending Childhood Obesity.* Geneva: WHO Document Production Services, 2016.

 connect To get the most out of your study of nutrition, go to McGraw-Hill's online resources: Connect www.mcgrawhillconnect.com, where you will find NutritionCalc Plus, LearnSmart, and many other dynamic tools.

Rate Your Plate

Getting Young Bill to Eat

Bill is 3 years old, and his mother is worried about his eating habits. He refuses to eat vegetables, meat, and dinner in general. Some days he eats very little food. He wants to eat snacks most of the time. Mealtime is a battle because Bill says he is not hungry, and his mother wants him to sit down and eat all of his lunch and dinner to make sure he gets all the nutrients he needs. He drinks five or six glasses of whole milk per day because that is the one food he likes.

When his mother prepares dinner, she makes plenty of vegetables, boiling them until they are soft, hoping this will appeal to Bill. Bill's dad waits to eat his vegetables last, regularly telling the family that he eats them only because he has to. He also regularly complains about how dinner has been prepared. Bill saves his vegetables until last and usually gags when his mother orders him to eat them. Bill has been known to sit at the dinner table for an hour until the war of wills ends. Bill's mother serves casseroles and stews regularly because they are convenient. Bill likes to eat breakfast cereal, fruit, and cheese, and regularly requests these foods for snacks. However, his mother tries to deny his requests, so that he will have an appetite for dinner. Bill's mother comes to you and asks you what she should do to get Bill to eat.

© McGraw-Hill Education/Jill Braaten, photographer

Analysis

1. List four mistakes Bill's parents are making that contribute to Bill's inadequate eating pattern.

   _____

   _____

   _____

2. List four strategies they might try to promote good eating habits in Bill.

   _____

   _____

   _____

© Digital Vision/PunchStock

Student Learning Outcomes

Chapter 20 is designed to allow you to:

20.1 Discuss demographic trends among adults in North America and how they impact health care.

20.2 List several hypotheses about the causes of aging.

20.3 Describe how physiological changes of aging affect nutritional status of adults.

20.4 Compare the dietary intake of adults with current recommendations.

20.5 Identify nutrition-related health conditions of the adult years and describe the prevention and treatment options.

20.6 List several nutritional programs available to help meet nutritional needs of older adults.

20.7 Compare benefits of moderate alcohol use to the risks of alcohol abuse.

Chapter 20
Nutrition During Adulthood

What Would You Choose?

At age 62, you have suffered for years with frequent heartburn and you've been taking an acid-reducing medication to reduce your symptoms. Recently, you began feeling weak, fatigued, and short of breath. Blood tests revealed macrocytic anemia due to vitamin B-12 deficiency. Due to reduced stomach-acid secretion, your absorption of vitamin B-12 has been impaired. What would you choose to boost your vitamin B-12 status?

a Leafy, green vegetables

b Beef pot roast

c Cheerios® cereal

d Centrum® Silver® Adults 50+ dietary supplement

Think about your choice as you read this chapter, then see What the Dietitian Chose at the end of the chapter.

Eating is one of our great pleasures. Guided by common sense and moderation, eating well is also a means to good health. Most of us want a long, productive life, free of illness. Unfortunately, many people from early middle age onward suffer from obesity, cardiovascular disease, hypertension, stroke, type 2 diabetes, osteoporosis, and other chronic diseases. We can slow the development of—and in some cases, even prevent—these diseases by following a dietary pattern such as that exemplified by MyPlate or the Mediterranean Diet. The effect of such a dietary pattern is most profitable if we begin early and continue throughout adulthood. We serve ourselves best—as individuals and as a nation—by striving to maintain vitality even in the later decades of life. This concept was first explored in Chapter 1 and is discussed again in this chapter, in light of the nutritional needs of adults.

Keep in mind that today's behaviors can significantly influence your health years from now. Although genes do play a role, as discussed in Section 3.11, many of the health problems that occur with age are not inevitable; they result from diet-related disease processes that influence physical health. Much can be learned from healthy older people whose attention to healthy dietary and activity patterns—along with a little help from heredity—keeps them active and vibrant well beyond typical retirement years. Successful aging is the goal. Age quickly or slowly: it is partly your choice.

20.1 The Graying of North America

Due to advances in health care and sanitation, the demographics of developed countries are shifting so that, as a population, we are getting older. In North America, the group constituting those aged 85+ years is the fastest growing segment. Between 1997 and 2050, the population aged 85+ years in the United States is expected to increase from 3.4 to 19 million (Fig. 20-1). Even more amazing, 1 million or more people in the United States could be over 100 years old in 2050.

This "graying" of North America poses some problems. Although people older than age 65 account for just 13% of the U.S. population, they account for more than 25% of all prescription medications used, 40% of acute hospital stays, and 50% of the federal health budget. Hip fractures alone cost the nation about $12 billion per year. Of older persons, 80% or more have chronic conditions, such as cardiovascular disease, type 2 diabetes, hypertension, and osteoporosis.

Postponing these chronic diseases for as long as possible will help control health care costs. Health and independence contribute quality—not just quantity—to life and lessen the load on an already overburdened health care system. Keep in mind that aging is not a disease. Furthermore, diseases that commonly accompany old age—osteoporosis and atherosclerosis, for example—are not an inevitable part of aging. Many can be prevented or managed. Some people *do* die of old age, not as a direct result of disease.

THE CAUSES OF AGING

Adulthood, the longest stage of the life cycle, begins when an adolescent completes his or her physical growth. Unlike earlier stages of the life cycle, nutrients are used primarily to maintain the body rather than support physical growth. (Pregnancy is the only time during adulthood when substantial amounts of nutrients are used for growth.) As adults get older, nutrient needs change. For example, vitamin D needs increase for older adults.

Aging can be defined as the time-dependent physical and physiological changes in body structure and function that occur normally and progressively throughout adulthood as humans mature and become older. One view of aging describes it as a process of slow cell death,

aging Time-dependent physical and physiological changes in body structure and function that occur normally and progressively throughout adulthood as humans mature and become older.

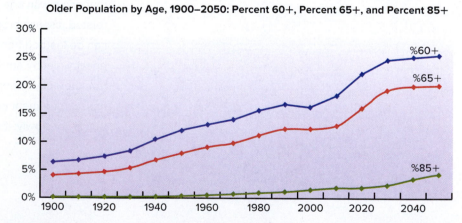

Older Population by Age, 1900–2050: Percent 60+, Percent 65+, and Percent 85+

FIGURE 20-1 ▲ **Growth of the U.S. Population of Older Adults.** This chart shows that the proportion of the total U.S. population composed of older adults has been steadily increasing over the past century and how these trends are expected to continue. The 85+ demographic group (green line), although still the smallest group in total numbers, is experiencing the most rapid rate of growth. Enhancements in health care and sanitation, as well as the baby boom that occurred after World War II, are contributing to the graying of North America. Conversely, most demographic groups under the age of 45 are shrinking as a percentage of overall population (not shown here). This means that fewer young people will be available to care for a growing population of older adults in years to come.

Source: U.S. Administration on Aging.

beginning soon after fertilization. When we are young, aging is not apparent because the major metabolic activities are geared toward growth and maturation. We produce plenty of active cells to meet physiological needs. During late adolescence and adulthood, the body's major task is to maintain cells. From the beginning of adulthood until age 30 or so, the body operates at peak performance: stature, stamina, strength, endurance, efficiency, and health are at their lifetime highs. Rates of cell synthesis and breakdown are balanced in most tissues.

Inevitably, though, cells age and die. After about age 30, the rate of cell breakdown slowly begins to exceed the rate of cell renewal, leading to a gradual decline in organ size and efficiency. Eventually, the body cannot adjust to meet all physiological demands, and body functioning begins to decrease (Fig. 20-2). Still, body systems and organs usually retain enough **reserve capacity** to handle normal, everyday demands throughout one's entire lifetime. Problems caused by diminished capacity typically do not arise unless severe demands are placed on the aging body. For example, alcohol intake can overtax an aging liver. The stress of shoveling a snow-covered sidewalk can exceed the capacity of the heart and lungs. Coping with an illness also can push an older body beyond its capacity.

The causes of aging remain a mystery. Most likely, the physiological changes of aging are the sum of automatic cellular changes, lifestyle practices, and environmental influences, as listed in Table 20-1. Even with the most supportive environment and healthy lifestyle, cell structure and function still decline over time. The eventual death of deteriorating cells is actually beneficial because it likely prevents diseases such as cancer. Unfortunately, there are negative consequences to this natural cell progression because, as more and more cells in an organ die, organ function decreases. For example, **kidney nephrons** are continually lost as we age. In some people, this loss exhausts the kidneys' reserve capacity and ultimately leads to kidney failure. Most people, however, maintain sufficient kidney function throughout life.

The diseases and degenerative processes commonly observed in older people have long been assumed to be unavoidable consequences of aging. Certainly, some of the declines we blame on aging may be inevitable, such as gradual reductions in tissue and organ cell numbers, graying hair, and reduced lung capacity. However, many of the so-called usual or degenerative age-related changes can, in fact, be minimized, prevented, and/or reversed by healthy lifestyles (e.g., eating a nutritious diet, exercising regularly, and getting enough sleep) and avoiding adverse environmental factors (e.g., excessive exposure to sunlight and cigarette smoke). These discoveries have led researchers to introduce the concepts of "usual aging" and "successful aging."

▲ The baby boom turned 70 in 2016, resulting in an increase in demand for attention to the health concerns of this aging population.
© Royalty-Free/Corbis

reserve capacity The extent to which an organ can preserve essentially normal function despite decreasing cell number or cell activity.

kidney nephrons The units of kidney cells that filter wastes from the bloodstream and deposit them into the urine.

USUAL AND SUCCESSFUL AGING

Body cells age, no matter what health practices we follow. However, to a considerable extent, you can choose how quickly you age throughout your adult years. *Usual aging* refers to

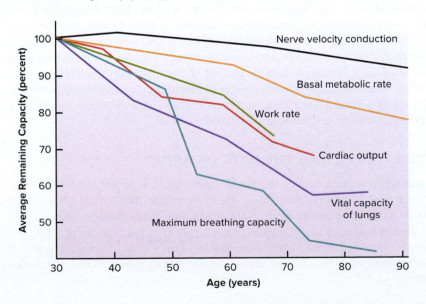

FIGURE 20-2 ◄ Declines in physiological function seen with aging. The decline in many body functions is especially evident in sedentary people.

▲ Adopting diet and lifestyle practices that minimize a decline in body function is an investment in your future health. Visit www.nia.nih.gov for many free resources on healthy aging. © Stockbyte/Getty Images

glycosylation The process by which glucose attaches to (glycates) other compounds, such as proteins.

TABLE 20-1 ■ **Current Hypotheses About the Causes of Aging**

Errors occur in copying the genetic blueprint (DNA).
Once sufficient errors in DNA copying accumulate, a cell can no longer synthesize the major proteins needed to function, and it therefore dies.

Connective tissue stiffens.
Parallel protein strands, found mostly in connective tissue, cross-link to each other. This decreases flexibility in key body components.

Electron-seeking compounds damage cell parts.
Electron-seeking free radicals can break down cell membranes and proteins.

Hormone function changes.
The blood concentration of many hormones, such as testosterone in men, falls during the aging process.

Glycosylation of proteins.
Blood glucose, when chronically elevated, attaches to (glycates) various blood and body proteins, decreasing their function and encouraging immune system attack on them.

The immune system loses some efficiency.
With advancing age, the immune system is less able to recognize and counteract foreign substances, such as viruses, that enter the body.

Autoimmunity develops.
Autoimmune reactions occur when white blood cells and other immune system components begin to attack body tissues, such as in arthritis.

Death is programmed into the cell.
Each human cell can divide only about 50 times after which the cell automatically succumbs.

Excess calorie intake speeds body breakdown.
Laboratory animals underfed by about 30% have been shown to live longer than their well-fed counterparts. Calorie restriction is the only proven way to substantially slow the aging process (see Further Readings 6 and 15).

Keep in mind that extending life without delaying onset of chronic disease prolongs suffering in many cases. In addition, the greater number of disabled years is costly to all North Americans. For these reasons, prolonging life without compressing the number of disabled years is called the "failure of success."

compression of morbidity Delay of the onset of disabilities caused by chronic disease.

life span The potential oldest age a person can reach.

life expectancy The average length of life for a given group of people born in a specific year.

those changes commonly thought to be a typical or expected part of aging, such as increasing body fatness, decreasing lean body mass, rising blood pressure, declining bone mass, and increasingly poor health. Researchers point out that many of these changes really represent an acceleration of the aging process induced by unhealthy lifestyle choices, adverse environmental exposures, and/or chronic disease. For instance, blood pressure does not tend to rise with age among people whose diets are traditionally low in sodium. Also, lean body mass is maintained much better in older people who exercise than in those who do not.

Successful aging, on the other hand, describes physical and physiological function declines that occur only because one grows older, not because lifestyle choices, environmental exposures, and chronic disease have assaulted body tissues. Those who are successful agers experience age-related declines at a slower rate and the onset of chronic disease symptoms at a later age than usual agers. Striving to have the greatest number of healthy years and the fewest years of illness is often referred to as **compression of morbidity.** In other words, a person tries to delay the onset of disabilities caused by chronic disease and to compress significant sickness related to aging into the last few years—or months—of life.

FACTORS AFFECTING THE RATE OF AGING

Life span refers to the maximum number of years a human can live. As far as we know, this has not changed in recorded time. The longest human life documented to date is 122 years for a woman and 116 years for a man. **Life expectancy,** alternatively, is the time an average person born in a specific year can expect to live. Life expectancy in North America is about 76 years for men and about 81 years for women, with a span of "healthy years" of about 64. Furthermore, most people who survive to age 80 can expect to live an additional 7 to 10 years.

The rate at which one ages is individual; it is determined by genetics, lifestyle, and environment. With the exception of genetics, most of the factors that influence the rate of aging are directly linked to choices that are under our control.

Genetics Living to an old age tends to run in some families. If your parents and grandparents lived a long time, you are likely to have the potential to live to an old age, too. Studies of twins indicate that about 20% to 30% of longevity can be attributed to genetics.

One of the most obvious genetic characteristics influencing longevity is gender. In the case of humans, as well as most other species, females tend to live longer than males. Another genetic characteristic that may influence longevity is metabolic efficiency. Some researchers hypothesize that individuals with a **thrifty metabolism** require fewer calories for metabolic processes and are able to store body fat more easily than those with faster metabolic rates. Throughout history, it was the individuals with thrifty metabolism who tended to live the longest because they efficiently stored fat during times of plenty and thus had the energy stores needed to survive frequent periods of food scarcity. In today's environment of labor-saving devices and abundant, energy-dense foods, however, a thrifty metabolism may actually reduce longevity. Accumulation of excessive body fat increases the risk of developing health problems that reduce life expectancy (e.g., heart disease, hypertension, and certain cancers).

Genetics remain largely unchangeable, but let us examine how you can exert control over your lifestyle and environment.

thrifty metabolism A genetic tendency toward efficient use of energy that results in below-average energy requirements and increased storage of calories as fat.

Lifestyle Lifestyle is one's pattern of living; it includes food choices, physical activity patterns, and substance use (e.g., alcohol, drugs, and tobacco). Lifestyle choices can have a major impact on health and longevity, partly by regulating gene expression. If an individual has a family history of premature heart disease, along with getting medical care, he can adjust his dietary and activity patterns, and decrease tobacco use to slow the progression of the disease and possibly extend his lifetime. The converse is true, too. That is, lifestyle choices (e.g., high-fat diet and sedentary lifestyle) can increase susceptibility to diseases that hasten the rate of aging, ultimately shortening life expectancy, even if a person is free from a genetic predisposition to disease.

In an effort to unlock the secrets to living a long and healthy life, researchers have been very interested in studying lifestyle patterns of communities in which life expectancy is higher than average. Several communities in which people quite often live to see their 90th and 100th birthdays include Okinawa, Japan; some parts of the Mediterranean region; and areas of California that are home to members of the Seventh-day Adventist religious denomination.

Worldwide, the highest average life expectancy (86 years for women and 78 years for men) is in Okinawa, southern Japan. The Okinawan dietary pattern is based on rice, fish, vegetable protein sources, fruits, vegetables, tea, herbs for seasonings, and small amounts of meat. Alcohol and salt intake is minimal. The low energy density translates into a generally low calorie intake, and the average BMI is 21. A desire to mimic their weight management success, compression of morbidity, and longevity has given rise to several popular books and websites that promote Okinawan dietary practices.

Followers of the traditional Mediterranean diet enjoy some of the lowest recorded rates of chronic disease in the world. Described in detail in Section 2.3, the Mediterranean diet features abundant daily intake of fruits, vegetables, whole grains, beans, nuts, and seeds. Olive oil, a source of heart-healthy monounsaturated fat, is the main dietary fat. Beans and fish are emphasized as sources of protein, whereas dairy products, eggs, poultry, and meats are used less frequently. Daily exercise is a way of life. In addition, many Mediterraneans partake of wine in moderation at mealtimes.

Loma Linda, California, is a town with a large population of Seventh-day Adventists, a Christian religious denomination that emphasizes stewardship of the mind and body as a way to honor God. Men in this group live about 7 years longer and women live about 4 years longer than average Americans. About 30% of Seventh-day Adventists follow a vegetarian dietary pattern, but even for those who occasionally consume animal products, the focus is on unprocessed plant foods. In particular, regular consumption of nuts and whole grains have emerged as dietary factors that predict the lower rates of chronic diseases observed

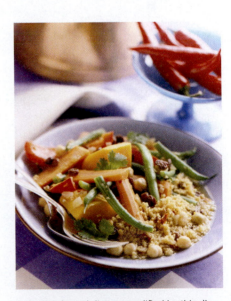

▲ A plant-based diet, exemplified by this dinner of couscous, chickpeas, and vegetables, is a common feature among populations who enjoy long, healthy lives. © Getty Images/Jonelle Weaver

Besides having other long-lived family members, people who live to 100 years generally:

- Do not smoke and do not drink heavily
- Gain little weight in adulthood
- Eat many fruits and vegetables
- Perform daily physical activity
- Challenge their minds
- Have a positive outlook
- Maintain close friendships
- Are (or were) married (especially true for men)
- Have a healthy rate of HDL-cholesterol production

in this population. Unlike the Mediterraneans, most Seventh-day Adventists avoid alcohol. Other salient aspects of the Seventh-day Adventist lifestyle that are associated with longevity include daily physical activity, avoidance of tobacco, strong faith, and strong social support within a tight-knit community.

Did you notice some common behaviors among these groups of people who enjoy extended quality and quantity of life? They all tend to focus on unprocessed, fiber-rich foods, healthy sources of fat (e.g., vegetable oils and fish), and lean sources of protein. Besides diet, physical activity is a major part of their daily routines. Compare these lifestyle choices with those of typical North Americans.

Environment Income, education level, health care, shelter, and psychosocial factors are some aspects of the environment that exert a powerful influence on the rate of aging. For instance, being able to purchase nutritious foods, quality health care, and safe housing helps decrease the rate of aging. Having the education needed to earn a sufficient income, as well as the knowledge required to select nutritious food and beverages and make wise lifestyle choices, also can slow the aging process. In addition, the willingness to seek health care promptly when it is needed, the capacity to follow the instructions of a health care provider, and the desire to accept the responsibility for one's own health can slow the rate of aging. Likewise, shelter that protects individuals from physical danger, climate extremes, and sun exposure helps slow the aging process. Allowing people to make at least some decisions for themselves and control their own activities (autonomy), and providing psychosocial support (informational and emotional resources) promote successful aging and psychological well-being. In contrast, aging is likely to accelerate if any or all of the converse are true—that is, insufficient income, low education level, lack of health care, inadequate shelter, and/or lack of autonomy and psychosocial support.

Newsworthy Nutrition

Low Animal Protein Intake Is Associated with a Major Reduction in Mortality

Caloric restriction (CR) without malnutrition has consistently shown to increase longevity in a variety of animal models. However, the effect of CR on the lifespan of humans remains controversial. The aim of this study was to combine epidemiological data with both animal and cellular study results to understand the link between protein intake, aging, disease, and mortality. Over 6380 U.S. adults, aged 50 and older, from the National Health and Nutrition Examination Survey (NHANES), were included in the sample. Mortality data was available for NHANES III participants through 2006 and covered an 18-year span. After follow-up, respondents, aged 50 to 65, with a high protein intake (>20% calories) had a 75% increase in overall mortality and a fourfold increase in cancer death. In respondents over 65, however, high protein intake was associated with reduced cancer and overall mortality. It is believed that these results are related to regulation of circulating insulin and inflammation. The authors speculate that vulnerable and often underweight seniors are more susceptible to protein malnourishment. It is also possible that other factors, such as inflammation or genetics, may contribute to the varying protein sensitivity in the elderly subjects. These results align with those of other studies showing that the amount of proteins derived from animal sources accounted for a significant proportion of the negative associations between overall protein intake and mortality. The authors are clear to point out that plant-based proteins are likely to maximize health benefits in all age groups and should not be avoided. In summary, these results suggest that low animal protein intake (<10% calories) during middle age followed by moderate to high protein consumption in old adults may optimize health span and longevity.

Source: Levine ME and others: Low protein intake is associated with a major reduction in IGF-1, cancer, and overall mortality in the 65 and younger but not older population. *Cell Metabolism* 19:407, 2014.

1. Describe three current hypotheses about the causes of aging.
2. What is the difference between *usual* and *successful* aging?
3. Discuss how genetics, lifestyle, and environment influence aging.

20.2 Nutrient Needs During Adulthood

The challenge of the adult years is to maintain the body, preserve its function, and avoid chronic disease; that is, to age successfully. A healthy diet can help achieve this goal. One blueprint for a healthy diet comes from the 2015–2020 Dietary Guidelines for Americans, discussed in Section 2.2. The advice from those guidelines included the following goals:

1. Follow a healthy eating pattern across the life span.
2. Focus on variety, nutrient density, and amount.
3. Limit calories from added sugars and saturated fats and reduce sodium intake.
4. Shift to healthier food and beverage choices.

Overall, good nutrition benefits adults in many ways. Meeting nutrient needs delays the onset of certain diseases; improves the management of some existing diseases; speeds recovery from many illnesses; increases mental, physical, and social well-being; and often decreases the need for and length of hospitalization (see Further Reading 2). As you know, American adults are fairly well nourished, although some dietary excesses and inadequacies do exist. For instance, common dietary excesses are calories, fat, sodium, and, for some, alcohol. The diets of adult women tend to fall short of the recommended amounts of vitamins D and E, folate, magnesium, calcium, zinc, and fiber. The diets of adult men tend to be low in the same nutrients, except vitamin D, which does not become problematic until age 50 (see Further Reading 19). The iron intake of most women during their childbearing years (19 to 50) is insufficient to meet their needs; however, due to a reduced iron need after **menopause,** older women do get enough iron.

People age 65 and up, particularly those in long-term care facilities and hospitals, are the single largest group at risk of malnutrition. They may become underweight and show signs of numerous micronutrient deficiencies (e.g., vitamins B-6 and B-12 and folate). To pinpoint those over age 65 at risk of nutrient deficiencies, the American College of Physicians, American Academy of Family Physicians, the Academy of Nutrition and Dietetics (formerly the American Dietetic Association), and the National Council on Aging developed the Nutrition Screening Initiative checklist (Fig. 20-3). Older Americans, family members, and health care providers can use the checklist to identify those at nutritional risk before health deteriorates significantly. Registered dietitian nutritionists can offer professional and personalized advice to help adults achieve a healthful dietary pattern.

The DRIs for adults (see Appendix G) are divided by gender and by age: ages 19 to 30, 31 to 50, 51 to 70, and beyond 70 years of age. The intervals encompassing ages 19 through 50 are often referred to as *young adulthood,* 51 to 70 as *middle adulthood,* and beyond 70 years of age as *older adulthood.* These changes in nutrient needs take into consideration aging-related physiological alterations in body composition, metabolism, and organ function.

menopause The cessation of the menstrual cycle in women, usually beginning at about 50 years of age.

KILOCALORIES

After age 30 or so, total kilocalorie needs of physically inactive adults fall steadily throughout adulthood. There are a variety of explanations for the lower kilocalorie requirements of older adults. Basal metabolic rate declines by about 2% per decade after age 30, such that overall energy needs of a 70-year-old man are reduced by 100 to 150 kcal per day compared to those of a 30-year-old man. Losses of lean mass and decreases in physical activity also tend to accompany aging. To a considerable extent, adults can exert control over this

FIGURE 20-3 ▶ A nutrition checklist for older adults.

Source: From the Nutrition Screening Initiative, a project of the American Academy of Family Physicians, the Academy of Nutrition and Dietetics (formerly the American Dietetic Association), and the National Council on Aging, Inc., and funded in part by a grant from Abbott Nutrition (formerly Ross Products Division, Abbott Laboratories). View online at the American College of Physicians website.

Nutrition Checklist for Older Adults: DETERMINE Mnemonic

Here's a nutrition check for anyone over age 65. Circle the number of points for each statement that applies. Then compute the total and check it against the nutritional score.

Possible Problem	Points	
Disease	2	1. The person has a chronic illness or current condition that has changed the kind or amount of food eaten.
Eating Poorly	3	2. The person eats fewer than two full meals per day.
	2	3. The person eats few fruits, vegetables, or milk products.
	2	4. The person drinks three or more servings of beer, liquor, or wine almost every day.
Tooth Loss\Mouth Pain	2	5. The person has tooth or mouth problems that make eating difficult.
Economic Hardship	4	6. The person does not have enough money for food.
Reduced Social Contact	1	7. The person eats alone most of the time.
Multiple Medications	1	8. The person takes three or more different prescription or over-the-counter drugs each day.
Involuntary Weight Loss\Gain	2	9. The person has unintentionally lost or gained 10 pounds within the last 6 months.
Needs Assistance In Self Care	2	10. The person cannot always shop, cook, or feed himself or herself.
Total		

Nutritional score:

0–2: Good. Recheck in 6 months.

3–5: Marginal. A local agency on aging has information about nutrition programs for the elderly. The National Association of Area Agencies on Aging can assist in finding help; call (800) 677-1116. Recheck in 6 months.

6 or more: High risk. A doctor should review this test and suggest how to improve nutritional health.

reduction in calorie need by exercising. Exercise can halt, slow, and even reverse reductions in lean body mass and subsequent declines in energy needs. Being able to consume more kilocalories makes it much easier to meet micronutrient needs without dietary supplements.

PROTEIN

The protein intake of adults of all ages in North America typically exceeds the current RDA (0.8 gram per kilogram of body weight) and falls within the recommended range of 10% to 35% of total kilocalories. However, several studies indicate that consuming protein in amounts slightly higher than the RDA (in the range of 1.0 to 1.3 grams per kilogram of body weight) may help preserve muscle and bone mass among older adults (see Further Readings 1 and 7). As with kilocalorie needs, protein requirements should be determined in relation to routine physical activity.

Furthermore, current research is focusing on the benefits of older adults consuming an adequate amount (25–30 grams) of high-quality protein at each meal, which, in combination with physical activity, may delay the onset of muscle loss, slow its progression, and reduce the magnitude of its functional consequences. Breakfast provides the best opportunity for improvement in protein intake because many individuals, including older adults, typically start their day with a meal that is low in protein and dominated by carbohydrate.

It is hypothesized that an even distribution of protein throughout the day along with physical activity will promote anabolism in older adults (see Further Reading 14).

Inclusion of animal proteins may be important because they generally have a higher proportion of the amino acid leucine, which plays a key role in stimulating muscle protein growth. Adults who have limited food budgets, have difficulty chewing meat, or are lactose intolerant may not get enough protein, especially animal protein. Recall from Section 6.7, that any protein consumed in excess of that needed for the maintenance of body tissue will be broken down and used as energy or stored as fat. The waste products of metabolism of protein must be removed by the kidneys; excessive protein intake may accelerate kidney function decline.

FAT

The fat intake of adults of all ages is often at or above the 20% to 35% of total kilocalories recommended by the Food and Nutrition Board. It is a good idea for almost all adults to reduce their fat intake because of the strong link between high-fat diets and obesity, heart disease, and certain cancers. In addition, reducing fat intake "frees up" some calories that can be better "spent" on complex carbohydrates (see Further Readings 11 and 16). The 2015–2020 Dietary Guidelines describe a healthy eating pattern as one that includes oils (27 grams or 5 teaspoons per day) and limits saturated fats and *trans* fats. A key recommendation is to consume less than 10% of kilocalories per day from saturated fats.

CARBOHYDRATES

The total carbohydrate intake of adults of all ages in North America is often lower than recommended. In addition, many adults need to shift the carbohydrate composition of their diets to emphasize complex carbohydrates while minimizing intake of sugary, simple carbohydrates. Remember that the healthy eating pattern described in the 2015–2020 Dietary Guidelines limits added sugars to 10% of kilocalories per day, but emphasizes the following carbohydrates:

- A variety of vegetables from all of the subgroups: dark green, red and orange, legumes (beans and peas), starchy, and other
- Fruits, especially whole fruits
- Grains, at least half of which are whole grains
- Fat-free or low-fat dairy, including milk, yogurt, cheese, and/or fortified soy beverages

While intakes of grains are generally adequate, only about 35% of Americans follow the advice to "make half your grains whole grains." A diet rich in complex carbohydrates helps us achieve nutrient needs and stay within calorie bounds because many highly sweetened foods are low in nutrients and high in calories. Replacing sweets and refined carbohydrates with foods rich in complex carbohydrates also improves blood glucose management. This is particularly helpful because inactivity and increasing body fatness are connected to insulin resistance. Dysfunctions of carbohydrate metabolism are so common that more than 25% of those age 65 years or older have diabetes. A diet rich in fiber helps adults reduce their risk of colon cancer and heart disease, lower their blood cholesterol levels, and avoid constipation. The typical American adult gets slightly more than half the recommended amount of dietary fiber.

WATER

Many adults, especially those in the later years, fail to consume adequate quantities of water. In fact, many are in a constant state of mild dehydration and at risk of electrolyte imbalances. Low fluid intakes in older adults may be caused by a fading sensitivity to thirst sensations, chronic diseases, and/or conscious reductions in fluid intake in order to reduce the frequency of urination. Some also may have increased fluid output because they are taking certain medications (i.e., diuretics and laxatives), have an **ostomy,** and/or experience an

ostomy Surgically created short circuit in intestinal flow where the end point usually opens from the abdominal cavity rather than the anus; for example, a colostomy. Short circuiting the intestinal flow means more water is lost in fecal matter than would be if the intestinal tract were intact.

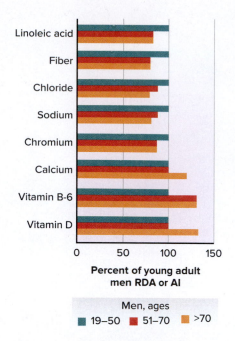

Men, ages
■ 19–50 ■ 51–70 ■ >70

FIGURE 20-4 ▲ Relative nutrient requirements for aging adult men. Only nutrients that vary by age are shown.

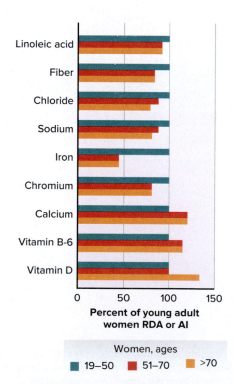

Women, ages
■ 19–50 ■ 51–70 ■ >70

FIGURE 20-5 ▲ Relative nutrient requirements for aging adult women. Only nutrients that vary by age are shown.

age-related decline in the kidneys' ability to concentrate urine. Dehydration is very dangerous and, among other symptoms, can cause disorientation and mental confusion, constipation, fecal impaction, and death.

MINERALS AND VITAMINS

Dietary requirements for many nutrients change throughout the adult years (Figs. 20-4 and 20-5). The micronutrients that need special attention because they tend to be present in less than optimal amounts in the diets of many adults are calcium, vitamin D, iron, zinc, magnesium, folate, and vitamins B-6, B-12, and E. Adults with impaired absorption or who are unable to consume a nutritious diet may benefit from mineral or vitamin supplements matched with their needs. In fact, many nutrition experts recommend a daily balanced multivitamin and mineral supplement for older adults, especially for those 70 years of age and older (see AARP's guide to supplements at http://www.aarp.org/health/drugs-supplements/info-09-2010/vitamins_from_a_to_z.html). Supplements or fortified foods can be especially helpful when it comes to meeting vitamin D and vitamin B-12 needs.

Calcium and Vitamin D These bone-building nutrients tend to be low in the dietary patterns of all adults. They become particularly problematic after age 50. Inadequate intake of these nutrients, combined with their reduced absorption, the reduced synthesis of vitamin D in the skin, and the kidneys' decreased ability to put vitamin D in its active form, greatly contributes to the development of osteoporosis. Getting enough of these nutrients is a challenge for many older adults because food sources of vitamin D are limited, and the major sources—fatty fish and fortified milk—are not widely consumed by older adults. Plus, with increasing age, lactase production frequently decreases. As you know, one of the richest and most absorbable sources of these nutrients—milk—contains lactose. To get the vitamin D and calcium needed, many with lactose intolerance can consume small amounts of milk at mealtime with no ill effects. Calcium-fortified foods, cheese, yogurt, fish eaten with bones (e.g., canned sardines or salmon), and dark, green leafy vegetables can help those with lactose intolerance meet calcium needs—but these foods often do not provide vitamin D. Just 10 to 15 minutes per day of sunlight can make a large difference in vitamin D status.

Iron Iron deficiency is the most common type of malnutrition during the adult years. Recall from Section 13.5 that iron deficiency can impair red blood cell synthesis, which leads to weakness, fatigue, shortness of breath, and "brain fog." Iron deficiency is found most frequently in women in their reproductive years because their dietary patterns do not provide enough iron to compensate for the iron lost monthly during menstruation. Other common causes of iron deficiency in adults of all ages include digestive tract injuries that cause bleeding (i.e., bleeding ulcers or hemorrhoids) and the use of medicines, such as aspirin, that cause blood loss. Impaired iron absorption due to age-related declines in stomach-acid production may contribute to iron deficiency in older adults. Remember that iron deficiency can be present before the actual signs of anemia.

Zinc In addition to less than optimal dietary zinc intake during adulthood, zinc absorption declines as stomach-acid production diminishes with age. Poor zinc status may contribute to the taste sensation losses, mental lethargy, declines in immune function, and delayed wound healing many elderly adults experience.

Magnesium This mineral tends to be low in the adult diet. Inadequate magnesium intakes may contribute to the bone loss, muscular weakness, and mental confusion seen in some elderly adults. It also can lead to sudden death from poor heart rhythm and is linked to cardiovascular disease, osteoporosis, and diabetes. The best source of magnesium is the food, because supplements can cause diarrhea.

Sodium Average sodium intakes of American adults are about 3400 milligrams per day—more than two times the AI (see Further Reading 9). A heavy reliance on processed foods and meals prepared in restaurants is mostly to blame for the high sodium intakes of Americans. The latest data from the What We Eat in America, National Health and Nutrition Examination Survey 2009–2010 indicates that sandwiches are major contributors of sodium in the dietary patterns of American adults (see Further Reading 18).

The declining sense of taste that typically accompanies aging could also contribute to a preference for highly salted foods. The Dietary Guidelines advise adults to consume less than 2300 milligrams of sodium per day. For adults over age 50; those with existing hypertension, prehypertension, diabetes, or kidney diseases; and all African-Americans, the upper limit is even lower: 1500 milligrams per day. These groups of people are especially sensitive to the effects of sodium on blood pressure. Less than 10% of adults, however, keep their sodium intakes below the UL. Recall that there are specific AIs for young, middle-aged, and older adults (see box). The most widely recognized consequence of high sodium intake is hypertension (see Section 9.9), but high sodium intake has also been linked to osteoporosis (increased calcium excretion in the urine) and may overtax the poorly functioning kidneys of older adults.

Even though excessive sodium receives most of the attention, low blood sodium (hyponatremia) is also a concern for older adults. Adults older than age 70, especially those who take diuretic medications or who have poor kidney function, are at increased risk for hyponatremia. The consequences of mild hyponatremia include lightheadedness, confusion, and unsteady gait, which can certainly increase the risk for falls among older adults. Other problems include fatigue, muscle cramps, and lack of appetite. There is no reason to severely restrict sodium among older adults who do not have kidney disease, but lowering sodium intakes closer to the AI would improve health for most adults.

Folate and Vitamins B-6 and B-12 Sufficient folate, because of its role in prevention of neural tube defects, is very important to women during the childbearing years. In later years, folate and vitamins B-6 and B-12 are especially important because they are required to clear homocysteine from the bloodstream. Elevated blood concentrations of homocysteine are associated with the increased risk of cardiovascular disease, stroke, bone fracture, and neurological decline seen in some elderly people. Vitamin B-12 is a particular problem for the older population because a deficiency may exist even when intake appears to be adequate. As people age, the stomach slows its production of acid and intrinsic factor, which leads to poor absorption of vitamin B-12. If vitamin B-12 is depleted, anemia and nerve damage could result. Adults age 51 years and older must meet vitamin B-12 needs with supplements or fortified foods, because synthetic vitamin B-12 is more readily absorbed than natural forms of B-12.

Vitamin E The dietary intake of most of the population falls short of recommendations for vitamin E. Low vitamin E intake means that the body has a reduced supply of antioxidants, which may increase the degree of cell damage caused by free radicals, promote the progression of chronic diseases and cataracts, and speed aging. In addition, low vitamin E levels can lead to declines in physical abilities.

Carotenoids Dietary intakes of certain carotenoids have been shown to have a variety of important antiaging and health protective effects. Specifically, lutein and zeaxanthin have been linked with the prevention of cataracts and age-related macular degeneration. Diets high in fruit and vegetables, the major sources of carotenoids and other beneficial phytochemicals, are consistently shown to be protective against a wide variety of age-related conditions.

ARE ADULTS FOLLOWING CURRENT DIETARY RECOMMENDATIONS?

In general, adults in North America are trying to follow many of the dietary recommendations described in this chapter. Since the mid-1950s, they have consumed less saturated fat as more people substitute fat-free and low-fat milk for cream and whole milk. However, they

Sodium

AI

  9–50 years: 1500 milligrams

  51–70 years: 1300 milligrams

  >70 years: 1200 milligrams

DV: 2400 milligrams

UL: 2300 milligrams

▲ Sodium needs for older adults are 1200 to 1300 milligrams per day. Older adults routinely consume at least this much sodium. Potassium needs are 4700 milligrams per day. Many older adults do not meet this goal. © Blend Images/Getty Images

▲ How does this breakfast of whole-grain cereal, fruit, and milk compare to MyPlate?
© Image Source/Corbis

eat more cheese, usually a concentrated form of saturated fat. Since 1963, they have eaten less butter, fewer eggs, less animal fat, and more vegetable oils and fish. These changes generally comply with recommendations to reduce the intake of saturated and *trans* fat in favor of unsaturated fat choices. Animal breeders are raising much leaner cattle and hogs than those produced in 1950, which also helps reduce saturated fat intake.

Other aspects of the average adult diet are still in need of improvement. The latest nutrition survey of eating habits in the United States shows that the major contributors of calories to the adult dietary pattern are white bread, beef, doughnuts, cakes and cookies, soft drinks, milk, chicken, cheese, alcoholic beverages, salad dressing, mayonnaise, potatoes, and sugars/syrups/jams. If Americans were truly lowering their intakes of sugar, saturated fat, and sodium while increasing their intakes of fiber, many of these foods would not appear at the top of the list.

> ✓ **CONCEPT CHECK 20.2**
>
> 1. Is the current adult RDA for protein appropriate for older adults? Why or why not?
> 2. Which nutrients should be limited in the dietary patterns of most American adults? Suggest three specific dietary changes that would help to limit these food components.
> 3. Name three nutrients that are commonly lacking in the dietary patterns of adults. Suggest one rich food source of each of these nutrients.

20.3 Factors Related to Nutritional Status of Adults

glycemic index (GI) The blood glucose response of a given food, compared to a standard (typically, glucose or white bread). Glycemic index is influenced by starch structure, fiber content, food processing, physical structure, and macronutrients in the meal such as fat.

Dietary adequacy is influenced by physiological, psychosocial, and economic factors. Table 20-2 summarizes the nutritional implications of many of the physiological changes that occur during adulthood. Some of the changes listed (e.g., tooth loss and changes in perceptions of taste and smell) can directly influence dietary intake. Other changes (e.g., loss of lean body tissue) can alter nutrient and/or kilocalorie needs. Some body changes (e.g., reduced stomach acidity, diminished kidney function) can affect nutrient utilization.

TABLE 20-2 ■ Coping with Physiological Changes of Aging

Physiological Changes	Recommended Responses
ⓘ Appetite	• Monitor changes in weight over time. • Eat small, frequent meals throughout the day. • Use supplemental nutritional drinks, such as Boost® and Ensure Plus®. • Choose energy-dense foods, such as plant sources of fat.
ⓘ Sense of taste and smell	• Vary the colors and textures of foods. • Experiment with sodium-free herbs and spices.
ⓘ Chewing or swallowing ability	• Work with a dentist or speech therapist to maximize chewing and swallowing ability. • Modify food consistency as necessary.
ⓘ Sense of thirst	• Monitor fluid intake. • Stay alert for evidence of dehydration (e.g., minimal or dark-colored urine).
ⓘ Stomach acidity	• Include some lean meats and iron-fortified foods in the dietary pattern. • Ask health care team to monitor iron status. • Consume a source of vitamin C to enhance absorption of nonheme iron from foods. • Choose foods fortified with vitamin B-12 or use a supplemental source of vitamin B-12.

TABLE 20-2 ■ (continued)

⬇ Bowel function	• Emphasize fruits, vegetables, and whole-grain breads and cereals, which are good sources of fiber. • Meet fluid needs.
⬇ Lactase production	• Limit milk serving size at each use. • Substitute yogurt or cheese for milk. • Use reduced-lactose or lactose-free products. • Seek nondairy calcium sources (see Section 11.11).
⬇ Liver function	• Consume alcohol in moderation, if at all (see Section 20.5). • Avoid consuming dietary supplements that contain more than 100% of the Daily Value of nutrients, especially vitamin A.
⬇ Insulin function	• Maintain healthy body weight. • Choose carbohydrates with low **glycemic index** (see Section 4.5). • Perform regular physical activity.
⬇ Kidney function	• If necessary, work with primary care provider and registered dietitian nutritionist to modify protein and other nutrients in diet.
⬇ Immune function	• Meet nutrient needs, especially protein, vitamin E, vitamin B-6, and zinc. • Perform regular physical activity.
⬇ Lung function	• Avoid tobacco products. • Perform regular physical activity.
⬇ Vision	• Choose a dietary pattern rich in fruits, vegetables, and whole-grain breads and cereals, which are natural sources of carotenoids, vitamin C, vitamin E, and zinc. • Regularly consume fatty fish, a source of omega-3 fatty acids. • Wear sunglasses in sunny conditions. • Avoid tobacco products. • Perform regular physical activity to improve insulin sensitivity. • In the case of diagnosed moderate macular degeneration, talk with a primary care provider about following a protocol of zinc, copper, vitamin E, vitamin C, and beta-carotene supplementation.
⬇ Lean tissue	• Meet nutrient needs, especially protein and vitamin D. • Perform regular physical activity, including strength training.
⬇ Cardiovascular function	• Achieve and maintain a healthy body weight. • Choose a dietary pattern based on fruits, vegetables, whole-grain breads and cereals, plant sources of protein, and fatty fish, which are good sources of soluble fiber, vitamin E, magnesium, and omega-3 fatty acids. • Adhere to prescribed medications to keep blood lipids and blood pressure within desirable ranges. • Stay physically active.
⬇ Bone mass	• Meet nutrient needs, especially protein, calcium, and vitamin D (regular sun exposure helps meet needs for vitamin D). • Perform regular physical activity, especially weight-bearing exercise. • Women should consider use of approved osteoporosis medications at menopause. • Aim to maintain a healthy body weight (i.e., BMI between 18.5 and 24.9).
⬇ Mental function	• Choose a dietary pattern rich in fruits, vegetables, whole grains, beans, and legumes, which are natural sources of antioxidant nutrients (see Section 13.7). • Consume seafood, a source of omega-3 fatty acids, twice per week. • Discuss the possible need for vitamin B-12 supplements with a primary care provider. • Strive for lifelong learning. • Perform regular physical activity. • Obtain adequate sleep.
⬇ Fat stores	Avoid overeating. • Perform regular physical activity.

Furthermore, chronic diseases and the medications used to manage them may influence food intake and nutrient needs. The following section details the influences of several of these factors on nutritional status during adulthood.

BODY COMPOSITION

The primary changes in body composition that occur with aging are diminished lean body mass, increased fat stores, and decreased body water. A focus on exercise, as detailed in a later section, can attenuate many of these unwanted changes.

The loss of lean body mass is termed **sarcopenia.** Some muscle cells shrink and others are lost as muscles age; some muscles lose their elasticity as they accumulate fat and collagen. Loss of muscle mass leads to a decrease in basal metabolism, muscle strength, and energy needs. Less muscle mass also leads to lower physical activity, which makes the prognosis for maintaining muscle even worse. Clearly, it is best to avoid this downward spiral.

As lean tissue declines with age, body fat often increases, a condition called **sarcopenic obesity** (see Further Reading 4). Much of this increase in body fat results from overeating and limited physical activity, although even athletic men and women typically gain some degree of midsection fat after age 50. A small fat gain in adulthood may not compromise health, but large gains are problematic. Recall that obesity increases risks for hypertension, cardiovascular disease, type 2 diabetes, osteoarthritis, and many other serious chronic conditions. Ultimately, these changes in body composition may diminish a person's ability to perform daily tasks, such as getting up from a chair and climbing a flight of stairs.

On the other hand, decreases in body weight can also be a problem for adults age 70 and older. About 2% of older adults are underweight (BMI less than 18.5). Unintended weight loss increases the risk of undernutrition, which alters an individual's ability to cope with illnesses and injuries and could ultimately lead to death. Potential causes for unintended weight loss among older adults (many of which can be detected using the nutrition screening tool in Figure 20-3) include:

- Illness
- Depression/social isolation
- Side effects of medications
- Changes in taste or smell
- Reduced chewing ability
- Limited financial resources
- Decreased dexterity or strength

BONES AND JOINTS

Recall from Section 11.2 that some bone loss is an expected consequence of aging. In women, bone loss rapidly occurs after menopause. For men, bone loss is slow and steady from middle age throughout later life. Many older adults may suffer from undiagnosed **osteomalacia,** a condition mainly caused by insufficient vitamin D. Osteoporosis can limit the ability of older people to shop, prepare food, and exercise. Consuming adequate vitamin D, calcium, and protein; not smoking; drinking alcohol moderately or not at all; and engaging in weight-bearing exercises can help preserve bone mass. Medications also can help lessen bone loss.

There are over 100 forms of arthritis, a disease that causes the degeneration and roughening of the cartilage that covers and cushions the joints. Such changes in the joints cause them to ache and become inflamed and painful to move. Severe arthritis can cause permanent joint changes, and some types of arthritis affect the heart, eyes, lungs, kidneys, and skin in addition to the joints. Over 50 million U.S. adults suffer from some type of arthritis. **Osteoarthritis,** which affects about 27 million U.S. adults, is the leading cause of disability among older persons. **Rheumatoid arthritis,** which affects about 1.5 million U.S. adults, is more prevalent in younger adults. **Gout,** a very painful form of arthritis that comes on suddenly and can be related to changes in the diet, affects about 6 million men and 2 million women in the United States.

Although precise causes or cures are unknown, many unproven arthritis "remedies" have been publicized. Unusual diets, food restrictions, and nutrient supplements are some of the

---

sarcopenia In general, loss of muscle tissue. Among older adults, this loss of lean mass greatly increases their risk of illness and death.

sarcopenic obesity Loss of muscle mass accompanied by gains in fat mass.

Researchers believe that maintaining lean muscle mass may be the most important strategy for successful aging, because doing so:

- Maintains basal metabolic rate, which helps to decrease the risk of obesity
- Keeps body fat low, which helps in the management of blood lipids and blood glucose
- Maintains body water, which decreases the risk of dehydration and improves body temperature regulation

osteomalacia Adult form of rickets. The bones have low mineral density and subsequently are at risk for fracture.

osteoarthritis A degenerative joint condition caused by a breakdown of cartilage in joints. It often results from "wear and tear" due to repetitive motions or the pressure of excess body weight.

rheumatoid arthritis A degenerative joint condition resulting from an autoimmune disease that causes inflammation in the joints and other sites of the body.

gout A form of arthritis caused by the buildup of uric acid crystals in the joints.

more popular treatments. Maintaining a healthy weight, which reduces stress on painful arthritic joints, is the best evidence-based diet-related strategy to offer relief from arthritis. Although no special diet, food, or nutrient has been proven to reliably prevent, relieve, or cure arthritis in humans, some research shows that a dietary pattern (e.g., Mediterranean diet) that is rich in antioxidant nutrients, anti-inflammatory phytochemicals, and omega-3 fatty acids can help to reduce the inflammation that underlies these conditions (see Further Reading 13 and Ask the RDN). As far as supplements go, glucosamine and/or chondroitin have been most extensively studied in relation to arthritis. Results remain controversial, but some studies demonstrate that these supplements can relieve pain, slow the progression of joint degeneration, or rebuild cartilage.

ASK THE RDN   Anti-Inflammatory Diet

Dear Author: My mother has been battling osteoarthritis for several years and wonders if Dr. Weil's Anti-Inflammatory Diet can help her cope with her disease. How is Dr. Weil's plan different from the Mediterranean diet?

In Section 10.2, we discussed the problem of chronic inflammation. When you are sick or injured, the inflammatory process is necessary: increased temperature, blood flow, and inflammatory factors help the white blood cells begin the healing process. However, chronic inflammation wreaks havoc on the body and is now thought to be at the root of many chronic diseases, including heart disease, Alzheimer's disease, and arthritis.

There is good evidence that an anti-inflammatory eating pattern may reduce inflammation, the risk of chronic diseases, and some symptoms of arthritis. The basic principles of an anti-inflammatory eating plan include:

- Eating plenty of fruits and vegetables
- Limiting or avoiding saturated and *trans* fats
- Including good sources of omega-3 fatty acids
- Eating plenty of whole grains
- Choosing lean sources of protein instead of red or processed meats
- Avoiding refined carbohydrates and highly processed foods
- Including herbs and spices with known anti-inflammatory effects

To ease arthritis, the #1 thing you can do is to keep your weight within a healthy range. Although Dr. Weil's plan is not aimed at weight loss, it is not surprising that when individuals consume a primarily plant-based diet and reduce their intakes of solid fats and highly processed foods, they often drop some pounds. Not only does weight loss reduce the compressive forces on stressed arthritic joints, research shows that it also reduces inflammation throughout the body.

Carbohydrates make up 40% to 50% of daily kilocalories on Dr. Weil's plan. Whole or cracked grains (e.g., brown rice, oatmeal, and bulgur wheat), beans, and abundant fruits and vegetables (e.g., winter squash and sweet potatoes) are recommended. When it comes to selecting produce, go for a wide variety of colorful fruits and vegetables. Many of the phytochemicals in colorful plant foods have anti-inflammatory effects.

Dr. Weil also emphasizes healthy fats, which should account for about 30% of your daily calories. He recommends seeking out sources of omega-3 fatty acids, which are found in foods like avocados; nuts and nut butters; fortified eggs; flaxseeds; hemp seeds; and fish such as salmon, sardines, black cod, and herring. Margarine and omega-6-rich oils (e.g., safflower, sunflower, or corn oil) are discouraged. Extra-virgin olive oil is the preferred oil for cooking and flavoring foods.

Protein should make up 20% to 30% of your daily calories on Dr. Weil's plan, but he stresses the importance of plant sources of protein. In fact, he recommends limiting most animal proteins to two servings per week. Instead, choose beans and products made from soybeans along with fish as sources of protein.

If the Anti-Inflammatory Diet sounds a lot like the Mediterranean diet you read about in Section 2.3 and Section 5.7, that's because Dr. Weil based his plan on this healthy dietary pattern! Although Dr. Weil's Anti-Inflammatory Diet has not been tested in clinical trials, it relies on evidence from epidemiological studies focusing on dietary patterns and inflammation. He adds

EXERCISE

Many physical changes of aging can be traced back to a sedentary lifestyle. As you might predict, an active lifestyle helps preserve muscle mass and decrease body fat. Physical activity increases muscle strength and mobility, improves balance and decreases the risk of falling, eases daily tasks that require some strength, improves sleep, slows bone loss, and increases joint movement, thus reducing injuries. It also has a positive impact on a person's mental outlook. Ideally, an active lifestyle should be maintained throughout life and include activities to build endurance, strength, balance, and flexibility. The 2008 Physical Activity Guidelines for Americans (see Section 2.2) provide the following guidelines specifically for older adults.

Aerobic Exercise All adults should engage in moderate-intensity aerobic exercise for at least 150 minutes per week, vigorous-intensity aerobic exercise for 75 minutes per week, or an equivalent combination of the two. This amount of aerobic activity improves endurance and aids in prevention of chronic diseases. A longer duration of daily exercise may be required for weight loss or weight maintenance. Weight-bearing exercises are particularly helpful for preservation of bone mass. For older adults who have not been physically active, it is important to increase the pace gradually. Even small bouts (e.g., 10 minutes) of physical activity are better than no exercise at all!

Strength Training To maintain lean tissue and basal metabolic rate, strength training should include 8 to 10 different exercises (each with two sets of 8 to 15 repetitions), performed two to three times per week. Exercises that involve the large muscle groups (e.g., arms, back, and legs) and exercises that enhance grip strength should be emphasized. Start slowly, concentrate on breathing, rest between sets, avoid locking joints in the arms and legs, and stop an exercise if it becomes painful.

Balance Exercises For those over age 65 who are at risk for falling, exercises that improve balance are recommended. Tai chi and yoga are a few types of exercise that can improve balance, but even standing on one foot or getting up from a chair without using hands can be a good start.

Flexibility Exercises Stretching exercises for each major muscle group should accompany aerobic or strength exercises at least 2 days per week. Improving flexibility can make it easier to perform many simple tasks, such as tying one's shoes.

All older adults should avoid inactivity. Having an exercise plan, developed with a health professional to accommodate individual health risks and needs, will enhance success for older adults. Men older than age 40; women older than age 50; those with heart conditions, diabetes, or joint problems; and anyone who has been sedentary should consult a primary care provider before beginning an exercise program. The Go4Life campaign from the National Institute of Aging encourages older adults to become more active and provides many practical tips for exercising safely. Learn more at go4life.nia.nih.gov and see Further Reading 5.

▲ Endurance, strength, balance, and flexibility are the four elements of the Go4Life campaign from the National Institute on Aging. Download a free copy of Exercise and Physical Activity: Getting Fit for Life at www.nia.nih.gov.
© Anne Smith

DIGESTIVE SYSTEM

As you recall from Section 3.9, digestion begins in the mouth. About 25% of older adults have no natural teeth, and many more are missing some teeth. The problem of tooth loss is worse among low-income populations. Even with properly fitting dentures, chewing ability may be limited. Older adults with poor dentition may avoid meats or crunchy fruits and vegetables, thereby missing out on important nutrients such as protein, iron, and zinc (from meat) as well as potassium and fiber (from fruits and vegetables). Ground meats and cooked vegetables are easier options for older adults with chewing problems (see Further Reading 20).

Further along the GI tract, the production of HCl, intrinsic factor, and some digestive enzymes (e.g., lactase) declines with advancing age (see Further Reading 17). In addition, some medications affect acid production. As a result of low acid production, absorption of some minerals, such as iron, is impaired. Low levels of acid and intrinsic factor reduce the digestion and absorption of vitamin B-12. Thus, even with adequate intakes of iron and vitamin B-12, older adults may become anemic. Symptoms of lactose intolerance can lead to avoidance of dairy products, which can limit the availability of bone-building nutrients. Fortified foods or supplements can help older adults overcome these problems with digestion and absorption of nutrients.

Constipation is the main intestinal problem for older people. To prevent constipation, older people should meet fiber needs, drink enough fluids, and exercise. Fiber supplements, such as Metamucil® or Phillip's Fiber Good® Gummies, may be useful when overall food consumption does not allow for adequate fiber intake. Because some medications can be habit forming, a primary care provider should be consulted to determine if a laxative or stool softener is needed.

In addition to changes in the GI tract, the functions of the accessory organs decline as we age. For instance, the liver functions less efficiently. A history of significant alcohol consumption or liver disease will intensify any existing problems with liver function. As liver efficiency declines, its ability to detoxify many substances, including medications, alcohol, and vitamin and mineral supplements, drops. The possibility for vitamin toxicity increases.

The gallbladder also functions less efficiently in later years. Gallstones can block the flow of bile out of the gallbladder into the small intestine, thereby interfering with fat digestion. Obesity is a major risk factor for gallbladder disease, especially in older women. A low-fat diet or surgery to remove the gallbladder may be necessary.

Although pancreatic function may decline with age, this organ has a large reserve capacity. One sign of a failing pancreas is high blood glucose, although this can occur as the result of several conditions. The pancreas may be secreting less insulin, or cells may be resisting insulin action (as is commonly seen in obese people with upper-body fat storage). Where appropriate, improved nutrient intake, regular physical activity, and loss of excess body weight can improve insulin action and blood glucose regulation.

NERVOUS SYSTEM

A gradual loss of nerve cells that transmit signals may decrease taste and smell perceptions and impair neuromuscular coordination, reasoning, and memory. Both hearing and vision decline with age. Hearing impairment is the greatest in those who have been exposed constantly to loud noises, such as urban traffic, aircraft noise, and music. Because they cannot hear well, older people may avoid social contacts, which increases their risk of inadequate dietary intake.

Declining eyesight, frequently caused by retina degeneration and cataracts, can affect a person's abilities to grocery shop, locate desired foods, read labels for nutritional content, and prepare foods at home. Vision losses also may cause people to curtail social contacts, reduce physical activity, and not practice daily personal health and grooming routines. Age-related macular degeneration, a common cause of failing eyesight in old age, affects about 11 million U.S. adults. A major risk factor is cigarette smoking. Diets rich in carotenoids and omega-3 fatty acids help to reduce the risk of certain eye diseases among older adults (see Further Reading 3).

▲ Poor dentition contributes to decreased food intake and digestive problems. Serve softer, easier-to-chew foods and allow extra time for chewing and swallowing. © Stockbyte/PunchStock

▲ Immune function declines with age, so food safety becomes increasingly important for older adults. Section 17.8 provides advice on this topic, such as washing one's hands and work surfaces before preparing food. © Photodisc/Getty Images

Neuromuscular coordination losses may make it difficult to shop for and prepare food. Physical tasks as simple as opening food packages can become so difficult that individuals restrict dietary intake to foods that require little preparation and depend on others to provide food that is ready to eat. Eating may become difficult, too. Loss of coordination makes it a challenge to grasp cup handles and manipulate eating utensils. As a result, older adults may avoid foods that can be easily spilled (e.g., soups and juices) or that need to be cut (e.g., meats, large vegetable pieces). Some may even withdraw from social interaction and eat alone, which often means eating less.

IMMUNE SYSTEM

With age, the immune system often operates less efficiently. Consuming adequate protein, vitamins (especially folate and vitamins A, D, and E), iron, and zinc helps maximize immune system function (see Chapter 13). Recurrent sicknesses and delayed wound healing are warning signs that nutrient deficiencies (especially of protein and zinc) may be hindering immune function. On the other hand, overnutrition appears to be equally harmful to the immune system. For example, obesity and excessive fat, iron, and zinc intakes can suppress immune function.

ENDOCRINE SYSTEM

As adulthood progresses, the rate of hormone synthesis and release can slow. Declining thyroid hormone production, for example, can decrease basal metabolic rate, leading to unexplained weight gain. A decrease in insulin release or sensitivity to insulin, for instance, means that it takes longer for blood glucose levels to return to normal after a meal. Maintaining a healthy weight, exercising regularly, adhering to a dietary pattern that is low in fat and high in fiber, and avoiding foods with a high glycemic index can enhance the body's ability to use insulin and restore elevated blood glucose levels to normal after a meal.

CHRONIC DISEASE

The prevalence of obesity, heart disease, osteoporosis, cancer, hypertension, and diabetes rises with age. More than 8 of every 10 older adults have one of these chronic and potentially debilitating diseases. Half of all elderly people have at least two chronic conditions. Chronic diseases may have a strong impact on dietary intake. For instance, obesity, heart disease, and osteoporosis may impair physical mobility to the extent that victims are unable to shop for and prepare food. Chronic disease also can influence nutrient and calorie needs. Cancer, for example, boosts both nutrient and calorie needs. Hypertension may indicate a need to lower sodium intake. Nutrient utilization can be affected by chronic disease, too. For instance, diabetes alters the body's ability to utilize glucose. In addition, the effects of heart disease on the kidneys may impair their ability to reabsorb glucose, amino acids, and vitamin C.

DEPRESSION

A positive outlook on life and intact support networks help make food and eating interesting and satisfying. In contrast, social isolation, grief, chronic pain and infirmity, or a change in lifestyle can lead to depression, loss of appetite, lack of interest in food, and disability. Depression affects about 8% of adults in the United States. Left untreated, depression can lead to a continual decline in appetite, which results in weakness, undernutrition, mental confusion, and increased feelings of isolation and loneliness (Fig. 20-6). In contrast, some people cope by overeating, which can lead to obesity and its associated problems. Depression may signal an underlying illness and can also impair recovery from other illnesses or injuries. As many as 15% of cases end in suicide. For these reasons, early detection of depression is important. Depression is often treatable, but medication alone will not help those experiencing major life changes, such as the death of a spouse. Adequate social support and/or psychological intervention are also essential.

Social isolation; perhaps spouse has died.

Loses interest in food: diet deteriorates.

Poor diet leads to weakness; this increases a feeling of isolation and abandonment.

Further isolation can then decrease desire for self-care.

Health declines visibly; weakness remains.

Self-care is seriously hampered.

FIGURE 20-6 ◀ The decline of health often seen in older adults. A small change leads to a chain of events or "domino effect" that results in poor health. Early intervention can prevent declines in physical health related to psychosocial factors.

Just as depression affects diet, dietary intake may influence depression. As yet, there is insufficient evidence to make nutrition recommendations to alleviate symptoms of depression, but it has been linked to poor intakes of omega-3 fatty acids, vitamin D, and some B vitamins (review Section 13.7).

ALZHEIMER'S DISEASE

Alzheimer's disease is an irreversible, abnormal, progressive deterioration of the brain that causes victims to steadily lose the ability to remember, reason, and comprehend. About 5.1 million adults in the United States have the disease. Alzheimer's disease often takes a terrible toll on the mental and eventual physical health of older people.

Research on the roles of individual nutrients and overall dietary patterns in the prevention or treatment of Alzheimer's disease is ongoing. Recall from Section 13.7, the MIND diet—rich in antioxidants, nutrients, omega-3 fatty acids, and phytochemicals—is a promising dietary strategy to prevent cognitive decline (see Further Reading 8).

MEDICATIONS

Older adults are major consumers of medications (prescription and over-the-counter) and nutrient supplements. About 90% of older adults take at least one prescription medication daily, and half of all people over age 65 take several medicines each day. The rate of supplement use increases throughout adulthood such that by age 50, approximately half of all adults are using supplements daily. Physiological declines that occur during aging (e.g., reduced body water and reduced liver and kidney function) exaggerate and prolong the effects of medications and nutrient supplements in older adults.

Medications can eradicate infections and control chronic diseases, but some also adversely affect nutritional status, particularly of those who are older and/or take many different medications. For instance, some medications depress taste and smell acuity or cause anorexia or nausea that can blunt interest in eating and lead to reduced dietary intake. Some medications alter nutrient needs. Aspirin, for example, increases the likelihood of stomach bleeding, so long-term use may elevate the need for iron, as well as other nutrients. Antibiotics kill beneficial bacteria along with pathogens, so they can limit the amount of vitamin K that is synthesized by bacteria in the large intestine (see Section 13.2). Some medications may impair nutrient utilization; diuretics and laxatives may cause excessive excretion of water and minerals. Even vitamin and mineral supplements may have unanticipated effects on nutritional status. Iron supplements taken in large doses can interfere with the functioning of zinc and copper. Folate supplements can mask vitamin B-12 deficiencies.

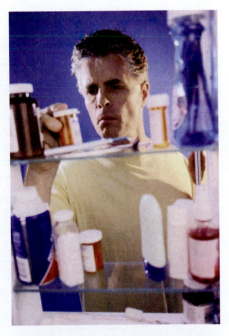

▲ About one-third of older adults take eight or more medications each day. In some cases, drugs can affect nutrient status. For example, certain diuretics may increase excretion of minerals in the urine. Other times, nutrients and other food components can impact the effectiveness of drugs. Vitamin K, for example, can affect the action of anticlotting medications. © Ingram Publishing

People who must take medications should eat nutrient-dense foods and avoid any specific food or supplement that interferes with the function of their medications. For example, vitamin K can reduce the action of oral anticoagulants, aged cheese can interfere with certain drugs used to treat hypertension and depression, and grapefruit can interfere with medications such as tranquilizers and those that lower cholesterol levels. A registered dietitian nutritionist can help to plan a dietary pattern that meets nutritional needs while avoiding harmful food/medication interactions.

COMPLEMENTARY AND ALTERNATIVE MEDICINE

At least half of adults report using some kind of dietary or herbal supplement. Recall from Section 8.5 that the safety, purity, and effectiveness of dietary supplements are not tightly monitored by FDA. Table 20-3 reviews some popular herbal products used by older adults. Note from the table that these products can pose health risks in certain people. In addition, they may be expensive—in some cases, more than $100 per month—and are not covered by health insurance plans. In recent years, the use of many herbal products has declined because of expense and questionable benefits. Instead, consumers are opting to spend their money on tried-and-true products, such as multivitamins, vitamin D, omega-3 fatty acids, fiber, and probiotics.

TABLE 20-3 ■ **A Closer Look at Some Popular Herbal Products**

Product	Purported Effects[a]	Side Effects	Vulnerable Population Groups
Black cohosh	• Mild reduction of postmenopausal symptoms (shown to be effective in some studies; use should not go beyond 6 months)	• Nausea • Liver damage	• Women who have had breast cancer • Pregnant women • Anyone taking estrogen, hypertension medications, or blood-thinning medications[b] • Anyone with abnormal liver function
Chondroitin sulfate	• Pain relief from osteoarthritis (possibly effective)	• GI tract upset • Swelling • Hair loss • Irregular heartbeat	• People with asthma • Men with prostate cancer • Anyone who takes blood-thinning medications
Cranberry	• Prevention or treatment of urinary tract infections (possibly effective) • Prevention of *Helicobacter pylori* infections of the stomach, with the aim of reducing the risk for ulcers (some evidence of efficacy)	• Gastrointestinal upset and diarrhea • Use of concentrated tablets may increase the risk of kidney stones	• People susceptible to kidney stones • Anyone taking antidepressants or prescription painkillers • Anyone taking blood thinners
Echinacea	• Prevention or treatment of colds or other infections (possibly effective)	• Nausea • Skin irritation • Allergic reactions • Minor GI tract upset • Increased urination	• Anyone with an autoimmune disease • Pre- or postsurgical patients • Anyone with allergies to daisies
Garlic	• Antifungal properties (possibly effective) • Reduction of blood cholesterol or blood pressure (possibly effective)	• GI tract upset (e.g., heartburn, flatulence) • Unpleasant odor • Allergic reactions	• Pre- or postsurgical patients • Perinatal women • Anyone taking blood-thinning medications or AIDS medications
Ginger	• Relief of nausea and vomiting (possibly effective)	• Heartburn • Diarrhea • Increased menstrual bleeding	• Pregnant women should proceed with caution due to possible risks for bleeding • People with bleeding disorders or who take blood-thinning medications • Anyone with a heart condition • People taking blood glucose-lowering medications

TABLE 20-3 ■ (continued)

Product	Purported Effects[a]	Side Effects	Vulnerable Population Groups
Ginkgo biloba	• Increased circulation (possibly effective) • Improvement of memory (especially for people with Alzheimer's disease; low evidence of efficacy)	• Mild headache • GI tract upset • Allergic reactions • Irritability • Reduced blood clotting • Seizures (if contaminated with toxic ginkgo seeds)	• People with bleeding disorders • Pre- or postsurgical patients • Anyone with allergies to the plant • Concurrent use of feverfew, garlic, ginseng, dong quai, or red clover • Anyone taking diabetes medications, blood-thinning medications, vitamin E supplements, antidepressants, or diuretics
Ginseng	• Lowering blood sugar (possibly effective) • Increased energy (possibly ineffective)	• Hypertension • Asthma attacks • Irregular heartbeat • Hypoglycemia • Insomnia • Headache • Nervousness • GI tract upset • Reduced blood clotting • Menstrual irregularities and breast tenderness	• Anyone who takes a prescription drug • Women who have had breast cancer • Anyone with chronic GI tract disease • Anyone with uncontrolled hypertension
Glucosamine sulfate	• Prevention and treatment of osteoarthritis (likely effective)	• GI tract upset	• People with asthma or shellfish allergies
St. John's wort	• Alleviation of mild to moderate depression (likely effective)	• Mild GI tract upset • Rash • Tiredness • Restlessness • Increased sensitivity to sunlight	• Anyone who takes a prescription drug • People with UV sensitivity, including that induced by medications or other treatments[c] • People with bipolar disorder, major depression, schizophrenia, and Alzheimer's disease • Anyone recovering from a graft or organ transplant
Turmeric	• Pain relief from osteoarthritis (possibly effective)	• GI tract upset • Dizziness	• People with gallbladder problems • People with GERD • Pre- or postsurgical patients
Valerian	• Alleviation of insomnia (possibly effective) • Reduction of anxiety (insufficient evidence to rate effectiveness)	• Impaired attention • Headache • Morning grogginess • Irregular heartbeat • GI tract upset • Disagreeable odor • Withdrawal delerium	• Anyone taking anesthetics or central nervous system depressants[d] • Anyone who drinks alcohol • People about to operate heavy machinery or drive

Pregnant or breastfeeding women, children under 2 years of age, anyone over the age of 65 years, and anyone with a chronic disease should never take supplements unless under the guidance of a primary care provider. A concern has been raised with regard to patients who abruptly end alternative medicines at the start of hospital treatments or deny that they are using alternative therapy. Interactions between alternative therapies and pharmaceutical drugs can be drastic and include complications such as delirium, clotting abnormalities, and rapid heartbeat, resulting in the need for intensive care. Full disclosure of all prescription and nonprescription treatments aids in prevention of such complications. Experts recommend that, if time permits, patients stop taking herbal products for about a week before a scheduled surgery or otherwise take all original supplement containers to the hospital, so that the anesthesiologist can evaluate what was taken.

[a]Ratings of effectiveness from MedlinePlus and/or NCCAM.

[b]Coumadin®, aspirin, Heparin®, Lovenox®, or Fragmin®.

[c]Sulfa medications, anti-inflammatory medications, or acid-reflux medications

[d]Valium, halcion, seconal

When it comes to herbal products, proceed with caution. Significant health risks—including death—have been associated with the use of some herbal products. FDA advises anyone who experiences adverse side effects from an herbal product to contact a primary care provider. Clinicians are then encouraged to report adverse events to FDA, state and local health departments, and consumer protection agencies.

If you decide to consume an herbal product, only ingest one product at a time, keep a diary of symptoms, and definitely check with your primary care provider before discontinuing any prescribed medication. In particular, be alert for the following herbal ingredients:

Chaparral	Kava kava	Paraguay tea	Stephania
Comfrey	Kombucha tea	Penny-royal	Tung shueh
Germander	Lobelia	Pokeroot	Willow bark
Hai gen fen	Magnolia	Sassafras	Yohimbe
Jin bu huan	Mandrake	Senna	

✓ CONCEPT CHECK 20.3

1. What is sarcopenia? What diet and lifestyle changes would you suggest to avoid this condition?

2. Describe three ways aging affects the processes of digestion, absorption, and utilization of nutrients.

3. How does depression influence nutritional status?

4. List two types of complementary and alternative medicine adults may use to improve immune function. List two that adults may use to cope with arthritis.

20.4 Ensuring a Healthful Diet for the Adult Years

Recommended dietary practices for later years would be to increase the diet's nutrient density and to make sure fiber and fluid intakes are adequate. In addition, some protein should come from lean meats to help meet protein, vitamin B-6, vitamin B-12, iron, and zinc needs.

Singles of all ages face logistical problems with food: purchasing, preparing, storing, and using food with minimal waste are challenging. Value-priced packages of meats and vegetables are normally too large to be useful for a single person. Many singles live in small dwellings, some without kitchens and freezers. Creating a diet to accommodate a limited budget and facilities and a single appetite requires special considerations. The following are some practical suggestions for diet planning for singles:

- If you have access to a freezer, cook large amounts, divide into single-serve portions, and freeze.
- Buy only what you will use; small containers may be expensive, but letting food spoil is also costly.
- Ask the grocer to divide family-sized packages of wrapped meat or fresh vegetables, separate, and wrap into smaller units.
- Buy smaller amounts of fruit—perhaps one ripe, one medium-ripe, and one unripe—so that the fruit can be eaten over a period of several days.
- Keep a box of dry milk handy to add nutrients to recipes for baked foods and other foods for which this addition is acceptable.

Table 20-4 provides more ideas for healthful eating in later years.

Nutritional deficiencies and protein-calorie malnutrition have been identified among some aging populations, particularly those in hospitals, nursing homes, or long-term care facilities. The Nutrition Checklist for Older Adults shown in Figure 20-3 can be used to

TABLE 20-4 ■ Guidelines for Healthful Eating in Later Years

- Eat regularly; small, frequent meals may be best. Use nutrient-dense foods as a basis for menus.

- Use labor-saving cooking methods and some healthier convenience foods, but try to incorporate some fresh foods into daily menus.

- Try new foods, new seasonings, and new ways of preparing foods. Use canned goods in moderation or choose those low in sodium.

- Keep easy-to-prepare foods on hand for times when you feel tired.

- Have a treat occasionally, perhaps an expensive cut of fish or a favorite fresh fruit.

- Eat in a well-lit or sunny area; serve meals attractively; and experiment with different flavors, colors, shapes, textures, and smells.

- Arrange kitchen and eating area so that food preparation and cleanup are simple.

- Eat with friends, relatives, or at a senior center when possible.

- Share cooking responsibilities with a neighbor or close friend.

- Use community resources for help with shopping and other daily care needs.

- Stay physically active.

- If possible, take a walk before eating to stimulate the appetite.

- When necessary, chop, grind, or blend hard-to-chew foods. Softer, protein-rich foods (e.g., shredded meats, eggs) can be substituted for whole pieces of meat when poor dentition prevents normal food intake. Prepare soups, stews, cooked whole-grain cereals, and casseroles.

- If your dexterity is limited, cut or chop the food ahead of time (perhaps with the help of a friend or family member), use utensils with deep sides or handles, and obtain more specialized utensils if needed.

identify older adults at nutritional risk. Malnutrition increases the risk for infections and bed sores (pressure ulcers) and compromises recovery from illness and surgery. Friends, relatives, and health care professionals should monitor nutrient intake in all older people, including those who live in long-term care facilities. Family members can play a valuable role in making sure nutrient needs are met by looking for weight maintenance based on regular, healthful meal patterns. If problems arise in consuming a healthful dietary pattern, a registered dietitian nutritionist can assess nutrition concerns and offer professional and personalized advice.

Older adults benefit from good nutrition in many ways. Meeting nutrient needs delays the onset of some diseases; improves the management of some existing diseases; hastens recovery from many illnesses; increases mental, physical, and social well-being; and often decreases the need for and length of hospitalization. MyPlate is a useful guide for planning healthy meals, but older adults must be sure to emphasize certain nutrients: potassium, calcium, vitamin D, vitamin B-12, and fiber. In 2016, Tufts University released an updated MyPlate for Older Adults that illustrates nutrient-dense food choices that are accessible and appealing for this population group (Figure 20-7). The graphic also affirms the importance of adequate fluid intake and modified physical activity goals. In some cases, dietary supplementation may be appropriate to address the unique needs of older adults.

Obtaining enough food may be difficult for some older persons, especially if they are unable to drive and relatives do not live close enough to help with cooking or shopping. For an older person, a request for help may be equated to a loss of independence. Pride or fear of hiring strangers may stand in the way of much-needed aid. In these cases, friends can be a big help. Special transportation arrangements may also be available through community agencies, local transit companies, or taxi services. Indeed, many eligible older people are missing meals and are poorly nourished because they do not realize that programs are

FIGURE 20-7 ▶ MyPlate for Older Adults. "MyPlate for Older Adults" Copyright 2016 Tufts University, all rights reserved. "MyPlate for Older Adults" graphic and accompanying website were developed with support from AARP Foundation. "Tufts University" and "AARP Foundation" are registered trademarks and may not be reproduced apart from their inclusion in the "MyPlate for Older Adults" graphic without express permission from their respective owners.

MyPlate for Older Adults

Fruits & Vegetables
Whole fruits and vegetables are rich in important nutrients and fiber. Choose fruits and vegetables with deeply colored flesh. Choose canned varieties that are packed in their own juices or low-sodium.

Healthy Oils
Liquid vegetable oils and soft margarines provide important fatty acids and some fat-soluble vitamins.

Herbs & Spices
Use a variety of herbs and spices to enhance flavor of foods and reduce the need to add salt.

Fluids
Drink plenty of fluids. Fluids can come from water, tea, coffee, soups, and fruits and vegetables.

Grains
Whole grain and fortified foods are good sources of fiber and B vitamins.

Dairy
Fat-free and low-fat milk, cheeses and yogurts provide protein, calcium and other important nutrients.

Protein
Protein rich foods provide many important nutrients. Choose a variety including nuts, beans, fish, lean meat and poultry.

Remember to Stay Active!

Tufts UNIVERSITY · JEAN MAYER USDA HUMAN NUTRITION RESEARCH CENTER ON AGING · HNRCA · AARP Foundation

available to help them. Irregular meal patterns and weight loss are warning signs that malnutrition may be developing. An effort should be made to identify poorly nourished seniors and inform them of community services.

COMMUNITY NUTRITION SERVICES FOR OLDER ADULTS

Health care advice and services for older people can come from clinics, private practitioners, hospitals, and health maintenance organizations (see Further Reading 10). Home health care agencies, adult day-care programs, adult overnight-care programs, and **hospice care** (for the terminally ill) also provide daily care for those who qualify.

One in five adults (about 11 million) are served by the Older Americans Act (OAA), which was reauthorized in 2015. Originally enacted in 1965, the OAA supports a range of home and community-based services, including Meals on Wheels and other nutrition programs. The OAA nutrition programs serve about 242 million meals each year to U.S. adults over the age of 60. Federal standards mandate that these meals supply at least one-third of adult energy and nutrient requirements.

Some meals (e.g., Meals on Wheels) are delivered directly to older adults in their homes. Although home-delivered meals can make a valuable contribution to the nutritional status of home-bound older adults, services are usually limited to one or two meals per day. If a recipient has a poor appetite, the food may end up stored for later or simply thrown away. If foods are not eaten on delivery and not stored properly, risk for foodborne illness could be a concern. Other meals are provided by congregate meal programs, which usually serve lunch at a central location. With congregate meals, the social aspect of eating tends to improve nutritional intake. However, programs generally provide just one meal per day on 5 days per week. Where can older adults with limited resources find additional nutrition assistance?

In addition to congregate and home-delivered meals, federal commodity distribution is available in some areas of the United States to low-income older people. Such individuals whose incomes are below the poverty level can benefit from the SNAP program (previously known as "food stamps"; see Section 16.3 for details on these programs). The Senior Farmers Market Nutrition Program (SFMNP) provides low-income seniors with coupons

hospice care A program offering care that emphasizes comfort and dignity at the end of life.

To learn more about resources available for older adults in your area, check out the following websites:

Food Assistance Programs for Seniors
www.nutrition.gov/food-assistance-programs

Elder Care Locator
www.eldercare.gov

National Institute on Aging
www.nia.nih.gov

American Geriatrics Society
www.americangeriatrics.org

Administration on Aging
www.aoa.gov

CASE STUDY   Dietary Assistance for an Older Adult

Frances is a 78-year-old woman who suffers from macular degeneration, osteoporosis, and arthritis. Since her husband died a year ago, she has moved from their family house to a small one-bedroom apartment. Her eyesight is progressively getting worse, making it hard to go to the grocery store or even to cook (for fear of burning herself). She is often lonely; her only son lives 1 hour away and works two jobs, but he visits her as often as he can. Frances has lost her appetite and, as a result, often skips meals during the week. She has resorted to eating mostly cold foods. These are simple to prepare but seriously limit the variety and palatability of her diet. Also, she wears dentures and has trouble chewing tough meats and foods with crisp textures. She is slowly losing weight as a result of her dietary changes and loss of appetite.

   Her typical diet usually consists of a breakfast that may include 1 slice of wheat toast with margarine, honey, and cinnamon, and 1 cup of hot tea. If she has lunch, she normally has a can of peaches, half of a turkey and cheese sandwich, and a glass of water. For dinner, she might have half of a tuna fish sandwich made with mayonnaise and 1 cup of iced tea. She usually includes one or two cookies at bedtime.

   Answer the following questions and check your responses at the end of this chapter.

© Getty Images

1. What nutrients are likely to be inadequate in Frances's current diet?
2. What potential effects will Frances's limited dietary pattern have on her health status?
3. Which physiological changes of aging will add to the effects of her inadequate dietary intake (review Table 20-2)?
4. What other questions would you ask Frances to get a better sense of her nutrition status?
5. What services are available in the community that could help Frances improve her diet?
6. What other convenience foods could be included in her diet to make it more healthful and more varied?

that can be exchanged for eligible foods (fruits, vegetables, honey, and fresh-cut herbs) at farmers markets, roadside stands, and community-supported agriculture (CSA) programs. Food cooperatives and a variety of clubs and religious and social organizations provide additional aid.

✓ CONCEPT CHECK 20.4

1. Gerald is a 76-year-old man whose wife recently passed away. He now lives alone for the first time in his life and is not accustomed to preparing meals for himself. What three pieces of advice would you give Gerald about eating well?
2. List three possible nutrition resources for an older adult with limited financial means.

20.5 Nutrition and Your Health
Nutrition Implications of Alcohol Consumption

© Getty Images/Digital Vision

in excess of moderate drinking. **Binge drinking,** introduced in the Section 1.8, is characterized by drinking so much within a short period of time (usually within 2 hours) that blood alcohol concentration (BAC) rises above the legal limit of 0.08 gram per deciliter. This usually correlates to five or more drinks in a row for men or four or more drinks in a row for women. Although binge drinking is certainly linked to negative effects on physical and emotional health, it is not necessarily an alcohol use disorder, which will be discussed next.

Moderate consumption of alcohol by a person of legal drinking age is an acceptable practice and even has some health benefits (see Further Reading 12). However, only about half of alcohol consumed is done so in moderation. About one in five people over the age of 12 report binge drinking in the last 30 days. Problem drinking that becomes severe is given the medical diagnosis of **alcohol use disorder.** About 18 million people in the United States suffer from alcohol use disorders (often referred to as *alcoholism*). By far, alcohol is the most commonly abused drug.

How Alcoholic Beverages Are Produced

The basis of alcohol production is fermentation, a process by which microorganisms break down simple sugars (e.g., glucose or maltose) to alcohol, carbon dioxide, and water in the absence of oxygen. High-carbohydrate foods encourage the growth of yeast, the microorganism responsible for alcohol production. Wine is formed by the fermentation of grape or other fruit juices. Beer is made from malted cereal grain. Distilled spirits (e.g., vodka, gin, and whiskey) are made from any number of fruits, vegetables, and grains. Production temperatures, the composition of the food used for fermentation, and aging techniques determine the characteristics of the product.

> Alcohol proof represents twice the volume of alcohol in percentage terms. Thus, 80 proof vodka is 40% alcohol.

Given the wide spectrum of alcohol use and abuse, knowledge of alcohol consumption and its relationship to overall health is essential to the study of nutrition. Alcoholic beverages contain the chemical form of alcohol known as **ethanol.** Although not a nutrient per se, alcohol is a source of kilocalories (about 7 kcal per gram). Approximately half of American adults drink alcohol. On average, alcohol accounts for about 3% of total calories in the average North American diet (Table 20-5).

A "standard drink" contains about 14 grams alcohol. For beer or wine coolers, this equates to a 12-fluid-ounce serving. Most cans of beer are 12 fluid ounces, but some cans or bottles may contain as much as 40 fluid ounces. Malt liquor has a slightly higher alcohol content than beer, so the standard drink size is 8 to 9 fluid ounces. For wine, a 5-fluid-ounce glass is standard. A standard drink of hard liquor, such as whiskey or rum, is the size of a shot glass—1.5 fluid ounces. Standard drink sizes are depicted in Figure 20-8.

Now that you know what a standard drink is, let us define some commonly referenced patterns of drinking. **Moderate drinking** is defined by single-day and weekly amounts. To be classified as a moderate drinker, an individual must meet both criteria. For men, moderate drinking is no more than 4 drinks in 1 day AND no more than 14 drinks per week. For women, moderate drinking is no more than 3 drinks in 1 day AND no more than 7 drinks per week. **Heavy drinking** encompasses all patterns of alcohol consumption

ethanol Chemical term for the form of alcohol found in alcoholic beverages.

moderate drinking For men, consuming no more than 4 drinks in 1 day AND no more than 14 drinks per week; for women, consuming no more than 3 drinks in 1 day AND no more than 7 drinks per week.

heavy drinking Any pattern of alcohol consumption in excess of 4 drinks in 1 day or 14 drinks per week for men or 3 drinks in 1 day or 7 drinks per week for women.

binge drinking Drinking sufficient alcohol within a 2-hour period to increase blood alcohol content to 0.08 grams per deciliter or higher; for men, consuming 5 or more drinks in a row; for women, consuming 4 or more drinks in a row.

alcohol use disorder A psychiatric disorder characterized by a problematic pattern of alcohol use that leads to significant impairment or distress.

TABLE 20-5 ■ Approximate Alcohol, Carbohydrate, and Calorie Content of Alcoholic Beverages*

Beverage	Amount (fluid ounces)	Alcohol (grams)	Carbohydrates (grams)	Calories (kcal)
Beer				
Regular	12	13	13	146
Light	12	11	5	99
Distilled Spirits				
Gin, rum, vodka, bourbon, whiskey (80 proof)	1.5	15	—	105
Wine				
Red/white/rosé	5	15	4	125
Dessert and sweet	5	23	17	225
Other Alcohol Drinks				
Daiquiri	7	20	33	259
Martini	3	27	—	189
Whiskey sour	3	13	14	147
Hard lemonade	11.2	13	34	228
Cream liqueur (34 proof)	1.5	6.5	10	154

*There is little to no fat or protein contribution to calorie content.

Source: USDA.

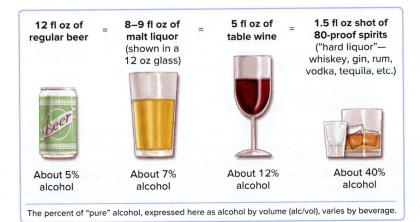

12 fl oz of regular beer = **8–9 fl oz of malt liquor** (shown in a 12 oz glass) = **5 fl oz of table wine** = **1.5 fl oz shot of 80-proof spirits** ("hard liquor"—whiskey, gin, rum, vodka, tequila, etc.)

About 5% alcohol   About 7% alcohol   About 12% alcohol   About 40% alcohol

The percent of "pure" alcohol, expressed here as alcohol by volume (alc/vol), varies by beverage.

FIGURE 20-8 ◄ What is a "standard drink"? The standard drink sizes shown provide about 14 grams of alcohol. Keep in mind that alcoholic beverages served in bars and restaurants can be 20% to 45% larger than a standard drink.

Source: NIAAA.

Absorption and Metabolism of Alcohol

Alcohol requires no digestion. It is absorbed rapidly from the GI tract by diffusion, making it the most efficiently absorbed of all calorie sources. Once absorbed, alcohol is freely distributed into all the fluid compartments within the body. About 1% to 3% of alcohol is excreted via urine and about 1% to 5% evaporates via the breath, the basis for the breathalyzer test. Most alcohol (90% to 98%), however, is metabolized. The liver is the primary site for alcohol metabolism, and some may also be metabolized by the cells lining the stomach. The main pathway of alcohol metabolism involves the enzymes **alcohol dehydrogenase** and **acetaldehyde dehydrogenase.** Alcohol cannot be stored in the body, so it takes absolute priority over other energy sources for metabolism.

As a person's alcohol consumption exceeds the body's capacity to metabolize it, blood alcohol concentration rises, the brain is exposed to alcohol, and symptoms of intoxication appear (Table 20-6). Absorption and metabolism of alcohol depend on numerous factors: genetics, gender, body size, physical condition, meal composition, gastric emptying rate, the alcohol content of the beverage, use of certain drugs, chronic alcohol use, and even how much sleep one has had. Women absorb and metabolize alcohol

alcohol dehydrogenase An enzyme used in alcohol (ethanol) metabolism that converts alcohol into acetaldehyde.

acetaldehyde dehydrogenase An enzyme used in ethanol metabolism that eventually converts acetaldehyde into carbon dioxide and water.

TABLE 20-6 ■ Blood Alcohol Concentration and Symptoms

Concentration[a]	Sporadic Drinker	Chronic Drinker	Hours for Alcohol to Be Metabolized[b]
50 (0.05%)	Congenial euphoria, decreased tension, and noticeable impairment in driving and coordination	No observable effect	2–3
75 (0.075%)	Gregarious	Often no effect	3–4
80–100 (0.08%–0.1%)	Uncoordinated, 0.08% is legal driving limit in U.S. and Canada	Minimal signs	4–6
125–150 (0.125%–0.15%)	Unrestrained behavior, episodic uncontrolled behavior	Pleasurable euphoria or beginning of uncoordination	6–10
200–250 (0.2%–0.25%)	Alertness lost, lethargic	Effort is required to maintain emotional and motor control	10–24
300–350 (0.3%–0.35%)	Stupor to coma	Drowsy and slow	10–24
>500 (>0.5%)	Some will die	Coma	>24

[a]Milligrams of alcohol per 100 milliliters of blood.

[b]For a social drinker; alcohol metabolism is somewhat faster in chronic alcohol abusers.

Source: Modified from Goldman L, Schafer AI: *Goldman's Cecil Medicine.* 24th edition. Philadelphia: Elsevier Health Sciences, 2012.

less efficiently than men. The amount of alcohol metabolized by the cells lining the stomach is greater in men than in women. Women also have less body water in which to dilute the alcohol than do men. Overall, women develop chronic alcohol-related ailments, such as cirrhosis of the liver, more rapidly than men do with the same alcohol-consumption habits.

Benefits of Moderate Alcohol Use

When used in moderation, alcohol is linked to several health benefits. Benefits of alcohol use are associated with specific intakes of no more than two drinks per day for men and no more than one drink per day for women. Socialization and relaxation are among the intangible benefits of moderate alcohol use by people of legal drinking age. In terms of physiological benefits, moderate drinkers experience lower risk of developing cardiovascular diseases and type 2 diabetes. Previous consumers of alcohol no longer experience the benefits of alcohol when consumption ceases. See Table 20-7 for additional benefits of moderate alcohol consumption.

Risks of Heavy Drinking

An alcohol use disorder is a formal psychiatric diagnosis defined in the latest edition of the *Diagnostic and Statistical Manual of Mental Disorders (DSM-5)* as a problematic pattern of alcohol use leading to significant impairment or distress. This new definition integrates both alcohol abuse and alcohol dependence into a single disorder with mild, moderate, and severe sub-classifications. According to *DSM-5,* diagnosis depends on meeting two or more of the following criteria within the past year:

- Use of alcohol in larger amounts or over a longer period than intended
- Persistent desire or unsuccessful efforts at cutting down or controlling alcohol use
- Spending a great deal of time obtaining, using, and recovering from the effects of alcohol
- Experiencing cravings for alcohol
- Repeated use of alcohol that results in failure to fulfill major obligations at school, work, or home
- Continued use of alcohol despite personal problems created by the effects of heavy drinking
- Avoiding social, occupational, or recreational activities due to use of alcohol
- Recurrent alcohol use in situations in which it is physically hazardous
- Continuing to use alcohol even after realizing one has a problem caused by heavy drinking

▲ Of all the alcohol sources, red wine in moderation is often singled out as the best choice because of the added bonus of the many phytochemicals present (e.g., resveratrol). These are leached out from the grape skins as the red wine is fermented. Dark beer is also a source of phytochemicals.

- Developing a **tolerance** to the effects of alcohol
- Experiencing symptoms of **withdrawal** in the absence of alcohol use

Alcohol use disorders affect about 17% of adult men and about 8% of adult women at some point in their lives. Studies suggest that about 40% of a person's risk for developing these disorders is genetic. Therefore, people with a family history of heavy drinking, particularly children of alcoholics, should be especially aware of their alcohol consumption.

Early diagnosis of alcohol use disorders can prevent multiple health problems and save millions in health care costs. Asking a person about the quantity and frequency of alcohol consumption is an important means of detecting problematic behaviors (see CAGE questionnaire in box). Observable warning signs of an alcohol use disorder may include an alcohol odor on the breath, flushed face and reddened skin, nervous system disorders (such as tremors), unexplained work absences, frequent accidents, and falls or injuries of vague origin. Laboratory evidence (e.g., impaired liver function, enlarged red blood cells, and elevated triglycerides) is also helpful for diagnosis of alcohol use disorders.

Despite the few benefits of regular, moderate use, the risks of heavy drinking are more numerous and harmful. Although it is one of the most preventable health problems, excessive consumption of alcohol contributes significantly to 5 of the 10 leading causes of death in North America: heart failure, certain forms of cancer, **cirrhosis** of the liver, motor vehicle and other accidents, and suicides (Table 20-7 lists additional health risks). In the United States, about $225 billion is spent annually in terms of lost productivity, medical care, and property damage associated with alcohol use disorders. Overall, alcohol use disorders typically reduce a person's life expectancy by 15 years.

Alcohol is the most damaging to the liver. **Cirrhosis** develops in up to 20% of cases of alcohol use disorders and is the second leading reason for liver transplants, affecting about 2 million people in the United States. This chronic and usually relentlessly progressive disease is characterized by fatty infiltration of the liver. Fatty liver occurs in response to increased synthesis of fat and decreased use of it for energy by the liver. Eventually, the enlarged fat deposits choke off the blood supply, depriving the liver cells of oxygen and nutrients. Liver cells can accumulate so much fat that they burst, die, and are replaced by connective (scar) tissue. At this stage, the liver is deemed cirrhotic (Fig. 20-9). Early stages

FIGURE 20-9 ▲ Effects of alcohol on the liver. Alcohol is particularly damaging to this organ. Pictured are (a) a healthy liver, and (b) a liver with cirrhosis. There is no cure for this disease except a liver transplant. © Science Source

of alcoholic liver injury are reversible, but advanced stages are not. Once a person has cirrhosis, there is a 50% chance of death within 4 years, a far worse prognosis than many forms of cancer. While no specific level of alcohol consumption guarantees cirrhosis, some evidence suggests that damage is caused by a dose as low as 40 grams per day for men (3 beers) and 20 grams per day for women (1.5 beers).

Alcoholic beverages have little nutritional value and, thus, nutrient deficiencies are a common result of alcohol use disorders. The protein and vitamin content is extremely low, except in beer, where it is marginal at best. Iron content varies widely between drinks, with red wine ranking especially high in iron. Deficiencies arise mainly from poor nutrient intakes, but increased urinary losses and fat malabsorption (linked to poor pancreatic function) also contribute. Vitamins most susceptible to depletion from heavy drinking include vitamins A, D, E, and K; thiamin; niacin; folate; vitamins B-6 and B-12; and vitamin C. Mineral deficiencies of calcium, phosphorus, potassium, magnesium, zinc, and iron are also possible. Conversely, vitamin and mineral toxicity is also of concern with heavy drinking. Damage to the GI tract and liver, as well as high levels of some minerals in alcoholic beverages, may lead to toxicity of

tolerance Needing more of a substance to achieve the desired effect (e.g., intoxication) or experiencing diminished effects of a given amount of a substance after repeated use.

withdrawal Physical symptoms related to cessation of substance use, such as sweating, rapid pulse, shakiness, insomnia, nausea and vomiting, anxiety, and even seizures.

cirrhosis A loss of functioning liver cells, which are replaced by nonfunctioning connective tissue. Any substance that poisons liver cells can lead to cirrhosis. The most common cause is a chronic, excessive alcohol intake. Exposure to certain industrial chemicals also can lead to cirrhosis.

cirrhosis A loss of functioning liver cells, which are replaced by nonfunctioning connective tissue. Any substance that poisons liver cells can lead to cirrhosis. The most common cause is a chronic, excessive alcohol intake. Exposure to certain industrial chemicals also can lead to cirrhosis.

CRITICAL THINKING

For many people, drinking and smoking go hand in hand. What health problems arise from the combination of these behaviors?

CAGE QUESTIONNAIRE

The CAGE questionnaire is used to identify alcohol use disorders. More than one positive response suggests an alcohol problem.

C: Have you ever felt you ought to *cut* down on drinking?

A: Have people *annoyed* you by criticizing your drinking?

G: Have you ever felt bad or *guilty* about your drinking?

E: Have you ever had a drink first thing in the morning to steady your nerves or get rid of a hangover (an *eye-opener*)?

TABLE 20-7 ■ Effects of Moderate Versus Heavy Drinking

	Moderate Drinking	Heavy Drinking
Coronary heart disease	Decreased risk of death in those at high risk for coronary heart disease–related death, primarily by increasing HDL-cholesterol, decreasing blood clotting, and relaxing blood vessels	Heart rhythm disturbances, heart muscle damage, increased blood triglycerides and blood clotting
Hypertension and stroke	Mild decrease in blood pressure, lower rates of ischemic stroke in people with normal blood pressure	Increased blood pressure (hypertension), more ischemic and hemorrhagic stroke
Peripheral vascular disease	Decreased risk due to reduced blood clotting	No benefit
Blood glucose regulation and type 2 diabetes	Decreased risk of developing type 2 diabetes, decreased risk of death from cardiovascular disease among those diagnosed with diabetes	Hypoglycemia, reduced insulin sensitivity, and damage to pancreas (site of insulin production)
Bone and joint health	Some increase in bone mineral content in women, linked to estrogen output	Loss of active bone-forming cells and eventual osteoporosis (nutrient deficiencies also contribute to this problem), increased risk of gout
Brain health	Enhanced brain function and decreased risk of dementia by increasing brain blood circulation	Brain tissue damage and decreased memory
Skeletal muscle health	No benefit	Skeletal muscle damage
Cancer	Decreased risk of colon, basal cell, ovarian, and prostate cancers (likely due to phytochemicals in red wine)	Increased risk of oral, esophageal, stomach, liver, lung, colorectal, and breast cancers (especially if the diet is deficient in folate)
Liver function	No benefit	Fatty infiltration and eventual liver cirrhosis (especially if a person is also infected with hepatitis C), iron toxicity
GI tract health	Decreased risk of certain bacterial infections in the stomach	Inflammation of the stomach (and pancreas), absorptive cell damage leading to malabsorption of nutrients
Immune system function	No benefit	Reduced function and increased infections
Nervous system function	No benefit	Loss of nerve sensation and nervous system control of muscles
Sleep disturbances	Some relaxation	Fragmented sleep patterns; worsens sleep apnea
Impotence and decreased libido	No benefit	Contributes to the problem in both men and women
Obesity	No benefit	Increased abdominal fat deposition; contributes to weight gain as calories from alcoholic beverages quickly add up
Dietary intake	May supply some B vitamins, phytochemicals, and iron	Leads to numerous nutrient deficiencies: protein, vitamins, and minerals
Fetal health	No benefit	Variety of toxic effects on the fetus when alcohol is consumed by pregnant women (see Section 18.2)
Socialization and relaxation	Provides some benefit to socialization and leads to relaxation by increasing brain neurotransmitter activity	Contributes to violent behavior and agitation

▲ The limit for alcohol intake for older adults is one drink per day. © Steve Mason/Getty Images

vitamin A, iron, lead, or cobalt. In nutritional treatment of alcohol use disorders, the immediate aim is eliminating alcohol intake, followed by restoration of nutrient stores.

Older adults are uniquely vulnerable to alcohol use disorders, perhaps due to an abundance of free time, social events involving drinking, interactions with medications, loneliness, or depression. Common symptoms of alcohol use disorders—trembling hands, slurred speech, sleep problems, memory loss, and unsteady gait—can be easily overlooked as signs of aging. Slower alcohol metabolism and decreased body water allow older adults to become intoxicated from a smaller amount of alcohol than their younger counterparts. Even moderate alcohol consumption can exacerbate some chronic health conditions, such as diabetes and osteoporosis. As well, even small amounts of alcohol can react negatively with various medications used by older persons. The adverse health effects of drinking may be amplified in older adults, so people over the age of 65 should limit alcohol consumption to no more than one drink per day.

Once a diagnosis of an alcohol use disorder is established, a primary care provider can arrange appropriate treatment and

Ethnicity plays an important role in both the probability of becoming a heavy drinker and the negative health risks associated with heavy drinking. Native Americans suffer the highest rates of unintentional injuries, suicide, homicide, and domestic abuse related to alcohol use. African-Americans with alcohol use disorders are at greater risk than other racial groups for tuberculosis, hepatitis C, HIV/AIDS, and other infectious diseases. Hispanic Americans are at particular risk for cirrhosis-related death.

counseling for the person and his or her family. Treatment often includes the use of targeted medications, counseling, and social support. Total abstinence must be the ultimate objective. Alcoholics Anonymous (AA) or other reputable therapy programs can support those struggling with alcohol use disorders and their families as they recover from this devastating disease.

Guidance Regarding Alcohol Use

No government agencies recommend drinking alcohol. The 2015–2020 Dietary Guidelines for Americans provide the following advice regarding use of alcoholic beverages:

- If alcohol is consumed, it should be in moderation—up to one drink per day for women and up to two drinks per day for men—and only by adults of legal drinking age.
- For those who choose to drink, moderate alcohol consumption can be incorporated within the calorie limits of most healthy eating patterns.
- The Dietary Guidelines do not recommend that individuals who do not drink alcohol start drinking for any reason;
- Many individuals should not consume alcohol, including individuals who are taking certain over-the-counter or prescription medications or who have certain medical conditions, those who are recovering from alcoholism or are unable to control the amount they drink, and anyone younger than 21 years.
- Individuals should not drink if they are driving, planning to drive, or are participating in other activities requiring skill, coordination, and alertness. Note the National Transportation Safety Board is calling for states to lower BAC limits from 0.08 to 0.05 gram per deciliter.
- Women who are or who may be pregnant should not drink. Drinking during pregnancy, especially in the first few months of pregnancy, may result in negative behavioral or neurological consequences in the offspring. Women who are breastfeeding should consult with their health care provider regarding alcohol consumption.

As the understanding of the relationship between drinking alcohol and health grows, registered dietitian nutritionists and other health professionals can promote healthy lifestyle—not by encouraging indiscriminate drinking, but by reassuring adults that moderate alcohol consumption may have beneficial health outcomes.

To learn more about alcohol use disorders, visit these websites:

- National Institute on Alcohol Abuse and Alcoholism: www.niaaa.nih.gov
- American Society of Addiction Medicine: www.asam.org
- Centers for Disease Control and Prevention: www.cdc.gov/alcohol

Summary (Numbers refer to numbered sections in the chapter.)

20.1 Although maximum life span has not changed, life expectancy has increased dramatically over the past century. For many societies, this means that an increasing proportion of the population is over 65 years of age. As health care costs rise, the goal of delaying disease becomes ever important.

The physiologic changes of aging are the sum of cellular changes, lifestyle practices, and environmental influences. Many of these changes can be minimized, prevented, and/or reversed by healthy lifestyles. Usual aging refers to the age-related physical and physiological changes that are commonly thought to be typical of aging. Successful aging describes the declines in physical and physiological function that occur because one grows older. Striving to have the greatest number of healthy years and the fewest of illness is referred to as compression of morbidity.

20.2 A dietary pattern based on MyPlate and the Dietary Guidelines for Americans can help one to preserve body function, avoid chronic disease, and age successfully. American adults are fairly well nourished, although common dietary excesses are calories, fat, sodium, and, for some, alcohol. Common dietary inadequacies include vitamins D and E, folate, magnesium, calcium, zinc, and fiber. People ages 65 and older, particularly those in long-term care facilities and hospitals, are at risk for malnutrition. The DETERMINE Nutrition Checklist for Older Adults can help to identify older adults at risk of nutrient deficiencies. The DRIs for adults are divided by gender and age to reflect how nutrient needs change as adults grow older. These changes in nutrient needs take into consideration the aging-related physiological alterations in body composition, metabolism, and organ function.

20.3 Chronic diseases, changes in body composition, and declining function of body systems can influence nutritional status. Of particular concern is sarcopenia, or loss of muscle mass that frequently accompanies aging. The use of medications and supplements can improve health and quality of life, but some also adversely affect nutritional status. Herbal products should be used with caution.

20.4 Dietary patterns for adults should be based on nutrient-dense foods and need to be individualized for existing health problems, physical abilities, the presence of drug-nutrient interactions, possible depression, and economic constraints. Community nutrition assistance programs, including congregate or home-delivered meal systems, SNAP, commodity distribution, and farmers markets make wholesome, nutritious foods accessible for low-income and older adults.

20.5 Alcohol requires no digestion and is metabolized primarily in the liver. The benefits of alcohol use are associated with low to moderate alcohol consumption. These benefits include the pleasurable and social aspects of alcohol use, a reduction in various forms of cardiovascular disease, increase in insulin sensitivity, and protection against some harmful stomach bacteria. Heavy drinking, however, contributes significantly to 5 of the 10 leading causes of death in North America. If alcohol is consumed, it should be consumed in moderation with meals. Women (and older adults, in general) are advised to drink no more than 3 drinks in 1 day and no more than 7 drinks per week; men should drink no more than 4 drinks in 1 day and no more than 14 drinks per week.

Check Your Knowledge (Answers are available at the end of this question set.)

1. The reason the incidence of obesity increases with age is that
   a. the basal metabolic rate decreases with age.
   b. physical activity often decreases with age.
   c. energy intake exceeds energy expenditure.
   d. any of these can occur.

2. Congregate meal programs provide
   a. 100% of nutrient needs.
   b. a social atmosphere for eating.
   c. food stamps.
   d. all of these.

3. Among the older population of the United States, the age of the fastest growing segment is _____ years.
   a. 65
   b. 74
   c. 79
   d. 85+

4. Which of the following accurately portrays a theory about the causes of aging?
   a. Increases in testosterone and estrogen affect cell processes.
   b. Blood sugar decreases, failing to supply adequate energy to brain cells.
   c. Inadequate calorie intake speeds body breakdown.
   d. Excess free radicals damage cell components.

5. The immune system becomes less efficient with age, so it is especially important to consume adequate _____ and _____, nutrients that contribute to immune function.
   a. vitamin A, potassium
   b. protein, zinc
   c. zinc, iodide
   d. vitamin A, vitamin K

6. Which of the following is a useful strategy to prevent or delay the onset of Alzheimer's disease?
   a. Avoid stressing the brain with challenging mental tasks.
   b. Limit intake of dairy products.
   c. Consume adequate B vitamins, such as folate, B-6, and B-12.
   d. Increase the ratio of omega-6 to omega-3 fatty acids in the diet.

7. To maintain optimal nutritional status and healthy weight, the diet of an older person should have a _____ nutrient density and be _____ in energy content.
   a. low, high
   b. low, low
   c. high, moderate
   d. high, high

8. Donald has been diagnosed with cirrhosis. To cope with his impaired liver function, he will need to
   a. take high doses of vitamin and mineral supplements.
   b. minimize alcohol intake.
   c. limit his intake of dietary fiber.
   d. do all of these.

9. Alcohol is digested in the
   a. stomach.
   b. small intestine.
   c. liver.
   d. None of these is correct, because alcohol requires no digestion.

10. Alcohol is most damaging to the
    a. brain cells, because alcohol can be used as an energy source even before glucose.
    b. kidney cells, because this is where alcohol is excreted.
    c. cells of the gastrointestinal tract, because they are in direct contact with ingested alcohol.
    d. liver cells, because this is where alcohol is metabolized.

Study Questions (Numbers refer to Learning Outcomes)

1. What is the difference between life span and life expectancy? **(LO 20.1)**

2. Describe two hypotheses proposed to explain the causes of aging, and note evidence for each in your daily life experiences. **(LO 20.2)**

3. List four organ systems that can decline in function in later years, along with a diet/lifestyle response to help cope with the decline. **(LO 20.3)**

4. Defend the recommendation for regular physical activity during older adulthood, including some resistance activity (weight training). **(LO 20.5)**

5. List four warning signs of undernutrition in older people that are part of the acronym DETERMINE. Briefly justify the inclusion of each. **(LO 20.2)**

6. List three important points made by the Dietary Guidelines for Americans for the general population and give an example of why each one may be difficult for older adults to implement. What are some suggestions for overcoming these barriers? **(LO 20.4)**

7. How might the nutritional needs of older people differ from those of younger people? How are their needs similar? Be specific. **(LO 20.4)**

8. List three common herbal remedies. What are the possible benefits and risks of each one? If your grandmother were considering using any of these herbal remedies, what advice would you give her? **(LO 20.6)**

9. What three resources in a community are widely available to aid older adults in maintaining nutritional health? **(LO 20.6)**

10. List two benefits of moderate alcohol intake. List two risks of heavy drinking. Should a nondrinker take up drinking for the health benefits? **(LO 20.7)**

What the Dietitian Chose

As far as nutrient deficiencies go, vitamin B-12 deficiency is relatively common. About 6% of older adults are deficient in vitamin B-12, and many more likely have marginal vitamin status. Older adults are at particular risk of vitamin B-12 deficiency because stomach production of acid and intrinsic factor, which are required for vitamin B-12 absorption, tends to decline with age. In addition, certain medications can reduce acid production and thereby affect B-12 absorption.

As you learned in Section 13.4, foods of animal origin are the only natural sources of vitamin B-12. Although the leafy green vegetables would be an excellent source of folate—another B vitamin that is required for red blood cell health—they are not a good food source of vitamin B-12.

A 3-ounce serving of pot roast provides about 100% of the 2.4 micrograms of vitamin B-12 needed per day. However, recall that stomach acid is needed to cleave vitamin B-12 from protein in food sources. Even though beef is a rich source of vitamin B-12,

© LWA/Dann Tardif/age fotostock

with reduced stomach-acid secretion, not much of the vitamin B-12 will be absorbed.

Synthetic vitamin B-12—the form found in dietary supplements and fortified foods—is actually better absorbed than the natural form of the vitamin. This is because synthetic vitamin B-12 does not have to be cleaved from food proteins before it can bind with intrinsic factor and be absorbed in the ileum of the small intestine. A fortified breakfast cereal, such as Cheerios®, provides about 80% of the RDA for vitamin B-12, and because this vitamin B-12 is not protein bound, it is efficiently absorbed. Thus, the Cheerios would be a good way to boost vitamin B-12 status.

A dietary supplement formulated for older adults, such as Centrum® Silver® Adults 50+, provides 25 micrograms of efficiently absorbed, synthetic vitamin B-12. That's 10 times the RDA! Is it a problem to consume this megadose of vitamin B-12? Actually, no

Upper Level has been set for vitamin B-12 and no toxicity has ever been reported. To correct your existing vitamin B-12 deficiency, the high dose of vitamin B-12 in this supplement would be most effective. After your nutrition status is back to normal, you could switch to a fortified food, such as breakfast cereal, to keep your red blood cells healthy with adequate B-12 and other micronutrients.

CASE STUDY SOLUTION — Dietary Assistance for an Older Adult

1. Frances's typical dietary pattern is low in many nutrients, including protein, calcium, iron, zinc, and vitamins B-12 and D, as well as fiber.
2. Her inadequate diet will cause a decline in her lean tissue and bone mass. With low intakes of iron and vitamin B-12, she may experience anemia. Her low intake of fiber may lead to problems with constipation.
3. Physiological changes that will tend to worsen her appetite include decreases in senses of taste and smell, diminished sense of thirst, and poor chewing ability (related to tooth loss). Bowel function tends to decline with age, which would only be further complicated by her low fiber intake. Low production of stomach acid and intrinsic factor might increase her risk of anemia, which is already a concern due to low intakes of iron and vitamin B-12.
4. It would be helpful to have additional information about her medical history, including any current diagnoses and medications. Medical conditions, such as high blood cholesterol, would likely affect diet recommendations. Many prescription and over-the-counter medications can affect appetite and nutrient availability. Also, knowing her height and weight could assist in setting kilocalorie goals. Information regarding her economic resources could be useful

when making dietary recommendations that she can actually follow.
5. Frances could contact a local government agency that offers congregate meal programs at a central location. She could inquire about location and availability of transportation to the site. This would give her social contact with other older adults, probably an important element missing in her life. This could help alleviate her loneliness. She could also request Meals on Wheels (if available) to provide one hot meal per day, which may also be what she needs to help stimulate her appetite. If her funds are limited, she may qualify for nutrition assistance from SNAP or local food pantries.
6. Nutrient-dense yet convenient foods that could improve her nutrient intake include milk, peanut butter, fortified breakfast cereals, canned chicken or deli meats, yogurt, sliced cheese, cottage cheese, calcium-fortified orange juice, canned or frozen fruits and vegetables, and some fresh fruits and vegetables that do not require preparation, such as prewashed lettuce and bananas. A further possibility is a nutrition bar or liquid nutritional supplement, such as a can of Ensure Plus®. The resulting increase in her nutrient intake would help prevent disease in the future and increase her sense of well-being.

Further Readings

1. Berner LA and others: Characterization of dietary protein among older adults in the United States: Amount, animal sources, and meal patterns. *Journal of the Academy of Nutrition and Dietetics* 113:809, 2013.

2. Bernstein M and others: Position of the Academy of Nutrition and Dietetics: Food and nutrition for older adults: Promoting health and wellness. *Journal of the Academy of Nutrition and Dietetics* 112:1255, 2012.

3. Broadhead GK and others: Dietary modification and supplementation for the treatment of age-related macular degeneration. *Nutrition Reviews* 73:448, 2015.

4. Buch A and others: Muscle function and fat content in relation to sarcopenia, obesity and frailty of old age—an overview. *Experimental Gerontology* 16(10), 2016.

5. Chodzko-Zajko WJ and others: American College of Sports Medicine Position Stand: Exercise and physical activity for older adults. *Medicine and Science in Sports and Exercise* 41:1510, 2009.

6. Esposito K and others: Long-term effect of Mediterranean-style diet and calorie restriction on biomarkers of longevity and oxidant stress in overweight men. *Cardiology Research and Practice* 2011:1, 2010.

7. Genaro P and others: Dietary protein intake in elderly women: Association with muscle and bone mass. *Nutrition in Clinical Practice* 30:283, 2015.

8. Getz L: The Mediterranean diet and cognition. *Today's Dietitian* 16:26, 2014.

9. Institute of Medicine: Sodium intake in populations: Assessment of evidence. National Academy of Sciences. May 2013. www.iom.edu/Reports/2013/Sodium-Intake-in-Populations-Assessment-of-Evidence.aspx. Accessed February 2, 2016.

10. Kamp BJ and others: Position of the American Dietetic Association, American Society for Nutrition, and Society for Nutrition Education: Food and nutrition programs for community-residing older adults. *Journal of the American Dietetic Association* 110:463, 2010.

11. Kushi LH and others: American Cancer Society guidelines on nutrition and physical activity for cancer prevention: Reducing the risk of cancer with healthy food choices and physical activity. *CA: A Cancer Journal for Clinicians* 62:30, 2012.

12. National Institute on Alcohol Abuse and Alcoholism: *Rethinking drinking: alcohol and your health.* December 2015. http://pubs.niaaa.nih.gov/publications/RethinkingDrinking/Rethinking_Drinking.pdf. Accessed February 4, 2016.

13. Oliviero F and others: How the Mediterranean diet and some of its components modulate inflammatory pathways in arthritis. *Swiss Medical Weekly* 145:w14190, 2015.

14. Paddon-Jones D and others: Protein and healthy aging. *American Journal of Clinical Nutrition* 101:s1339, 2015.

15. Redman LM and others: Caloric restriction in humans: Impact on physiological, psychological, and behavioral outcomes. *Antioxidants & Redox Signaling* 14:275, 2011.

16. Riediger ND and others: A systemic review of the roles of n-3 fatty acids in health and disease. *Journal of the American Dietetic Association* 109:668, 2009.

17. Scarlata K: Digestive wellness: The link between aging and digestive disorders. *Today's Dietitian* 17(7):12, 2015.

18. Sebastian RS and others: Sandwiches are major contributors of sodium in the diets of American adults: Results from What We Eat in America, National Health and Nutrition Examination Survey 2009-2010. *Journal of the Academy of Nutrition and Dietetics* 115:272, 2015.

19. Thalheimer JC: Nutrition and healthy aging for men. *Today's Dietitian* 17(6):44, 2015.

20. Touger-Decker R, Mobley C: Position of the American Academy of Nutrition and Dietetics: Oral health and nutrition. *Journal of the Academy of Nutrition and Dietetics* 113:693, 2013.

 To get the most out of your study of nutrition, go to McGraw-Hill's online resources: Connect www.mcgrawhillconnect.com, where you will find NutritionCalc Plus, LearnSmart, and many other dynamic tools.

ChooseMyPlate.gov

I. Am I Aging Healthfully?

Take Control of Your Aging by Dr. William B. Malarkey (Wooster Book Co., Wooster, OH, 1999) includes a plan that incorporates various diet and lifestyle factors associated with successful aging. Indicate the degree to which you are following such a plan (or alternatively, fill this out with a parent or another older relative in mind).

Physical: Do you eat a well-balanced diet, exercise on a regular basis, remain free of illness, abstain from smoking, refrain from drinking alcohol excessively, and experience refreshing sleep?

_____

_____

Intellectual: Are you analytical, do you read regularly, do you learn new things each day, do you engage your mental ability at work (or at school), and do you often reflect on your life?

_____

_____

_____

Emotional: Are you at peace, do you like who you are, are you optimistic, and do you laugh and relax regularly?

_____

_____

_____

Relational: Are you a good listener, do you feel supported by friends, do you attend social functions, do you talk with family members often, and do you feel close to coworkers (or fellow students)?

_____

_____

_____

Spiritual: Do you appreciate nature, give to or serve others, meditate or seek religious worship, and feel life has meaning?

_____

_____

_____

The more of these factors that you include in your life, the more well rounded your plan is for maintaining overall health. Any one of the five areas in which you are not achieving success should show you characteristics to work on in the future.

© Royalty-Free/Corbis

II. Helping Older Adults Eat Better

During their lifetimes, most people usually eat meals with families or loved ones. As people reach older adulthood, many of them are faced with living and eating alone. In a study of the diets of 4400 older adults in the United States, one man in every five living alone and over age 55 ate poorly. One of four women between the ages of 55 and 64 years followed a low-quality diet. These poor dietary patterns can contribute to deteriorating mental and physical health. Consider the following example of the living situation of an older adult.

© Mel Curtis/Getty Images

Neal, a 70-year-old man, lives alone in his home in a local suburb. His wife died 1 year ago. He does not have many friends; his wife was his primary confidante. His neighbors across the street and next door are friendly, and Neal used to help them with yard projects in his spare time. Neal's health has been good, but he has had trouble with his teeth recently. His diet has been inadequate, and in the past 3 months, his physical and mental vigor has deteriorated. He has been slowly lapsing into a depression, so he keeps the shades drawn and rarely leaves his house. Neal keeps very little food in the house because his wife did most of the cooking and shopping, and he just is not that interested in food.

If you were one of Neal's relatives and learned of Neal's situation, what six things could you do or suggest to help improve his nutritional status and mental outlook? Look back into this chapter to get some ideas.

1. _____
2. _____
3. _____
4. _____
5. _____
6. _____

Appendix A

Daily Values Used on Food Labels

Daily Values Used on Food Labels in the United States, with a Comparison to the Latest RDAs and Other Nutrient Standards*

Dietary Constituent	Unit of Measure	Current Daily Values for People Over 4 Years of Age	RDA or Other Current Dietary Standard	
			Males 19–30 Years Old	Females 19–30 Years Old
Total fat[†]	g	<65	—	—
Saturated fatty acids[†]	g	<20	—	—
Protein[†]	g	50	56	46
Cholesterol[§]	mg	<300	—	—
Carbohydrate[†]	g	300	130	130
Dietary fiber	g	25	38	25
Vitamin A	µg Retinol activity equivalents	1000	900	700
	International units	5000	3000	2300
Vitamin D	International units	400	600	600
Vitamin E	International units	30	22–33	22–33
Vitamin K	µg	80	120	90
Vitamin C	mg	60	90	75
Folate	µg	400	400	400
Thiamin	mg	1.5	1.2	1.1
Riboflavin	mg	1.7	1.3	1.1
Niacin	mg	20	16	14
Vitamin B-6	mg	2	1.3	1.3
Vitamin B-12	µg	6	2.4	2.4
Biotin	µg	300	30	30
Pantothenic acid	mg	10	5	5
Calcium	mg	1000	1000	1000
Phosphorus	mg	1000	700	700
Iodine	µg	150	150	150
Iron	mg	18	8	18
Magnesium	mg	400	400	310
Copper	mg	2	0.9	0.9
Zinc	mg	15	11	8
Sodium[‡]	mg	<2400	1500	1500
Potassium[‡]	mg	3500	4700	4700
Chloride[‡]	mg	3400	2300	2300
Manganese	mg	2	2.3	1.8
Selenium	µg	70	55	55
Chromium	µg	120	35	25
Molybdenum	µg	75	45	45

*Daily Values are generally set at the highest nutrient recommendation in a specific age and gender category. Many Daily Values exceed current nutrient standards. This is in part because aspects of the Daily Values were originally developed in the early 1970s using estimates of nutrient needs published in 1968. The Daily Values have yet to be updated to reflect the current state of knowledge.

[†]These Daily Values are based on a 2000-kcal diet, instead of RDAs, with a caloric distribution of 30% from fat (and one-third of this total from saturated fat), 60% from carbohydrate, and 10% from protein.

[§]Based on recommendations of U.S. federal agencies.

[‡]The considerably higher Daily Values for sodium and chloride are there to allow for more diet flexibility, but the extra amounts are not needed to maintain health.

Appendix B

Diabetes Menu-Planning Tools

Lists, Choices, and Exchanges: Making Sense of Meal Planning for Diabetes

Registered dietitian nutritionists and other diabetes educators work closely with their patients to help them understand how the foods they eat directly impact their day-to-day quality of life. **Food lists** (also known as *exchange lists*) are one way diabetes educators can help people to plan their dietary patterns to better manage their blood sugar. The first exchange lists for people with diabetes were developed by the American Dietetic Association (now the Academy of Nutrition and Dietetics), American Diabetes Association, and U.S. Public Health Service over 50 years ago. Since then, they have been revised to reflect advances in nutrition recommendations and the ever-expanding variety of foods in the marketplace. The most recent version, *Choose Your Foods: Food Lists for Diabetes,* was published in 2014.

Food lists organize the many details of the nutrient composition of foods into a manageable framework based on calorie and macronutrient content. In the *Food Lists for Diabetes,* individual foods are placed into three broad groups: carbohydrates, proteins, and fats. Within these groups are lists that contain foods of similar macronutrient composition: various types of milk and milk substitutes, fruits, vegetables, starches, other carbohydrates, proteins, and fats. There are even lists that show how to account for alcohol, combination foods (e.g., casseroles), and a wide variety of fast foods. These lists are designed so that, when the given serving size is observed, each food on a list provides roughly the same amount of carbohydrate, protein, fat, and kilocalories. The patient and a registered dietitian nutritionist first tailor a healthy eating pattern to meet the client's energy and specific macronutrient needs. Then, the client can select **choices** (i.e.,*exchanges*) from each of the various lists that fit into the plan without having to look up or memorize the nutrient values of numerous foods.

Table B-1 summarizes the basic nutrient composition of foods in each food list. The serving sizes of individual foods in a list may vary, but general estimates are given. The protein and milk and milk substitutes lists are divided into subclasses, which vary in fat content and, thus, in the amount of kilocalories they provide. You can see that each food list is unique in the kilocalories and macronutrients it supplies. A healthy meal plan should include foods from each of the lists to ensure nutrient adequacy. Study Table B-1 to become familiar with the food groupings, the approximate size of choices on each food list, and the amounts of carbohydrate, protein, fat, and kilocalories per choice.

Because the *Food Lists for Diabetes* offer a quick way to estimate the calorie, carbohydrate, protein, and fat content in any food or meal, they are a valuable menu-planning tool for individuals without diabetes, as well. In fact, the Academy of Nutrition and Dietetics and the American Diabetes Association have published a related guide, *Choose Your Foods: Food Lists for Weight Management.*

Recognize that the *Food Lists for Diabetes* group foods somewhat differently than MyPlate. For the *Food Lists,* we care more about nutrient composition and the food's eventual physiological effect on blood sugar than its plant or animal origin. For example, the starch list includes not only bread, dry cereal, cooked cereal, rice, and pasta but also baked beans, corn on the cob, and potatoes. Although potatoes and corn are vegetables, their macronutrient composition resembles that of bread more than that of broccoli. In addition, many foods that would traditionally be categorized as dairy products do not appear with the milk and milk substitutes list. Instead, cheeses are grouped as proteins, whereas cream and cream cheese show up on the fats lists.

food lists A system for classifying foods into numerous lists based on the foods' macronutrient composition, and establishing serving sizes, so that one serving of each food on a list contains the same amount of carbohydrate, protein, fat, and calorie content; also called *exchange lists.*

choice The serving size of a food on a specific exchange list; formerly called exchange.

TABLE B-1 ■ Approximate Nutrient Composition of Food Choices from *Choose Your Foods: Food Lists for Diabetes, 2014*

Groups/Lists	Household Measures*	Carbohydrate (g)	Protein (g)	Fat (g)	Energy (kcal)
Carbohydrates					
Starch (e.g., bread, cereal, pasta, rice, crackers, and beans)	1 slice, ¾ cup raw, or ½ cup cooked	15	3	1 or less†	80
Fruits	1 small/medium piece	15	—	—	60
Milk and milk substitutes	1 cup				
Fat free, low fat		12	8	0–3†	100
Reduced fat		12	8	5	120
Whole		12	8	8	160
Nonstarchy vegetables	1 cup raw or ½ cup cooked	5	2	—	25
Sweets, desserts, and other carbohydrates	Varies	15	Varies	Varies	Varies
Proteins	1 ounce	—	7	2	45
Lean		—	7	5	75
Medium fat		—	7	8	100
High fat		Varies	7	Varies	Varies
Plant based					
Fats	1 teaspoon	—	—	5	45
Alcohol	Varies	Varies	—	—	100

Source: *Choose Your Foods: Food Lists for Diabetes,* 2014 which is the basis of a meal planning system designed by a committee of the American Diabetes Association and the Academy of Nutrition and Dietetics.

*An estimate; see food lists for actual amounts.

†Calculated as 1 gram for purposes of calorie contribution.

In some instances, a food counts for more than one choice at a time. In the category of sweets, desserts, and other carbohydrates, you will find a variety of snack items and condiments that count as carbohydrates and fats. The food lists also provide the user with some guidance on accounting for a wide variety of combination foods, such as pizza, casseroles, and soups. A list of free foods includes choices such as reduced-fat or fat-free foods, condiments, seasonings, and sugar-free drinks that, when consumed in moderation, have little or no impact on energy intake and blood sugar.

USING THE *FOOD LISTS* TO DEVELOP DAILY MENUS

Now let us use the *Food Lists* to plan a 1-day menu. Our kilocalorie target will be 2000 kcal, with 55% derived from carbohydrates (1100 kcal), 15% from protein (300 kcal), and 30% from fat (600 kcal). This can be achieved with 2 reduced-fat milk choices, 3 nonstarchy vegetable choices, 5 fruit choices, 11 starch choices, 4 lean protein choices, and 6 fat choices (Table B-2). This is just one of many possible combinations; the *Food Lists* offer great flexibility. For example, more protein choices could be included if less milk were used.

Table B-3 arbitrarily distributes these choices into breakfast, lunch, dinner, and a snack. Breakfast includes 1 reduced-fat milk choice, 2 fruit choices, 2 starch choices, and 1 fat choice. Drawing from the food lists, this plan could be achieved with ¾ cup of a ready-to-eat breakfast cereal, 1 cup of reduced-fat milk, 1 slice of bread with 1 teaspoon margarine, and 1 cup of orange juice.

TABLE B-2 ■ Possible Food Choice Patterns That Yield 55% of Calories as Carbohydrate, 30% as Fat, and 15% as Protein

Food List	1200*	1600*	2000	2400	2800	3200	3600
Milk (reduced fat)	2	2	2	2	2	2	2
Nonstarchy vegetable	3	3	3	4	4	4	4
Fruit	3	4	5	6	8	9	9
Starch	5	8	11	13	15	18	21
Protein (lean)	4	4	4	5	6	7	8
Fat	2	4	6	8	10	11	13

*Calorie intakes of 1200 and 1600 kcal contain 20% of calories as protein and 50% of calories as carbohydrate to allow for greater flexibility in diet planning.

TABLE B-3 ■ **Sample 1-Day 2000-kcal Menu Based on the Food Lists for Diabetes Plan***

Breakfast	
1 reduced-fat milk choice	1 cup reduced-fat milk (some on cereal)
2 fruit choices	1 cup orange juice
2 starch choices	¾ cup ready-to-eat breakfast cereal and 1 piece whole-wheat toast
1 fat choice	1 teaspoon soft margarine on toast
Lunch	
4 starch choices	2 slices whole-wheat bread and 6 graham crackers (2½ inches by 2½ inches)
2 fat choices	1 slice bacon, 1 teaspoon mayonnaise
1 nonstarchy vegetable choice	1 sliced tomato
2 fruit choices	1 banana (9 inches)
1 reduced-fat milk choice	1 cup reduced-fat milk
Snack	
1 starch choice	¾ ounce pretzels
Dinner	
4 lean protein choices	4 ounces lean steak (well trimmed)
2 starch choices	1 medium baked potato
1 fat choice	1 teaspoon soft margarine
2 nonstarchy vegetable choices	1 cup cooked broccoli
1 fruit choice	1 kiwi fruit
	Coffee (if desired)
Snack	
2 starch choices	1/2 large bagel
2 fat choices	2 tablespoons regular cream cheese

*The target plan was a 2000-kcal intake, with 55% of calories from carbohydrate, 15% from protein, and 30% from fat. Computer analysis indicates that this menu yielded 2040 kcal, with 53% of calories from carbohydrate, 16% from protein, and 31% from fat—in close agreement with the targeted goals.

This 1-day menu is only one of endless possibilities with the *Food Lists for Diabetes*. Apple juice could replace the orange juice; two apples could be exchanged for the banana. For simplicity, we have used a variety of individual foods to achieve the total number of choices for this healthy eating plan. However, the *Food Lists* also include some commonly used combination foods. For instance, a 1-cup serving of lasagna typically provides 2 medium-fat meat choices plus 2 carbohydrate choices. With practice, you will be able to estimate the choices from complex foods on your own (Fig. B-1). For now, using individual foods makes learning the *Food Lists* much easier. Finally, you might want to prove to yourself that the food choices listed in Table B-3 really fulfill the plan set forth in Table B-2.

Food List	Total Food Choices to Be Consumed Daily	Food Choices Consumed at Each Meal			
		Breakfast	Lunch	Dinner	Snacks
Milk and milk substitutes					
Nonstarchy vegetables					
Fruits					
Starch					
Proteins					
Fats					

FIGURE B-1 ◀ Record the *Food Lists for Diabetes* pattern you have chosen in the left-hand column. Then distribute the food choices throughout the day, noting the food to be used and the serving size.

Examples of Food Choices from *Food Lists for Diabetes*

In this section, you will find just a few examples of the many food choices that are included in the most recent edition of *Choose Your Foods: Food Lists for Diabetes* from the American Diabetes Association. For complete information, you can order your own copy of the booklet at http://www.shopdiabetes.org.

Starches

Starches provide 15 grams of carbohydrate, 0 to 3 grams of protein, 0 to 1 gram of fat, and about 80 kcal per serving. Keep in mind that the serving sizes for starch choices on these food lists are usually smaller than those recommended by MyPlate. Also, some foods with high fat content may be counted as 1 starch plus 1 or 2 fats. Beans, peas, and lentils count as 1 starch plus 1 lean protein choice.

BREAD

Serving Size	Food
¼	Bagel, large (about 4 oz)
1 slice	Bread
½	English muffin
1	Pancake (4-inch diameter)
1	Tortilla, flour (6-inch diameter)
⅓	Tortilla, flour (10-inch diameter)
3¼-inch square	Naan
½	Hamburger bun

CEREALS

Serving Size	Food
½ cup	Cooked cereal (e.g., oatmeal)
¼ cup	Granola cereal
1½ cups	Puffed cereal (e.g., puffed rice)
½ cup	Sweetened cereal (e.g., Frosted Flakes®)
¾ cup	Unsweetened ready-to-eat cereal (e.g., Cheerios®)

GRAINS

Serving Size	Food
⅓ cup	Rice, cooked (e.g., white and brown)
⅓ cup	Pasta, cooked
½ cup	Wild rice, cooked
⅓ cup	Quinoa, cooked

STARCHY VEGETABLES

Serving Size	Food
½ cup	Corn
1 cup	Mixed vegetables (e.g., corn, peas, and carrots)
½ cup	Spaghetti sauce
¼ large	Potato, baked
½ cup	Potatoes, mashed
1 cup	Winter squash (e.g., acorn and butternut)
½ cup	Sweet potato

CRACKERS AND SNACKS

Serving Size	Food
8	Animal crackers
3 2½-inch squares	Graham crackers
6	Saltines
6	Butter crackers (e.g., Ritz®; count as 1 starch + 1 fat)
3 cups	Popcorn (no fat added)
¾ ounce	Pretzels
8	Baked snack chips
13	Tortilla or potato chips (count as 1 starch + 2 fats)

BEANS, PEAS, AND LENTILS
(count as 1 starch and 1 lean protein)

Serving Size	Food
⅓ cup	Baked beans
½ cup	Beans, cooked or canned (e.g., black, garbanzo, and kidney)
½ cup	Lentils, cooked
½ cup	Peas, cooked (e.g., black-eyed and split)

Fruits

One choice from the Fruits list provides 15 grams of carbohydrate, 0 grams of protein, 0 grams of fat, and 60 kcal. Typically, 1 fruit choice is equal to ½ cup of canned or frozen fruit, 1 small fresh fruit, ½ cup of unsweetened fruit juice, or 2 tablespoons of dried fruit. Recognize that the fruit you buy at the grocery store may amount to more than one fruit choice; a large banana, for example, counts for 2 fruit choices. The serving sizes of fruit juices and dried fruit are small because these are more concentrated sources of carbohydrates and energy.

FRUITS

Serving Size	Food		Serving Size	Food
1 small	Apple (about 4 oz)		½ cup	Kiwi, sliced
½ cup	Applesauce, unsweetened		1 medium	Orange
1 extra small	Banana (about 4 inches)		½ cup	Pineapple, canned
1 cup	Blackberries		3	Prunes
¾ cup	Blueberries		½ cup	Pomegranate seeds (arils)
12	Cherries		1¼ cup	Strawberries, whole
17	Grapes		1¼ cup	Watermelon, diced
1 cup	Honeydew melon, diced			

FRUIT JUICE

Serving Size	Food
½ cup	Apple juice or apple cider
⅓ cup	Grape juice
½ cup	Orange juice
⅓ cup	Prune juice

Milk and Milk Substitutes

Milk and milk substitutes are divided into subcategories based on their fat content. All milk and yogurt products provide 12 grams of carbohydrate and 8 grams of protein but may vary in fat content from 0 to 8 grams per choice. The subcategory of other milk foods and milk substitutes includes some products that may be used in place of milk in the diet (e.g., soy milk), but have a slightly different nutrient profile than traditional milk and yogurt products. Those foods, as indicated below, are counted as a combination of carbohydrate (15 grams of carbohydrate, 70 kcal) and fat (5 grams of fat, 45 kcal) choices. Please note that other products used as dairy alternatives (e.g., almond milk) are listed with fat choices.

FAT-FREE (SKIM) AND LOW-FAT MILK AND YOGURT
(12 grams of carbohydrate, 8 grams of protein,
0–3 grams of fat, and 100 kcal)

Serving Size	Food
1 cup	Fat-free (skim) milk, 1% milk, or buttermilk
½ cup	Canned, evaporated, fat-free milk
⅔ cup	Yogurt (fat-free plain or fat-free Greek, unsweetened or artificially sweetened)

REDUCED-FAT (2%) MILK AND YOGURT
(12 grams of carbohydrate, 8 grams of protein, 5 grams of fat, and 120 kcal)

Serving Size	Food
1 cup	2% milk, acidophilus milk, or kefir
⅔ cup	Yogurt (reduced fat, plain)

WHOLE MILK AND YOGURT
(12 grams of carbohydrate, 8 grams of protein, 8 grams of fat, and 160 kcal)

Serving Size	Food
1 cup	Whole milk, buttermilk, or goat's milk
½ cup	Evaporated whole milk
1 cup	Yogurt (whole milk, plain)

OTHER MILK FOODS AND MILK SUBSTITUTES

Serving Size	Food	Choices
⅓ cup	Eggnog (made from whole milk)	1 carbohydrate + 1 fat
1 cup	Rice drink, plain, fat free	1 carbohydrate
1 cup	Rice drink, flavored, low fat	2 carbohydrates
1 cup	Soy milk, plain, low fat	½ carbohydrate + ½ fat
1 cup	Soy milk, regular, plain	½ carbohydrate + 1 fat
⅔ cup	Yogurt with fruit, low fat	1 fat-free milk + 1 carbohydrate

Nonstarchy Vegetables

Nonstarchy vegetables still provide carbohydrates, but not as much as their starchy counterparts. One nonstarchy vegetable provides 5 grams of carbohydrate, 2 grams of protein, 0 grams of fat, and 25 kcal. Typically, a choice is equal to ½ cup of cooked vegetables or 1 cup of raw vegetables. Large servings of nonstarchy vegetables (i.e., three choices) should be counted as one carbohydrate choice (15 grams of carbohydrate, 70 kcal) rather than multiple nonstarchy vegetables. Because of their low carbohydrate content, salad greens (e.g., iceberg, romaine, and endive) actually count as free foods. To comply with advice from the Dietary Guidelines for Americans, it is important to select a variety of starchy and nonstarchy vegetables each day because each has a distinct micronutrient and phytochemical profile. Take extra care to select vegetables with deep colors, such as spinach, carrots, and beets.

Serving Size	Food
½ cup	Asparagus, cooked
1 cup	Baby carrots, raw
½ cup	Beets, cooked
½ cup	Broccoli, cooked
½ cup	Collard greens, cooked
1 cup	Cucumber, raw slices
½ cup	Green beans, cooked
½ cup	Summer squash, cooked
½ cup	Tomatoes, stewed

Sweets, Desserts, and Other Carbohydrates

Foods on this list may not match the nutrient profiles of other starches, but they are commonly consumed and must be accounted for in diet planning. Sweetened beverages, desserts, and sweeteners and condiments that we add to foods can be counted as a combination of carbohydrate (15 grams of carbohydrates, 70 kcal) and fat (5 grams of fat, 45 kcal) choices.

BEVERAGES, SODA, AND SPORTS DRINKS

Serving Size	Food	Choices
½ cup	Cranberry juice cocktail	1 carbohydrate
1 cup	Fruit drink or lemonade	2 carbohydrates
1 can (12 oz)	Soft drink, regular	2½ carbohydrates
1 cup	Sports drink (e.g., Gatorade®)	1 carbohydrate

BROWNIES, CAKE, COOKIES, GELATIN, PIE, AND PUDDING

Serving Size	Food	Choices
1¼-inch square	Brownie, unfrosted	1 carbohydrate + 1 fat
1/12 cake	Angel food cake, unfrosted	2 carbohydrates
2-inch square	Cake, frosted	2 carbohydrates + 1 fat
2	Chocolate chip cookies	1 carbohydrate + 2 fats
5	Vanilla wafers	1 carbohydrate + 1 fat
½ cup	Gelatin, regular	1 carbohydrate
1/8 pie	Pumpkin pie	1½ carbohydrates + 1½ fats
½ cup	Pudding, regular, made with 2% milk	2 carbohydrates

CANDY, SPREADS, SWEETS, SWEETENERS, SYRUPS, AND TOPPINGS

Serving Size	Food	Choices
5	Chocolate kisses	1 carbohydrate + 1 fat
2 tbsp	Liquid nondairy coffee creamer	1 carbohydrate
1 tbsp	Honey	1 carbohydrate
1 tbsp	Jam or jelly, regular	1 carbohydrate
1 tbsp	Pancake syrup, regular	1 carbohydrate

CONDIMENTS AND SAUCES

Serving Size	Food	Choices
3 tbsp	Barbecue sauce	1 carbohydrate
½ cup	Gravy	½ carbohydrate + ½ fat
3 tbsp	Salad dressing, fat free, cream based	1 carbohydrate

DOUGHNUTS, MUFFINS, PASTRIES, AND SWEET BREADS

Serving Size	Food	Choices
1	Glazed doughnut	2 carbohydrates + 2 fats
1 (4 oz)	Muffin, regular	4 carbohydrates + 2½ fats
1 (2½ oz)	Danish	2½ carbohydrates + 2 fats

FROZEN BARS, FROZEN DESSERTS, FROZEN YOGURT, AND ICE CREAM

Serving Size	Food	Choices
1 (3 oz)	Frozen 100% fruit juice bar	1 carbohydrate
½ cup	Ice cream, no sugar added	1 carbohydrate + 1 fat
½ cup	Ice cream, regular	1 carbohydrate + 2 fats
½ cup	Sherbet	2 carbohydrates
½ cup	Greek frozen yogurt, low fat	1½ carbohydrates

Protein

Similar to the choices on the Milk and Milk Substitutes list, protein choices vary in fat and kilocalorie content. Lean protein choices, such as egg whites and skinless poultry, provide 0 grams of carbohydrate, 7 grams of protein, 2 grams of fat, and 45 kcal. Medium-fat protein choices, such as whole eggs and poultry with skin, provide 0 grams of carbohydrate, 7 grams of protein, 5 grams of fat, and 75 kcal. High-fat protein choices, including many types of sausage and bacon, provide 0 grams of carbohydrate, 7 grams of protein, 8 grams of fat, and 100 kcal. Plant-based protein choices usually contain some carbohydrates, so they count as a combination of carbohydrate or starch and protein choices. Note that choices are very small; a typical hamburger would count as 3 or 4 protein choices.

LEAN PROTEIN (0 grams of carbohydrate, 7 grams of protein, 2 grams of fat, and 45 kcal)

Serving Size	Food
1 oz	Beef with 10% or lower fat (e.g., round and sirloin)
1 oz	Cheese with 3 grams of fat or less (e.g., fat-free mozzarella)
1 oz	Fish, not fried (e.g., catfish, cod, and tuna canned in water)
2	Egg whites
1 oz	Wild game (e.g., buffalo and venison)
1 oz	Lean pork (e.g., ham and tenderloin)
1 oz	Poultry, without skin
1 oz	Deli meats with 3 grams of fat or less per serving (e.g., turkey and ham)
1 oz	Shellfish (e.g., shrimp and crab)

MEDIUM-FAT PROTEIN (0 grams of carbohydrate, 7 grams of protein, 5 grams of fat, and 75 kcal)

Serving Size	Food
1 oz	Beef with 15% or lower fat (e.g., rib roast and ground beef)
1 oz	Cheese with 4 to 7 grams of fat per ounce (e.g., feta and mozzarella)
1	Egg
1 oz	Fish, fried
1 oz	Pork (e.g., cutlet and shoulder roast)
1 oz	Poultry, with skin

HIGH-FAT PROTEIN (0 grams of carbohydrate, 7 grams of protein, 8 grams of fat, and 100 kcal)

Serving Size	Food
2 slices	Bacon, pork
1 oz	Cheese (e.g., American, cheddar, Parmesan, and Swiss)
1	Hot dog
1 oz	Deli meats with 8 grams of fat or more per serving (e.g., bologna and salami)
1 oz	Sausage (e.g., bratwurst and summer sausage)

PLANT-BASED PROTEIN

Serving Size	Food	Choices
⅓ cup	Baked beans	1 starch + 1 lean protein
½ cup	Beans, cooked or canned (e.g., black, kidney, and pinto)	1 starch + 1 lean protein
½ cup	Edamame, shelled	½ carbohydrate + 1 lean protein
⅓ cup	Hummus	1 carbohydrate + 1 medium-fat protein
3 oz	Meatless burger, soy based	½ carbohydrate + 2 lean proteins
½ cup	Tofu	1 medium-fat protein

Fats

One fat choice is 5 grams of fat and 45 kcal. Fats are subdivided into unsaturated fats, which come mainly from plant sources, and saturated fats, which come mainly from animal sources. In line with recommendations from other major health authorities, the *Food Lists for Diabetes* advises people to choose unsaturated fats in place of saturated fats and to avoid *trans* fats.

UNSATURATED FATS – MONOUNSATURATED FATS (5 grams of fat and 45 kcal)

Serving Size	Food
1 cup	Almond milk, unsweetened
2 tbsp	Avocado
1½ tsp	Nut butter (e.g., almond and peanut)
6	Almonds
10	Peanuts
16	Pistachios
1 tsp	Oil (e.g., canola and olive)

UNSATURATED FATS – POLYUNSATURATED FATS (5 grams of fat and 45 kcal)

Serving Size	Food	Serving Size	Food
1 tbsp	Low-fat vegetable oil spread	1 tsp	Oil (e.g., corn, safflower, and sunflower)
1 tsp	Margarine	2 tbsp	Salad dressing, reduced fat (may contain carbohydrate)
1 tbsp	Low-fat mayonnaise	1 tbsp	Salad dressing, regular
1 tsp	Mayonnaise	1 tbsp	Flaxseed, ground

SATURATED FATS (5 grams of fat and 45 kcal)

Serving Size	Food	Serving Size	Food
1 slice	Bacon	1 tsp	Butter, regular
1 tbsp	Butter, reduced fat	2 tbsp	Coconut, shredded

Free Foods

A *free food* is any food or drink that contains less than 20 kcal or less than 5 grams of carbohydrate per serving. When eaten in small amounts throughout the day, these foods have little impact on blood sugar. Foods with a serving size listed should be limited to 3 servings per day. Foods listed without a serving size (indicated with a *) can be eaten as often as you like. However, many free foods are high in sodium, so moderation is important.

LOW-CARBOHYDRATE FOODS

Serving Size	Food	Serving Size	Food
1 piece	Candy, hard or sugar free	*	Sugar substitutes
2 tsp	Jam or jelly, light or no-sugar-added type	½ cup	Raw nonstarchy vegetables (e.g., broccoli, carrots, cucumber, and tomato)
*	Gelatin, sugar free	¼ cup	Cooked nonstarchy vegetables (e.g., carrots, cauliflower, and green beans)
*	Salad greens (no dressing)		

REDUCED-FAT OR FAT-FREE FOODS

Serving Size	Food	Serving Size	Food
1 tbsp	Cream cheese, fat free	1 tbsp	Mayonnaise, fat free
4 tsp	Coffee creamer, liquid, sugar free, flavored	1 tbsp	Salad dressing, fat free
1 tsp	Margarine spread, reduced fat	2 tbsp	Whipped topping, light or fat free

CONDIMENTS

Serving Size	Food	Serving Size	Food
2 tsp	Barbecue sauce	1 tbsp	Parmesan cheese, grated
1 tbsp	Ketchup	1½	Dill pickles (medium)
	Hot pepper sauce	1 tbsp	Soy sauce
	Mustard (e.g., brown, Dijon, or yellow)		

DRINKS/MIXES

Serving Size	Food	Serving Size	Food
*	Bouillon or broth	*	Coffee, unsweetened or artificially sweetened
*	Club soda	*	Water
*	Diet soft drinks, sugar free	*	Water, flavored, sugar free

SEASONINGS

Serving Size	Food
*	Garlic, fresh or powder
*	Herbs, fresh or dried
*	Spices

Combination Foods

These foods contain a mixture of ingredients and cannot be grouped into one food list. Many of these foods are high in sodium.

ENTREES

Serving Size	Food	Choices
1 cup (8 oz)	Casserole-type entrees (e.g., tuna noodle, lasagna, and spaghetti with meatballs)	2 carbohydrates + 2 medium-fat proteins
1 cup (8 oz)	Stews (meat and vegetables)	1 carbohydrate + 1 medium-fat protein + 0 to 3 fats

FROZEN MEALS/ENTREES

Serving Size	Food	Choices
1 (5 oz)	Burrito (beef and bean)	3 carbohydrates + 1 lean protein + 2 fats
9–12 oz	Dinner-type healthy meal (less than 400 kcal)	2 to 3 carbohydrates + 1 to 2 lean proteins + 1 fat
¼ of a 12-inch	Pizza with thin crust and meat toppings	2 carbohydrates + 2 medium-fat proteins + 1½ fats
1 (4½ oz)	Pocket sandwich	3 carbohydrates + 1 lean protein + 1 to 2 fats

SALADS (DELI-STYLE)

Serving Size	Food	Choices
½ cup	Coleslaw	1 carbohydrate + 1½ fats
½ cup	Macaroni salad	2 carbohydrates + 3 fats
½ cup (3½ oz)	Tuna salad or chicken salad	½ carbohydrate + 2 lean proteins + 1 fat

SOUPS

Serving Size	Food	Choices
1 cup (8 oz)	Bean, lentil, or split pea soup	1½ carbohydrates + 1 lean protein
1 cup (8 oz)	Chowder (made with milk)	1 carbohydrate + 1 lean protein + 1½ fats
1 cup (8 oz)	Ramen noodle soup	2 carbohydrates + 2 fats
1 cup (8 oz)	Tomato soup (made with water)	1 carbohydrate
1 cup (8 oz)	Broth-based soups with vegetables and meat	1 carbohydrate + 1 lean protein

Fast Foods

Fast foods are high in sodium and fat. These should be consumed in moderation, if at all. It is much easier to control carbohydrate, fat, sodium, and kilocalorie intake when you prepare your own foods at home rather than relying on restaurants.

MAIN DISHES/ENTREES

Serving Size	Food	Choices
1 (7 oz)	Chicken breast, breaded and fried	1 carbohydrate + 6 medium-fat proteins
6	Chicken nuggets or tenders	1 carbohydrate + 2 medium-fat proteins + 1 fat
1 (2 oz)	Chicken wing, breaded and fried	½ carbohydrate + 2 medium-fat proteins
⅛ of 14-inch	Pizza, thick crust with or without meat toppings	2½ carbohydrates + 1 high-fat protein + 1 fat

ASIAN

Serving Size	Food	Choices
1 cup (6 oz)	Meat with vegetables in sauce	1 carbohydrate + 2 lean proteins + 1 fat
1 (3 oz)	Egg roll with meat filling	1½ carbohydrates + 1 lean protein + 1½ fats
1 cup	Fried rice, meatless	2½ carbohydrates + 2 fats
1 cup	Lo mein or chow mein	2 carbohydrates + 2 fats

MEXICAN

Serving Size	Food	Choices
1 (6 oz)	Burrito with beans and cheese	3½ carbohydrates + 1 medium-fat protein + 1 fat
8	Nachos with cheese	2½ carbohydrates + 1 high-fat protein + 2 fats
1 (3 oz)	Crisp taco with meat and cheese	1 carbohydrate + 1 medium-fat protein + ½ fat
1 lb	Taco salad with chicken and tortilla bowl	3½ carbohydrates + 4 medium-fat proteins + 3 fats

SANDWICHES

Serving Size	Food	Choices
1 (4 oz)	Breakfast burrito with sausage, egg, and cheese	1½ carbohydrates + 2 high-fat proteins
1 (7 oz)	Grilled chicken sandwich	3 carbohydrates + 4 lean proteins
1 (5 oz)	Fried fish fillet sandwich with cheese and tartar sauce	2½ carbohydrates + 2 medium-fat proteins + 1 ½ fats
1 (8 oz)	Cheeseburger (4 oz) with condiments	3 carbohydrates + 4 medium-fat proteins + 2½ fats
1 6-inch	Submarine sandwich (no cheese or sauce)	3 carbohydrates + 2 lean proteins + 1 fat

SIDES/APPETIZERS

Serving Size	Food	Choices
1 medium (5 oz)	French fries	3½ carbohydrates + 3 fats
8 (5 oz)	Onion rings	3½ carbohydrates + 4 fats
1 small	Side salad (no cheese, croutons, or dressing)	1 nonstarchy vegetable

BEVERAGES AND DESSERTS

Serving Size	Food	Choices
12 fl oz	Coffee, latte, with fat-free milk	1 fat-free milk
16 fl oz	Milkshake	7 carbohydrates + 4 fats
1 small	Ice cream cone	2 carbohydrates + ½ fat

Alcohol

For people with diabetes, up to 1 or 2 drinks per day for women and men, respectively, can safely fit into a healthy eating plan. Alcohol itself does not raise blood glucose, but alcoholic drinks often contain carbohydrates that must be counted. One alcohol equivalent provides 100 kcal. One carbohydrate choice provides 15 grams of carbohydrate and 70 kcal. Alcohol should be consumed with a meal to lower the risk of hypoglycemia.

Serving Size	Drink	Choices
12 fl oz	Beer, regular	1 alcohol equivalent + 1 carbohydate
1½ fl oz	Distilled spirits (e.g., rum and vodka)	1 alcohol equivalent
5 fl oz	Champagne	1 alcohol equivalent
3½ fl oz	Dessert wine	1 alcohol equivalent + 1 carbohydrate

Appendix C

Dietary Assessment

Although it may seem overwhelming at first, it is easy to track the foods you eat. One tip is to record all foods and beverages as soon as possible after consumption.

I. **Fill in the food record form that follows.** Appendix C contains a blank copy, Table C-2 (see the completed example in Table C-1). Your instructor may ask you to record one day or several days. To get a good estimate of your usual nutrient intake, it is best to record several days (e.g., two weekdays and one weekend day). As you record your intake for use on the nutrient analysis form that follows, consider the following tips:
- Measure and record the amounts of foods eaten in portion sizes of cups, teaspoons, tablespoons, ounces, slices, or inches (or convert metric units to these units).
- Record brand names of all food products, such as "Quick Quaker Oats®."
- Measure and record all those little extras, such as gravies, salad dressings, taco sauces, pickles, jelly, sugar, ketchup, and margarine.
- For beverages:
  - List the type of milk, such as whole, fat free, 1%, evaporated, chocolate, or reconstituted dry.
  - Indicate whether fruit juice is fresh, frozen, or canned.
  - Indicate type for other beverages, such as fruit drink, fruit-flavored drink, Kool-Aid®, and hot chocolate made with water or milk.
- For fruits:
  - Indicate whether fresh, frozen, dried, or canned.
  - If whole, record number eaten and size with approximate measurements (such as 1 apple—3 inches in diameter).
  - Indicate whether processed in water, light syrup, or heavy syrup.
- For vegetables:
  - Indicate whether fresh, frozen, dried, or canned.
  - Record as portion of cup, teaspoon, or tablespoon, or as pieces (such as carrot sticks—4 inches long, ½ inch thick).
  - Record preparation method.
- For cereals:
  - Record cooked cereals in portions of tablespoon or cup (a level measurement after cooking).
  - Record dry cereal in level portions of tablespoon or cup.
  - If margarine, milk, sugar, fruit, or something else is added, measure and record amount and type.
- For breads:
  - Indicate whether whole wheat, rye, white, and so on.
  - Measure and record number and size of portion (biscuit—2 inches across, 1-inch thick; slice of homemade rye bread—3 inches by 4 inches, ¼-inch thick).
  - Sandwiches: list all ingredients (lettuce, mayonnaise, tomato, and so on).
- For meat, fish, poultry, and cheese:
  - Give size (length, width, and thickness) in inches or weight in ounces after cooking for meat, fish, and poultry (such as cooked hamburger patty—3 inches across, ½-inch thick).
  - Give size (length, width, and thickness) in inches or weight in ounces for cheese.
  - Record measurements only for the cooked, edible part—without bone or fat left on the plate.
  - Describe how meat, poultry, or fish was prepared.

- For eggs:
  - Record as soft or hard cooked, fried, scrambled, poached, or omelet.
  - If milk, butter, or drippings are used, specify types and amount.
- For desserts:
  - List commercial brand or "homemade" or "bakery" under brand.
  - Purchased candies, cookies, and cakes: specify kind and size.
  - Measure and record portion size of cakes, pies, and cookies by specifying thickness, diameter, and width or length, depending on the item.

TABLE C-1 ■ **Example of a One-Day Food Record**

Time	Minutes Spent Eating	M or S*	H† (0–3)	Activity While Eating	Place of Eating	Food and Quantity	Others Present	Reason for Choice
7:10 a.m.	15	M	2	Standing, fixing lunch	Kitchen	Orange juice, 1 cup	—	Health
						Crispix cereal, 1 cup		Habit
						Nonfat milk, ½ cup		Health
						Sugar, 2 tsp		Taste
						Black coffee, 1 cup		Habit
10:00 a.m.	4	S	1	Sitting, taking notes	Classroom	Diet cola, 12 oz	Class	Weight control
12:15 p.m.	40	M	2	Sitting, talking	Student union	Chicken sandwich with lettuce and mayonnaise (3 oz chicken, 2 slices of white bread, and 2 tsp mayonnaise)	Friends	Taste
						Pear, 1 medium		Health
						Nonfat milk, 1 cup		Health
2:30 p.m.	10	S	1	Sitting, studying	Library	Regular cola, 12 oz	Friend	Hunger
6:30 p.m.	35	M	3	Sitting, talking	Kitchen	Pork chop, 1	Boyfriend	Convenience
						Baked potato, 1		Health
						Margarine, 2 tbsp		Taste
						Lettuce and tomato salad, 1 cup		Health
						Ranch dressing, 2 tbsp		Taste
						Peas, ½ cup		Health
						Whole milk, 1 cup		Habit
						Cherry pie, 1 piece		Taste
						Iced tea, 12 oz		Health
9:10 p.m.	10	S	2	Sitting, studying	Living room	Apple, 1 medium	—	Weight control
						Water, 1 cup		Weight control

*M or S: Meal or snack.

†H: Degree of hunger (0 none; 3 maximum).

TABLE C-2 ■ **One-Day Food Record**

Time	Minutes Spent Eating	M or S*	H† (0–3)	Activity While Eating	Place of Eating	Food and Quantity	Others Present	Reason for Choice

*M or S: Meal or snack.

†H: Degree of hunger (0 none; 3 maximum).

II. **Enter all the foods and beverages you consumed into your NutritionCalc Plus software** (see Figure C-1). If you have not already done so, you will need to create a profile in NutritionCalc Plus before you begin. For each food or drink, select the meal or snack and the appropriate serving size. If you have data for more than one day, be sure to enter your foods and beverages on separate days. If the NutritionCalc Plus database does not contain the exact food or drink you consumed, you may need to enter a reasonably close substitute. For example, the chicken sandwich from the student union in the food record example in Table C-1 was entered as a Subway® 6" chicken sandwich on white bread.

FIGURE C-1 ▶ Entering food and beverage intake data using NutritionCalc Plus.

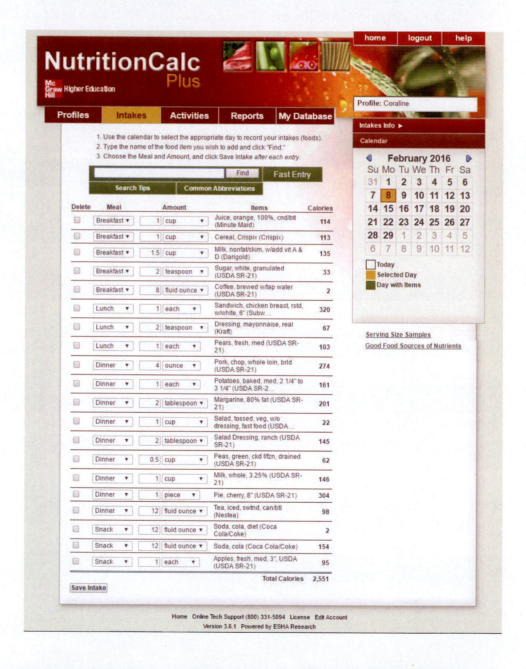

III. **Use NutritionCalc Plus to generate a report of your nutrient intake** (see Figure C-2) After you have finished entering all the foods and beverages you consumed, save your intake data and click on the **Reports** tab. Select **Bar Graph** to see a report of your nutrient intake for a particular day or several days compared to your nutrient needs.

Be sure to select the day(s) and meal(s) you would like to analyze, then click **Update Preview.** You may save your report, print it, or email it as an attachment to yourself or your instructor.

FIGURE C-2 ◀ Sample Bar Graph Report from NutritionCalc Plus.

Bar Graph Report

The Bar Graph Report displays graphically the amount of the nutrient consumed and compares that to the dietary intake recommendations.

Profile Info

Personal: Coraline   Female   20 yrs   5 ft 7 in   140 lb

Student Info: Coraline

Day(s): 2016 Feb 8 (All)

Activity Level: Low Active   (Strive for an Active activity level.)

BMI: 21.9   Normal is 18.5 to 25.

Weight Change: None   Best not to exceed 2 lbs per week.

Nutrient	Value	DRI Goal	Percent
Basic Components			
Calories	2,550.94	2,265.28	113 %
Calories from Fat	795.17	634.28	125 %
Calories from SatFat	210.19	203.88	103 %
Protein (g)	91.45	50.80	180 %
Carbohydrates (g)	359.90	311.48	116 %
Sugar (g)	198.50		
Dietary Fiber (g)	24.57	31.71	77 %
Soluble Fiber (g)	3.07		
InSoluble Fiber (g)	14.98		
Fat (g)	88.35	70.48	125 %
Saturated Fat (g)	23.35	22.65	103 %
Trans Fat (g)	4.49		
Mono Fat (g)	30.26	25.17	120 %
Poly Fat (g)	20.00	22.65	88 %
Cholesterol (mg)	177.85	300.00	59 %
Water (g)	2,107.35	2,700.00	78 %
Vitamins			
Vitamin A - RAE (mcg)	806.51	700.00	115 %
Vitamin B1 - Thiamin (mg)	2.89	1.10	263 %
Vitamin B2 - Riboflavin (mg)	2.62	1.10	238 %
Vitamin B3 - Niacin (mg)	20.21	14.00	144 %
Vitamin B6 (mg)	2.51	1.30	193 %
Vitamin B12 (mcg)	4.11	2.40	171 %
Vitamin C (mg)	179.10	75.00	239 %
Vitamin D - mcg (mcg)	7.22	15.00	48 %
Vitamin E - Alpha	5.93	15.00	40 %
Folate (mcg)	427.29	400.00	107 %
Minerals			
Calcium (mg)	866.26	1,000.00	87 %
Iron (mg)	21.72	18.00	121 %
Magnesium (mg)	188.62	310.00	61 %
Phosphorus (mg)	1,018.75	700.00	146 %
Potassium (mg)	3,282.85	4,700.00	70 %
Sodium (mg)	2,597.88	2,300.00	113 %
Zinc (mg)	8.11	8.00	101 %
Other			
Omega-3 (g)	1.87		
Omega-6 (g)	17.95		
Alcohol (g)	0.00		
Caffeine (mg)	212.72		

IV. **Use NutritionCalc Plus to compare your dietary pattern to the dietary pattern recommended by the Dietary Guidelines for Americans** (see Figure C-3).On the **Reports** tab, choose **MyPlate.** Select the day(s) and meal(s) you would like to analyze, then click **Update Preview.** You may save your report, print it, or email it as an attachment to yourself or your instructor.

FIGURE C-3 ▶ Sample MyPlate Report from NutritionCalc Plus.

V. **Evaluate your dietary pattern.** Answer the following questions about the results of your own dietary assessment and suggest ways that you could improve your dietary pattern.

1. How did your kilocalorie intake compare to the goal recommended by NutritionCalc Plus? If it was much higher or lower than your goal, what specific changes could you make to adjust your energy intake?

2. Do your meals usually resemble MyPlate? If not, what specific changes could you make to improve your meal planning?

3. Use the worksheet below to calculate your fat intake as a percentage of total kilocalories. How does this compare to the Acceptable Macronutrient Distribution Range (AMDR) of 20% to 35% of total kilocalories from fat (review Chapter 5, Section 5.7)? If your fat intake does not fall within the AMDR, what specific changes could you make?

Calculating Percent of Kilocalories from Fat:

_____ grams of fat × 9 kcal per gram = _____ kcal from fat

_____ kcal from fat / _____ total kcal = _____ % of kcal from fat

4. Use the worksheet below to calculate your saturated fat intake as a percentage of total kilocalories. How does this compare to the Dietary Guidelines' recommendation to limit saturated fat to 10% of total kilocalories? If your intake of saturated fat was higher than 10% of total kcal, what specific dietary changes could you make to lower your intake of saturated fat?

Calculating Percent of Kilocalories from Saturated Fat:

_____ grams of saturated fat × 9 kcal per gram = _____ kcal from saturated fat

_____ kcal from saturated fat / _____ total kcal = _____ % of kcal from saturated fat

5. The Dietary Guidelines advise Americans to limit their consumption of added sugars. What were some sources of added sugars in your diet on the days you recorded? List several nutrient-dense food choices you could use to replace sources of added sugars in your dietary pattern.

6. What was your average fiber intake for the 3 days? How close did you come to meeting the AI for fiber? If your intake of fiber was lower than the AI, what specific dietary changes could you make to improve your intake of fiber?

7. How did your average intake of sodium compare to your AI and UL for sodium? If your sodium intake was higher than the UL, what specific dietary changes could you make to lower your intake of sodium?

8. Are your intakes of any vitamins or minerals less than 75% of the RDA or AI? Choose one of these nutrients and discuss how you could change your _dietary_ habits to increase your intake of this nutrient.

9. Besides sodium, do your intakes of any vitamins or minerals exceed the UL? (Also consider any micronutrients consumed in supplement form.) If so, what negative consequences could this have for your health?

10. If you consume alcohol, are your drinking habits consistent with the Dietary Guidelines' recommendations to limit alcohol to 1 drink per day (women) or 2 drinks per day (men)? List one potential benefit of moderate alcohol consumption. List one negative consequence of excessive alcohol consumption.

Appendix D

Chemical Structures Important In Nutrition

Amino Acids

Histidine (His)
(essential)

Tryptophan (Trp)
(essential)

Glycine (Gly)

Methionine (Met)
(essential)

Leucine (Leu)
(essential)

Alanine (Ala)

Arginine (Arg)
(essential in infancy)

Lysine (Lys)
(essential)

Proline (Pro)

Glutamic Acid (Glu)

Aspartic Acid (Asp)

Serine (Ser)

Phenylalanine (Phe)
(essential)

Isoleucine (Ile)
(essential)

Tyrosine (Tyr)

Glutamine (Gln)

Asparagine (Asn)

Threonine (Thr)
(essential)

Valine (Val)
(essential)

Cysteine (Cys)

Vitamins

Vitamin A: retinol

Beta-carotene

Vitamin E

Vitamin K

7-Dehydrocholesterol

1,25-Dihydroxy-vitamin D₃ (calcitriol)

Carbon #25

Carbon #1

Active vitamin D (calcitriol) and its precursor 7-dehydrocholesterol

Thiamin

Niacin (nicotinic acid and nicotinamide)

Nicotinic acid

Nicotinamide

Riboflavin

Pyridoxine

Pyridoxal

Pyridoxamine

Vitamin B-6 (a general name for three compounds—pyridoxine, pyridoxal, and pyridoxamine

Biotin

Pantothenic acid

Folate (folic acid form)

Vitamin C (ascorbic acid)

Vitamin B-12 (cyanocobalamin) The arrows in this diagram indicate that the spare electrons on the nitrogens are attracted to the cobalt atom.

$$CH_3 - \overset{\overset{\displaystyle O}{\|}}{C} - CH_3$$

Acetone

CO_2

$$CH_3 - \overset{\overset{\displaystyle O}{\|}}{C} - CH_2 - \overset{\overset{\displaystyle O}{\|}}{C} - OH$$

Acetoacetic acid

$2H^+$

$$CH_3 - \overset{\overset{\displaystyle OH}{|}}{CH} - CH_2 - \overset{\overset{\displaystyle O}{\|}}{C} - OH$$

ß-Hydroxybutyric acid

Ketone bodies

Point of cleavage to yield
ADP and energy release

Triphosphate

Ribose
(a sugar)

Adenine

**Adenosine triphosphate
(ATP)**

Appendix E

Sources of Nutrition Information

Consider the following reliable sources of food and nutrition information:

Journals That Regularly Cover Nutrition Topics

American Family Physician*
American Journal of Clinical Nutrition
American Journal of Epidemiology
American Journal of Medicine
American Journal of Obstetrics and
*   Gynecology*
American Journal of Public Health
American Scientist
Annals of Internal Medicine
Annual Review of Medicine
Annual Review of Nutrition
Appetite
Archives of Disease in Childhood
British Journal of Nutrition
BMJ (British Medical Journal)
Canadian Journal of Dietetic Practice
*   and Research*
Cancer Research
Clinical Nutrition
Critical Reviews in Food Science
*   and Nutrition*
Current Opinion in Clinical Nutrition
*   and Metabolic Care*
Current Opinion in Endocrinology,
*   Diabetes and Obesity*

Diabetes
Diabetes Care
Food and Chemical Toxicology
Gastroenterology
International Journal of Behavioral
*   Nutrition and Physical Activity*
International Journal of Obesity
Journal of the American College
*   of Nutrition**
Journal of the Academy of Nutrition and
*   Dietetics**
Journal of the American Geriatrics Society
JAMA (Journal of the American
*   Medical Association)*
Journal of Clinical Investigation
Journal of Food Science
Journal of Functional Foods
Journal of Human Nutrition and Dietetics
JNCI (Journal of the National
*   Cancer Institute)*
Journal of Nutrition
Journal of Nutrition Education and
*   Behavior**
Journal of Nutrition in Gerontology
*   and Geriatrics*

Journal of Pediatrics
The Lancet
Maternal and Child Health
Medicine & Science in Sports & Exercise
Nature
The New England Journal of Medicine
Nutrition
Nutrition & Dietetics
*   Nutrition in Clinical Practice**
Nutrition Journal
Nutrition, Metabolism and Cardiovascular
*   Diseases*
Nutrition Research Reviews
Nutrition Reviews
Nutrition Today*
Obesity
Pediatric Obesity
Pediatrics
Proceedings of the Nutrition Society
Public Health Nutrition
Science
Science News*
Scientific American
Today's Dietitian*

The majority of these journals are available in college and university libraries or in a specialty library on campus, such as one designated for health sciences. Most of them are now available online. As indicated, a few journals will be filed under their abbreviations, rather than the first word in their full name. A reference librarian can help you locate any of these sources. The journals with an asterisk (*) are ones you may find especially interesting and useful because of the number of nutrition articles presented each month or the less technical nature of the presentation.

Magazines for the Consumer That Cover Nutrition Topics

Better Homes and Gardens
Good Housekeeping

Health
Men's Health

Parents
Self

Textbooks and Other Sources for Advanced Study of Nutrition Topics

Erdman JW, MacDonald IA, Zeisel SH: *Present knowledge in nutrition.* 10th ed. Washington, DC: International Life Sciences and Wiley-Blackwell, 2012.

Gropper SS, Smith JL: *Advanced nutrition and human metabolism.* 6th ed. Belmont, CA: Wadsworth, Cengage, 2012.

Mahan LK, Escott-Stump S, Raymond JL: *Krause's food and the nutrition care process,* 13th ed. St. Louis: Elsevier Saunders, 2011.

Rodwell VW and others: *Harper's illustrated biochemistry.* 30th ed. New York: McGraw-Hill Education, 2015.

Ross AC and others: *Modern nutrition in health and disease.* 11th ed. Philadelphia: Lippincott, Williams & Wilkins, 2012.

Stipanuk MH, Caudill MA: *Biochemical, physiological, and molecular aspects of human nutrition.* 3rd ed. St. Louis: Philadelphia: Elsevier Saunders, 2012.

Newsletters That Cover Nutrition Issues on a Regular Basis

Berkeley Wellness
University of California at Berkeley
www.berkeleywellness.com

Consumer Health Digest
www.consumerhealthdigest.com

Environmental Nutrition
www.environmentalnutrition.com

Harvard Health Letter (and others)
Harvard Medical School
www.health.harvard.edu/newsletters

Health & Nutrition Letter
Tufts University
www.nutritionletter.tufts.edu

Mayo Clinic Health Letter
Mayo Clinic
healthletter.mayoclinic.com

Nutrition Action Healthletter
Center for Science in the Public Interest
www.cspinet.org

ENC Blog
Egg Nutrition Center
www.eggnutritioncenter.org/blog

Soy Connection
United Soybean Board
www.soyconnection.com

Women's Nutrition Connection Newsletter
Weill Cornell Medical College
www.womensnutritionconnection.com

Professional Organizations

Academy of Nutrition and Dietetics
www.eatright.org

American Academy of Pediatrics
www.aap.org

American Cancer Society
www.cancer.org

American College of Sports Medicine
www.acsm.org

American Dental Association
www.ada.org

American Diabetes Association
www.diabetes.org

American Geriatrics Society
www.americangeriatrics.org

American Heart Association
www.heart.org

American Institute for Cancer Research
www.aicr.org

American Medical Association
www.ama-assn.org

American Public Health Association
www.apha.org

American Society for Nutrition
www.nutrition.org

Canadian Diabetes Association
www.diabetes.ca

Canadian Nutrition Society
www.cns-scn.ca

Dietitians of Canada
www.dietitians.ca

Environmental Working Group
www.ewg.org

Food and Nutrition Board of the Institute of Medicine
https://iom.nationalacademies.org/
    About-IOM/Leadership-Staff/IOM-
    Staff-Leadership-Boards/Food-and-
    Nutrition-Board.aspx

Institute of Food Technologists
www.ift.org

National Council on Aging
www.ncoa.org

National Osteoporosis Foundation
www.nof.org

Society for Nutrition Education and Behavior
www.sneb.org

Professional Organizations with a Commitment to Nutrition Issues

Bread for the World Institute
www.bread.org

Food Research & Action Center
frac.org

Institute for Food and Development Policy
foodfirst.org

La Leche League International
www.llli.org

March of Dimes
www.marchofdimes.org

National Council Against Health Fraud
www.ncahf.org

National WIC Association
www.nwica.org

Overeaters Anonymous
www.oa.org

Oxfam America
www.oxfamamerica.org

Local Resources for Advice on Nutrition Issues

Registered Dietitian Nutritionists
    (RDNs) in health care, city, county,
    or state agencies, as well as in private
    practice
Cooperative extension agents in county
    extension offices
Nutrition faculty affiliated with depart-
    ments of food and nutrition, and
    dietetics

Government Agencies Concerned with Nutrition Issues or That Distribute Nutrition Information

United States

Agricultural Research Service
United States Department of Agriculture
www.ars.usda.gov

Food and Drug Administration
www.fda.gov

Food Safety and Inspection Service
United States Department of Agriculture
www.fsis.usda.gov

MyPlate
www.choosemyplate.gov

National Agricultural Library
www.nal.usda.gov

National Cancer Institute
www.cancer.gov

National Center for Health Statistics
www.cdc.gov/nchs

National Heart, Lung, and Blood Institute
www.nhlbi.nih.gov

National Institute on Aging
www.nia.nih.gov

Federal Citizen Information Center
publications.usa.gov

U.S. Government Publishing Office
www.gpo.gov

Canada

Canadian Food Inspection Agency
www.inspection.gc.ca

Health Canada
www.hc-sc.gc.ca

United Nations

Food and Agriculture Organization
www.fao.org

World Health Organization
www.who.int

Trade Organizations and Companies That Distribute Nutrition Information

Abbott Nutrition
abbottnutrition.com

American Institute of Baking
www.aibonline.org

American Meat Institute
www.meatinstitute.org

Beech-Nut Nutrition
www.beechnut.com

Campbell Soup Company
www.campbells.com/campbell-soup

Dannon Company
www.dannon.com

Del Monte Foods
www.delmonte.com

DSM Nutritional Products
www.dsm.com

General Mills/Pillsbury
www.generalmills.com

Gerber
www.gerber.com

H.J. Heinz
www.heinzbaby.com

Idaho Potato Commission
idahopotato.com

Kellogg Company
www.kelloggs.com

Kraft Foods Group, Inc.
www.kraftrecipes.com

Mead Johnson Nutrition
www.meadjohnson.com

National Dairy Council
www.nationaldairycouncil.org

Sunkist Growers
www.sunkist.com

Appendix F

English-Metric Conversions And Metric Units

Metric-English Conversions

LENGTH

English (USA)	Metric
inch (in)	= 2.54 cm, 25.4 mm
foot (ft)	= 0.30 m, 30.48 cm
yard (yd)	= 0.91 m, 91.4 cm
mile (statute) (5280 ft)	= 1.61 km, 1609 m
mile (nautical) (6077 ft, 1.15 statute mi)	= 1.85 km, 1850 m

Metric	English (USA)
millimeter (mm)	= 0.039 in (thickness of a dime)
centimeter (cm)	= 0.39 in
meter (m)	= 3.28 ft, 39.37 in
kilometer (km)	= 0.62 mi, 1091 yd, 3273 ft

WEIGHT

English (USA)	Metric
grain	= 64.80 mg
ounce (oz)	= 28.35 g
pound (lb)	= 453.60 g, 0.45 kg
ton (short—2000 lb)	= 0.91 metric ton (907 kg)

Metric	English (USA)
milligram (mg)	= 0.002 grain (0.000035 oz)
gram (g)	= 0.04 oz (1/28 of an oz)
kilogram (kg)	= 35.27 oz, 2.20 lb
metric ton (1000 kg)	= 1.10 tons

VOLUME

English (USA)	Metric
cubic inch	= 16.39 cc
cubic foot	= 0.03 m^3
cubic yard	= 0.765 m^3
teaspoon (tsp)	= 5 ml
tablespoon (tbsp)	= 15 ml
fluid ounce	= 0.03 liter (30 ml)*
cup (c)	= 237 ml
pint (pt)	= 0.47 liter
quart (qt)	= 0.95 liter
gallon (gal)	= 3.79 liters

Metric	English (USA)
milliliter (ml)	= 0.03 oz
liter (L)	= 2.12 pt
liter	= 1.06 qt
liter	= 0.27 gal

1 liter ÷ 1000 = 1 milliliter or 1 cubic centimeter (10^{-3} liter)
1 liter ÷ 1,000,000 = 1 microliter (10^{-6} liter)

*Note: 1 ml = 1 cc.

Metric and Other Common Units

Unit/Abbreviation	Other Equivalent Measure
milligram/mg	1/1000 of a gram
microgram/μg	1/1,000,000 of a gram
deciliter/dl	1/10 of a liter (about ½ cup)
milliliter/ml	1/1000 of a liter (5 ml is about 1 tsp)
International Unit/IU	Crude measure of vitamin activity generally based on growth rate seen in animals

Fahrenheit-Celsius Conversion Scale

To convert temperature scales:
Fahrenheit to Celsius °C = (°F 2 32) × 5/9
Celsius to Fahrenheit °F = 9/5 (°C) + 32

Household Units

3 teaspoons	= 1 tablespoon	= 15 grams
4 tablespoons	= ¼ cup	= 60 grams
5 ⅓ tablespoons	= ⅓ cup	= 80 grams
8 tablespoons	= ½ cup	= 120 grams
10 ⅔ tablespoons	= ⅔ cup	= 160 grams
16 tablespoons	= 1 cup	= 240 grams
1 tablespoon	= ½ fluid ounce	= 15 milliliters
1 cup	= 8 fluid ounces	= 15 milliliters
1 cup	= ½ pint	= 240 grams
2 cups	= 1 pint	= 480 grams
4 cups	= 1 quart	= 960 grams = 1 liter
2 pints	= 1 quart	= 960 grams = 1 liter
4 quarts	= 1 gallon	= 3840 grams = 4 liters

DIETARY REFERENCE INTAKES (DRIs): RECOMMENDED INTAKES FOR INDIVIDUALS, VITAMINS

Food and Nutrition Board, Institute of Medicine, National Academies

Life Stage Group	Vitamin A (µg/d)[a]	Vitamin C (mg/d)	Vitamin D (µg/d)[b,c]	Vitamin E (mg/d)[d]	Vitamin K (µg/d)	Thiamin (mg/d)	Riboflavin (mg/d)	Niacin (mg/d)[e]	Vitamin B-6 (mg/d)	Folate (µg/d)[f]	Vitamin B-12 (µg/d)	Pantothenic Acid (mg/d)	Biotin (µg/d)	Choline (mg/d)[g]
Infants														
0–6 mo	400*	40*	10	4*	2.0*	0.2*	0.3*	2*	0.1*	65*	0.4*	1.7*	5*	125*
7–12 mo	500*	50*	10	5*	2.5*	0.3*	0.4*	4*	0.3*	80*	0.5*	1.8*	6*	150*
Children														
1–3 y	300	15	15	6	30*	0.5	0.5	6	0.5	150	0.9	2*	8*	200*
4–8 y	400	25	15	7	55*	0.6	0.6	8	0.6	200	1.2	3*	12*	250*
Males														
9–13 y	600	45	15	11	60*	0.9	0.9	12	1.0	300	1.8	4*	20*	375*
14–18 y	900	75	15	15	75*	1.2	1.3	16	1.3	400	2.4	5*	25*	550*
19–30 y	900	90	15	15	120*	1.2	1.3	16	1.3	400	2.4	5*	30*	550*
31–50 y	900	90	15	15	120*	1.2	1.3	16	1.3	400	2.4	5*	30*	550*
51–70 y	900	90	15	15	120*	1.2	1.3	16	1.7	400	2.4[h]	5*	30*	550*
>70 y	900	90	20	15	120*	1.2	1.3	16	1.7	400	2.4[h]	5*	30*	550*
Females														
9–13 y	600	45	15	11	60*	0.9	0.9	12	1.0	300	1.8	4*	20*	375*
14–18 y	700	65	15	15	75*	1.0	1.0	14	1.2	400[i]	2.4	5*	25*	400*
19–30 y	700	75	15	15	90*	1.1	1.1	14	1.3	400[i]	2.4	5*	30*	425*
31–50 y	700	75	15	15	90*	1.1	1.1	14	1.3	400[i]	2.4	5*	30*	425*
51–70 y	700	75	15	15	90*	1.1	1.1	14	1.5	400	2.4[h]	5*	30*	425*
>70 y	700	75	20	15	90*	1.1	1.1	14	1.5	400	2.4[h]	5*	30*	425*
Pregnancy														
≤18 y	750	80	15	15	75*	1.4	1.4	18	1.9	600[j]	2.6	6*	30*	450*
19–30 y	770	85	15	15	90*	1.4	1.4	18	1.9	600[j]	2.6	6*	30*	450*
31–50 y	770	85	15	15	90*	1.4	1.4	18	1.9	600[j]	2.6	6*	30*	450*
Lactation														
≤18 y	1200	115	15	19	75*	1.4	1.6	17	2.0	500	2.8	7*	35*	550*
19–30 y	1300	120	15	19	90*	1.4	1.6	17	2.0	500	2.8	7*	35*	550*
31–50 y	1300	120	15	19	90*	1.4	1.6	17	2.0	500	2.8	7*	35*	550*

mg = milligram, mg = microgram

NOTE: This table (taken from the DRI reports; see www.nap.edu) presents Recommended Dietary Allowances (RDAs) in **bold type** and Adequate Intakes (AIs) in ordinary type followed by an asterisk (*). RDAs and AIs may both be used as goals for individual intake. RDAs are set to meet the needs of almost all (97 to 98%) individuals in a group. For healthy breastfed infants, the AI is the mean intake. The AI for other life stage and gender groups is believed to cover needs of all individuals in the group, but lack of data or uncertainty in the data prevents being able to specify with confidence the percentage of individuals covered by this intake.

[a] As retinol activity equivalents (RAEs). 1 RAE = 1 µg retinol, 12 µg β-carotene, 24 µg α-carotene, or 24 µg β-cryptoxanthin. To calculate RAEs from REs of provitamin A carotenoids in foods, divide the REs by 2. For preformed vitamin A in foods or supplements and for provitamin A carotenoids in supplements, 1 RE = 1 RAE.

[b] cholecalciferol. 1 µg cholecalciferol = 40 IU vitamin D.

[c] In the absence of adequate exposure to sunlight.

[d] As α-tocopherol. α-Tocopherol includes RRR-α-tocopherol, the only form of α-tocopherol that occurs naturally in foods, and the 2R-stereoisomeric forms of α-tocopherol (RRR-, RSR-, RRS-, and RSS-α-tocopherol) that occur in fortified foods and supplements. It does not include the 2S-stereoisomeric forms of α-tocopherol (SRR-, SSR-, SRS-, and SSS-α-tocopherol), also found in fortified foods and supplements.

[e] As niacin equivalents (NE). 1 mg of niacin = 60 mg of tryptophan; 0–6 months = preformed niacin (not NE).

[f] As dietary folate equivalents (DFE). 1 DFE = 1 µg food folate = 0.6 µg of folic acid from fortified food or as a supplement consumed with food = 0.5 µg of a supplement taken on an empty stomach.

[g] Although AIs have been set for choline, there are few data to assess whether a dietary supply of choline is needed at all stages of the life cycle, and it may be that the choline requirement can be met by endogenous synthesis at some of these stages.

[h] Because 10 to 30% of older people may malabsorb food-bound B-12, it is advisable for those older than 50 years to meet their RDA mainly by consuming foods fortified with B-12 or a supplement containing B-12.

[i] In view of evidence linking folate intake with neural tube defects in the fetus, it is recommended that all women capable of becoming pregnant consume 400 µg from supplements or fortified foods in addition to intake of food folate from a varied diet.

[j] It is assumed that women will continue consuming 400 µg from supplements or fortified food until their pregnancy is confirmed and they enter prenatal care, which ordinarily occurs after the end of the periconceptional period—the critical time for formation of the neural tube.

Adapted from the Dietary Reference Intakes series, National Academies Press. Copyright 1997, 1998, 2000, 2001, 2011, by the National Academy of Sciences. The full reports are available from the National Academies Press at www.nap.edu.

DIETARY REFERENCE INTAKES (DRIs): RECOMMENDED INTAKES FOR INDIVIDUALS, ELEMENTS
Food and Nutrition Board, Institute of Medicine, National Academies

Life Stage Group	Calcium (mg/d)	Chromium (µg/d)	Copper (µg/d)	Fluoride (mg/d)	Iodine (µg/d)	Iron (mg/d)	Magnesium (mg/d)	Manganese (mg/d)	Molybdenum (µg/d)	Phosphorus (mg/d)	Selenium (µg/d)	Zinc (mg/d)
Infants												
0–6 mo	200*	0.2*	200*	0.01*	110*	0.27*	30*	0.003*	2*	100*	15*	2*
7–12 mo	260*	5.5*	220*	0.5*	130*	11	75*	0.6*	3*	275*	20*	3
Children												
1–3 y	700	11*	340	0.7*	90	7	80	1.2*	17	460	20	3
4–8 y	1000	15*	440	1*	90	10	130	1.5*	22	500	30	5
Males												
9–13 y	1300	25*	700	2*	120	8	240	1.9*	34	1250	40	8
14–18 y	1300	35*	890	3*	150	11	410	2.2*	43	1250	55	11
19–30 y	1000	35*	900	4*	150	8	400	2.3*	45	700	55	11
31–50 y	1000	35*	900	4*	150	8	420	2.3*	45	700	55	11
51–70 y	1000	30*	900	4*	150	8	420	2.3*	45	700	55	11
>70 y	1200	30*	900	4*	150	8	420	2.3*	45	700	55	11
Females												
9–13 y	1300	21*	700	2*	120	8	240	1.6*	34	1250	40	8
14–18 y	1300	24*	890	3*	150	15	360	1.6*	43	1250	55	9
19–30 y	1000	25*	900	3*	150	18	310	1.8*	45	700	55	8
31–50 y	1000	25*	900	3*	150	18	320	1.8*	45	700	55	8
51–70 y	1200	20*	900	3*	150	8	320	1.8*	45	700	55	8
>70 y	1200	20*	900	3*	150	8	320	1.8*	45	700	55	8
Pregnancy												
≤18 y	1300	29*	1000	3*	220	27	400	2.0*	50	1250	60	12
19–30 y	1000	30*	1000	3*	220	27	350	2.0*	50	700	60	11
31–50 y	1000	30*	1000	3*	220	27	360	2.0*	50	700	60	11
Lactation												
≤18 y	1300	44*	1300	3*	290	10	360	2.6*	50	1250	70	13
19–30 y	1000	45*	1300	3*	290	9	310	2.6*	50	700	70	12
31–50 y	1000	45*	1300	3*	290	9	320	2.6*	50	700	70	12

NOTE: This table presents Recommended Dietary Allowances (RDAs) in **bold type** and Adequate Intakes (AIs) in ordinary type followed by an asterisk (*). RDAs and AIs may both be used as goals for individual intake. RDAs are set to meet the needs of almost all (97 to 98%) individuals in a group. For healthy breastfed infants, the AI is the mean intake. The AI for other life stage and gender groups is believed to cover needs of all individuals in the group, but lack of data or uncertainty in the data prevents being able to specify with confidence the percentage of individuals covered by this intake.

Sources: Dietary Reference Intakes for Calcium, Phosphorus, Magnesium, Vitamin D, and Fluoride (1997); Dietary Reference Intakes for Thiamin, Riboflavin, Niacin, Vitamin B-6, Folate, Vitamin B-12, Pantothenic Acid, Biotin, and Choline (1998); Dietary Reference Intakes for Vitamin C, Vitamin E, Selenium, and Carotenoids (2000); Dietary Reference Intakes for Vitamin A, Vitamin K, Arsenic, Boron, Chromium, Copper, Iodine, Iron, Manganese, Molybdenum, Nickel, Silicon, Vanadium, and Zinc (2001); and Dietary Reference Intakes for Calcium and Vitamin D (2011). These reports may be accessed via www.nap.edu.

Adapted from the Dietary Reference Intake series, National Academies Press. Copyright 1997, 1998, 2000, 2001, and 2011 by the National Academy of Sciences. The full reports are available from the National Academies Press at www.nap.edu.

DIETARY REFERENCE INTAKES (DRIs): RECOMMENDED INTAKES FOR INDIVIDUALS, MACRONUTRIENTS
Food and Nutrition Board, Institute of Medicine, National Academies

Life Stage Group	Carbohydrate (g/d)	Total Fiber (g/d)	Fat (g/d)	Linoleic Acid (g/d)	α-Linolenic Acid (g/d)	Protein[a] (g/d)
Infants						
0–6 mo	60*	ND	31*	4.4*	0.5*	9.1*
7–12 mo	95*	ND	30*	4.6*	0.5*	**11.0**
Children						
1–3 y	**130**	19*	ND[b]	7*	0.7*	**13**
4–8 y	**130**	25*	ND	10*	0.9*	**19**
Males						
9–13 y	**130**	31*	ND	12*	1.2*	**34**
14–18 y	**130**	38*	ND	16*	1.6*	**52**
19–30 y	**130**	38*	ND	17*	1.6*	**56**
31–50 y	**130**	38*	ND	17*	1.6*	**56**
51–70 y	**130**	30*	ND	14*	1.6*	**56**
>70 y	**130**	30*	ND	14*	1.6*	**56**
Females						
9–13 y	**130**	26*	ND	10*	1.0*	**34**
14–18 y	**130**	26*	ND	11*	1.1*	**46**
19–30 y	**130**	25*	ND	12*	1.1*	**46**
31–50 y	**130**	25*	ND	12*	1.1*	**46**
51–70 y	**130**	21*	ND	11*	1.1*	**46**
>70 y	**130**	21*	ND	11*	1.1*	**46**
Pregnancy						
14–18 y	**175**	28*	ND	13*	1.4*	**71**
19–30 y	**175**	28*	ND	13*	1.4*	**71**
31–50 y	**175**	28*	ND	13*	1.4*	**71**
Lactation						
14–18 y	**210**	29*	ND	13*	1.3*	**71**
19–30 y	**210**	29*	ND	13*	1.3*	**71**
31–50 y	**210**	29*	ND	13*	1.3*	**71**

NOTE: This table presents Recommended Dietary Allowances (RDAs) in **bold type** and Adequate Intakes (AIs) in ordinary type followed by an asterisk (*). RDAs and AIs may both be used as goals for individual intake. RDAs are set to meet the needs of almost all (97 to 98%) individuals in a group. For healthy breastfed infants, the AI is the mean intake. The AI for other life stage and gender groups is believed to cover needs of all individuals in the group, but lack of data or uncertainty in the data prevents being able to specify with confidence the percentage of individuals covered by this intake.

[a]Based on 0.8g protein/kg body weight for reference body weight.

[b]ND = not determinable at this time.

Sources: Dietary Reference Intakes for Energy, Carbohydrate, Fiber, Fat, Fatty Acids, Cholesterol, Protein, and Amino Acids (2002). This report may be accessed via www.nap.edu.

Adapted from the Dietary Reference Intake series, National Academies Press. Copyright 1997, 1998, 2000, 2001, by the National Academy of Sciences. The full reports are available from the National Academies Press at www.nap.edu.

D

DIETARY REFERENCE INTAKES (DRIs): RECOMMENDED INTAKES FOR INDIVIDUALS, ELECTROLYTES AND WATER
Food and Nutrition Board, Institute of Medicine, National Academies

Life Stage Group	Sodium (mg/d)	Potassium (mg/d)	Chloride (mg/d)	Water (L/d)
Infants				
0–6 mo	120*	400*	180*	0.7*
7–12 mo	370*	700*	570*	0.8*
Children				
1–3 y	1000*	3000*	1500*	1.3*
4–8 y	1200*	3800*	1900*	1.7*
Males				
9–13 y	1500*	4500*	2300*	2.4*
14–18 y	1500*	4700*	2300*	3.3*
19–30 y	1500*	4700*	2300*	3.7*
31–50 y	1500*	4700*	2300*	3.7*
51–70 y	1300*	4700*	2000*	3.7*
>70 y	1200*	4700*	1800*	3.7*
Females				
9–13 y	1500*	4500*	2300*	2.1*
14–18 y	1500*	4700*	2300*	2.3*
19–30 y	1500*	4700*	2300*	2.7*
31–50 y	1500*	4700*	2300*	2.7*
51–70 y	1300*	4700*	2000*	2.7*
>70 y	1200*	4700*	1800*	2.7*
Pregnancy				
14–18 y	1500*	4700*	2300*	3.0*
19–50 y	1500*	4700*	2300*	3.0*
Lactation				
14–18 y	1500*	5100*	2300*	3.8*
19–50 y	1500*	5100*	2300*	3.8*

NOTE: The table is adapted from the DRI reports. See www.nap.edu. Adequate Intakes (AIs) are followed by an asterisk (*). These may be used as a goal for individual intake. For healthy breastfed infants, the AI is the average intake. The AI for other life stage and gender groups is believed to cover the needs of all individuals in the group, but lack of data prevent being able to specify with confidence the percentage of individuals covered by this intake; therefore, no Recommended Dietary Allowance (RDA) was set.

Source: Dietary Reference Intakes for Water, Potassium, Sodium, Chloride, and Sulfate (2005). This report may be accessed via www.nap.edu.

ACCEPTABLE MACRONUTRIENT DISTRIBUTION RANGES

Macronutrient	Range (percent of energy)		
	Children, 1–3 y	Children, 4–18 y	Adults
Fat	30–40	25–35	20–35
omega-6 polyunsaturated fats (linoleic acid)	5–10	5–10	5–10
omega-3 polyunsaturated fats[a] (α-linolenic acid)	0.6–1.2	0.6–1.2	0.6–1.2
Carbohydrate	45–65	45–65	45–65
Protein	5–20	10–30	10–35

[a]Approximately 10% of the total can come from longer-chain n-3 fatty acids.

SOURCE: Dietary Reference Intakes for Energy, Carbohydrate, Fiber, Fat, Fatty Acids, Cholesterol, Protein, and Amino Acids (2002). The report may be accessed via www.nap.edu.

Adapted from the Dietary Reference Intakes series, National Academies Press. Copyright 1997, 1998, 2000, 2001, 2011, by the National Academy of Sciences. The full reports are available from the National Academies Press at www.nap.edu.

DIETARY REFERENCE INTAKES (DRIs): TOLERABLE UPPER INTAKE LEVELS (UL[a]), VITAMINS
Food and Nutrition Board, Institute of Medicine, National Academies

Life Stage Group	Vitamin A (µg/d)[b]	Vitamin C (mg/d)	Vitamin D (µg/d)	Vitamin E (mg/d)[c,d]	Vitamin K	Thiamin	Riboflavin	Niacin (mg/d)[d]	Vitamin B-6 (mg/d)	Folate (µg/d)[d]	Vitamin B-12	Pantothenic Acid	Biotin	Choline (g/d)	Carotenoids[e]
Infants															
0–6 mo	600	ND[f]	25	ND	ND	ND	ND	ND	ND	ND	ND	ND	ND	ND	ND
7–12 mo	600	ND	38	ND	ND	ND	ND	ND	ND	ND	ND	ND	ND	ND	ND
Children															
1–3 y	600	400	63	200	ND	ND	ND	10	30	300	ND	ND	ND	1.0	ND
4–8 y	900	650	75	300	ND	ND	ND	15	40	400	ND	ND	ND	1.0	ND
Males, Females															
9–13 y	1700	1200	100	600	ND	ND	ND	20	60	600	ND	ND	ND	2.0	ND
14–18 y	2800	1800	100	800	ND	ND	ND	30	80	800	ND	ND	ND	3.0	ND
19–70 y	3000	2000	100	1000	ND	ND	ND	35	100	1000	ND	ND	ND	3.5	ND
>70 y	3000	2000	100	1000	ND	ND	ND	35	100	1000	ND	ND	ND	3.5	ND
Pregnancy															
≤18 y	2800	1800	100	800	ND	ND	ND	30	80	800	ND	ND	ND	3.0	ND
19–50 y	3000	2000	100	1000	ND	ND	ND	35	100	1000	ND	ND	ND	3.5	ND
Lactation															
≤18 y	2800	1800	100	800	ND	ND	ND	30	80	800	ND	ND	ND	3.0	ND
19–50 y	3000	2000	100	1000	ND	ND	ND	35	100	1000	ND	ND	ND	3.5	ND

[a]UL = The maximum level of daily nutrient intake likely to pose no risk of adverse effects. Unless otherwise specified, the UL represents total intake from food, water, and supplements. Due to lack of suitable data, ULs could not be established for vitamin K, thiamin, riboflavin, vitamin B-12, pantothenic acid, biotin, or carotenoids. In the absence of ULs, extra caution may be warranted in consuming levels above recommended intakes.

[b]As preformed vitamin A only.

[c]As α-tocopherol; applies to any form of supplemental α-tocopherol.

[d]The ULs for vitamin E, niacin, and folate apply to synthetic forms obtained from supplements, fortified foods, or a combination of the two.

[e]β-Carotene supplements are advised only to serve as a provitamin A source for individuals at risk of vitamin A deficiency.

[f]ND = Not determinable due to lack of data of adverse effects in this age group and concern with regard to lack of ability to handle excess amounts. Source of intake should be from food only to prevent high levels of intake.

SOURCES: Dietary Reference Intakes for Calcium, Phosphorus, Magnesium, Vitamin D, and Fluoride (1997); Dietary Reference Intakes for Thiamin, Riboflavin, Niacin, Vitamin B-6, Folate, Vitamin B-12, Pantothenic Acid, Biotin, and Choline (1998); Dietary Reference Intakes for Vitamin C, Vitamin E, Selenium, and Carotenoids (2000); and Dietary Reference Intakes for Vitamin A, Vitamin K, Arsenic, Boron, Chromium, Copper, Iodine, Iron, Manganese, Molybdenum, Nickel, Silicon, Vanadium, and Zinc (2001). These reports may be accessed via www.nap.edu.

Adapted from the Dietary Reference Intakes series, National Academies Press. Copyright 1997, 1998, 2000, 2001, 2011, by the National Academy of Sciences. The full reports are available from the National Academies Press at www.nap.edu.

E

DIETARY REFERENCE INTAKES (DRIs): TOLERABLE UPPER INTAKE LEVELS (UL[a]), ELEMENTS AND ELECTROLYTES[b,c]
Food and Nutrition Board, Institute of Medicine, National Academies

Life Stage Group	Arsenic[b]	Boron (mg/d)	Calcium (g/d)	Copper (μg/d)	Fluoride (mg/d)	Iodine (μg/d)	Iron (mg/d)	Magnesium (mg/d)[d]	Manganese (mg/d)	Molybdenum (μg/d)	Nickel (mg/d)	Phosphorus (g/d)	Selenium (μg/d)	Vanadium (mg/d)[e]	Zinc (mg/d)	Sodium (mg/d)	Chloride (mg/d)
Infants																	
0–6 mo	ND[f]	ND	1	ND	0.7	ND	40	ND	ND	ND	ND	ND	45	ND	4	ND	ND
7–12 mo	ND	ND	1.5	ND	0.9	ND	40	ND	ND	ND	ND	ND	60	ND	5	ND	ND
Children																	
1–3 y	ND	3	2.5	1000	1.3	200	40	65	2	300	0.2	3	90	ND	7	1500	2300
4–8 y	ND	6	2.5	3000	2.2	300	40	110	3	600	0.3	3	150	ND	12	1900	2900
Males, Females																	
9–13 y	ND	11	3	5000	10	600	40	350	6	1100	0.6	4	280	ND	23	2200	3400
14–18 y	ND	17	3	8000	10	900	45	350	9	1700	1.0	4	400	ND	34	2300	3600
19–70 y	ND	20	2.5[g]	10000	10	1100	45	350	11	2000	1.0	4	400	1.8	40	2300	3600
>70 y	ND	20	2	10000	10	1100	45	350	11	2000	1.0	3	400	1.8	40	2300	3600
Pregnancy																	
≤18 y	ND	17	3	8000	10	900	45	350	9	1700	1.0	3.5	400	ND	34	2300	3600
19–50 y	ND	20	2.5	10000	10	1100	45	350	11	2000	1.0	3.5	400	ND	40	2300	3600
Lactation																	
≤18 y	ND	17	3	8000	10	900	45	350	9	1700	1.0	4	400	ND	34	2300	3600
19–50 y	ND	20	2.5	10000	10	1100	45	350	11	2000	1.0	4	400	ND	40	2300	3600

[a]UL = The maximum level of daily nutrient intake that is likely to pose no risk of adverse effects. Unless otherwise specified, the UL represents total intake from food, water, and supplements. Due to lack of suitable data, ULs could not be established for arsenic, chromium, and silicon. In the absence of ULs, extra caution may be warranted in consuming levels above recommended intakes.

[b]Although a UL was not determined for arsenic, there is no justification for adding arsenic to food or supplements.

[c]Although silicon has not been shown to cause adverse effects in humans, there is no justification for adding silicon to supplements.

[d]The ULs for magnesium represent intake from a pharmacological agent only and do not include intake from food and water.

[e]Although vanadium in food has not been shown to cause adverse effects in humans, there is no justification for adding vanadium to food and vanadium supplements should be used with caution. The UL is based on adverse effects in laboratory animals and this data could be used to set a UL for adults but not children and adolescents.

[f]ND = Not determinable due to lack of data of adverse effects in this age group and concern with regard to lack of ability to handle excess amounts. Source of intake should be from food only to prevent high levels of intake.

[g]Upper Limit declines to 2 after age 50.

SOURCES: Dietary Reference Intakes for Calcium and Vitamin D (2011); Dietary Reference Intakes for Calcium, Phosphorus, Magnesium, Vitamin D, and Fluoride (1997); Dietary Reference Intakes for Thiamin, Riboflavin, Niacin, Vitamin B-6, Folate, Vitamin B-12, Pantothenic Acid, Biotin, and Choline (1998); Dietary Reference Intakes for Vitamin C, Vitamin E, Selenium, and Carotenoids (2000); Dietary Reference Intakes for Vitamin A, Vitamin K, Arsenic, Boron, Chromium, Copper, Iodine, Iron, Manganese, Molybdenum, Nickel, Silicon, Vanadium, and Zinc (2001); and Dietary Reference Intakes for Water, Potassium, Sodium, Chloride, and Sulfate (2004). These reports may be accessed via www.nap.edu.

Adapted from the Dietary Reference Intakes series, National Academies Press. Copyright 1997, 1998, 2000, 2001, 2011, by the National Academy of Sciences. The full reports are available from the National Academies Press at www.nap.edu.

F

Glossary

1,25-dihydroxyvitamin D₃ (calcitriol)
Biologically active form of vitamin D.

25-hydroxyvitamin D₃ (calcidiol or calcifediol) Form found in blood. Sometimes shortened to 25(OH)D₃.

7-dehydrocholesterol Precursor of vitamin D found in the skin.

absorption The process by which substances are taken up from the GI tract and enter the bloodstream or the lymph.

absorptive cells Also known as *enterocytes;* the intestinal cells that line the villi and participate in nutrient absorption.

Acceptable Daily Intake (ADI) Estimate of the amount of a sweetener that an individual can safely consume daily over a lifetime. ADIs are given as milligrams per kilogram of body weight per day.

acesulfame-K Alternative sweetener that yields no energy to the body; 200 times sweeter than sucrose.

acetaldehyde dehydrogenase An enzyme used in ethanol metabolism that eventually converts acetaldehyde into carbon dioxide and water.

acid group In chemistry, a functional group that consists of a carbon atom that shares bonds with two oxygen atoms. This is the site where fatty acids are linked to glycerol to form triglycerides.

action potential Change in the electrical charge of the nerve cell membrane resulting in an electrical signal that can be transmitted from one nerve cell to the next.

active absorption Movement of a substance across a semipermeable membrane from an area of lower solute concentration to an area of higher solute concentration. This type of transport requires energy and a carrier.

adaptive thermogenesis This term encompasses the ability of humans to regulate body temperature within narrow limits (thermoregulation). Two visible examples of thermogenesis are fidgeting and shivering when cold.

additives Substances added to foods, either intentionally or incidentally.

adenosine diphosphate (ADP) A breakdown product of ATP. ADP is synthesized into ATP using energy from foodstuffs and a phosphate group (abbreviated Pᵢ).

adenosine triphosphate (ATP) The main energy currency for cells. ATP energy is used to promote ion pumping, enzyme activity, and muscular contraction.

Adequate Intake (AI) Nutrient intake amount set for any nutrient for which insufficient research is available to establish an RDA. AIs are based on estimates of intakes that appear to maintain a defined nutritional state in a specific life stage.

adipose tissue Connective tissue made up of cells that store fat and also cushions and insulates the body.

adjustable gastric banding A restrictive procedure in which the opening from the esophagus to the stomach is reduced by a hollow gastric band.

aerobic Requiring oxygen.

aging Time-dependent physical and physiological changes in body structure and function that occur normally and progressively throughout adulthood as humans mature and become older.

air displacement A method for estimating body composition that makes use of the volume of space taken up by a body inside a small chamber. This tool is also known as air displacement plethysmography.

alcohol Ethyl alcohol or ethanol (CH_3CH_2OH) is the compound in alcoholic beverages.

alcohol dehydrogenase An enzyme used in alcohol (ethanol) metabolism that converts alcohol into acetaldehyde.

alcohol use disorder A psychiatric disorder characterized by a problematic pattern of alcohol use that leads to significant impairment or distress.

alcohol-related birth defects (ARBDs) One or more birth defects (e.g., malformations of the heart, bones, kidneys, eyes, or ears) related to confirmed alcohol exposure during gestation.

alcohol-related neurodevelopmental disorders (ARNDs) One or more abnormalities of the central nervous system (e.g., small head size, impaired motor skills, hearing loss, or poor hand-eye coordination) related to confirmed alcohol exposure during gestation.

aldosterone A hormone produced by the adrenal glands when blood volume is low. It acts on the kidneys to conserve sodium (and therefore water) to increase blood volume.

allergen A foreign protein, or antigen, that induces excess production of certain immune system antibodies; subsequent exposure to the same protein leads to allergic symptoms. Whereas all allergens are antigens, not all antigens are allergens.

allergy A hypersensitive immune response that occurs when immune bodies produced by us react with a protein we sense as foreign (an antigen).

alpha-linolenic acid An essential omega-3 fatty acid with 18 carbons and three double bonds.

amenorrhea Absence of menstrual periods in a woman of reproductive age.

amino acid The building block for proteins containing a central carbon atom with nitrogen and other atoms attached.

amphetamine A group of medications that induce stimulation of the central nervous system and have other effects in the body. Abuse is linked to physical and psychological dependence.

amylase Starch-digesting enzyme produced by the salivary glands and the pancreas.

amylopectin A digestible branched-chain type of starch composed of glucose units.

amylose A digestible straight-chain type of starch composed of glucose units.

anaerobic Not requiring oxygen.

anal sphincters A group of two sphincters (inner and outer) that help control expulsion of feces from the body.

anaphylaxis A severe allergic response that results in lowered blood pressure and respiratory distress. This can be fatal.

anemia A decreased oxygen-carrying capacity of the blood. This can be caused by many factors, such as iron deficiency or blood loss.

anencephaly Birth defect characterized by the absence of some or all of the brain and skull.

angiotensin A hormone produced by the liver and activated by enzymes from the kidneys. It signals the adrenal glands to produce aldosterone also and directs the kidneys to conserve sodium (and therefore water). Both of these actions have the effect of increasing blood volume.

animal model Use of animals to study disease to understand more about human disease.

anorexia nervosa An eating disorder characterized by extreme restriction of energy intake relative to requirements leading to significantly low body weight.

anthocyanins Flavonoid plant pigments that appear red, purple, or blue and are found in berries, grapes, and red cabbage.

anthropometric assessment Measurement of body weight and the lengths, circumferences, and thicknesses of parts of the body.

antibody Blood protein that binds foreign proteins found in the body.

antibody-mediated immunity A process in which one type of lymphocyte produces antibodies that bind to specific antigens, thus marking foreign proteins or pathogens for destruction by other white blood cells.

antidiuretic hormone (ADH) A hormone that is secreted by the pituitary gland when blood concentration of solutes is high. It causes the kidneys to decrease water excretion, which increases blood volume.

antigen Any substance that induces a state of sensitivity and/or resistance to microorganisms or toxic substances after a lag period; a foreign substance that stimulates a specific aspect of the immune system.

antioxidant A substance that has the ability to prevent or repair the damage caused by oxidation.

anus Last portion of the GI tract; serves as an outlet for the digestive system.

appetite The primarily psychological (external) influences that encourage us to find and eat food, often in the absence of obvious hunger.

arachidonic acid (AA) An omega-6 fatty acid made from linoleic acid with 20 carbon atoms and four carbon-carbon double bonds.

aril Clear, ruby-colored fruit or seed pod that surrounds a tiny, crisp seed inside a pomegranate.

artery A blood vessel that carries blood away from the heart.

ascending colon Segment of the large intestine that carries feces from the cecum, up the right side of the abdomen, to the transverse colon.

aseptic processing A method by which food and container are separately and simultaneously sterilized; it allows manufacturers to produce boxes of milk that can be stored at room temperature.

aspartame Alternative sweetener made of two amino acids and methanol; about 200 times sweeter than sucrose.

atherosclerosis A buildup of fatty material (plaque) in the arteries, including those surrounding the heart.

atopic disease A condition involving an inappropriate immune response to environmental allergens; examples include asthma, eczema, and seasonal allergies.

atypical anorexia nervosa A subthreshold eating disorder in which a person meets most of the criteria for diagnosis of anorexia nervosa, except weight is within a normal range.

avoidant/restrictive food intake disorder (ARFID) Eating disorder characterized by failure to meet energy or nutrient needs, resulting in significant weight loss, nutritional deficiencies, or dependence on tube or intravenous feeding; the eating disturbance is not better explained by lack of available food, a medical problem, or another eating disorder.

bacteria Single-cell microorganisms; some produce poisonous substances, which cause illness in humans. Bacteria can be carried by water, animals, and people. They survive on skin, clothes, and hair, and thrive in foods at room temperature. Some can live without oxygen and survive by means of spore formation.

bariatrics The medical specialty focusing on the treatment of obesity.

basal metabolism The minimal amount of calories the body uses to support itself in a fasting state when resting and awake in a warm, quiet environment. It amounts to roughly 1 kcal per kilogram per hour for men and 0.9 kcal per kilogram per hour for women; these values are often referred to as *basal metabolic rate (BMR)*.

basophil The white blood cell that controls inflammation; level increases with poisoning.

benign Noncancerous; tumors that do not spread.

beriberi The thiamin-deficiency disorder characterized by muscle weakness, loss of appetite, nerve degeneration, and sometimes edema.

beta-carotene The orange-yellow pigment in carrots; beta-carotene is the only carotenoid that can be sufficiently absorbed and converted into retinol in the body.

BHA, BHT Butylated hydroxyanisole and butylated hydroxytoluene: two common synthetic antioxidants added to foods.

bile A liver secretion stored in the gallbladder and released through the common bile duct into the first segment of the small intestine. It is essential for the digestion and absorption of fat.

bile acid A compound produced by the liver. Bile acids are the main component of bile, which aids in emulsification of fat during digestion in the small intestine.

binge drinking Drinking sufficient alcohol within a 2-hour period to increase blood alcohol content to 0.08 grams per deciliter or higher; for men, consuming 5 or more drinks in a row; for women, consuming 4 or more drinks in a row.

binge eating Consuming an abnormally large amount of food within a short time period (e.g., 2 hours).

binge-eating disorder An eating disorder characterized by recurrent episodes of binge eating that are associated with marked distress and lack of control over behavior, but not followed by inappropriate compensatory behaviors to prevent weight gain.

binge-eating disorder of limited duration A form of other specified feeding or eating disorders in which a person meets all of the criteria for diagnosis of binge-eating disorder—except the duration of the disordered eating behavior is less than 3 months.

binge-eating disorder of low frequency A form of other specified feeding or eating disorders in which a person meets all of the criteria for diagnosis of binge-eating disorder—except the frequency of binges is less than once per week.

bioavailability The degree to which an ingested nutrient is absorbed and available to be utilized by the body.

biochemical assessment Measurement of biochemical functions (e.g., concentrations of nutrient by-products or enzyme activities in the blood or urine) related to a nutrient's function.

bioelectrical impedance The method to estimate total body fat that uses a low-energy electrical current. The more fat storage a person has, the more impedance (resistance) to electrical flow will be exhibited.

biological pest management Control of agricultural pests by using natural predators, parasites, or pathogens. For example, ladybugs can be used to control an aphid infestation.

biotechnology A collection of processes that involves the use of biological systems for altering and, ideally, improving the characteristics of plants, animals, and other forms of life.

bisphosphonates Drugs that bind minerals and prevent osteoclast breakdown of bone. Examples are alendronate (Fosamax) and risedronate (Actonel).

body mass index (BMI) Weight (in kilograms) divided by height (in meters) squared; a value of 25 and above indicates overweight and a value of 30 and above indicates obesity.

bolus A moistened mass of food swallowed from the oral cavity into the pharynx.

bomb calorimeter An instrument used to determine the calorie content of a food.

bond A linkage between two atoms formed by the sharing of electrons, or attractions.

bone marrow The spongy tissue in flat bones and trabecular bone that contains stem cells.

bone mineral density Total mineral content of bone at a specific bone site divided by the width of the bone at that site, generally expressed as grams per cubic centimeter.

bone remodeling The chemical process by which bone is broken down and replaced by new bone.

branched-chain amino acids Amino acids with a branching carbon backbone; these are leucine, isoleucine, and valine. All are essential amino acids.

brown adipose tissue A specialized form of adipose (fat) tissue that produces large amounts of heat by metabolizing energy-yielding nutrients without synthesizing much useful energy for the body. The unused energy is released as heat.

buffer Compounds that cause a solution to resist changes in acid–base conditions.

bulimia nervosa An eating disorder characterized by recurrent episodes of binge eating followed by inappropriate compensatory behaviors to prevent weight gain.

bulimia nervosa of limited duration A form of other specified feeding or eating disorders in which a person meets all of the criteria for diagnosis of bulimia nervosa—except the duration of the disordered eating behavior is less than 3 months.

bulimia nervosa of low frequency A form of other specified feeding or eating disorders in which a person meets all of the criteria for diagnosis of bulimia nervosa—except the frequency of binge-compensate cycles is less than once per week.

cancer A condition characterized by uncontrolled growth of abnormal cells.

capillary A microscopic blood vessel that connects the smallest arteries and veins; site of nutrient, oxygen, and waste exchange between body cells and the blood.

capillary bed Network of one-cell-thick vessels that create a junction between arterial and venous circulation. It is here that gas and nutrient exchange occurs between body cells and the blood.

carbohydrate A compound containing carbon, hydrogen, and oxygen atoms. Most are known as *sugars, starches,* and *fibers.*

carbohydrate loading A process in which a high-carbohydrate diet is consumed for 6 days before an athletic event while tapering exercise duration in an attempt to increase muscle glycogen stores.

carbon footprint The greenhouse gas emissions caused by an organization, event, product, or individual.

carbon skeleton Amino-acid structure that remains after the amino group ($—NH_2$) has been removed.

cardiovascular disease A general term that refers to any disease of the heart and circulatory system. This disease is generally characterized by the deposition of fatty material in the blood vessels (hardening of the arteries), which in turn can lead to organ damage and death. Also termed coronary heart disease (CHD), as the vessels of the heart are the primary sites of the disease.

cardiovascular system The body system consisting of the heart, blood vessels, and blood. This system transports nutrients, waste products, gases, and hormones throughout the body and plays an important role in immune responses and regulation of body temperature.

carotenoids Precursors of vitamin A found in plant foods.

case-control study A study in which individuals who have a disease or condition, such as lung cancer, are compared with individuals who do not have the condition.

catalase Antioxidant enzyme system that converts harmful reactive oxygen species (peroxides) into less harmful products (water and oxygen).

cecum A pouch at the first part of the large intestine that houses many bacteria.

celiac disease Chronic, immune-mediated disease precipitated by exposure to dietary gluten in genetically predisposed people.

cell The structural basis of plant and animal organization. In animals it is bounded by a cell membrane. Cells have the ability to take up compounds from and excrete compounds into their surroundings.

cell nucleus An organelle bound by its own double membrane and containing chromosomes, the genetic information for cell protein synthesis and cell replication.

cell-mediated immunity A process in which certain white blood cells come in contact with the invading cells to destroy them.

cellular differentiation The process of a less-specialized cell becoming a more specialized type. Think of stem cells in the bone marrow becoming red and white blood cells.

cellulose An undigestible, nonfermentable, straight-chain polysaccharide made of glucose molecules.

cerebrovascular accident (CVA) Death of part of the brain tissue due typically to a blood clot. Also termed a *stroke.*

ceruloplasmin Copper-containing protein in the blood; functions in the transport of iron.

chain-breaking Breaking the link between two or more behaviors that encourage overeating, such as snacking while watching television.

chemical reaction An interaction between two chemicals that changes both chemicals.

chlorosis In traditional medical terminology, a form of iron-deficiency anemia characterized by pale or greenish skin, weakness, fatigue, and shortness of breath. In modern medical literature, chlorosis is termed *hypochromic anemia.*

choice The serving size of a food on a specific exchange list; formerly called *exchange.*

cholesterol A waxy lipid found in all body cells. It has a structure containing multiple chemical rings that is found only in foods that contain animal products.

chromosome A single, large DNA molecule and its associated proteins; contains many genes to store and transmit genetic information.

chronic Long-standing, developing over time. When referring to disease, this term indicates that the disease process, once developed, is slow and lasting. A good example is cardiovascular disease.

chylomicron Lipoprotein made of dietary fats surrounded by a shell of cholesterol, phospholipids, and protein. Chylomicrons are formed in the absorptive cells of the small intestine after fat absorption and travel through the lymphatic system to the bloodstream.

chyme A mixture of stomach secretions and partially digested food.

cirrhosis A loss of functioning liver cells, which are replaced by nonfunctioning connective tissue. Any substance that poisons liver cells can lead to cirrhosis. The most common cause is a chronic, excessive alcohol intake. Exposure to certain industrial chemicals also can lead to cirrhosis.

cis **fatty acid** A form of an unsaturated fatty acid that has the hydrogens lying on the same side of the carbon-carbon double bond.

clinical assessment Examination of general appearance of skin, eyes, and tongue; evidence of rapid hair loss; sense of touch; and ability to cough and walk.

coagulation Formation of a blood clot.

coenzyme An organic compound that combines with an inactive enzyme to form a catalytically active form. In this manner, coenzymes aid in enzyme function.

cofactor An inorganic compound (e.g., mineral) that combines with an inactive enzyme to form a catalytically active form.

cognitive behavioral therapy Psychological therapy in which the person's assumptions about dieting, body weight, and related issues are confronted. New ways of thinking are explored and then practiced by the person. In this way, an individual can learn new ways to control disordered eating behaviors and related life stress.

cognitive restructuring Changing one's frame of mind regarding eating; for example, instead of using a difficult day as an excuse to overeat, a person would substitute other pleasures for rewards, such as a relaxing walk with a friend.

collagen Hard, insoluble and fibrous protein found in connective tissue, bone, teeth, tendons, and blood vessels.

colostrum The first fluid secreted by the breast during late pregnancy and the first few days after birth. This thick fluid is rich in immune factors and protein.

community supported agriculture (CSA) Partnership between local food producers and community members. Farmers offer a share of foods to individuals, families, or companies that have pledged support to the CSA either financially and/or by working for the CSA.

compensatory behaviors Actions taken to rid the body of excess calories and/or to alleviate guilt or anxiety associated with a binge; examples include vomiting, misuse of laxatives, or excessive exercise.

complementary proteins Two food protein sources that make up for each other's inadequate supply of specific essential amino acids; together, they yield a sufficient amount of all nine and so provide high-quality (complete) protein for the diet.

complex carbohydrate Carbohydrate composed of many monosaccharide molecules. Examples include glycogen, starch, and fiber.

compression of morbidity Delay of the onset of disabilities caused by chronic disease.

conditionally essential amino acids Amino acids that must be made from essential amino acids if insufficient amounts are eaten.

congenital hypothyroidism A birth defect that impairs thyroid hormone synthesis. If untreated, this can lead to mental retardation and stunting of growth.

congenital lactase deficiency Birth defect resulting in the inability to produce lactase, such that a lactose-free diet is required from birth.

connective tissue Protein tissue that holds different structures in the body together. Some body structures are made up of connective tissue—notably, tendons and cartilage. Connective tissue also forms part of bone and the nonmuscular structures of arteries and veins.

constipation A condition characterized by infrequent bowel movements.

contingency management Forming a plan of action to respond to a situation in which overeating is likely, such as when snacks are within arm's reach at a party.

control group Participants in an experiment who are not given the treatment being tested.

cortical bone The compact or dense bone found on the outer surfaces of bone.

creatine An organic (i.e., carbon-containing) molecule in muscle cells that serves as part of a high-energy compound (termed creatine phosphate or phosphocreatine) capable of synthesizing ATP from ADP.

Creutzfeldt-Jakob disease A rare, degenerative, invariably fatal brain disorder. Symptoms include problems with muscular coordination, personality changes including progressive and severe mental impairment, impaired vision that may lead to blindness, and involuntary muscle jerks.

cross-contamination Process by which bacteria or other microorganisms are unintentionally transferred from one substance or object to another, with harmful effect.

cytokines Chemical messengers that regulate immune responses.

cytoplasm The fluid and organelles (except the nucleus) in a cell.

dehydration Inadequate intake of water to replace losses.

Delaney Clause A clause to the 1958 Food Additives Amendment of the Pure Food and Drug Act in the United States that prevents the intentional (direct) addition to foods of a compound shown to cause cancer in laboratory animals or humans.

dementia A general loss or decrease in mental function.

denaturation Alteration of a protein's three-dimensional structure, usually because of treatment by heat, enzymes, acid or alkaline solutions, or agitation.

dental caries Erosions in the surface of a tooth caused by acids made by bacteria as they metabolize sugars.

deoxyribonucleic acid (DNA) The site of hereditary information in cells; DNA directs the synthesis of cell proteins.

depolarization During nerve impulse transmission, the process in which the resting state of the nerve cell membrane (slightly negative inside the cell membrane) is temporarily disrupted.

descending colon Segment of the large intestine that carries feces from the transverse colon, down the left side of the abdomen, to the sigmoid colon.

diabetes A group of diseases characterized by high blood glucose. Type 1 diabetes involves insufficient or no release of the hormone insulin by the pancreas and therefore requires daily insulin therapy. Type 2 diabetes results from either insufficient release of insulin or general inability of insulin to act on certain body cells, such as muscle cells. Persons with type 2 diabetes may or may not require insulin therapy.

diastolic blood pressure The pressure in the arterial blood vessels when the heart is between beats.

dietary assessment Estimation of typical food choices relying mostly on the recounting of one's usual intake or a record of one's previous days' intake.

dietary fiber Fiber found in food.

Dietary Reference Intakes (DRIs) Term used to encompass nutrient recommendations made by the Food and Nutrition Board of the Institute of Medicine. These include RDAs, AIs, EERs, and ULs.

digestion Process by which large ingested molecules are mechanically and chemically broken down to produce basic nutrients that can be absorbed across the wall of the GI tract.

digestive system System consisting of the gastrointestinal tract and accessory structures (liver, gallbladder, and pancreas). This system performs the mechanical and chemical processes of digestion, absorption of nutrients, and elimination of wastes.

diglyceride A breakdown product of a triglyceride consisting of two fatty acids bonded to a glycerol backbone.

direct calorimetry A method of determining a body's energy use by measuring heat released from the body. An insulated chamber is typically used.

disaccharide Class of sugars formed by the chemical bonding of two monosaccharides.

disordered eating Mild and short-term changes in eating patterns that occur in relation to a stressful event, an illness, or a desire to modify one's diet for a variety of health and personal appearance reasons.

diuretic A substance that increases the volume of urine.

diverticula Pouches that protrude through the exterior wall of the large intestine.

diverticulitis An inflammation of the diverticula caused by acids produced by bacterial metabolism inside the diverticula.

diverticulosis The condition of having many diverticula in the large intestine.

docosahexaenoic acid (DHA) An omega-3 fatty acid with 22 carbons and six carbon-carbon double bonds. It is present in large amounts in fatty fish and is slowly synthesized in the body from alpha-linolenic acid. DHA is especially present in the retina and brain.

double-blind study An experimental design in which neither the participants nor the researchers are aware of each participant's assignment (test or placebo) or the outcome of the study until it is completed. An independent third party holds the code and the data until the study has been completed.

dual energy X-ray absorptiometry (DEXA) A scientific tool used to measure bone mineral density.

duodenum First segment of the small intestine that receives chyme from the stomach and digestive juices from the pancreas and gallbladder. This is the site of most chemical digestion of nutrients; approximately 10 inches in length.

early childhood caries Tooth decay that results from formula or juice (and even human milk) bathing the teeth as the child sleeps with a bottle in the mouth. The upper teeth are mostly affected as the lower teeth are protected by the tongue; formerly called *nursing bottle syndrome* and *baby bottle tooth decay*.

eating disorder Severe alterations in eating patterns linked to physiological changes. The alterations are associated with food restriction, binge eating, inappropriate compensatory behaviors, and fluctuations in weight. They also involve a number of emotional and cognitive changes that affect the way a person perceives and experiences his or her body.

eclampsia A severe form of gestational hypertension characterized by protein in the urine and seizures (formerly called *toxemia*).

edema The buildup of excess fluid in extracellular spaces.

eicosanoids A class of hormone compounds, including the prostaglandins, derived from the essential polyunsaturated fatty acids. These signaling compounds are involved in cellular activity that affects practically all important functions in the body.

eicosapentaenoic acid (EPA) An omega-3 fatty acid with 20 carbons and five carbon-carbon double bonds. It is present in large amounts in fatty fish and is slowly synthesized in the body from alpha-linolenic acid.

electrolyte A mineral that separates into positively or negatively charged ions in water. They are able to transmit an electrical current.

elimination diet A restrictive diet that systematically tests foods that may cause an allergic response by first eliminating them for 1 to 2 weeks and then adding them back, one at a time.

embryo In humans, the developing offspring in utero from about the beginning of the third week to the end of the eighth week after conception.

emulsifier A compound that can suspend fat in water by isolating individual fat droplets, using a shell of water molecules or other substances to prevent the fat from coalescing.

endocrine gland A hormone-producing gland.

endocrine system The body system consisting of the various glands and the hormones these glands secrete. This system has major regulatory functions in the body, such as reproduction and cell metabolism.

endometrium The membrane that lines the inside of the uterus. It increases in thickness during the menstrual cycle until ovulation occurs. The surface layers are shed during menstruation if conception does not take place.

endoplasmic reticulum (ER) An organelle composed of a network of canals running through the cytoplasm. Part of the endoplasmic reticulum contains ribosomes.

endorphins Natural body tranquilizers that may be involved in the feeding response and function in pain reduction.

energy balance The state in which energy intake, in the form of food and beverages, matches the energy expended, primarily through basal metabolism and physical activity.

energy density A comparison of the calorie (kcal) content of a food with the weight of the food. An energy-dense food is high in calories but weighs very little (e.g., potato chips), whereas a food low in energy density has few calories but weighs a lot (e.g., an orange).

enterohepatic circulation A continual recycling of compounds such as bile acids between the small intestine and the liver.

environmental assessment Includes details about living conditions, education level, and the ability of the person to purchase, transport, and cook food. The person's weekly budget for food purchases is also a key factor to consider.

enzyme A compound that speeds up the rate of a chemical reaction but is not altered by the reaction. Almost all enzymes are proteins (some are made of genetic material).

eosinophil This white blood cell is a type of phagocyte that increases in number during allergic reactions.

epidemiology The study of how disease rates vary among different population groups.

epigenetics Heritable changes in gene function that are independent of DNA sequence. For example, malnutrition during pregnancy may modify gene expression in the fetus and affect long-term body weight regulation in the offspring.

epigenome A network of chemical compounds surrounding DNA that modify the genome without altering the DNA sequences and have a role in determining which genes are active (expressed) or inactive (silenced) in a particular cell.

epiglottis The flap that folds down over the trachea during swallowing.

epinephrine A hormone also known as *adrenaline;* it is released by the adrenal glands (located on each kidney) at times of stress. It acts to increase glycogen breakdown in the liver, among other functions.

epithelial tissue The surface cells that line the outside of the body and all external passages within it.

ergogenic Work-producing. An ergogenic aid is a mechanical, nutritional, psychological, pharmacological, or physiological substance or treatment intended to directly improve exercise performance.

erythrocyte Mature red blood cell. These have no nucleus and a life span of about 120 days; they contain hemoglobin, which transports oxygen and carbon dioxide.

erythropoiesis Formation of red blood cells.

erythropoietin A hormone secreted mostly by the kidneys that enhances red blood cell synthesis and stimulates red blood cell release from bone marrow.

esophagus A tube in the GI tract that connects the pharynx with the stomach.

essential amino acids The amino acids that cannot be synthesized by humans in sufficient amounts or at all and therefore must be included in the diet; there are nine essential amino acids. These are also called *indispensable amino acids.*

essential fatty acids Fatty acids that must be supplied by the diet to maintain health. Currently, only linoleic acid and alpha-linolenic acid are classified as essential.

essential nutrient In nutritional terms, a substance that, when left out of a diet, leads to signs of poor health. The body either cannot produce this nutrient or cannot produce enough of it to meet its needs. If added back to a diet before permanent damage occurs, the affected aspects of health are restored.

Estimated Energy Requirement (EER) Estimate of the energy (kcal) intake needed to match the energy use of an average person in a specific life stage.

ethanol Chemical term for the form of alcohol found in alcoholic beverages.

exercise Physical activities that are planned, repetitive, and intended to improve physical fitness.

extracellular fluid Fluid found outside the cells; it represents about one-third of body fluid.

extracellular space The space outside cells; represents one-third of body fluid.

facilitated diffusion Movement of a substance across a semipermeable membrane from an area of higher solute concentration to an area of lower solute concentration. This type of transport does not require energy, but it does require a carrier.

failure to thrive Condition of inadequate growth during infancy or early childhood caused by poor nutritional intake, inefficient nutrient absorption, or excessive energy expenditure; commonly defined as weight-for-age below the fifth percentile on multiple occasions or weight declining two or more major percentile lines on a standardized growth chart.

famine An extreme shortage of food, which leads to massive starvation in a population; often associated with crop failures, war, and political unrest.

fat adaptation Manipulating the diet and physical training regimen so that muscles become more efficient at metabolizing fat as fuel during aerobic activity.

fat-soluble Soluble in fats, oils, or fat solvents.

fat-soluble vitamins Vitamins that dissolve in fat and such substances as ether and benzene but not readily in water. These vitamins are A, D, E, and K.

fecal impaction The presence of a mass of hard, dry feces that remains in the rectum as a result of chronic constipation.

feces Mass of water, fiber, tough connective tissues, bacterial cells, and sloughed intestinal cells that passes through the large intestine and is excreted through the anus; also called *stool.*

female athlete triad A condition characterized by disordered eating, lack of menstrual periods (amenorrhea), and osteoporosis.

fermentation The conversion of carbohydrates to alcohols, acids, and carbon dioxide without the use of oxygen.

ferritin A protein that stores iron and releases it in a controlled manner. Acts as a buffer against iron deficiency and iron overload.

fetal alcohol spectrum disorders (FASDs) A group of irreversible physical and mental abnormalities in the infant that result from the mother's consuming alcohol during pregnancy.

fetal alcohol syndrome (FAS) Severe form of FASD that involves abnormal facial features and problems with development of the nervous system and overall growth as a result of maternal alcohol consumption during pregnancy.

fetal origins hypothesis A theory that links nutritional and other environmental insults that occur during gestation to the future health of the offspring.

fetus The developing life form from about the beginning of the ninth week after conception until birth.

fiber Substances in plant foods not digested in the human stomach or small intestine. These add bulk to feces. Fiber naturally found in foods is also called *dietary fiber.*

flavonoids Most common group of polyphenol phytochemicals; found in citrus fruits, berries, red onion, tea, red wine, and dark chocolate.

fluorosis Discoloration of tooth enamel sometimes accompanied with pitting due to consuming a large amount of fluoride for an excessive period.

foam cells Lipid-loaded white blood cells that have surrounded large amounts of a fatty substance, usually cholesterol, on the blood vessel walls.

FODMAPs **F**ermentable **o**ligosaccharides, **d**isaccharides, **m**onosaccharides, **and** **p**olyols. These carbohydrates may be poorly digested and lead to GI symptoms such as bloating, gas, and diarrhea in some people.

folate term to describe a variety of forms of this B vitamin found in foods and in the body.

food allergy An adverse reaction to food that involves an immune response; also called *food hypersensitivity.*

food deserts Urban neighborhoods and rural towns without ready access to fresh, healthy, and affordable food.

food insecure The state of being without reliable access to a sufficient quantity of affordable, nutritious food.

food insecurity A condition of anxiety regarding running out of either food or money to buy more food.

food intolerance An adverse reaction to food that does not involve an allergic reaction.

food jag A period of time (usually a few days or weeks) during which a person will eat only a limitied variety of foods.

food lists A system for classifying foods into numerous lists based on the foods' macronutrient composition, and establishing serving sizes, so that one serving of each food on a list contains the same amount of carbohydrate, protein, fat, and calorie content; also called *exchange lists.*

foodborne illness Sickness caused by the ingestion of food containing harmful substances.

foodborne infection Occurs when a person eats food containing harmful microorganisms, which then grow in the intestinal tract and cause illness.

foodborne intoxication Results when a person eats food containing toxins that cause illness.

free radical An unstable atom with an unpaired electron in its outermost shell; also called *reactive oxygen species.*

fructose A six-carbon monosaccharide that usually exists in a ring form; found in fruits and honey; also known as *fruit sugar.*

fruitarian A person who primarily eats fruits, nuts, honey, and vegetable oils.

functional fiber Fiber added to foods that has been shown to provide health benefits.

functional foods Foods that have health benefits beyond basic nutrition.

fungi Simple parasitic life forms, including molds, mildews, yeasts, and mushrooms. They live on dead or decaying organic matter. Fungi can grow as single cells, like yeast, or as a multicellular colony, as seen with molds.

galactose A six-carbon monosaccharide that usually exists in a ring form; closely related to glucose.

gallbladder An organ attached to the underside of the liver; site of bile storage, concentration, and eventual secretion.

gastroesophageal reflux disease (GERD) Disease that results from stomach acid backing up into the esophagus. The acid irritates the lining of the esophagus, causing pain.

gastrointestinal (GI) tract The main sites in the body used for digestion and absorption of nutrients. It consists of the mouth, esophagus, stomach, small intestine, large intestine, rectum, and anus. Also called the *digestive tract.*

gastroplasty Gastric bypass surgery performed on the stomach to limit its volume to approximately 30 milliliters. Also referred to as stomach stapling.

gender and development (GAD) approach Understanding the roles and responsibilities of both men and women in the process of sustainable development.

gene A specific segment on a chromosome. Genes provide the blueprint for the production of cell proteins.

gene expression Use of DNA information on a gene to produce a protein. Thought to be a major determination of cell development.

generally recognized as safe (GRAS) A list of food additives that in 1958 were considered safe for consumption. Manufacturers were allowed to continue to use these additives, without special clearance, when needed for food products. FDA bears responsibility for proving they are not safe, and can remove unsafe products from the list.

genes A specific segment on a chromosome. Genes provide the blueprint for the production of all body proteins.

genetic engineering Manipulation of the genetic makeup of any organism with recombinant DNA technology.

genetically modified organism (GMO) Any organism created by genetic engineering.

genomics The study of the function and structure of the complete set of DNA within a single cell of an organism, known as the genome.

gestation The period of intrauterine development of offspring, from conception to birth; in humans, normal gestation is 38 to 42 weeks.

gestational diabetes A high blood glucose concentration that develops during pregnancy and returns to normal after birth; one cause is the placental production of hormones that antagonize the regulation of blood glucose by insulin.

gestational hypertension Blood pressure greater than 140/90 mmHg that is first diagnosed after 20 weeks of gestation. This may evolve into preeclampsia or eclampsia.

global maternal mortality ratio The number of maternal deaths per 100,000 live births.

glucagon A hormone made by the pancreas that stimulates the breakdown of glycogen in the liver into glucose; this ends up increasing blood glucose. Glucagon also increases the generation of glucose from non-carbohydrate substances.

glucose A six-carbon sugar that exists in a ring form; found as such in blood, and in table sugar bound to fructose; also known as *dextrose,* it is one of the simple sugars.

glutathione peroxidase An antioxidant enzyme system that converts certain free radicals (peroxides) into less harmful compounds (alcohols and water).

glycemic index (GI) The blood glucose response of a given food, compared to a standard (typically, glucose or white bread). Glycemic index is influenced by starch structure, fiber content, food processing, physical structure, and macronutrients in the meal such as fat.

glycerol A three-carbon alcohol used to form triglycerides.

glycogen A carbohydrate made of multiple units of glucose with a highly branched structure. It is the storage form of glucose in humans and is synthesized (and stored) in the liver and muscles.

glycosylation The process by which glucose attaches to (glycates) other compounds, such as proteins.

goiter An enlargement of the thyroid gland; this is often caused by insufficient iodine in the diet.

Golgi complex The cell organelle near the nucleus that processes newly synthesized protein for secretion or distribution to other organelles.

gout A form of arthritis caused by the buildup of uric acid crystals in the joints.

green revolution Refers to increases in crop yields that accompanied the introduction of new agricultural technologies in less-developed countries, beginning in the 1960s. The key technologies were high-yielding, disease-resistant strains of rice, wheat, and corn; greater use of fertilizer and water; and improved cultivation practices.

gruel A thin mixture of grains or legumes in milk or water.

gums Polysaccharides occurring naturally that cause an increase in viscosity; used as thickeners, gels, emulsifiers, and stabilizers.

gut-associated lymphoid tissues (GALT) Clusters of lymphoid cells located throughout the gastrointestinal tract that destroy pathogens.

hard water Water that contains high levels of calcium and magnesium.

hazard Chance that injury will result from use of a substance.

heart attack Rapid fall in heart function caused by reduced blood flow through the heart's blood vessels. Often part of the heart dies in the process. Technically called a myocardial infarction.

heavy drinking Any pattern of alcohol consumption in excess of 4 drinks in 1 day or 14 drinks per week for men or 3 drinks in 1 day or 7 drinks per week for women.

helminth Parasitic worm that can contaminate food, water, feces, animals, and other substances.

hematocrit The percentage of blood made up of red blood cells.

heme iron Iron provided from animal tissues in the form of hemoglobin and myoglobin. Approximately 40% of the iron in meat is heme iron; it is readily absorbed.

hemicellulose A nonfermentable fiber containing xylose, galactose, glucose, and other monosaccharides bonded together.

hemochromatosis A disorder of iron metabolism characterized by increased iron absorption and deposition in the liver and heart. This eventually poisons the cells in those organs.

hemoglobin The iron-containing part of the red blood cell that carries oxygen to the cells and carbon dioxide away from the cells. The heme iron portion is also responsible for the red color of blood.

hemolytic uremic syndrome (HUS) Disease characterized by anemia caused by destruction of red blood cells (hemolytic), acute kidney failure (uremic), and a low platelet count.

hemopoietic Stem cells in the bone marrow that are capable of developing into blood cells.

hemorrhage An escape of blood from blood vessels.

hemorrhagic stroke Damage to part of the brain resulting from rupture of a blood vessel and subsequent bleeding within or over the internal surface of the brain.

hemorrhoid A pronounced swelling of a large vein, particularly veins found in the anal region.

hemostasis The process of stopping blood loss.

hepatic portal circulation The portion of the circulatory system that uses a large vein (portal vein) to carry nutrient-rich blood from capillaries in the intestines and portions of the stomach to the liver.

hepatic portal vein Large vein leaving the intestine and stomach and connecting to the liver.

high-density lipoprotein (HDL) The lipoprotein in the blood that picks up cholesterol from dying cells and other sources and transfers it to the other lipoproteins in the bloodstream, as well as directly to the liver; low HDL increases the risk for cardiovascular disease.

high-fructose corn syrup (HFCS) Corn syrup that has been manufactured to contain between 42% and 90% fructose.

high-intensity interval training (HIIT) Short, intense aerobic workout that alternates short periods of intense anaerobic exercise with less-intense recovery periods to provide improved athletic capacity and condition, improved glucose metabolism, and improved fat burning.

high-quality (complete) proteins Dietary proteins that contain ample amounts of all nine essential amino acids.

homocysteine An amino acid that arises from the metabolism of methionine. Vitamin B-6, folate, vitamin B-12, and choline are required for its metabolism. Elevated levels are associated with an increased risk of cardiovascular disease.

hospice care A program offering care that emphasizes comfort and dignity at the end of life.

human immunodeficiency virus (HIV) The virus that leads to acquired immune deficiency syndrome (AIDS).

hunger The primarily physiological (internal) drive to find and eat food.

hydrogenation The addition of hydrogen to a carbon-carbon double bond, producing a single carbon-carbon bond with two hydrogens attached to each carbon.

hydrolyzed protein formula Infant formula in which the proteins have been broken down into smaller peptides and amino acids to improve digestibility and reduce exposure to potential food allergens; sometimes called *predigested* or *hypoallergenic infant formula.*

hydroxyapatite Crystalline compound containing calcium, phosphorus, and sometimes fluoride, also known as bone mineral.

hygiene hypothesis Assumption that reduced exposure to microorganisms in the environment (e.g., as a result of overuse of antibacterial soaps and antibiotics) impairs proper development of the immune system, making a person more susceptible to allergies and autoimmune diseases.

hyperglycemia High blood glucose, above 125 milligrams per 100 milliliters of blood.

hypertension A condition in which blood pressure remains persistently elevated. Obesity, inactivity, alcohol intake, excess salt intake, and genetics may each contribute to the problem.

hypertonic Having high concentration of solutes.

hypochromic Pale in color (in reference to red blood cells), as could occur with inadequate hemoglobin content.

hypoglycemia Low blood glucose, below 40 to 50 milligrams per 100 milliliters of blood for nondiabetics.

hyponatremia Dangerously low blood sodium level.

hypothalamus A region at the base of the brain that contains cells that play a role in the regulation of energy intake, respiration, body temperature, satiety, and other body functions.

hypotheses Tentative explanations by a scientist to explain a phenomenon.

hypotonic Having low concentration of solutes.

identical twins Two offspring that develop from a single ovum and sperm and, consequently, have the same genetic makeup.

ileocecal sphincter The ring of smooth muscle between the end of the small intestine and the beginning of the large intestine.

ileum Last segment of the small intestine; approximately 5 feet in length.

immunoglobulins Proteins found in the blood that bind to specific antigens; also called antibodies. The five major classes of immunoglobulins play different roles in antibody-mediated immunity.

incidental food additives Additives that appear in food products indirectly, from environmental contamination of food ingredients or during the manufacturing process.

indirect calorimetry A method to measure energy use by the body by measuring oxygen uptake and carbon dioxide output. Formulas are then used to convert this gas exchange value into energy use, estimating the proportion of energy nutrients that are being oxidized for energy in the fuel mix.

infertility Inability of a couple to conceive after 1 year of unprotected intercourse.

inflammatory response A response that occurs when tissues are injured, causing the damaged cells to release chemicals that result in blood vessels leaking fluid into the tissues, causing swelling and inflammation.

inorganic Any substance lacking carbon atoms bonded to hydrogen atoms in the chemical structure.

insulin A hormone produced by the pancreas. One of insulin's roles is to increase the synthesis of glycogen in the liver and the movement of glucose from the bloodstream into body cells.

intentional food additives Additives knowingly (directly) incorporated into food products by manufacturers.

intracellular fluid Fluid contained within a cell; it represents about two-thirds of body fluid.

intrinsic factor A proteinlike compound produced by the stomach that enhances vitamin B-12 absorption.

ion A positively or negatively charged atom.

irradiation A process in which radiation energy is applied to foods, creating compounds (free radicals) within the food that destroy cell membranes, break down DNA, link proteins together, limit enzyme activity, and alter a variety of other proteins and cell functions of microorganisms that can lead to food spoilage. This process does not make the food radioactive.

isoflavones Phytochemicals produced in legumes, with soybeans being the most common source of isoflavones in food.

isotonic Having equal concentration of solutes.

jejunum Middle segment of the small intestine; approximately 4 feet in length.

ketone bodies Partial breakdown products of fat that contain three or four carbons.

ketosis The condition of having a high concentration of ketone bodies and related breakdown products in the bloodstream and tissues.

kidney nephrons The units of kidney cells that filter wastes from the bloodstream and deposit them into the urine.

kilocalorie (kcal) Heat energy needed to raise the temperature of 1000 grams (1 L) of water 1 degree Celsius.

kwashiorkor A disease occurring primarily in young children who have an existing disease and consume a marginal amount of calories and insufficient protein in relation to needs. The child generally suffers from infections and exhibits edema, poor growth, weakness, and an increased susceptibility to further illness.

kyphosis Abnormally increased bending of the spine.

lactase An enzyme made by absorptive cells of the small intestine; this enzyme digests lactose to glucose and galactose.

lactation The period of milk secretion following pregnancy; typically called *breastfeeding*.

lacteal Lymphatic vessels that absorb fats from the small intestine.

lactic acid A three-carbon acid formed during anaerobic cell metabolism; a partial breakdown product of glucose; also called *lactate*.

lactic acid bacteria Strains of bacteria that produce lactic acid from fermentation of dairy products; may confer health benefits when consumed as probiotics.

Lactobacillus bifidus factor A protective factor secreted in the colostrum that encourages growth of beneficial bacteria in the newborn's intestines.

lactoovovegetarian A person who consumes plant products, dairy products, and eggs.

lactose intolerance A condition in which symptoms such as abdominal gas and bloating appear as a result of severe lactose maldigestion.

lactose Glucose bonded to galactose; also known as *milk sugar*.

lactovegetarian A person who consumes plant products and dairy products.

lanugo Downlike hair that appears after a person has lost much body fat through semistarvation. The hair stands erect and traps air, acting as insulation for the body to compensate for the relative lack of body fat, which usually functions as insulation.

laxative A medication or other substance that stimulates evacuation of the intestinal tract.

lean body mass Body weight minus fat storage weight equals lean body mass. This includes organs such as the brain, muscles, and liver, as well as bone and blood and other body fluids.

lecithin A group of phospholipid compounds that are major components of cell membranes.

leptin A hormone made by adipose tissue in proportion to total fat stores in the body that influences long-term regulation of fat mass. Leptin also influences reproductive functions, as well as other body processes, such as release of the hormone insulin.

let-down reflex A reflex stimulated by infant suckling that causes the release (ejection) of milk from milk ducts in the mother's breasts; also called *milk ejection reflex*.

leukocyte White blood cell; cell of the immune system.

life expectancy The average length of life for a given group of people born in a specific year.

life span The potential oldest age a person can reach.

lignin A nonfermentable fiber made up of a multiringed alcohol (noncarbohydrate) structure.

limiting amino acid The essential amino acid in lowest concentration in a food or diet relative to body needs.

linoleic acid An essential omega-6 fatty acid with 18 carbons and two double bonds.

lipase Fat-digesting enzyme produced by the salivary glands, stomach, and pancreas.

lipid A compound containing much carbon and hydrogen, little oxygen, and sometimes other atoms. Lipids do not dissolve in water and include fats, oils, and cholesterol.

lipoprotein lipase An enzyme attached to the cells that form the inner lining of blood vessels; it breaks down triglycerides into free fatty acids and glycerol.

lipoprotein A compound found in the bloodstream containing a core of lipids with a shell composed of protein, phospholipid, and cholesterol.

lobules Saclike structures in the breast that store milk; also called *alveoli*.

locavore Someone who eats food grown or produced locally or within a certain radius such as 50, 100, or 500 miles.

long-chain fatty acid A fatty acid that contains 12 or more carbons.

low birth weight (LBW) Referring to any infant weighing less than 2.5 kilograms (5.5 pounds) at birth; most commonly results from preterm birth.

low-density lipoprotein (LDL) The lipoprotein in the blood containing primarily cholesterol; elevated LDL is strongly linked to cardiovascular disease risk.

lower esophageal sphincter A circular muscle that constricts the opening of the esophagus to the stomach. Also called the *gastroesophageal sphincter* or the *cardiac sphincter*.

lower quality (incomplete) proteins Dietary proteins that are low in or lack one or more essential amino acids.

lower-body obesity The type of obesity in which fat storage is primarily located in the buttocks and thigh area. Also known as gynoid or gynecoid obesity.

lumen The hollow opening inside a tube, such as the GI tract.

lymph A clear fluid that flows through lymph vessels; carries most forms of fat after their absorption by the small intestine.

lymph nodes Clusters of lymphoid tissue, situated along the lymph vessels, that trap and destroy pathogens.

lymphatic system A system of vessels and lymph that accepts fluid surrounding cells and large particles, such as products of fat absorption. Lymph eventually passes into the bloodstream from the lymphatic system.

lymphocyte The white blood cell responsible for the immune response; regulates antibody production.

lymphoid tissue Specialized cells that participate in the immune response; includes the thymus, spleen, lymph nodes, and white blood cells.

lysosome A cellular organelle that contains digestive enzymes for use inside the cell for turnover of cell parts.

lysozyme An enzyme produced by a variety of cells; it can destroy bacteria by rupturing their cell membranes.

macrocytic (megaloblastic) Large cell size.

macronutrient A nutrient needed in gram quantities in a diet.

macrophages Large white blood cells that arise from monocytes; one of several types of white blood cells that phagocytize pathogens and signal other white blood cells to mount an immune response.

major mineral Vital to health, a mineral that is required in the diet in amounts greater than 100 milligrams per day.

malignant Malicious; in reference to a tumor, the property of spreading locally and to distant sites.

malnutrition Failing health that results from longstanding dietary practices that do not coincide with nutritional needs.

maltase An enzyme made by absorptive cells of the small intestine; this enzyme digests maltose to two glucoses.

maltose Glucose bonded to glucose.

marasmus A disease resulting from consuming a grossly insufficient amount of protein and calories; one of the diseases classed as protein-calorie malnutrition. Victims have little or no fat stores, little muscle mass, and poor strength. Death from infections is common.

market basket Food the FDA buys, prepares, and analyzes as part of the ongoing Total Diet Study (TDS), which monitors levels of about 800 contaminants and nutrients in the average U.S. diet; the number varies slightly from year to year. About 280 kinds of foods and beverages from representative areas of the country are included four times a year.

megadose Large intake of a nutrient beyond estimates of needs or what would be found in a balanced diet; 2 to 10 times human needs is a starting point.

megaloblast A large, immature red blood cell that results from the inability of the cell to divide normally (*megalo* = large; *blast* = primitive or immature).

megaloblastic (macrocytic) anemia Anemia characterized by the presence of abnormally large red blood cells.

Menkes syndrome An inherited X-linked recessive pattern disorder that affects copper levels in the body.

menopause The cessation of the menstrual cycle in women, usually beginning at about 50 years of age.

metabolic syndrome A condition in which a person has poor blood glucose regulation, hypertension, increased blood triglycerides, and other health problems. This condition is usually accompanied by obesity, lack of physical activity, and a diet high in refined carbohydrates. Also called Syndrome X.

metabolic water Water formed as a by-product of carbohydrate, lipid, and protein metabolism.

metabolism Chemical processes in the body by which energy is provided in useful forms and vital activities are sustained.

metastasize The spreading of disease from one part of the body to another, even to parts of the body that are remote from the site of the original tumor. Cancer cells can spread via blood vessels, the lymphatic system, or direct growth of the tumor.

methotrexate A drug used to treat cancer, because it interferes with the growth of cells that reproduce quickly.

methyl group In chemistry, a carbon atom that shares bonds with three hydrogen atoms. The methyl group is the omega end of a fatty acid.

microbiome Entire collection of microorganisms, their genes, and their environment.

microbiota Community of microorganisms living in a particular region; with regard to our discussion of probiotics, the community of microorganisms coexisting on and within the human body.

microcytic Small cell size.

micronutrient A nutrient needed in milligram or microgram quantities in a diet.

microvilli Extensive folds on the muscosal surface of the absorptive cells.

mineral Element used in the body to promote chemical reactions and to form body structures.

mitochondria Organelles that are the main sites of energy production in a cell. They contain the pathway for oxidizing fat for fuel, among other metabolic pathways.

moderate drinking For men, consuming no more than 4 drinks in 1 day AND no more than 14 drinks per week; for women, consuming no more than 3 drinks in 1 day AND no more than 7 drinks per week.

moderate-intensity aerobic physical activity Aerobic activity that increases a person's heart rate and breathing to some extent (4–6 on RPE scale). Examples include brisk walking, dancing, swimming, or bicycling on level terrain.

monocyte The white blood cell that ingests foreign cells; also called a phagocyte.

monoglyceride A breakdown product of a triglyceride consisting of one fatty acid attached to a glycerol backbone.

monosaccharide Simple sugar, such as glucose, that is not broken down further during digestion.

monounsaturated fatty acid A fatty acid containing one carbon-carbon double bond.

motility Generally, the ability to move spontaneously. It also refers to movement of food through the GI tract.

mucilage A viscous fiber consisting of chains of galactose, mannose, and other monosaccharides; characteristically found in seaweed.

mucus A thick fluid secreted by many cells throughout the body. It contains a compound that has both carbohydrate and protein parts. It acts as a lubricant and means of protection for cells.

multiple sclerosis An unpredictable disease of the central nervous system that can range from relatively benign to somewhat disabling to devastating, as communication between the brain and other parts of the body is disrupted.

muscle tissue A type of tissue adapted to contract, to cause movement.

muscle-strengthening activity Physical activity that increases skeletal muscle strength, power, endurance, and mass. Examples include lifting weights, using weight machines, and calisthenics (e.g., push-ups).

myelin A lipid and protein combination (lipoprotein) that covers nerve fibers.

myocardial infarction Death of part of the heart muscle. Also termed a *heart attack*.

myoglobin Iron-containing protein that binds oxygen in muscle tissue.

negative energy balance The state in which energy intake is less than energy expended, resulting in weight loss.

negative protein balance A state in which protein intake is less than related protein losses, such as often seen during acute illness.

neotame General-purpose, nonnutritive sweetener that is approximately 7000 to 13,000 times sweeter than table sugar. It has a chemical structure similar to aspartame.

nervous system The body system consisting of the brain, spinal cord, nerves, and sensory receptors. This system detects sensations, directs movements, and controls physiological and intellectual functions.

nervous tissue Tissue composed of highly branched, elongated cells that transport nerve impulses from one part of the body to another.

neural tube defect A defect in the formation of the neural tube occurring during early fetal development. This type of defect results in various nervous system disorders, such as spina bifida. Folate deficiency in the pregnant woman increases the risk that the fetus will develop this disorder.

neuron The structural and functional unit of the nervous system. Consists of a cell body, dendrites, and an axon.

neurotransmitter A compound made by a nerve cell that allows for communication between it and other cells.

neutrophil A common white blood cell that fights infections; levels rise during bacterial or fungal infections.

night blindness Vitamin A deficiency disorder that results in loss of the ability to see under low-light conditions.

night eating syndrome Eating a lot of food in the late evening and nocturnal awakenings with ingestion of food.

nitrosamine A carcinogen formed from nitrates and breakdown products of amino acids; can lead to cancer.

nonceliac gluten sensitivity (NCGS) One or more of a variety of immune-related conditions with symptoms similar to celiac disease that are precipitated by the ingestion of gluten in people who do not have celiac disease.

nonessential amino acids Amino acids that can be synthesized by a healthy body in sufficient amounts; there are 11 nonessential amino acids. These are also called *dispensable amino acids.*

nonfermentable fiber A fiber that is not easily metabolized by intestinal bacteria; also called *insoluble fiber.*

nonheme iron Iron provided from plant sources and animal tissues other than in the forms of hemoglobin and myoglobin. Nonheme iron is less efficiently absorbed than heme iron; absorption is closely dependent on body needs.

nonspecific immunity Defenses that stop the invasion of pathogens; requires no previous encounter with a pathogen; also called *innate immunity.*

norepinephrine A neurotransmitter from nerve endings and a hormone from the adrenal gland. It is released in times of stress and is involved in hunger regulation, blood glucose regulation, and other body processes.

NSAIDs Nonsteroidal anti-inflammatory drugs; include aspirin, ibuprofen (Advil®), and naproxen (Aleve®).

nutrient density The ratio derived by dividing a food's nutrient content by its calorie content. When the food's contribution to our nutrient need for that nutrient exceeds its contribution to our calorie need, the food is considered to have a favorable nutrient density.

nutrients Chemical substances in food that contribute to health, many of which are essential parts of a diet. Nutrients nourish us by providing calories to fulfill energy needs, materials for building body parts, and factors

to regulate necessary chemical processes in the body.

nutrigenetics Study of the effects of genes on nutritional health, such as variations in nutrient requirements and responsiveness to dietary modifications.

nutrigenomics Study of how food impacts health through its interaction with our genes and its subsequent effect on gene expression.

nutrition security Secure access to a nutritious diet coupled with a sanitary environment and adequate health services and care.

nutritional genomics Study of interactions between nutrition and genetics; includes nutrigenetics and nutrigenomics.

nutritional state The nutritional health of a person as determined by anthropometric measurements (height, weight, circumferences, and so on), biochemical measurements of nutrients or their by-products in blood and urine, a clinical (physical) examination, a dietary analysis, and economic evaluation; also called nutritional status.

obesity Disorder involving excessive body fat that increases the risk of health problems.

oleic acid An omega-9 fatty acid with 18 carbons and one double bond.

omega-3 (ω-3) fatty acid An unsaturated fatty acid with the first double bond on the third carbon from the methyl end ($-CH_3$).

omega-6 (ω-6) fatty acid An unsaturated fatty acid with the first double bond on the sixth carbon from the methyl end ($-CH_3$).

organ A group of tissues designed to perform a specific function; for example, the heart, which contains muscle tissue, nerve tissue, and so on.

organ system A collection of organs that work together to perform an overall function.

organelles Compartments, particles, or filaments that perform specialized functions within a cell.

organic food Food grown without use of pesticides, synthetic fertilizers, sewage sludge, genetically modified organisms, antibiotics, hormones, or ionizing radiation.

osmosis The passage of water through a membrane from a less concentrated compartment to a more concentrated compartment.

osteoarthritis A degenerative joint condition caused by a breakdown of cartilage in joints. It often results from "wear and tear" due to repetitive motions or the pressure of excess body weight.

osteoblast Bone cells that initiate the synthesis of new bone.

osteocalcin Small protein in the organic matrix of bone.

osteoclast Bone cells that break down bone and subsequently release bone minerals into the blood.

osteocyte Osteoblast embedded into the bone matrix.

osteomalacia Adult form of rickets. The bones have low mineral density and subsequently are at risk for fracture.

osteopenia A bone disease defined by low mineral density.

osteoporosis The presence of a stress-induced fracture or a T-score of -2.5 or lower. The bones are porous and fragile due to low mineral density.

ostomy Surgically created short circuit in intestinal flow where the end point usually opens from the abdominal cavity rather than the anus; for example, a colostomy. Short circuiting the intestinal flow means more water is lost in fecal matter than would be if the intestinal tract were intact.

overnutrition A state in which nutritional intake greatly exceeds the body's needs.

ovum The egg cell from which a fetus eventually develops if the egg is fertilized by a sperm cell.

oxalic acid (oxalate) An organic acid found in spinach, rhubarb, beet greens, chard, and sweet potatoes. It can depress the absorption of certain minerals, such as calcium, but only in the food itself.

oxidation The process of losing an electron during a chemical reaction.

oxidative stress Imbalance between the production of reactive compounds and the body's ability to protect against their adverse effects.

oxidize In the most basic sense, the loss of an electron or gain of an oxygen by a chemical substance. This change typically alters the shape and/or function of the substance.

oxytocin A hormone secreted by the pituitary gland. It causes contraction of the musclelike cells surrounding the ducts of the breasts and the smooth muscle of the uterus.

parasite An organism that lives in or on another organism and derives nourishment from it.

parathyroid hormone (PTH) A hormone made by the parathyroid glands that increases synthesis of the vitamin D hormone and aids calcium release from bone and calcium conservation by the kidneys, among other functions.

Parkinson's disease Disease that belongs to a group of conditions called motor system disorders, which are the result of the loss of dopamine-producing brain cells. The four primary symptoms of PD are tremor, or trembling in hands, arms, legs, jaw, and face; rigidity, or stiffness of the limbs and trunk; bradykinesia, or slowness of movement; and postural instability, or impaired balance and coordination.

passive diffusion Movement of a substance across a semipermeable membrane from an area of higher solute concentration to an area of lower solute concentration. This type of transport does not require a carrier and does not require energy.

pasteurizing The process of heating food products to kill pathogenic microorganisms and reduce the total number of bacteria.

pectin A viscous fiber containing chains of galacturonic acid and other monosaccharides; characteristically found between plant cell walls.

pellagra Niacin-deficiency disease characterized by dementia, diarrhea, and dermatitis, and possibly leading to death.

pepsin A protein-digesting enzyme produced by the stomach.

peptide bond A chemical bond formed between amino acids in a protein.

percentile Classification of a measurement of a unit into divisions of 100 units.

perforation A hole made by boring or piercing. With reference to the gastrointestinal tract, the hole is in the wall of the esophagus, stomach, intestine, rectum, or gallbladder. Complications include bleeding and infection.

periodization Cycling the volume, intensity, and activities of workouts throughout the training season.

periosteum A specialized connective tissue covering all bones and having bone-forming potential.

peristalsis A coordinated muscular contraction used to propel food down the gastrointestinal tract.

pernicious anemia The anemia that results from a lack of vitamin B-12 absorption; it is pernicious because of associated nerve degeneration that can result in eventual paralysis and death.

peroxisome A cell organelle that destroys toxic products within the cell.

pH A measure of relative acidity or alkalinity of a solution. The pH scale is 0 to 14. A pH of 7 is neutral; a pH below 7 is acidic; a pH above 7 is alkaline.

phagocytes Immune cells (e.g., neutrophils and macrophages) that engulf substances.

phagocytosis A process in which a cell forms an indentation, and solid particles enter the indentation and are engulfed by the cell.

pharynx The organ of the digestive tract and respiratory tract located at the back of the oral and nasal cavities, commonly known as the throat.

phenylketonuria (PKU) Disease caused by a defect in the liver's ability to metabolize the amino acid phenylalanine into the amino acid tyrosine; untreated, toxic by-products of phenylalanine build up in the body and lead to mental retardation.

phlebotomy Therapeutic blood removal, as a blood donation, for the purpose of ridding the body of excess iron.

phosphocreatine (PCr) A high-energy compound that can be used to reform ATP. It is used primarily during bursts of activity, such as lifting and jumping.

phospholipid Any of a class of fat-related substances that contain phosphorus, fatty acids, and a nitrogen-containing component. Phospholipids are an essential part of every cell.

photosynthesis Process by which plants use energy from the sun to synthesize energy-yielding compounds, such as glucose.

physical activity Any movement of skeletal muscles that requires energy.

physical fitness The ability to perform moderate to vigorous activity without undue fatigue.

physiological anemia The normal increase in blood volume in pregnancy that dilutes the concentration of red blood cells, resulting in anemia; also called *hemodilution*.

phytic acid (phytate) A constituent of plant fiber that chemically binds minerals and prevents their absorption. Phytic acid can depress calcium absorption from other foods present in the GI tract.

phytochemical A chemical found in plants. Some phytochemicals may contribute to a reduced risk of cancer or cardiovascular disease in people who consume them regularly.

pica The practice of eating nonfood items, such as dirt, laundry starch, or clay.

pinocytosis A process in which a cell forms an indentation, and fluid enters the indentation and is engulfed by the cell.

placebo Generally, an inactive medicine or treatment used to disguise the treatments given to the participants in an experiment.

placenta An organ that forms in the uterus in pregnant women. Through this organ, oxygen and nutrients from the mother's blood are transferred to the fetus, and fetal wastes are removed. The placenta also releases hormones that maintain the state of pregnancy.

plaque A cholesterol-rich substance deposited in the blood vessels; it contains various white blood cells, smooth muscle cells, various proteins, cholesterol and other lipids, and eventually calcium.

plasma The fluid, extracellular portion of blood.

platelet A protoplasmic disc smaller than a red blood cell that promotes coagulation; also called *thrombocyte*.

polycystic ovary syndrome (PCOS) A condition of hormonal imbalance (e.g., elevated testosterone and insulin) in a woman that can lead to infertility, weight gain in the abdominal region, excessive growth of body hair, and acne.

polypeptide A group of 10 to 2000 or more amino acids bonded together to form proteins.

polysaccharides Carbohydrates containing many glucose units, from 10 to 1000 or more.

polyunsaturated fatty acid A fatty acid containing two or more carbon-carbon double bonds.

pool The amount of a nutrient stored within the body that can be mobilized when needed.

positive energy balance The state in which energy intake is greater than energy expended, generally resulting in weight gain.

positive protein balance A state in which protein intake exceeds related protein losses, as is needed during times of growth.

prebiotic Selectively fermented ingredient that results in specific changes in the composition and/or activity of the gastrointestinal microbiota, thus conferring benefits upon the host.

preeclampsia A form of gestational hypertension characterized by protein in the urine.

preservatives Compounds that extend the shelf life of foods by inhibiting microbial growth or minimizing the destructive effect of oxygen and metals.

preterm An infant born before 37 weeks of gestation; also referred to as *premature*.

primary hypertension Blood pressure of 140/90 mmHg or higher with no identified cause; also called *essential hypertension*.

primary lactose maldigestion Develops after early childhood, at about age 3 to 5 years, when the production of the enzyme lactase decreases.

probiotic Live microorganisms that, when administered in adequate amounts, confer health benefits on the host.

progression Incremental increase in frequency, intensity, and time spent in each type of physical activity over several weeks or months.

prolactin A hormone secreted by the pituitary gland that stimulates the synthesis of milk in the breast.

prostate gland A solid, chestnut-shaped organ surrounding the first part of the urinary tract in the male. The prostate gland secretes substances into the semen.

protein Food and body compounds made of more than 100 amino acids; proteins contain carbon, hydrogen, oxygen, nitrogen, and sometimes other atoms in a specific configuration. Proteins contain the form of nitrogen most easily used by the human body.

protein equilibrium A state in which protein intake is equal to related protein losses; the person is said to be in protein balance.

protein turnover The process by which cells break down old proteins and resynthesize new proteins. In this way, the cell will have the proteins it needs to function at that time.

protein-calorie malnutrition (PCM) A condition resulting from regularly consuming insufficient amounts of calories and protein. The deficiency eventually results in body wasting, primarily of lean tissue, and an increased susceptibility to infections. Also known as *protein-energy malnutrition (PEM)*.

proton pump inhibitor A medication that inhibits the ability of gastric cells to secrete hydrogen ions. Low doses of this class of medications are also available without prescription (e.g., omeprazole [Prilosec]R).

protozoa One-celled animals that are more complex than bacteria. Disease-causing protozoa can be spread through food and water.

provitamin A A substance that can be converted into vitamin A.

purging disorder An eating disorder characterized by repeated purging (e.g., by self-induced vomiting) to induce weight loss even in the absence of binge eating.

pyloric sphincter Ring of smooth muscle between the stomach and the small intestine.

pyruvic acid A three-carbon compound formed during glucose metabolism; also called *pyruvate*.

R-proteins Proteins produced by the salivary glands that bind to free vitamin B-12 in the stomach and protect it from stomach acid.

radiation Literally, energy that is emitted from a center in all directions. Various forms of radiation energy include X rays and ultra-violet rays from the sun.

rancid Containing products of decomposed fatty acids that have an unpleasant flavor and odor.

receptor A site in a cell at which compounds (such as hormones) bind. Cells that contain receptors for a specific compound are partially controlled by that compound.

recombinant DNA technology A test tube technology that rearranges DNA sequences in an organism by cutting the DNA, adding or deleting a DNA sequence, and rejoining DNA molecules with a series of enzymes.

Recommended Dietary Allowance (RDA) Nutrient intake amount sufficient to meet the needs of 97% to 98% of the individuals in a specific life stage.

rectum Terminal portion of the large intestine.

reduction The process of gaining an electron during a chemical reaction.

registered dietitian (RD) A person who has completed a baccalaureate degree program approved by the Accreditation Council for Education in Nutrition and Dietetics (ACEND), performed at least 1200 hours of supervised professional practice, passed a registration examination, and complies with continuing education requirements.

registered dietitian nutritionist (RDN) The RDN is the updated credential formerly abbreviated RD. The credential was updated to better reflect the scope of practice of the dietitian and to align with the new name of the professional organization for dietitians, the Academy of Nutrition and Dietetics.

relapse prevention A series of strategies used to help prevent and cope with weight-control lapses, such as recognizing high-risk situations and deciding beforehand on appropriate responses.

repolarization During nerve impulse transmission, the restoration of the resting state of the nerve cell membrane.

reserve capacity The extent to which an organ can preserve essentially normal function despite decreasing cell number or cell activity.

resorption The process of losing substance. Bone resorption is part of the initial process for remodeling and growth.

resting metabolism The amount of calories the body uses when the person has not eaten in 4 hours and is resting (e.g., 15 to 30 minutes) and awake in a warm, quiet environment. It is usually slightly higher (10%) than basal metabolism due to the less strict criteria for the test; often referred to as *resting metabolic rate (RMR)*.

retina A light-sensitive lining in the back of the eye. It contains retinal.

retinal Aldehyde form of vitamin A.

retinoic acid Acid form of vitamin A.

retinoids Chemical forms of preformed vitamin A; one source is animal foods.

retinol Alcohol form of vitamin A.

retinyl Storage form of vitamin A.

rheumatoid arthritis A degenerative joint condition resulting from an autoimmune disease that causes inflammation in the joints and other sites of the body.

ribonucleic acid (RNA) The single-stranded nucleic acid involved in the transcription of genetic information and translation of that information into protein structure.

ribosomes Cytoplasmic particles that mediate the linking together of amino acids to form proteins; may exist freely in the cytoplasm or attached to endoplasmic reticulum.

rickets A disease characterized by poor mineralization of newly synthesized bones because of low calcium content. Arising in infants and children, this deficiency is caused by insufficient amounts of the vitamin D hormone in the body.

risk factors A term used frequently when discussing the factors contributing to the development of a disease. A risk factor is an aspect of our lives, such as heredity, lifestyle choices (e.g., smoking), or nutritional habits.

saccharin Alternative sweetener that yields no energy to the body; 300 times sweeter than sucrose.

safety Relative certainty that a substance will not cause injury.

saliva Watery fluid, produced by the salivary glands in the mouth, that contains lubricants, enzymes, and other substances.

sarcopenia In general, loss of muscle tissue. Among older adults, this loss of lean mass greatly increases their risk of illness and death.

sarcopenic obesity Loss of muscle mass accompanied by gains in fat mass.

satiety A state in which there is no longer a desire to eat; a feeling of satisfaction.

saturated fatty acid A fatty acid containing no carbon-carbon double bonds.

scavenger cells Specific form of white blood cells that can bury themselves in the artery wall and accumulate LDL. As these cells take up LDL, they contribute to the development of atherosclerosis.

scurvy The vitamin C deficiency disease characterized by weakness, fatigue, slow wound healing, opening of previously healed wounds, bone pain, fractures, sore and bleeding gums, diarrhea, and pinpoint hemorrhages on the skin.

secondary hypertension Blood pressure of 140/90 mmHg or higher as a result of disease (e.g., kidney dysfunction or sleep apnea) or drug use.

secondary lactose maldigestion Occurs when production of the enzyme lactase declines for no apparent reason. When significant symptoms develop after lactose intake, it is then called *lactose intolerance.*

secretory vesicles Membrane-bound vesicles produced by the Golgi complex; contain protein and other compounds to be secreted by the cell.

self-monitoring Tracking foods eaten and conditions affecting eating; actions are usually recorded in a diary, along with location, time, and state of mind. This is a tool to help people understand more about their eating habits.

sequestrants Compounds that bind free metal ions. By so doing, they reduce the ability of ions to cause rancidity in foods containing fat.

serum Protein-rich portion of blood that separates out when blood coagulates.

set-point Theory of weight status that refers to the close regulation of body weight. It is not known what cells control this set point or how it functions in weight regulation. There is evidence, however, that complex mechanisms exist that help regulate weight.

sickle cell disease (sickle cell anemia) An illness that results from a malformation of the red blood cell because of an incorrect structure in part of its hemoglobin protein chains.

sigmoid colon Last segment of the large intestine that carries feces from the descending colon to the rectum.

simple sugar Monosaccharide or disaccharide in the diet.

sleeve gastrectomy Surgical reduction of stomach by about 75% (to about the size of a banana). Also known as the gastric sleeve.

small for gestational age (SGA) Referring to infants who weigh less than the expected weight for their length of gestation.

This corresponds to less than 2.5 kilograms (5.5 pounds) in a full-term newborn. A preterm infant who is also SGA will most likely develop some medical complications.

soft water   Water that contains a high level of sodium.

solvent   A liquid substance in which other substances dissolve.

sorbitol   Alcohol derivative of glucose that yields about 3 kcal/g but is slowly absorbed from the small intestine; used in some sugarless gums and dietetic foods.

specific immunity   Function of white blood cells directed at specific antigens; also called *adaptive immunity*.

spina bifida   Birth defect resulting from improper closure of the neural tube during embryonic development. The spinal cord or fluid may bulge outside the spinal column.

spleen   Lymphoid organ located near the stomach that filters aged and dead cells and foreign proteins out of blood.

spontaneous abortion   Cessation of pregnancy and expulsion of the embryo or nonviable fetus prior to 20 weeks' gestation. This is the result of natural causes, such as a genetic defect or developmental problem; also called *miscarriage*.

starch   A carbohydrate made of multiple units of glucose attached together in a form the body can digest; also known as *complex carbohydrate*.

sterol   A compound containing a multi-ring (steroid) structure and a hydroxyl group (–OH). Cholesterol is a typical example.

stevia   Alternative sweetener derived from South American shrub; 100 to 300 times sweeter than sucrose.

stimulus control   Altering the environment to minimize the stimuli for eating (e.g., removing foods from sight by storing them in kitchen cabinets).

stress fracture   A fracture that occurs from repeated jarring of a bone. Common sites include bones of the foot.

stroke   A decrease or loss in blood flow to the brain that results from a blood clot or other change in arteries in the brain. This in turn causes the death of brain tissue. Also called a *cerebrovascular accident*.

stromal   Stem cells that can produce bone, cartilage, and fat.

subclinical   Stage of a disease or disorder not severe enough to produce symptoms that can be detected or diagnosed.

sucralose   Alternative sweetener that has chlorines in place of 3 hydroxyl (–OH) groups on sucrose; 600 times sweeter than sucrose.

sucrase   An enzyme made by absorptive cells of the small intestine; this enzyme digests sucrose to glucose and fructose.

sucrose   Fructose bonded to glucose; table sugar.

sugar   A simple carbohydrate with the chemical composition $(CH_2O)n$. The basic unit of all sugars is glucose, a six-carbon ring structure. The primary sugar in the diet is sucrose, which is made up of glucose and fructose.

superoxide dismutase   Antioxidant enzyme system that converts certain free radicals (superoxide anions) into less damaging products (oxygen and hydrogen peroxide).

sustainable agriculture   Agricultural system that provides a secure living for farm families; maintains the natural environment and resources; supports the rural community; and offers respect and fair treatment to all involved, from farm workers to consumers to the animals raised for food.

sustainable development   Economic growth that will simultaneously reduce poverty, protect the environment, and preserve natural capital.

symptom   A change in health status noted by the person with the problem, such as stomach pain.

synapse   The space between one neuron and another neuron (or cell).

synbiotic   Combination of pro- and prebiotics taken to confer health benefits on the host.

systolic blood pressure   The pressure in the arterial blood vessels associated with the pumping of blood from the heart.

teratogen   A compound (natural or synthetic) that may cause or increase the risk of a birth defect. Exposure to a teratogen does not always lead to a birth defect; its effects on the fetus depend on the dose, timing, and duration of exposure.

tetany   A body condition marked by sharp contraction of muscles and failure to relax afterward; usually caused by abnormal calcium metabolism.

theory   An explanation for a phenomenon that has numerous lines of evidence to support it.

thermic effect of food (TEF)   The increase in metabolism that occurs during the digestion, absorption, and metabolism of energy-yielding nutrients. This represents 5% to 10% of calories consumed.

thrifty metabolism   A genetic tendency toward efficient use of energy that results in below-average energy requirements and increased storage of calories as fat.

thrombocyte (platelet)   A protoplasmic disc smaller than a red blood cell; promotes coagulation.

thymus   Lymphoid organ located near the heart that participates in maturation of white blood cells.

thyroid hormones   Hormones produced by the thyroid gland that regulate growth and metabolic rate.

tissue saturation   The limited storage capacity of water-soluble vitamins in the tissues.

tissues   Collections of cells adapted to perform a specific function.

tocopherols   The chemical name for some forms of vitamin E. The alpha form is the most potent.

Tolerable Upper Intake Level (UL)   Maximum chronic daily intake level of a nutrient that is unlikely to cause adverse health effects in almost all people in a specific life stage.

tolerance   Needing more of a substance to achieve the desired effect (e.g., intoxication) or experiencing diminished effects of a given amount of a substance after repeated use.

total parenteral nutrition   The intravenous feeding of all necessary nutrients, including the most basic forms of protein, carbohydrates, lipids, vitamins, minerals, and electrolytes.

toxicity   Capacity of a substance to produce injury or illness at some dosage.

toxicology   Scientific study of harmful substances.

toxin-mediated infection   Occurs when a person eats food containing harmful bacteria. While in the intestinal tract, the bacteria produce toxins that cause illness.

toxins   Poisonous compounds produced by an organism that can cause disease.

trabecular bone   The less dense, more open structure bone found in the inner layer of bones.

trace mineral   Vital to health, a mineral that is required in the diet in amounts less than 100 milligrams per day.

***trans* fatty acid**   A form of an unsaturated fatty acid, usually a monounsaturated one when found in food, in which the hydrogens on both carbons forming the double bond lie on opposite sides of that bond.

transcription   Process by which genetic information stored as DNA within the nucleus is copied to RNA during protein synthesis.

transferrin   Iron-binding protein; controls the level of free iron in blood.

transgenic organism   Organism that contains genes originally present in another organism.

translation   Process by which genetic information copied into RNA dictates the amino acid sequence to form a protein.

transverse colon   Segment of the large intestine that carries feces from the ascending colon, from right to left across the top of the abdomen, to the descending colon.

triglyceride   The major form of lipid in the body and in food. It is composed of three fatty acids bonded to glycerol.

trimesters   Three 13- to 14-week periods into which the normal pregnancy (on average, 40 weeks) is divided somewhat arbitrarily for purposes of discussion and analysis. Development of the offspring, however, is continuous throughout pregnancy, with no specific physiological markers demarcating the transition from one trimester to the next.

trypsin A protein-digesting enzyme secreted by the pancreas to act in the small intestine.

tumor Mass of cells; may be cancerous (malignant) or noncancerous (benign).

type 1 diabetes A form of diabetes characterized by total insulin deficiency due to destruction of insulin-producing cells of the pancreas. Insulin therapy is required.

type 1 osteoporosis Porous trabecular bone characterized by rapid bone demineralization following menopause.

type 2 diabetes A form of diabetes characterized by insulin resistance and often associated with obesity. Insulin therapy can be used but is often not required.

type 2 osteoporosis Porous trabecular and cortical bone observed in men and women after the age of 70.

ulcer Erosion of the tissue lining, usually in the stomach or the upper small intestine. As a group these are generally referred to as peptic ulcers.

ultra-high temperature (UHT) processing Method of sterilizing food by heating it above 275 °F (135 °C) for 1 to 2 seconds. Also called *ultra-heat treatment*.

ultratrace mineral A mineral present in the human diet in trace amounts but that has not been shown to be essential to human health.

umami A brothy, meaty, savory flavor in some foods. Monosodium glutamate enhances this flavor when added to foods.

undernutrition Failing health that results from a longstanding dietary intake that is not enough to meet nutritional needs.

underwater weighing Also known as hydrostatic weighing, this is a method of estimating total body fat by weighing the individual on a standard scale and then weighing him or her again submerged in water. The difference between the two weights is used to estimate total body volume.

underweight A body mass index below 18.5. The cutoff is less precise than for obesity because this condition has been less studied.

upper-body obesity The type of obesity in which fat is stored primarily in the abdominal area; defined as a waist circumference more than 40 inches (102 centimeters) in men and more than 35 inches (88 centimeters) in women; closely associated with a high risk for cardiovascular disease, hypertension, and type 2 diabetes. Also known as android obesity.

urea Nitrogenous waste product of protein metabolism; major source of nitrogen in the urine.

ureter Tube that transports urine from the kidney to the urinary bladder.

urethra Tube that transports urine from the urinary bladder to the outside of the body.

urinary system The body system consisting of the kidneys, urinary bladder, and the ducts that carry urine. This system removes waste products from the circulatory system and regulates blood acid-base balance, overall chemical balance, and water balance in the body.

vasoconstriction The narrowing of blood vessels. As part of hemostasis, this temporarily reduces the flow of blood to the site of injury while a clot is being formed.

vegan A person who eats only plant foods.

vein A blood vessel that carries blood to the heart.

very-low-calorie diet (VLCD) Known also as *protein-sparing modified fast (PSMF)*, this diet allows a person less than 800 calories per day, often in liquid form. Of this, 120 to 480 calories are typically from carbohydrate, and the rest are mostly from high-quality protein.

very-low-density lipoprotein (VLDL) The lipoprotein created in the liver that carries cholesterol and lipids that have been taken up or newly synthesized by the liver.

vigorous-intensity aerobic physical activity Aerobic activity that greatly increases a person's heart rate and breathing (7–8 on RPE scale). Examples include jogging, singles tennis, swimming continuous laps, or bicycling uphill.

villi (singular, villus) The fingerlike protrusions into the small intestine that participate in digestion and absorption of food.

virus The smallest known type of infectious agent, many of which cause disease in humans. A virus is essentially a piece of genetic material surrounded by a coat of protein. They do not metabolize, grow, or move by themselves. They reproduce only with the aid of a living cellular host.

viscous fiber A fiber that is readily fermented by bacteria in the large intestine; also called *soluble fiber*.

vitamin An essential organic (carbon-containing) compound needed in small amounts in the diet to help regulate and support chemical reactions and processes in the body.

vitamin D-2 (ergocalciferol) Form found in nonanimal sources, such as in some mushrooms.

vitamin D₃ (cholecalciferol) Previtamin form found naturally in some animal sources, including fish and egg yolks.

vulnerable employment Employment status groups that are less likely to have formal work arrangements, and are therefore more likely to lack decent working conditions, adequate social security, and "voice" through effective representation by trade unions and similar organizations. Vulnerable employment is often characterized by inadequate earnings, low productivity, and difficult conditions of work that undermine workers' fundamental rights.

water The universal solvent; chemically, H_2O. The body is composed of about 60% water. Water (fluid) needs are about 9 (women) or 13 (men) cups per day; needs are greater if one exercises heavily.

water intoxication Potentially fatal condition that occurs with a high intake of water, which results in a severe dilution of the blood and other fluid compartments.

water-soluble vitamins Vitamins that dissolve in water. These vitamins are the B vitamins and vitamin C.

water-soluble Capable of dissolving in water.

white blood cells One of the formed elements of the circulating blood system; also called *leukocytes*. White blood cells are able to squeeze through intracellular spaces and migrate. They phagocytize bacteria, fungi, and viruses, as well as detoxify proteins that may result from allergic reactions, cellular injury, and other immune system cells.

whole grains Grains containing the entire seed of the plant, including the bran, germ, and endosperm (starchy interior). Examples are whole wheat and brown rice.

Wilson's disease A genetic disorder that results in accumulation of copper in the tissues; characterized by damage to the liver, nervous system, and other organs.

withdrawal Physical symptoms related to cessation of substance use, such as sweating, rapid pulse, shakiness, insomnia, nausea and vomiting, anxiety, and even seizures.

xerophthalmia Hardening of the cornea and drying of the surface of the eye, which can result in blindness.

xylitol Alcohol derivative of the five-carbon monosaccharide xylose.

zoochemicals Chemicals found in animal products that have health-protective actions.

zygote The fertilized ovum; the cell resulting from the union of an egg cell (ovum) and sperm until it divides.

Index